Integrated Basic Surgical Sciences

Integrated Basic Surgical Sciences

James Toouli
MB BS PhD FRACS
Professor, Department of General and Digestive Surgery, Flinders
University, Flinders Medical Centre, Bedford Park, South Australia,
Australia

Chris Russell
MS FRCS
Consultant Surgeon, Middlesex Hospital and King Edward VII
Hospital for Officers, London, UK

Peter Devitt
MS FRACS
Consultant Surgeon, Department of Surgery, Royal Adelaide
Hospital, Adelaide, South Australia, Australia

Celia Ingham Clark
MChir FRCS
Consultant General Surgeon, Department of Surgery, Whittington
Hospital, London, UK

A member of the Hodder Headline Group
LONDON • SYDNEY • AUCKLAND
Co-published in the USA by
Oxford University Press, Inc., New York

Published in Great Britain in 2000 by
Arnold, a member of the Hodder Headline Group,
338 Euston Road, London NW1 3BH

http://www.arnoldpublishers.com

Co-published in the USA by
Oxford University Press Inc.,
198 Madison Avenue, New York, NY 10016
Oxford is a registered trademark of Oxford University Press

Whilst the advice and information in this book are believed to be true and
accurate at the date of going to press, neither the authors nor the publisher
can accept any legal responsibility or liability for any errors or omissions
that may be made. In particular (but without limiting the generality of the
preceding disclaimer) every effort has been made to check drug dosages;
however, it is still possible that errors have been missed. Furthermore,
dosage schedules are constantly being revised and new side-effects
recognized. For these reasons the reader is strongly urged to consult the
drug companies' printed instructions before administering any of the drugs
recommended in this book.

British Library Cataloguing in Publication Data
A catalogue record for this book is available from the British Library

Library of Congress Cataloging-in-Publication Data
A catalog record for this book is available from the Library of Congress

ISBN 0 340 700912

1 2 3 4 5 6 7 8 9 10

Publisher: Annalisa Page / Nick Dunton
Project Editor: Melissa Morton
Production Editor: Wendy Rooke
Production Controller: Sarah Kett

Typeset in 10/12 pt Minion by J&L Composition Ltd, Filey, North Yorkshire
Printed and bound in Spain by Mateu Chromo Sa

What do you think of this book? Or any other Arnold title?
Please send your comments to feedback.arnold@hodder.co.uk

Contents

List of Contributors

Anselm O. Agwunobi
MB BS FRCS
Clinical Fellow, Intestinal Failure Unit, Hope Hospital, Salford, Manchester, UK

Iain D. Anderson
BSc MD FRCS
Hillsborough Tutor in Critical Care and Consultant Surgeon, Hope Hospital, Salford, Manchester, UK

Åke Andrén-Sandberg
MD PhD
Chairman and Professor, Department of Surgery, Haukeland University Hospital, Bergen, Norway

Stephen G.E. Barker
MB BS BSc MS FRCS
Consultant Vascular and General Surgeon, Academic Vascular Unit, Department of Surgery, Middlesex Hospital, University College London Hospitals, London, UK

David Belford
BMed Sc MB BS PhD
Senior Research Scientist, Cooperative Research Centre for Tissue Growth and Repair, Adelaide, South Australia, Australia

Roger Bell
MB BS FRACS
Consultant Surgeon and Head of Vascular Surgery, Sir Charles Gairdner Hospital, Perth, Western Australia, Australia

David A.R. Bessant
FRCOphth
Specialist Registrar, Moorfields Eye Hospital, London, UK

Hilary A. Blacklock
MB ChB FRACP FRCPA
Haematologist, Department of Haematology, Middlemore Hospital and Clinical Reader, Department of Molecular Medicine, School of Medicine, Auckland, New Zealand

John Blennerhassett
MB ChB FRCPA
Consultant Pathologist, Dunedin Hospital and Emeritus Professor, University of Otago, Dunedin, New Zealand

Nikolai Bogduk
MD PhD DSc DipAnat FAFRM
Profesor of Anatomy and Musculoskeletal Medicine, University of Newcastle, Royal Newcastle Hospital, Newcastle, New South Wales, Australia

Stephen G. Bown
MD FRCP
Professor of Laser Medicine and Surgery, National Medical Laser Centre, Department of Surgery, Royal Free and University College Medical School, London, UK

D. John Brazier
FRCS FRCOphth
Consultant Ophthalmic Surgeon, University College Hospitals, University of London, London, UK

Kevin G. Burnand
MS FRCS
Professor of Vascular Surgery, United Medical and Dental Schools of Guy's and St Thomas's Hospitals and Consultant Surgeon, St Thoma's Hospital, London, UK

Anthony J. Buzzard
MB BS FRACS FRCS FACS
Senior Lecturer, Department of Surgery, Alfred Hospital, Monash University, Melbourne, Australia

Christopher M.J. Cain
MB BS MD FRACS FA Orth A
Senior Visiting Medical Specialist, Royal Adelaide Hospital and Flinders Medical Centre, Bedford Park, and Department of Orthopaedic Surgery and Trauma, Faculty of Medicine, University of Adelaide, Adelaide, South Australia, Australia

Gordon L. Carlson
BSc MB ChB MD FRCS
MRC Senior Clinical Fellow and Honorary Consultant Surgeon, Department of Surgery, Hope Hospital, Salford, Manchester, UK

Thomas W.G. Carrell
MA FRCS
Lecturer in Surgery, Department of Surgery, St Thoma's Hospital, London, UK

Laurie Catley
MB BS
Haematology Registrar, Department of Haematology, Institute of Medical and Veterinary Science, Adelaide, South Australia, Australia

Ian Civil
MB ChB FRACS FACS
Director of Trauma Services, Department of Surgery, Auckland Hospital, Auckland, New Zealand

Matthew A. Clark
MB ChB FRACS
General Surgical Registrar, Department of Surgery, Middlemore Hospital, Auckland, New Zealand

George G. Collee
MB ChB FRCA
Consultant Anaesthetist, Royal Free Hospital, London, UK

John P.V. Collins
MD MCH FRCS FRACS
Associate Professor of Surgery, Faculty of Medicine and Health Science, Middlemore Hospital, Auckland, New Zealand

W. Bruce Conolly
FRCS FRACS FACS
Associate Professor of Hand Surgery, Department of Surgery and Associate Professor of Hand Surgery, University of Sydney, University of New South Wales and Director of Hand Surgery, St Luke's Hospital Complex, Potts Point, New South Wales, Australia

Rodney D. Cooter
MB BS MD FRACS
Head, Plastic and Reconstructive Surgery, Department of Surgery, University of Adelaide, Royal Adelaide Hospital, Adelaide, South Australia, Australia

Maria Crotty
MPH PhD FAFRM
Senior Lecturer in Rehabilitation Medicine, Flinders University Department of Rehabilitation and Aged Care, Repatriation General Hospital, Daw Park, South Australia, Australia

D. Wynne L. Davies
MB BCh DRCOG DCH FRCA
Consultant Anaesthetist, Department of Anaesthesia, Middlesex Hospital, London, UK

Ken Davis
FIBMS
Chief Medical Scientist, Transfusion Medicine Unit and Haematology, Institute of Medical and Veterinary Science, Adelaide, South Australia, Australia

Bren Dorman
MB ChB FRACS
Otolaryngologist Head and Neck Surgeon, Department of Otolaryngology, Green Lane Hospital, Auckland, New Zealand

Friedericke Eben
MRCOG
Consultant Obstetrician and Gynaecologist, Whittington Hospital, London, UK

Andrew M. Ellis
MB BS FRACS (Orth)
Senior Lecturer in Orthopaedic and Traumatic Surgery, Department of Orthopaedics, University of Sydney, Royal North Shore Surgery Hospital, St Leonards, New South Wales, Australia

Mark Emberton
BSc MD FRCS (Urol)
Senior Lecturer in Urology, Institute of Urology and Nephrology, University College London Medical School, London, UK

Hamish P. Ewing
FRACS
Associate Professor of Surgery, Department of Surgery, University of Melbourne, The Northern Hospital, Epping, Victoria, Australia

Irwin Faris
MD FRACS
Professor of Surgery, Department of Surgery, University of Melbourne, The Geelong Hospital, Geelong, Victoria, Australia

Kingsley Faulkner
MB BS FRACS
Consultant Surgeon and Head of the Department of General Surgery, Sir Charles Gairdner Hospital, Perth, Western Australia, Australia

Kenneth C.H. Fearon
MD FRCS
Professor of Surgical Onocology and Consultant Colorectal Surgeon, Department of Surgery, University of Edinburgh, Royal Infirmary, Edinburgh, UK

Paul Finucane
MSc FRCPI FRACP
Professor of Rehabilitation and Aged Care, Flinders University Department of Rehabilitation and Aged Care, Repatriation General Hospital, Daw Park, South Australia, Australia

Sheila E. Fisher
MSc FDS FFD FRCS
Consultant Maxillofacial Surgeon, Department of Maxillofacial Surgery, Queen's Medical Centre, Nottingham, UK

Robert D. Fraser
MB BS MD FRACS FAOrthA
Clinical Professor and Head of Spinal Unit, Department of Orthopaedics and Trauma, Faculty of Medicine, University of Adelaide, Adelaide, South Australia, Australia

Peter Freeman
MB ChB FRCS FFAEM FACEM
Director of Emergency Medicine, Auckland Hospital, Auckland, New Zealand

O. James Garden
MD FRCS
Regius Professor of Surgery, Department of Surgery, University of Edinburgh, Royal Infirmary, Edinburgh, UK

Robert George
MA MD FRCP
Director, Palliative Care Centre, Camden and Islington Community Trust, and Royal Free and University College Medical School, London, UK

Alison R. Gillams
MRCP FRCR
Senior Lecturer, Radiology Department, Middlesex Hospital, London, UK

Grant Gillett
D Phil (Oxon) FRACS
Professor of Medical Ethics, Otago Bioethics Centre, University of Otago Medical School, Dunedin, New Zealand

Scott M. Graham
MB BS(Hons) FRACS
Associate Professor, Department of Otolaryngology – Head and Neck Surgery, University of Iowa Hospitals and Clinics, Iowa City, Iowa, USA

Hugh Greville
MB BS B Med Sci FRACP
Senior Consultant Respiratory Physician, Department of Thoracic Medicine, Royal Adelaide Hospital, Adelaide, South Australia, Australia

John C. Hall
MS DS FRACS
Head of Surgery, University of Western Australia and Professor, University Department of Surgery, Royal Perth Hospital, Perth, Western Australia

James Hamill
MBChB FRACS
Trauma Fellow, Auckland Hospital, Auckland, New Zealand

Geoffrey S. Hebbard
MB BS BMed Sci PhD FRACP
Consultant Gastroenterologist, Gastroenterology Department, Repatriation General Hospital, Daw Park, South Australia, Australia

Joseph L. Hegarty
MD
Chief Resident in Otolaryngology, Department of Otolaryngology – Head and Neck Surgery, University of Iowa Hospitals and Clinics, University of Iowa, Iowa City, Iowa, USA

David G. Hill
MB ChB FRCS FRACS
Director of Cardiothoracic Surgery, Department of Cardiothoracic Surgery, The Geelong Hospital, Geelong, Victoria, Australia

Anthony K. House
MS FRCS FRACS
Professor of Surgery, University of Western Australia, Senior Transplant Surgeon, Sir Charles Gairdner Hospital, Perth, Western Australia, Australia

Michael Hulme-Moir
MBChB FRACS
Surgical Registrar, Auckland Hospital, Auckland, New Zealand

Raja L.A. Jayaweera
MA LLB MB BS DA FRCA
Consultant Anaesthetist, Department of Anaesthesia, Whittington Hospital, London, UK

Norman Johnson
MD FRCP
Consultant Respiratory Physician and Honorary Senior Lecturer, Director of Research and Development, Chest Department, Whittington Hospital, London, UK

Nigel R. Jones
DPhil FRACS
Michell Professor of Neurosurgery, University of Adelaide, Royal Adelaide Hospital, Adelaide, South Australia, Australia

Robert M. Jones
FRACS FRCS
Director, Liver Transplant Unit, Austin Repatriation Medical Centre, Melbourne, Australia

Suchitra Kanagasundaram
FRCA FANZCA
Consultant Anaesthetist, Department of Anaesthesia, The Whittington Hospital, London, UK

Anthony Kierath
MB BS FRCS FRACS
General Surgeon, West Perth, Western Australia, Australia

Chris Kneebone
MB BS FRACP
Senior Visiting Neurologist, Department of Neurology, Royal Adelaide Hospital, Adelaide, South Australia, Australia

Suren Krishnan
MB BS FRACS
Consultant Otorhinolaryngologist, Otorhinolaryngology Unit, Royal Adelaide Hospital, Adelaide, South Australia, Australia

Brian R. Landers
MB BS FRACS
Senior Visiting Urologist, The Queen Elizabeth Hospital, Woodville, South Australia, Australia

David J. Leaper
MD ChM FRCS(Glas) Ed FRCS(Eng) FACS
*Professor of Surgery, University of Newcastle upon Tyne, North
Tees Hospital, Stockton on Tees, UK*

John V. Lloyd
MB BS MD PhD FRACP
*Senior Specialist Haematologist, Division of Haematology,
Institute of Medical and Veterinary Science, Adelaide, South
Australia, Australia*

Bryony E. Lovett
MChir FRCS
*Specialist Registrar, Department of Surgery, Middlesex Hospital,
London, UK*

John Ludbrook
MD DSc CRM FRCS FRACS
*Professorial Fellow, University of Melbourne Department of
Surgery, Royal Melbourne Hospital, Melbourne, Victoria,
Australia*

Donald G. MacLellan
BSc MD FRACS
*Professor of Surgery, Canberra Clinical School, University of
Sydney, Canberra, Australia*

Leo Mahar
MB BS FRACP
*Cardiologist, Department of Cardiology, Royal Adelaide
Hospital, Adelaide, South Australia, Australia*

Villis R. Marshall
MD FRACS
*Professor and Chairman, Department of Surgery, Flinders
Medical Centre, Bedford Park, South Australia, Australia*

Jenepher Ann Martin
MB BS MS MEd FRACS
*Coordinator of Surgical Education, Royal Australasian College
of Surgeons, Melbourne, Australia*

John Miller
MB BS FRACS
*Senior Lecturer in Urology, University of Adelaide and
Consultant Urologist, The Queen Elizabeth Hospital, Woodville,
South Australia, Australia*

Michael Muller
MB BS FRACS
*General and Burn Surgeon, Division of Surgery, Royal Brisbane
Hospital, Brisbane, Queensland, Australia*

Anthony R. Mundy
MS FRCP FRCS
*Professor of Urology and Director of the Institute of Urology and
Nephrology, Institute of Urology, Middlesex Hospital, London,
UK*

The late Mervyn G. Neely
MB BS FRCS FRACS FACS
*Surgeon, Honorary Associate Professor of the University of
Queensland, Mater Medical Centre, South Brisbane,
Queensland, Australia*

John P. Neoptolemos
MA MB BChr MD FRCS
*Professor and Head of Department, Department of Surgery,
Royal Liverpool University Hospital, Liverpool, UK*

James D. Palmer
MS FRCS
Consultant Neurosurgeon, Derriford Hospital, Plymouth, UK

John E. Payne
MS FRCS FRACS FACS
*Senior Lecturer, Department of Surgery, University of Sydney,
Sydney, New South Wales, Australia*

Mario Penta
MB BS MS FRACS
*Consultant Orthopaedic Surgeon, Department of Orthopaedic
Surgery, Royal Adelaide Hospital, Adelaide, South Australia,
Australia*

Michael C. Pietroni
MB BS FRCS
*Consultant Surgeon, Whipps Cross Hospital, Leytonstone,
London, UK*

Miklós J. Pohl
FRCS FRACS
*Clinical Senior Lecturer and Senior Visiting Plastic Surgeon,
Royal Hobart Hospital, Hobart, Tasmania, Australia*

Julia M. Potter
BMed Sc MB BS PhD FRCPA
*Clinical Professor, University of Queensland and Director of
Chemical Pathology, The Prince Charles Hospital and Chemical
Pathologist, Royal Brisbane Hospital, Department of Chemical
Pathology, The Prince Charles Hospital, Chermside,
Queensland, Australia*

David Ralph
BSc MS FRCS (Urol)
*Consultant Urologist, St Peter's Hospital, Middlesex Hospital,
London, UK*

Crichton F. Ramsay
MB ChB MRCP
*Consultant Chest Physician, Department of Respiratory
Medicine, Norfolk and Norwich Hospital, Norwich, UK*

Nicholas Rieger
MB MS FRACS
*Senior Lecturer in Surgery, Department of Surgery, The Queen
Elizabeth Hospital, Woodville, South Australia, Australia*

Peter C. Robinson
MB BS FRACP
Senior Consultant Physician, Thoracic Medicine Unit, Royal Adelaide Hospital, Adelaide, South Australia, Australia

Michael Rodgers
MB ChB FRACS
General Surgeon, Auckland Hospital, Auckland, New Zealand

Margaret Schnitzler
MB BS PhD FRACS
Associate Professor of Surgery, Department of Surgery, Royal North Shore Hospital, St Leonards, New South Wales, Australia

Jonathan W. Serpell
MB BS MD FRACS
Specialist Surgeon, Breast, Endocrine and Surgical Oncology Unit and Honorary Senior Lecturer, Department of Surgery, Alfred Hospital, Monash University and Specialist Endocrine, Oncological and General Surgeon and Head of General Surgery Unit, Frankston Hospital, Melbourne, Australia

Jean Simpson
BSc MSc
Public Health Specialist, Department of Public Health, Ealing, Hammersmith and Hounslow Health Authority, Southall, Middlesex, UK

Gabriella Slapak
MB BS MRCP
Specialist Registrar, University Department of Medicine, Royal Free Hospital, London, UK

John Slavin
MB BS MS FRCS
Senior Lecturer and Honorary Consultant Surgeon, Department of Surgery, Royal Liverpool Hospital, Liverpool, UK

John M.B. Smith
MSc PhD
Associate Professor and Head, Department of Microbiology, School of Medical Sciences, University of Otago, Dunedin, New Zealand

Justine R. Smith
MB BS BA PhD FRACO FRACS
Lecturer and Consultant Ophthalmologist, Department of Ophthalmology, Flinders University of South Australia and Flinders Medical Centre, Bedford Park, South Australia, Australia

Alan M.F. Stapleton
PhD FRACS
Consultant Urologist, Senior Lecturer in Surgery, Urology Unit, Division of Surgery, Repatriation General Hospital, Daw Park, South Australia, Australia

Gordon G. Stuart
FRACS
Director of Neurosurgery, Department of Neurosurgery, Royal Brisbane Hospital, Herston, Queensland, Australia

David W. Thomas
MB BS BMed Sc FRACP FRCPA MAABCB
Professor of Chemical Pathology, Department of Chemical Pathology, Women and Children's Hospital, North Adelaide, South Australia, Australia

William E.G. Thomas
MS FRCS
Surgical Skills Tutor, Royal College of Surgeons of England and Consultant Surgeon, Royal Hallamshire Hospital, Sheffield, UK

Philip D. Thompson
MB BS PhD FRACP
Professor of Neurology, Department of Medicine, Royal Adelaide Hospital, Adelaide, South Australia, Australia

James Toouli
MB BS PhD FRACS
Professor and·Head, Department of General and Digestive Surgery, Flinders University, Flinders Medical Centre, Bedford Park, South Australia, Australia

Christian H. Wakefield
BSc MD FRCS
Lecturer in Surgery, University Department of Surgery, Royal Infirmary, Edinburgh, UK

John A. Walsh
MD FRACS
Consultant Vascular Surgeon, Flinders Medical Centre, Bedford Park, South Australia, Australia

David I. Watson
MB BS MD FRACS
Senior Consultant Surgeon, University of Adelaide Department of Surgery, Royal Adelaide Hospital, Adelaide, South Australia, Australia

David Wattchow
BM BS PhD FRACS
Associate Professor/Senior Consultant in Surgery, Department of Surgery, Flinders Medical Centre, Bedford Park, South Australia, Australia

Douglas E. Whitelaw
MB ChB MRCP
Consultant Gastroenterologist, Queen Elizabeth Hospital, Welwyn Garden City, UK

Robin G. Woolfson
MD FRCP
Consultant and Honorary Senior Lecturer, Department of Nephrology, Institute of Urology and Nephrology, UCLMS, Middlesex Hospital, London, UK

Jennifer G. Worrall
MD MRCP
Consultant Rheumatologist, Department of Rheumatology, Whittington Hospital, London, UK

Foreword

This book, which has been edited by Mr Chris Russell from the Middlesex Hospital, Mrs Celia Ingham Clark from the Whittington Hospital, Professor Jim Toouli from the Flinders University Medical Centre and Mr Peter Devitt from the Royal Adelaide Hospital, has set itself a very specific target for readership. This consists of young surgeons in their basic surgical training years, particularly in the UK and the Australian and New Zealand systems.

The book is divided into two parts, the first of which addresses clinical problems with a discussion of the scientific principles underlying the cause of the problem, its diagnosis and management. The second part of the book deals with clinical practice, and covers the scientific basis of various investigations used in different areas of surgical practice, as well as the principles of pre-operative assessment, anaesthesia, surgery and, in particular, the use of surgical tools such as diathermy during surgery. Again this part concentrates on the basic scientific principles on which clinical practice and surgical techniques are based.

Thus this new book, produced under the auspices of the Royal Australasian College of Surgeons, does present a novel approach to discussion of the scientific principles underlying surgical problems and surgical practice at a level suitable for basic surgical trainees in their early years of training. It should also help them to prepare for the appropriate examinations at the end of their basic training. Although primarily directed at such trainees, I would be surprised if the book does not prove to have an even wider appeal.

Peter J. Morris FRS FRCS FRACS FACS
Nuffield Professor of Surgery
University of Oxford

Preface

The methods of educating doctors are changing in tune with the recognition that we have moved from the 'industrial age' to the 'information age'. Medical teachers have appreciated this change and are responding with curricula which are designed to promote lifelong learning habits. Problem-based learning has formed the focus for these curricula and has generated enthusiasm in both students and teachers.

Problem-solving is not foreign to surgeons. Indeed, it might be argued that the surgical 'mind' could best be described as 'problem-solving focused'. Hence it was a logical move when we set about the task of designing a book for students of surgery that we should choose a problem-based format.

Integrated Basic Surgical Sciences is organized into two major parts. The first part, entitled 'Clinical Problems', aims to provide an understanding of common surgical problems as they might be presented by a patient to a clinician. The authors have endeavoured to describe the anatomy, physiology and pathophysiology of each problem with the aim of providing an understanding of why each clinical syndrome is produced. As a consequence of this, the reader will not be exposed to an exhaustive list of pathological causes for each problem, but instead will gain an understanding of the mechanisms which underpin the development of the symptoms. We would hope that the reader will use this understanding and apply it in the development of an appropriate diagnosis for an individual patient.

The second part of the book is entitled 'Clinical Practice'. Here we have abandoned the problem-based approach. The chapters in this section are designed to provide a basic knowledge of topics which are crucial in underpinning the practice of surgery.

The book has been developed to support the learning objectives of the trainee surgeons in their basic year of surgical training. However, it will also provide a ready reference for surgical students enrolled in medical schools with problem-based learning curricula.

The Editors have welded together their experience in education of surgical students and trainees in Australia, New Zealand and the UK. In itself this background is unique, and we believe that it gives the book much depth. Consequently, the contributing authors reflect a similar geographical distribution and have been invited to participate because of their commitment to education and their enthusiasm for this new approach. We are deeply indebted to them and grateful that they have delivered their chapters promptly so as to ensure the currency of all aspects of the book.

We wish to dedicate this book to our surgical students. We hope that you find this book as interesting and stimulating to read and use as we have found it to be during its gestation and birth.

James Toouli
Chris Russell
Peter Devitt
Celia Ingham Clark

Part 1

Clinical Problems

An overview of pain

Nikolai Bogduk

Introduction

When a patient reports pain, they do not know and cannot tell what is causing it. At best they may be able to describe what the pain feels like and where it *seems* to be coming from. It is then the surgeon's professional responsibility to determine, as best he or she can, what the cause is and to do something about it. Fundamental to these responsibili-ties is an understanding of the mechanisms of pain. Anatomy establishes the neural circuitry of pain. Physiology describes how it operates, but also provides the basis for how pain might be treated either pharmaco-logically or surgically.

DEFINITION

In its definition of pain, the International Association for the Study of Pain states that pain is 'an unpleasant sensory and emotional experience' (Merskey and Bogduk, 1994: p. 210). This definition emphasizes that pain is neither tangible nor peripheral. It is not a sensation like touch or temperature. It is an emotional experience in the patient's mind that can be evoked in a variety of ways.

The definition goes on to elaborate as follows: '... experience, associated with actual or potential tissue damage, or described in terms of such damage'. The first of these two clauses describes pain as traditionally understood – that it is an experience evoked by disease or injury to structures or organs of the body. The second clause recognizes that some patients may complain of pain but exhibit no apparent tissue damage, and enables the introduction of terms such as psychogenic pain, abnormal illness behaviour and somatoform disorder. These concepts accept that the patient does suffer pain, but imply that tissue injury or disease is not the cause.

When elaborated in terms of the physiological mech-anisms involved, this definition allows pain to be classi-fied as nociceptive, neurogenic or psychogenic (Figure 1.1.1). Nociceptive pain is the archetypal mechanism whereby the psychic experience of pain is evoked by damage to somatic or visceral tissues. This type of pain may be perceived as local pain, or it may be referred. Neurogenic pain arises not from peripheral stimulation but from abnormal activity in the nerves that normally transmit nociceptive pain. Psychogenic pain is believed to arise from influences in the patient's mind, such as memory and association with past stressful events; technically, it also includes malingering.

NOCICEPTION

The human body is endowed with nerves designed to detect tissue damage. These nerves do not transmit pain, but they do transmit information about noxious stimuli – hence the term 'nociception'. This information may evoke pain when it reaches the cerebral cortex, but not unless and until it does so will the patient experience pain.

Physiologically, nociception involves four processes,

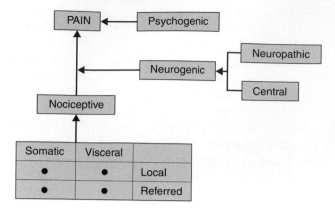

Figure 1.1.1 The classification of pain by mechanism. As a psychic experience, pain may be evoked by psychogenic, neurogenic or nociceptive means. Nociceptive pain may be somatic or visceral in origin, and may even be local or referred.

namely transduction, peripheral transmission central transmission, and modulation. The details of each process are pertinent to both the interpretation of pain and its treatment.

TRANSDUCTION

Tissue damage is detected by free nerve endings that are distributed throughout the external epithelial tissues of the body, and all fibrous connective tissues, including skeletal and smooth muscles. They are absent from the parenchyma of solid viscera, but are present in their capsules. In hollow viscera, they are absent from the serosa, but are present under the epithelium and in the muscularis.

Transduction involves the production in the free nerve endings of a generator potential, or receptor potential, that is proportional to the intensity of stimulation. If and once this generator potential is of sufficient magnitude, it will evoke an action potential in the nerve fibre that subtends the free nerve ending.

Nociceptive free nerve endings can be stimulated either chemically or mechanically. The most common algogenic chemicals are hydrogen ions, potassium ions, bradykinins and serotonin. These are substances typically liberated by damaged cells, or produced by the inflammatory response to tissue damage. Hydrogen ions from lactic acid, together with metabolites of adenosine triphosphate, are algogenic substances that accumulate in tissues that have been rendered 'ischaemic' by obstruction of venous outflow by muscle contraction or spasm.

As a class, the prostaglandins do not evoke pain when applied to nerve endings. However, prostaglandins sensitize nerve endings and facilitate the action of other algogenic compounds on nociceptive nerve endings. Substance P is a polypeptide, found in nociceptive

nerves, that is released in the periphery when these nerves are stimulated. However, it is not algogenic in the periphery. Rather, its role is to promote vasodilatation and to enhance the inflammatory response to injury.

The mechanism of mechanical nociception is poorly understood because it is difficult to study at the microscopic level *in vivo*, but it is clearly apparent at the clinical level. Mechanical nociception occurs whenever collagenous tissues are stretched. Examples include the rapid expansion of the capsules of solid viscera, the expansion of periosteum by underlying blood, infection or tumour, and the strain of ligaments, joint capsules and tendons in biomechanical disorders of the musculoskeletal system. By inference, the transduction mechanism appears to involve compression of free endings woven through the lattice-work of collagen in these tissues, as this lattice-work is deformed under tension.

PERIPHERAL TRANSMISSION

There are no specialized nociceptive nerve fibres in the human body. Nociception is mediated by nerves that otherwise subserve other functions. Nevertheless, all nociceptive neurones belong to the Aδ or C classes of peripheral neurones.

Certain, but not all, Aδ fibres that normally mediate mechanical sensations can be nociceptive. At low intensities of stimulation they convey the sensation of pressure. At higher intensities they evoke pain. Similarly, Aδ and C fibres that normally mediate temperature sensation can evoke pain when the stimulus exceeds 45°C. The difference between innocuous and noxious stimuli is coded by an increasing frequency of discharge in the fibres that detect the stimuli. In humans, all C fibres are polymodal in that they can respond to mechanical, thermal and chemical stimuli. Some are responsive only in the noxious range while others are silent under normal conditions and only become active when peripheral tissues have been sensitized by chemicals released by tissue damage or inflammation.

Most nociceptive afferents enter the spinal cord through dorsal roots, although some undertake a peculiar, circuitous route through ventral roots. In the context of nociceptive afferents from the viscera, although in the periphery these travel along with sympathetic efferents in splanchnic nerves, they none the less enter the cord through dorsal roots. This distinction apart, as a rule they enter the same spinal cord segment as that which supplies the efferents to the organ from which the nociceptive fibres arise.

Upon entering the cord, nociceptive afferents do not immediately enter the grey matter. They are first distributed rostrally and caudally along the cord in the dorsolateral tract. From here, multiple collaterals from each individual nociceptive afferent enter the dorsal column of grey matter (Figure 1.1.2). As a result, any one nociceptive afferent will ramify in the dorsal horns of segments anywhere between one to three levels rostral and caudal to the segment of entry.

Nociceptive afferents ramify in laminae I, II and III of the dorsal horn. In these lamina they assume a diversity of simple and complex connections with interneurones and second-order neurones that reside in the grey matter. The details of these connections are not of immediate relevance to surgeons in general, but they are perhaps pertinent to neurosurgeons and orthopaedic surgeons who may be called upon to interpret the vagaries of certain pain problems and their treatment by drugs and acupuncture. However, a teleological question prompts a critical perception about the circuitry of pain at this stage. Why should there be a synapse?

If transmission of information is all that is required, it is redundant to interrupt a nociceptive neurone with a synapse. Nor is it simply an architectural idiosyncrasy that somewhere peripheral neurones are obliged to hand over to central neurones. The answer lies in the fact, ubiquitous in the nervous system, that synapses are produced wherever there is a need and the opportunity for control. In the nociceptive system, the junction between peripheral afferents and second-order transmission neurones in the dorsal horn is the first site of such control.

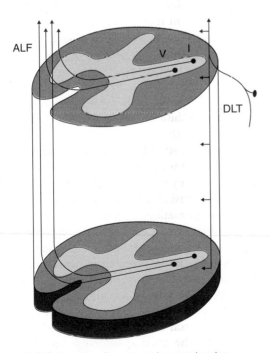

Figure 1.1.2 Primary afferents and second-order nociceptive neurones in the spinal cord. Primary afferents ascend and descend in the dorsolateral tract (DLT), sending collaterals into the dorsal horns of several spinal cord segments, where they synapse with neurones in laminae I and V, whose axons form anterolateral funiculus (ALF).

CENTRAL TRANSMISSION

Resident in the dorsal horn are large neurones in lamina I, known as marginal neurones. These are nociceptive specific, and transmit only nociceptive information which they receive from nociceptive afferents.

Resident in lamina V of the dorsal horn are large neurones that are capable of transmitting information about pressure and touch as well as nociceptive information. Accordingly they are referred to as wide-dynamic-range neurones. Their axons receive a direct input from collaterals of fibres in the posterior columns that transmit non-noxious information. They are also connected to nociceptive afferents through interneurones that reside in lamina II and lamina III. These interneurones allow controls to be exerted (as described below under Modulation).

First synapse

At the synapses between nociceptive afferents and second-order neurones, the principal transmitter substances involved are glutamate and substance P, and the receptors are the AMPA, NMDA and NK-1 receptors (**a**mino hydroxy-**m**ethyl-isoxazole-**p**ropionic **a**cid receptor, **N**-**m**ethyl-**D**-**a**spartate receptor, and **neu**rokinin-**1** receptor). The complexities of these receptors, their operation and their interactions have been the focus of much intensive research in recent years. The details are not of immediate relevance to surgeons in practice, but certain principles are pertinent to surgeons in training because they foreshadow how pain might be treated in the near future.

Glutamate acts on the AMPA receptor to produce a brief depolarization of the post-synaptic membrane (Figure 1.1.3). However, the principal target of glutamate is the NMDA receptor, but its calcium channel is blocked by magnesium. Previous stimulation of the AMPA receptors is required to remove the magnesium by a voltage-gated mechanism. Once the channel is opened, and provided that glutamate is still being released, the NMDA receptor can respond. It causes a strong depolarization of the post-synaptic membrane and permits the influx of calcium. Substance P has a very slow onset of action. It acts on NK-1 receptors to produce a very strong, prolonged depolarization, but it also initiates several intracellular events. Activation of G protein and phospholipase C in the cell membrane results in the conversion of phosphatidyl inositol to inositol triphosphate and diacylglycerol. Inositol triphosphate acts on the endoplasmic reticulum to release calcium into the cytosol. Diacylglycerol, in association with calcium, activates protein kinase C which translocates in the cell membrane and facilitates the action of the NMDA receptor. Thus if glutamate is still being

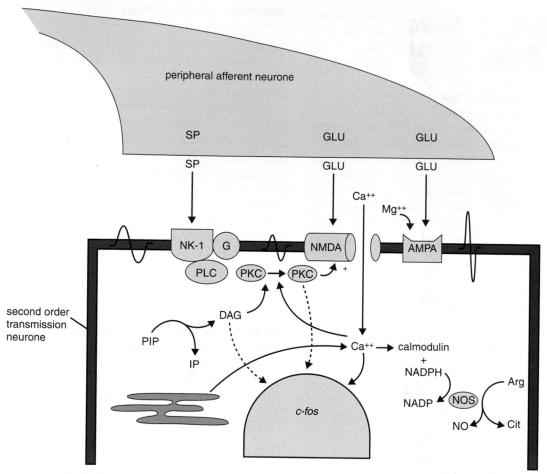

Figure 1.1.3 Events in the first nociceptive synapse. AMPA, amino-hydroxy-methyl-isoxazole-propionic acid receptor; NMDA, *N*-methyl, D-aspartate receptor; NK-1, neurokinin-1 receptor; GLU, glutamate; SP, substance P; G, G protein; PLC, phospholipase C; PIP, phosphatidyl inositol phosphate; IP, inositol triphosphate; DAG, diacylglycerol; PKC, protein kinase C; NOS, nitric oxide synthetase; Arg, arginine; Cit, citrulline; NO, nitric oxide.

produced, the post-synaptic membrane continues to be depolarized, and more strongly. Diacylglycerol, protein kinase C and calcium promote the expression of proto-oncogenes such as *c-fos*. Intracellular calcium, in combination with calmodulin and NADPH, activates nitric oxide synthetase to produce nitric oxide.

This seemingly complex series of events serves to filter and amplify nociceptive transmission. A trivial noxious stimulus will not evoke a strong central response, because it causes only a small release of glutamate, which can act only on the AMPA receptor. For the NMDA receptor to be activated, there needs to be a sustained release of glutamate. Moreover, only if glutamate continues to be released can the NMDA receptor take advantage of the late facilitation provided by substance P. However, once these conditions are satisfied, the post-synaptic membrane responds in a strong and sustained manner, with the response far outlasting the original stimulus. Thus any serious noxious stimulus causes the central nervous system to respond in an alarming manner,

which is appropriate to the threat that the noxious stimulus poses.

The normal function of the intracellular effects of NMDA and NK-1 receptors is not understood. In other systems the expression of *c-fos* is regarded simply as a marker of cell activity. However, it has been postulated that in chronic pain states, certain products of *c-fos* activity are deleterious to the cell and cause hyperexcitability. The continued production of nitric oxide produces hyperalgesia, which is manifested as increased sensitivity to cutaneous and deep mechanical stimulation, which spreads beyond the original site of pain.

Ascending tracts

The axons of marginal neurones and wide-dynamic-range neurones leave the grey matter and mainly cross the midline in the anterior white commissure to form the anterolateral funiculus. A minority ascend in ipsilateral pathways (Figure 1.1.4).

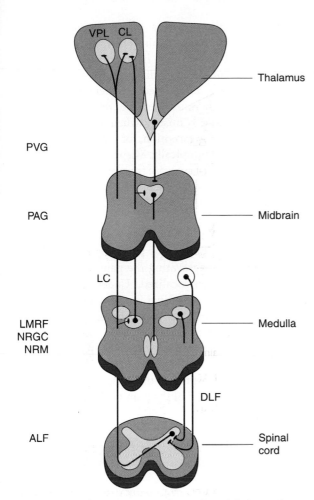

Figure 1.1.4 Central transmission and modulation pathways of the nociceptive system. ALF, anterolateral funiculus; VPL, ventral posterior lateral nucleus; CL, central lateral nucleus; NRGC, nucleus reticularis gigantocellularis; PAG, periaqueductal grey matter; LC, locus coeruleus; LMRF, lateral medullary reticular formation; NRM, nucleus raphe magnus; PVG, periventricular grey matter; DLF, dorsolateral funiculus.

The anterolateral funiculus constitutes what were previously known as the anterior and lateral spinothalamic tracts. Modern research has demonstrated that the functional segregation ascribed to these tracts is no longer tenable. The axons of wide-dynamic-range neurones are dispersed throughout the regions occupied by these classical pathways. Consequently, both touch and nociception are conveyed by both pathways.

Ascending axons have two primary destinations (Figure 1.1.4). Those of the neospinothalamic system relay to the ventral posterior lateral (VPL) and central lateral (CL) nuclei of the thalamus. From the VPL nucleus the information is conveyed to the parietal lobe, and this connection appears to be responsible for conveying the location of the origin of the stimulus. The CL nucleus projects through the reticular formation of the thalamus to the limbic system, and it is this pathway that is responsible for evoking the aversive and emotional nature of the pain experience.

Axons of the paleospinothalamic system relay to the reticular formation of the brainstem, principally to the nucleus reticularis gigantocellularis (NRGC). There they are also joined by collaterals of the neospinothalamic system. Ascending projections from the reticular formation reinforce the aversive effect of the CL nucleus, but local projections activate modulating influences.

MODULATION

Various nuclei in the brainstem exert a tonic inhibitory effect on the spinal cord. Essentially they prevent the spinal cord and central nervous system from becoming overloaded with sensory information. However, by modulating this inhibition, the nervous system can admit and enhance information in which it is interested, and suppress parallel information that might interfere with or obscure the perception of desired information. Noxious stimuli are clearly events in which the nervous system should be interested. Consequently, upon receiving nociceptive information, the nervous system modulates the descending inhibition in order to enhance the clarity of nociceptive information.

Ascending nociceptive axons activate the NRGC, which in turn activates the nucleus raphe magnus (NRM), the periaqueductal grey matter, and other sites such as the locus coeruleus and the lateral medullary reticular formation (LMRF). From these sites neurones descend into the spinal cord, where they exert inhibitory effects on afferent traffic (Figure 1.1.4). These effects are exerted directly on second-order nociceptive neurones and on interneurones that inhibit primary afferents or second-order neurones. This negative feedback produces centre-surround inhibition (or lateral inhibition). The inhibition is directed not at the segment through which nociception is being conveyed but to adjacent segments. By suppressing the activity of adjacent segments, the descending inhibition enhances the perception of the incoming signal. In essence, centre-surround inhibition increases the signal-to-noise ratio in the nociceptive system.

Neurones descending from the NRM use serotonin as their transmitter substance, and those from the locus coeruleus and LMRF use noradrenalin. The interneurones involved use enkephalin and GABA as their transmitter substances. Many, if not most, of the techniques used to produce analgesia rely on capturing the inhibitory effects of modulation in the nociceptive system, usually by mimicking the effects of its transmitter substances.

REFERRED PAIN

Referred pain is pain which is perceived in a location innervated by nerves other than those that innervate the actual source of pain. For many years physiologists sought the mechanism for referred pain. However, the concept can best be explained by reversing the question. Localized pain is the exception; referred pain is not.

The nociceptive system is poorly organized somatotopically. There is generally a poor correlation between the site of stimulation and the neurone that transmits information about it in the central nervous system. This is particularly the case for pain evoked from deep tissues. Deep tissues are innervated in a convergent manner. Peripheral nerves from various sites converge on and synapse with the same second-order neurone. In turn, many second-order neurones converge on the one third-order neurone in the thalamus. Without any other information about the source of a stimulus, the thalamic neurone cannot stipulate which second-order neurone stimulated it, or which peripheral nerve stimulated the second-order neurone. As a result, the parietal lobe cannot specify precisely the origin of the stimulus. Its information is, at best, limited to ± 1 segment about the spinal cord segment from which it received the signal. Unable to specify the exact source, the parietal lobe registers the pain as arising from somewhere among the tissue innervated by those segments. As a result, deep pain is perceived over a wide area with indistinct boundaries, but nevertheless centred over a particular region of the body.

This may seem to be an inefficient design, but it makes teleological sense. Although it may be pertinent for an organism to know that it is suffering deep pain, it is not material to know its exact location, for there is nothing that the organism could do about the pain even if it did know the exact location of its source. The organism cannot escape or avoid the pain of pancreatitis or of peptic ulceration. Therefore, it is redundant to have the nervous system wired to detect the exact source. In the limbs, knowing whether the pain arises from the thigh or the knee makes no difference if the only recourse is to rest the injured limb.

In contrast, it is worthwhile to know the exact location of a noxious stimulus to skin. The skin is the external surface of the body, and a noxious stimulus to it implies an external threat which might be avoided. The threatened part of the body can be withdrawn from the stimulus. Consequently, the skin is innervated in a highly organized somatotopic manner. Moreover, noxious stimuli to the skin are also likely to stimulate touch fibres whose distribution is precisely registered in the parietal lobe. For these various reasons, pain arising from the skin is virtually always well localized.

These realizations resolve the distinction between referred pain and localized pain. The distinction lies not in a special mechanism, but in the difference between deep pain and cutaneous pain. Deep tissues are poorly innervated somatotopically because there is no purpose in their being richly innervated. Therefore deep pain is poorly localized and is misconstrued as being referred. Cutaneous pain is the exception, for there is a purpose in innervating it somatotopically. Misperceptions about the mysteries of referred pain arise from assuming that cutaneous pain should be the archetype. They are removed by the realization that deep pain is the archetype and cutaneous pain is the special case.

Some attempt at localizing deep pain can be made by the patient or by a surgeon by palpating for tenderness. If they succeed in aggravating the pain, the source will appear to have been localized. Under those circumstances, however, additional information is being applied to the perception of pain. The external surface of the body is being touched. Therefore, the parietal lobe receives parallel information from the skin. The cutaneous information is well localized and, when associated with aggravation of pain, it is the cutaneous information that allows the location of the pain to be inferred.

APPLICATION

When a patient reports deep pain arising from a viscus or from a somatic structure, they will indicate a body region. What a surgeon contributes under these circumstances is the ability to recognize that region as a body segment to which a number can be ascribed. The patient's pain will be arising from one or other of the structures innervated by the same spinal cord segments that innervate that part of the body wall in which the pain is perceived. By recognizing the segments involved, and by knowing what other structures are innervated by those segments, the surgeon can formulate a differential diagnosis of the source of pain.

For that purpose, a comprehensive knowledge of the segmental innervation of the body wall, the viscera and limbs is required. To that end, several succinct rules and helpful maps apply.

In the thorax, the segmental innervation of the body wall is indicated by the ribs. The segmental nerves are distributed in the intercostal space of the same segmental number. Thus pain mediated by the T3 segment will approximately follow the T3 intercostal space. Pain from midline structures innervated by T3 will be perceived over the sternum opposite the T3 intercostal spaces.

In the abdomen, the same pattern applies – but without the local benefit of ribs. However, the segmental pattern is predicated by the projection of the lower six ribs.

If the costal cartilages are ignored, the lower six ribs point into the abdominal region, and their respective segmental nerves pass in the same direction in which those nerves project. In that regard, the umbilicus belongs to the T10 segment because the tenth rib points to the umbilicus. The location of other segments can be derived. Given that the sixth rib is the last to reach the sternum, the T7 to T9 segments are evenly dispersed in parallel from the sternum to the umbilicus. The T11 to L1 segments are dispersed from the umbilicus to the pubis.

A report of pain in any one (or more) of these segmental regions implies a source in the bones, joints, ligaments, muscles or viscera innervated by the spinal cord segment of the same number. The bones, joints and muscles can be readily identified as those of the vertebral column and ribs with the same segmental numbers as the body segment. However, viscera do not bear obvious segmental numbers, but their segmental innervation can be summarized in diagrammatic form (Figure 1.1.5), and can also be worked out from a short series of simple rules.

The thoracic viscera are all innervated by the T1–4 or T1–5 segments. The terminal oesophagus and proximal stomach are innervated by T5,6. The duodenum and organs stemming from it are innervated by segments T7,8 ($\pm$ 1). The jejunum is innervated by T9. The ileum and ileocolic region are innervated by T10. The colon is progressively innervated by T11, T12 and L1,2. The proximal parts of the urinary tract are innervated by T12 $\pm$ 1, and its distal parts are innervated by L1 $\pm$ 1.

At this point, two traditional misconceptions need to be dispelled. First, pain is not referred to dermatomes. It is referred deeply to segments of the body wall or limbs. It is just fortuitous, although distracting, that over the abdomen and thorax, the dermatome overlies the body wall segment of the same number. However, in the limbs and in the head this relationship does not exist. In those regions pain is clearly referred in a deep pattern, not according to dermatomes.

Secondly, a report of pain in a given region of the abdomen or thorax does not imply a source in the viscera underlying that region. Epigastric pain is often regarded as an indication of a possible source in the stomach, duodenum or pancreas, all of which lie in the epigastric region of the abdomen. However, the reason why these viscera are possible sources of epigastric pain is that they are innervated by the T6 to T9 segments of the spinal cord, which also happen to innervate the abdominal wall in the epigastric region. Appendicial pain is referred to the umbilicus not because of the T10 dermatome, but because the umbilicus lies in the T10 body wall segment. The transverse colon may lie in the epigastrium, but because it is innervated by T12, referred pain from the transverse colon will be perceived in the suprapubic region.

In the limbs, the pattern of segmental distribution is twisted and blended, and there is no distinct band of tissue that corresponds to a particular neural segment. However, a reasonable and clinically useful approximation can be constructed on the basis of the segmental innervation of muscles. Deep pain in the limbs will be approximately perceived in those muscles that are innervated by the same segments that innervate the source of pain. The segmental innervation of the muscles of the limbs is summarized in Figure 1.1.6.

NEUROGENIC PAIN

In a sense, neurogenic pain is not 'natural'. The nociceptive system is designed to detect damage in peripheral tissues. However, damage to the nerves of the nociceptive system can also evoke pain. The pain is real and has a physiological basis, but instead of arising from the tissues or regions in which it is perceived, it is evoked from the nerves that innervate these regions.

The term 'neurogenic pain' explicitly denotes pain arising from nerves. As such, it embraces pain evoked from a variety of sites. Nociceptive activity arising from the axons of peripheral nerves is referred to as neuropathic pain, which means pain due to a disorder of a

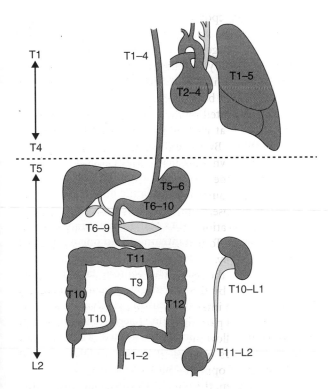

Figure 1.1.5 A schematic summary of the segmental innervation of the thoracic and abdominal viscera.

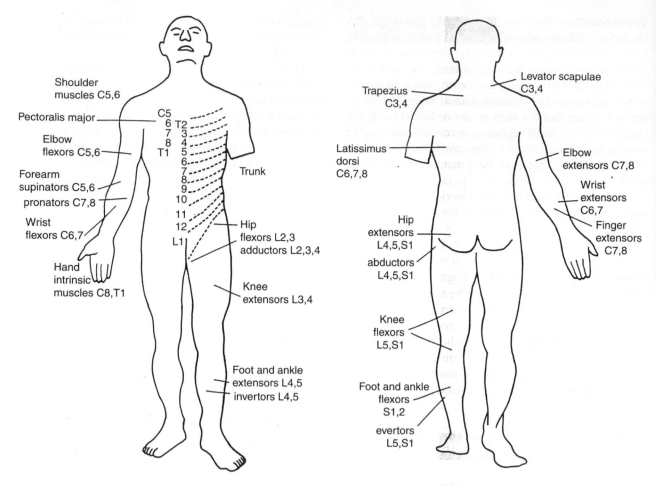

Figure 1.1.6 A schematic summary of the segmental innervation of the muscles of the limbs.

nerve (implicitly a peripheral nerve). Pain evoked from the central nervous system is referred to as central pain, in order to make clear that the source lies in the central nervous system, not in the periphery.

Neuropathic pain may be caused by a peripheral neuropathy, as in diabetic neuropathy and post-herpetic neuralgia, or by a neuroma. The mechanisms of pain in peripheral neuropathy are incompletely understood and differ according to aetiology. Hypotheses include ectopic discharge in the diseased axons or from their cell bodies, or loss of inhibition, in the spinal cord, of nociceptive neurones by non-nociceptive neurones.

The mechanisms of pain from neuromata are better understood. When a nerve is transected, axon sprouts emerge within hours, attempting to regenerate the nerve. If these sprouts fail to reach the distal stump of the severed nerve, they form a tangle that constitutes the neuroma. These neuromata are exquisitely sensitive to mechanical stimulation and to circulating noradrenaline. As a result they are spontaneously active and are aggravated by touch. The discharge that they produce elicits a complaint of pain.

Central pain occurs when second-order or third-order neurones in the nociceptive system become spontaneously active. Archetypally this occurs when these neurones lose their accustomed afferent input. Hence a synonym for central pain is 'deafferentation pain'. The most common clinical examples are the pain of brachial plexus avulsion, the pain of chronic post-herpetic neuralgia, and spinal cord injury pain. More classical – but rarer – is thalamic pain, which occurs as a result of infarction of cells that inhibit nociceptive thalamic nuclei.

When deafferentated, central nervous system neurones alter the characteristics of their membranes. It is as if the neurone throws a tantrum – if no one is speaking to it any more, it no longer bothers to maintain the apparatus with which to listen. The neurone fails to manufacture receptors, and its membrane becomes unstable, as a result of which the neurone discharges spontaneously. Paradoxically, the pain is perceived as arising in the region that is manifestly denervated. This does not make it false or imagined. In fact, any fallacy lies in expecting all pain to have a somatic or visceral source. In the case of central pain, the source lies half-way up the nociceptive system, but the patient has no way of knowing this.

PSYCHOGENIC PAIN

There are no positive diagnostic criteria for psychogenic pain. This is a concept, not an entity. It assumes that some patients can experience pain as a result of influences in their mind in the absence of peripheral input. Technically, psychogenic pain is a central pain but one that arises in the patient's forebrain or temporal lobe. Without objective access to the patient's cerebral cortex, the biological basis for this concept cannot be tested.

A label of psychogenic pain is ascribed by some practitioners to patients who ostensibly lack evidence of nociceptive or neurogenic pain. By that token it is a default diagnosis, but therein lies its liability. Use of the term 'psychogenic pain' (or any of its synonyms) may reflect the surgeon's inability to diagnose, or the lack of means to diagnose, true nociceptive or neurogenic pain whose mechanism has yet to be determined. Less than 50 years ago psychiatry textbooks referred to ulcerative colitis and rheumatoid arthritis as psychosomatic disorders. Less than 20 years ago the pain of spinal cord injury was considered to be psychogenic, and less than 10 years ago peptic ulceration was blamed on stress.

THERAPEUTIC IMPLICATIONS

The anatomy and physiology of nociception underlie the basis of conventional and alternative methods of pain treatment. Their relationship to the four components of nociception is summarized in Figure 1.1.7

The ideal method of relieving pain is to resolve the disorder that is causing it. However, infection treated by antibiotics is the only pure example of this option. The suppression of inflammation by steroids is a cognate example, but steroids do not cure the cause of the inflammation. Surgical options are to excise the diseased and painful organ (if it can be sacrificed), to repair it or to replace it.

NSAIDs are useful for post-operative analgesia, and it is attractive to explain their action in terms of inhibition of the facilitatory effect of prostaglandins on nerves in areas of tissue damage. However, the analgesic potency of NSAIDs is not related to their ability to inhibit prostaglandins. It is more likely that the cardinal mechanism by which NSAIDs afford analgesia operates in the central nervous system. NSAIDs have no peripheral action on mechanical nociception, and they offer no greater analgesia than paracetamol in chronic musculoskeletal disorders.

Local anaesthetics can be used to anaesthetize the peripheral nerves that transmit nociception. However, they are not curative. Nevertheless, a series of blocks can

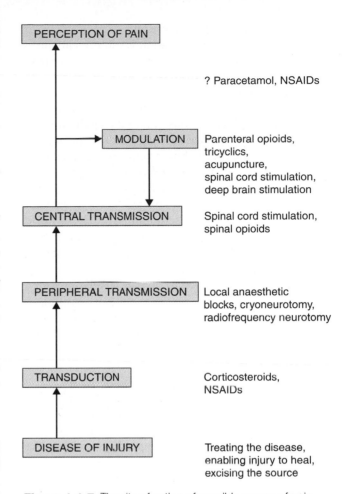

Figure 1.1.7 The site of action of possible means of pain management related to the physiology of nociception.

be useful for providing analgesia while natural healing occurs, e.g. after certain fractures or for surgical wounds. Peripheral nerves can also be frozen (cryoneurotomy) or coagulated (radiofrequency neurotomy) to secure anaesthesia of a painful part of the body for periods longer than the possible duration of action of local anaesthetics.

In some quarters, transcutaneous electrical nerve stimulation (TENS) is used for pain control. This technique is believed to produce analgesia by stimulating large-diameter afferent nerve fibres that inhibit small-diameter, nociceptive afferents. However, the technique appears to work well only in those instances where the electrodes can be interposed between the source of pain and the central nervous system, e.g. in painful conditions of the distal upper limb. In other instances, such as back pain and obstetric pain, controlled trials have shown that the effect of TENS is no greater than that of a placebo.

Most other techniques of pain management in some way interfere with descending modulation of nociception. Low-dose opioids (oral or injected) act by a peculiar effect on descending inhibition. They do not block nociception, but instead they reduce tonic descending inhibition. This corrupts centre-surround inhibition and decreases the signal-to-noise ratio of nociception. In effect, the nociceptive information is still present and is being transmitted through the central nervous system, but it is obscured by surrounding noise. Obscuring the signal obtunds the response.

On the other hand, opioids injected in high concentrations, although at low doses, into the epidural space (or intrathecally) exert a direct effect on the spinal cord, where they mimic the inhibitory action of enkephalin on primary afferents and second-order neurones, and thereby interrupt nociception. Tricyclic antidepressants are believed to exert a similar analgesic effect by enhancing the inhibitory action of serotonin in the dorsal horn. The mechanism of action of simple analgesics such as paracetamol is unknown, but is thought to be located in the central nervous system.

Acupuncture is believed to operate largely through a process known as diffuse noxious inhibitory control, in which the noxious acupuncture stimulus evokes widespread activation of descending inhibition to all segments of the spinal cord, thereby inhibiting any ongoing nociceptive traffic. Thus acupuncture operates on the same system as opioids, but in an opposite sense.

Spinal cord stimulation involves the implantation in the epidural space of wires that stimulate ascending and descending tracts. This stimulation interferes with the transmission of nociception, perhaps by corrupting the nociceptive signal, replacing it with a tingling sensation, and perhaps also by evoking descending inhibition.

Deep brain stimulation is an advanced technique of pain management in which electrodes are inserted under stereotactic control into the periventricular grey matter and used to increase descending inhibition to all segments of the spinal cord. A variant of this method involves stimulating nociceptive tracts just below the VPL and CL nuclei of the thalamus in order to corrupt the nociceptive signal.

Because the neurones involved lack receptors, central pain is difficult to treat. It is temporarily responsive to intravenous infusions of lignocaine, and may be controlled with oral doses of mexiletine if the latter is toler-ated. Surgically, spontaneously active neurones can be destroyed by radiofrequency coagulation in a procedure known as dorsal root entry zone (DREZ) lesioning.

Possible techniques of pain management that are currently being explored include the development of NMDA-receptor blockers and nitric-oxide blockers, and intrathecal administration of adrenoreceptor blockers.

FURTHER READING

Bonica JJ (ed.). 1990: *The management of pain. Vols I and II*. Philadelphia, PA: Lea & Febiger.

Coderre TJ, Katz J, Vaccarino AL, Melzack R. 1993: Contribution of central neuroplasticity to pathological pain: review of clinical and experimental evidence. *Pain* **52**, 259–85.

Guyton AC. 1991: *Textbook of medical physiology*, 8th edn. Philadelphia, PA: Saunders.

McMinn RMH. 1990: *Last's anatomy*, 8th edn. Edinburgh: Churchill Livingstone.

Merskey H, Bogduk N (eds). 1994: *Classification of chronic pain. Descriptions of chronic pain syndromes and definition of pain terms*, 2nd edn. Seattle: IASP Press.

National Health and Medical Research Council, Health Care Committee. 1989: *Report of Working Party on Acupuncture*. Canberra: National Health and Medical Research Council.

Siddall PJ, Cousins MJ. 1998: Introduction to pain mechanisms: implications for neural blockade. In Cousins MJ, Bridenbaugh PO (eds), *Neural blockade in clinical anaesthesia and management of pain*, 3rd edn. Philadelphia, PA: Lippincott-Raven, 675–99.

Wilcox GL. 1991: Excitatory neurotransmitters and pain. In Bond MR, Charlton JE, Woolf CJ (eds), *Proceedings of the Fifth World Congress on Pain*. Amsterdam: Elsevier, 97–117.

Headache

Chris Kneebone, Gordon G. Stuart and Philip D. Thompson

Introduction

Headache is a common complaint and a frequent reason for medical consultation. It is estimated that 80% of the population, encompassing all age groups, experience headache at some time, and that approximately 17% of females and 6% of males experience migraine. While patients may refer to their headaches in terms such as 'a normal headache', 'eye strain', 'sinus headache' or a 'sick headache', there is also an understanding that headache may be the presenting symptom of serious pathology, engendering a level of anxiety in those who present for medical review. Although the vast majority will have a benign explanation, the risk of missing serious and treatable causes demands a detailed and appropriately directed history and examination. This should determine the need for further investigation, but it is worth remembering that a normal computed tomogram of the head is not sufficient to exclude all forms of serious pathology presenting as headache, e.g. temporal arteritis, benign intracranial hypertension and various forms of meningeal irritation. Before discussing the topic of headache in greater detail, the pain sensitivity of cranial structures and the anatomy of innervation of pain-sensitive cranial structures will be reviewed briefly.

SOURCES OF HEAD PAIN

The most important sources of intracranial pain are the blood vessels, particularly the proximal parts of the cerebral arteries, the large veins and venous sinuses, and the dura near meningeal blood vessels. Pain may also arise from the periosteum and scalp muscles. Direct stimulation or injury of the brain itself does not cause pain. The skull bone, pia arachnoid and choroid plexus are also insensitive to pain.

PATHWAYS OF PAIN TRANSMISSION

Noxious stimuli to the pain-sensitive areas described above excite pain receptors which transmit signals to the brain via small myelinated and unmyelinated nerve fibres carried in the three divisions of the trigeminal nerve and via the dorsal roots of the second and third cervical nerves. The trigeminal fibres enter the pons and descend in the ipsilateral descending tract and nucleus of the trigeminal nerve, merging with the substantia gelatinosa region of the upper cervical cord, which also receives fibres from the upper cervical sensory nerve roots (Figure 1.2.1).

DISTRIBUTION OF PAIN REFERRED FROM CRANIAL STRUCTURES

Pain from the anterior and middle cranial fossae (including the tentorium cerebelli) is transmitted by the ophthalmic and maxillary divisions of the trigeminal nerve and is felt in the region of the eye and orbit, forehead or temporal regions, respectively. Overlap of cranial and cervical pain fibres in the cervical cord can lead to

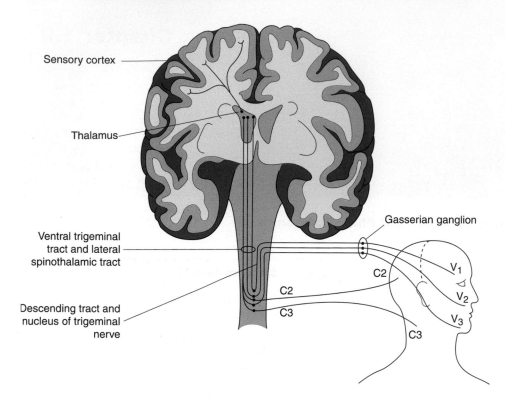

Sensory cortex

Thalamus

Gasserian ganglion

Ventral trigeminal tract and lateral spinothalamic tract

C2

C2

V₁

C2

V₂

C3

V₃

Descending tract and nucleus of trigeminal nerve

C3

Figure 1.2.1 Illustration of the major pain pathways from the head and cervical spine, and the central projections of pain fibres.

referral of pain arising in upper cervical structures to the frontal or orbital region, in addition to the occipital and upper cervical regions.

HISTORY

A detailed account of the characteristics and evolution of the headache is crucial when differentiating between the various causes of headache, and a complete history is the most important and useful clinical tool. Most diagnoses will be evident or suspected from the history before the examination. Important features to elicit in the history are listed in Table 1.2.1. As a general rule, headaches of recent origin are more likely to reflect underlying pathology. Neurological symptoms accompanying the headache, particularly if progressive, should alert the clinician to an underlying structural cause. In the patient presenting with a new type of headache it is important to determine exactly how it commenced. Most varieties of headache, even those with a rapid onset, build up in intensity over a period of time that may range from minutes to days. In contrast, the headache of subarachnoid haemorrhage is instantaneously severe at the onset – a sensation similar to being struck on the head. Of concern is the history of a recent-onset headache that has progressively worsened over time. Most forms of benign headache are either episodic or wax and wane in intensity. The onset of a new type of headache after the age of 50 years should lead to consideration of the possibility of temporal arteritis, which is frequently associated with

symptoms of systemic illness and, less commonly, retinal or cerebral ischaemia.

EXAMINATION

A convenient way to begin the examination is to ascertain whether the patient is unwell or distressed by headache at the time of presentation. The patient with a febrile or systemic illness should be assessed for evidence of meningeal irritation (due to haemorrhage or infection) by examining for neck stiffness and impairment of straight leg raising (Kernig's sign). Drowsiness or impairment of consciousness suggest depression of cerebral function which could be due to encephalitis, drug effects or a cerebral mass (tumour or haematoma) causing raised intracranial pressure and brainstem compression. Examination of the optic fundi for papilloedema is essential. A search should be made for neurological signs such as dysphasia, altered higher mental function, hemianopia, weakness, imbalance or cortical sensory loss. Such findings suggest an underlying structural lesion.

A patient presenting during the course of a migraine will generally appear pale and unwell with photophobia, nausea and possibly vomiting, and will not wish to be disturbed. There should be no evidence of fever or neck stiffness. When assessing the well patient, additional features that should be sought include assessment of the cervical spine, sinuses and teeth or other sources of head pain. In addition to the neurological examination, significant hypertension should be excluded.

Table 1.2.1 Important points in the clinical history of a headache

Exact description of mode of onset of presenting headache	
Sudden	
Stepwise	
Gradual, progressive	

Length of history
Have different varieties of headache occurred in the past?
Age at onset and duration of each type of headache

Presenting headache

Location	Variable
	Stereotyped
Quality	Throbbing, stabbing, pulsating
	Dull constant pressure
	Tightness on or around the head
	Continuous deep boring sensation
Intensity	Continuous
	Steadily worsening
	Variable intensity

Frequency and periodicity

Duration of each headache

Warning symptoms prior to the onset of headache

Time of onset	Variable
	Stereotyped
	Day or night
	In relation to the menstrual cycle

Precipitants

Exacerbating factors	Coughing, straining, postural change
	Noise, bright lights
Relieving factors	Medication
Associated symptoms	Nausea
	Vomiting
	Photophobia and other visual disturbances
	Neck pain and stiffness

General health

Family history

Papilloedema

Papilloedema is a cardinal sign of raised intracranial pressure (see Plate 1.2.1 in the colour plate section). Fully developed papilloedema following sustained raised intracranial pressure is easily recognized by the disappearance of the physiological cup, blurring of disc margins and a greyish discoloration of the surrounding retina. The retinal vessels appear to be elevated by the disc swelling and the veins are enlarged compared to the arteries. Haemorrhages and exudates may also appear. Visual field testing may reveal enlargement of the blind spots and some constriction of the peripheral field. Early papilloedema can be difficult to diagnose with certainty, and is often recognized by the conjunction of the features listed in Table 1.2.2.

INVESTIGATION OF HEADACHE

A progressive history of a new headache, the presence of neurological symptoms or neurological signs on examination, and the recent onset of headache in a patient over the age of 50 years are indications for investigation. This should begin with brain imaging, a full blood count, determination of sedimentation rate and a search for evidence of fever or other systemic disease.

DIAGNOSIS OF HEADACHE

The causes of headache can be classified into primary headache syndromes, without any structural, vascular, infective or systemic disease, and those which are secondary to an identifiable cause (Table 1.2.3). Diagnosis of primary headache syndromes is aided by a long history

Table 1.2.2 Ophthalmoscopic features of early papilloedema

1. **Disc hyperaemia** (particularly if the disc becomes pinker over the course of serial examinations) note the normal variation in disc colour

2. **Blurring of disc margins** (nasal, upper and lower poles affected before temporal margin) and blurring of the detail of the physiological cup. Isolated blurring of disc margins is not diagnostic of papilloedema, and may be seen with hypermetropia

3. **Overfilling of retinal veins**. Distention of retinal veins is an important early sign of papilloedema, particularly if venous pulsation cannot be discerned after light pressure on the globe

4. **Disc border haemorrhages** (radial linear red streaks on the surface of the nerve fibres overlying the margin of the disc) are a reliable sign of early papilloedema

Table 1.2.3 Classification of primary and secondary headache syndromes

> **Primary headache syndromes**
> Migraine
> Tension-type headache
> Cluster headache and chronic paroxysmal hemicrania
> Ice-pick headache and stabbing headache
> Benign cough, exertional and sex headache
>
> **Secondary headache syndromes**
> Head trauma
> Vascular disorders
>   Subarachnoid haemorrhage
>   Temporal arteritis
>   Cerebral venous thrombosis
>   Systemic hypertension
> Changes in intracranial pressure
>   Raised intracranial pressure
>   Low intracranial pressure
> Infective causes
>   Intracranial infection
>   Systemic infection
> Drug-induced and drug-withdrawal headaches
> Metabolic disorders
> Headache associated with disorders of neck, cranial or
>   extracranial structures

of recurrent stereotyped headaches with symptom-free intervals. These headaches can be further classified according to their individual characteristics.

CLINICAL CHARACTERISTICS OF PRIMARY HEADACHE SYNDROMES

MIGRAINE

Migraine is the commonest cause of episodic disabling headache and may occur with or without a preceding aura. Migraine without aura is the commonest form, and should be considered whenever there is a recurring pattern of unilateral, throbbing or pounding headache, associated with nausea, photophobia and sensitivity to noise, that is severe enough to interfere with normal activities. Most migrainous headaches last for between 4 and 48 h and recur with variable frequency, interspersed with symptom-free intervals. In migraine with aura, which is present in 25% of migraneurs, the onset of headache is preceded by or coincides with an aura. The commonest aura is an evolving visual disturbance beginning in one or both visual fields, consisting of scintillating or shimmering elements, accompanied by visual distortion, obscuration and scotomata. Typically, the

pattern is an expanding sequence of zigzag lines referred to as a 'fortification spectrum'. The visual disturbance may evolve into a patchy visual loss, a hemianopia or near-complete visual loss. Other common forms of aura include speech disturbance and unilateral positive sensory symptoms (tingling or pins and needles, rather than loss of feeling). Typically, the sensory disturbance spreads over a period of several minutes. In some patients the visual aura will give way to speech difficulties and then to sensory symptoms as the disturbance spreads anteriorly from the occipital lobes. This pattern of evolving sequential deficits helps to distinguish migrainous symptoms from those associated with cerebrovascular disease or epilepsy.

Pathophysiology of migraine

The pathophysiological mechanisms which underlie the development of migraine remain unclear. There is frequently a positive family history of migraine, and susceptibility to migraine may be genetically based (inherited mutations in neuronal voltage-gated ion channels are found in some families with familial hemiplegic migraine). The headache of migraine arises in the cerebral and extracranial blood vessels. A cascade of chemical events in the wall of affected blood vessels produces a sterile inflammatory response. These responses can be blocked by serotonin or serotonin-like agonists which bind to serotonin 1B and D receptors.

The aura of migraine is thought to reflect the cortical phenomenon known as 'spreading depression'. This was first identified more than 50 years ago in anaesthetized animals as a slowly spreading suppression of electroencephalographic activity of the cerebral cortex. In the mouse, spreading cortical depression is associated with the release of calcitonin gene-related peptide and nitrous oxide, neurotransmitters which have been closely associated with the development of migraine headache. Functional imaging studies in patients during a migrainous aura have shown spreading oligaemia advancing forward over the occipital cortex at a rate of approximately 3 mm/min, similar to that of spreading depression. Oligaemia is thought to be secondary to reduced neuronal metabolic demand rather than a primary ischaemic phenomenon. Accordingly, the aura of migraine is no longer viewed as a consequence of vasospasm, nor is the headache simply associated with vascular dilatation. A brief outline of the approaches used to treat migraine is given in Table 1.2.4.

TENSION-TYPE HEADACHE

Tension headaches tend to be bilateral and are often described as a tightness or pressure around the head. Episodic tension headaches are usually associated with

Table 1.2.4 Brief outline of the treatment of migraine

1. **Preventative measures**
   Avoid known precipitants

2. **Management of the acute attack**
   Simple analgesics plus anti-emetic (metaclopramide)
   Ergot alkaloids (ergotamine, dihydroergotamine)
   Selective serotonin type 1 receptor agonists
      ('triptans')

3. **Prophylactic or interval therapy (frequency > 2 per month)**
   Beta-blockers (propranolol, metoprolol, atenolol)
   Serotonin antagonists (pizotifen, cyproheptadine)
   Ergot derivatives (ergotamine, methysergide)

stress or mental and physical fatigue. Chronic tension headache, by definition, occurs 15 or more times a month, and is frequently present on a continuous or daily basis. Its underlying basis remains uncertain. This type of headache is the commonest cause of a chronic, semi-continuous persistent daily headache, and frequently responds to small doses of a tricyclic antidepressant.

CLUSTER HEADACHE, CHRONIC PAROXYSMAL HEMICRANIA AND OTHER CRANIAL PAINS

Cluster headache derives its name from recurrent headaches occurring in clusters, each lasting a month or two, followed by a symptom-free interval lasting from months to years. During a cluster the patient, typically a middle-aged man, experiences episodes of severe orbital or peri-orbital pain several times a day, each episode lasting from 15 min to 3 h. The pain is accompanied by lacrimation, rhinorrhoea and nasal congestion on the affected side. During the cluster the patient is commonly woken at about the same time during the night with an attack. Chronic paroxysmal hemicrania is a similar condition. In contrast to cluster headache, it more commonly affects women, the episodes of pain are briefer (lasting several minutes) and the frequency of attacks is higher (several per day). These headaches may also be accompanied by autonomic phenomena. A dramatic response to treatment with indomethacin is characteristic.

A variety of other patterns of headache may be reported, particularly by patients with migraine. These include idiopathic stabbing ('ice-pick') headaches, consisting of brief sharp pain in various cranial locations (especially ocular and peri-ocular).

COUGH, EXERTIONAL AND SEX HEADACHES

Benign cough, exertional and sex or orgasmic headaches all raise concern about an intracranial lesion. These headaches are described as severe, generalized, exploding or throbbing, and begin in a crescendo fashion over a period of a few minutes. Cough headaches tend to be brief, lasting only minutes, but exertional and sex headaches may last several hours. An Arnold-Chiari malformation or other transient obstruction to the flow of spinal fluid should be excluded in cough and exertional headache. The sudden onset of headache during sexual intercourse raises the possibility of a ruptured berry aneurysm and a subarachnoid haemorrhage. When there is no past history of similar stereotyped episodes, it may be necessary to exclude a subarachnoid haemorrhage with brain imaging and spinal fluid examination.

CLINICAL CHARACTERISTICS OF SECONDARY HEADACHE SYNDROMES

HEADACHE ASSOCIATED WITH HEAD TRAUMA

Headache commonly follows a head injury with or without concussion, but may also signal the potentially serious consequence of intracranial bleeding. Chronic post-traumatic headache is defined by the persistence of headache for more than 8 weeks, and often appears to be multifactorial in origin.

HEADACHE AND SUBARACHNOID HAEMORRHAGE

Rupture of an intracranial aneurysm or arteriovenous malformation characteristically presents with headache. The majority (70%) of subarachnoid haemorrhages are due to rupture of an aneurysm, 10% are due to arteriovenous malformations, 10% are hypertensive in origin and in 10% the cause is never established. In the case of aneurysm rupture, the headache is instantaneous in onset and severe. There may be loss of consciousness, and typically the onset is associated with prostration, nausea, vomiting and photophobia. The headache may radiate to the neck with severe neck pain and neck stiffness on examination. It is estimated that 40% of subarachnoid haemorrhages are preceded by a warning leak during which the headache is often not as dramatic or disabling. Patients may delay seeking medical advice and wait to see whether the headache will resolve. If it persists, they may present a week or two later and fail to describe the apoplectic onset of the headache, particularly if it occurred during sexual activity or while they were straining on the toilet. The development of sciatica a few days after a severe headache is suggestive of a subarachnoid haemorrhage with subarachnoid blood irritating the lumbar and sacral nerve roots. Early diagnosis and appropriate management at this stage are associated with a good outcome in 85% of cases. The risk of re-bleeding leading to death or severe disability demands that this history is actively sought.

HEADACHE AND TEMPORAL ARTERITIS

Patients over the age of 50 years who present with a new type of headache require careful consideration, including exclusion of giant cell or temporal arteritis. Early recognition and treatment are important, since the arteritis may lead to optic nerve ischaemia and blindness or stroke. Symptoms of systemic disease, e.g. lethargy, malaise and weight loss, are often present, the temporal arteries may be firm and tender to palpation, and the sedimentation rate is elevated. The headache settles rapidly with steroid treatment.

HEADACHE AND CEREBRAL VENOUS THROMBOSIS

The large cerebral veins and venous sinuses are pain sensitive, and thrombosis within the cerebral venous system is associated with headache. Venous sinus thrombosis may also result in raised intracranial pressure. Haemorrhagic infarction within the cortex leads to focal neurological deficits. Seizures are common. Thrombosis within cerebral veins is well demonstrated by magnetic resonance imaging.

HEADACHE AND SYSTEMIC HYPERTENSION

Headache may accompany severe hypertension or a sudden rise in blood pressure as may occur in patients with malignant hypertension, eclampsia or a phaeochromocytoma.

HEADACHE ASSOCIATED WITH CHANGES IN INTRACRANIAL PRESSURE

Raised intracranial pressure

Obstructive hydrocephalus is produced by lesions obstructing the flow of cerebrospinal fluid. This may occur anywhere from the lateral ventricles through the foramina of Monro, within the third ventricle, the aqueduct of Sylvius, the outlets of the fourth ventricle (the foramina of Magendie and Luschka), within the fourth ventricle, or by passage through the subarachnoid space or absorption via arachnoid granulations into superior sagittal sinus. The headache of raised intracranial pressure is most troublesome when the patient is lying down. It is worse on waking in the morning, and will fre-

quently disturb sleep. It is aggravated by manoeuvres which increase central venous pressure, such as coughing, sneezing, straining, or bending down or forward. When raised intracranial pressure is related to a mass lesion, there may also be focal symptoms or focal headache due to traction on blood vessels and dura. A lesion in the anterior third ventricle, such as a colloid cyst, may obstruct the foramen of Monro intermittently, producing sudden rises in intracranial pressure, acute severe headache, loss of muscle tone and drop attacks. Craniocervical junction malformations may obstruct the flow of spinal fluid when venous pressure is raised, causing cough headaches. Similar headaches with papilloedema and other evidence of raised intracranial pressure occur in benign intracranial hypertension, where there is no evidence of any mass effect or obstruction to cerebrospinal fluid circulation. In such cases it is important to exclude occult venous sinus thrombosis.

Low intracranial pressure

Low cerebrospinal fluid pressure is usually caused by persistent leakage of spinal fluid after an intentional or inadvertent dural puncture, e.g. during lumbar puncture or myelography, or as a complication of epidural anaesthesia, neurosurgical procedures or trauma. Low-pressure headaches may be accompanied by neck stiffness and are very sensitive to changes in posture, being worse on standing and improved by lying down. Such headaches are thought to be related to a reduction in support for the brain and increased traction on dural blood vessels.

INTRACRANIAL INFECTION

Meningitis and encephalitis are accompanied by severe headache associated with evidence of meningeal irritation. Fever, photophobia, neck stiffness and a positive Kernig's sign are generally prominent. A cerebral abscess may be associated with a headache related to a mass effect and raised intracranial pressure.

INTRACRANIAL NEOPLASIA

Headache is a relatively uncommon presentation of intracranial tumours, whether extrinsic to the brain (meningioma) or primary or secondary intracerebral. Headache may be a result of raised intracranial pressure caused by complications of the neoplasm, such as haemorrhage or obstruction to the CSF pathway. Otherwise, it is not until the tumour reaches a considerable size that it produces sufficient mass effect to displace and cause traction on blood vessels and dura, such that a headache results. The headache is generally dull and lateralized to the side of pathology.

HEADACHE ASSOCIATED WITH SUBSTANCES OR THEIR WITHDRAWAL

Headache can be an adverse side-effect to many medications. It is commonly seen with vasodilator agents, including the nitrates, nitrites and calcium-channel blockers. It is also often seen after exposure to agents such as carbon monoxide and volatile hydrocarbons such as solvents. Frequent or daily use of medication for treating headache can also induce a chronic headache as a rebound phenomenon. This is notoriously true of ergotamine, but has also been more frequently recognized as a problem when taking analgesia on a daily basis, particularly those preparations which contain some form of opiate. Caffeine withdrawal has a similar effect.

HEADACHE ASSOCIATED WITH NON-CEPHALIC INFECTION

Headache frequently accompanies systemic febrile illness, whether it is viral or bacterial. It is usually present with influenza-like illnesses, and can be a persistent and troublesome symptom with infectious mononucleosis. A viral illness may at times be associated with meningism without evidence of meningitis on CSF examination.

HEADACHE ASSOCIATED WITH METABOLIC DISORDERS

A range of metabolic disorders, such as hypoxia, hypercapnia, and hypoglycaemia may be associated with headache.

HEADACHE OR FACIAL PAIN ASSOCIATED WITH DISORDERS OF NECK, CRANIAL OR EXTRACRANIAL STRUCTURES

Headaches that arise in the cervical spine, eyes, ears, nose and sinuses, teeth, jaws and temporomandibular joints are generally located over the affected stuctures. Headaches of joint or musculoskeletal origin are typically tender to palpation of the affected part and exacerbated by movement. Sinus headaches are made worse by bending forward.

Painful eye

Justine R. Smith

Introduction

Ocular pain is an extremely common complaint which is distressing for the patient, and which may signify sight-threatening disease. Generally it is possible to make the diagnosis from an account of the pain, including any associated symptoms, and a basic clinical examination. A primary determinant of the pain experience is the tissue location of the pathology. The nasociliary branch of the ophthalmic division of the trigeminal nerve provides all somatic sensory innervation to the eye, but the various ocular structures receive very different supplies. The cornea has one of the densest sensory networks of any body tissue, no doubt reflecting its role as the necessarily exposed, essential refracting surface of the visual system. Corneal lesions may be exquisitely painful, often being likened to a foreign body on the eye. The sclera also receives significant sensory innervation, but the conjunctiva contains few nerve endings and is rarely a source of significant ocular discomfort. Both the iris and the choroid are sparsely innervated, while the ciliary body contains a dense sensory plexus. The retina has essentially no somatic sensory innervation. Consequently, retinal conditions such as age-related macular degeneration, diabetic retinopathy and retinal detachment are associated with painless visual loss. Similarly, as the lens contains no sensory nerves, cataract does not cause ocular pain. The orbital tissues are well innervated by various branches of the ophthalmic and maxillary nerves.

SIGNIFICANT CAUSES OF A PAINFUL EYE TABLES 1.3.1 AND 1.3.2

INFECTIOUS KERATITIS

The commonest corneal infections are viral. Herpes simplex virus most often produces a dendritic ulcer, although other corneal lesions, including the relatively larger geographic ulcer and stromal keratitis without ulceration, are also possible sequelae. Infection is acquired through close physical contact with an individual who is shedding virus, typically from vesicles on the lips. The primary ocular infection is frequently subclinical, but may also present as blepharoconjunctivitis. With clinical resolution, the virus moves along the ophthalmic nerve to the trigeminal ganglion, where it remains dormant. Situations of physical or psychological stress trigger its return to the eye. The dendritic ulcer has a characteristic branching pattern, best seen when the eye is stained with fluorescein 2% eyedrops and viewed with a cobalt blue light (see Plate 1.3.1 in the colour plate section). Examination may also reveal reduced corneal sensation. Without treatment, 50% of dendritic lesions heal without complication. However, this rate improves to almost 100% if a topical antiviral agent such as aciclovir 3% ointment is used. Topical corticosteroids are strictly contraindicated for dendritic ulceration, as these drugs enhance viral replication and may lead to worsening of the disease.

Table 1.3.1 Significant causes of a painful eye

Ocular causes
1. Ocular trauma
2. Infectious keratitis (viral, bacterial)
3. Scleritis
4. Acute anterior uveitis
5. Angle-closure glaucoma (primary, neovascular)
6. Endophthalmitis

Orbital causes
1. Orbital trauma
2. Orbital cellulitis
3. Orbital inflammatory syndrome
4. Optic neuritis

Like herpes simplex virus, the varicella-zoster virus may also lodge in the trigeminal ganglion following primary infection, in this case, chicken-pox. Reactivation, often related to Hodgkin's lymphoma, early HIV infection or immunosuppression, causes herpes zoster ophthalmicus. In addition to the characteristic vesicular rash presenting in the distribution of the ophthalmic nerve, inflammation involves the eye in about 50% of cases. A reasonably reliable sign of ocular involvement is extension of the skin rash on to the nasal tip, which is also supplied by the nasociliary nerve. Keratitis is one of the commonest complications, and a variety of corneal lesions are possible. Late disease is often neurotrophic rather than inflammatory. Other significant sequelae include anterior uveitis and scleritis (see below). A course of oral aciclovir should be instituted within 72 h of disease onset in order to reduce the incidence of ocular complications. The value of topical antiviral treatment remains controversial. However, topical corticosteroids are often useful for controlling the inflammatory complications.

Ordinarily, antimicrobial agents in the tear film, conjunctiva-associated lymphoid tissue and an intact epithelium protect the cornea from bacterial or fungal keratitis. Such infection is usually associated with a predisposing condition such as dry eyes, contact-lens wear, chronic lid or lacrimal infection, corneal disease and immunosuppression. On examination, a corneal ulcer is associated with opaque stromal suppuration (see Plate 1.3.2 in the colour plate section). *Staphylococcus aureus, Streptococcus pneumoniae* and *Pseudomonas aeruginosa* are the most common pathogens, but the causative microbe cannot be deduced from the clinical picture. Scrapings must be obtained for microscopy with stains and culture. Fortified topical antibiotics are initially instilled hourly. Cephazolin 5% has been widely employed for Gram-positive infections, and gentamicin 1.4% for Gram-negative infections. However, newer antibiotics are becoming increasingly popular, including the topical quinolones, which are active against many

Table 1.3.2 Clinical features which distinguish different causes of 'red eye'

Condition	Characteristic symptoms	Characteristic signs
Conjunctivitis	If infective, contact If allergic, hay fever Sticky eyes	Bilateral Palpebral injection Ocular discharge
Corneal abrasion	History of trauma Foreign-body pain	Irregular corneal epithelial defect
Bacterial corneal ulcer	Predisposing eye condition Severe foreign-body pain	Deep corneal defect Stromal opacification
Dendritic corneal ulcer	Previous attacks Foreign-body pain	Branching corneal epithelial defect Reduced corneal sensation
Acute anterior uveitis	Related medical condition Previous attacks Photophobia	Ciliary injection Small, irregular pupil
Episcleritis	Isolated red eye	Sectorial injection
Anterior scleritis	Related medical condition Severe aching pain	Violet discoloration Eye injected despite phenylephrine 10% Globe tenderness
Primary angle-closure glaucoma	Nausea and vomiting Severe aching pain	Cloudy cornea Flat anterior chamber Fixed mid-dilated pupil

Gram-negative bacterial species. Filamentous fungi and yeasts are uncommon causes of microbial keratitis, and are treated with topical ketoconazole 1% and amphotericin B 1%, respectively. Acanthamoeba keratitis is a disease of contact-lens wearers. Diagnosis is difficult, and eradication of the organism may require penetrating keratoplasty as well as a variety of topical antiparasitic agents.

SCLERITIS

Scleral inflammation causes aching pain that is severe enough to prevent sleep. Most patients are older adults, frequently diagnosed with rheumatoid arthritis or other collagen vascular diseases. When the disease involves the anterior sclera, congestion of the scleral vascular plexus produces a violet discoloration of this tissue. In some cases the entire anterior sclera is involved, while in others only a sector is inflamed. There may be a scleral nodule (see Plate 1.3.3 in the colour plate section). By slit-lamp examination it is often possible to distinguish the deep scleral vascular plexus from overlying conjunctival and episcleral vessels. A useful clue is that these deeper vessels cannot be constricted by topical phenylephrine 10%. The eyeball is tender to touch, but visual acuity is often normal, and the pupil should react normally. Posterior scleritis is far less common. The eye may not be red, and clinical signs relate to extension of the inflammation inward to involve the retina, choroid and optic nerve, or outward to involve orbital structures. Ocular ultrasound demonstrates thickening of the posterior eye wall. The most serious complication of untreated scleritis is ocular perforation. If oral non-steroidal anti-inflammatory drugs do not settle the inflammation, systemic corticosteroids or other immunosuppressive agents are employed. Episcleritis is a painless benign condition that is sometimes confused with anterior scleritis.

ACUTE ANTERIOR UVEITIS

Acute anterior uveitis is an inflammatory disorder of the iris and/or ciliary body, also commonly referred to as acute iritis or acute iridocyclitis. Most patients first present in adulthood, and up to 50% of these individuals will suffer from a related systemic disease. Common associations are the seronegative HLA B27-linked arthropathies, including ankylosing spondylitis, Reiter's syndrome, psoriatic arthritis and arthritis associated with inflammatory bowel disease, and sarcoidosis. Photophobia (ocular pain on exposure to light) is a prominent symptom. This is produced by movements of the inflamed anterior uveal tissues in response to light. Blood from these structures drains partly via the anterior ciliary veins, producing a hyperaemia which is maximal at the limbus, known as ciliary injection. The pupil is small due to spasm of the iris sphincter, and often irregular as a result of posterior synechiae (adhesions between the iris and the anterior lens surface) (see Plate 1.3.4 in the colour plate section). The disease lasts for about 6 weeks, but recurrent episodes are common. Treatment is essential in order to prevent permanent structural damage to the eye, such as cataract, glaucoma and cystoid macular oedema. Fortunately, acute anterior uveitis can usually be successfully managed with topical corticosteroids and cycloplegics.

ANGLE-CLOSURE GLAUCOMA

Glaucoma refers to any condition in which elevated intra-ocular pressure damages the optic nerve, producing visual field loss. Primary angle-closure glaucoma occurs in individuals with narrowed anterior chamber angles, as is seen in hypermetropia (long-sightedness), and may also occur with ageing as the lens size increases. Slight forward movement of the peripheral iris may close the angle and obstruct aqueous outflow at the trabeculum. In the face of continuing aqueous production, the intra-ocular pressure quickly rises from about 20 mmHg to 50–100 mmHg. This causes sudden and severe aching ocular pain, often associated with profuse sweating, nausea and vomiting. Visual acuity is markedly reduced. There is ciliary injection, and the cornea is cloudy due to pressure-induced oedema. The pupil is mid-dilated and fixed as a result of iris ischaemia (see Plate 1.3.5 in the colour plate section). Oblique pen-light illumination will reveal shallow anterior chambers bilaterally. If left untreated, complete and irreversible visual loss rapidly ensues. A reduction in pressure is generally achieved by suppressing aqueous secretion using intravenous acetazolamide and topical timolol 0.5%. In severe cases, hyperosmotic agents such as mannitol may be needed. Pilocarpine eyedrops, which normally constrict the pupil, are not useful while the iris is ischaemic and paralysed. Further attacks can be prevented by laser peripheral iridotomy, and the second eye is also treated prophylactically.

Neovascular glaucoma is a secondary form of angle-closure glaucoma which may also cause marked ocular aching. In this condition, ocular ischaemia leads to the release of angiogenic factors within the eye. As a result, a fibrovascular membrane grows across the surface of the iris and on to the anterior chamber angle, preventing aqueous outflow. Most cases of neovascular glaucoma are attributable to either central retinal vein occlusion or proliferative diabetic retinopathy. The intra-ocular pressure is 50 mmHg or more, and, apart from a deep anterior chamber, clinical findings are similar to those for primary angle-closure glaucoma. However, in addition, slit-lamp examination reveals rubeosis iridis (new blood vessels on the surface of the iris) and in some cases a spontaneous hyphaema (blood in the anterior chamber). Treatment is notoriously difficult. Drainage surgery is the only option. In some cases the intra-ocular pressure cannot be controlled, and enucleation may finally be required to control pain in a blinded eye.

ENDOPHTHALMITIS

Endophthalmitis, an infection that involves the ocular cavities and globe wall, is uncommon but potentially blinding. Usually an exogenous infection follows surgery or trauma. Infrequently, haematogenous spread of micro-organisms to the eye may result in endogenous endophthalmitis. The organism most commonly isolated post-operatively is *Staphylococcus epidermidis*, but *Staphylococcus aureus*, *Pseudomonas aeruginosa* and various streptococcal species are also frequently responsible. These pathogens reside in the patient's conjunctival sac. Endophthalmitis with *Propionibacterium acnes* is peculiar to intra-ocular lens implantation. Bacteria lodge around the lens, causing chronic inflammation with a delayed presentation. In post-traumatic endophthalmitis, environmental organisms are isolated as well as conjunctival flora. Typically, the patient presents within the first 48 h following surgery or injury. There is severe ocular pain and poor vision, lid oedema, conjunctival injection and chemosis (conjunctival oedema), a cloudy cornea and a hypopyon (pus in the anterior chamber) (see Plate 1.3.6 in the colour plate section). Vitritis causes a poor red reflex. Aqueous and vitreous specimens are collected for microbiological analysis, and broad-spectrum antibiotics are injected intravitreally. Often cephazolin and gentamicin will cover the offending organism. Recently, vancomycin has been used in preference to cephazolin to ensure cover for methicillin-resistant *Staphylococcus* species, and ceftazidime has been employed to avoid the retinal toxicity associated with aminoglycosides. Vitrectomy is considered if visual acuity is severely reduced. Intensive fortified topical antibiotics are also administered, the choice being dictated by Gram stain and culture results. Broad-spectrum topical antibiotics, often chloramphenicol 0.5%, are used routinely during the first post-operative week in order to reduce the incidence of endophthalmitis.

ORBITAL CELLULITIS

It is essential to distinguish between orbital cellulitis and the more common preseptal cellulitis. The latter does not penetrate the orbital septum which separates the structures of the lids from the orbital contents. Orbital infection commonly spreads from the nasopharynx or paranasal sinuses. Pathogens include *Haemophilus influenzae*, *Streptococcus pneumoniae*, *Staphylococcus aureus*, aerobic Gram-negative bacteria and anaerobes. Introduction of the *Haemophilus influenzae* type b vaccine has greatly reduced the incidence of infection due to this organism. Deeply penetrating lid trauma may introduce environmental organisms. The patient is usually a child or young adult, presenting with sepsis with unilateral eye pain, lid oedema, conjunctival infection and chemosis, restricted ocular motility and proptosis. Normal motility and absence of ocular displacement suggest preseptal cellulitis. If left untreated, this condition may be fatal as a result of cavernous sinus thrombosis, meningitis, extradural abscess and/or brain abscess. Treatment is often empirical. Nasal and conjunctival cultures are rarely positive, although blood cultures may be helpful. The cellulitis generally responds to cefotaxime and flucloxacillin administered intravenously. An orbital or subperiosteal abscess should be suspected if there is no response to the antibiotics or there is a relapse on treatment. Such collections demand drainage, and may be localized by orbital CT scanning. Follow-up of sinus disease is indicated.

OPTIC NEURITIS

Inflammation of the optic nerve commonly occurs in the context of multiple sclerosis, and is the presenting feature in about 25% of cases. Many patients are therefore young adult women. There is sudden unilateral visual loss, associated with ocular pain that is exacerbated by eye movements and pressure on the eye. On examination, visual acuity is variably reduced, and there is a relative afferent pupillary defect. Because of selective involvement of the papillomacular bundle within the optic nerve, visual field testing reveals a central scotoma and colour vision is severely affected. The eye itself appears normal, with a normal optic disc, because the site of involvement lies behind the globe. The natural history is for slow recovery to occur over the ensuing 6 weeks. The authors of the Optic Neuritis Treatment Trial recommend that brain magnetic resonance imaging (MRI) scanning be performed immediately, in order to identify demyelination suggestive of multiple sclerosis. If plaques are present and the patient has been seen early, a 3-day course of intravenous methylprednisolone, followed by high-dose oral prednisolone, should be considered. This was shown to reduce the 2-year rate of developing further symptoms related to multiple sclerosis by more than 50%. For the optic neuritis, there is no long-term benefit of such therapy, and troublesome pain may be managed effectively with non-steroidal anti-inflammatory drugs.

ORBITAL INFLAMMATORY SYNDROME

Pseudotumour or orbital inflammatory syndrome is characterized by infiltration of the orbit by lymphocytes, often simulating an orbital neoplasm. Acute forms cause significant ocular pain. Involvement may be diffuse or localized, when it may affect the anterior orbit, one or more extra-ocular muscles, the lacrimal gland or the orbital apex. In the Tolosa-Hunt syndrome, inflammation involves the cavernous sinus. The disease most commonly occurs in middle-aged adults who present with an acute onset of unilateral ocular pain, often related to eye movement. Examination may reveal lid swelling, conjunctival infection and chemosis, proptosis, ophthalmoplegia or a palpable mass, depending on the site of involvement. There may be intra-ocular inflammation, and visual acuity may be impaired if there is optic nerve inflammation. Orbital computed tomography (CT) imaging is useful for localizing the areas involved. Symptoms frequently respond rapidly to high doses of an oral corticosteroid such as prednisolone, which is then tapered slowly over many months. Unresponsive disease is an indication for biopsy in order to exclude lymphoproliferative disease. Occasionally other treatments, such as alternative immunosuppressive agents or radiotherapy, are required. Thyroid eye disease is a common differential diagnosis, but this condition is typically painless.

OCULAR AND ORBITAL TRAUMA

Corneal trauma is the commonest cause of ocular pain presenting for assessment. Corneal abrasions are best highlighted by instillation of fluorescein 2% eyedrops and illumination with cobalt blue light (see Plate 1.3.7 in the colour plate section). A broad-spectrum antibiotic ointment such as chloramphenicol 0.5% is instilled into the conjunctival sac, and two pads are firmly applied in order to close the lids. The eye is checked daily until healing is complete in order to exclude infection. Poor healing with inadequate adhesion between the epithelium and basement membrane may result in a recurrent corneal erosion. The erosion typically occurs as the lids are first opened on waking. Treatment involves long-term use of a topical lubricant after the lesion has healed with patching. A corneal foreign body is obvious (see Plate 1.3.8 in the colour plate section), but the lid must be everted to identify an upper tarsal foreign body which is producing painful vertical scratches across the cornea. After instillation of a topical anaesthetic such as amethocaine 0.5%, the foreign body can often be removed with either a moistened cotton bud or a 25-G needle. If the particle is metallic, rust may remain in the cornea (see Plate 1.3.9 in the colour plate section). This can also be removed with a needle. However, such procedures should be performed under slit-lamp control in order to avoid ocular perforation. After removal of the foreign body, topical antibiotics and eye padding are indicated. Flash burns due to exposure to ultraviolet light are visible as tiny punctate ulcers across the central cornea. These are managed as a corneal abrasion. The most serious chemical burn is that due to alkali, which readily penetrates the cornea to access the eye (see Plate 1.3.10 in the colour plate section). Copious irrigation at the scene is essential. Conjunctival pH is monitored by means of an indicator strip, and should be $\leqslant 7.5$. Subsequent management aimed at preventing corneal scarring remains controversial.

Blunt ocular trauma causes a wide range of pathology, including lid haematomas, subconjunctival haemorrhage, corneal oedema, acute iritis, hyphaema (see Plate 1.3.11 in the colour plate section), mydriasis, iris disinsertion, lens dislocation and cataract, vitreous haemorrhage, retinal oedema, haemorrhage, tears and detachment, choroidal rupture, optic nerve contusion, orbital haematoma and globe rupture. There may also be associated orbital wall fractures. Anterior segment conditions are often painful, but the majority resolve spontaneously. A hyphaema is associated with a risk of rebleeding during the subsequent week, as well as angle-recession glaucoma in the long term. The more sinister posterior ocular lesions are frequently painless. Medial lid lacerations may involve the lacrimal drainage system, and complicated repair with intubation is required in order to avoid subsequent epiphora (tearing). Conjunctival lacerations heal readily without the need for suturing, but deeper damage must be excluded. Penetrating eye injuries will show an entry wound and a variety of other injuries depending on the path followed by the object responsible (see Plate 1.3.12 in the colour plate section). A foreign body may be present, which can often be localized by CT scanning. These injuries require broad-spectrum antibacterial coverage, tetanus prophylaxis and anti-emetics prior to prompt repair with removal of any foreign material.

ACKNOWLEDGEMENTS

Slit lamp photographs are provided courtesy of Ms. Angela Chappell, Ophthalmic Photographer, Flinders University of SA and Flinders Medical Centre.

FURTHER READING

Kanski JJ. 1999: *Clinical ophthalmology. A systematic approach*, 4th edn. Oxford: Butterworth-Heinemann.

Spalton DJ, Hitchings RA, Hunter PA. 1994: *Atlas of clinical ophthalmology*, 2nd edn. London: Mosby-Year Book Europe Ltd.

Tang RA, Pardo G. 1996: *Ocular and periocular pain. Focal points. Clinical modules for ophthalmologists. Vol. 14 (2).* San Francisco, CA: American Academy of Ophthalmology.

Chest pain

David G. Hill

Introduction

Chest pain presents in a myriad of ways in patients whose anxiety is possibly mirrored by those around them, further complicating the task of the doctor, who must extract enough information on assessment to formulate a suitable treatment plan.

As 75% of severe chest pain is caused by ischaemic heart disease or other life-threatening conditions, such as dissecting aortic aneurysm, the pattern of the pain must be carefully analysed.

CARDIAC PAIN

PAIN IN MYOCARDIAL INFARCTION

Pain during myocardial infarction is classically described as a centrally located, crushing sensation in the chest, sometimes radiating to the medial side of the left arm, or less commonly into the neck and mandible. However, interrogation and observation will show a pattern of evolving pain commencing with a true visceral pain which is later transmitted as referred pain. The patient will describe a pain of variable intensity but associated with a feeling of constriction, making breathing difficult. This visceral pain is not well localized, but rather dull and aching behind the sternum and accompanied by a strong autonomic reaction. These responses include nausea and vomiting, sweating, circulatory changes in blood pressure and increased pulse rate. As the ischaemia becomes prolonged, deep referred pain develops. Deep referred pain has a more exact localizing pattern that is felt behind the sternum, spreading to muscle and bone on one or both sides of the chest and sometimes radiating down the arms, more commonly the left

arm, or into the jaw. Superficial referred pain occurs in about 20% of cases as cutaneous dysaesthesia in the dermatomes C8–T1.

The pathophysiological mechanisms underlying cardiac pain are not fully understood, but possibly the initial pain is induced by stimulation of mechanoreceptors following the loss of contractility in the distorted or distended ventricular muscle, or results from coronary arterial vasoreceptors responding to hypotension distal to a coronary artery lesion. Secondary causes of pain are due to biochemical substances produced following tissue or platelet breakdown. Lactic acid, potassium ions and kinins are implicated, causing stimulation of afferent C fibres. Ischaemic neuropathy of cardiac nerves may further contribute to prolonged pain, because myelinated fibres are considered to be more susceptible to ischaemia, allowing unbalanced pain transmissions to pass through central gate-control mechanisms.

PAIN IN ANGINA

The pain of *stable angina* is dominated by deep referred pain with muscular tenderness. Visceral pain is present, but it is less intense. The pain lasts from 30 s to 30 min, and may be accompanied by autonomic reflexes, including nausea and vomiting. It usually follows exertion and is aggravated by cold weather, heavy meals and emotion. It is frequently relieved by nitroglycerine. The sense of fear which accompanies acute myocardial infarction is not usually a feature of stable angina.

Unstable angina occurs with more intensity, in response to little exertion and even at rest. It responds poorly to conservative management, and may progress to myocardial infarction.

A variant type of angina (*Prinzmetal's angina*) occurs at rest and is caused by *coronary artery spasm. Atypical angina* remains a problem, as it can occur anywhere in the chest or epigastrium, and is difficult to differentiate from *functional angina*. Clues suggesting the latter diagnosis include pain that is described as stabbing or piercing, pinpointed in the precordial area. Caution should be exercised in making this diagnosis, even in the presence of a normal coronary angiogram.

Other cardiac diseases, such as cardiomyopathy and aortic stenosis, cause angina. Endocarditis and myocarditis may cause dull chest pain and are usually associated with signs of infection. In the early stages of mitral stenosis there may be a dull left-sided posterior chest pain, which is thought to be caused by distension of the left atrium.

PRE-OPERATIVE CARDIAC PAIN

A common problem confronting surgeons and their residents is the management of patients whose medical history includes chest pain typical of angina complicating the symptoms of their surgical problem. In many instances a referral for a cardiological opinion may be the best approach, but a number of general guidelines have been developed to minimize peri-operative myocardial complications.

1. The Canadian Cardiovascular Society has described an anginal classification which assesses the level of angina.

   Class 0:   No angina.

   Class I: 'Ordinary physical activity does not cause angina.' Rapid, strenuous, prolonged exertion produces pain.

   Class II: 'Slight limitation of ordinary activity.' Walking more than two blocks, climbing more than one flight of stairs, or performing physical activity under stressed conditions (e.g. after meals, in the cold or wind, or immediately after waking) produces pain.

   Class III: 'Marked limitation of ordinary activity.' Pain occurs with activity in normal conditions and at normal pace.

   Class IV: 'Inability to carry on any physical activity without discomfort – anginal syndrome may be present at rest.'

2. All patients who have atherosclerotic disease in one region should be assessed with regard to:

   (a) risk factors, e.g. hypertension, obesity, lipid levels, diabetes and smoking habits;

   (b) symptoms of atherosclerosis elsewhere, e.g. cerebral, cardiac, peripheral vessels;

   (c) evidence of comorbid diseases, e.g. respiratory function, renal impairment, haematological disorders.

3. The American College of Cardiology/American Heart Association Task Force has described a method for peri-operative cardiovascular evaluation for non-cardiac surgery. Clinical predictors of increased peri-operative cardiovascular risk (myocardial infarction, congestive heart failure, death) are described (see Table 1.4.1).

In addition, the cardiac risks stratification for non-cardiac surgical procedures describes high-risk, intermediate and low-risk procedures (see Table 1.4.2).

In emergency cases the clinician's best approach is to provide recommendations for peri-operative management and surveillance.

In cases where the degree of urgency is less, further assessment of cardiovascular risk should be undertaken.

1. Patients with major clinical predictors of increased peri-operative cardiovascular risk should have a full cardiovascular evaluation.

2. Patients with intermediate clinical predictors of increased peri-operative cardiovascular risk should be further stratified according to functional capacity. This can be expressed in metabolic equivalent (MET) levels (see Table 1.4.3). Functional capacity has been classified as excellent (> 7 METs), moderate (4–7 METs) or poor (< 4 METs). Patients with poor functional capacity and those with moderately reduced functional capacity who are to undergo high-risk procedures should have further cardiovascular evaluation.

3. Non-cardiac surgery is generally safe for patients with minor or no clinical predictors, and with moderate or excellent functional capacity regardless of the surgical type.

Table 1.4.1 Clinical predictors of increased peri-operative cardiovascular risk

Major:
Unstable coronary syndromes
● Recent myocardial infarction* with evidence of important ischaemic risk by clinical symptoms or non-invasive study
● Unstable or severe angina† (Canadian Class III or IV)‡
Decompensated congestive heart failure
Significant arrhythmias
● High-grade atrioventricular block
● Symptomatic ventricular arrhythmias in the presence of underlying heart disease
● Supraventricular arrhythmias with uncontrolled ventricular rate
Severe valvular disease

Intermediate:
Mild angina pectoris (Canadian Class I or II)
Prior myocardial infarction by history or pathological Q-waves
Compensated or prior congestive heart failure
Diabetes mellitus

Minor:
Advanced age
Abnormal electrocardiogram (ECG) (left ventricular hypertrophy, left bundle branch block, S-T abnormalities)
Rhythm other than sinus (e.g. atrial fibrillation)
Low functional capacity (e.g. inability to climb a flight of stairs with a bag of groceries)
History of stroke
Uncontrolled systemic hypertension

* The American College of Cardiology National Database Library defines *recent myocardial infarction* as more than 7 days but less than or equal to 1 month (30 days).
† May include 'stable' angina in patients who are unusually sedentary.
‡ Campeau L. 1976: Grading of angina pectoris. *Circulation* **54**, 522–3.
Reprinted with permission from the American College of Cardiology. Eagle KA, Brundage BH, Chaitman BR *et al.* 1996: Guidelines for perioperative cardiovascular evaluation for noncardiac surgery. Report of the American College of Cardiology/American Heart Association Task Force on Practice Guidelines (Committee on Perioperative Cardiovascular Evaluation for Noncardiac Surgery). *Journal of the American College of Cardiology* **27**, 910–948.

NON-CARDIAC CHEST PAIN

DISEASE OF THE THORACIC AORTA

Aortic dissection typically presents with sudden onset of excruciating central chest pain, often described as a tearing or ripping feeling, which may cause the patient to writhe in agony. The pain may gradually subside (in contrast to ischaemic cardiac pain, which usually waxes and wanes), and may move to the back as the dissection propagates distally. Transoesophageal echocardiography is the most useful investigation, and will delineate the site of the tear, the length of the aorta dissected, the true and false lumens, and the competency of the aortic valve.

Non-dissecting aneurysms of the thoracic aorta can cause a steady boring pain because of erosion of adjacent musculoskeletal structures or stimulation of aortic end organs. The dilated aorta may be visible on chest X-ray with a widened mediastinum, but the diagnosis will be better established with a CT scan or MRI.

PULMONARY EMBOLUS

Pulmonary embolism has a number of clinical presentations, characteristically occurring 5 to 10 days postoperatively, and it can be difficult to distinguish from myocardial infarction. Dyspnoea is usually the first and most predominant symptom. Chest pain is dull and occurs only with major emboli (the pain of pulmonary infarction is delayed and is pleuritic in nature).

The pathophysiological events following a major embolus depend on the extent of pulmonary vascular obstruction and whether vasoactive humeral agents, such as serotonin and thromboxane A2, are released from activated platelets. The right ventricle dilates, which may cause the pain. Because there is reduced left ventricular filling and reduced coronary blood flow, the

Table 1.4.2 Cardiac risk* stratification of non-cardiac surgical procedures

---

High (reported cardiac risk often >5%)
- Emergency major operations, particularly in the elderly
- Aortic and other major vascular procedures
- Peripheral vascular procedures
- Anticipated prolonged surgical procedures associated with large fluid shifts and/or blood loss

Intermediate (reported cardiac risk generally <5%)
- Carotid endarterectomy
- Head and neck procedures
- Intraperitoneal and intrathoracic procedures
- Orthopaedic procedures
- Prostate procedures

Low[†] (reported cardiac risk generally <1%)
- Endoscopic procedures
- Superficial procedures
- Cataract procedures
- Breast procedures

---

*Combined incidence of cardiac death and non-fatal myocardial infarction.

†Do not generally require further pre-operative cardiac testing.

Reprinted with permission from the American College of Cardiology (see footnote to Table 1.4.1 for reference).

pain may be angina. However, the symptoms are improved by Trendelenberg tilting, in contrast to the situation with left ventricular failure.

The most useful investigation for a patient presenting with suspected pulmonary embolus is an arterial blood gas determination on room air. The chest X-ray is usu-ally not diagnostic in the acute stage, but is necessary to exclude other problems. Patients who are well enough should have a lung scan (ventilation-perfusion (VQ) scan). The first step involves the patient inhaling technetium-labelled gas (Technegas), and images are taken of the ventilation phase. Technetium macro-aggregates of albumin are then given intravenously and the perfusion phase is imaged. A defect on the perfusion scan which is not present on the ventilation scan – the so-called mismatched defect – is associated with a high probability of a diagnosis of pulmonary embolus (Figure 1.4.1), although unfortunately the test is not highly sensitive. Echocardiography, particularly transoesophageal echo, is very useful in more severe cases. Pulmonary angiography may be performed in complicated cases, but is mainly of historical interest. The possible roles of magnetic resonance pulmonary angiography, spiral CT and plasma D-dimer measurement are currently being evaluated.

PERICARDITIS

Pericardial pain, if present, may be one of two types. The first is the dull, aching, nauseous, poorly localized 'visceral' type, involving the precordium and easily confused with myocardial infarction. It probably results from stretching of the pericardial sac. The second type is a sharp, stabbing, referred type of pain, localized to the left chest, shoulder, neck or scapula. It is exacerbated by lying down and relieved by bending forward. This represents inflammation of the mediastinal or diaphragmatic pleura.

The most characteristic sign of pericarditis is a friction rub; signs of cardiac tamponade are occasionally present. The electrocardiographic changes are as follows:

Table 1.4.3 Estimated energy requirements for various activities*

1 MET ↕ 4 METs	Can you take care of yourself? Eat, dress or use the toilet? Walk indoors around the house? Walk a block or two on level ground at 2–3 miles/h or 3.2–4.8 km/h? Do light work around the house such as dusting or washing dishes?	4 MET ↕ 10 METs	Climb a flight of stairs or walk up a hill? Walk on level ground at 4 miles/h or 6.4 km/h? Run a short distance? Do heavy work around the house such as scrubbing floors or lifting or moving heavy furniture? Participate in moderate recreational activities such as golf, bowling, dancing, doubles tennis, or throwing a baseball or football? Participate in strenuous sports such as swimming, singles tennis, football, basketball, or skiing

*Adapted from the Duke Activity Status Index and American Heart Association Exercise Standards.

MET, metabolic equivalent.

Reprinted with permission from the American College of Cardiology (see footnote to Table 1.4.1 for reference).

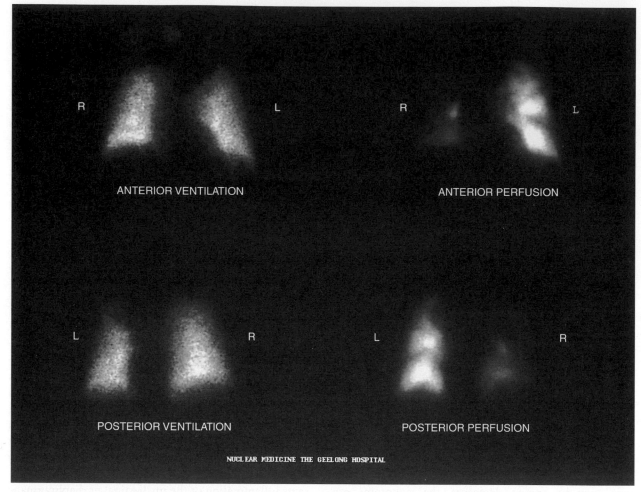

ANTERIOR VENTILATION

ANTERIOR PERFUSION

POSTERIOR VENTILATION

POSTERIOR PERFUSION

NUCLEAR MEDICINE THE GEELONG HOSPITAL

Figure1.4.1 Lung scan showing pulmonary emboli. There are multiple emboli in both lungs. These are illustrated by comparing the perfusion phase with the corresponding scans in the ventilation phase. Multiple defects are identified.

1. low voltage;
2. S-T elevation without a reciprocal relationship between leads I and III; and
3. diffuse T-wave inversion.

MEDIASTINITIS/MEDIASTINAL TUMOURS AND CYSTS

Mediastinitis produces central chest discomfort associated with fever and often rigors. Movements of the neck may be painful if the infection has tracked into this area, and there may be cough or dysphagia indicating tracheal or oesophageal involvement. The chest X-ray may be normal, or there may be bulging of the mediastinal borders with displacement of the trachea and oesophagus. Air in the mediastinum or tracking up the fascial planes in the neck may be seen, especially if the cause is oesophageal perforation.

Between one-third and one-half of mediastinal tumours and cysts are asymptomatic, and they are most frequently discovered by chest X-ray. Tumours such as thymoma, retrosternal goitre and lymphadenopathy may cause retrosternal pain, particularly if there is malignant change. This is usually a consequence of compression or invasion of other mediastinal structures. The pain is dull and aching and may be associated with non-specific signs of weight loss, weakness and fever.

OESOPHAGEAL PAIN

Gastrointestinal causes account for up to 50% of patients who have central chest pain once cardiac ischaemia has been excluded. It is a true visceral pain and can be a formidable challenge to the clinician, as it may mimic cardiac pain perfectly, e.g. in radiating to the arm and jaw. Differentiating features are that oesophageal pain is felt more posteriorly, may be relieved by milk and antacids, and can be associated with other symptoms, such as dysphagia and waterbrash.

The causes of oesophageal pain are as follows.

1. *Mechanical stimulation by abnormal contractions.* This pain is present in motility disorders, such as achalasia, diffuse oesophageal spasm, lower oesophageal sphincter dysfunction and oesophageal stenosis, particularly with malignant disease. Lesions in the upper third of the oesophagus have referred pain in the upper sternum, lesions in the distal third produce pain behind the lower sternum, and those in the middle third give rise to referred pain in either area.

2. *Inflammation.* This occurs in patients with oesophagitis, gastroesophageal reflux and peptic ulcer of the oesophagus. The pain presents as a very unpleasant deep burning feeling behind the sternum at the level of the xiphoid process. When associated with hiatus hernia, the pain is aggravated in the horizontal position.

Inflammation of abdominal structures can cause visceral pain which is felt mainly in the chest. This includes gastric ulcers, pancreatitis, cholecystitis and colonic distension of the splenic flexure.

Barium swallow, endoscopy and motility studies are the most important methods for investigating oesophageal disease. CT and MRI scans are used mainly in malignant disease to detect spread in the mediastinum. Ultrasonography can be used for pre-operative staging of oesophageal carcinoma.

PLEURAL PAIN

Pleuritic pain is sharp and localized, and its hallmark is that it is worsened by respiratory movements and coughing. It is usually unilateral, is aggravated by movement and is therefore more severe in the lower chest because of increased motion of the lower costal margin. It is caused by irritation and inflammation of the parietal pleura (the visceral pleura does not have pain receptors and does not cause pain). The common causes of pleural pain are pleurisy of viral origin, pneumonia and pulmonary infarction. The pace of onset varies with the cause; in the case of pulmonary infarction it is usually sudden, but with pneumonia it may be more gradual. Pleural inflammation involving the central tendon of the diaphragm is transmitted by the phrenic nerves (C3 and C4) and referred to the shoulder. In apical pleurisy the pain is posterior, in the interscapular area.

Pneumothorax presents as either spontaneous or traumatic. The symptoms vary according to the cause, but with primary spontaneous pneumothorax, the most common type, the usual presentation is sharp unilateral chest pain accompanied by shortness of breath. In two-thirds of patients breathlessness is minimal, but if severe dyspnoea is present in a previously healthy subject, this usually indicates that the pneumothorax is under tension. The pain in pneumothorax is continuous, but is exacerbated by deep inspiration or by postural change.

Physical signs may be absent, or there may be diminished breath sounds and a crepitus sound may be heard over the anterior chest wall.

The chest X-ray is the chief diagnostic tool in pneumothorax, and the characteristic finding is a convex lung edge with a surrounding lucent zone separating it from the chest wall.

Pleural effusions may cause pain of sudden onset which can be intense initially, but then gradually subsides when the effusion increases in size. There may be dull chest discomfort if the effusion becomes infected and an empyema develops, and there may be a feeling of heaviness on that side of the chest if the effusion is large.

Primary tumours of the pleura, e.g. mesothelioma or metastases involving the pleura, cause severe chronic pain which may disturb sleep.

The *lung parenchyma* has no pain receptors and therefore there is no lung pain. Approximately 40% of patients with lung cancer have chest pain, and much of this may be because of pleural involvement. Patients with a lung abscess may have pleuritic pain or a deep-seated aching discomfort over the area of the lesion.

Generalized pleural pain accompanied by fever and malaise may be caused by Coxsackie B viral infection (Bornholm's disease).

CHEST WALL PAIN

Chest wall pain can be easily confused with pleural pain, and there are many and diverse causes. The pain may be generalized, localized or confined to a segmental dermatome. Chronic breathlessness due to asthma or emphysema may cause generalized chest wall pain, as can collagen diseases such as polymyalgia rheumatica and dermatomyositis.

Other causes of localized chest wall pain are muscular strain related to coughing or unusual exertion, chest trauma (including fractured ribs and sternum), costochondral dislocation and pathological fractures (more common in the elderly because of osteoporosis or malignancy). There is usually tenderness in the area of the pain. Local pain over the costochondral and costosternal joints associated with swelling and tenderness is Tietze's disease.

Pain in the distribution of a dermatome may be due to the prevesicular phase of herpes zoster, invasion of intercostal nerves by tumour (Pancoast's syndrome, mesothelioma) or spinal problems such as cervicodorsal arthritis or spinal nerve compression resulting from vertebral collapse.

FURTHER READING

Eagle KA, Brundage BH, Chaitman BR *et al.* 1996: Guidelines for perioperative cardiovascular evaluation for noncardiac surgery. Report of the American College of Cardiology/American Heart Association Task Force on Practice Guidelines (Committee on Perioperative Cardiovascular Evaluation for Noncardiac Surgery).

Journal of the American College of Cardiology **27**, 910–948.

Seaton A, Seaton D, Leitch AG. 1989: *Crofton and Douglas's respiratory diseases*, 4th edn. Oxford: Blackwell Scientific Publications.

Wall, PD, Melzack R. 1984: *Textbook of pain.* Edinburgh: Churchill Livingstone.

Abdominal and pelvic pain

Margaret Schnitzler

Introduction

Acute abdominal pain is the cause of presentation in up to 10% of patients who are seen in the emergency department, and it is the most common surgical emergency, with the exception of trauma. In at least one-third of cases, a precise cause for the pain is not identified and no particular treatment is required. Based on the analysis of large numbers of patients in developed countries, acute appendicitis is by far the most common specific diagnosis in patients requiring operation for acute abdominal pain, accounting for about 15–30% of the total. Acute cholecystitis, small bowel obstruction and gynaecological conditions are the next most frequently diagnosed conditions,

together representing about 15–20% of cases requiring operation. Variation in the pattern of disease is observed with age. In children, over 90% of cases are due to either non-specific abdominal pain, including mesenteric adenitis, or acute appendicitis. In older patients, cholecystitis is the most common cause of acute abdominal pain, and diverticulitis, pancreatitis, cancer, vascular conditions and complications of hernia are much more commonly observed than in patients under the age of 50 years. Some of the possible causes of abdominal or pelvic pain are listed in Table 1.5.1 and illustrated in Figure 1.5.1.

PATHOPHYSIOLOGY

Abdominal and pelvic pain can be broadly classified as either visceral or somatic in origin. Somatic pain is usually perceived as fairly superficial, and is due to stimulation of pain fibres in the parietal peritoneum, which is innervated by spinal nerves T7 to L1. This type of pain is mediated by myelinated A-delta fibres associated with somatic nerves to the overlying abdominal wall and skin, and it tends to be sharp and relatively well localized. Irritation of the parietal peritoneum, e.g. by blood, bile or bacterial inflammation, will result in somatic pain.

Visceral pain, on the other hand, is mediated primarily by afferent C fibres in the capsule or muscle wall of the abdominal or pelvic viscera. These fibres usually travel with the splanchnic afferent nerves, except those from the proximal oesophagus and the rectum, cervix,

bladder and prostate, which accompany the parasympathetic nerves. Pain originating in visceral organs is caused by increased wall tension as a result of either contraction or distension, or by chemical irritation or ischaemia. It is usually perceived as dull, deep-seated and poorly localized, and is generally felt in the midline because of the bilateral sensory supply of the spinal cord. Pain associated with foregut structures, e.g. the stomach, duodenum and pancreatico-biliary tree, is felt in the epigastrium, while that of the midgut is localized to the periumbilical region. Hindgut pain, such as that arising from the left colon and rectum, is felt in the hypogastrium (Table 1.5.1).

Referred pain is that which is perceived at a site removed from the origin of the pain, e.g. testicular pain associated with a ureteric calculus, or shoulder tip pain due to diaphragmatic irritation. It is mediated by the same nerve segment that supplies the affected organ, and

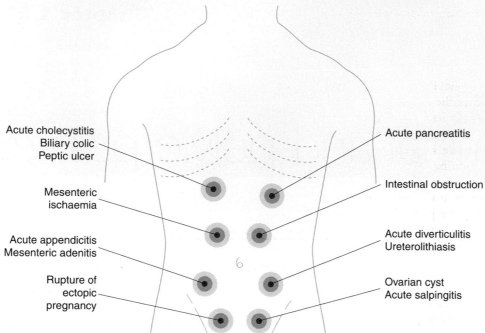

Acute cholecystitis
Biliary colic
Peptic ulcer

Acute pancreatitis

Mesenteric
ischaemia

Intestinal obstruction

Acute appendicitis
Mesenteric adenitis

Acute diverticulitis
Ureterolithiasis

Rupture of
ectopic
pregnancy

Ovarian cyst
Acute salpingitis

Figure 1.5.1 Location of common causes of abdominal and pelvic pain.

Table 1.5.1 Innervation of the abdominal and pelvic viscera

Organ	Segmental innervation
Stomach and duodenum	T5–7
Biliary tree	T6–8
Small intestine	T8–10
Colon	T10–L1
Kidney	T10–L1
Cervix	S2–4
Bladder	S2–4
Rectum	S2–4

reflects the fact that afferent neurones from different peripheral sites are mediated by the same central pathway.

CLINICAL ASSESSMENT

It is apparent that the ability to perform an appropriate assessment of a patient with acute abdominal pain is an important skill for the general surgeon. Much has been written about this subject, including the classic text by Sir Zachary Cope, which highlights the importance of the history and clinical signs in the early diagnosis of the acute abdomen. Needless to say, since Cope's monograph was published in 1921, many advances in diagnos-

tic testing and imaging have been made. Changes have also occurred in the spectrum of disease and the patient population that are now likely to be encountered by surgeons. Despite this, the basic approach to the patient with abdominal pain has changed little, and consists of a careful history and physical examination, appropriate radiological and other investigations, formulation of a likely diagnosis and a decision regarding operative or non-operative management.

HISTORY

The importance of the clinical history has been shown in studies examining the use of a structured data sheet to collect information from patients who present with abdominal pain. Eliciting all of the relevant history enhances overall diagnostic accuracy and also results in fewer inappropriate admissions and operations or other management errors. The following factors should be considered in the history.

Mode of onset and progression

Pain which is severe and very sudden in onset suggests perforation, torsion or rupture of an intra-abdominal or pelvic structure, such as a ruptured aortic aneurysm, perforated peptic ulcer or torted ovarian cyst. Pain which is vague and poorly localized at first, but which becomes more severe and localized over a period of several hours, typically occurs in conditions such as acute appendicitis or diverticulitis, which are characterized by peritoneal irritation.

Severity and nature

Intermittent or crampy pain (colic) is typical of obstruction of a hollow viscus such as the intestine, Fallopian tube or ureter. The pain usually lasts for minutes at a time and then eases for a variable period. It is often severe, and is associated with restlessness and sometimes with sweating, nausea and vomiting. It should be noted that the pain caused by obstruction of the biliary tree, although termed biliary colic, is usually constant rather than intermittent. Constant severe pain which lasts for hours or more without subsiding suggests ischaemia or inflammation.

Location and shifting

Perhaps the best example of the importance of a shift in the location of pain is provided by the typical change in the pain of acute appendicitis from the periumbilical region to the right lower quadrant. The general location of the pain can provide a guide to its possible causes, but is by no means invariably accurate. For example, acute sigmoid diverticulitis may present with hypochondrial or right lower quadrant pain depending on the position of the sigmoid colon.

Radiation

Although pain due to parietal irritation is usually well localized, that of visceral origin is often perceived as a diffuse and deep-seated pain. Some patterns of radiation of visceral pain are commonly observed. Pain of biliary origin frequently radiates to the right subscapular region, while that due to pancreatitis more commonly penetrates straight through to the back. Small intestinal (and appendiceal) colic is perceived in the periumbilical region, while colonic colic is referred to the hypogastrium.

Precipitating and relieving factors

The patient should be asked about the effect of movement, coughing, eating or other activities, which may indicate peritoneal inflammation or specific conditions such as pancreatitis, which are typically relieved by sitting forward.

Associated features

Symptoms such as anorexia, nausea, vomiting, diarrhoea or fever can provide clues about the cause of pain, although they are non-specific. Vomiting may be a reflex phenomenon associated with severe pain, in which case it usually occurs after the onset of the pain. Fever is common in inflammatory conditions, but can be absent, particularly in the elderly. Other more specific features such as haematemesis, jaundice or urinary symptoms are relevant in some cases.

Other relevant history

The patient should be asked about previous similar episodes of pain, and any previous abdominal surgery or other past or intercurrent illnesses. Other factors, such as the use of medication, alcohol intake and a history of trauma, should be considered. In women, details of menstrual and obstetric history should also be sought.

PHYSICAL EXAMINATION

General points

The examination commences with careful general observation, noting features such as pallor, diaphoresis, tachycardia, fever or hypotension. The demeanour and posture of the patient may also provide clues to the diagnosis, e.g. the restlessness of the patient with renal colic or the person with appendicitis who lies still with their legs flexed. It is useful to ask the patient to indicate the site of pain prior to commencing palpation. An exacerbation of pain produced by coughing indicates likely peritoneal irritation. The patient should be positioned comfortably lying supine, and a thorough abdominal examination performed, including examination of the hernial orifices and pelvis.

Inspection

A careful examination should be made for previous surgical scars, herniae, skin changes or abnormal veins. Visible masses, peristalsis or pulsations may also be observed.

Auscultation

The complete absence of bowel sounds suggests peritonitis or other causes of ileus, while high-pitched 'tinkling' sounds characteristically occur with intestinal obstruction. However, it should be recognized that the presence of normal bowel sounds does not exclude significant intra-abdominal pathology.

Percussion

This may be useful to distinguish gaseous distension from other causes, and to detect the presence of ascites. Loss of the usual liver dullness may be detected in patients with a large amount of free intraperitoneal gas. Gentle percussion over the abdomen is also the best way to demonstrate peritoneal irritation, and is much less distressing to the patient than the eliciting of rebound or release tenderness.

Palpation

Gentle palpation should commence as far as possible from the site of maximal pain indicated by the patient. This is particularly important in children, as causing distress initially will prevent a thorough examination. Asking the patient to breathe deeply helps to distinguish voluntary muscle guarding from the true guarding associated with peritonitis. Deeper palpation may be required to elicit mild localized tenderness or to identify a mass.

Other techniques

Specific manoeuvres can be used to assist in the diagnosis of particular conditions. Extension or rotation of the right hip may cause pain in a patient with retrocaecal or pelvic appendicitis. Tenderness on inspiration during palpation beneath the right costal margin (Murphy's sign) is suggestive of acute cholecystitis.

Rectal examination may be useful in the identification of pelvic tenderness or masses. In women with lower abdominal pain, vaginal examination should be performed in order to identify any uterine or adnexal pathology, or abnormal discharge.

INVESTIGATIONS

Laboratory and radiological investigations are not always necessary in the evaluation of the patient with abdominal or pelvic pain, and will only rarely establish a definite diagnosis. For example, the management of an otherwise healthy young adult male with symptoms and clinical signs of acute appendicitis will not be altered by the finding of a normal white blood cell count and abdominal X-ray. On the other hand, appropriate investigations can provide valuable information which aids assessment of the patient and subsequent management.

LABORATORY TESTS

A full blood count may reveal evidence of neutrophil leucocytosis, which is suggestive of acute bacterial infection or inflammation. However, the absence of this finding does not exclude an acute inflammatory condition, and should be regarded only as an adjunct to the clinical signs. This is particularly true in patients who are elderly or immunocompromised, in whom leucocytosis may not develop.

Red cell indices may indicate acute or chronic anaemia or suggest dehydration.

Serum electrolytes, urea and creatinine are also useful for assessing the extent and effect of fluid losses, and should be measured in patients who are acutely unwell or who have experienced vomiting and diarrhoea. In patients with pain of suspected pancreatic or biliary origin, measurement of liver enzymes and serum amylase or lipase should be performed. A markedly increased amylase or lipase level is highly suggestive of acute pancreatitis, although moderate elevations may also be observed in patients with other acute conditions, such as intestinal obstruction or ischaemia.

Urinalysis is easy to perform, and may provide useful information, e.g. about the presence or absence of red cells in a patient with suspected renal colic. White blood cells can be found in the urine in patients with retroperitoneal or pelvic inflammatory conditions, such as appendicitis or diverticulitis, as well as in those with urinary tract infection.

Other laboratory investigations, such as blood gas analysis, lactic acid measurement or a pregnancy test, should be performed when clinically indicated.

RADIOLOGICAL TESTS

Erect and supine X-rays of the abdomen and an erect chest X-ray should be performed in patients with suspected intestinal obstruction, perforation or ischaemia. The presence of free intraperitoneal or retroperitoneal air is usually an indication for urgent surgical intervention. Dilated loops of bowel and air fluid levels indicate intestinal obstruction or ileus, while mural or mucosal thickening are suggestive of intestinal ischaemia or inflammation. A chest X-ray will occasionally identify lower-lobe pneumonia as a cause of acute upper abdominal pain. These investigations can also identify radio-opaque calculi in the urinary tract, vascular or pancreatic calcification or foreign bodies. Although simple and readily available, it is inappropriate to perform plain radiographs routinely in patients with abdominal pain, as is sometimes recommended. These tests are unlikely to be useful in patients with uncomplicated acute appendicitis, gynaecological conditions or biliary tract disease, for example, and should only be ordered if they are likely to alter the diagnosis or management in a particular patient.

Ultrasound is playing an increasing role in the assessment of patients with abdominal and pelvic pain, and has the advantages of being relatively inexpensive, widely available and non-invasive. In some institutions, appropriately trained surgeons or resident staff use this diagnostic modality in the emergency department, with good results. It is particularly useful for evaluation of the biliary system, and is the best way to identify calculi in the gall bladder, or to confirm the diagnosis of acute cholecystitis. Imaging of the uterus, Fallopian tubes and ovaries is also best performed by ultrasonography, using the abdominal or transvaginal route.

Computerized tomography (CT) is another very useful modality for the investigation of selected patients with abdominal pain. It is by far the best way to evaluate the retroperitoneum, particularly the pancreas, and it is also a sensitive technique for the identification of colonic and small bowel inflammation, hepatic and splenic pathology and free intraperitoneal fluid or gas.

OTHER INVESTIGATIONS

A variety of other specific tests may be indicated in particular circumstances. An electrocardiogram should be performed in older patients with upper abdominal pain, as acute myocardial ischaemia may present in this way. Upper and lower gastrointestinal endoscopy is sometimes helpful, e.g. in the diagnosis of peptic ulcer disease or inflammatory bowel disease. Radioisotope scanning can be used to confirm the diagnosis of acute cholecystitis if ultrasonography is inconclusive.

Diagnostic laparoscopy also has a role, particularly in the evaluation of gynaecological pathology such as salpingitis, tubal pregnancy or complicated ovarian cysts, and in the differentiation of these conditions from acute appendicitis.

MANAGEMENT

Once a thorough clinical evaluation and appropriate investigations have been conducted, it should be possible to formulate a working diagnosis on which subsequent management can be based. Perhaps the most important initial decision is whether or not immediate laparotomy is required, which will be the case in only a small minority of patients with acute abdominal pain. In most other circumstances, even when surgery is required, expedient laparotomy can be performed after a brief period of assessment, investigation and resuscitation. Most patients who present with acute abdominal or pelvic pain will not require urgent surgery, and in many cases the initial management will involve a period of observation, investigation and clinical review. Where possible, this review should be performed by the same clinician, so that subtle changes in the condition of the patient can be detected. The interval between assessments must be chosen according to the clinical situation, but should be no more than several hours initially.

Appropriate analgesia should be provided promptly to all patients who are in pain, and should not be withheld while the patient is awaiting review by a member of the surgical team. The belief that significant clinical signs will be masked by analgesia is incorrect, and it is inappropriate to deny pain relief on that basis. In many circumstances, the administration of analgesia will actually facilitate accurate assessment, particularly in children or those who are very distressed. Pain which is not relieved by narcotic analgesia should be regarded seriously, and should raise the index of suspicion for ischaemia as a cause of the pain.

IMMEDIATE OR URGENT OPERATION

The main indication for immediate operation is haemodynamic instability associated with bleeding, e.g. following rupture of an aortic or visceral aneurysm, or an ectopic pregnancy.

Even when a definitive diagnosis cannot be made pre-operatively, it is vital that the need for urgent surgery is recognized in a patient showing signs of peritonitis, progressive sepsis or mesenteric ischaemia. Generalized tenderness and rigidity, increasing distension, haemodynamic instability or a strangulated hernia are all features which indicate the need for operation within hours of presentation.

NON-URGENT OPERATION

When the cause of the pain is uncertain and the clinical features which indicate the need for urgent intervention are absent, a period of observation is appropriate. There is no evidence that the incidence of complications is increased by observation of selected patients, and the rate of negative laparotomies is reduced by this approach. During the observation period, any fluid and electrolyte abnormalities should be corrected, and any necessary investigations can be performed. Where indicated, e.g. in patients with acute cholecystitis, antibiotic therapy should be commenced. Nasogastric intubation should be performed in patients with intestinal obstruction. Depending on the clinical course of the patient, and the results of radiological or other investigations, the need for operation may become evident over a period of hours or days. This may occur, for example, in patients with small intestinal obstruction which fails to resolve with non-operative treatment, or in the case of acute diverticulitis with worsening signs of sepsis or peritonitis.

In many cases, however, continued non-operative management is appropriate even when the cause of pain has been recognized, and operation is reserved for management of complications. For example, this is the case in most patients with acute pancreatitis, endometriosis or inflammatory bowel disease. In some circumstances it will be important to arrange follow-up investigations or review in order to evaluate further the underlying cause of the pain. For instance, a patient with presumed acute sigmoid diverticulitis should undergo endoscopic or radiological investigation of the colon after the pain has resolved, in order to define the extent of the disease and to exclude a neoplasm.

NON-OPERATIVE MANAGEMENT

A large number of patients who present with acute abdominal or pelvic pain will not have a specific cause for the pain identified, and will not require surgical intervention either urgently or electively. In addition to this group, there will be some patients in whom a non-surgical cause of the pain is identified and appropriately treated. Such patients include those with acute myocardial infarction, pneumonia, hepatitis, pyelonephritis or gastroenteritis. Other specific conditions should be considered in particular circumstances, e.g. bacterial peritonitis in patients undergoing peritoneal dialysis, or neutropenic enterocolitis in those receiving cytotoxic chemotherapy. Rare causes of pain, such as sickle-cell crisis, diabetic ketoacidosis or familial Mediterranean fever, should also be borne in mind.

SUMMARY

Abdominal or pelvic pain is a common cause of presentation to surgeons, and a rational approach to the diagnosis and management of this problem is essential. The symptoms may be caused by a vast range of pathophysiological conditions, although the majority of cases are due to a relatively small number of common conditions. While most patients will not require surgical interven-

tion, it is important to identify those in whom urgent operation is indicated, in order to avoid unnecessary morbidity or mortality. The selective use of laboratory, radiological and other investigations, combined with careful clinical observation, will guide management in the remaining cases.

FURTHER READING

Attard AR, Corlett MJ, Kidner NJ *et al.* 1992: Safety of early pain relief for acute abdominal pain. *British Medical Journal* **305**, 554–6.

Boey J. 1994: The acute abdomen. In Way LW (ed.), *Current surgical diagnosis and treatment*. Norwalk, CT: Appleton and Lange, 441–52.

Irvin TT. 1989: Abdominal pain: a surgical audit of 1190 emergency admissions. *British Journal of Surgery* **76**, 1121–5.

Ness TJ, Gebhart GF. 1990: Visceral pain: a review of experimental studies. *Pain* **41**, 167–234.

Paterson-Brown S. 1990: Modern aids to clinical decision-making in the acute abdomen. *British Journal of Surgery* **77**, 13–18.

Rapkin AJ. 1990: Neuroanatomy, neurophysiology and neuropharmacology of pelvic pain. *Clinics in Obstetrics and Gynaecology* **33**, 119–29.

Silen W. 1990: *Cope's early diagnosis of the acute abdomen*. New York: Oxford University Press.

Perineal/anal pain

Margaret Schnitzler

Introduction

Pain in the perineal or anal regions is a common symptom which usually has a readily identifiable cause. Despite this, errors of diagnosis are frequently made by those who are unfamiliar with the assessment of this problem. Although the conditions which cause anal or perianal pain are rarely life-threatening, they can cause considerable distress and inconvenience. Similarly, appropriate diagnosis and treatment can afford great relief to the patient.

HISTORY

The diagnosis can often be made on the basis of the history alone. Factors to be considered include the age of the patient, the onset, severity and duration of the pain, the effect of defecation and the presence of any associated bleeding or palpable mass. A history of prior perianal symptoms, inflammatory bowel disease or sexually transmitted disease should also be sought. The general medical condition of the patient must also be ascertained, as certain perianal conditions are more likely to occur in association with underlying diseases such as diabetes or human immunodeficiency virus (HIV) infection.

PHYSICAL EXAMINATION

Examination of the area must be conducted gently and skilfully in order to elicit the necessary information without causing distress. The patient should be positioned in the left lateral or prone jacknife position, and adequate lighting must be used. The perianal skin should first be inspected for any swelling, inflammation, ulceration or other lesions. Gentle palpation around the anus will identify a region of tenderness or induration. Prior to performing a rectal examination, the anus should be carefully examined by slight traction on the perianal skin, in order to identify an anal fissure. The presence of marked sphincter spasm on attempting digital rectal examination is highly suggestive of an acute anal fissure or ulcer. Further examination should not be performed immediately if there is severe pain and sphincter spasm. If an anal fissure is suspected, appropriate therapy can be initiated, and further examination can then be performed on a subsequent occasion. If the diagnosis is uncertain, an examination under anaesthesia should be performed in order to evaluate the problem fully.

Unless examination is too painful, proctoscopy should be performed in order to identify pathology within the anal canal. This may reveal a chronic fissure, internal haemorrhoids or ulceration associated with infection or malignancy. The presence of purulent discharge within the anal canal or identification of an internal fistula opening can aid the evaluation of anorectal sepsis. A sigmoidoscopic examination should also be performed in order to detect any evidence of inflammatory bowel disease or other abnormality within the rectum. Other relevant examination, e.g. of the abdomen and inguinal lymph nodes, should be performed where appropriate.

ANORECTAL ABSCESS

Most abscesses in the anorectal region do not have an identifiable predisposing cause, and are thought to arise from obstruction and subsequent infection of glands in the anal canal. The condition can occur at any age, but is most common in men aged between 20 and 50 years. About 50% of all anorectal abscesses occur in the perianal region and are relatively superficial. The remainder are located in the ischiorectal fossa, the intersphincteric region or above the levator muscles (Figure 1.6.1).

The most common symptom is perianal pain, which is usually of gradual onset and increasing severity over hours or days. The pain is constant and may keep the patient awake at night. It can generally be localized to a particular area, and the patient often notices a lump or firm area in the region of the pain. There may be associated fever and systemic symptoms.

Examination usually reveals an area of localized tenderness and induration in the perianal region. There is often some cellulitis overlying the abscess, but the skin may also appear completely normal. The presence of cellulitis and induration of the perianal skin almost invariably indicates that there is an underlying abscess which requires drainage. Treatment with antibiotic therapy alone is inadequate, and only results in prolongation of the symptoms. Rectal examination in a patient with an obvious anorectal abscess is uncomfortable and usually non-contributory. In patients who present with severe anal pain but show no external evidence of an abscess, rectal examination is essential. In such cases an intersphincteric abscess may be recognized as a tender submucosal swelling, and a supralevator abscess can sometimes be identified. Examination under anaesthesia is usually required to identify and treat these more complex anorectal abscesses adequately.

Drainage of the abscess may be performed under local or general anaesthesia, depending on the size and complexity of the abscess, the facilities available and the preference of the patient. The incision should be sufficient to allow complete drainage of the cavity, and should be positioned over the region of maximal induration, as close to the anus as is feasible. This is done so that subsequent fistulotomy, if required, can be performed without creating a large wound. If the presence or location of an abscess is uncertain, aspiration with a needle and syringe may be helpful in planning the site of the incision. It is not necessary to make a cruciate incision, or to excise skin, unless there is evidence of necrosis. A gauze pack may be inserted to aid haemostasis; this can be removed by the patient in a bath the following day. Further packing of the cavity is not usually necessary, unless it is very large or complex. Some surgeons recommend the insertion of a catheter or drain into the cavity, but this is not required to obtain adequate drainage. Successful treatment of perianal and ischiorectal abscesses by means of incision, curettage and primary closure has also been reported.

Parenteral antibiotic therapy should be used in immunocompromised patients and those with extensive cellulitis or tissue necrosis, but is not usually necessary following drainage of a simple abscess. Culturing of the

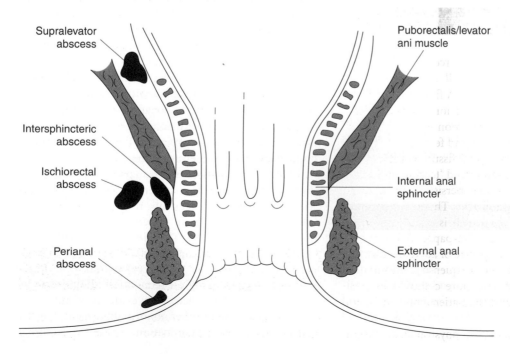

Figure 1.6.1 Diagram indicating the location of anorectal abscesses and fistulae.

Supralevator abscess

Intersphincteric abscess

Ischiorectal abscess

Perianal abscess

Puborectalis/levator ani muscle

Internal anal sphincter

External anal sphincter

pus obtained is appropriate if the patient is immuno-compromised or likely to require antibiotic therapy, so that a suitable agent can be selected. It has also been demonstrated that the nature of the causative organism can help to predict the likelihood of subsequent fistula development. If only non-enteric organisms are identi-fied, the probability of later fistula occurrence is very low. Approximately half of the patients who present with an anorectal abscess will be found to have a fistula. There is controversy as to whether a fistula should be defini-tively treated or even sought at the time of abscess drainage. In the case of a simple perianal abscess with an obvious low-lying fistula, immediate fistulotomy can be safely performed, but in complex cases or those with extensive sepsis, simple abscess drainage is preferable. The patient should be warned of the possibility of an underlying fistula, and advised to seek medical attention if there is persistent drainage from the perianal region.

Special consideration should be given to the immunocompromised patient with anorectal sepsis, in whom the clinical features may be atypical. Patients who are receiving chemotherapy and those with haematolog-ical malignancies, human immunodeficiency virus (HIV) infection or diabetes are at increased risk of sepsis in the perineal region. Pain is the main symptom, but there may be relatively little abnormality on physical examination, and localized abscess formation will not occur if there is pronounced leucopenia. Examination under anaesthesia is usually required to clarify the situa-tion, with drainage of any collections and biopsy of abnormal tissue which help to confirm the diagnosis of malignancy or opportunistic infection.

ANAL FISSURE

This common condition can be a source of great distress, to the extent that the patient will avoid defecation because of the severity of the pain. A fissure is a split in the anoderm, usually in the posterior midline. It can occur at any age, but is most common in young adults, with an equal incidence in males and females.

The patient with an acute anal fissure complains of pain which is often sharp, severe and 'tearing' in nature during defecation. The pain may persist for minutes or hours afterwards as a deep dull ache. There is often asso-ciated bright rectal bleeding which is usually small in amount and noticed on the toilet-paper. A history of these symptoms is highly suggestive of an acute anal fis-sure, although the patient will frequently attribute the problem to 'haemorrhoids'. In more chronic cases the pain is often less severe, and the patient may notice an associated skin tag.

The most consistent finding on physical examination

is of anal sphincter spasm, which often precludes digital examination. A fissure may be seen when the anus is effaced. The most usual site is the posterior midline, fol-lowed by the anterior midline, and less commonly later-ally. The triad of an anal fissure, hypertrophic anal papilla and prominent skin tag may be observed in chronic cases.

The exact aetiology of anal fissures is unknown, although they are commonly attributed to the passage of a hard stool. This precipitating factor is not always pre-sent, and many patients report that the pain began after an apparently normal bowel movement, or following an episode of diarrhoea. Both clinical examination and manometric studies have confirmed that patients with an anal fissure have increased resting anal sphincter tone, although the exact association between this finding and the presence of a fissure is unclear. There is some exper-imental evidence to suggest that ischaemia of the anal canal due to a relative deficiency in the blood supply to the posterior portion of the spastic sphincter is responsi-ble for persistence of the fissure. It is well recognized that effective treatment of an anal fissure is based on a reduc-tion in internal sphincter tone, which produces both relief of the pain and healing of the fissure in the major-ity of cases.

Depending on the duration and severity of the symp-toms, a variety of management strategies can be employed. In many cases an acute fissure will heal spon-taneously without specific treatment. Stool-softening agents and topical anaesthetic agents are frequently rec-ommended and may provide symptomatic relief while healing occurs. If the fissure fails to heal, or if the pain is severe, lateral internal sphincterotomy is very effective in relieving pain and healing the fissure. There is a small but definite incidence of impaired continence, particu-larly for flatus, after this procedure. Other surgical pro-cedures, such as posterior sphincterotomy, fissurectomy and sphincter stretch, have been shown to be associated with more complications than lateral internal sphinc-terotomy. Recently, two alternatives to surgical sphinc-terotomy have been reported. Glyceryl-trinitrate ointment acts as a nitric-oxide donor and produces relaxation of the internal anal sphincter, while botu-linum toxin has a similar effect due to neuromuscular blockade. Each of these agents produces a 'chemical' sphincterotomy which results in a reduction in pain and healing of the fissure in a certain proportion of cases.

PROLAPSED THROMBOSED INTERNAL HAEMORRHOIDS

Although anal pain of various types is frequently attrib-uted to haemorrhoids, they are not painful unless they are thrombosed. Thrombosis is most likely to occur in prolapsing haemorrhoids, which may then become irreducible and eventually gangrenous. This causes severe pain and requires immediate therapy. On examination the diagnosis is usually obvious, with a mass of oedematous, thrombosed haemorrhoids which cannot be reduced into the anal canal (Figure 1.6.2). The patient should be admitted to hospital and given adequate analgesia. Bed rest, ice packs and topical ointments are often prescribed, but their efficacy is questionable. The optimal management is surgical haemorrhoidectomy, which should be performed as soon as is practicable unless there is a contraindication to the procedure. When it is performed using the correct surgical technique, the morbidity of urgent haemorrhoidectomy in this setting is no higher than that of elective haemorrhoidectomy.

PERIANAL HAEMATOMA

Often referred to as a thrombosed external haemorrhoid, a perianal haematoma is due to thrombosis of a subcutaneous vein. It presents with acute pain and a palpable lump in the perianal region. On examination the lesion

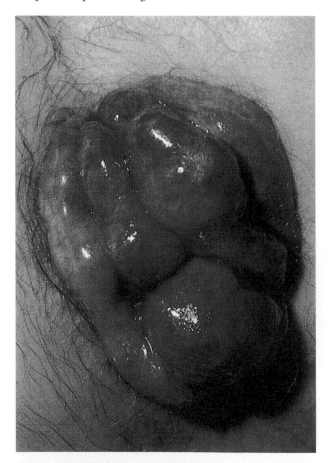

Figure 1.6.2 Prolapsed thrombosed internal haemorrhoids. (Reproduced courtesy of Dr Mark Killingback, Sydney.)

is easily seen, and it sometimes appears bluish in colour. Although pain may be severe in the early stages of this condition, it resolves over a period of several days if left untreated. Occasionally the haematoma discharges spontaneously, resulting in a small amount of bleeding. If the patient presents with acute pain in the early stages of the condition, surgical treatment of the lesion is appropriate, as this shortens the duration of the pain. Often, however, the patient does not present for several days, by which time the symptoms have started to resolve, and continued conservative management is then preferable. If surgical treatment is performed, the lesion should be excised, rather than simply being incised with evacuation of the clot. This ensures that recurrence does not occur at that site, and it also prevents the formation of a large skin tag which may be troublesome. The procedure can be performed under local anaesthesia if suitable facilities are available, and the wound may be left open or closed primarily. Occasionally the thrombosis extends into the anal canal, or involves an internal haemorrhoid which has prolapsed. In such cases general anaesthesia is preferred in order to ensure adequate exposure to the anal canal.

PRURITUS ANI

Although not a cause of severe pain, pruritus ani deserves mention as it is a very common condition which causes irritation and discomfort in the perianal region. The cause of the condition is unknown, and it may have a relapsing and remitting course. The patient presents with intense itchiness and sometimes a burning sensation in the perianal skin. Scratching exacerbates the irritation and may result in excoriation of the skin, with consequent bleeding and pain. Often the patient will attempt to solve the problem by frequent cleansing of the area, which unfortunately tends to worsen the condition. Stopping the use of soap or lotions, and the avoidance of scrubbing are often all that is needed to alleviate the symptoms. The use of topical hydrocortisone ointment is helpful in more severe cases, but care must be taken to ensure that it is not used for prolonged periods of time, as atrophy of the perianal skin may result.

FOURNIER'S GANGRENE

This rare condition of necrotizing infection of the perineum may complicate otherwise minor anorectal sepsis, surgery or urinary infection, particularly in immunocompromised patients. Severe perineal pain, fever and systemic toxicity are the usual presenting features, and the development of these symptoms, particularly in a susceptible patient, requires urgent assessment and treatment. Inspection of the perineum reveals marked swelling, and necrosis of the skin and underlying tissues develops rapidly if therapy is delayed. High-dose parenteral antibiotic therapy should be instituted immediately, and surgical debridement of all necrotic tissue must be performed without delay. Bacterial culture usually reveals a mixture of flora – both aerobic and anaerobic. The fulminant nature of this infection means that extensive skin and soft-tissue excision is often required, necessitating later reconstruction. Despite appropriate therapy, the mortality of this condition remains significant.

ANAL CARCINOMA

Although not common, anal carcinoma is an important cause of anal pain which should be considered in certain individuals. It is most common in those over the age of 50 years, but it can occur at an earlier age, particularly in immunosuppressed patients. There has been a marked increase in the incidence of anal carcinoma in young homosexual men, particularly those with HIV.

In addition to anal pain, the patient may notice bleeding, pruritus, discharge or a palpable mass.

If the lesion is arising from the perianal skin, it will usually be readily identified on inspection of the anus. More commonly the tumour lies within the anal canal, where it can be palpated as a firm indurated or ulcerating lesion. Proctosigmoidoscopy and biopsy are best performed under anaesthesia in order to assess adequately the local extent of the tumour. Most anal canal malignancies are squamous-cell or cloacogenic carcinomas, which are treated with a combination of chemotherapy and radiotherapy, rather than by surgery.

Neck and back pain

Christopher M.J. Cain and Robert D. Fraser

Introduction

Up to 80% of the population will experience an episode of neck or back pain of sufficient severity to prevent them from performing their normal work, sporting or social activities at some stage in their life. In the majority of cases the symptoms are the result of degenerative changes, and episodes of pain will usually settle spontaneously. In cases where symptoms persist or are of sufficient magnitude to

warrant intervention, the origin of the pain should be identified before contemplating operative intervention.

The clinical features of common neck and back complaints will be described. The differential diagnosis, indications for radiological investigation and their timing, the place of the 'physical therapies' and the indications to proceed with operative intervention will also be discussed.

NECK PAIN

CERVICAL BRACHALGIA

Cervical brachalgia refers to symptoms of neck and shoulder discomfort associated with referred pain extending into the upper limb which follows the distribution of a cervical nerve root. Symptoms usually develop as the result of a disc prolapse or the extrusion of disc material into the spinal canal, which results in the compression or irritation of the exiting nerve root.

The symptoms are slightly more common in males than in females (1.4:1), and may be associated with heavy lifting or a jarring injury, but symptoms may also develop without a specific precipitating event.

Pain often radiates to the scapular region and sometimes the occiput. Clinically, the patient may present with a torticollis, and may have tender trigger points in the posterior cervical musculature.

Movements are restricted and painful, but movement in at least one direction is usually full and painless in all

but the most severe cases. There may be weakness of the muscle groups innervated by the affected nerve root, sensory changes in the affected dermatome and reflex changes that aid identification of the site of the pathology.

The foramenal compression test is often positive, the neck is positioned in slight extension and tilted towards the side that is causing pain. Axial compression is applied to the top of the skull and pain is produced, which is referred into the shoulder and arm along the affected dermatome. The C6 and C7 cervical roots are most commonly involved.

Differential diagnosis

This should include the following.

Cervical rib: usually affects the C8 and T1 roots.

Carpal tunnel syndrome: neck movements are painless and symptoms are usually confined to the hand.

Supra-spinatus tendon lesions or other shoulder pathology: pain does not extend below the elbow and there is no neurological abnormality.

Tumours of the cervical spine or adjacent region: may present with radicular symptoms; usually found in older individuals, and associated with other features of malignancy.

Cervical spine infection: will usually be associated with a systemic illness, fever and malaise; typical radiographic features may be delayed by several weeks.

Brachial neuritis: pain is often of sudden onset and severe, but with multiple levels involved.

Investigation

Plain radiographs will often demonstrate the loss of the normal cervical lordosis. Degenerative changes are often evident, but these changes may not be the cause of the patient's symptoms.

As a general rule, plain radiographs are of limited value in the assessment of cervical brachalgia and are not usually indicated in the initial assessment of this condition.

If a neoplastic process is suspected, plain radiographs may identify an infiltrative process, and a bone scan may be of value to confirm the presence of disseminated disease.

A CT scan will demonstrate spinal canal or foramenal stenosis that may or may not be related to the patient's symptoms. It may also demonstrate the presence of a localized disc protrusion, but the relative lack of epidural fat and artefact produced by the shoulders often results in difficulty in differentiating the dural sac and its contents from the intervertebral disc. A CT scan therefore has a relatively low yield in the assessment of cervical brachalgia.

An MRI scan is the investigation of choice in the assessment of cervical brachalgia, but should only be requested if operative intervention is being considered.

CT myelography has been largely replaced by MRI, but may still have a place in the assessment of symptoms of brachalgia in association with multiple-level degeneration to identify the site or sites of neural compromise.

Treatment

Resolution of symptoms will usually occur spontaneously within 6 to 12 weeks in 80–85% of cases. Rest will often be of some benefit in the initial stages of the condition, but should be limited to no more than 3 to 4 days. The short-term use of a cervical support may enable the individual to remain active during the initial period of discomfort. Use of an external brace continually for more than 1 to 2 weeks should be discouraged, as it will lead to weakness of cervical musculature and prolong the recovery phase of the condition.

Analgesics and anti-inflammatory medication can be utilized, but are only of value if they enable the individual to resume activity.

Cervical traction may provide relief of symptoms, but this is usually only short term, with symptoms recurring once traction has been removed. Traction may be of value in the management of severe acute symptoms, but should not exceed 5 kg (the approximate weight of the head).

Massage, ultrasound, interferential and other local therapeutic modalities may also provide symptomatic relief and assist in the restoration of function, but are unlikely to alter the natural history of the condition significantly if function cannot be restored in the first 4 to 6 weeks.

If symptoms are severe and refractory operative intervention may be considered, but usually not until symptoms have been present for at least 6 and more often 12 weeks. If there is evidence of progressive neurological deterioration or spinal cord compression, operative decompression should be undertaken, and this is usually performed via an anterior approach. The success rate for surgery of this type is of the order of 90–95% relief of referred pain to the upper limb. However, neck discomfort may persist in some cases, due to adjacent degenerative changes.

CERVICAL SPONDYLOSIS

Cervical spondylosis refers to degenerative disease of the subaxial cervical spine associated with loss of disc height, lipping of vertebral bodies, the formation of spondylophytes and degeneration of facet and unco-vertebral joints.

More than 80% of the UK population over 55 years of age have features of cervical spondylosis, but less than 5% will undergo operative intervention in the treatment of this condition. The majority of those who do have surgery are treated for cervical brachalgia or myelopathy due to associated foramenal or spinal canal stenosis.

Patients are usually over 40 years of age and complain of neck pain of gradual onset, which is often worse in the morning. Pain may radiate widely to the occiput, shoulder and arm. The first movement to be lost is extension, and there may also be marked limitation of lateral flexion when upright, which improves on lying down.

Symptoms of paraesthesia, weakness and clumsiness are occasionally reported and, rarely, signs of a cervical myelopathy such as brisk reflexes, increased tone and increased urinary frequency or urgency will be evident.

Investigation

Plain radiographs will usually identify the presence of degenerative disease, but it is important to remember to treat the patient and not the radiograph. It is also a well-accepted fact that there is no direct correlation between the extent of degeneration that is evident radiographically and discomfort.

A plain radiograph may be requested if symptoms do not respond to simple analgesics, anti-inflammatory medication and local therapeutic modalities after 2 to 4 weeks, in order to exclude other significant pathology.

A bone scan may be indicated to identify a localized area of degeneration that may respond to a steroid injection, or to exclude a neoplastic process.

A CT or MRI scan is only indicated if operative intervention is being considered to treat localized disease, or to relieve neural compromise.

Treatment

Rest, avoidance of aggravating activities, and the use of analgesics and anti-inflammatories are the mainstay of treatment. A cervical collar may be of value during acute episodes of pain, but the long-term use of a collar should be discouraged. Physiotherapy and local therapeutic modalities may also result in symptomatic relief, but this is usually short-lived. If cervical spondylosis is associated with radicular symptoms or myelopathy, surgical decompression may be indicated and may be performed via an anterior or posterior approach, depending on the location of the pathology and the sagittal alignment of the cervical spine.

In some cases, a cervical fusion may be indicated for the treatment of neck pain in the absence of radicular symptoms. However, the surgical treatment of neck pain, in the absence of a neurological deficit and discrete radicular symptomatology, does not significantly alter the natural history of this degenerative process.

BACK PAIN

The intervertebral disc has a blood supply up to the age of 8 years, after which time the intervertebral disc becomes the largest avascular structure in the body. Nutrition is thereafter provided by diffusion from the adjacent end-plate and the outer annulus.

Kirkaldy-Willis recognized that all spines degenerate, and divided the process of degeneration into the following three stages.

1. *Dysfunction* (15–45 years), characterized by circumferential and radial tears in the annulus with localized facet joint synovitis.

2. *Instability* (35–70 years), characterized by internal disc disruption, disc resorption, degeneration of facet joints with capsular laxity, subluxation and joint erosion (disc herniation is a complication of stages 1 and 2).

3. *Stabilization* (> 60 years), characterized by progressive development of hypertrophic bone about

the disc and facet joints, leading to segmental stiffening or ankylosis.

Disc degeneration may result from an injury that causes an annular tear, and which may or may not be associated with the prolapse of nuclear material. Degeneration is also influenced by environmental factors such as manual work and smoking, but the single most important factor is the genetic make-up of the disc and the vertebral end-plate. Mechanical back pain is the term used to describe pain that is aggravated by loading the spine and intervertebral discs. The load on the discs is greatest during lifting and bending activities and when maintaining a seated posture, and is least when lying down. Pain may be described as discogenic if it is generally worse on sitting and bending and is relieved by standing, walking and lying down. There may also be a component of facet irritation, which is characterized by increased discomfort on extension, lateral flexion or rotation in a particular direction. However, pain on extension may also be due to a central posterior disc protrusion or annular tear.

This degenerative process does not always result in pain, which is likely to be related to variations in the innervation of the spine, and in the support provided by the paravertebral musculature during various activities.

Approximately 80% of the population will suffer from back pain due to degenerative disease at some stage in their life, and back pain is slightly more common in males than it is in females. Back pain is the reason for approximately 2% of GP presentations, but as symptoms settle spontaneously in the majority of cases, or can be controlled medically, only 1–2% of those with back pain will subsequently undergo surgical intervention.

INVESTIGATION

No investigations are indicated in the assessment of 'mechanical back pain' in the absence of a history of significant trauma, in which case plain radiographs will usually exclude a significant bony injury.

A CT scan may demonstrate features of degeneration, but these changes may not be responsible for the patient's symptoms. More often than not, the CT will be considered to be normal or near normal for the patient's age and sex, and it is not a very useful or cost-effective investigation in the assessment of mechanical back pain.

Where facet pain appears to predominate, facet joint injections may be of value both diagnostically and therapeutically, but are unlikely to result in permanent or long-term relief of symptoms.

An MRI scan is the investigation of choice. It will demonstrate the anatomy of the lumbar spine in detail, and it may identify localized disc of degeneration.

If degeneration is localized and symptoms are sufficiently severe for operative intervention to be contemplated, lumbar discography may be requested in order to identify the disc or discs responsible for symptoms. Discography is by no means a panacea and remains the subject of controversy, but at present it is the only investigation available that enables the identification of a painful intervertebral disc.

SPINAL FUSION

Spinal fusion remains a controversial area in spinal surgery. The indications for spinal fusion are considered dubious by some, and there have been no reliable comparative trials evaluating its efficacy compared to the non-operative approach.

Surgery of this type requires an extended recovery time, and should only be contemplated if the origin of the pain has been identified with some degree of certainty. It is also important that the patient understands the likelihood of success and provides their full informed consent to the procedure.

Macnab has stated that the surgical treatment of low back pain is rarely indicated, and that virtually all back pain due to degenerative disc disease will settle to a tolerable level if stress is taken off the spine by weight loss, strengthening of the abdominal muscles, and modification of activities.

The outcome of spinal fusion surgery for one or two level degenerative disc disease is 70–80% good or excellent results, with 20–25% of cases being no better, and up to 5% being worse off at the completion of treatment than they were prior to surgery. Surgery for more extensive degenerative disease is associated with a lower likelihood of success.

Spinal fusion should therefore be considered as the last resort in the treatment of degenerative disc disease.

DISC 'PROLAPSE' AND 'SCIATICA'

The term 'disc bulge' is used to describe a diffuse expansion of the annular margin which usually develops in association with degeneration of the disc and loss of disc height. A 'disc protrusion or prolapse' results from the development of an annular tear. The integrity of the inner annulus is disrupted and nuclear material protrudes through, resulting in a focal protrusion of the outer annulus.

Both disc bulges and protrusions are common, with up to 15% of asymptomatic lumbar discs showing evidence of a disc bulge or protrusion on MRI or CT investigations. These changes are likely to be of no significance unless the distribution of symptoms correlates with the site and size of the disc pathology that is evident.

An 'extruded' disc fragment is one that has erupted through the outer annulus into the spinal canal, but part of the disc fragment remains within the confines of the annulus or disc space. A 'sequestered' disc fragment is one that has been expelled from the disc and lies free within the spinal canal. An extruded or sequestered fragment is more likely to result in symptoms of nerve root or cauda equina compression.

Around 95% of disc protrusions, extrusions or sequestra occur at the L4–5 or L5–S1 levels, and about 65% occur at L4–5.

Sciatica refers to the distribution of the pain, and is not a diagnosis of the cause of the pain. Pain follows the distribution of the sciatic nerve, which comprises the L4, L5 and S1 nerve roots. Leg and/or buttock pain is more pronounced than back pain, and the patient will usually display positive nerve root tension signs, such as a positive straight leg raise or bow-string test. Nerve root irritation is characterized by the presence of myotomal pain. Nerve root compression is characterized by the presence of weakness, and reduced sensitivity to light touch or pin-prick and reflex changes.

Patients with sciatica are usually aged between 20 and 40 years, and the first severe attack may be precipitated by a relatively minor back strain. Back discomfort may precede the onset of leg pain by days or even weeks. Severe back, buttock and leg pain then develops while lifting, stooping, coughing, sneezing or straining, which results in the development of a disc prolapse, extrusion or sequestrum. Backache and sciatica will usually be exaggerated by sitting, bending, lifting, coughing or straining, and are relieved, at least to some extent, by lying down.

Cauda equina compression, with the development of bladder and bowel dysfunction, may occur rarely. In this case, surgical decompression becomes an emergency in order to avoid or limit any permanent deficit.

Investigation

Plain radiographs may exclude significant bony pathology, but are generally not cost-effective in the evaluation of sciatica.

A CT scan will often identify a disc protrusion or sequestrum, particularly in slim individuals. In obese patients and those with a greater body mass, the definition of tissue planes becomes less distinct and the results may be inconclusive.

An MRI scan will provide greater anatomical detail, and it remains the investigation of choice in the assessment of disc pathology. However, it should be regarded as a pre-operative investigation and be requested by a specialist if he or she is considering surgical intervention. Myelography now has a limited role in the assessment of sciatica, but may be requested if an MRI scan cannot be performed.

Treatment

Symptoms will settle spontaneously in the majority of cases, and operative intervention is rarely indicated. Treatment should therefore be symptomatic in the first instance. Rest should not extend beyond 3 days, as extended rest delays restoration of function and resolution of symptoms.

Non-steroidal anti-inflammatories are usually of little value in the acute management of sciatica, and there is little or no place for the use of muscle relaxants, oral corticosteroids or antidepressants in the management of acute back and leg pain.

Physiotherapy may result in short-term pain relief, but there is no evidence to suggest that it alters the natural history of the condition. Exercises to strengthen the abdominal and extensor muscles are of benefit once symptoms have started to settle, and the emphasis of 'physical therapy' should be the restoration of function.

The epidural injection of local anaesthetic and steroid (Cilestone chronodose) is useful in the acute stage of sciatica and results in short-term relief in 60–85% of cases and up to 6 months relief in 30–40% of cases. The effect appears to be related to the acceleration of the natural history, or at least the temporary relief of symptoms while the natural history becomes evident.

Indications for surgery

These are as follows:

1. cauda equina compression with bladder and/or bowel involvement;

2. failure of conservative treatment extending over at least 6 and usually 12 weeks;

3. progressive neurological deficit.

Surgical intervention usually takes the form of a partial discectomy, and satisfactory results can be expected in 90–95% of cases. There is a 5% incidence of recurrent disc protrusion, the rate of which does not appear to be affected by the extent of disc clearance at operation. There is also a 5% incidence of significant mechanical back pain, but the incidence of back pain is not significantly different in patients who have surgery compared to those who do not.

SPINAL CANAL STENOSIS

Spinal canal stenosis is a common complaint among the elderly population, and is characterized by narrowing of the spinal or nerve root canal and intervertebral foramen. Developmental or congenital stenosis in isolation is rare, and symptoms usually develop as a result of a combination of congenital narrowing of the canal and degenerative disease or other pathology. Stenosis may be central, or involve the lateral recess or foramen, and it is not uncommon to see features of all three in the same patient.

Stenosis most commonly affects the third, fourth and fifth motion segments of the lumbar spine, and symptoms do not usually develop until the seventh decade of life.

The smallest cross-sectional area of the lumbar spinal canal is usually at the level of the facet joints, which are usually narrowest at the L3–4 level. The narrowest AP diameter is usually from the posterior vertebral wall to the upper border of the spinous process. Verbiest defined absolute lumbar spinal canal stenosis as less than 10 mm and relative stenosis as less than 12 mm.

Patients usually report experiencing pain in the buttocks and thighs when walking or standing, and this pain is often associated with feelings of heaviness, weakness and sometimes numbness in the legs. Back pain may also be associated with these symptoms, and leg symptoms may be unilateral or bilateral.

The symptoms are usually rapidly relieved by rest, particularly sitting or flexion of the lumbar spine. A neurological deficit may develop with activity, but a lack of clinical signs on examination is not uncommon, and root tension signs are usually negative. Spinal canal stenosis is considered to be a vascular phenomenon due to its claudicant nature, and it has been postulated that it is due to either a vascular steal or venous congestion and stasis.

The following features differentiate spinal canal stenosis from vascular claudication:

1. pain is maximal in the thighs rather than in the calves;

2. it is associated with paraesthesia and weakness after walking;

3. stopping and keeping the back extended will not relieve the pain;

4. walking with the back flexed increases the walking distance (e.g. pushing a shopping trolley).

Investigations

Plain radiographs will usually reveal extensive degenerative changes involving the intervertebral discs and facet joints. The presence of a degenerative spondylolisthesis should alert the observer to the presence of possible canal compromise.

A CT scan will usually provide adequate detail of the bony margins of the spinal canal, but definition of neural structures, the disc and ligamentum flavum is often inadequate.

Myelography is a pre-operative investigation and will demonstrate the levels involved and the extent of surgery required. It has now been largely replaced by MRI scanning, but is of value in selected cases to assist in the planning of operative intervention.

MRI is playing an increasingly important role in the assessment of spinal canal stenosis. It is non-invasive, can be performed as an out-patient procedure, and provides good visualization of the extent of canal compromise and neurological involvement.

Treatment

Modifications in activity will often result in the patient being able to cope with their symptoms. An epidural injection may also produce clinical improvement and enable the individual to avoid operative intervention. This is particularly appealing in the very old or those who are considered to be a high anaesthetic risk.

Analgesics and anti-inflammatories may be of value, particularly when symptoms of canal stenosis are associated with degenerative back and buttock pain due to facet arthritis. The patient's quality of life remains the key factor in deciding when to consider surgical intervention. Decompression can be expected to result in relief of leg pain, but may not improve back pain. Where a degenerative spondylolisthesis is evident and there are features of degenerative back pain, particularly if the facet joints are sagittal in their orientation, a spinal fusion may be considered necessary. Instrumentation in these circumstances is associated with an increased fusion rate, but the presence of osteoporosis, which is not uncommon in this group of patients, may result in early loosening of the implants, loss of fixation and the subsequent need for further intervention.

A good or excellent outcome can be expected in 80–85% of cases after decompression. About 10–15% of patients will develop features of recurrent stenosis at the same or other levels in the lumbar spine, yet few of them require further surgery, and 15–20% complain of increased degenerative back pain after decompression without fusion.

SPONDYLOLISTHESIS

This refers to the forward shift of one vertebra on another, and is derived from the Greek *spondl*, meaning spine, and *olisthesis*, meaning a downward slipping. It is most commonly seen at L4–5 or L5–S1, and is evident in *c.* 4.4% of the population aged 6 years compared to *c.* 6% in adulthood. Spondylolisthesis has not been identified in individuals at or soon after birth, and it appears to develop after vertical ambulation has commenced.

Classification

Spondylolisthesis may be classified as follows:

1. congenital or dysplastic (males < females) (20%);

2. degenerative (males < females) (25%);
3. isthmic or lytic (males > females) (50%);
4. traumatic or pathological (5%).

Lytic spondylolisthesis is the commonest form, and is more common in males than in females, but the condition is more likely to progress and become symptomatic in females than in males. Females are also four times more likely to develop a degenerative slip than males. There is seldom a history of severe injury, and the pars defect usually develops as a result of repetitive stress. Shear stresses are greatest in the pars interarticularis when the spine is extended, and these lesions are more common in individuals who sustain repetitive extensor strains. There is an increased incidence in individuals with thoraco-lumbar Scheuermann's disease, which is thought to be associated with a compensatory increase in the lumbar lordosis of these patients. There is also an increased incidence in family members of affected individuals, gymnasts, fast bowlers, members of certain Eskimo tribes, and in individuals with sacral spina bifida and sacralization of the fifth lumbar vertebra.

Clinically, there may be no external sign of the underlying lesion. In more severe cases there is increased lumbar lordosis, a protruding abdomen and prominent buttocks. Adolescents or adults usually present with backache, or the presence of a lysis or spondylolisthesis may be an incidental finding on a radiograph taken for another reason. A step can often be felt in the spinous processes of the lumbar vertebrae. Girls are more prone to severe deformity, and more often display clinical symptoms than boys. Symptoms are relatively uncommon in children, and are rarely severe enough in adolescents for medical attention to be sought.

Investigation

Plain radiographs will usually reveal the lesion, and oblique films demonstrate the classical sign of a collar on the 'Scotty dog'. Disc height may be reduced and slips of greater than 50% are often associated with a significant lumbo-sacral kyphosis.

CT scans with reverse obliquity of the gantry will demonstrate the lysis more clearly, and a bone scan may be useful for identifying whether the spondylolysis is active, which may influence treatment.

A myelogram or MRI scan may be indicated if there is a neurological deficit.

Treatment

Rest and analgesics are indicated for acute episodes of pain, but the emphasis should be on abdominal toning, modification of activity and the avoidance of hyperextension of the lumbar spine.

Where the bone scan is active, the 'stress fracture' may

be of recent onset, in which case healing may be possible. Here the use of a brace may be considered for 3 months, after which time activity modification may enable the healing of the lesion. Where there is an established non-union there is little point in using a brace, and rehabilitation should commence immediately. Facet or pars injections may ease symptoms and allow greater involvement in rehabilitation activities.

Patients should be counselled against a vocation that involves lifting or strenuous activity, and individuals with a slip of greater than 25% are thought to be at greater risk of back injury during contact sports.

Adolescents with a slip of less than 25% do not generally require surgical treatment, and surgery should only be considered if the pain is persistent and prevents work and social pursuits, where there is associated neurological compromise, or if there is significant or progressive deformity. In general, the development of a spondylolysis, with or without listhesis, does not cause pain in most patients. In the majority of cases, a child with either a spondylolysis or spondylolisthesis can be permitted to enjoy a normal childhood and adolescence without restriction of activities, fear of progressive slip or disabling pain.

Limb pain

John A. Walsh

Introduction

Limb pain may have vascular, musculoskeletal, neurological or rare unusual aetiologies. The characteristics and site of the pain may lead one to the most probable cause with the aid of physical examination and appropriate non-invasive and invasive investigations. For example, in the first instance it is important to establish whether the pain is related to exercise or is present at rest.

LEG PAIN ON WALKING

Calf muscle pain which occurs after walking a predictable distance, e.g. 100 m, and which is made worse by walking uphill or up stairs, is characteristic of *intermittent claudication*. Typically it is relieved by rest, e.g. for 5 min, and the patient can then walk again. Clues to the presence of peripheral vascular disease narrowing or occluding the superficial femoral artery are gained from a history of the presence of one or more of the five principal risk factors, namely smoking, hypertension, diabetes mellitus, elevated cholesterol and obesity, and examination may reveal reduced or absent peripheral pulses. The definitive non-invasive investigations are ankle/brachial Doppler pressure index with or without exercise and colour duplex scanning of arterial inflow into the affected limb. Arteriography remains the gold standard. Treatment options include conservative, endovascular or bypass procedures.

If these investigations are normal, then other causes to consider include the following.

Pseudoclaudication from spinal canal stenosis Investigations include X-ray of the lumbo-sacral spine, CT myelogram or MRI. The treatment options are physiotherapy, epidural steroids or surgical decompression.

Compartment syndrome This usually involves the anterior compartment, i.e. the tight compartment containing the tibialis anterior muscle. Measurement of the intra-compartmental pressure before and after exercise is the investigation of choice, and the pressure may rise as high as 100 mmHg after exercise in a severe compartment syndrome. Surgical decompression by slitting open the investing deep fascia is the treatment of choice.

Stress fracture This usually involves the lower one-third of the tibia. Pain is made worse by activity and is confined to the shin. The diagnosis is made by nuclear scan.

Periostitis This usually involves the length of the tibia on the medial aspect. A nuclear scan will highlight the area of periostitis and differentiate it from a stress fracture.

Torn muscle A history of trauma or sudden pain from tearing of the affected muscle together with local tenderness with or without swelling in an otherwise normal leg are clues to making the diagnosis.

Chronic venous insufficiency In this condition the patient complains of a bursting pain and swelling on walking. The aetiology is severe restriction of venous outflow from the limb following a deep vein thrombosis, and excessive fibrosis and narrowing of the deep veins, producing 'venous claudication'. Wearing a tight bandage or stocking may exacerbate the symptoms. Examination of the limb should reveal changes consistent with the post-phlebitic syndrome, namely swelling, post-phlebitic varicose veins, varicose pigmentation, eczema, *atrophie blanche*, lipodermatosclerosis and possible ulceration in the garter area. Non-invasive investigations include colour duplex scanning, air plethysmography, photo-plethysmography and minimally invasive measurement of ambulatory venous pressure and venography. Treatment is difficult, but cross-over femoro-femoral venous bypass is sometimes feasible.

Joint disease A history of knee or ankle pain with localized tenderness with or without swelling will easily differentiate joint problems from the other causes of leg pain on walking.

THIGH AND LEG PAIN ON WALKING

Calf muscle and thigh pain which occur on walking a predictable distance, e.g. 100 m, are characteristic of intermittent claudication due to peripheral vascular disease affecting more proximal vessels, i.e. iliac vessels, or the aorta if the pain is bilateral. With occlusion or stenosis of an internal iliac artery, the symptom complex includes buttock claudication in addition to thigh and calf claudication.

Physical examination usually reveals a weak or absent femoral pulse, and after exercise the ankle/brachial Doppler pressure index should fall to low levels. Arteriography is indicated with a view to endovascular (i.e. balloon angioplasty with or without stent) or arterial reconstruction (e.g. ilio-femoral bypass or extra-anatomical femoro-femoral cross-over bypass).

In the presence of normal arterial circulation, the differential diagnosis includes the following:

1. spinal canal stenosis;

2. sciatica – with characteristic posterior midline thigh and calf pain exacerbated by movement, including straight leg raising;

3. muscle strain;

4. referred pain from viscera;

5. inguinal hernia;

6. hip joint disease, e.g. osteoarthritis, capsulitis;

7. meralgia paraesthetica – entrapment of the lateral cutaneous nerve of the thigh as it passes beneath the inguinal ligament; the main symptom is disturbed sensation over the lateral aspect of the upper thigh;

8. ilio-psoas strain;

9. polymyalgia rheumatica, characterized by pain and stiffness in multiple joints (upper and lower limbs); associated with a high ESR (e.g. 100 mm/h) and a dramatic therapeutic response to prednisolone, which is then titrated to control symptoms and ESR.

LOWER LIMB PAIN AT REST

A clinical presentation of chronic severe burning pain in the foot which is exacerbated by warmth (e.g. the blankets in bed), so that the patient sleeps with the foot exposed or sleeps in a chair, suggests *critical ischaemia* of the rest pain type. This may progress to ulceration and gangrene depending on the severity of underlying peripheral vascular disease, the pathological process being thrombosis on atheromatous plaques.

On examination the affected foot is cold with pallor and venous guttering on elevation and dependent rubor (positive Buerger's test). Lower limb pulses are reduced or absent, and the resting ankle-brachial pressure index is well below 0.50, and usually less than 0.25.

This clinical picture indicates a 'threatened limb', so early arteriography with a view to vascular reconstruction is the management option of choice. If revascularization is not feasible, then a major amputation (below or above the knee) may well be the outcome. Sympathectomy is an option, although a good sustained result is unlikely. However, the lumbar neurolytic sympathectomy technique using 10% phenol in contrast medium under image-intensifier control is well established, has been validated, and can be performed safely on elderly patients by Pain-Unit anaesthetists.

Sudden onset of a cold, painful lower extremity presents quite a different clinical picture to the above chronic presentation. The classical acute onset of all the P's (pain, pallor, paralysis, pulseless, paraesthesiae) indicates acute embolus or acute thrombosis. The findings of arrhythmia (especially atrial fibrillation), normal contralateral pulses and perfusion and no history suggestive of chronic peripheral vascular disease favour a diagnosis of embolus, whereas a past history of claudication in either limb, together with reduced pulses on the contralateral side and sinus rhythm, favour acute thrombosis as an extension of chronic peripheral arterial atheroma. This dilemma can be solved by arteriography. The therapeutic options for a lower limb embolus include thrombolysis or embolectomy usually via the common femoral artery, followed by heparin and long-term warfarin treatment. Acute thrombosis is amenable to thrombolysis with streptokinase, urokinase or tissue plasminogen activator as a precursor to a more definitive endovascular or surgical reconstructive procedure to correct the underlying arterial problem that caused the acute (or chronic) thrombosis. In addition, thrombolysis may well clear propagated thrombus to such an extent that a more limited surgical procedure may be possible, e.g. limited endarterectomy rather than a long bypass.

PAIN AND BURNING SYMPTOMS WITH NORMAL ARTERIAL CIRCULATION

Many patients present with odd pains, burning sensations or 'pins and needles' in the feet and possibly legs as well, but with normal pulses, capillary return and normal non-invasive tests (Doppler, duplex).

The following conditions can be considered.

Diabetic neuropathy Symptoms of electric shock-like pains shooting from the foot up the leg are presumably due to the gradual demyelination of nerve sheaths. Eventually a bilateral ascending sensory neuropathy may develop, with loss of protective sensation and vulnerability to trauma. Once developed, the painful diabetic neuropathy is difficult to treat, but discomfort may be lessened by amitriptyline, carbamazepine, nifedipine or mexilitine. Prevention by encouraging tight control of diabetes is the aim in long-term management of diabetes mellitus.

Non-diabetic sensory neuropathy Various types of sensory neuropathy can develop as isolated problems, and may require sural nerve biopsy to make a definitive diagnosis.

Reflex sympathetic dystrophy Sympathetic overactivity syndromes may develop after relatively trivial trauma or following poliomyelitis or hemiparesis from a cerebrovascular accident.

The essential features of reflex sympathetic dystrophy are an extremity which is:

- cold;
- blue/pale;
- sweaty;
- swollen;
- painful;
- hypersensitive to touch; with
- loss of function.

Variants include shoulder-hand syndrome and Sudeck's atrophy, in which the disuse leads to demineralization of bone. The condition used to be called 'causalgia', but this relates more to brachial plexus injury. Treatment includes stellate ganglion block or cervico-thoracic sympathectomy.

Ekbom's syndrome (restless legs syndrome) This odd condition was first described in 1960 (by Ekbom) and is characterized by involuntary movements of the lower limbs, especially in bed at night. Fortunately, it responds to benzodiazepines, e.g. clonazepam. A variant of Ekbom's syndrome designated as *akathisia* is manifested as bizarre sensory symptoms of burning or icy cold feelings in the lower extremities, in the absence of any organic vascular or neurological abnormality.

Erythromelalgia Literally painful red extremities are characterized by hot and possibly swollen feet, including the toes. Patients describe the condition as like having cayenne pepper sprinkled on to a raw blistered area. There may be a history of physical or chemical trauma triggering the condition. The affected toes or foot indeed feel hot, and appear vasodilated. The symptoms are relieved by walking barefoot on cold tiles or immersing the extremities in ice-cold water. The condition is analogous to the triple response to histamine, i.e. antidromic vasodilatation in response to a noxious sensory stimulus. A diagnostic lumbar sympathectomy with bupivacaine will exacerbate the condition which is therefore the opposite to vasospasm in the physiological sense. Relief may sometimes be obtained by treatment with aspirin, non-steroidal anti-inflammatory drugs, colchicine, antihistamine or clonidine.

UPPER LIMB PAIN

OVERVIEW

There are two fundamental questions to be answered when a patient presents with upper limb pain.

1. Is the pain *unilateral* or *bilateral*?
2. Is there any evidence of ischaemia?

The answers to these two questions will narrow down the possible causes to a problem confined to one limb, e.g. arterial embolus or local musculoskeletal abnormality, as distinct from a more general problem, e.g. small-vessel disease or polymyalgia rheumatica affecting both limbs.

Unilateral ischaemic pain

Essentially there are four principal causes:

1. trauma;
2. embolism;
3. atheromatous occlusion (usually subclavian);
4. thoracic outlet syndrome.

A history of trauma, or sudden onset of embolic occlusion against a background of atrial fibrillation or the chronic nature of the atheromatous occlusion, should easily solve the differential diagnosis of the first three conditions above, aided by clinical and Doppler examination of pulses. However, the symptoms and signs of *thoracic outlet syndrome* are more difficult to diagnose.

For the arterial variety (as opposed to the neurological or venous type of thoracic outlet syndrome), the subclavian artery is caught in a pincer movement between the clavicle and the first rib (or a cervical rib or congenital band) when the shoulder is abducted. Disappearance of the radial pulses on shoulder abduction is unreliable, so duplex scanning with or without arteriography with the shoulder in the neutral and then abducted position is indicated in order to make a definitive diagnosis. Standard treatment is first rib resection with or without reconstruction of the subclavian artery if damaged and with or without cervico-thoracic sympathectomy for digital ischaemia.

The neurological variant of thoracic outlet syndrome results from traction on the lower cord of the brachial plexus producing symptoms and signs in the distribution of C8 and T1 nerve roots, and axillary-subclavian venous thrombosis is the venous manifestation of thoracic outlet syndrome. Again, first rib resection may be required and, with axillary-subclavian venous thrombosis, thrombolysis usually precedes first rib resection. However, there is a definite place for conservative treatment with heparin followed by 3 months of warfarin treatment.

Bilateral ischaemic pain

Bilateral ischaemic pain involving many digits suggests an underlying small-vessel disease or 'vasculitis'. However, where there is vasospasm only with the characteristic white to blue to red discoloration on exposure to cold, then a diagnosis of Raynaud's disease or primary Raynaud's phenomenon is likely. All screening tests must be normal before this benign condition (first described by Raynaud in 1862) can be diagnosed with confidence. If the fingertips show evidence of tissue necrosis, then secondary Raynaud's phenomenon due to an underlying systemic disorder is likely. The most common causes are scleroderma (including the CREST variant), rheumatoid arthritis and hyperviscosity states, e.g. polycythaemia and thrombocytosis. CREST syndrome (calcinosis, Raynaud's, oesophageal stenosis, sclerodactyly and telangiectasia) tends to run a protracted and relatively benign course. However, there are many other causes, including other collagen diseases, e.g. polyarteritis nodosa, vibrating tool use, drug overdose (e.g. ergot), disseminated intravascular coagulation, antigen–antibody reactions on the endothelium and systemic malignancy.

Investigations are aimed at narrowing down the above possible causes. They include full blood examination (FBE), erythrocyte sedimentation rate, antinuclear antibody, rheumatoid factor, serum electrophoresis, cryoglobulin and cold agglutinins. Treatment is essentially conservative, with avoidance of tobacco and cold exposure, vasodilatation with topical nitrobid, intra-arterial or intravenous regional guanethidine, stellate block and occasionally sympathectomy. Arteriography with macrofilms using the digital subtraction technique may clarify difficult diagnostic problems, as it will demonstrate digital artery occlusions.

Non-ischaemic upper limb pain

As with the lower limb, any musculoskeletal, traumatic or degenerative problem may lead to upper limb pain, and reflex sympathetic dystrophy is more common in the upper limb than the lower one.

Pain and/or sensory loss in the distribution of any of the C5–8, T1 nerve roots suggests a brachial plexus or cervical spine lesion. A sound knowledge of the upper limb dermatomes and also of the innervation of the hand is needed so that a plexus lesion can be differentiated from a peripheral nerve lesion.

Pain in the lateral three and a half fingers with or without wasting of the thenar muscles makes a carpal tunnel syndrome likely. Nerve conduction studies are useful for differentiating peripheral nerve lesions from musculoskeletal (including tendon sheath) abnormalities. Painful joints and 'torn ligaments' can be investigated by plain X-ray, ultrasound, MRI and arthroscopy, and a high ESR in a patient with multiple painful stiff joints may lead to a diagnosis of polymyalgia rheumatica.

FURTHER READING

The STILE Investigators. 1994: Results of a prospective randomized trial evaluating surgery versus thrombolysis for ischaemia of the lower extremity. The STILE Trial. *Annals of Surgery*, **220**, 251–68.

Clunie CJA, Tjandra JJ, Francis DMA. 1997: *Textbook of surgery. Section 11*. Melbourne: Blackwell Science.

Cousins MJ, Reeve TS, Glynn CJ, Walsh JA, Cherry DA. 1979: Neurolytic lumbar sympathetic blockade: duration of denervation and relief of rest pain. *Anaesthesia and Intensive Care* 7, 121–35.

Ekbom KA. 1960: Restless legs syndrome. *Neurology* **10**, 868–73.

Glynn CJ, Basedow RW, Walsh JA. 1981: Pain relief following post-ganglionic sympathetic blockade with intravenous guanethidine. *British Journal of Anaesthesia*, **53**, 1297–301.

Raynaud M. 1862: *De l'asphyxie locale et de la gangrène symétrique des extrémités*. Thesis. Paris: University of Paris.

Rob C, Smith R. 1997: Operative surgery. In Jamieson CW, Yao JST (eds), *Concise vascular surgery*. London: Chapman and Hall Medical.

Walsh JA, Glynn CJ, Cousins MJ, Basedow RW. 1984: Blood flow, sympathetic activity and pain relief following lumbar sympathetic blockade or surgical sympathectomy. *Anaesthesia and Intensive Care* **13**, 18–24.

Chapter 1.9

Painful hand

Miklós J. Pohl and W. Bruce Conolly

Introduction

Pain is a disagreeable sensation mediated by a complex system of afferent nerve stimuli which interact with the emotional state of the individual. The affected person's past experience, motivation and state of mind all modify pain.

The hand is one of the body's most sensitive structures, sensation being one of its major functions. Pain in the hand often reflects a disorder of one of its gliding parts, such as a tendon or a joint. Pain may be due to irritation of a peripheral nerve, lack of blood supply or infection.

Pain guards of the hand against injury, thus the con-genital absence of pain makes the hand susceptible to the stresses and injuries of everyday life. Lack of the pain-protective mechanism results in a reduction of blood supply, infection, gangrene and even amputation of those parts that are subjected to stress.

Past experience, tension, anxiety and emotional state may all influence the perception of pain. Pain destroys function more easily than any other derangement of the hand. Its adverse effects physically disable the whole extremity, and indeed disable the whole patient.

TYPES OF PAIN

ORGANIC AND FUNCTIONAL PAIN

Pain may be *organic* or *functional*. Organic pain may be peripheral/local or central/referred. Somatic or sympathetic nerve fibres may mediate pain. Pain in any region of the body may be nociceptive or neurogenic and each type may be local or referred.

Nociceptive pain is pain which arises within the somatic tissues of the body walls, limbs or viscera. The characteristic feature of nociceptive pain is that it is elicited by the stimulation of free nerve endings in the source tissue.

Neurogenic pain is pain that is not elicited by the stimulation of nerve endings, but is evoked by activity in nociceptive nerves generated somewhere along the nociceptive pathway, either in a peripheral nerve, the spinal cord or the thalamus. The pain is perceived to arise in the region innervated by the affected nerve, even though there is no lesion in the tissues of that region. A neuroma is a typical example of a lesion giving rise to neurogenic pain.

As mentioned above, pain may be peripheral or central. Peripheral pain may become central, and vice versa. Peripheral pain can be superficial or deep. Superficial pain is readily localized, usually within the skin, and provokes an immediate withdrawal of the stimulated part. It is often associated with tachycardia and palpitation. In contrast, deep pain is poorly localized, dull and oppressive, invoking bradycardia, hypotension and syncope. Central pain follows peripheral pain, and persists even after the peripheral stimuli have abated. Anxiety enhances and prolongs central pain.

Functional pain – occasionally, despite repeated examination and investigations, an organic cause for pain in the hand cannot be found. Patients in this category often have increased stress and anxiety levels, and are not infrequently involved in protracted medicolegal proceedings. Despite this, every effort should be made to examine and investigate the patient most thoroughly before this diagnosis is made.

ACUTE AND CHRONIC PAIN

Acute pain is pain that is experienced at the time of injury or which develops from other acute causes over a period of weeks or months. Usually, once treated, the pain disappears. This type of pain must be differentiated from *chronic pain* and *chronic pain syndrome*. Chronic pain is pain that persists beyond 6 months despite conventional therapy, but which is organic in nature. Chronic pain syndrome, on the other hand, is functional in origin, nearly always associated with minimal objective findings, and falls into the 'compensation seeking' category. Patients belonging to this group often try to manipulate the surgeon, their family and their environment for financial or emotional gain.

ANATOMICAL BASIS FOR PAIN IN THE HAND

THE TISSUES

Each of the different tissues affected expresses pain in a unique way. In general, the greater the distance from the periphery, the more diffuse is the distribution of sensory organs in the tissues.

Skin

Skin is a sensitive shield that protects the body. It is the most frequently injured tissue in the hand. Pain is produced by specific injury to the skin, such as excessive tension from tight wound closure, or focal pressure from poorly applied splints and dressings. Fixation of skin to bone resulting from insufficient subcutaneous padding, e.g. as in some amputation stumps, predisposes the tissues to minimal pressure and may result in localized ischaemic pain.

Fascia

The fascia has a sensory network of finely beaded terminals; in other words, it has its own pain receptors. Being inelastic, it is pressure sensitive, and therefore an expanding compartment in the hand or forearm will cause persistent throbbing pain and is a signal to consider urgent fasciotomy.

Muscle pain

This is less localized than pain in highly sensitive tissues such as skin and periosteum, but more distinctly localized than visceral pain. A painful muscle reacts by protective spasm. Compression or contraction and stretching (either acute or chronic) can cause muscle pain, as in myosotis or ischaemia.

Tendon

Pain sensation in tendons is usually poorly localized and of low intensity, except when it occurs in a fibrous compartment.

Bone pain

This arises from the blood vessels via the sympathetic fibres as well as the sensory fibres from the peripheral nerves, which accompany them. The marrow cavity has a sensory supply, making the bone sensitive to intraosseous pressure.

Periosteum

This is extremely sensitive, and periosteal pain can be the presenting symptom in fractures, periosteal contusion and periostitis. However, a benign bone tumour with an intact periosteum and absence of increased interosseous pressure may be painless.

Joint pain

This arises from synovial membrane, fibrous capsule and ligaments, as well as from the vasomotor supply to the joint (sympathetic).

Articular cartilage

This is insensitive, as no sensory nerve fibres have been found within it. Since there are no blood vessels in cartilage, there are no sympathetic fibres penetrating it. However, subchondryl bone and synovitis can cause pain in conditions associated with damaged cartilage. Painful crepitation on joint movement indicates an irregular joint surface. A stiff joint from a shortened capsule or ligament can also cause joint pain.

Neurogenic pain

Peripheral nerve trauma, especially that involving sensory nerves, can also affect the sympathetic nerves in surrounding tissue and cause a painful reflex vasomotor condition known as complex regional pain syndrome (CRPS), previously also called reflex sympathetic dystrophy (RSD) or causalgia.

GENERAL PRINCIPLES

Peripheral nerve injury causing pain

Peripheral nerve injury is often followed by a variable degree of pain, and this is followed by reactive anaesthesia which protects the part for several minutes or hours. This anaesthesia may persist or be replaced by a variety of painful sensations, e.g. hot shooting sharp pain. After 2 to 4 weeks, dysaesthesia manifests as a neuroma and nerve regeneration with a positive Tinel sign.

In the absence of normal regeneration, an indefinable period of fixed pain may lead to the development of CRPS.

Nerve compression

This may cause diffuse pain, paraesthesia or numbness in an anatomically recognized distribution. The type of pain is frequently intermittent, depending on the degree of oedema and compression, as in carpal tunnel syndrome, ulnar tunnel syndrome and radial tunnel syndrome. However, experimental compression of peripheral nerves and nerve roots does not cause pain, but produces paraesthesia as a result of ischaemia and conduction block.

Nerves may be compressed in a variety of ways, e.g. osteophytes in cervical spondylosis, intervertebral disc protrusion and nerves within a tight osseo-ligamentous compartment.

Neuritic pain

This may be due to inflammatory, metabolic or nutritional causes. An example of a viral inflammatory cause is the neuritic pain caused by herpes zoster. Pain may also be caused by irritation in the central nervous system and/or spinal chord.

Referred pain

Pain may be referred to the hand from the apical thorax and brachial plexus by tumours causing compression there (Pancoast syndrome).

Vascular pain

Lack of blood supply to muscles due to ischaemia following trauma or application of a tight dressing or plaster may cause pain that constitutes a surgical emergency. Occasionally a vascular tumour (e.g. glomus tumour) may be painful, especially if it is subungual. Ischaemic pain is usually constant and severe, and more than would be expected from the type of injury that has occurred. It is not relieved by painkillers and does not subside if a splint is applied or removed. When this type of pain is caused by ischaemic muscle, the stretch test is useful for detecting an increase in compartment pressure (Volkmann's contracture).

Pain may also occur in the fingertips as a result of ischaemia, e.g. in Raynaud's disease, embolus to the digital artery, and frostbite.

CLINICAL APPROACH TO HAND PAIN

HISTORY

Site and radiation

Pain felt in the hand and radiating proximally up the limb usually arises from the hand itself. For example, in carpal tunnel syndrome, pain may radiate to the neck but there are no physical signs proximal to the wrist. Pain originating in the neck, as in cervical spondylitis, is usually referred down the limb.

Type of pain

A *throbbing* pain usually indicates venous or lymphatic congestion due to oedema, most commonly caused by inflammation. External compression from a bandage or plaster may also cause this type of pain. *Local burning* pain usually indicates pressure caused by a tight plaster or dressing over a bony prominence. *Persistent generalized burning* pain is found in CRPS.

Pain from nerve compression may also be described as burning, but there is a strong element of paraesthesia, and the pain is *intermittent*. *Sharp*, *shooting* and very localized pain on contact may signify a neuroma.

Onset and aggravation

Movement aggravates the pain of any inflamed tissue (e.g. tenosynovitis). Pain and numbness that wake the patient from sleep are characteristic of carpal tunnel syndrome.

Pattern of pain

Intermittent pain is characteristic of nerve compression, and is exacerbated by excessive or repetitive movements and pregnancy. *Continuous* pain occurs in CRPS. Salicylates are said to alleviate the pain of an osteoma with dramatic effect.

Exacerbating and relieving factors

Resting the arm in a splint and elevation relieve the pain in most instances.

Associated symptoms

These include crepitation, clicking, functional impairment and loss of strength.

Subjective evaluation

This involves an evaluation of overall emotional state.

PHYSICAL EXAMINATION

Examination begins from the moment the patient enters the room and shakes hands. Many clues can be gained by carefully observing the patient while they are undressing, especially if the injury was work related or the patient is awaiting compensation. The whole patient must be examined, paying particular attention to the neck and cervical spine and the whole of the upper limb, culminating with the wrist and hand. Remember that *both* limbs must be examined and compared.

Inspection

The skin may show old or new scars, some surgical and some self-inflicted. Note the pattern of scars, which may hint at the diagnosis, such as burn scars in the median nerve distribution suggesting anaesthesia and injury to the median nerve. A scar may be the site of a painful neuroma, and one particular digit may show less dirt staining than the rest of the hand, indicating lack of use.

Odd patterns of scarring may reveal self-inflicted injuries, such as transverse scars across the volar wrist and forearm of the non-dominant limb.

The skin may also reflect vasomotor and trophic changes, such as onycholysis and lack of sweating. Vascular changes may also indicate the presence of CRPS or Raynaud's disease.

The pattern of skin creases and calluses should also be noted. Look for contour change that is swelling from regional oedema, e.g. as in de Quervain's tenosynovitis. Swelling may also be noted in the arthritides in cases of cellulitis or infection and tumours. Note muscle wasting. The pattern of wasting may indicate specific nerve compression or pathology that is not in the hand but originates in the cervical spine.

Palpation

During palpation of a patient's hand note the degree of the withdrawal response. A patient with a very tender neuroma will withdraw his or her hand very briskly (fifth-degree withdrawal response) whereas a patient with mild carpal tunnel syndrome may only pull away gently (first-degree response). Ask the patient to point to the most painful area first. Then proceed to palpate the non-tender areas of the hand, proceeding to 'the area' that the patient complains of most, confirming this by reproducing the pain on palpation and/or movement. Passive manipulation of certain joints will confirm diseases in the trapezio-metacarpal, piso-triquetral and third carpo-metacarpal joints.

When localizing pain, ask the following questions.

1. Is this the point at which you normally feel the pain?
2. Does the pain radiate anywhere?

Localization of the pain is extremely important for forming an accurate diagnosis and formulating appropriate treatment. Not infrequently patients are unable to localize their pain, which may be dull and ill-defined.

Movement

Ask the patient to reproduce the movement that provokes the pain. Distinguish *passive* movements that cause pain (e.g. osteoarthritis) from *active* movements that cause pain (e.g. trigger finger).

Specific tests

The *Allan test* is used to test the circulation and patency of both radial and ulnar arteries in the hand. First palpate each artery at both wrists. Then occlude both arteries by direct pressure. Ask the patient to pump each hand to exsanguinate it. Release one artery and note the distribution of its reactive hyperaemia, and the time of its appearance in the palm and fingertips. Repeat the process with release of the opposite artery.

The *Phalen test* is used for carpal tunnel syndrome (CTS) median nerve compression at the wrist. With the forearm supported, ask the patient to flex each wrist. Two-thirds of patients with CTS will complain of paraesthesia and numbness in the median nerve distribution within 60 s. The rapidity of onset of symptoms often indicates the severity of compression.

The *Watson scaphoid shift test* is used to assess scapholunate instability (SLI). With your thumb on the scaphoid tubercle and your index finger on the proximal pole of the scaphoid dorsally, ask the patient to deviate his or her wrist radially and ulnarwards. This will reproduce pain and a click in SLI.

The *Finkelstein test* is used to detect de Quervain's tenosynovitis. Ask the patient to grip his or her thumb into the palm. Active or passive ulnar deviation of the wrist will cause pain at the radial side of the wrist in the first extensor compartment.

Examination under anaesthetic block Lignocaine 0.5% may be injected with a 25-G needle into trigger points. If this relieves pain, it may confirm a diagnosis such as neuroma. If injection does not relieve the pain, then further investigations may be necessary.

INVESTIGATIONS

The more clear-cut the diagnosis after a thorough history and examination, the fewer the investigations that will need to be performed. For more complex conditions, and in cases involving workers' compensation and medico-legal proceedings, it is important to have objective evidence such as grip dynamometry, gonyometry and nerve conduction studies. Even in a clinically obvious case of CTS, nerve conduction studies are advisable if the cause is thought to be work related, especially in view of the fact that 10% of patients may not make a full recovery following surgery.

1. *X-ray* is the most frequently performed investigation in cases where a skeletal cause of pain is suspected, or when it is felt that the skeletal architecture may be altered secondarily, e.g. by tumour. Special

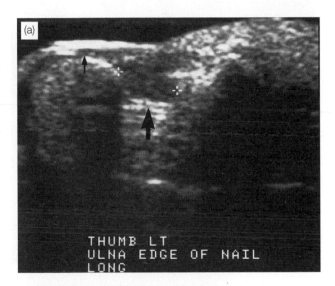

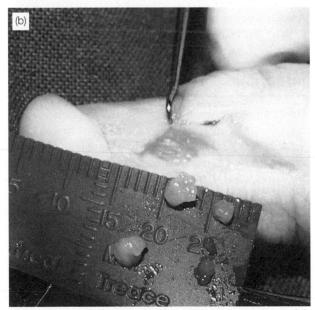

Figure 1.9.1 A 55-year-old man had persisting pain beneath his left thumbnail apparatus. A glomus tumour was suspected on ultrasound (a) and confirmed by surgical exploration (b). Two glomus tumours were found.

projections and dynamic studies may need to be undertaken, such as stress views for a suspected ligamentous rupture, or angiograms for suspected vascular malformations.

2. *Isotope bone scanning* should be performed when a skeletal cause of pain is suspected and the X-ray was normal. A scan may also be positive in CRPS, and in wrist and hand arthropathies. A negative bone scan will usually exclude a skeletal cause of pain.

3. *Ultrasound imaging* is most helpful in showing even tiny radiolucent foreign bodies, tumours, e.g. glomus tumour (Figure 1.9.1), and tenosynovitis. An ultrasound video recording will demonstrate dynamic disorders of joints and tendons.

4. *CT and MRI scanning* occasionally provide valuable information enabling the diagnosis of difficult rare conditions such as osteochondritis, osteoma and fractured hook of hamate (Figure 1.9.2).

5. *Doppler* is useful in vascular conditions that affect the hand, such as aneurysms.

6. *Electrodiagnostic studies*, including nerve conduction studies and electromyography, are helpful in determining the degree and level of nerve compression and medical neurological conditions such as polymyalgia and viral neuritis.

7. *Special tests* are used to investigate diabetes and arthropathies such as gout and rheumatoid arthritis.

8. *Arthroscopy* is especially helpful in wrist conditions where there may be ligamentous tears or injuries in the triangular fibrocartilage.

9. *Needle aspiration of fluid* – joint aspiration may identify causes of synovitis and effusions.

THE MANAGEMENT OF HAND PAIN

ACUTE PAIN

The aim here is to control pain caused by injury, and this means reduction of fractures and decompression of tight compartments following internal vascular trauma to the forearm and hand. Splinting and elevation, with maintenance of good circulation and control of oedema and prevention of infection, should be the aims of treatment. Ice treatment for acute soft-tissue injury may be helpful in alleviating acute pain, swelling and haematoma formation. Occasionally, local anaesthetic injection can relieve acute pain. Psychological support and recognition and relief of anxiety can be as important as analgesia itself.

Narcotics may be given in acute hand trauma. However, the staff should be cautioned not to give repeated doses without first checking the tightness of

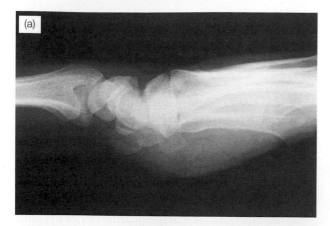

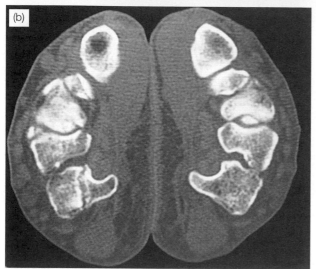

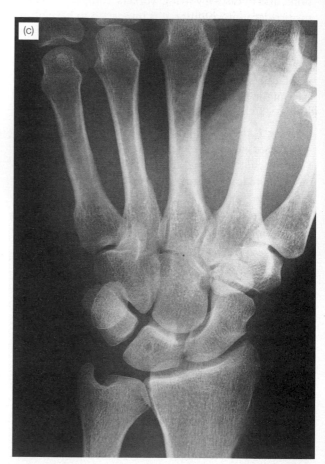

Figure 1.9.2 A 40-year-old right-handed golfer had persisting pain in the hypothenar eminence. This patient had resection of the hook of hamate with relief of pain and tenderness, and a return to full golfing activities after 10 weeks. (a) and (b) Plain X-rays PA and lateral views show no abnormality. (c) A CT scan shows the fractured hook of hamate.

dressings, swelling, peripheral circulation and sensation in the injured limb. Once these causes of pain have been excluded and it is established that the pain is from the injury itself, repeated injection of narcotics may be given cautiously.

POST-OPERATIVE PAIN

Localized burning pain suggests pressure of a splint over a bony prominence, and throbbing pain indicates congestion caused by a constrictive dressing or plaster. *When there is persistent pain, the splint and dressing should always be immediately removed and the wound and limb examined by the surgeon.*

Narcotics may mask complications of ischaemia, congestion, sepsis and localized pressure post-operatively.

INFECTION

Infection causes congestion and irritation of nerve endings, resulting in pain. Splintage and intravenous antibiotics and oral analgesics should relieve the pain. Narcotics are not usually necessary. Suppuration should be suspected if there is a history of 2 to 5 days of progressive throbbing pain or pain preventing sleep. This usually necessitates surgical drainage. Pain that persists after drainage may indicate incompleteness of drainage or the presence of a foreign body.

NON-TRAUMATIC PAINFUL CONDITIONS

Musculo-tendinous pain

In an acute situation, splint the part, prescribe anti-inflammatory medication and consider the injection of corticosteroid intralesionally, as in de Quervain's tenosynovitis, medial epicondylitis (golfer's elbow) and lateral epicondylitis (tennis elbow).

In cases of tendonitis and tenovaginitis where there is crowding of structures within a narrow space, surgical release is the best option once conservative measures have failed.

Vascular pain

Arterial blockage by embolus or thrombus may cause pain in the hand, and may require embolectomy and anticoagulation.

For the pain in vasospastic states such as Raynaud's disease and the inadvertent intra-arterial injection of drugs, sympathetic block may be of value.

Bone and joint pain

For arthritis, splintage and basic physiotherapy measures are the first line of treatment. Medication such as the anti-inflammatories and analgesics follow. Joint replacement is employed in cases where conservative measures have failed and where there is loss of use, pain and progressive deformity.

Infective arthritis is treated with intravenous antibiotics, rest and elevation for 24 h. If the pain and inflammation have not improved or dissipated, then surgical drainage must be employed.

Nerve compression syndromes

Compression of the median nerve at the wrist is a frequent cause of pain in the hand. Median nerve compression at the wrist must be distinguished from referred pain from the neck. A detailed history with regard to past trauma to the upper limb and neck and degenerative disease must be sought.

Conservative measures may be employed initially, including rest splinting and steroid injections, but most cases proceed to carpal tunnel release, by either open or endoscopic methods.

The ulnar nerve may be compressed at the elbow (cubital tunnel) or more distally at the wrist (Guyon's canal). Again conservative measures are employed first, but most cases proceed to surgery. At the elbow the ulnar nerve is transposed to the anterior compartment of the forearm, whereas compression at the wrist is treated by releasing Guyon's canal.

Numerous other nerve compressions have been described in the upper limb, but they are beyond the scope of this chapter.

TUMOURS IN THE HAND

A ganglion may present acutely as a tender swelling, or rarely it may press on a nerve in a confined space, e.g. in the carpal tunnel or Guyon's canal. Ganglia may be aspirated or excised.

Bone cysts

The bones of the wrist joint are subject to neoplastic and metabolic changes. A cyst in a confined space, e.g. in the carpal tunnel, may cause ache or pain and require excision and bone grafting.

Osteoid osteoma

Characteristically this causes pain in the wrist, which is worse at night and relieved by aspirin. Osteoid osteomas often occur in the carpus or in one of the phalanges. They have a characteristic X-ray appearance and are best excised and bone-grafted (Figure 1.9.3).

Other benign and malignant tumours

These may arise in any of the tissues of the hand, and they are treated on their own merits, but a description is beyond the scope of this chapter. Any space-occupying lesion in the hand may cause pain either by direct pressure on a nerve or by stretching ligamentous, capsular or fascial structures around it.

SYMPATHETICALLY MEDIATED PAIN

Complex regional pain syndrome is described in detail in Chapter 1.1.

MISCELLANEOUS CAUSES

These include heterotropic calcification of soft tissues around the wrist, e.g. flexor carpi ulnaris, and may need curettage.

Repetitive strain injury (RSI)

This is also known as regional upper limb pain syndrome, cumulative trauma disorder (CTD), or work-related over-use syndrome, all of which refer to an upper limb pain that appears to be caused by repetitious activity. The muscles may become fatigued and in some instances there may be an organic tissue problem.

The best definition of RSI is a syndrome that affects the muscular skeletal system and is associated with excessive repetitive or eccentric stresses, rather than a disease process as such. It may also be regarded as a combination of soft-tissue and articular disorders

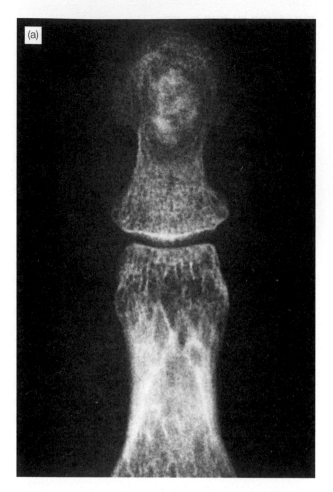

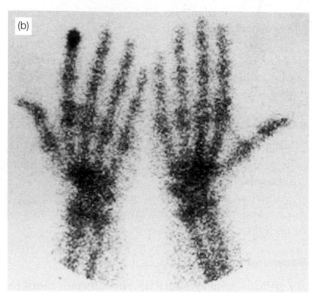

Figure 1.9.3 A 26-year-old woman had persisting pain in her left index finger tip for several years before a plain X-ray (a) showed the classic features of an osteoid osteoma with a central circumscribed nidus of the sclerotic bone and a circumferential osteopenic area in the distal phalanx. A bone scan (b) showed increased uptake. Photograph courtesy of Dr Douglass Wheen.

associated with prolonged static postures or excessive movement demands. The location, distribution and progression of systems can be explained in terms of the biomechanically integrated function of the neuromuscular articular system. It is important to exclude organic causes of pain such as tendonitis and carpal tunnel syndrome. Unfortunately, most cases of RSI are related to patients seeking workers' compensation benefits.

SYNOPSIS OF TREATMENT FOR PAIN

1. Diagnosis – recognize and treat the cause with the appropriate modalities, which range from rest, elevation and splintage to intravenous antibiotics and surgery.

2. Assess the psychological, social and economic state of the patient.

3. In general terms, in the presence of trauma, rest is the single factor of most importance in getting the patient healed and pain free. The patient must maintain hand activity, and this involves specialized hand physiotherapists and rehabilitation workers.

4. The different modalities for treating hand pain may include:

   (a) drugs – anti-inflammatory agents, tranquillizers, antidepressants and sedatives, to mention just a few;

   (b) physical treatment – physiotherapy may include splints (either static or dynamic), hot packs, paraffin wax, ultrasound, desensitization and mobilization.

5. Patients who are resistant to conventional modes of treatment may need to be referred to a multi-disciplinary pain clinic staffed by pain therapists, including anaesthetists, psychiatrists, psychologists, hand therapists and rehabilitation physicians. The patient may ultimately just have to accept their pain and adjust to it, but during this process they will need a large amount of emotional and physical support.

Analgesics

Julia M. Potter

Introduction

A logical approach to analgesics is best founded on our current understanding of pain and the factors which modulate its perception. The diagram in Figure 1.10.1 illustrates how in many cases the same factors may result in either inflammation or pain, and are inextricably linked. Thus the drugs which are used in the treatment of pain have been broadly divided into four categories (see Table 1.10.1). As well as the pharmacological treatment of pain, there are other valuable adjuncts, such as neurocutaneous stimulation.

The WHO Cancer Pain Relief Program (Table 1.10.2) is one approach that is promoted in the management of severe chronic pain.

Pain is the unpleasant perception of a noxious stimulus,

and has both objective and subjective components. In developing a framework for discussing analgesia, one can use a very simple model to illustrate most of the important points, such as that shown in Figure 1.10.1.

When a noxious stimulus acts on a receptor, the action potential that is generated is transmitted along the neurone (e.g. C fibres). Both the initial stimulus and the action potential which it generates are subject to modulation by chemical and/or neuronal input. The net perception in the subject may then be quite different, depending on the circumstances. In the presence of inflammation, chemical mediators of pain include serotonin (or 5-hydroxytryptamine), histamine and various kinins (e.g. bradykinin). If the pain is primarily due to ischaemia (e.g. following thrombosis), the mediators include the accumulated metabolic products (e.g. lactate). Prostanoids, such as prostaglandins E and F, play a role in both inflammatory and ischaemic pain, particularly in sensitizing the pain receptors and hence potentially amplifying the noxious stimulus. Within the nociceptive pathway itself, the neurotransmitters include the amino acid glutamate, and neuropeptides such as substance P.

The pathway is subject to both positive and negative

Table 1.10.1 Drugs used in the treatment of pain

Opioids
Non-steroidal anti-inflammatory drugs (NSAIDs)
Adjunctive agents used in palliative care (e.g. antidepressants)
Drugs used in pain syndromes (e.g. carbamazepine)

Table 1.10.2 WHO Pain Relief Program

Severity of pain	Primary drug	Potential concurrent therapy	
Level 1	Non-opioid	± Adjuvant	
Level 2 Pain persisting or increasing	Weak opioid	± Non-opioid	± Adjuvant
Level 3 Pain persisting or increasing	Strong opioid	± Non-opioid	± Adjuvant

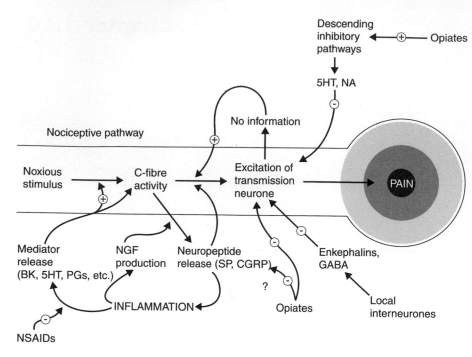

Descending
inhibitory ←— ⊕ — Opiates
pathways

↓

5HT, NA

⊖

No information

Nociceptive pathway

⊕

Excitation of
transmission
neurone

PAIN

Noxious
stimulus → C-fibre
activity

⊕

Mediator
release
(BK, 5HT, PGs, etc.)

NGF
production

Neuropeptide
release (SP, CGRP)

Enkephalins,
GABA

⊖

?

INFLAMMATION

⊖

Opiates

Local
interneurones

⊖

NSAIDs

Figure 1.10.1 Summary of modulatory mechanisms in the nociceptive pathway. (Reproduced with permission from Rang HP, Dale MM, Ritter JM. 1995: *Pharmacology*, 3rd edn. Edinburgh: Churchill Livingstone, p. 610.)

modulation. As shown in the diagram, opiates act both within the central nervous system and in the periphery. In the CNS, opiates result in inhibition of the pathway via release of 5-hydroxytryptamine and noradrenalin in the descending inhibitory pathways. In the periphery, opiates decrease presynaptic neurotransmitter release (and thus are inhibitory), as well as reducing neuropeptide release, and thus having an effect on the inflammation. Conversely, by enhancing the release of substance P, inflammation amplifies the neuronal contribution to pain.

OPIOIDS

An opioid or opiate is any substance which produces morphine-like effects. In order to satisfy the criteria for an opioid, the morphine-like agonist effects must be blocked by specific antagonists such as naloxone. The pharmacological group of opioids includes all of the naturally occurring neuropeptides (e.g. beta-endorphin), morphine itself, and synthetic analogues of morphine, some of which bear little apparent chemical resemblance to morphine (e.g. methadone). The term 'opioid' is derived from 'opium', a crude extract of the juice of the poppy *Papaver somniferum*. The term 'narcotic' is best not used, both because it has legal connotations, and because it only addresses a small part of the spectrum of pharmacological effects of these compounds.

There are three true opioid receptor subtypes (mu, delta and kappa) (see Table 1.10.3). The fourth subtype (sigma) is not a specific opioid receptor and binds other psychomimetic drugs as well. The opioid receptors are G-protein receptors, but the main agonist effects appear to link the G-protein directly to ion channels, without an apparent need for a second messenger. Opioid agonists cause K^+ channels to open (with hyperpolarization of the membrane) and decrease neurotransmitter release (due to decreased calcium entry into the cell). Table 1.10.3 provides a summary of the major properties of individual receptors, and examples of agonists and antagonists.

Although the production of analgesia is paramount, the other effects attributed to receptor stimulation produce significant and clinically relevant side-effects. Opioids act both centrally and peripherally, but they are less useful in pain syndromes which are neuropathic in origin (e.g. phantom pain). Opioids produce euphoria, which makes an important contribution to the subjective component of pain relief. Whilst the respiratory depression is generally regarded as being a problem of high-dose administration, it may occur at therapeutic doses if the dose is administered too rapidly. With regard to the use of opioids for analgesia, suppression of the cough reflex may cause problems, with inability to remove bronchial secretions adequately and with unprotected airways. However, suppression of the cough reflex may be advantageous in some patients, and cough linctus may contain opioids such as codeine. In patients who suffer from asthma, the use of morphine (or heroin) may

Table 1.10.3 Properties and effects of opioid receptors and drugs

Receptor subtype	Mu	Delta	Kappa	Sigma
Properties				
Analgesia	Supraspinal/spinal		Spinal	–
Respiratory depression	++		–	–
Pupil	Constricts		–	Dilates
Gastrointestinal tract motility	Decreased		–	–
Smooth muscle spasm	++		–	–
Behaviour/effect	Euphoria ++		Dysphoria +	Dysphoria ++
	Sedation ++		Sedation +	Psychomimetic
Physical dependence	++		+	–
Opioids				
Peptides:				
Endorphin	+++	+++	+++	–
Drugs:				
Agonists: Morphine	+++	+	++	–
Fentanyl	+++	+	–	–
Partial/mixed agonists:				
Pentazocine	Antagonist	+	Partial agonist	+
Buprenorphine	Partial agonist	–	–	–
Antagonists:				
Naloxone	+++	++	++	–

precipitate bronchoconstriction. This is due to histamine release from mast cells, the other effect of which may be urticaria or evidence of skin itching and scratching, often seen in drug users. The use of opioids results in a large number of side-effects in the gastrointestinal system. Nausea and/or vomiting may occur in up to 40% of patients and is due to central stimulation of the chemoreceptor trigger zone. In general, tachyphylaxis occurs with this side-effect, and with chronic dosing the symptoms become less troublesome. However, that is not the case for the increased smooth muscle tone and decreased motility of the smooth muscle of the gut, and constipation is common in those who use opioids chronically. The increase in smooth muscle tone may also result in worsening symptoms of biliary colic. In patients with pancreatitis the choice of analgesic can be very difficult, and increased plasma activity of amylase and lipase may accompany the use of morphine. Increased smooth muscle tone may also cause symptoms in the urinary tract, and contribute to urinary retention in the post-operative patient.

One of the most important pharmacological properties of the opioids is the production of tolerance and dependence. Tolerance is the requirement for increased doses of drug in order to produce the same pharmacological effect. In the case of opioids, tolerance is detectable within 24 h and develops to a significant degree within days. Dependence has two components. The first is physical dependence, which is characterized by the production of an abstinence or withdrawal syndrome. Opioid withdrawal has given rise to the term 'cold turkey', which is a description of the profound piloerection which accompanies its withdrawal. The complete withdrawal syndrome has elements of high sympathetic nervous system output, with tachycardia, anxiety, sweating and nausea, as well as influenza-like symptoms and fever, diarrhoea and insomnia. These symptoms are common to all withdrawal syndromes, differing only in degree. The second component of dependence is subjective or psychological dependence. This is best described as a profound 'craving'. The development of tachyphylaxis and dependence is ascribed to receptor changes. Although the primary effects of the opiate receptor (e.g. analgesia) are not thought to depend on a second messenger, tolerance and dependence have been explained in terms of upregulation of adenylate cyclase (i.e. increased activity of the intracellular enzyme with subsequent decreases in cAMP, a second messenger). The physical craving is less well explained, and may be due to the involvement of secondary neuronal pathways and neurotransmitter release (e.g. catecholamines). The symptoms of withdrawal may be precipitated by use of antagonists such as naloxone.

How does one choose an opioid for clinical use? Table 1.10.4 compares the potencies of some of the opioids with respect to morphine, and some of their pharmacokinetic properties. Fentanyl, which is the most potent example of the opioids shown, is only administered parenterally, and has a very short duration of effect. Its use is therefore limited to circumstances in which either a very short-term effect is required, or frequent bolus administration or a constant infusion is convenient (e.g. during anaesthesia or in intensive care). The oral bioavailability of opioids is generally poor, the best-absorbed opioid being methadone. There are other important differences in the pharmacokinetics of the opioids. Morphine is glucuronidated in the liver, and the glucuronides are excreted via the kidney. The metabolite morphine-6-glucuronide is also a potent analgesic. This is useful therapeutically, but it also means that in renal impairment, if the dosing of morphine is not reduced, accumulation may occur. For instance, in a patient with shock or acute or chronic renal failure, due to the decreased clearance of the glucuronide, he or she may become obtunded even after administration of standard doses of morphine. The short half-life of morphine has in the past limited its usefulness in circumstances in which chronic and high doses have been required. Now slow-release preparations of oral morphine have been developed particularly for use in chronic pain and palliative care. Although chronic dosing of morphine can cause significant side-effects due to metabolite accumulation, as mentioned above, methadone can cause a similar problem, but due to accumulation of the drug itself. Its metabolism is saturable in the therapeutic dosing range (similar to the saturation observed with other drugs, e.g. phenytoin). Thus judicious care is required when increasing the dose. Methadone has tended to have a role in cases in which a longer duration of effect would be desirable, e.g. in the treatment of burns, or in the maintenance treatment of drug addicts. However, the former role is becoming less important with the advent of the slow-release preparations of morphine described above. Another opioid for which metabolite accumulation may cause troublesome side-effects is pethidine. Its metabolite, norpethidine, is hallucinogenic and may produce convulsions.

Two of the opioids are prodrugs, i.e. the parent drug itself is not active, but its conversion *in vivo* results in pharmacological activity. Codeine is one such drug, being metabolized to morphine itself. The metabolism of codeine depends on the cytochrome P4502D6

Table 1.10.4 Properties of opioids: relative analgesic potencies and pharmacokinetics

	Relative potency	Parenteral dose (mg)*	Oral dose (mg)*	Plasma half-life	Comments
Agonists:					
Heroin: diacetylmorphine	1.5	5	60	30 min	Prodrug: monoacetylmorphine and morphine active
Morphine	1	10	60	2 h	Also morphine-6-glucuronide
Fentanyl	60	50 µg/kg	–	3 h	Duration 30 min for single dose
Pethidine	0.2	75	–	3–4 h	
Methadone	1	10	20	15–40 h	Saturable kinetics
Codeine: 3-methylmorphine	0.1	–	30	–	Prodrug: morphine active
d-propoxyphene	0.06	–	65	6–12 h	
Partial agonists/agonists:					
Buprenorphine	30	0.3	0.4†	6–8 h	
Pentazocine	0.5	30	180	4 h	
Antagonists:					
Naloxone	–	0.4–0.8	–	30 min	Repeated dosing if necessary

*Assuming not tolerant/non-habituated.
†Sublingual administration.

isozyme (CyP2D6). The activity is genetically determined, and in subjects with low activity (designated 'slow metabolizers') the conversion of codeine to morphine may be so small as to be negligible, and the subject will gain no benefit from administration of codeine. This is important in practical terms, because a number of compound analgesic preparations contain codeine. A significant number of patients derive little benefit from using these preparations. The usual response is to increase the dose, but clearly there would be little advantage to this in the group of patients with the 'slow-metabolizer' phenotype. The second example of a prodrug is heroin (or diacetylmorphine). It is metabolized very rapidly to acetylmorphine initially, and then to morphine itself, within the CNS. The increase in potency of heroin compared to that of morphine is due to its rapid passage across the blood–brain barrier. It must be remembered that heroin is a regulated substance in many countries, and its possession for any reason may be illegal.

The use of opioids is accompanied by significant side-effects. In patients in whom chronic dosing is necessary, these may be so great that the benefits of analgesia are outweighed by the problems of the side-effects. Likewise, the pharmacokinetics may impose rigid and generally short dosing schedules. Recently, the advent of the slow-release preparations has greatly assisted in this area. However, an alternative approach which has an important place in both analgesia and anaesthesia is intrathecal administration of opioids. The basis of its development was an attempt to decrease exposure of opioid receptors which lay outside the CNS, and so to decrease systemic side-effects, while at the same time ensuring adequate or high-dose delivery rapidly into the CNS. It must be appreciated that, in so doing, side-effects such as respiratory depression are not diminished, and that extra-CNS exposure does occur because the opioids move bidirectionally across the blood–brain barrier. However, this technique, coupled with constant infusion pump delivery, has provided many patients with good analgesia.

Another technique that is dependent on a pump delivery system is that which may be used post-operatively, in which the opioid dose and rate of administration are determined by the patient according to their analgesic requirements. Although the introduction of this system was a matter of concern in many centres, as was the use of a low-dose intravenous infusion, in units in which the system is used, the median total cumulative dose per patient has actually decreased.

A section on opioids would not be complete without a brief consideration of opioid antagonists. At the beginning of the section, it should have become apparent that the definition of an opioid includes antagonist effects. However, in a more practical role, it is important to be aware of the potential use of true antagonists such as naloxone in reversing the respiratory depression and hypotension of opioid overdose. Due to the shorter half-life of naloxone compared to those of agonists, it may be necessary not only to administer a large dose of naloxone in order to reverse respiratory depression, for instance, but also to give several doses over time.

NON-STEROIDAL ANTI-INFLAMMATORY DRUGS (NSAIDS)

The NSAIDs are a group of chemically distinct families of compounds which share the common properties of being anti-inflammatory, analgesic and antipyretic. The central mechanism of action of all three pharmacological effects is inhibition of arachidonate cyclo-oxygenase (COX). However, some drugs (e.g. paracetamol) are relatively poor inhibitors of COX and function primarily as free-radical scavengers. Thus their anti-inflammatory effect is due at least in part to diminished tissue damage. The precursors of the inflammatory mediators include the eicosanoids, which are derived from membrane phospholipids, principally arachidonic acid. COX catalyses the conversion of arachidonic acid to eicosanoids, which give rise to the prostaglandin and leukotriene series (Table 1.10.5)

Prostanoid products have important physiological roles in normal homeostasis (e.g. in vascular responses). The prostanoid produced in an individual cell type is

Table 1.10.5 Eicosanoid derivatives in inflammation

Substrate	Enzyme	Product
Membrane phospholipid	Phospholipase A2	Arachidonic acid Lyso-glyceryl-phosphorylcholine
Arachidonic acid	Cyclo-oxygenase (COX-1, COX-2)	Prostaglandins
Arachidonic acid	Lipoxygenase (multiple forms)	Leukotrienes
Lyso-glyceryl-phosphorylcholine		Platelet aggregating factor (PAF)

specific for that cell (e.g. prostacyclin in vascular endothelium, thromboxane A2 (TXA2) in platelets). Each of the prostanoids acts on one of five main prostanoid receptor types, which have been given the name of the natural agonist prostanoids (e.g. TXA2 acts on receptors, causing vasoconstriction, platelet aggregation and bronchoconstriction). The half-lives of prostanoids released into plasma are generally very short (less than 1 min). The clearance is the result of two different mechanisms. First, for many prostanoids there is an active carrier-mediated uptake into cells followed by enzymatic degradation. This mechanism is particularly active in lung tissue. Secondly, in comparison, TXA2 hydrolyses rapidly ($< 30\,s$) in plasma to an inactive product TXB2. By having local tissue production and very short half-lives, the effects of prostanoid release are kept relatively specific and confined within an individual organ or tissue. However, if antagonists of synthesis are introduced therapeutically, the possibility of widespread, non-organ-specific side-effects is very real. There are two forms of cyclo-oxygenase, which is an intracellular enzyme bound to the endoplasmic reticulum. COX-1 is a constitutive enzyme (i.e. it is always present) which is found in most cells. COX-2 is induced in inflammatory cells by the inflammatory stimulus.

Inflammation is always accompanied by prostaglandin release, the most common prostaglandin being PGE_2, which is released from local tissues, blood vessels, and in chronic inflammation from monocytes and macrophages. PGI_2 and PGD_2 are also involved, the latter being released from mast cells. They are powerful precapillary vasodilators, causing redness and increased blood flow. They are synergistic with bradykinin and histamine in producing vasodilatation, but importantly they are synergistic in capillary permeability and potentiating the pain which results from bradykinin release (i.e. they sensitize the afferent C fibres). The E series is also associated with the production of high fever, possibly via the mediating effects of endogenously released interleukin-1 (IL-1). The antipyretic effect of the NSAIDs is partly due to inhibition of PGE_2 synthesis in the hypothalamus. NSAIDs will only reduce body temperature if it is raised; the drugs do not cause hypothermia. Although the emphasis here is on the E series producing inflammation, PGE_2 also has several anti-inflammatory roles. This is probably important in modulating inflammatory cells *in vivo*, i.e. a form of product inhibition.

Lipoxygenases are cytosolic enzymes which are found particularly in lung tissue, platelets, mast cells and leucocytes. They, too, have specific identified receptors through which their effects are mediated. There are numerous end-products. For example, leukotriene B4 (LTB4) is a potent chemotactic compound which attracts neutrophils and macrophages. It produces up-regulation of cell-adhesion molecules and increases free-radical and cytokine production, with consequent increases in cellular proliferation.

The third arm of the phospholipid metabolite pattern (Table 1.10.5) is platelet aggregating factor (PAF). Acting through specific receptors, this also produces vasodilatation and increased vascular permeability, as well as initiating the platelet changes which gave rise to its name. In addition, it is a potent chemotactic agent, particularly for eosinophils, and in high concentration it produces hyperalgesia.

Individual members of the NSAIDs have become associated with specific therapies and uses. Some of these developments are based on known drug effects, while others are based on traditional practice alone. Aspirin has become a very important agent in its role as an antiplatelet drug. Aspirin is unique among the NSAIDs in this role, which arose because it alone inhibits COX-1 irreversibly. COX-1 activity in the cell can only be restored by synthesis of new protein. The platelet lacks this synthetic capability, being a small collection of membrane-bound cytoplasm, and hence the cohort of platelets that is exposed to aspirin will remain unable to synthesize TXA2 for the rest of its natural life. The balance in the cardiovascular system between platelets and vascular endothelium, whose COX-1 complement will have been restored (i.e. between TXA2 and prostacyclin), will then be in favour of reduced platelet aggregation and small-vessel vasodilatation.

The side-effects of NSAIDs are significant (Table 1.10.6). Individual compounds have been identified as being more likely to cause side-effects, but this is also very variable between patients. In the gastrointestinal system, indigestion and epigastric pain are common, particularly with aspirin and indomethacin. The pain is due to mucosal damage which is caused by a reduction in prostaglandin synthesis within the stomach. Prostaglandins afford protection to the mucosa by increasing mucous and bicarbonate secretion, decreasing proton secretion and vasodilating the mucosal vessels, thus enabling acid removal. The mucosal damage may proceed to erosions and frank ulceration. NSAIDs are a common cause of iron deficiency anaemia due to chronic blood loss among elderly patients who take these drugs. Haematemesis and melaena are less common but important consequences.

The renal side-effects of NSAIDs are also important. Normal homeostasis in the kidney depends upon prostaglandin secretion causing local vasodilatation. This mechanism protects glomerular and medullary blood flow when total renal perfusion is decreased and there are high concentrations of circulating systemic vasoconstrictors (e.g. angiotensin II and noradrenaline in cardiac failure or in shock). If prostaglandin synthesis is blocked, the initial renal change will be reflected in sodium and water retention (which is common in the

Table 1.10.6 Properties of some common NSAIDs

NSAID	Plasma half-life	Properties	Inhibition of COX isozymes‡	Comments
Aspirin*	3–5 h low dose >12 h high dose	A, I, P†	1	Irreversible enzyme inhibition Antiplatelet effects
Diclofenac	1–2 h	A, I, P		Raised transaminases. Duration of effect > plasma half-life? Due to decreased arachidonic acid
Ibuprofen	2 h	A, I, P	1 > 2	Relatively low incidence of side-effects
Indomethacin	2 h	I >> A, P	1	High side-effect profile
Ketoprofen	2 h	A, I, P		Beware high dose; use post-operatively
Mefanamic acid	4 h	A, P	1 > 2	Most often used for dysmenorrhoea
Naproxen	13 h	I > A, P	1 = 2	
Paracetamol	2–4 h	A, P	1 = 2, but weak	Hepatotoxic in overdose
Piroxicam	45 h	I > A, P	1 > 2	

*Aspirin, acetylsalicylic acid.
†A, analgesic; I, anti-inflammatory; P, antipyretic.
‡Relative inhibition of the two identified COX enzymes.

patient with incipient heart failure). The syndrome may progress to acute renal insufficiency or failure, and the patient will require renal dialysis. An historic and specific problem associated with chronic NSAID use was the occurrence of analgesic nephropathy (papillary necrosis). Although phenacetin was responsible in the past, it is unclear whether the chronic combination therapies that are currently in use may lead to the same problem.

NSAIDs may precipitate asthma and other allergic conditions such as urticaria. This is due to a relative increase in leukotriene production as well as a decrease in the synthesis of prostaglandins, some of which are bronchodilators. Aspirin is most commonly associated with these problems.

Other side-effects are specifically associated with individual NSAIDs. The first of these is the hepatic damage which may result from paracetamol toxicity. It is well known that liver toxicity may result from paracetamol taken in an acute overdose. However, it is important to recognize that in subjects in whom liver function is already compromised, and particularly in patients with liver enzyme induction (e.g. by alcohol or anticonvulsants), therapeutic doses of paracetamol may cause the same syndrome. The second specific problem is becoming less important, namely the syndrome which accompanies high-dose usage of salicylate. Symptomatically the patient is said to be suffering from 'salicylism', with tinnitus and deafness, but there is also a metabolic acidosis which may cause diagnostic confusion. Aspirin is

also not generally recommended for use in children, due to its apparent association with Reye's syndrome and a high mortality.

NEUROPATHIC PAIN

It was noted above that opiates are often unsuccessful in the treatment of neuropathic or phantom pain. Neuropathic pain, such as the pain of diabetic neuropathy or herpes zoster infection (shingles), is thought to be caused by the spontaneous discharge of sensory neurones, the trigger for which is not understood. The pain may respond to drugs such as mexilitene, which has membrane properties similar to those of local anaesthetics such as lignocaine. However, mexilitene has the advantage that it can be administered orally.

Trigeminal neuralgia may also be considered within this category of neuropathic pain. It also is due to paroxysmal neuronal discharges. Carbamazepine is one of the classical anticonvulsant drugs, but in addition it has an important role in the treatment of trigeminal neuralgia. It decreases membrane excitability by blocking the fast sodium channels, again like local anaesthetics. The net effect is a decrease in action potential formation. The drug is much more effective in neurones which are firing repetitively, particularly at high frequency.

A third pain syndrome which could be included in this category is that of migraine. Although the underlying cause(s) remain(s) fiercely debated, there is consensus that the transmitter 5-hydroxytryptamine is involved, and that inflammatory factors contribute to the syndrome. Many of the drugs used in the treatment of migraine are active at the serotonin receptors, either as agonists in the case of drugs used in an acute attack (e.g. ergotamine or sumatriptan) or as antagonists in a prophylactic role (e.g. methysergide or cyproheptadine). However, NSAID administration will abort an attack if administered early in the prodrome, and if necessary administered with metoclopramide to improve gastrointestinal absorption.

ADJUNCTIVE THERAPY AND PALLIATIVE CARE

In patients with chronic pain syndromes (e.g. in malignancy), not only are high-dose opiates employed, but frequently a combination of medications is used to assist with the analgesia (e.g. the WHO Cancer Pain Relief Program). The drugs include antidepressants and anxiolytics. With regard to their mechanism of action, they are not considered to be acting 'non-specifically'. Drugs such as the tricyclic antidepressants have multiple receptor properties, and decrease the reuptake of bioamines into the presynaptic membranes. Thus they will increase the local concentrations of neurotransmitters such as noradrenaline and serotonin, and are thought to enhance directly the spinal inhibitory pathways, as shown in Figure 1.10.1. The benzodiazepines (e.g. diazepam) modulate sensory input and alter perceptions.

The contribution of transcutaneous electrical nerve stimulation (TENS) and acupuncture can also be considered here. Although both produce analgesia which is segmental in nature, the underlying mechanisms are different. Acupuncture produces an increase in endorphin concentration in cerebrospinal fluid (CSF). TENS does not produce any measurable change in endorphin release, and the resultant analgesia is not reversed by naloxone. The differences also extend to potential areas of use, with TENS being more efficacious in neuropathic pain.

FURTHER READING

Marshall KA. 1996: Managing cancer pain: basic principles and invasive treatments. *Mayo Clinic Proceedings* **71**, 472–7.

Perkins M, Dray A. 1996: Novel pharmacological strategies for analgesia. *Annals of the Rheumatic Diseases* **55**, 715–22.

Stein C. 1995: The control of pain in peripheral tissue by opioids. *New England Journal of Medicine* **332**, 1685–90.

Vane JR, Botting RM. 1998: Mechanism of nonsteroidal drugs. *American Journal of Medicine* **104**, 2S–8S.

Zacny JP. 1996: Should people taking opioids for medical reasons be allowed to work and drive? *Addiction* **91**, 1581–4.

Zech DF, Grond S, Lynch J, Hertel DI, Lehmann KA. 1995: Validation of World Health Organization guidelines for cancer pain relief: a 10-year prospective study. *Pain* **63**, 65–76.

Shock

Iain D. Anderson

Introduction

Shock can be defined as tissue perfusion and oxygenation which are inadequate for the body's needs at that particular moment in time. Without treatment, hypoxic cells quickly die – hence the description of shock as 'a pause in the act of dying'. It is important to state at the outset that the typical clinical picture of shock, namely the ashen, cool and sweaty patient with tachycardia, pallor and profound hypotension, represents the final stages of shock, and that many patients with clinically important shock have much more subtle signs, and indeed a proportion are normoten-sive. In considering shock clinically, it is important to focus on the concept of tissue perfusion and oxygenation rather than a specific value of blood pressure. You should aim to identify and treat shock at an early stage. If shock is not treated promptly, a series of potentially irreversible changes occur in the circulation, causing sequential multiple organ failure which is often fatal. The successful treatment of shock depends on adequately supporting the patient until the underlying cause can be treated. This often requires prompt surgical intervention.

THE CAUSES OF SHOCK

The causes of shock are shown in Figure 2.1.1. Clinical signs can give pointers to the cause of shock, and certain mechanisms are common to one or more forms of shock apart from the common underlying abnormality of tissue hypoxia and hypoperfusion.

HYPOVOLAEMIC SHOCK

Hypovolaemia is the commonest cause of shock in surgical practice. It ranges in severity from rapid exsanguination to very subtle and often unrecognized forms of subacute tissue hypoperfusion. It is useful to consider haemorrhagic shock separately for two reasons. First, it is a useful model around which to discuss the basic pathophysiological changes of shock, and secondly, it often requires prompt surgery to stop the flow of blood, in addition to resuscitative therapies.

Haemorrhagic shock

Haemorrhagic shock occurs in four common circumstances in surgical practice. Trauma, post-surgical bleeding, ruptured aortic aneurysms and gastrointestinal haemorrhage (typically from a peptic ulcer) account for the majority of cases. Bleeding may be external and obvious, but more commonly it is internal and, all too often, hidden. Following injury, occult internal haemorrhage occurs, particularly within the thorax, abdomen and pelvis, but also in the soft tissues around fractured long bones and following maxillofacial trauma. After surgical operations, a very significant volume of internal bleeding may occur without any blood appearing in surgical drains. Empty drains are therefore no reassurance that haemorrhage is not occurring. Haemorrhage is associated with the classical signs of shock, which can be common to all forms of shock under certain circumstances.

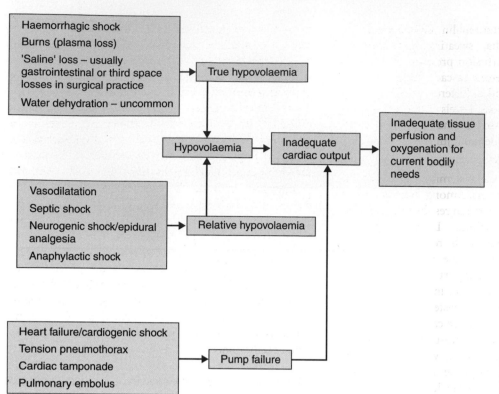

Figure 2.1.1 Common types and causes of shock in surgical practice.

Compensatory mechanisms

Clinical mechanisms When haemorrhage occurs, certain compensatory mechanisms are activated, and it is the activation of these mechanisms which produces many of the signs. There is considerable individual variation in the severity of haemorrhage required to bring about clinical signs, and it is important to remember that clinical signs are generally a late feature and will thus lead to the clinician underestimating the severity of shock. For hypotension and reproducible signs to be consistently observed, a circulatory volume deficit of about 30% is required. By the time an acute loss of 40% has been sustained, the patient is near death. Particularly in younger patients and those on medications, blood pressure may be maintained until a sudden near-terminal collapse occurs. The importance of diagnosing and acting on subtle findings cannot be overemphasized.

Neurogenic mechanisms The circulation possesses its own neurogenic compensatory mechanisms. Haemorrhage reduces venous return and hence cardiac output. Initially, diastolic pressure will rise, so reducing pulse pressure. At some point blood pressure will begin to fall, but this is often relatively late. The arterial baroreceptors begin to sense these changes when pulse pressure decreases, and they then cause reflex tachycardia and vasoconstriction. Vascular beds such as the heart, brain and kidney are relatively protected by their autoregulatory mechanisms, but the skin undergoes early changes. This brings about the cool, sweaty and pale peripheries

that are characteristic of haemorrhagic shock. It is important to remember that when the skin is underperfused the same is true for the intra-abdominal viscera. The volume of blood in the venous system falls and the peripheral veins collapse. Despite renal autoregulation, hypotension results in reduced renal blood flow and an increased filtration fraction. Fluid is conserved through sodium retention in particular, and little urine is formed.

Cellular mechanisms Changes also occur at the microcirculatory and cellular levels. Hypotension and the reduction in venous volume change the capillary pressure, thereby permitting fluid to move from the extracellular fluid compartment back into the circulating volume compartment. There is further movement of fluid from the intracellular compartment to maintain equilibrium with the extracellular compartment. Reduced peripheral perfusion results in metabolic (lactic) acidosis. This has several effects, including myocardial depression. At a later stage, hepatic synthesis of albumen is increased to restore plasma protein losses and erythropoietin is produced to replace the lost red cell mass. The loss of red blood cells at the time of haemorrhage contributes to hypoxia and this together with acidosis, stimulates the chemoreceptors to increase respiratory rate – another typical sign of terminal shock.

Endocrine mechanisms Certain endocrine changes characterize shock. Part of the baroreceptor response to hypotension is increased sympathetic activation via sympathetic nerves and also the adrenal medulla. Circulating levels of adrenalin and noradrenalin are increased. This contributes to tachycardia, sweating and hyperglycaemia. Reduced renal perfusion pressure activates the renin–angiotensin–aldosterone cascade. Angiotensin is a potent vasoconstrictor, and aldosterone causes sodium retention and potassium loss. Levels of vasopressin and glucocorticoids are increased in many shocked states, particularly following accidental injury.

Tissue damage The effects of reduced perfusion pressure, tissue hypoxia and the systemic response to this have effects on internal organs. Among these is the kidney, where prolonged hypotension results in acute tubular necrosis and renal failure. Lesser degrees of hypotension are associated with reversible uraemia. When one particular part of the body is rendered ischaemic, the perfusion of that part (often a limb) can result in an ischaemia-reperfusion injury which manifests as a worsening of the systemic shock state. Ischaemic and hypotensive damage can also take its toll on the heart and the brain, but most commonly effects are seen on the microcirculation, where the normal reflex responsiveness of the arterioles and venules is lost, the capillaries themselves become leaky and an irreversible shock state is reached (see below).

The existence of these powerful compensatory mechanisms explains why clinical response to shock is a relatively late phenomenon, and to this must be added individual variation in response. It is unwise to rely on a single clinical sign, such as blood pressure, not only for the reasons mentioned above, but also because the baseline blood pressure of any individual is usually unknown when they present acutely with shock. It is not known whether their normal blood pressure is usually well above or even significantly below the 'average' of 120/80 mmHg. When it is appreciated that intestinal hypoperfusion appears to contribute to a release of cytokines and other small molecules which precipitate the individual towards irreversible shock and multiple organ failure, it will be appreciated how important it is to diagnose shock at this stage, when the only visible signs relate to cutaneous underperfusion.

The most important step in the treatment of haemorrhagic shock is control of bleeding, and this usually requires some kind of surgical intervention. Intravenous fluid replacement, while essential, is of secondary importance except when the haemorrhage is minor, or in the rare event that it is caused primarily by coagulopathy. More often coagulopathy is a consequence of continued lower-grade haemorrhage, with replacement by cold transfused blood which is deficient in clotting factors. Here again surgical control of the bleeding source is the key. Furthermore, recently transfused blood is an inefficient transporter of oxygen to the tissues and carries the risk of virus transmission. When called to assess the shocked patient, the surgeon must immediately assess the urgency of the threat to life. External haemorrhage must be immediately controlled and the exsanguinating patient transferred to the operating theatre without delay. Only very rarely (e.g. for the patient with penetrating thoracic trauma who has arrested within the Emergency department) is surgery outwith the operating theatre indicated. By contrast, simple external pressure on a bleeding point is always indicated. Good vascular access (16 G or larger) is obtained at two sites and blood is drawn for cross-matching, baseline full blood count and biochemical analysis. The surgeon should assess the degree of haemorrhage and decide whether the patient requires un-cross-matched blood (group O), type-specific blood (cross-matched only for ABO), or whether they can wait for a full cross-match. In general, exsanguinating patients (i.e. those with marked pallor, loss of consciousness, blood pressure < 80 mmHg systolic or an obvious major source of haemorrhage) are candidates for un-cross-matched blood, particularly if the time course is short. Any shocked patient is likely to require type-specific blood and surgical intervention. Surgical intervention often requires an old-fashioned open surgical approach, but equally, depending on circumstances, it may require less invasive procedures, e.g. the application of an external fixator to a fractured pelvis, or injection sclerotherapy of a bleeding duodenal ulcer. Initial fluid resuscitation should be undertaken with warmed crystalloid solution. A reasonable initial bolus is 20 mL/kg, repeated if necessary, for the hypotensive patient. By the time 1500–2000 mL have been infused, blood should be available for further transfusion. Some authorities advocate the initial use of a colloid solution containing particles of larger molecular weight which remain within the circulation longer. There is no clear advantage to this, but those who advocate it would limit total colloid infused to no more than the volume of crystalloid infused or 1500 mL, whichever is less. Again, it is pointless to replace the patient's circulatory blood volume systematically with a circulatory volume consisting of clear fluids. Whichever intial fluid is used, the emphasis must be on early blood transfusion and the early control of haemorrhage in haemorrhagic shock. All colloids are associated with anaphylactic reactions and with occasional difficulties with cross-matching, although with modern solutions these problems are now uncommon. Care of the circulation forms just one part of patient resuscitation and it must follow – not precede – adequate management of the airway and breathing. This includes the administration of high-flow (12–15 L) oxygen therapy, preferably monitored by pulse oximetry.

Once immediate therapy – including surgical intervention if indicated – has been started, attention can then be turned in less severe cases to identification of the source of haemorrhagic shock. This may require investigation, which must be carried out in a safe manner with adequate medical support and monitoring. The same is true for interventions (e.g. by embolization) performed in the radiology suite rather than in the operating theatre, and it is the surgeon's duty to ensure that this mobile critical care takes place.

The importance of pulse oximetry has been referred to above, and at an early stage blood should be drawn for arterial blood gases and a urinary catheter inserted to monitor urine output, as this is one of the more reliable indicators of the adequacy of resuscitative therapy. The patient must be kept warm and transferred to a high-dependency unit or intensive care area as quickly as possible, or to the operating theatre if necessary.

Other types of hypovolaemic shock

Other forms of hypovolaemic shock will give rise to similar clinical features and systemic responses, except that pallor will not be so marked in many cases, as the haemoglobin level will be normal. However, the other features of peripheral and visceral hypoperfusion and hypoxia will be evident, and the treatment principles remain the same, except that such early recourse to blood-component therapy will not be indicated. In surgical practice, most hypovolaemic patients will have lost either modified saline solution (intestinal obstruction, peritonitis, etc.) or plasma (burns). Fluid replacement is again by means of normal saline or Ringer's lactate solution. As with haemorrhagic shock, the clinical signs of the underlying condition will be evident, and once the patient has been resuscitated, definitive treatment of the underlying condition will be necessary, often with considerable urgency.

SEPTIC SHOCK

In septic shock there is a basic difference in underlying pathophysiology. Here the release of cytokines and other small chemical mediators results in vasodilatation. This increases the capacity of the circulation, and the relative hypovolaemia that results leads to hypotension and hypoxia. Because of the vasodilatation, the patient's peripheries are often warm and pink. The mediators also cause capillary leakage, and tissue fluid (oedema) develops rapidly in severe cases. This oedema increases the distance from the erythrocyte in the capillary to the tissue cells, so contributing to cellular hypoxia. Numerous mediators are involved in the septic process. Molecules of the bradykinin cascade, the complement system, the numerous metabolites of arachidonic acid and the cytokines released in response to sepsis, particularly endotoxin, are important. The key cytokines in the last pathway include interleukin-1 (IL-1), IL-6 and tumour necrosis factor alpha. Numerous other cytokines are involved, but these key cytokines undergo marked

amplification and result in a rapid escalation of the systemic response to a septic insult. When a second septic insult comes along (second-hit theory) the response is even greater, and severe septic shock is more likely to result. There is a continual gradation of severity of sepsis from common minor infective processes without systemic upset to the patient with multiple organ failure as a result of sepsis, but again the key is to look for subtle signs of failure to respond to early resuscitative measures. Once septic shock is advanced, the outlook is bleak whatever supportive therapy and definitive treatment are given. Occasionally, septic shock begins with a 'cold' phase where the peripheral features are those of hypothermia and vasoconstriction, akin to hypovolaemic shock. This may be because of the pattern of cytokine release, or because of the fluid changes and true hypovolaemia associated with the underlying cause, such as peritonitis. In these cases, it is only once fluid resuscitation has been started that the typical 'warm' shock picture emerges.

Once again the treatment of septic shock revolves around adequate resuscitation and prompt definitive treatment. Fluid resuscitation and oxygen therapy play an essential part, but early cultures from the bloodstream and from any identifiable source of sepsis should be obtained before antibiotic therapy is commenced. The rate of progression of septic shock is unpredictable, and treatment of the underlying cause may precipitate or alleviate shock in the short term. However, without appropriate treatment of the underlying cause, survival is very unlikely once septic shock has developed.

CARDIOGENIC SHOCK

The diagnosis of cardiogenic shock is an important one for the surgeon to make, primarily because the initial management is different. While oxygen therapy remains essential, the administration of large volumes of intravenous fluid will usually tend to aggravate the common form of cardiogenic shock (due to ischaemic heart disease, myocardial infarction or arrhythmia). The less frequently encountered forms of pump failure (due to tension pneumothorax, cardiac tamponade and pulmonary embolus) all respond to intravenous fluid infusion, but obviously need prompt treatment of the cause of the shock by chest drainage, pericardial aspiration and surgical drainage and anticoagulation, respectively. Further comments will be restricted to the common form of cardiogenic shock that is due to intrinsic cardiac disease. The pathophysiology of the failing heart is quite different to the normal heart, and several vicious circles interact to produce the shock state. Reduced cardiac performance, whether caused by arrhythmia, loss of muscle mass due to previous infarction, or inefficient cardiac activity due to some other factor, results in the cardiac output being inadequate. This inadequacy may be aggravated or first made apparent by the increased demands imposed by surgery, sepsis or hypovolaemia. Cardiogenic shock results in an increase in catecholamine release. This has the peripheral effects described above, but also increases the afterload against which the heart has to pump. This increased resistance to ejection further reduces cardiac performance. The reduction in cardiac performance has two effects. First, the amount of blood being pushed forward to perfuse the tissues is effectively reduced, and secondly, blood accumulates within the pulmonary circulation and pumonary oedema eventually occurs. Normally the heart responds to its filling pressure (pre-load) by increasing its stroke volume and output. The failing heart is less able to increase its output and is thus progressively less able to respond to increased pre-load. Furthermore, the failing heart responds to increased demand by an increase in rate rather than an increased stroke volume. This is less efficient, and as myocardial perfusion through the coronary arteries occurs during diastole, myocardial ischaemia tends to occur and, as with tachycardia, the time available for myocardial perfusion is reduced. The failing heart tends to be dilated. This increases myocardial wall tension which, together with the effects of the increased levels of circulating catecholamines, increases myocardial oxygen demand. These factors conspire to bring about myocardial ischaemia, which worsens cardiac performance.

Treatment of heart failure thus depends on the optimization of pre-load, cardiac function and after-load. Usually pre-load is inappropriately elevated, although the less common causes of pump failure mentioned above will respond to further increases in pre-load. When the pre-load is high it must be reduced by stopping intravenous fluid infusion and by the administration of diuretics and vasodilators. While pulmonary oedema can be reasonably treated by the simple administration of oxygen and diuretics, any patient with cardiogenic shock should be treated within a high-care unit with invasive monitoring and specialist input. Inappropriately elevated after-load can also be treated by vasodilators. Intrinsic cardiac function can be optimized by controlling the heart rate by treating any arrhythmia present. Myocardial oxygen supply can be optimized by the administration of high-flow oxygen, by correction of pre-load and after-load, and by inotrope therapy as indicated. It will thus be seen that the treatment of heart failure differs from the treatment of other forms of shock which are seen in surgical practice in that intravenous fluid therapy can be harmful; however, oxygen therapy remains a cornerstone.

Thus the patient in cardiogenic shock is also cold, clammy and cyanosed peripherally, has a tachycardia and may have a low blood pressure, but importantly they have an elevated jugular venous pressure and may well be dyspnoeic.

IDENTIFYING THE UNDERLYING CAUSE

The rapid assessment of the patient with attention to the ABCs (**A**irway, **B**reathing, **C**irculation) is designed to keep them alive long enough for the underlying cause to be determined and definitive treatment to be administered. It cannot be emphasized strongly enough that it is the administration of definitive treatment to the underlying cause that changes the natural history of the shock process. Simply resuscitating the patient will result in recurrent shock from which it will be all the more difficult to resuscitate the patient again. As the immediate management and resuscitation of the patient are effected, certain pointers to the diagnosis will emerge, and it will be clear from the above account that certain baseline tests will be important in every shocked patient on a surgical ward. These will include cross-matching, full blood count, biochemical analysis, chest X-ray and ECG. Often clotting analysis and blood cultures will be needed, and at a later stage arterial blood gases will be necessary. Except for the minority of patients who require immediate surgery, a more detailed clinical assessment of the patient can be made while the response to immediate resuscitative therapies is assessed. Information should be drawn from the patient's case notes, from the patient if they are alert and orientated, and from nursing staff and relatives depending on the case. It may be necessary to contact senior staff urgently. A full physical examination should be performed, and from this it is often possible to identify the type of shock and the source of the problem: there may be specific signs of haemorrhage, hypovolaemia, cardiac problems (e.g. chest pain) or a source of sepsis. It may then be possible to institute an appropriate therapeutic plan or, if doubt remains, selective investigations can be carried out, but again the importance of conducting these safely has been highlighted above. The timing of investigations and definitive therapy depends on the severity of the shock process but, given its very nature, time is usually of the essence and investigation and treatment should proceed whatever the hour. In the vast majority of surgical patients the problem usually lies not with the failure of the surgeon to establish the differential diagnosis and the final cause, but rather with his or her failure to appreciate the true severity and urgency of the shock state.

The baseline blood tests provide valuable information. The haemoglobin level will fall serially, although it may be normal at the start of a haemorrhagic episode. Haemoglobin will also fall as the hypovolaemic patient (without haemorrhage) is resuscitated, on account of haemodilution. A patient may typically exhibit a leucocytosis during sepsis, but leucopenia can also be seen, and haemorrhage, injury and surgery are all potent causes of leucocytosis as well. Thrombocytopenia will occur during haemorrhagic and septic shock, and can also indicate progressing multiple organ failure. Uraemia most frequently suggests renal compromise, and when the level of urea is elevated to a greater degree than that of creatinine, this suggests a pre-renal mechanism. Uraemia is also observed during gastrointestinal haemorrhage, due to absorption of blood products from the intestine. Hypokalaemia and hypomagnesaemia are often seen in shock, and both can contribute to reduced cardiac function. Hypocalcaemia usually reflects the dilutional hypoalbuminaemia that is a common manifestation of many forms of shock and critical illness. Abnormal liver function tests can indicate biliary or hepatic sepsis, and they also occur during multiple organ failure.

Plotting the rate of change of serial cardiac enzymes can confirm or refute the presence of a myocardial infarction within a matter of hours, even without the presence of diagnostic ECG changes.

ASSESSING THE RESPONSE TO TREATMENT

Shocked patients can usefully be categorized into three groups on the basis of their response to initial therapy. First of all, the patient who clearly does not respond to immediate resuscitation therapies will require immediate transfer to the intensive care unit (for septic or cardiogenic shock) or to the operating theatre (for haemorrhagic shock). These patients are relatively infrequent, but when they do present it is important that the surgeon is immediately prepared to transfer them appropriately. Delay is usually associated with the demise of the patient, and the urgency of the situation must be recognized. Secondly, the patient with a relatively minor insult who responds adequately to initial therapies might be one who has continued to ooze for several hours following operation, but in whom the problem is only diagnosed once shock has developed. In this case, replacement of blood and perhaps correction of mild coagulopathy may suffice. Another example would be the patient who develops sepsis following instrumentation of the urinary tract. Often there is a catastrophic episode of hypotension and cyanosis which resolves rapidly with the administration of oxygen, intravenous fluids and broad-spectrum antibiotics. However, any patient who has an episode of shock should be monitored closely for 12–24 h afterwards, and in many cases this monitoring will take place within a high-dependency environment. The level of observation will be greater if the patient is elderly, or has a complex surgical problem or underlying medical conditions. In these complex patients it is the ability of the surgeon to maintain watchfulness over multiple factors that governs the outcome. This attention to detail is a cornerstone of successful surgical critical care.

The next category of patient is the one who responds only temporarily to initial therapies. Such patients are challenging in that the magnitude of the problem may not be realized for some time. Initially, the patient may appear to respond well – hence the importance of continuing vigilance. However, the shock state gradually returns, either due to persistence of the underlying problem or because the initial therapy was not as complete as was first thought. Numerous examples of this should spring to mind, as there is not a surgeon practising who has not misjudged a shocked patient in this way on at least one occasion. Again, haemorrhage can provide a classic example. Signs of haemorrhage only become apparent once a significant volume deficit exists, and once this has been corrected it will be some time before it becomes apparent whether or not the haemorrhage is continuing at a significant rate. This is particularly true following operation, where there is often some reluctance to return the patient to the operating theatre. There is usually less of a problem following injury, where shock is a clear indication for surgical intervention, or with bleeding peptic ulcers, where again there are clear indications for endoscopic or surgical intervention. Another example of this temporary response due to progression of the shock process is provided by the septic patient. Here the multiple cascades of cytokines and other mediators continue to cause circulatory derangement. Again the patient will respond to early therapy with oxygen, fluids and antibiotics, but when his or her predisposition to cytokine activation is marked, or when the severity of the sepsis itself is great, then vasodilatation continues and, in combination with tissue hypoxia, sequential problems arise. Progressive hypotension may be seen, or alternatively oliguria (due to acute renal failure), dyspnoea (due to adult respiratory distress syndrome) or coagulopathy may become apparent. In order to prevent this, initial septic episodes which do not respond completely must be fully and promptly investigated and treated. This includes appropriate imaging, often by CT scanning and drainage of any collection by interventional radiology or surgery, in addition to antibiotic and fluid therapy. A temporary response may also be seen due to a mixed shock picture. A surgical patient with hypovolaemia but underlying ischaemic heart disease may respond well to fluid therapy intially, only to develop pulmonary oedema as resuscitation progresses.

REASSESSMENT AND MONITORING

It will be clear from all of the above that frequent clinical reassessment by senior staff is important. This clinical reassessment is supplemented by appropriate monitoring, and the importance of high-dependency-unit monitoring with hourly (or more frequent) recording of vital signs, including temperature, heart rate, pulse oximetry, blood pressure and urine output, is taken as standard. So far, no mention has been made of central venous pressure (CVP) monitoring. This is because the CVP line should be used only for monitoring, and not for primary resuscitation.

Blood pressure recording

Regular blood pressure recording is obviously an integral part of the assessment of shock. A common difficulty with patients who are admitted as emergencies is not knowing their baseline blood pressure. While a blood pressure of 70 mmHg systolic in a middle-aged individual is obviously low, a blood pressure of 110/70 mmHg may be proportionately reduced in the elderly and usually mildly hypertensive patient. While tissue perfusion is more important, once the mean arterial pressure falls below 70 mmHg, tissue beds which cannot autoregulate do suffer deleterious effects, however vasodilated the patient may be. Blood pressure monitoring can be undertaken either with a semi-automatic cuff machine or by direct intra-arterial beat-to-beat recording using an arterial cannula and a transducer. This also permits blood gas monitoring.

Central venous pressure (CVP) monitoring

Central venous pressure monitoring is indicated when there is doubt about the adequacy of circulatory filling, or when inotropes are indicated. Thus it should be emphasized that the clearly hypovolaemic patient does not require placement of a central line, but simply needs peripheral fluid resuscitation with appropriate fluids. The insertion of a central venous pressure line, even by a highly experienced clinician, runs the risk of potentially serious complications such as thoracic haemorrhage, pneumothorax or air embolism at a time when the patient is least able to tolerate them. It is usually accepted that a CVP of 8–12 cmH$_2$O is adequate, but this will vary from patient to patient, and a more accurate test is to give a small fluid bolus (e.g. 200 mL saline) and to see whether this causes a sustained increase in the CVP over a period of 30 min or so. If the CVP increases and remains elevated, then the circulation is probably full. CVP monitoring only indicates right-heart filling pressures, but it is the filling pressure of the left heart that primarily drives the circulation. This is particularly important in patients with lung and heart disease.

Urine output

Hour-to-hour or even more frequent assessment of urine output is vital. This is facilitated by urinary catheterization and the collection of urine in a graduated urimeter. In a patient with refractory oliguria, urinary sodium can be measured on a spot sample, but where oliguria is due a pre-renal mechanism, the urine sodium level is low as the body frantically attempts to conserve sodium and hence water in order to maximize circulating volume. Once renal failure is established, the tubules can no longer concentrate urine, and the urinary sodium content increases. Urine can also be cultured to look for a source of septic shock, and this should be done routinely, together with cultures of sputum and blood, when septic shock of unknown cause is suspected.

These investigations are commonly available on the surgical high-dependency unit, but a further common problem is for the junior surgeon to fail to seek timely expert help once his or her own diagnostic and therapeutic interventions are exhausted. If a patient fails to respond adequately to optimization of the central venous pressure, then further assessment and management by an intensivist are needed.

Cardiac output and related indices

When CVP measurement is insufficient for the shocked patient, assessment of cardiac output is required. This is usually the case in the patient with shock and profound cardiac disease, or in the patient with multiple organ failure who requires multiple inotropes to sustain cardiovascular function. The established technique of cardiac output measurement is with a pulmonary artery catheter. This measures cardiac output by a dilution technique. Ice-cold saline at a known temperature is injected into the right heart and sampled through a different catheter channel lying distally. The degree of temperature change indicates the amount by which the injected fluid has been diluted. The volume of injectate is known, and therefore the dilution indicates the cardiac output. This technique therefore requires certain assumptions and the measurement is not an absolute value. Such measurements have a 10–15% inherent inaccuracy. When cardiac output, central venous pressure, heart rate and blood pressure are known, numerous other cardiac indices can be calculated. These include measures of systemic vascular resistance (i.e. the degree of peripheral vasodilatation) and the whole-body consumption of oxygen by the tissues. Inotrope and vasodilator drugs can be employed to tailor specific aspects of cardiac function in tandem with intravenous fluid therapy in order to maximize cardiovascular function appropriately for an individual patient. This is a complex procedure and requires expertise and careful monitoring. It is generally carried out within the confines of the intensive-care unit.

Pulmonary artery catheters are highly invasive and carry their own risks of complications. For this reason, non-invasive techniques have been under investigation for some time. These techniques are generally slightly less accurate and clinically useful, but are of increasing value in certain circumstances. The cardiac output can be measured by transoesophageal Doppler using a device that resembles a slightly bulky orogastric tube. Another technique is that of transthoracic bioimpedance, where again fluid fluxes within the thorax are measured electronically, and from these readings mathematical calculations are performed in order to determine cardiac output. Gastric tonometry is a technique that measures gastric mucosal acidosis and hence provides some index of gastrointestinal perfusion. This type of regional technique may in time become an important advance because shock does not affect all tissue beds equally, as some possess inherent protection through autoregulatory mechanisms. Future monitoring techniques are likely to make increasing use of non-invasive and regional methods. It will be appreciated that none of these methods directly measure the degree of shock – namely the degree of tissue hypoxia that is present within the cells of the body. Traditional measures of cardiovascular adequacy, namely urine output, heart rate and blood pressure, and cardiac output, do not accurately reflect this either. The best measurements to date have proved to be oxygen consumption and possibly serum lactate levels, although opinions on this do vary. Advocates of oxygen consumption use intravenous fluids and inotropic therapy to increase cardiovascular function until oxygen consumption can be increased no further. They believe that until this point is reached a latent oxygen debt (and therefore shocked state) must exist in at-risk patients. The degree to which different experts would 'fill up' and drive the circulation varies considerably, but the underlying concept of a hidden or occult tissue oxygen debt is a useful one. There is considerable evidence that an occult tissue oxygen debt exists in many critically ill patients, and some consideration should be given to the possibility of treating this in line with local policies. The serum lactate level reflects tissue hypoxia, but unfortunately it is also elevated by liver dysfunction. Nevertheless, many intensivists use this as a marker for shock severity.

MULTIPLE ORGAN FAILURE

Multiple organ failure is the term that denotes sequential serious dysfunction of the body's vital systems one after the other. The term 'irreversible shock' has been used for many years, and multiple organ failure simply denotes a greater understanding of the pathophysiology involved. Once shock of any aetiology results in capillary leakage, a vicious cycle of increasing tissue hypoxia is entered. Systemic inflammation results in adult respiratory distress syndrome, while hypoperfusion results in renal failure and coagulopathy due to liver dysfunction. The cardiovascular system becomes unresponsive to its own neurohumoral control mechanisms, and then increasingly less responsive to exogenously administered catecholamines, and in at least 50% of patients with multiple organ failure, the outcome is fatal. Single organ failure is commonly survived, but patients with three or more failed organs very seldom survive. The pathological processes that result in multiple organ failure must be identified and treated before this stage is reached. This is achieved by good surgical critical care which leads to the identification of shock at an early stage, prompt and adequate resuscitation, rapid investigation and full treatment of the underlying cause.

Multiple organ failure also represents the end-point for the common pathophysiological processes of shock. Sepsis can very quickly result in capillary leakage, but hypovolaemia, haemorrhage, trauma, burns, pancreatitis and cardiogenic shock can also precipitate the activation of the cytokine and humoral cascades that ultimately result in multiple organ failure. Several stages of sepsis severity have been defined, and these have analogous conditions within the other aetiologies of shock. Importantly, these earlier conditions serve to remind us of the importance of early intervention. The systemic inflammatory response syndrome (SIRS) is the earliest stage. This is characterized by two or more of the following:

1. temperature above 38°C or below 36°C;

2. heart rate higher than 90 beats/min;

3. respiratory rate higher than 20 breaths/min or $PaCO_2$ lower than 4.3 kPa;

4. white blood count (WBC) higher than 12×10^9/L or lower than 4×10^9/L.

Sepsis is defined as systemic inflammatory response syndrome (SIRS) with a documented infection, while severe sepsis is deemed to be present when there is haemodynamic compromise. The multiple organ dysfunction syndrome is a state of physiological derangement in which organ function is not capable of maintaining homeostasis. This may involve the cardiovascular, respiratory, gastrointestinal, CNS, clotting, liver or endocrine systems. The features of multiple organ failure – the next and all too often final stage – have been described above.

The management of multiple organ failure still follows essentially the same principles as that of earlier stages of shock, as no specific therapies exist for multiple organ failure. The intensive care staff will still try to optimize cellular oxygenation by detailed support of cardiorespiratory function. When adult respiratory distress syndrome (ARDS) is severe, maintaining oxygenation is difficult and complex techniques of ventilation are required. Simply using a ventilator to breathe larger breaths at higher pressure results in increasing damage to the lungs (barotrauma and volutrauma), and it may be necessary to ventilate the patient in the prone position, to change the usual ratio between inspiration and expiration, or to permit carbon dioxide levels to rise (permissive hypercapnia). Circulatory support is usually maintained by a combination of inotropes. Noradrenalin is used primarily when the systemic vascular resistance is low, as typically occurs in septic shock. Combinations of adrenalin, dopamine and dobutamine are also used. While low-dose dopamine may be a reasonable therapy on the surgical high-dependency unit, more complex inotrope therapies should be restricted to the intensive care unit. It is always a prerequisite that the patient's circulation is full and that these agents are administered through a central line. Biochemical problems of renal failure are overcome by haemofiltration, a technique which puts less stress on the circulation, and haemodialysis, which simply supports the patient until renal function has recovered spontaneously. It is known that the starved intestine is more prone to atrophy and possibly to releasing endotoxins than the gut which continues to be used for feeding, and therefore enteral nutrition is considered important in the patient in the intensive care unit. Even relatively modest amounts of enteral nutrition can exert a protective effect, and certain specific foodstuffs, notably glutamine, may have a beneficial but as yet unproven role. Notwithstanding these supportive therapies, it is still essential to find the underlying cause of the shock state, particularly when this is septic in nature. The patient must be exhaustively investigated for occult intra-abdominal or intrathoracic sepsis by imaging and, if necessary, by exploratory surgery. Once in the intensive care unit, of course, the patient is easy prey to nosocomial pneumonia or line sepsis, either of which can compound the septic state. Joint management and continual reassessment are needed.

Fluids and electrolytes

Suchitra Kanagasundaram

Introduction

A rational approach to disturbances of fluid and electrolyte imbalance requires both knowledge of normal physiology and application of some basic principles.

The aim of this chapter is to outline such basic principles in their application to clinical situations that one is likely to encounter in the surgical ward.

FLUID COMPARTMENTS

To understand fluid balance, it is necessary to know from which compartment(s) fluid is being lost, and to which compartment fluids would be distributed when administered to the patient.

Total body water (TBW) constitutes 45–75% of the total body weight (45% in elderly women and 60% in elderly men). TBW is distributed between two main body compartments, namely the extracellular fluid (ECF) and the intracellular fluid (ICF). ECF is further divided into the interstitial space (ISS) and the intravascular space (IVS). Absolute volumes for a 70-kg man and relative size in relation to body weight (BW) are shown in Figure 2.2.1.

WATER DISTRIBUTION

Osmotic forces determine the distribution of water between the ICF space and the ECF space. The number of discrete particles in each compartment is responsible for osmotic activity. Figure 2.2.2 shows the solute composition on either side of the cell membrane, where sodium (Na^+) in the ECF and potassium (K^+) in the ICF are responsible for most of the osmotic activity of the respective compartments.

- The barrier between the two compartments is the cell membrane, which is freely permeable to water, but the membrane-sited Na^+/K^+ pump restricts the entry of sodium into cells.

- The osmolality is the same on each side of the compartment as water moves freely across to

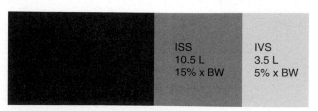

Figure 2.2.1 Distribution of TBW (42 L) in a 70-kg man.

ISS
10.5 L
15% x BW

IVS
3.5 L
5% x BW

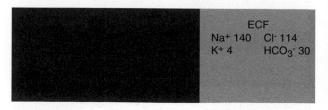

Figure 2.2.2 Solute composition of fluid compartments.

ECF
Na+ 140   Cl- 114
K+ 4   HCO₃- 30

Table 2.2.1 Electrolyte composition (mmol/L) and volume of body fluids

	Na⁺	K⁺	Cl⁻	Volume (L/day)
Saliva	15	19	40	1.5
Stomach	50	15	140	2.5
Bile, small bowel	130–145	5–12	70–100	4.2
Sweat – insensible	12	10	12	0.6

maintain equilibrium (normal osmolality of 280–290 mosm/kg).

- An acute change in the composition of the fluid compartments is accompanied by rapid equilibration as water moves to the compartment of higher osmolality.

For example, if the Na⁺ concentration in the ECF increases, water will move out of the intracellular space into the ECF to re-establish osmotic equilibrium.

The barrier between the IVS and the ISS is the capillary membrane, which is freely permeable to water and electrolytes, but not to proteins (colloids). As a result, the solute composition of the ISS and IVS is the same, but protein which is present at a higher concentration in the plasma exerts an osmotic effect known as colloid osmotic pressure (COP). The COP tends to draw fluid into the capillary, and the hydrostatic pressure difference between the capillary and the interstitium tends to push fluid out (Starling's forces; see Figure 2.2.3).

The distribution of water between the ISS and the IVS is dependent on a balance between hydrostatic pressure and colloid osmotic pressure.

Case 2.2.1 A 60-year-old woman (body weight 70 kg) is admitted with a 2-day history of abdominal pain and vomiting. On examination she presents with dry mucous membranes and tachycardia. Her abdomen is distended, and radiological investigation confirms small-bowel obstruction.

Which fluid would you choose to replace deficit, and how quickly should this be administered?

There are two considerations here:
- the fluid compartment that has suffered the loss;
- the extent of the deficit.

FLUID REPLACEMENT

Information about the electrolyte composition of body fluids (Table 2.2.1) helps to determine the compartment from which fluid has been lost and the choice of replacement fluid.

The composition of intravenous fluids influences their distribution in the fluid compartments (Table 2.2.2). The distribution of crystalloids after intravenous administration is determined by their Na⁺ concentration. Sodium is restricted to the ECF compartment, as

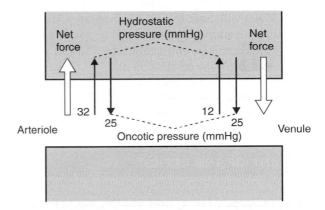

Figure 2.2.3 Hydrostatic forces across a capillary wall (Starling's forces). Reproduced with permission from Aitkenhead AR, Smith G (eds). 1990: *Textbook of anaesthesia*, 2nd ed Edinburgh: Churchill Livingstone.

Table 2.2.2 Content of crystalloid solutions

Solution	Electrolyte content (mmol/L)		Osmolality
0.9% Saline (normal saline)	Na⁺ Cl⁻	154 154	308
4% Glucose 0.18% Saline	Na⁺ Cl⁻ Glucose (mg/dL)	31 31 40	284
5% Glucose	Nil Glucose (mg/dL)	 50	278
Hartmann's solution	Na⁺ Cl⁻ K⁺ HCO₃⁻ Ca⁺⁺	131 112 5 29 4	278

Table 2.2.3 Estimation of percentage dehydration using patient's history and examination

	Body weight (%)	Volume of fluid (L/70 kg)	Signs/symptoms
Mild	>4	2–3	Thirst, reduced skin turgor, dry tongue
Moderate	5–8	4–6	Oliguria, orthostatic hypotension, tachycardia, in addition to the above
Severe	8–10	>7	Thready pulse, hypotension, cool peripheries

Na^+ cannot normally enter cells. Therefore solutions containing isotonic concentrations of this ion (e.g. normal saline) will only expand the ECF.

Intravenous administration of 5% glucose will result in a fall in ECF osmolality (glucose is rapidly metabolized). Water will move from the ECF to the ICF in order to maintain osmotic equilibrium. Therefore 1 L of 5% glucose will distribute throughout the TBW in proportion to the size of the compartments.

With regard to the above case, small-bowel losses result in contraction of the ECF space, and normal saline would be the most appropriate replacement fluid.

EXTENT OF THE DEFICIT

Consider pre-existing and continuing loss

In response to the above case, the patient's history and physical examination (see Table 2.2.3) would suggest that approximately 6% of the body weight is lost as water (4–5 L). The presence of orthostatic hypotension would confirm this.

Gradual replacement with 0.9% normal saline is preferable in the absence of hypovolaemic shock, and replacement of K^+ should be included. Adequacy of volume expansion and correction of fluid deficit are evaluated from physical findings and investigation. Skin turgor, peripheral perfusion, blood pressure, venous pressure and urine output should all improve.

How would you diagnose significant hypovolaemia and what is its cause?

It would be diagnosed on the basis of low blood pressure, poor peripheral perfusion and profound oliguria. Gastrointestinal losses through sequestration into the gut and vomiting lead to contraction of the ECF space by the very nature of the composition of the fluid that is lost. As plasma volume is part of the ECF space, any decrease in ECF will mean a decrease in circulating volume. Other causes, such as cardiac disease and sepsis, should be excluded.

Case 2.2.2 A 45-year-old man presents for elective cholecystectomy.

What are his daily fluid and electrolyte requirements?

His requirements are as follows (Table 2.2.4):

1. water – 2000–2500 mL/day (70-kg adult) or 30–35 mL/kg/day;

2. sodium – 1 mmol/kg/day;

3. potassium – 1 mmol/kg/day.

Maintenance fluid requirements can be administered intravenously as:

- 2500 mL 4% glucose/0.18% saline; or
- 2000 mL 5% glucose + 500 mL 0.9% saline; plus KCl, 1 g (13 mmol) added to each 500-mL bag.

What factors should be considered when planning his peri-operative fluid and electrolyte regime?

Maintenance and replacement of losses should be considered for the pre-, intra- and post-operative period.

Pre-operative period
A patient presenting for minor or moderate elective surgery does not usually require pre-operative fluids, as the loss suffered during the period of starvation can be replaced intra-operatively. (Patients who have suffered

Table 2.2.4 Normal intake and output of water for a 70-kg man

Input (mL)		Output (mL)	
Ingested	1500	Urine	1500
Solid food	700	Faeces	100
Metabolic	300	Skin	500
		Lungs	400
Total	2500		2500

fluid loss due to underlying pathology require fluid replacement prior to surgery.)

Intra-operative period

Intra-operative fluid administration includes the following:

- 1.5 mL/kg/h for the duration of pre-operative starvation; plus

- 1.5 mL/kg/h normal maintenance; plus

- 5 mL/kg/h operative insensible loss; plus

- blood loss – in excess of 15% of blood volume replaced by blood.

A combination of Hartmann's solution, colloid and blood may be used intra-operatively. Dextrose saline and 5% dextrose are hypotonic fluids, which are inappropriate for replacement of fluid loss from the ECF.

Post-operative period

The following factors should be considered when planning a post-operative fluid regimen.

1. The hormonal response to surgery, i.e. elevated levels of ADH and aldosterone, results in retention of both water and sodium. In addition, there is a reduction in the ability to excrete free water for 72 h post-operatively. The above responses influence the choice of fluid to be prescribed for the post-operative period. It is therefore inappropriate to prescribe large volumes of 5% glucose or glucose saline as the only replacement fluid. Such a fluid regime is usually responsible for the development of hyponatraemia.

2. In addition to maintenance fluids, additional fluid should be administered for post-operative losses. Again it is important to consider the ionic composition of the fluid loss and the respective compartment from which the fluid was lost (Table 2.2.5).

3. Renal perfusion must be maintained by close attention to fluid replacement, and any deterioration in renal function must be recognized early on. The importance of accurate fluid balance cannot be over-emphasized.

Table 2.2.5 Selection of replacement fluid

Loss	Compartment	Replacement
Gastrointestinal losses (nasogastric, colonic), third space	ECF	Normal saline
Sweating, diarrhoea	TBW	5% glucose/ glucose saline
Haemorrhage	IVS	Colloid, blood

4. Potassium should be avoided in the first 24 h, as immediate post-operative renal function is uncertain. Thereafter, 1 mmol/kg should be prescribed and subsequently increased depending on losses and plasma levels.

5. Patients with cardiac failure, sepsis syndrome, liver failure and renal dysfunction may need special consideration with regard to monitoring and fluid therapy.

> **Case 2.2.3** A 17-year-old male who was involved in a road traffic accident is transported to the Emergency Department. He is alert, with blood pressure of 70 mmHg systolic, and his pulse rate is 140 beats/min. He complains of pain on manual pelvic compression.

What is the cause of his low blood pressure?

It is caused by hypovolaemic shock due to acute loss of circulating blood.

What is the blood volume of this 70-kg adult male, and what percentage of his blood volume has he lost?

His blood volume is 70 mL/kg (5 L).

An assessment of blood loss may be made from the patient's history and measured loss, but more commonly one has to rely on clinical evaluation.

This patient's blood loss is about 30% of blood volume due to pelvic fracture and associated retroperitoneal haemorrhage (Table 2.2.6).

Which fluid would you use for initial resuscitation?

The choice of fluid for resuscitation from haemorrhagic shock remains controversial. Isotonic electrolyte solutions (Ringer's lactate or normal saline) provide transient expansion of the IVS, but because they are distributed throughout the entire ECF, 4 L of crystalloid are required to expand the IVS by 1 L. Advanced Trauma Life Support (ATLS) protocols adopt the 3:1 rule if using crystalloid (i.e. 300 mL of electrolyte solution for every 100 mL of blood loss).

Colloid solutions are initially confined to the IVS and expand this compartment. However, this effect is temporary and varies according to the colloid.

Although initial fluid resuscitation may include a combination of fluids, the main considerations are tissue perfusion and oxygenation. This requires frequent reassessment of the clinical state of the patient and appropriate revision of treatment.

Table 2.2.6 Estimation of fluid and blood requirements. Reproduced with permission from the ACS Committee on Trauma. 1997: *Advanced Trauma Life Support*® *Student Manual*. Chicago, IL: American College of Surgeons, p.108.

	Class I	**Class II**	**Class III**	**Class IV**
Blood loss (mL)	*c.* 750	750–1500	1500–2000	> 2000
Blood volume (%)	*c.* 15	*c.* 15–30	30–40	> 40
Pulse rate (beats/min)	< 100	> 100	> 120	> 140
Blood pressure	Normal	Normal	Decreased	Decreased
Respiratory rate (breaths/min)	14–20	20–30	30–40	> 35
Urine output (mL/h)	> 30	20–30	5–15	Negligible
CNS	–	–	Anxious	Confused
Fluid replacement	Crystalloid	Crystalloid	Crystalloid + blood	Crystalloid + blood

ELECTROLYTE IMBALANCE

SODIUM

Sodium is responsible for most of the osmotic pressure of the ECF. Sodium balance is therefore closely related to ECF volume and water balance.

Hyponatraemia

Hyponatraemia (Na < 135 mmol/L) can be due to sodium depletion, water retention, or both (Table 2.2.7). Evaluation of ECF volume (ECFV) is therefore important in diagnosis and management.

Symptoms of hyponatraemia

Plasma sodium concentration is the main determinant of plasma osmolality. Hyponatraemia is associated with a decrease in plasma osmolality, and the gradient across the cell membrane causes water to move into the intracellular fluid (ICF), resulting in intracellular overhydration. Symptoms (including headache, lethargy, nausea and vomiting, convulsions and coma) may not be evident until plasma sodium levels have fallen below 120 mmol/L.

Treatment

Treatment should be tailored to the clinical situation and a distinction should be made between acute and chronic development of hyponatraemia.

Chronic hyponatraemia, e.g. that due to congestive heart failure (CHF), is seldom symptomatic. Treatment should be directed at the underlying cause.

Acute hyponatraemia, if symptomatic, is an emergency and the patient may require transfer to the intensive-care unit.

Therapy is directed at increasing ECF tonicity in order to move water from the ICF to the ECF. Aim for a safe plasma level (120 mmol/L).

Hypertonic saline (308 mmol/L) should be used with caution. Infusion should be designed to raise Na$^+$ levels at a rate of 1 mmol/L/h until the patient becomes symptom free or plasma sodium has increased by 20–25 mmol/L, or a serum Na$^+$ level of 125–130 mmol/L is achieved.

Note that serial measurement of sodium is required to measure efficacy of treatment.

Hypernatraemia

Hypernatraemia (plasma Na$^+$ > 155 mmol/L) is treated by replacement of water orally or with 5% dextrose (Table 2.2.8).

POTASSIUM

K$^+$ is an intracellular ion, and plasma K$^+$ reflects approximately 2% of total body potassium. K$^+$ enters the body

Table 2.2.7 Causes of hyponatraemia

Decrease in ECFV

Renal loss:	Addison's disease, diuretics, renal tubular acidosis
Extrarenal loss:	Gastrointestinal, third space, severe sweating, burns, peritonitis

Increase in ECFV

Dilutional:	Congestive heart failure, cirrhosis, nephrotic syndrome, renal failure

Normal ECFV

	Inappropriate secretion of antidiuretic hormone (SIADH), hypothyroidism, renal failure, iatrogenic – IV therapy, transurethral resection of the prostate (TURP) syndrome (absorption of hypotonic fluids)

Table 2.2.8 Causes of hypernatraemia

Pure water loss	Fever, hot climate, thyrotoxicosis Diabetes insipidus (ADH) Cranial, nephrogenic
Hypotonic fluid loss	Gastrointestinal losses (water in excess of solute) Skin – sweating Osmotic diuresis
Salt gain	Iatrogenic – isotonic fluids given for hypotonic loss Drugs – steroids

via dietary ingestion (50–200 mmol/day) or intravenous administration. A decrease in the plasma concentration of potassium must involve decreased ingestion, increased loss or increased entry into cells.

$$\text{Diet}$$
$$\downarrow$$
$$\text{Plasma } K^+ \rightleftharpoons \text{Cells}$$
$$\uparrow$$
$$\text{Losses (faeces, urine, sweat)}$$

Hypokalaemia

Losses
Gastrointestinal losses include the following:

- vomiting, nasogastric suction;
- diarrhoea, laxative abuse;
- fistulae;
- villous adenoma of the rectum.

Renal losses include the following:

- hyperaldosteronism;
- diuretics, steroids;
- congestive heart failure;
- nephrotic syndrome;
- cirrhosis.

Increased entry and redistribution
These may be due to the following:

- insulin, beta-adrenergic agonists;
- alkalaemia.

Signs and symptoms include muscle weakness, fatigue, paralytic ileus and cardiac conduction defects which may be life-threatening.

ECG shows an increase in PR interval, ST-segment depression, reduced height of T-waves and, in severe cases, U-waves appear with a widened QRS complex.

Treatment
Most of the K^+ loss occurs from the ICF space (approximately 40% of the body weight (Figure 2.2.1).

$$K^+ \text{ deficit} = (\text{normal} - \text{measured } K^+) \times$$
$$0.4 \text{ body weight (kg)}$$

Mild hypokalaemia (3.0–3.5 mmol/L) is usually tolerated in the absence of digoxin therapy. Severe symptoms and ECG evidence of hypokalaemia suggest that treatment should be more aggressive. Rapid administration of potassium is dangerous, and infusion rates above 10–20 mmol/h should only be used in life-threatening situations and with ECG monitoring.

Hyperkalaemia

Increased intake
This may be due to oral intake or iatrogenic intravenous administration.

Reduced excretion
This may be due to acute renal failure, Addison's disease or hypoaldosteronism.

Redistribution and release from cells
This may be due to acidosis, catabolism, muscle injury, digoxin, suxamethonium, beta-blockers or haemolysis.

- The most important effect of hyperkalaemia is on the myocardium.

- ECG changes include tall T-waves and wide QRS. Cardiac arrest is possible at plasma levels higher than 7 mmol/L.

- Acute hyperkalaemia requires immediate correction.

FURTHER READING

Aveling W. 1991: Fluids, electrolytes and acid–base balance. In Adams AP, Cashman JP (eds), *Anaesthesia and analgesia and intensive care*. London: Edward Arnold, 81–94.

Hillman K. 1989: Fluid therapy. In Atkinson RS, Adams AP (eds), *Anaesthesia and Analgesia*. London: Churchill Livingstone, 105–23.

Rose BD. 1994: *Clinical physiology of acid–base and electrolyte disorders*. New York: McGraw-Hill.

Rosenthal M. 1995: Fluid and electrolyte therapy in patients during and after surgery. *Current Opinion in Critical Care* 1, 469–77.

Turner D. 1990: Fluid, electrolyte and acid–base balance. In Aitkenhead A, Smith G (eds), *Textbook of anaesthesia*. London: Churchill Livingstone, 389–98.

Willatts S. 1987: *Lecture notes on fluid and electrolyte balance*. Oxford: Blackwell Scientific Publications.

Abdominal fistulae

Anselm O. Agwunobi and Gordon L. Carlson

Introduction

A fistula is an abnormal connection between two epithelial surfaces. In the case of an abdominal fistula, it may be between two or more hollow viscera, when it is known as an internal fistula, or between a hollow viscus and the skin, when it is known as an external fistula (enterocutaneous fistula). An abdominal fistula may be termed 'simple' if there is a direct connecting tract or 'complex' if there is an associated abscess cavity or multiple tracts. An end fistula arises within the long axis of the bowel and is associated with loss of intestinal continuity, e.g. a duodenal stump after gastrectomy (Figure 2.3.1), whereas a lateral fistula arises from an otherwise continuous segment of bowel (Figure 2.3.2). As a guide to the physiological impact of a fistula on the patient, fistulae are further classified as 'low output' if they discharge less than 500 mL of intestinal contents in 24 h and 'high output' if the discharge is more than 500 mL, except in the case of pancreatic fistulae, which are defined as high output if fistula loss exceeds 200 mL a day.

AETIOLOGY

Approximately 80–85% of abdominal fistulae are due to post-operative complications resulting from unrecognized bowel injury or anastomotic leakage. Anastomotic leakage may be due to either local or systemic factors. Other causes of abdominal fistulae include inflammatory bowel diseases, malignancy, radiation and trauma (see Table 2.3.1).

MANAGEMENT

The majority of abdominal fistulae develop post-operatively, and therefore there is usually a history of recent abdominal surgery. An abdominal fistula may result in large fluid and electrolyte losses, especially if the fistula arises from the proximal gastrointestinal tract. Malnutrition and sepsis frequently develop and are associated with an unacceptably high mortality if they are

Table 2.3.1 Aetiology of abdominal fistulae

Aetiological factor	Comments
Anastomotic leakage	*Local factors*: poor surgical technique, poor blood supply to bowel ends, tension along suture lines, residual disease, distal obstruction
	Systemic factors: sepsis, malnutrition, immunosuppression
Inflammatory causes	Crohn's disease, diverticular disease, tuberculosis
Malignancy	Either direct invasion or perforation with abscess formation
Radiation	May manifest immediately or years later
Trauma	Blunt or penetrating trauma

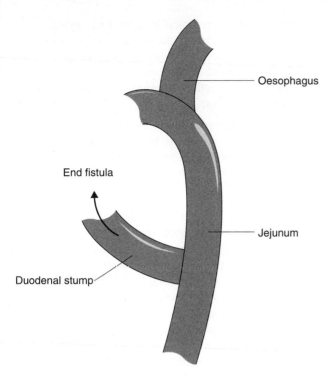

Figure 2.3.1 End fistula – Roux-en-Y loop of jejunum.

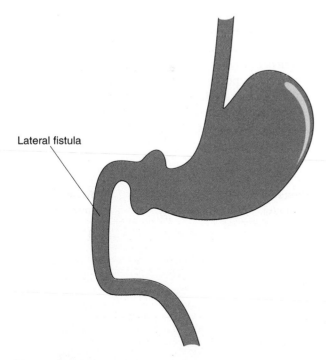

Figure 2.3.2 Lateral fistula.

not adequately treated. Fortunately, advances in nutritional and metabolic support, nursing and wound care and interventional radiology have revolutionized the overall management of abdominal fistulae. Thus the management of a patient with abdominal fistula involves a multidisciplinary team of nurses, stoma therapists, dietitians, physiotherapists, pharmacists and laboratory staff, as well as the clinicians.

In proximal high-output fistulae the integrity of the overlying skin may be threatened, and adequate protection of the skin must be ensured.

The outcome of management of abdominal fistulae mainly depends on how well these various associated complications are managed, and they will therefore be considered in more detail below.

CONTROL OF SEPSIS

Sepsis is the commonest cause of mortality among patients with abdominal fistulae. The majority of the abdominal fistulae that are seen in clinical practice are due to post-operative complications following anastomotic leakage, in some cases following multiple laparotomies. This invariably leads to the formation of adhesions which trap discharged intestinal contents with the formation of pockets of infection. Unless these are actively sought and adequately eradicated, all efforts to support the patient nutritionally will be in vain, as the current methods of nutritional support do not reverse the malnutrition and hypercatabolism induced by sepsis. Pointers to abdominal sepsis include persistently low albumin levels and inability to gain weight in the face of adequate nutritional and metabolic replacements. Leucocytosis or leucopenia, pyrexia, tachycardia and tachypnoea, either in isolation or in combination, may also be present. Although ultrasound and radiolabelled leucocyte scans can be used to diagnose intra-abdominal abscesses, contrast-enhanced computerized tomography (CT) is the most useful investigation for distinguishing fluid-filled abscess cavities from bowel loops. The majority of abscess cavities can then be drained percutaneously under CT or ultrasound guidance. Pus from the cavity should be sent for microbiological analysis. Antibiotics are only indicated in the presence of cellulitis or systemic illness. In some cases, control of sepis will necessitate laparotomy and the creation of stomas.

METABOLIC AND NUTRITIONAL CARE

The amount of fluid and electrolyte loss can best be appreciated by noting the amount and composition of various gastrointestinal secretions as shown in Table

2.3.2. For example, in a proximal jejuno-cutaneous fistula there are large losses of fluids and electrolytes, sometimes in excess of 4–5 L/day, with the potential for very significant fluid and electrolyte imbalances. These losses need to be replaced vigorously, generally with isotonic saline with added potassium. Daily estimation of plasma electrolytes, urea and haematocrit, as well as urinary sodium output (which may be a more sensitive indicator of sodium status than the plasma sodium concentration), should take place until satisfactory stabilization is achieved. At this stage twice weekly estimations should suffice.

Nutritional support should commence as soon as possible, preferably within 48 h in a patient with a high-output fistula, in order to avoid malnutrition and its attendant complications. An initial clinical and laboratory assessment should be performed to determine the best possible route for the delivery of nutritional support.

CLINICAL ASSESSMENT

This should include a detailed history to assess energy and protein intake and expenditure, taking into consideration the degree of stress. The history of the current illness and its effects on appetite, swallowing, absorption and fistula output should be noted. The patient's current weight, weight loss, evidence of muscle wasting, skinfold thickness and other anthropometric measurements should be recorded by a trained observer.

LABORATORY ASSESSMENT

This should include the following:

- a full blood count with differential analyses looking for evidence of anaemia, microcytosis (iron deficiency), macrocytosis (folate and vitamin B_{12} deficiency) and leucopenia;

- nutritional screen – total iron-binding capacity, creatinine and trace elements (magnesium, calcium, copper, zinc, iron and selenium) should be estimated; in sick surgical patients, albumin concentrations reflect illness severity rather than nutritional status;

- transferrin and pre-albumin levels are less easily measured, but are said to be a more sensitive indicator of body protein status than albumin because of their shorter half-lives;

- urinary nitrogen.

Armed with these baseline nutritional measurements, which should be repeated regularly to monitor the response to nutritional therapy, a decision should then be made about the best possible route for delivery of nutrition. In low-output distal ileal and colonic fistulae, enteral nutrition with a low-residue, high-protein diet may be administered orally. In proximal gastrointestinal fistulae, enteral nutrition may be given via a tube if access can be gained to the gut distal to the fistula. This is often technically difficult. In such cases parenteral nutrition is the best solution, because it provides adequate nutrition and total bowel rest, both of which are important for fistula closure. As mentioned above, allowances should be made for daily energy requirements as well as the increase in energy expenditure associated with stress. In general, 25 kcal/kg/day with 1 g of nitrogen/200 kcal will suffice for the majority of patients provided that sepsis is eradicated. Parenteral nutrition can be given via a peripheral vein, but use of this route is very limited due to its association with a high incidence of thrombophlebitis. Central venous catheters placed in the distal superior vena cava (SVC) to minimize the risk of venous thrombosis are preferable. They should be inserted under strict aseptic conditions using radiological screening to position the catheter tip correctly. Cuffed catheters such as Hickman or Broviac lines are used in cases where long-term intravenous feeding (more than 6 weeks) is anticipated. Central venous catheters that are

Table 2.3.2 Intestinal secretions and their composition

Type	Volume (L/day)	Sodium (mmol/L)	Potassium (mmol/L)	Chloride (mmol/L)	Bicarbonate (mmol/L)
Saliva	1.5	10	20–25	15–40	30
Gastric	1.5–2.5	50–100	10–15	100–140	0
Duodenum	2.0	130	5	90	0–10
Jejunum	3.0	140	5	100–105	15–30
Bile	0.8–1.0	145	5	100	70–115
Pancreas	0.8	145	5	100	15–35

used for feeding should be cared for by a dedicated nursing team. Such catheters should be used only for feeding and handled with strict aseptic technique. It has been repeatedly shown that provided a strict protocol is adhered to, line infection rates can be negligible.

SKIN CARE

The integrity of the skin at the fistula site is threatened even with the lowest-output fistulae. Skin protection is important, particularly in the case of gastric, duodenal and proximal jejunal fistulae, in which the output of activated digestive enzymes and extremely acid or alkaline fluid may lead to rapid digestion of the surrounding skin. This chemical erosion, in combination with bacterial invasion, can lead to extension of infection through fascial planes, subcutaneous tissues and muscle.

A large number of devices, barrier creams and pastes are now available to deal with these problems, and the advice of an experienced stoma therapist is therefore invaluable. Stomahesive sheets and drainage bags are the most commonly used methods. High-output fistulae may be troublesome for the patient, especially during the night, and in such cases 'megostomy' devices such as the Greensmith device (see Plate 2.3.1 in the colour plate section) are of value. If the fistula opening is within a large dehisced abdominal wound, the large Eakin bags (see Plate 2.3.2 in the colour plate section) will be more appropriate, because they can be fashioned to the desired size and shape of the wound. They can be connected to a suction catheter. Where this is not possible it may be better to create a proximal defunctioning stoma such as a loop jejunostomy to protect the skin. Although fluid and electrolytes losses are likely to be higher, a well-fashioned stoma is better for skin integrity than a poorly controlled fistula. Stoma output can frequently be controlled by reducing oral intake, and by the use of codeine phosphate and proton-pump inhibitors. Octreotide may be effective in high-output stomas, but it has not been shown to promote fistula closure.

PSYCHOLOGICAL ASSESSMENT

The development of an abdominal fistula in a patient is a major disappointment for the surgeon but more so for the patient. Coupled with this is the prospect of further surgery, a long stay in hospital and loss of earnings. All of these add to the anxiety and depression often observed among this group of patients, and psychotherapy should be part of their rehabilitation process.

DEFINITIVE TREATMENT

The surgery of abdominal fistulae is very complex, and timing is extremely important. Adequate investigations and treatment of any ongoing sepsis and nutritional support are critical to the eventual outcome. The majority of abdominal fistulae will close spontaneously within 4–6 weeks with conservative treatment, while a significant minority will not close for reasons such as the following:

- associated abscess cavity;
- distal obstruction;
- bowel discontinuity;
- mucocutaneous continuity;
- disease at the fistula site, e.g. Crohn's disease or cancer.

Two categories of surgical treatment can be identified in the management of abdominal fistulae, namely conservative and definitive surgical treatments.

CONSERVATIVE TREATMENT

This applies to procedures that are designed to eliminate practical problems of fistula management but which do not attempt fistula excision. They may help to accelerate fistula closure and they include the following:

- creation of a proximal stoma to divert intestinal contents away from the fistula, i.e. loop jejunostomy or a gastrostomy;
- open drainage of an intra-abdominal abscess where percutaneous drainage is not practically possible.

DEFINITIVE PROCEDURES

In the absence of adverse factors, a spontaneous closure rate of 60–70% can be expected within 4–6 weeks in patients with an enterocutaneous fistula with bowel rest and adequate nutritional support. For those fistulae that fail to close, a definitive procedure to excise the fistula may be required. The anatomy of the fistula must be thoroughly defined beforehand, and this is best achieved by a combination of fistulography and intestinal contrast studies. Imaging of the urinary and biliary systems may also be required, depending on the clinical circumstances. The surgical strategy should be individualized, as fistula characteristics vary from patient to patient. In general, however, adequate time should be allowed for the long and difficult dissections that often characterize fistula surgery. After fistula excision, primary anastomosis should only be attempted if local and systemic factors are favourable. Otherwise, the bowel ends should be exteriorized and anastomosis performed at a later date when conditions have improved. Abscess cavities should be curetted and anastomoses kept away from them because of the risk of further fistulation. Omentum can be used to pack abscess cavities for this purpose.

FURTHER READING

Berry SM, Fischer JE. 1996: Classification and pathophysiology of enterocutaneous fistulas. *Surgical Clinics of North America* **76**, 1009–18.

El-Bahar T, Irving M. 1988: Intestinal fistulae. In Russell RCG (ed.), *Recent advances in surgery. 13.* Edinburgh: Churchill Livingstone, 103–24.

Foster CE III, Lefor AT. 1996: General management of gastrointestinal fistulas. Recognition, stabilisation, and correction of fluid and electrolyte imbalances. *Surgical Clinics of North America* **76**, 1019–33.

Hill G. 1988: Nutrition in the surgical patient. In Cuschieri A, Giles GR, Moossa AR (eds), *Essential surgical practice.* Bristol: John Wright and Sons Ltd, 109–19.

Hill GL (ed.). 1992: *Disorders of nutrition and metabolism in clinical surgery.* Edinburgh: Churchill Livingstone.

Irving M. 1977: Local and surgical management of enterocutaneous fistulas. *British Journal of Surgery* **64**, 690–4.

Keighley MRB. 1993: Intestinal fistulas. In Keighley MRB, Williams NS (eds), *Surgery of the anus, rectum and colon.* London: W.B. Saunders, 2013–102.

McIntyre PB, Ritchie JK, Hawley PR *et al.* 1984: Enterocutaneous fistula – a review of 132 cases. *British Journal of Surgery* **71**, 293–6.

Meguid MM, Campos ACL. 1996: Nutritional management of patients with gastrointestinal fistulas. *Surgical Clinics of North America* **76**, 1035–80.

Smith JAR. 1992: Fluid balance and electrolyte disturbance. In Johnson CD, Taylor I (eds), *Recent advances in surgery. 15.* Edinburgh: Churchill Livingstone, 209–23.

Chapter 3.1

Anaemia and erythropoiesis

Hilary A. Blacklock

Introduction

Anaemia is common in surgical patients, either as a presenting clinical problem, as a consequence of ongoing pathology, or arising from blood loss before, during, or soon after any operative procedure. The type of anaemia may allow identification of the underlying diagnosis. Tests to verify the mechanism of the anaemia are necessary before the patient is given replacement therapy or a red cell transfusion, so that the underlying diagnosis is not obscured. This is particularly important in immune haemolytic anaemia and sickle cell disease, which may have implications for peri-operative management, and also in iron, B_{12} and folate deficiency. A complete work up is not always possible however, in a serious emergency such as a massive gastrointestinal haemorrhage in association with liver disease.

The need for pre-operative transfusion should be determined on an individual basis, taking into account cardiovascular status, operative blood loss and haemoglobin concentration (see also Chapter 28). Haematinics may be appropriate to improve the haemoglobin concentration, or to prevent the development of anaemia; for example iron supplements to raise the haemoglobin concentration after significant surgical blood loss and ongoing vitamin B_{12} therapy is necessary in all patients who have had a total ileal resection.

ERYTHROPOIESIS

As the erythroblast or nucleated red cell develops in the bone marrow, the cytoplasm becomes haemoglobinized, DNA activity is suppressed, the chromosomes condense, and the nucleus becomes pyknotic before being extruded by an active process involving cytoplasmic cleavage and cell movement. Each day approximately 2×10^{11} mature erythroid cells enter the circulation by squeezing through gaps in the marrow sinusoid walls. Release appears to be mediated mainly by the hormone erythropoietin (EPO). Red cells usually only enter the blood after the nucleus has been extruded, but when sinusoidal porosity is increased in situations of marrow stress, such as hypoxia, haemolysis or haemorrhage (also marrow infiltration and diseases such as myelofibrosis), immature or nucleated red cells may be present in the blood. Residual RNA remnants retained during cleavage (known as Howell-Jolly bodies) are normally removed when the cell passes through the spleen – these persist in the blood after splenectomy or in states of hyposplenism.

The newly released red cells can be counted after applying a supra-vital stain to reveal a reticulum of residual RNA. In a steady state, these reticulocytes, which make up about 1–2% of the red cell count (absolute value $c.$ $10–120 \times 10^9$/L), mature in the marrow for 1–2 days before entering the blood. If the marrow is under stress, the circulation maturation time may be prolonged up to 3 days – this should be considered when using the reticulocyte count as an indicator of marrow production.

REGULATION OF EYTHROPOIESIS

An erythropoietic stimulus maintains a relatively constant red cell mass, but also allows increased production in response to hypoxia and anaemia. The most important factors are EPO (*c.* 90% of which is produced in the kidney), which increases in response to a low local oxygen tension (Figure 3.1.1.), and the nutrients iron, vitamin B_{12} and folate. Other essential factors for red cell production are vitamin B_6 (pyridoxine), riboflavin, vitamin E, copper, proteins and carbohydrates. Several hormones – corticosteroids, growth hormone, thyroxine and testosterone (the latter is responsible for the higher haemoglobin levels in men) – also play a role in the regulation of erythropoiesis by enhancing the response of the developing red cell to EPO. Deficiencies of these result in anaemia, which corrects with hormone replacement. Cytokines other than EPO also influence erythropoiesis, the most important being interleukin-3, which acts on the least mature erythroid cells.

RED CELL LIFESPAN

The red cell, unique in retaining function after losing its nucleus, is a bag of haemoglobin programmed to survive approximately 120 days, after which the integrity and the deformability of its membrane wears out. Then, under the influence of a change in pH and a reduced glucose concentration in the splenic milieu, the red cell now with a more rigid membrane, is no longer capable of passing between sinus endothelial cells and is destroyed by phagocytosis. This removal from the circulation also occurs in other organs, including the liver and the marrow, especially in situations of hyposplenism. The components of the cells are then disassembled – the amino acids are returned to the protein pool and iron liberated from haem is recycled by transferrin back to the developing red cells. The breakdown of the protopor-

phyrin ring releases carbon, which is excreted from the lungs, and the remaining pyrrole ring is carried as bilirubin to the liver, where it is conjugated to glucuronide and excreted (Figure 3.1.2).

Red cell survival is reduced in blood loss and haemolysis. In the latter situation, haemoglobin released from damaged cells is bound to haptoglobin, and the ensuing complex is removed by hepatic parenchymal cells. The absence of serum haptoglobins is strongly suggestive of haemolysis as long as other causes are excluded, mainly megaloblastic anaemia and end-stage liver disease (where production is impaired). Additional supportive laboratory data include a raised bilirubin (unconjugated) and reticulocyte count, and a positive anti-globulin (direct Coombs) test if red cell antibodies are responsible (as in immune haemolytic anaemia).

ANAEMIA

Anaemia is a significant reduction in the oxygen-carrying haemoglobin, measured in g/L of blood, compared with a normal population of that age, sex and physiological state, e.g. pregnancy. When one or more of the factors regulating erythropoiesis are deficient, or when the marrow is significantly diseased, anaemia may result from decreased production of haemoglobin with a low reticulocyte count (Table 3.1.1). A low haemoglobin can also occur when there is increased destruction or loss of red cells, as in haemolysis or haemorrhage. In these situations, the reticulocyte count will be high if there is adequate marrow function and nutrients – indeed the marrow can increase production eight to tenfold in response to severe anaemia. When a missing haematinic is administered such as iron, a reticulocyte response should be evident in 5–7 days, and will continue until the haemoglobin reaches a 'normal' level for that individual.

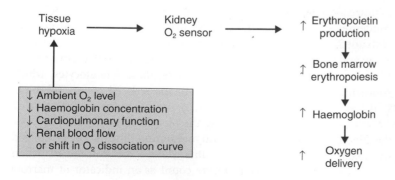

Figure 3.1.1. Erythropoietin production, which increases in response to renal hypoxia, stimulates erythropoiesis and thus increases oxygen delivery.

Table 3.1.1 Classification of anaemia by pathophysiology

Decreased production

Haemoglobin synthesis: iron deficiency, thalassaemia,
 anaemia of chronic disease, chronic renal failure
DNA synthesis: megaloblastic anaemia
Stem cell: aplastic anaemia, myeloproliferative leukaemia
Bone marrow infiltration: carcinoma, lymphoma
Toxic injury: radiotherapy, chemotherapy, viruses

Increased destruction

Blood loss: acute or chronic
Haemolysis (intrinsic)
    Membrane: hereditary spherocytosis, elliptocytosis
    Haemoglobin: sickle cell disease, unstable
      haemoglobin
    Glycolysis: pyruvate kinase deficiency, etc.
    Oxidation: G6PD deficiency
Haemolysis (extrinsic)
    Immune: warm antibody, cold antibody
    Microangiopathic: DIC, thrombotic thrombocytopenic
      purpura
    Haemolytic–uraemic syndrome, mechanical cardiac
      valve
    Infection: clostridial bacteraemia
Hypersplenism

CAUSE OF ANAEMIA

The cause of anaemia should always be pursued – indeed it may be the pointer to a serious underlying diagnosis. This process requires a careful history, clinical examination and further investigations, including blood tests (ESR, reticulocyte count, haptoglobins, renal and liver function tests, iron studies, B_{12} and folate assays) and sometimes additional tests such as a bone marrow biopsy. To help determine the cause of the anaemia, the mean cell volume (MCV), a red cell parameter measured directly by modern electronic cell counters, can give additional useful data (Table 3.1.2). However, in some clinical situations the parameters can be variable; for example in chronic blood loss, occult or otherwise, the MCV can be mildly raised from an increased reticulocytosis, normal, or low if iron deficiency has developed.

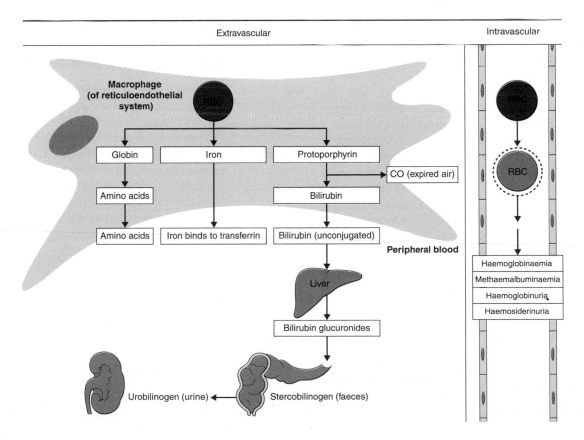

Fig. 3.1.2. Red cell breakdown.

Table 3.1.2 MCV as a clue to the cause of anaemia in the surgical patient

Type of anaemia	Further tests*	Causes
LOW–MCV (50–76 fL)		
Iron deficiency	I, R, O, E, U, G, +/-C	GI bleeds, gastric, duodenal, gynaecological disorders
Thalassaemia	I, E, HS	Genetic
Anaemia of chronic disease**	E, K, L, M, A, X, S, P,C,T	Cancers, infections, e.g. TB, autoimmune
NORMAL MCV (76–96 fL)		
Blood loss	R, U,O, G, C, +/-X	Trauma, surgery, GI disease, blood tests
Haemolysis	R, E, A,H, L	Immune-mediated, microangiopathic, membrane defects
INCREASED MCV (96–130+ fL)		
Alcohol, liver, renal, thyroid, drugs ***	L, K, R, C, T	Liver disease, hypothyroidism, etc.
Reticulocytosis***	R, H, V, L	Bleeding, haemolysis, marrow infiltration, hypoxia
Marrow disease	R, P, C,E, L,+/-A,B, +/-S	Marrow disorders, leukaemias, cancers
Folate deficiency	R, V, H	Anorexia, malabsorption, increased use (haemolysis)
B_{12} deficiency	R, V, H, A	Gastrectomy, ileal disease, pernicious anaemia

*Test codes: A, autoimmune serology; B, bone marrow; C, coagulation screen; E, ESR; G, GI endoscopy; H, haemolysis tests; HS, haemoglobinopathy screening; I, iron studies; K, kidney tests; L, liver functions; M, microbiology; O, faecal occult bloods; P, protein studies; R, reticulocyte count; S, bone scan; T, tissue biopsy; U, urinalysis; V, vitamin assays; X, X-rays.
** MCV not usually ≤ 70 fL.
*** MCV not usually > 115 fL.

ANAEMIA OF CHRONIC DISEASE VS. IRON DEFICIENCY

In surgical practice, anaemia of chronic disease (ACD), which occurs with chronic inflammation, infections and neoplasms, can be difficult to differentiate from iron deficiency. The red cell abnormalities in chronic disorders may depend on the duration and severity of the underlying disorder and other coexistent factors if present, such as renal failure, thalassaemia and additional iron deficiency. Indeed, ACD and iron deficiency often occur together. In chronic disorders, cytokines such as interleukin-1 and interferons mediate the immune or inflammatory response. Some of these patients may have increased EPO, but the usual finding is a level lower than expected for the haemoglobin. Relatively high levels of EPO are more likely to be associated with increased levels of other cytokines, including tumour necrosis factor. These can effect a number of symptoms such as weight loss, and blood changes, including a block in duodenal iron absorption, impaired mobilization of iron from reticulo-endothelial stores (producing a fall in serum iron even when marrow stores are adequate), a low reticulocyte count, a low, normal or reduced MCV (although not usually < 70 fL), and a slightly reduced red cell survival. Serum transferrin (TIBC) is often reduced and the serum ferritin falsely elevated – a rule of thumb is that in situations of chronic disease, a ferritin < 50 μg/L may represent coexistent iron deficiency, and a trial of

iron therapy is warranted. Iron deficiency is otherwise relatively easy to diagnose, classically with a raised TIBC and a serum ferritin below the reference range.

Investigation of the cause of iron defciency

If iron deficiency is confirmed and if there is no clear-cut cause such as haematuria, gastrointestinal blood loss should be pursued. The exact bleeding site is sought from the history and physical and rectal examination, by faecal occult blood tests and by the appropriate use of gastrointestinal endoscopies, which are often successful in detecting significant gastrointestinal pathology. Hookworm ova are looked for in stools of patients from areas where this infestation occurs. Rarely, a coeliac axis angiogram may be necessary to demonstrate angiodysplasia.

OTHER ANAEMIAS OF RELEVANCE TO SURGICAL PRACTICE

Hypersplenism may result in anaemia (and other cytopenias) from increased red cell pooling and decreased survival. The diagnosis, made in the presence of splenomegaly by exclusion of other causes of anaemia, is ultimately confirmed by a response to splenectomy. Hypersplenism should be considered in patients with chronic liver disease and portal hypertension.

Alcoholism produces anaemia by several mechanisms,

including a direct toxic effect of the ethanol on haem synthesis, folate deficiency from poor nutrition, hypersplenism and iron deficiency from bleeding varices.

Folate lack occurs from dietary deficiency (common in seriously ill or malnourished patients), from malabsorption (as in coeliac disease and tropical sprue) and from increased use or loss (as occurs in pregnancy, haemolysis, Crohn's disease and haemodialysis). Folate supplements should be given to all debilitated individuals and those unable to eat, such as intensive care patients. A serum B_{12} level should be checked when folate is started.

In surgical practice, *vitamin B_{12} deficiency* is most commonly due to acquired pernicious anaemia, total or partial gastrectomy, or intestinal causes such as the intestinal stagnant loop syndrome (including jejunal diverticulosis, ileo-colic fistula, anatomical blind-loop and intestinal stricture), ileal resection, Crohn's disease and tropical sprue. Ongoing parenteral supplements should be given routinely in those patients with extensive gastric and ileal resections.

Autoimmune haemolytic anaemia is often treated with splenectomy. The presence of one or more autoantibodies makes red cell cross-matching difficult and the transfusion more hazardous, and ongoing transfusion support is more likely to be problematic (the recipient may develop further antibodies). Transfusion should be avoided unless the risks of non-transfusion are greater than the risks of transfusion.

Sickle cell anaemia (HbS) should be excluded in black Americans and Africans and others from Saudi Arabia, India and Southern Europe who are being considered for surgery. Patients may present with a crisis resulting in splenic or bone infarcts (also osteomyelitis), cholelithiasis, hepatic infarcts, priapism, chronic skin ulcers and dactylitis. In homozygotes undergoing major surgery, it is advisable to reduce the level of HbS by transfusion to around 20%, and special attention is needed during the operation and anaesthetic with respect to hydration, acid–base balance and oxygenation. Complications are more common with regional anaesthesia than with other types of anaesthesia in these patients.

Thalassaemias are common genetic disorders occurring in a broad geographical region from the Mediterranean through the Middle East and India to Southeast Asia, and in other populations, including Polynesians. Four alpha genes (two on each chromosome) are responsible for the production of a normal component of alpha globin chains; individuals with *alpha thalassaemia* have a deletion of between one and three genes. The deletion of four, known as the Hb-Barts hydrops fetalis syndrome, is incompatible with life. This can occur in a child born to two parents with the (α, α/-, -) genotype. Genetic counselling and pre-natal diagnosis should be performed to prevent the maternal morbidity associated with the inevitable intrauterine death. The deletion of three alpha genes (α, - / -, -) known as HbH disease results in anaemia and organomegaly – some with this genotype require ongoing red cell transfusions.

In contrast, the *beta thalassaemias* are mainly the result of point mutations rather than gene deletions. These can be classified clinically into those who make no β chains (β^0) or those who make some (β^+ thalassaemia). In homozygous β^0, also known as beta-thalassaemia major, the severe clinical consequences can be suppressed by lifelong transfusions, or cured by bone marrow transplantation. The main difficulty in the surgical patient is to differentiate the genetic forms from iron deficiency. As iron deficiency makes the diagnosis of the milder forms difficult, tests should be delayed until any deficiency is corrected.

FURTHER READING

Carson JL, Duff A, Poses RM, *et al.* 1996: Effect of anaemia and cardiovascular disease on surgical mortality and morbidity. *Lancet* **348**, 1055–60.

Garden MS, Grant RE, Jebraili S. 1996. Peri-operative complications in patients with sickle cell disease. An orthopaedic perspective. *American Journal of Orthopaedics* **25**, 353-6.

Hoffbrand AV, Pettit J. 1994: Essential haematology. Oxford: Blackwell Science.

Koshy M, Weiner SJ, Miller ST, *et al.* 1995: Surgery and anesthesia in sickle cell disease. Cooperative Study of Sickle Cell Diseases. *Blood* **86**, 3676–84.

Means JT. 1995: Pathogenesis of the anaemia of chronic disease: a cytokine-mediated anaemia. *Stem Cells* **13**, 32–7.

Patel RI, Witt L, Hannallah RS. 1997: Pre-operative laboratory testing in children undergoing elective surgery. *Journal of Clinical Anesthesia* **9**, 569–75.

Rockey DC, Cello JP. 1993: Evaluation of the gastrointestinal tract in patients with iron deficiency anaemia. *New England Journal of Medicine* **329**, 1691–5.

Haemostasis and anticoagulation in surgery

Hilary A. Blacklock

Introduction

Surgery severely tests the complex haemostatic mechanism. Because of the arterial pressure, there needs to be instantaneous localized coagulation to minimize bleeding from vascular injury, without compromising general blood flow. Inhibitors are also essential to maintain blood fluidity, especially in the veins, where the flow is slow or intermittent. Bleeding is a major surgical complication of great interest to all surgeons – the operator needs to be responsible for haemostasis during and after any procedure. Good surgical techniques to minimize blood loss and exemplary management, with early ambulation and infection prophylaxis to prevent thromboses at unwanted sites, are essential, particularly in patients with coagulopathies or thrombophilia.

Pre-existing bleeding disorders may cause or aggravate the disease process and increase the surgical risk, especially if there is a significant past history of bleeding. In these situations, a careful history to assess the risk of bleeding is the surgeon's responsibility. Patients with congenital or acquired disorders that increase the risk of thrombo-embolism may present with a pathological process which requires surgery, such as a mesenteric artery thrombosis with bowel infarction. These individuals are at particular risk peri-operatively with the activation of clotting factors, especially if there is significant immobility or an increase in acute-phase reactants, particularly fibrinogen.

NORMAL HAEMOSTASIS

In order to maintain the integrity of the body and stop significant bleeding after vascular injury, the haemostatic mechanism is complex, involving activation and inhibition of pathways, and integrating blood vessels with platelets and humoral factors. Following vascular injury, a haemostatic plug (Figure 3.2.1) is formed with two main components:

1. a primary platelet plug;
2. a solid fibrin clot (the coagulation cascade).

PRIMARY PLATELET PLUG FORMATION

The blood vessel intima is covered with endothelial cells resting on a basement membrane. In larger vessels, particularly arteries, increasing amounts of elastin, innervated smooth muscle cells and collagen (essential for mechanical integrity) are found. Elastin allows the vessels to distend, aiding resealing following minor trauma (e.g. venepuncture). Smooth muscle cells that are vasoconstricting in response to sympathetic nerve stimulation or trauma immediately slow the blood flow to the injured area, minimizing blood loss. This, together with exposure of collagen and release of tissue factor, activates platelet secretion and adhesion and the coagulation cascade.

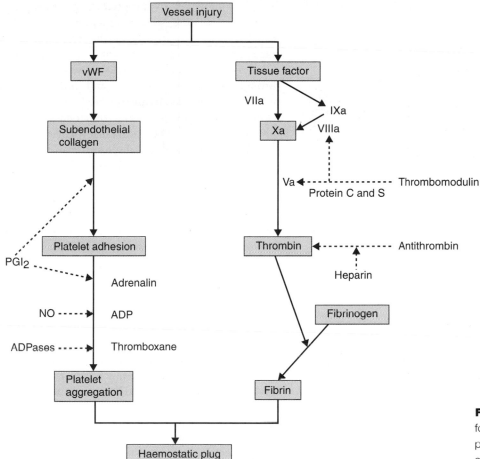

Figure 3.2.1 Clot formation involves the production of platelet aggregates and solid fibrin.

Endothelial cell function

The endothelial cells inhibit haemostasis by making, releasing and binding factors on their surface (Figure 3.2.2) including tissue plasminogen activators and inhibitors, antithrombin III, heparin-related molecules, platelet factor 4, protein S and thrombomodulin. Other substances that profoundly influence the platelet–vessel wall interaction include von Willebrand factor and prostacyclin. *Von Willebrand factor (vWF)*, which is made by endothelial cells and platelets, is essential for platelet adhesion to the sub-endothelial matrix. Thrombin, interleukin-I, adrenalin (most potent), vasopressin and insulin can all stimulate endothelial vWF release. Vigorous exercise and vessel occlusion are also effective in raising levels in individuals with mild deficiencies. Raised levels occur in many diseases, especially those of the liver. *Prostacyclin*, or prostaglandin I_2, which is synthesized by endothelial cells, is a potent vasodilator that inhibits and can also *reverse* platelet aggregation. Thrombin generation at the injury site stimulates adjacent endothelial prostacyclin synthesis, and this counteracts the platelet-aggregating activity of thrombin, localizing platelet plug formation.

Platelet structure and function

Platelets are biconvex discs with a diameter of 2–4 μm, a volume of 5–8 fL and containing cytoplasmic granules, namely mitochondria, alpha granules (the most frequent type) and the rarer dense bodies (Figure 3.2.3). The alpha granules contain chemicals, platelet-specific peptides or coagulation factors, which contribute to platelet function and aggregation, coagulation and a number of non-haemostatic defence mechanisms (chemotaxis, mitogenesis and vessel repair). Platelets activated by foreign surfaces or agonists (collagen, thrombin, adrenalin, ADP and thromboxane) rapidly lose their discoid shape, become spherical, extend pseudopodia and aggregate, releasing factor V and vWF. This primary plug formation on damaged vessel walls is then stabilized with an overlying clot.

Platelet production and lifespan

Platelets are cytoplasmic fragments of bone-marrow megakaryocytes. At the earliest recognizable platelet precursor stage, the nucleus divides (endomitosis), but the cell itself does not. This is associated with membrane

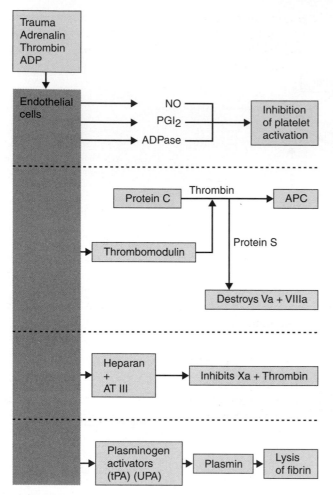

Figure 3.2.2 Endothelial cells synthesize prostaglandin I₂ (PGI₂), thrombomodulin, heparan and plasminogen activators which inhibit thrombus formation and maintain vascular patency.

formation and cytoplasmic maturation under the influence of various growth factors, including interleukin-11 and thrombopoietin. The cytoplasm has platelet features such as membrane glycoproteins, specific granules and lysosomes. The increasing membranes are accommodated by progressive invaginations that eventually become platelet membranes. A mature megakaryocyte, commonly at the eight-nucleus (8N) stage but up to 64N (as large as 60 μm in diameter), produces as many as 2000 platelets. Pseudopodia extend through the marrow sinusoids, and individual platelets or larger cytoplasmic fragments are broken off. The latter are carried to the pulmonary microcirculation where they break down into individual platelets. In some thrombocytopenias, the cytoplasm matures faster, so that even 4N cells produce platelets – these tend to be more active, and larger with an increased mean platelet volume (MPV).

Platelets usually survive for 8 to 14 days after marrow release. Splenic sequestration then occurs for 24–48 h before they enter the circulation. The platelet count is maintained relatively constant in the range 150–400 × 10⁹/L. Neonates have a slightly lower level, and 'adult' values are reached by about 3 months of age. There are no other significant age or sex differences except for a slight fluctuation in women, with the lowest levels occurring at or just before menstruation. Heavy exercise and adrenergic stimulation temporarily raise the count. There is also some racial variation. In Mediterranean races, the platelet count may be as low as 80 × 10⁹/L, but with an increase in size, the platelet mass remains unaltered.

FIBRIN CLOT FORMATION

Three vitamin K-dependent enzyme complexes control the reactions that lead to thrombin generation during coagulation. Each comprises a serine protease and a cofactor protein [tissue factor (TF), factor V or factor VIII, respectively] assembled on a membrane surface (Figure 3.2.4). This localization also helps limit the clotting process. The exposure of TF as a result of surgical or inflammatory endothelial damage initiates clotting via the formation of a catalytic complex between TF and factor VIIa (extrinsic Xase). This activates the serine protease components of both the intrin-

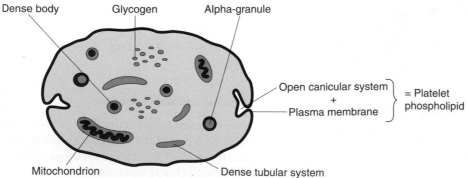

Figure 3.2.3 A diagrammatic representation of a blood platelet.

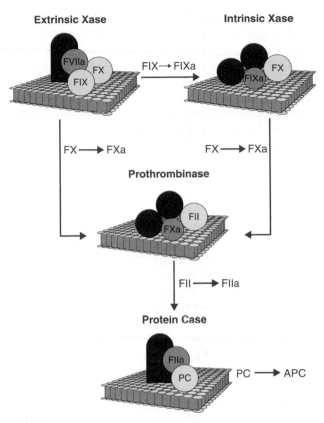

Figure 3.2.4 Each of the vitamin K-dependent enzyme complexes is shown schematically assembled on a phospholipid surface. The cofactors tissue factor (TF), activated factors VIII (FVIIIa), V (FVa) and thrombomodulin (TM) are each associated with a serine protease FVIIa, FIXa, FXa and thrombin (FIIa). The substrates of the complexes {FIX, FX, prothrombin (FII)} are also shown. The reactants and products associated with each reaction complex are indicated. APC, activated protein C. (Reproduced with permission from Mann KG, Lorand L. 1993.)

sic Xase (FIXa–FVIIIa) and prothrombinase (FXa–FVa) complexes, and the latter converts prothrombin to thrombin. The separation of the cascade into *intrinsic* and *extrinsic* components is useful for understanding the coagulation screening tests, but these terms are misleading. For example, the main stimulus for the *intrinsic* pathway is collagen, and TF or procoagulants enter the circulation.

Final common pathway

Factor Xa converts factor II (prothrombin) to IIa (thrombin) in a reaction that requires calcium and activated platelet membranes with factor V as an accelerator. Thrombin then converts fibrinogen to fibrin, which polymerizes and consolidates unstable primary platelet plugs into solid aggregates. Subsequent clot retraction helps to oppose damaged edges of endothelium. Thrombin, a focal point of coagulation, has several actions, including platelet aggregation and autostimulation by activating the intrinsic pathway. Thrombin activity is regulated by a number of mechanisms, antithrombin III being the main inhibitor.

The inhibitor system

Natural anticoagulants limit and localize clots to the site of injury. As well as being important in coagulation, thrombin also initiates anticoagulation and self-downregulates by forming a complex with vascular thrombomodulin. This complex activates the plasma zymogen protein C, and this activated form (APC) inhibits coagulation by proteolysis of cofactors Va and VIIIa. Protein S binds to protein C at the platelet surface acting as a cofactor (Figure 3.2.5). Receptors for thrombomodulin and protein C or activated protein C on vascular endothelium may be important in enhancing local anticoagulation.

Antithrombin III inactivates thrombin and the other serine proteases (XIIa, XIa, Xa, IXa) by irreversible binding. This inactivation is relatively slow, but when heparin binds to antithrombin, a conformational change in the latter immediately inactivates thrombin. Other thrombin inactivators exist but are less important physiologically.

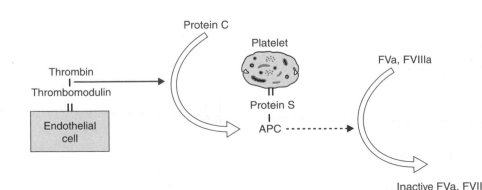

Figure 3.2.5 Protein C anticoagulant system. Thrombin bound to thrombomodulin on the endothelial surface activates protein C, which inactivates factors Va and VIIIa. APC, activated protein C.

FIBRINOLYSIS

The fibrinolytic system, which is also activated by vessel injury, is necessary to remove fibrin, and its impairment can be catastrophic, with haemorrhage and/or thrombosis. Components include plasminogen, tissue plasminogen activator (t-PA), anti-activators and fibrin degradation products (Figure 3.2.6). The most important component is plasmin, which is activated from the inactive precursor plasminogen. This activation can proceed from either the tissues (*extrinsic*) or the vessel wall (*intrinsic*), but mainly follows the release of t-PA from endothelium where it is produced and stored. Any t-PA leaking into plasma is quickly cleared by the liver, or inactivated by plasminogen activator inhibitor-1.

Venous occlusion, strenuous exercise, thrombin, adrenalin, vasopressin and analogues, e.g. synthetic 1-deamino-8-D-arginine vasopressin (DDAVP), markedly increase t-PA release. Its activity on plasminogen is negligible until it is fibrin bound, and it is then greatly potentiated. This effect is further enhanced by plasmin itself, which cleaves t-PA, allowing it to complex with plasminogen and fibrinogen more readily. This fibrin dependence strongly localizes t-PA plasmin generation to the clot. Circulating plasmin is inactivated by α2-antiplasmin and α2-macroglobulin, preventing widespread destruction of fibrinogen and other coagulation factors. Activated protein C stimulates fibrinolysis by destroying t-PA inhibitors. Recombinant t-PA is used for thrombolytic therapy, as are other fibrinolytic agents that convert plasminogen to plasmin (urokinase, produced mainly in the kidney, and streptokinase, a product of haemolytic streptococci).

Plasmin digests fibrinogen, fibrin, factor V, factor VIII and other proteins. Its activity can be inhibited by the antifibrinolytic agents, aminocaproic acid and tranexamic acid which block the plasminogen-binding sites. Cleavage of fibrin and fibrinogen produces a variety of degradation products. The largest of these, X, released from early digestion, retains thrombin-susceptible sites and is thus a competitive inhibitor of thrombin. A later smaller digestion fragment, Y, inhibits fibrin polymerization. Large amounts of the smallest fragments, D and E are detected in the plasma in disseminated intravascular coagulation.

SURGICAL BLEEDING RISK ASSESSMENT

The most important aspect of the assessment of surgical bleeding risk is an *accurate history* (Box 3.2.1). Patients with no suggestion of abnormal bleeding on history or physical examination are at low risk of having a significant coagulopathy. Laboratory tests are then generally not needed. With unreliable or incomplete histories or a suggestion of abnormal bleeding, a coagulation screen is recommended, including prothrombin time, activated partial thromboplastin time and a platelet count. Routine tests, which have been shown to be of no benefit in *healthy* people, are still requested by many surgeons before elective surgery, including tests in healthy children.

The *bleeding time* (BT) is used to screen for platelet dysfunction, e.g. von Willebrand disease and uraemia. However, the test has many inherent problems, the skin BT does not necessarily correlate with bleeding elsewhere, and there is no data currently available to prove that it predicts surgical bleeding. Dialysis, platelet or red-cell transfusions (or erythropoietin) and intravenous DDAVP can improve the BT in uraemia, but controlled studies are lacking. Until data is available to show that patients with prolonged BT have increased bleeding, correction of the BT should not be regarded as validated medical therapy. Similarly, the prediction of surgical bleeding from *in-vitro* platelet functional tests (replacing BTs in some laboratories) is not yet known.

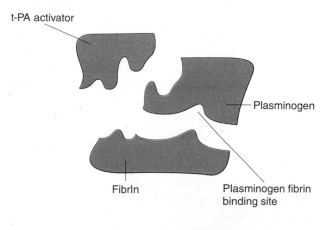

t-PA activator

Plasminogen

Fibrin

Plasminogen fibrin binding site

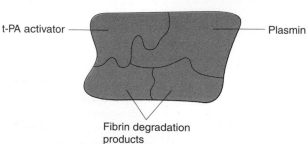

t-PA activator

Plasmin

Fibrin degradation products

Figure 3.2.6 Activation of fibrinolysis: the binding of plasminogen to fibrin permits the formation of the active form, plasmin. Plasmin degrades fibrin into degradation products.

BOX 3.2.1 PRE-OPERATIVE ASSESSMENT OF A BLEEDING RISK

History

- Previous surgery or dental bleeding; transfusions
- Easy bruising, bleeding after trauma, spontaneous haemorrhage (epistaxis, haemarthrosis), menorrhagia, obstetric bleeding
- Concurrent illnesses; renal, liver or myeloproliferative disorders
- Family history; medication, especially warfarin, aspirin
- Abnormal blood count

Examination Bruises, splenomegaly, liver disease, lymphadenopathy, joint deformities, rectal exam

Laboratory tests – use selectively

Level 1. Negative history, minor operation: no tests needed

Level 2. Negative history, major operation: routine coagulation screen:

- platelet count, prothrombin ratio (PR or INR), activated partial thromboplastin time (APTT)
- fibrinogen level or thrombin clotting time

Level 3. Suspicious history and/or major operation with major effect on haemostasis, e.g. cardiopulmonary bypass, neurosurgery:

- bleeding time (BT) and/or platelet function tests (see text)
- *special* coagulation tests*: factor assays, von Willebrand screen
- *miscellaneous*: renal, liver functions

---

*Reserve for those with a significant history and/or abnormality on routine coagulation screening.

DISORDERS OF HAEMOSTASIS RELEVANT TO SURGERY

INCREASED VASCULAR FRAGILITY (NON-THROMBOCYTOPENIC PURPURAS)

Manifestations Bleeding with normal platelet count, bleeding time and other screening tests – seldom serious, more likely to have ecchymoses, dependent petechiae, gum bleeding, gastrointestinal bleeds.

Causes Infections (e.g. meningococcal and subacute bacterial endocarditis which damage the endothelium), collagen problems (scurvy, Ehlers-Danlos syndrome), hereditary haemorrhagic telangiectasia, amyloidosis.

PLATELET DEFICIENCY (THROMBOCYTOPENIA)

Manifestations Immediate bleeding after trauma, increased risk of incisional bleeding when $< 80 \times 10^9$/L, increasing with lower counts, ecchymoses or bleeding from pathological sites, e.g. gastric ulcer, surgical wound $< 40 \times 10^9$/L; spontaneous bleeding $< 20 \times 10^9$/L (skin, epistaxis, gum bleeding, menorrhagia, CNS).

Causes Decreased production occurs in marrow diseases, AIDS, megaloblastosis, congenital causes, sepsis, drug reactions (e.g. chemotherapy) or idiosyncratic reactions (most commonly ethanol, quinine, thiazides). Increased destruction is caused by massive blood loss, disseminated intravascular coagulation (DIC), hypersplenism, auto-immune (idiopathic thrombocytopenia purpura, systemic lupus erythematosus), iso-immune disorders (post transfusion, fetal–maternal incompatibility), thrombotic thrombocytopenia purpura, haemolytic uraemic syndrome, haemangiomas.

PLATELET DYSFUNCTION

Manifestations Similar to but less severe bleeding than occurs with thrombocytopenia.

Causes Congenital disorders, uraemia, myeloproliferative disorders, aspirin and acquired storage pool disease (platelet release during cardiopulmonary bypass) and severe vasculitis resulting in non-functional platelets.

COAGULATION FACTOR DEFICIENCIES

Manifestations Deep muscle haematomas, as well as ecchymoses. Spontaneous haemarthroses usually occur only in severe haemophilia.

Causes Inherited factor deficiencies; antibody mediated (rare).

OTHER HAEMOSTATIC DEFECTS RELEVANT TO SURGERY

Disseminated intravascular coagulation (DIC) Increased clotting from tissue factor release into the blood (obstetric catastrophe, placental abruption), tissue injury (burns, surgery, trauma), malignancies (acute promyelocytic leukaemia, mucous adenocarcinoma, tumours of the pancreas and prostate), sepsis or endothelial damage (vasculitis – malignant hypertension, meningococcal or rickettsial disease), giant haemangiomas, and subsequent bleeding.

Manifestations If fibrin formation is severe, multiple organ failure can occur. The consumption of platelets, fibrinogen and factor VIII can result in bleeding, with activation of fibrinolysis as a secondary event. Intravascular fibrin damages erythrocytes, producing micro-angiopathic haemolytic anaemia. Therapy is aimed at treating the underlying disease. Consider the judicious use of low-dose heparin for thrombosis, with the addition of appropriate clotting factors if there is bleeding, although the latter should not normally be used without heparin.

Massive transfusion Platelet and coagulation factor loss, especially fibrinogen. Monitor haemostasis to allow specific replacement as needed: platelets, plasma, cryoprecipitate (best source of fibrinogen).

Vitamin K deficiency Acquired bleeding tendency.

1. *Diagnosis:* Prolonged prothrombin time (PT) and activated partial thromboplastin time (APTT) with normal thrombin time, non-correction *in vitro* with protamine, normal platelet count and normal Echis ratio.

2. *Causes:* Malabsorption (α1-antitrypsin deficiency, bile duct atresia, abeta-lipoproteinaemia, coeliac disease, chronic diarrhoea, cystic fibrosis, cholestasis), fasting, alcoholism, drugs (cephalosporins, β-lactams, vitamin E, salicylates).

Liver disease Bleeding in advanced disease is common due to oesophageal varices. Any part of haemostasis can be abnormal, including the following: impaired clotting from decreased synthesis of clotting factors, vitamin K deficiency; thrombocytopenia from hypersplenism, reduced thrombopoietin production; platelet function defects from impaired clearance of inhibitors; DIC from procoagulants from liver cells, endotoxins, reduced antithrombin III, protein C and clearance of activated factors; systemic fibrinolysis from reduced α2-antiplasmin and clearance fibrinolytic enzymes.

Aspirin Even at low doses, aspirin causes a mild bleeding tendency by irreversibly acetylating the enzyme cyclo-oxygenase which is involved in platelet aggregation. An effect may remain for the life of the platelet (7–10 days), although a major effect only persists for 3–5 days. Aspirin alone does not usually cause significant bleeding, but may aggravate coagulopathies, e.g. von Willebrand disease (vWD) or thrombocytopenia.

INCREASED THROMBO-EMBOLIC RISK IN THE SURGICAL PATIENT, AND RECOMMENDATIONS FOR PREVENTION AND TREATMENT

Patients undergoing major trauma or surgery, especially orthopaedic or abdominal surgery (Figure 3.2.7) have a high thrombosis risk due to the sustained activation of coagulation from vascular damage, aggravated by other factors, including immobility and activation of acute-phase reactants, especially fibrinogen (Box 3.2.2). *Thrombophilia* refers to familial or acquired disorders that promote thrombosis, and these usually increase the surgical risk. Deep vein thrombosis (DVT) in the lower limbs and superficial thrombophlebitis are the commonest primary events – subsequent pulmonary emboli are potentially life-threatening. Visceral, cerebral and upper limb venous thrombi are more rare.

ACQUIRED THROMBOTIC RISK FACTORS

Cancer is associated with increased venous and arterial thromboses. A low-grade DIC is often responsible, activated by a unique procoagulant or tissue factor. *Haematological disorders*, e.g. *polycythaemia vera* and *paroxysmal nocturnal haemoglobinuria*, have increased thromboses from abnormal platelets and/or hyperviscosity. Venous thrombosis may occur in unusual sites, such as the mesenteric or hepatic veins. Arterial thrombosis may manifest as large-vessel occlusions (stroke, myocardial infarction) or as microvascular events with painful burning in the peripheries. *Autoimmune haemolytic anaemia, lupus anticoagulant, anticardiolipin*

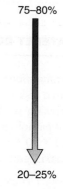

Spinal cord injury
Knee arthroplasty
Leg amputation
Hip fracture surgery
Hip arthroplasty
Lower limb fracture
Open prostatectomy
General abdominal surgery
Gynaecological surgery
Kidney transplantation
Non-cardiac thoracic surgery
Neurosurgery
Open meniscectomy

75–80%

20–25%

Figure 3.2.7 Risk groups in trauma and surgery in order of decreasing frequency of DVT without coagulation prophylaxis.

BOX 3.2.2 RISK FACTORS FOR SURGICAL THROMBO-EMBOLISM

- **Personal characteristics:** Age 40–60 years; 61–70 years (2 factors); . 70 (3 factors); obesity; pregnancy or post partum , 1 month

- **Past history:** Previous major surgery, past deep vein thrombosis or pulmonary embolism (3 factors); familial thrombophilia

- **Physical:** Trauma; immobilization (previous or present duration > 72 h); confining air or car travel (> 4 h within week of admission)

- **Surgical:** Elective operation . 2 h duration; major surgery especially coronary artery bypass grafting, renal transplant, splenectomy; laparoscopic surgery with pneumo-peritoneum

- **Coexistent pathology:** Malignancy (especially breast, uterus, bowel, lung, pancreas); blood disorders and acquired hypercoagulability states including lupus anti-coagulant/anti-phospholipid syndrome; myocardial infarction, congestive heart disease; severe pulmonary disease; inflammatory bowel disease; pelvic or long bone fracture, leg ulcer, oedema, stasis and/or varicose veins; severe sepsis

- **Treatment related:** Crystalloid IV infusion (. 0.5 L/24 h); central venous access; high-dose oestrogens

---

and the *antiphospholipid syndrome* are other disorders with increased thromboses. Delay surgery until disease control is achieved (if possible), and administer prophylactic anticoagulants. Other risk factors are listed in Box 3.2.2 and anticlotting prophylaxis is listed in Box 3.2.3.

Standard heparin (UFH) causes heparin-induced thrombocytopenia (HIT) in up to 10% of patients treated for a week or longer (there is a lower incidence with low-molecular-weight heparins). In a small number of these, severe thrombocytopenia occurs with a high incidence of arterial thrombosis, often in large vessels, e.g. iliac artery, aorta. Heparin-specific IgG antibodies bind to platelets, triggering aggregation and thrombocytopenia. Platelets must be monitored in heparin therapy lasting more than 5 days, and if the platelet count is $< 100 \times 10^9$/L with heparin-induced antibodies present, heparin must be discontinued, as ongoing therapy is often fatal. HIT is usually treated with danaparoid (dermatan, heparan and chondroitin sulphates).

BOX 3.2.3 RECOMMENDED ANTICLOTTING PROPHYLAXIS FOR SURGICAL PATIENTS

Effective prophylactic measures are available for patients at increased thrombotic risk during surgery

Low Risk (1 factor)

- early ambulation or gradient compression stockings (GCS) (optional)

Higher risk (> 2 factors)

- early ambulation, GCS, intermittent pneumatic compression, prophylactic anticoagulation

---

FAMILIAL CAUSES INCREASING SURGICALLY RELATED THROMBO-EMBOLISM

One or more biochemical defects may be identified in up to 60% of confirmed DVTs. A thrombophilia screen should be undertaken in young patients with unexpected thrombosis and in others with a family history of thrombosis. In hereditary forms, the first thrombosis often occurs between 15 and 40 years, precipitated in about 50% of cases by an event such as surgery or pregnancy. The commonest disorder (c. 40%) is a mutation of the factor V molecule (factor V Leiden), which renders it resistant to degradation by activated protein C (APC resistance). However, there are no data demonstrating an increased surgical thrombotic risk in this disorder. Deficiencies of protein C or protein S account for about 10% of hereditary thrombophilia. Rarer conditions include fibrinogen mutations (1%), plasminogen (1–2%) and antithrombin III deficiency (5%). The latter may also be acquired (heparin, DIC, thrombosis, liver disease, surgery, pregnancy, nephrotic syndrome). The familial thrombophilias described more recently include a prothrombin 20210A allele (increased DVTs) and hyperhomocystinaemia (arterial and venous thromboses).

By the age of 45 years, thrombosis has occurred in approximately 50% of those with protein C or S deficiency. (Other causes of low levels include extensive thrombosis, inflammation, pregnancy, liver disease, DIC, vitamin K deficiency and warfarin.) Double heterozygotes for protein S and factor V Leiden have a 70% risk of thrombosis, and any combination of familial defects increases the risk. Moreover, there is increased thrombosis from interactions between inherited risks (e.g. the prothrombin mutation) and acquired risks (e.g. contraceptives).

HEPARINS: MODE OF ACTION

Low-molecular-weight heparins (LMWHs) are now replacing standard unfractionated heparin (UFH). Causing a configurational change in antithrombin III, heparin's interaction with thrombin and activated factor X (factor Xa) is accelerated by about 1000-fold. Unlike UFH, which has equivalent activity against Xa and thrombin, the main activity of LMWHs is against Xa (100%, compared to about 30% with UFH). With less binding to plasma proteins (including acute-phase reactants), endothelium and macrophages, LMWHs provide more predictable anticoagulation, better bioavailability, and a dose-independent clearance mechanism; their half-life is 2–4 times that of UFH, ranging from 2 to 4 h after intravenous injection and from 3 to 6 h after subcutaneous injection. Laboratory monitoring (anti-Xa levels) is unnecessary except in cases of renal failure (creatinine > 0.30 mmol/L), body weight > 100 kg, pregnancy or significant bleeding. About 50% of cases with DVTs can be treated safely with LMWHs as out-patients, with the advantages of reduced monitoring, subcutaneous injections and the lower risk of HIT.

RECOMMENDED ANTICOAGULANT PROPHYLAXIS FOR HIGH-RISK SURGICAL PROCEDURES (TABLE 3.2.1)

General surgery

Low-dose UFH (5000 U administered subcutaneously 2 h before surgery and every 8 to 12 h post-operatively) provides safe, effective prophylaxis, reducing the risk of DVT and fatal pulmonary embolism by 70% and 50%, respectively, with minimal bleeding. Like UFH, LMWHs are also given subcutaneously 2 to 12 h before surgery, but only once daily post-operatively. LMWHs are marginally more effective than low-dose UFH in preventing thrombo-embolism, with fewer wound and injection site haematomas, less HIT and less monitoring required.

Lower limb orthopaedic surgery

DVTs occur in total hip replacements and hip fracture surgery (50–70% without prophylaxis). LMWHs are safe and effective in reducing DVTs (range of risk reduction, 31–79%) without increasing bleeding. LMWHs have a small advantage over warfarin and UFH. A recent trial suggests that recombinant hirudin, a thrombin-specific inhibitor, is more effective than enoxaparin.

Total knee replacement

In six trials LMWHs were found to be superior to warfarin, although the DVT incidence remained high (25–30%, 25% of which were proximal). Give LMWH more than 12 h post-operatively in order to minimize bleeding.

Hip fracture surgery

Low-dose UFH, LMWH and warfarin all reduce DVTs by 45%. Treatment with LMWH should be started pre-operatively if a delay in surgery is expected. Warfarin is less effective because surgical times are difficult to predict.

Acute spinal cord injury

DVT and pulmonary embolism may occur in 14.5% and 4.6% of cases, respectively, during the first fortnight after injury, with a cumulative risk of up to 40%. Two small trials suggest that LMWHs are effective. Intermittent pneumatic compression combined with low-dose UFH and elastic stockings also appear to be effective prophylaxis.

Multiple trauma

A randomized study of major trauma patients with no intracranial bleeding compared low-dose UFH with LMWH starting within 36 h after the injury. LMWH reduced DVTs from 44% to 31%, and reduced proximal thromboses from 15% to 6%. Major bleeding occurred in six cases (1.7%), five treated with LMWH.

Femoropopliteal bypass grafts

A study showed that 1-year graft survival was significantly better with LMWH (78%) than with aspirin and dipyridamole (64%).

WARFARIN TREATMENT

Warfarin is monitored with the prothrombin time (PT), which responds to reduced levels of vitamin K-dependent clotting factors II, VII and X. The PT is converted into an international normalized ratio (INR) from the international sensitivity index of the laboratory reagent. This inter-laboratory standardization allows patients to be monitored at any laboratory. During the first 48 h of treatment, anticoagulation is mainly due to reduced factor VII (half-life 6 h). Because the half-life of vitamin K-dependent protein C is similar, the anticoagulation can be counteracted by a procoagulant effect (from the reduced protein C). In contrast, warfarin's *antithrombotic* effect (caused mainly by a reduced factor II) is delayed by as long as 60 h. This provides the rationale for administering heparin and warfarin concurrently for 5 days, stopping heparin when the INR is therapeutic for 2 consecutive days. The use of a 5-mg loading dose of warfarin may be better than 10 mg, avoiding the

Table 3.2.1 Advantages of low-molecular-weight heparins and recommended doses for the prevention and treatment of thrombosis

Indication	Advantages of LMWH	Recommended doses*
Prevention General surgery	At least as effective as low-dose UFH but can be given once daily and causes fewer haematomas at injection sites	*Low risk†:* Dalteparin, 2500 U 1–2 h before and once daily after surgery Enoxaparin, 2000 U 1–2 h before and once daily after surgery Nadroparin, 3100 U 2 h before and once daily after surgery Tinzaparin, 3500 U 2 h before and once daily after surgery *High risk†:* Dalteparin, 5000 U 10–12 h before and once daily after surgery Enoxaparin, 4000 U 10–12 h before and once daily after surgery
Orthopaedic surgery	More effective than low-dose UFH; more effective than warfarin in total knee joint replacement, and monitoring is usually not necessary. Hirudin may be more effective than enoxaparin in total hip joint replacement	Ardeparin, 50 U/kg twice daily starting 12–24 h after surgery Dalteparin, 5000 U 8–12 h before and once daily, starting 12 h after surgery Enoxaparin, 3000 U twice daily starting 12–24 h after surgery, or 4000 U once daily starting 10–12 h before surgery Nadroparin, 40 U/kg starting 2 h before surgery and once daily after surgery for 3 days; the dose is then increased to 60 U/kg once daily Tinzaparin, 50 U /kg 2 h before and once daily after surgery, or 75 U/kg once daily starting 12–24 h after surgery
Acute spinal injury	Apparently effective, whereas low-dose UFH heparin is not, and higher doses of UFH cause excessive bleeding	Enoxaparin, 3000 U twice daily
Multiple trauma	More effective than low-dose UFH	Enoxaparin, 3000 U twice daily
Medical conditions	As effective as low-dose UFH, but can be given once daily	Dalteparin, 2500 U once daily Enoxaparin, 2000 U twice daily
Treatment Venous thromboembolism	At least as safe and effective as UFH, but can be given subcutaneously without laboratory monitoring, thereby allowing home therapy	Dalteparin, 100 U/kg twice daily Enoxaparin, 100 U/kg twice daily Nadroparin, 90 U/kg twice daily Tinzaparin, 175 U/kg once daily

*Doses in anti-FXa units. The prophylactic doses for each LMWH are slightly different (lower doses for low-risk general surgical or medical patients and higher doses for high-risk general or orthopaedic surgical patients). Higher doses started pre-operatively are given 10–12 h before surgery to avoid excessive bleeding. Lower doses of LMWH can be given 1–2 h pre-operatively. The doses for treating venous thromboembolism are higher than those for prophylaxis, with similar regimens for each LMWH.
† Low risk: uncomplicated abdominal or pelvic surgery lasting 30 minutes or more.
High risk: abdominal or pelvic surgery for cancer or in those with previous venous thromboembolism.
(Adapted from Weitz JI. 1997.)

hypercoagulability from the rapid fall in protein C and an excessive bleeding risk in high-risk patients.

SURGICAL PROCEDURES IN PATIENTS ON ANTICOAGULANTS

Anticoagulated patients are managed in the context of current doses with laboratory testing, treatment cessation and reversal of the coagulopathy where appropriate,

depending on the clinical problem, the urgency and type of surgery. It should also be considered whether the anticoagulant is responsible for some or all of the presenting problem(s). For patients on *warfarin*, minor procedures can be performed safely by allowing the INR to drift towards normal (e.g. < 1.5) with subsequent replacement of missing doses. For major procedures, warfarin should be stopped 4–7 days before surgery (some studies suggest that warfarin pretreatment may be beneficial in cardiac surgery) and patients with a high thrombotic risk should receive heparin in the interim. High-dose LMWH should not be given within 12 h and UFH within 4 h of major elective surgery. LMWH should not be given within 24 h of cardiac surgery. In emergencies, reversal of *heparin* anticoagulation may be necessary using protamine for LMWH and UFH, and vitamin K_1 and/or plasma (start with 2 U) or prothrombinex (50 IU of factor IX/kg body weight) for warfarin. If warfarin is to be stopped, 5–10 mg of vitamin K_1 can be given, but this dose causes warfarin resistance for 7–14 days; if warfarin is to continue, give only 1–2 mg. After vitamin K_1 has been administered, the maximal effect occurs at 24 h, with a partial response usually occurring after 8 h. With plasma or factor concentrates the anticoagulant effect starts immediately, and then declines over 24 h. Recheck the INR and give further plasma or factor concentrates if required. The latter are more effective in achieving adequate levels of factor IX, and should be used in orally anticoagulated patients with life-threatening haemorrhage. *Aspirin* should be stopped 3–4 days before surgery where normal haemostasis is important (e.g. CNS, ophthalmic surgery). If the proposed operation is urgent, transfusion of platelets may be effective when the last aspirin dose has cleared from the circulation (< 90 min), or the surgeon may operate anyway, relying on meticulous surgical haemostasis.

ANTIFIBRINOLYTIC AGENTS

Aminocaproic acid (EACA) and tranexamic acid (TA) both inhibit fibrinolysis by blocking the plasminogen fibrin binding sites and preventing plasmin formation (Table 3.2.2).

Table 3.2.2 Recommended dosage and administration of antifibrinolytic agents

	Loading dose	Maintenance dose
EACA	100 mg/kg IV or PO	500–1000 mg/h IV or PO
Tranexamic acid	10 mg/kg IV	10 mg/kg IV q 6–8 h 25 mg/kg PO q 6–8 h

CLINICAL USE OF ANTIFIBRINOLYTIC AGENTS IN SURGERY

Antifibrinolytic agents (AFAs) stop or prevent bleeding by blocking systemic and/or local fibrinolysis at sites of vascular injury.

Treatment to block systemic fibrinolysis

1. *Bleeding after thrombolysis*: Occasionally warranted for acute catastrophic bleeding, particularly if surgery is immediate, but seldom needed because thrombolytic agents have a short half-life (< 30 min). Persistent bleeding is likely to be due to clotting factor depletion, platelet function defects or structural lesions rather than to systemic fibrinolysis.

2. *Rare catastrophic events associated with systemic fibrinolysis*: Examples include amniotic fluid embolism and heat stroke.

3. *Bleeding after cardiopulmonary bypass*: AFAs effectively reduce bleeding in cardiopulmonary bypass, and are commonly used in prolonged surgical procedures or in those who bleed following bypass termination (bleeding in this setting can also be due to platelet dysfunction).

Inhibition of Local Fibrinolysis

Local fibrinolysis, a normal slow response to thrombosis, usually occurs without haemorrhage at the site of vascular injury. However, if there is a coexisting coagulopathy (e.g. haemophilia) or excessive local fibrinolysis, surgical bleeding can persist. Systemic AFAs or local application can block local fibrinolysis.

1. *Oral and upper respiratory tract bleeding:* Oral EACA can substitute for clotting factor infusions in children and adults who are undergoing dental extractions. Topical TA has been successfully used for dental surgery in patients with artificial cardiac valves on warfarin. EACA and TA can control nasal and oral bleeding in patients with coagulopathies, as in myelodysplasia.

2. *Gastrointestinal haemorrhage*: AFAs are ineffective in massive bleeding, but they may control chronic oozing in patients with coagulopathies, or in those who are not surgical candidates. Use AFAs carefully in inflammatory bowel disease (thrombosis risk already increased).

3. *Uterine bleeding*: After standard approaches, AFAs may be useful in refractory menorrhagia, excessive bleeding after cone biopsy, or haemorrhage secondary to intrauterine contraceptive devices.

4. *Haematuria*: Avoid AFAs in upper urinary tract bleeding (risk of potential ureteric clotting). Severe prostatic bleeding can be treated effectively, and in trials AFAs reduced bleeding by approximately 50%.

FURTHER READING

Davie EW, Fujikawa K, Kisiel W. 1991: The coagulation cascade: initiation, maintenance, and regulation. *Biochemistry* **30**, 10363–70.

De Stefano V, Finazzi G, Mannucci PM. 1996: Inherited thrombophilia: pathogenesis, clinical syndromes and management. *Blood* **87**, 3531–44.

Erikkson BI, Wille-Jorgensen P, Kalebo P *et al.* 1997: A comparison of recombinant hirudin with a low-molecular-weight heparin to prevent thrombo-embolic complications after total hip replacement. *New England Journal of Medicine* **337**, 1329–35.

Goldhaber S. 1994: Epidemiology of pulmonary embolism and deep vein thrombosis. In Bloom AL, Forbes CD, Thomas DP, Tuddenham EGD (eds), *Haemostasis and thrombosis*, 3rd edn. Edinburgh: Churchill Livingstone, 1327–33.

Harrison L, Johnston M, Massicotte P, Crowther M, Moffat K, Hirsh J. 1997: Comparison of 5-mg and 10-mg loading doses in initiation of warfarin therapy. *Annals of Internal Medicine* **6**, 133–6.

Lind SE. 1991: The bleeding time does not predict surgical bleeding. *Blood* **77**, 2547–52.

Mann KG, Lorand L. 1993: Introduction: blood coagulation. *Methods in Enzymology* **222**, 1–10.

Mannucci PM. 1998: Haemostatic drugs. *New England Journal of Medicine* **339**, 245–53.

Messmore HL, Godwin MJ. 1994: Medical assessment of bleeding in the surgical patient. *Medical Clinics of North America* **78**, 625.

Patel RI, De Witt L, Hannallah RS. 1997: Preoperative laboratory testing in children undergoing elective surgery. *Journal of Clincal Anesthesia* **9**, 569–75.

Sindet-Perdersen S, Ramstrom G, Bernvil S, Blomback M. 1989: Haemostatic effect of tranexamic acid mouthwash in anticoagulant-treated patients undergoing oral surgery. *New England Journal of Medicine* **320**, 840–3.

Weitz JI. 1997: Low-molecular-weight heparins. *New England Journal of Medicine* **337**, 688–98.

Epistaxis

Bren Dorman

Introduction

Most patients who develop bleeding from the nose are able to deal with the problem without medical intervention. This chapter outlines the evaluation, investigations and management of those patients who need or seek further help in controlling their nasal bleeding problem. Epistaxis can be minor and merely a nuisance, but it can also be severe, and if not managed correctly may also result in life-threatening cardiorespiratory changes.

EPIDEMIOLOGY

Anterior epistaxis is more common in children and posterior epistaxis is more common in the older patient. There are often seasonal fluctuations, with a higher incidence in the winter. This may be related to the higher incidence of upper respiratory tract infections at this time, as well as greater temperature variations. The presence of infection or tumours in the nose and sinuses, nasal or facial trauma and foreign bodies in the nose can all cause epistaxis. Inherited conditions such as hereditary haemorrhagic telangiectasia involving a lack of contractile elements in the vessel walls can lead to significant bleeding and prove difficult to control. Some systemic disorders and diseases result in blood dyscrasias and subsequent coagulopathy which can lead to epistaxis. The history should identify those patients who are on medication that may affect blood clotting or platelet function.

Common presentations for epistaxis include the following:

Intermittent epistaxis in a child or adult This may resolve spontaneously or with local pressure. The cause may be related to digital manipulation of the anterior nose or it may be truly spontaneous. The commonest area of involvement is the anterior inferior aspect of the septum where there is a plexus of vessels in the mucosa (Little's area). Bleeding can occur when the patient becomes hot during exercise or physical work. Dryness of the mucosa with crusting can also be a factor.

Significant epistaxis in an older patient This may be spontaneous, but it also occurs as a result of local trauma, e.g. a fall. There can be significant blood loss and it may be difficult to control. Some older patients are on aspirin and others are on anticoagulants, so enquiry about medication is important. The bleeding site can be variable, being located either anteriorly on the septum or posteriorly on the lateral nasal wall near the posterior aspect of the middle turbinate. Posterior bleeding is often more difficult to identify and control. Many older patients are hypertensive and, although this can result in a greater and more prolonged epistaxis, it is not the cause of it.

Epistaxis following trauma (e.g. in contact sport, a road traffic accident, a fall or following an assault) Usually local pressure and ice have been applied to the nose at the time. One should be aware of the possibility of nasal and even facial fractures in these patients.

Epistaxis following nasal surgery Depending on the complexity and nature of the surgery, the bleeding that may occur can be severe. Septal surgery and, in particular, turbinate surgery can result in arterial haemorrhage that can be very frightening to the patient and a challenge to control. The bleeding may occur immediately following the procedure, or about 7–10 days later. In the latter situation it is likely that there has been some infection in the nose. Bleeding can also occur from the margins of a septal perforation which may have developed from previous nasal surgery, or from chronic decongestant or cocaine use.

VASCULAR ANATOMY

The blood supply to the nose and sinuses is from branches of the external and internal carotid arteries.

The external carotid artery branches that are of importance to the nose are the maxillary artery (with its terminal branch, the sphenopalatine artery, entering the nose through the foramen at the posterior end of the middle turbinate) and the facial artery (with its superior labial branch). The internal carotid artery branch of importance is the ophthalmic artery which supplies the nose via the anterior and posterior ethmoidal arteries.

The lateral nasal wall is supplied by the lateral branches of the anterior and posterior ethmoidal arteries, the lateral branch of the sphenopalatine artery and the greater palatine artery (Figure 3.3.1).

The septum is supplied by the septal branches of the anterior and posterior ethmoidal arteries, the septal branches of the sphenopalatine artery, the greater palatine artery and the septal branches of the superior labial artery (Figure 3.3.2).

Little's area is located in the anterior inferior septum where there is a confluence of the terminal branches of the anterior ethmoidal, sphenopalatine and superior labial arteries called Kiesselbach's plexus. This is the site of most anterior nosebleeds, representing about 90% of all epistaxis.

MANAGEMENT STRATEGIES

This section outlines the management of epistaxis in those patients who present to a medical practitioner for help in controlling the bleeding. This may be as a primary care situation or in a hospital or clinic environment. The immediate steps in management of acute epistaxis are discussed first, and attention is then focused on the investigations required to attempt to determine the underlying cause of the bleeding. Chronic intermittent epistaxis is not usually so urgent, and can be investigated and managed on an out-patient basis.

Management depends on the following.

- *Disease factors*: the severity of the bleeding, the need for resuscitation, the nature of the onset of the bleeding (spontaneous or trauma related), and the presence of associated conditions such as nasal or facial injuries.

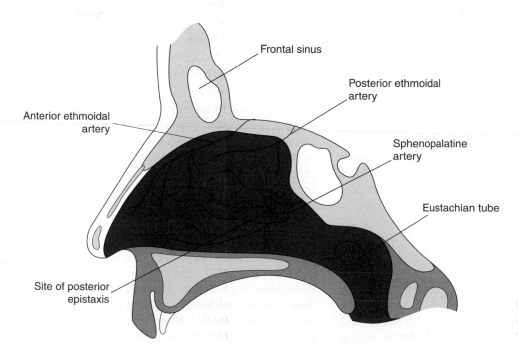

Figure 3.3.1 Vascular supply to the lateral wall of the nose.

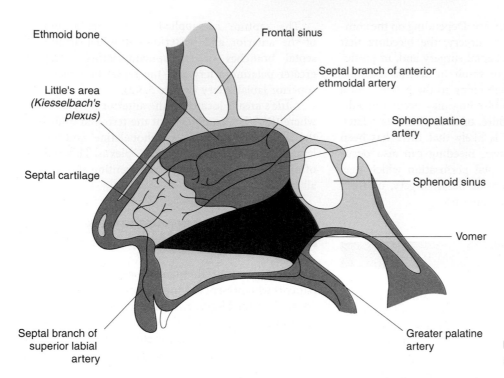

Figure 3.3.2 Vascular supply to the septum.

- *Patient factors*: the age of the patient, their social circumstances, the presence of any known underlying medical conditions, and the type of medication that the patient is taking.

- *Logistic factors*: the availability of medical expertise and equipment, and the proximity of in-patient care.

ACUTE EPISTAXIS

The acute management of epistaxis may be carried out by a variety of people, especially in the trauma situation or in the case of a minor bleed at home. This section looks at the management carried out by medical staff in an accident and emergency department, in an out-patient clinic or as an in-patient in hospital. Equipment requirements include a headlight (so that both hands are free to examine the nose and deal with the bleeding), an assistant (usually the clinic nurse), appropriate instruments to examine the nose, local anaesthetic (both topical and injectable), a satisfactory nasal suction, and a range of nasal packing materials.

Flexible and rigid nasal endoscopes are excellent for examination of the nose and nasopharynx when searching for the site of the bleeding, but these are usually only available in the otolaryngology clinic.

The technique for dealing with the bleeding is described below.

Intermittent spontaneous epistaxis in a child or adult This is usually a chronic intermittent problem that is

annoying to the patient and from time to time can be quite distressing. It is best evaluated in an out-patient environment where a thorough examination can be carried out with nasal application of local anaesthetic followed by chemical or electrocautery of the bleeding site. If there is crusting and drying of the nasal mucosa, then application of an antibiotic ointment to the area can help to prevent recurrence.

Significant epistaxis in an older patient Some assessment should be made of the amount of blood loss and whether resuscitative measures are required. An IV line should be placed in a patient with significant blood loss. It is not uncommon for elderly patients with epistaxis to have marked elevation of their blood pressure, so it may need to be lowered.

Epistaxis following trauma (e.g. in contact sport, a road traffic accident, a fall or following an assault) If the epistaxis has occurred secondarily to physical trauma in a healthy adult, then local pressure and the application of ice may control the bleeding. One should be aware of the possibility of associated nasal or facial fractures, so X-rays may be required. If there are lacerations present, then antibiotics are usually required to prevent secondary infection.

Epistaxis following nasal surgery This may be due to bleeding from the septum or from the inferior turbinates. It may occur immediately after the procedure (primary haemorrhage) or several days later (secondary haemorrhage). In the latter case antibiotics are necessary.

INITIAL MANAGEMENT

The technique for immediate management is as follows.

1. Using appropriate equipment, the nose is suctioned and the blood crusts and any fresh blood removed.

2. The nose is then packed with cotton wool or gauze soaked in a *local anaesthetic solution* (4% xylocaine and adrenalin 1:1000 in the ratio 3:1). Cocaine can be used instead.

3. After 5–10 min this pack is removed and the nose is carefully examined.

4. The use of rigid or flexible endoscopes is invaluable in these situations, as it enables close examination of the anterior and posterior areas of the septum and the lateral walls of the nose. If there is no further bleeding, then this is easily undertaken and the bleeding point may be identified.

5. The bleeding point can be cauterized with AgNO$_3$ sticks or with electrocautery. Antibiotic ointment is then applied.

6. If there is continued haemorrhage from the nose when the initial local anaesthetic pack has been removed, a further pack may be placed. Further local anaesthesia can be achieved by injecting xylocaine and adrenalin into the septum, the dorsum, the infra-orbital nerves and the greater palatine nerves.

Nasal packing is usually only required if the bleeding continues from a site despite cautery, if there is a large area that is bleeding, or if it is originating from the posterior aspect of the nose and is inaccessible to cautery. Antibiotic cover is required if packing is used, and in nearly all situations the patient is observed in hospital.

Anterior and posterior nasal packing may include ribbon gauze, a preformed nasal sponge pack or an epistaxis balloon, but other material can also be used. The pack can be inserted into the anaesthetized nose with appropriate instruments. If the anterior packing fails to control the bleeding, then a posterior pack should be considered. This is usually an inflatable balloon device which is passed into the nasopharynx, inflated and then brought forward in the nose so that the balloon fits snugly against the posterior choanae of the nose. Anterior nasal packing is then placed and the balloon is held forward with anterior traction. Some balloon devices are contoured so that anterior traction is minimal or not required at all. Posterior packs require special expertise to insert them correctly. There are various risks with the use of a posterior nasal pack, including respiratory changes, cardiac rhythm changes, avascular necrosis of the palate, otitis media, sinusitis and possibly septicaemia. The failure rate of nasal packing is estimated to be about 25%, and it carries a complication rate of over 60%.

FURTHER MANAGEMENT

In cases where the nasal packing has not controlled the epistaxis, other measures must be instigated. *Selective arterial embolization* of the maxillary artery and its terminal branches has been used successfully, but it requires an experienced radiologist to carry out the procedure. The success rate for controlling the bleeding is about 90%, with a 0.1% complication rate. The vascular anatomy is displayed by the digital subtraction angiography as part of the technique. Embolization may also be needed if the middle meningeal artery contributes to the nasal blood supply.

Ligation of the arterial branches supplying the nose may be required if there is continued bleeding despite other measures. It is not intended to devascularize the nose completely, but to drop the blood pressure enough to allow clotting and cessation of the epistaxis.

If the bleeding is from the superior or anterior aspect of the nose, then consideration should be given to *ligation of the ethmoidal arteries*. The anterior and posterior arteries should both be ligated with a suture or a vascular clip after exposing the vessels in the orbit as they cross the medial wall to enter the ethmoid sinus.

If the bleeding is from the posterior aspect of the nose, then *maxillary artery or external carotid artery ligation* should be considered. The maxillary artery can be ligated via the antrum or via the oral cavity.

Under general anaesthesia, the pterygopalatine fossa is accessed via a Caldwell-Luc procedure and removal of the posterior wall of the maxillary antrum. This exposes the third part of the maxillary artery and its branches. All of the branches should be clipped with vascular clips. Contraindications to the transantral approach include sinusitis, facial fractures, tumours and developmental abnormalities of the sinus. This approach is also not usually possible in children.

The alternative approach to the maxillary artery is intra-orally, where access is gained to the first and second parts of the maxillary artery via an incision in the gingivobuccal sulcus opposite the third molar and extending down to the ramus of the mandible. The artery is clipped once it has been visualized through the buccal fat pad and the temporalis muscle.

If these steps are not successful in controlling the bleeding, then ligation of the external carotid artery or its branches may have to be considered. The neck is explored, the external carotid artery and its branches are identified and the appropriate branches are then ligated.

INVESTIGATIONS

When the acute epistaxis has been controlled and the patient is stable, further investigations are usually required. These include a full blood count, a coagulation screen and liver function tests. More detailed investigations depend on the possible aetiology of the epistaxis. For instance, if a nasal or nasopharyngeal tumour is suspected, then CT or MRI scanning would be appropriate.

FURTHER READING

Cummings CW. 1993: *Otolaryngology – head and neck surgery*. St Louis, MO: Mosby Publishing.

Haemoptysis

Hugh Greville

Introduction

The lung is a very vascular organ and is therefore suscep-tible to bleeding. By definition, any blood coughed up from the lungs is haemoptysis and warrants serious considera-tion. The definition covers small amounts of blood, as may be seen in acute bronchitis, to massive life-threatening vol-umes of blood, as may be seen in the erosion of a pul-monary artery by a tumour. The definition of massive haemoptysis varies from author to author, ranging from 200 to 600 mL over a 24-h period. The latter figure is the one most commonly used.

ANATOMY AND PHYSIOLOGY

The lung and the airways have a dual blood supply, namely the bronchial and pulmonary systems. Anatomically, the pulmonary artery arises from the right ventricle and then bifurcates into the right and left pulmonary arteries. These main vessels then divide, and branches follow the airways accompanying them to the primary lobules. These vessels terminate in the alveolar capillary network. The pulmonary veins which drain the alveolar capillaries run in the interlobular septa, at a dis-tance from the bronchovascular bundle, before empty-ing into the left atrium. The main function of the pulmonary vascular system is to deliver the deoxygenated blood from the right ventricle to the alveolar capillaries and then to return the oxygenated blood to the left heart. It must be able to accommodate all of the cardiac output from the right heart under a range of conditions, from rest to high cardiac output states associated with exer-cise. The right heart does not need to generate such high pressures as the systemic (left) heart, as it only needs to be able to perfuse to the apex of the lung. The pul-monary artery is a low-pressure system. The lung capillar-ies are not as well supported as systemic vessels, and high pressures and high flow rates can result in damage to the alveolar capillaries.

The bronchial vascular system arises from the sys-temic circulation. There are many configurations for the bronchial circulation. The most common is for there to be one artery to the right lung and two to the left. The right bronchial artery arises from the first right inter-costal artery (the internal mammary and right subcla-vian arteries are other common origins). The two left bronchial arteries usually arise from the descending tho-racic aorta. The bronchial arteries form a network of ves-sels around the hilum with branches following the major bronchi. These vessels form a plexus around the bronchi with branches to an inner submucosal plexus. The bronchial artery capillary plexus in the region of the ter-minal bronchiole is also supplied by branches of the pul-monary artery, and this is one site where there is communication between the two circulations. From this area of the lung, the venous drainage of the bronchial artery system is through the pulmonary veins into the left atrium. In the more central regions of the lungs there are distinct bronchial veins which drain into the azygous, hemiazygous or intercostal veins, all of which drain into the right atrium. The main function of the bronchial circulation is to supply nutrition to the lungs and airways. Other proposed functions include temperature regulation and lung fluid balance. It is a high-pressure system with systemic pressures, and it has been suggested that the high pressures and muscular arteries may add structural support to the lung parenchyma. In contrast to the pulmonary artery system, which accommodates the entire cardiac output, only approximately 1% of the cardiac output goes through the bronchial arterial system.

The two circulatory systems are not independent, but show both anatomical connections and functional interdependence. The anatomical connections occur at three levels:

1. bronchopulmonary anastomoses between the bronchial artery and the pulmonary artery;

2. between the capillary drainage of the bronchial plexus and the end-capillary vessels of the alveolar capillary bed;

3. between the bronchial plexus vessels that drain into the pulmonary veins.

Functionally, the two circulations are able to complement each other in the event of the loss or impairment of one of them. This interaction accounts for the uncommon occurrence of pulmonary infarction, even with total blockage of a pulmonary artery. Under these circumstances, the blood flow through the bronchial artery system increases. In lung transplantation the bronchial arterial system is severed, but the viability of the lungs and airways is preserved by increases in pulmonary artery blood flow.

AETIOLOGIES

Bleeding from the bronchial vessels is the most common cause of haemoptysis (95% of cases in some series). Haemoptysis resulting from involvement of the pulmonary vessels is less common but no less dramatic. The common aetiologies will depend on the regional distribution of diseases. In some regions tuberculosis will clearly be the most common cause. In other areas tuberculosis will be uncommon and other aetiologies, such as carcinoma of the lung, will have a higher incidence. The age of the individual will also be a contributing factor, carcinoma of the lung being very uncommon in the younger population. Other local factors need to be considered, e.g. in areas with a high incidence of HIV disease the major causes will be infection or pulmonary Kaposi's

sarcoma. Table 3.4.1 lists many of the common and less common causes of haemoptysis, and Table 3.4.2 the usual causes of massive haemoptysis.

A history is taken with two objectives. The first is to establish the likely cause and diagnosis of the haemoptysis, and the second is to determine as accurately as possible the blood loss, which is an indicator of the

Table 3.4.1 Causes of haemoptysis

Infective
Acute tracheobronchitis
Bacterial pneumonia
Tuberculosis
Atypical mycobacteria
Lung abscess
Aspergillosis and aspergilloma
Bronchiectasis
Pneumocystis carinii pneumonia
Fungal pneumonia
Septic pulmonary emboli

Neoplastic
Bronchogenic carcinoma
Endobronchial metastases
Carcinoid tumour
Haematoma
Endometriosis

Cardiovascular
Pulmonary oedema
Mitral stenosis
Pulmonary hypertension
Pulmonary embolus/infarct
Arteriovenous malformation

Immune
Systemic lupus erythematosus
Wegener's granulomatosis
Goodpasture's syndrome
Bechet's disease

Trauma
Chest trauma
Vascular catheter insertion
Transbronchial biopsy

Bleeding disorders
Anticoagulants
Coagulation disorders
Thrombocytopenia

Miscellaneous
Intrabronchial foreign body
Pulmonary haemosiderosis
Bronchiolithiasis

Table 3.4.2 Causes of massive haemoptysis

Bronchial carcinoma
Tuberculosis
Bronchiectasis
Lung abscess
Aspergilloma
Arteriovenous malformations

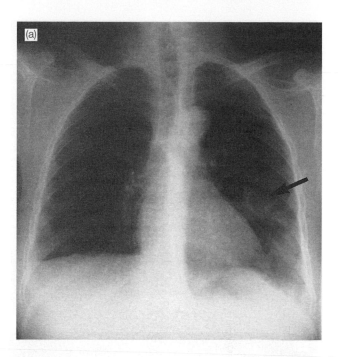

likely prognosis. While the diagnostic possibilities for haemoptysis are wide-ranging, the history should be directed at making a differential diagnosis. The history needs to establish whether this is an acute or chronic problem. A history suggestive of an acute pneumonia should also be sought. Anaerobic lung infections and abscess formation may occur in patients at risk of aspiration (e.g. alcoholics, epileptics). Such patients may have few respiratory symptoms and often present with minor fevers, weight loss or debility (Figure 3.4.1) Preceding systemic symptoms with cough, weight loss and fevers may suggest tuberculosis, particularly if there is a known contact with pulmonary TB or the individual has risk factors for developing TB. Risk factors for human immunodeficiency virus (HIV) infection should also be sought because of the number of causes of haemoptysis associated with this infection. Haemoptysis in a patient with diabetic ketoacidosis, with the appropriate chest roentgenogram, should suggest mucormycoses. A smoking history is clearly important, as carcinoma of the lung is the most common cause of massive haemoptysis in smoking populations. Indeed, haemoptysis is a common presenting symptom in a significant number of patients who are finally diagnosed with lung cancer. Metastatic cancer to the lung may be suggested from the history. In HIV-positive individuals, Kaposi's sarcoma involving the airways should be considered. Chronic bronchitis is a very common cause of minor haemoptysis, often with some blood streaking of the sputum. However, because of the common association between chronic bronchitis, cigarette smoking and lung cancer, the latter should always be considered.

A history of preceding interstitial lung disease (particularly one which can cause cavitary lesions), old TB or sarcoid may alert the physician to the possibility of a mycetoma, particularly with the appropriate radiological findings (Figure 3.4.2).

While rheumatic heart disease with mitral valve stenosis and pulmonary hypertension is not common in affluent societies, the possibility should be considered in an older individual or in underdeveloped countries. Pulmonary hypertension with any cause

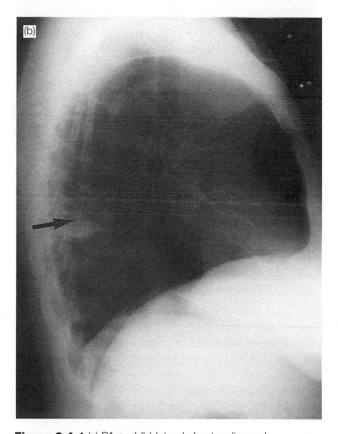

Figure 3.4.1 (a) PA and (b) lateral chest radiograph demonstrating a thin-walled cavitating lesion (arrows) in the apical segment of the left lower lobe. This 58-year-old woman was an alcoholic and presented with massive haemoptysis. Despite administration of appropriate antibiotics, the haemoptysis continued and she required a left lower lobectomy to resect the anaerobic abscess.

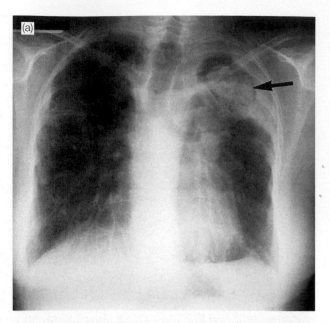

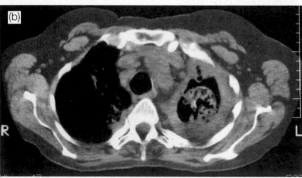

Figure 3.4.2 (a) A PA chest radiograph in a 69-year-old man with haemoptysis demonstrating an aspergilloma in a cavity in the left upper lobe (arrow). He had had pulmonary tuberculosis in the past. (b) The CT scan shows considerable pleural thickening at the left apex with a necrotic intra-cavitary fungal ball in the cavity. Intra-cavity amphotericin was instilled through a percutaneous catheter inserted under CT guidance with good results.

may also give rise to haemoptysis (Figure 3.4.3). Left ventricular failure with pulmonary vascular congestion is a common cause of minor haemoptysis.

Bronchiectasis is a common cause of haemoptysis, including massive haemoptysis (Figure 3.4.3). It has many aetiologies, including previous severe bacterial pneumonia, measles or pertussis. In some centres cystic fibrosis will be the most common cause of bronchiectasis. Acute pulmonary vasculitis due to autoimmune disease, particularly systemic lupus erythematosus, may present with massive haemoptysis, as may Wegener's granulomatosis and other necrotizing vasculitidies.

Generalized coagulopathies (including anticoagulants) and bleeding disorders need to be considered in the differential diagnosis.

EXAMINATION

The physical examination has two major components in patients with haemoptysis: first, to determine the need for stabilization and resuscitation, and secondly, to confirm the clinical diagnosis or expand the differential diagnosis.

DIAGNOSIS

CHEST ROENTGENOGRAM

Postero-anterior (PA) and lateral films are essential when investigating any patient with haemoptysis. The radiological appearances can be diagnostic both in localizing the likely site of bleeding and in providing the most likely diagnosis. The chest roentgenogram may be normal in a certain proportion of patients. In one retrospective study including in-patients and out-patients, plain roentgenograms were normal in 50% of cases. It is uncommon for the roentgenogram to be normal in patients with massive haemoptysis.

Diagnostic appearances include tumours and apical lesions such as an aspergilloma. Care should be taken not to confuse the appearance of blood in the lungs with the primary pathology. It is not always possible to distinguish blood in the lungs from consolidation or atelectasis. Gravity will determine the distribution of extravasated blood, and abnormalities are more common in the lower and dependent zones.

The chest roentgenogram may not always be of help in patients with pre-existing respiratory disease or radiological abnormalities. This is the case for many patients with cystic fibrosis presenting with haemoptysis. However, it is still our practice to give these patients a plain chest roentgenogram in the initial assessment, as intervening infection cannot be excluded on clinical grounds.

BRONCHOSCOPY

Bronchoscopy is essential for all patients with haemoptysis, in order to localize the site of bleeding and to establish a diagnosis. It may also be used to control bleeding in some instances. There is some debate as to whether a rigid or fibre-optic bronchoscope (FOB) should be used in patients with massive haemoptysis. The debate in this instance is related to the difficulties in performing an adequate examination of the bronchi in the presence of bleeding, and the technical difficulties involved in aspirating large volumes of blood through the narrow suction channels of a FOB. On the other hand, most physicians are more experienced in the use of FOBs.

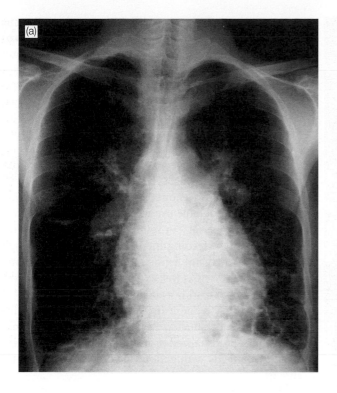

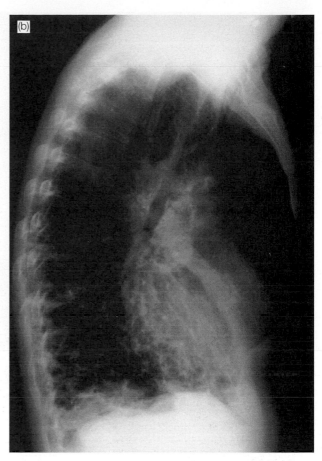

Figure 3.4.3 (a) PA and (b) lateral chest radiographs of a 62-year-old man with cystic bronchiectasis and pulmonary hypertension. There are generalized cystic changes throughout the lung fields, which are most apparent in the lower zones on these radiographs. The right pulmonary artery is enlarged, consistent with pulmonary hypertension. The patient's haemoptysis responded to intravenous antibiotics.

It is usual practice to bronchoscope all patients with haemoptysis, even those with normal chest roentgenograms. This is done mainly to exclude bleeding sites in the large central airways, in particular bronchial carcinoma (Figure 3.4.4). Bronchoscopy should be performed even in young patients because of the possibility of benign tumours, particularly adenomas (Figure 3.4.5). Although they are uncommon, malignant tumours (often metastatic) also need to be considered in this age group. These tumours are often located in the central airways and are not visible on plain chest roentgenograms. Many patients will have nothing more than evidence of chronic bronchitis with a markedly inflamed, hyperaemic mucosa which bleeds easily on contact with the bronchoscope and when biopsied. The incidence of carcinoma in patients with normal chest roentgenograms is low, and is generally quoted as being between 5% and 15%. The incidence will depend on how vigorous the physician is in investigating patients with haemoptysis.

Bronchoscopy should be used in conjunction with other diagnostic modalities. At bronchoscopy the usual diagnostic samples should be taken. These must include bronchial washings or bronchoalveolar lavage, brushings and biopsies of suspicious areas. Specimens should be sent for routine examination, including microbiological testing (aerobic and anaerobic cultures), special stains and special cultures, including *Mycobacterium* and fungi. Specimens should be examined for abnormal cytology, and biopsies sent for histopathological examination.

COMPUTED TOMOGRAPHY (CT)

CT scans are an important investigational tool in the diagnosis and management of haemoptysis. They are able to locate and define the anatomy of lung lesions more accurately than plain chest roentgenograms. The definition of the lung parenchyma can also be of use in diagnosing lung disease. There is still some debate as to the place of CT scanning in the routine investigation of haemoptysis, particularly in patients with a normal chest

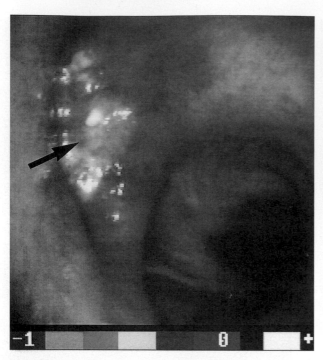

Figure 3.4.4 The appearance at bronchoscopy of a recurrence of tumour in the stump of the left main bronchus (arrowed). This 48-year-old man had a long history of tobacco smoking and had undergone a left pneumonectomy for a squamous-cell carcinoma 2 years previously.

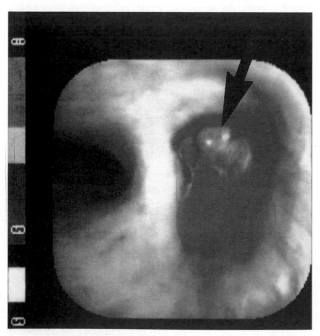

Figure 3.4.5 Bronchoscopic view of a tumour (arrowed) completely occluding the right main bronchus in a 27-year-old non-smoking woman presenting with haemoptysis. Biopsies showed a carcinoid tumour. A right pneumonectomy was performed.

roentgenogram. In one restrospective study, CT scans were considered to be of more diagnostic value than bronchoscopy. However, in that study the most common diagnosis was bronchiectasis. The present data suggest that it does not add significantly to bronchoscopy in the diagnosis of patients with lung cancer and a normal chest roentgenogram. In a patient with a high risk of tumour, a normal chest roentgenogram and bronchoscopy, a CT scan should be considered. The main risk factor that needs to be considered is a history of smoking. In low-risk patients a CT scan is rarely useful.

The use of intravenous contrast with CT scanning may be of considerable use in the detection and definition of pulmonary arteriovenous shunts. It is useful for defining both the feeding and draining vessels. Although this modality may not define the anatomy of the feeding and draining vessels as well as angiography, it is less invasive and is more readily available.

CT scanning is more useful than bronchoscopy for the diagnosis of smaller, more peripheral carcinomas that cannot be visualized bronchoscopically, but it is less useful in patients with endobronchial lesions in central airways.

High-resolution CT scans are the best method of diagnosing bronchiectasis and determining the extent of the disease. Typical radiological patterns are found in interstitial disease and disease of peripheral airways, such as bronchiolitis obliterans. Haemoptysis due to interstitial lung disease is uncommon but well recognized.

Helical CT scans can create images of the airways making it possible to detect intrabronchial lesions. At present it is not likely that this technique will replace bronchoscopic examination of the airways. Helical CT scans are being more widely used in the diagnosis of pulmonary thrombo-embolic disease, and are of most help when the more central vessels are involved.

ANGIOGRAPHY

Selective angiography of the pulmonary and bronchial vasculature can be of use in identification of the site of haemorrhage. Angiography is also important for defining the anatomy of the structures involved, including feeding and draining vessels (Figure 3.4.6). It is uncommon for angiography to demonstrate active extravasation, but there are other indicators to suggest the area of bleeding. The effects of chronic lung disease and chronic inflammation will result in many of the pathological changes which can be demonstrated by angiography. These include localized hypervascularity, tortuosity, arteriovenous formations and aneurysmal formations. The chronic changes may also result in increased blood flow and anastomoses between the bronchial (or systemic) circulation and the pulmonary vessels. These

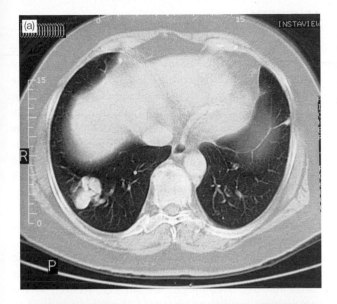

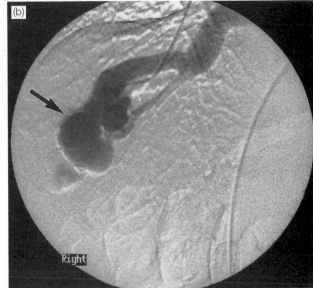

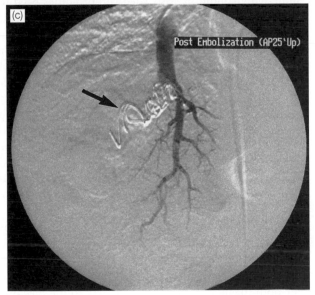

Figure 3.4.6 This 60-year-old woman had presented with haemoptysis and dyspnoea. The chest radiograph showed a coin lesion close to the diaphragm. (a) The CT scan demonstrated a lobulated vascular lesion in the right lower lobe. Smaller lesions were visible in other CT slices. (b) A selective angiogram demonstrated the arteriovenous malformation (AVM, arrow). (c) Embolization of the AVM at the time of angiography was performed using coils (arrow). The patient's symptoms resolved.

communications may be visualized or filling of the pulmonary vessels demonstrated with angiography. It is important to note that systemic arteries (particularly the intercostal, subclavian and internal mammary vessels) may be the main feeder vessels to the bleeding site, and it may be necessary to cannulate and angiogram these vessels in the search for the bleeding site. If the site of bleeding is identified, then local treatment, embolization, can be instituted.

NUCLEAR MEDICINE STUDIES

Nuclear medicine studies are not of great use in the investigation of most patients with haemoptysis. The main application of nucleotide studies in patients with haemoptysis is in the diagnosis of pulmonary embolus and infarction. In the presence of embolus there should be a high-probability scan with an anatomical unit of a pulmonary segment or greater that has ventilation and no perfusion (ventilation/perfusion mismatch).

MANAGEMENT

There has recently been significant progress in the management of haemoptysis. A few years ago there were essentially only two methods for treating haemoptysis, namely conservative treatment and surgery. With the advent of invasive radiology, a very useful therapeutic technique has been added to the management of haemoptysis.

Massive haemoptysis is a frightening experience for both patient and physician. Patients with massive haemoptysis die from asphyxiation due to the blood in the airways and air spaces, and not from the effects of blood loss. The immediate management of a patient with uncontrolled massive haemoptysis is to maintain an airway and protect the non-bleeding lung. The patient should be placed with the bleeding lung dependent and with the head lower than the feet. If bleeding continues and there is a clear need for resuscitation, an endotracheal tube should be inserted. Intubation allows the airways in the good lung to be protected from flooding, and the patient can be mechanically ventilated with supplemental oxygen to help maintain adequate oxygenation. A variety of double-lumen endotracheal tubes is available. The advantage of these tubes is that each main bronchus is intubated and the right and left lung can also be independently ventilated or suctioned. Inflation of the cuffs can prevent blood from flooding into the contralateral lung, but even when well placed there may not be complete protection of the contralateral lung. Double-lumen endotracheal tubes require a skilled operator to pass and position them properly, and are best used under controlled conditions with the patient anaesthetized and paralysed. The lumen diameters of most of these tubes are not sufficient to allow introduction of a bronchoscope, and are easily occluded by a blood clot. A single-lumen endotracheal tube can also be used. If the site of bleeding is in the right lung, the left mainstem bronchus can be intubated and the cuff inflated. When the site of bleeding is known to be in the left lung, the right mainstem bronchus can be intubated, although this approach is not usually satisfactory because there will be occlusion of the right upper lobe bronchus. As with the use of a double-lumen tube intubation, this procedure needs to be performed by an experienced and skilled operator. The placement of a single-lumen endotracheal tube can best be achieved using a fibre-optic bronchoscope. The endotracheal tube is placed over the FOB, which is then passed into the airways. This allows for direct visualization of the airways and correct placement.

Following the localization of the bleeding site and diagnosis of the underlying disorder, a treatment decision needs to be made. The options include conservative medical treatment, local treatment under bronchoscopic vision, obliteration or embolization under radiological control, or surgical management. There are no recognized guidelines to aid this decision. One author has recommended that surgical intervention should be considered when haemoptysis exceeds 1000 mL/24 h, non-surgical approaches with blood loss of 500–1000 mL/24 h, and observation with appropriate diagnostic work-up for haemoptysis of less than 500 mL/24 h. A major problem in the management of patients with haemoptysis is that massive life-threatening bleeding can occur despite encouraging clinical improvement and no blood loss for prolonged periods.

SURGERY

It is clear that surgery can be a life-saving and definitive therapy for massive haemoptysis. The mortality rate from surgery will depend on patient selection, and the figures vary up to 50%, but are generally below 10%. In the presence of active haemoptysis, the mortality rate increases dramatically and is 30–50% in most series. The data comparing surgical and medical outcomes are difficult to interpret. The underlying diseases have changed over the years, and there is now a greater range of medical options, including embolization. The management of patients and resuscitation, and particularly intensive-care management, have also improved in recent years.

The usual criteria for selecting patients for thoracic surgery need to be employed when selecting patients with massive haemoptysis for surgery. As well as the underlying condition, associated comorbidities need to be considered. Surgery is clearly not indicated in patients with multiple or bilateral bleeding sites. Patients need to be clinically stable both haemodynamically and from a respiratory point of view. Importantly, the patient must have sufficient respiratory reserve to be able to tolerate loss of lung parenchyma without the surgery resulting in respiratory failure. The usual rule of thumb is that the estimated post-operative FEV_1 should exceed 800–1000 mL. If previous spirometry or current results are not available, best judgement should be exercised from the history of premorbid exercise tolerance and activity levels.

LOCAL TREATMENT

The use of either a rigid bronchoscope or a FOB allows for both diagnosis of and local therapy to the bleeding site, or isolation of the bleeding segment.

Local therapies that have been used include local application of vasoconstricting agents including adrenalin. This agent is most commonly used in patients with bleeding following bronchial or transbronchial lung biopsies, and its place in the management of other causes of haemoptysis is unclear. Thrombosing agents, e.g. thrombin and fibrinogen-thrombin can be applied topically.

Irrigation of the bleeding area with cold saline has been effective in some series. Intrabronchial balloons can be used to isolate the bleeding segment or tamponade the bleeding site. Fogarty catheters can be placed through a bronchoscope (either rigid or a FOB). The balloon is left inflated for 24–48 h. Once the catheter is in place, a coagulant solution can be injected through the lumen of the Fogarty catheter distal to the occluding balloon.

LASER TREATMENT

These measures appear to be more than temporizing, and the rebleeding rate is low. However, the numbers of patients in most of the studies that have used these techniques are small, and more definitive treatments should still be considered.

LOCAL INSTALLATION OF ANTIFUNGAL AGENTS

In some centres the placement of antifungal agents directly into cavities with fungus balls (mycetomas) has met with success. The catheter can be placed either through the airways or percutaneously.

EMBOLIZATION

Embolization is a very useful technique, and is considered by some to be the first line of treatment for massive haemoptysis. It is useful in patients who are not suitable for surgery but who need control of their haemoptysis. It can be used for managing patients with multiple bleeding sites or arteriovenous malformations, for those patients who have medical comorbidities which would preclude surgery, and for those whose respiratory disease would not allow lung resection. Patients with inoperable carcinoma of the lung with massive bleeding are an example of a relevant application of this procedure. The procedure can also be repeated if there is rebleeding in either the short or long term. This makes it a very useful technique in the management of haemoptysis in patients for whom the latter is a long-term problem, e.g. such a patient with cystic fibrosis.

The technique of embolizing pulmonary bleeding sites through arterial catheters has been available since the late 1970s. It has not been widely used until the last few years, when catheter technology improved, making the catheterization of the bronchial arteries easier. A major advantage of the technique is that the embolization can be performed at the same time as the diagnostic angiogram. Once the abnormal feeding artery or arteries have been identified, the decision can then be made as to whether embolization should be performed. With the catheter in the arterial vessel, embolic material is injected to thrombose the vessel (Figure 3.4.6 (c)). The materials used include gels, coils, balloons or various combinations.

The immediate success rate of embolization is 75–90%. In the mid-term there is a rebleed in approximately 20% of cases, and the long term rebleed rate is 50% in some series. It is likely that the long-term rebleed rate is dependent on the underlying pathologies. If embolization fails to stop the bleeding, it is recommended that other systemic arterial supplies to the bleeding site be sought (see section on angiography above).

Embolization is not without possible complications. The main problems are related to embolization of systemic arteries associated with the bronchial arteries. These vessels include arteries to the spinal cord, oesophagus, trachea, and the vaso vasorum of the aorta. Spinal cord ischaemia with paralysis is a well-recognized complication of bronchial artery embolization. On occasion, particularly with large arteriovenous malformations, thrombotic emboli can result in cerebral artery ischaemia and stroke. However, in experienced centres the complication rate of embolization is low.

Chapter 3.5

Haematemesis/melaena/ rectal bleeding/anaemia

Hamish P. Ewing

Introduction

Like so much of surgery, gastrointestinal bleeding makes for an interesting detective story. Very often the clue to the source of blood loss is to be found either in the patient's past history or in their current symptoms. A systematic approach and listening carefully to the described history will often lead you to the answer more directly.

Bleeding can of course arise from any part of the alimentary tract but, as is the case elsewhere in medicine, common things are common. This chapter is intended to highlight these most common sources of bleeding, and will also mention those 'less likely, but always to be remembered' sources.

ANATOMY

Where does all of the anatomy learned in the past fit into this picture?

1. When considering a peptic ulcer, any lesion which lies in the vicinity of a named artery is very likely to rebleed (or fail to stop in the first instance), so surgery becomes a relative indication.

2. Conversely, small and unnamed vessels, such as those feeding a patch of angiodysplasia or found at the neck of a colonic diverticulum, will normally stop bleeding spontaneously. This again will dictate the management approach.

The relationship of the third part of the duodenum to the aorta is an essential ingredient in the formation of an aorto-duodenal fistula.

Similarly, an understanding of the portal circulation and its potential for bleeding from the developed porto-systemic shunts is necessary. However, with regard to bleeding, anatomy is 'where you find it' and does not necessarily follow the rules, especially when one consid-

ers the multitude of pathologies which might lead to gastrointestinal bleeding.

PATHOLOGY

A very clear understanding of the physiology of response to fluid loss (see Chapter 2.2) is essential for the proper management of gastrointestinal bleeding.

Gastrointestinal bleeding is a relatively common problem constituting 100 per 100 000 acute hospital admissions in the UK. Interestingly, of these, about 60% are due to peptic ulcer disease. Thus an understanding of gastric mucosal protection is needed when considering peptic ulceration.

Anorectal physiology needs to be understood (see Chapter 30.4) when considering the development of haemorrhoids or diverticular disease, both of which can in turn be a source of gastrointestinal blood loss.

Gastrointestinal bleeding appears to fall into one of four symptom patterns:

1. haematemesis;

2. melaena;
3. rectal bleeding;
4. occult blood loss/anaemia.

HAEMATEMESIS

Definition Haematemesis is the vomiting of blood, be it bright or 'coffee grounds' which implies conversion of haemoglobin to methaemoglobin by gastric acid.

The causes of haematemesis are summarized in Table 3.5.1.

A large volume of bright blood with no melaena is most commonly due to bleeding varices, although a chronic peptic ulcer penetrating a named vessel (gastro-duodenal artery, splenic artery or a branch of the left gastric artery on the lesser curve) could be a possibility, as could an aorto-duodenal fistula.

Smaller volumes could obviously be due to any of the sources listed above.

MELAENA

Definition Melaena is the passage of offensive-smelling black tarry stool. This black colour results from prolonged contact of blood with gastric juices, which leads to the formation of haematin.

Melaena is a distinct entity which essentially infers upper gastrointestinal bleeding. Melaena is a term commonly used loosely and occasionally misleadingly by medical and nursing staff. The only way to be sure of this diagnosis is to perform a rectal examination *personally* and to examine the contents present. In the

Table 3.5.1 Causes of haematemesis with or without melaena

Most common causes
- Haemorrhagic gastritis
- Peptic ulcer disease
- Reflux oesophagitis
- Oesophageal varices

Less common or rare causes
- Mallory-Weiss tear
- Malignancy of oesophagus or stomach
- Swallowed blood (e.g. epistaxis)
- Vascular abnormality of the stomach (e.g. angiodysplasia/telangiectasia)
- Leiomyoma of the stomach
- Aorto-duodenal fistula
- Haematobilia
- Duodenal diverticulum (often fourth part)

acute setting, melaena indicates upper gastrointestinal bleeding, while red blood per rectum is a much more challenging symptom, as the source could be any point in the gastrointestinal tract.

The most common cause of melaena without haematemesis is bleeding due to duodenal ulceration. The combination of haematemesis and melaena obviously includes all of the sources listed in the Haematemesis section (see Table 3.5.1).

As the diagnostic clues for haematemesis and melaena are essentially the same, I shall now consider them under one heading.

Historical clues

1. *Oesophageal varices* may have been documented previously or there may be chronic liver disease evident. Remember, however, that *one-third* of patients who bleed with documented varices will have a source of bleeding other than varices.

2. A past history of ulcer disease, symptoms of indigestion, or the ingestion of ulcerogens (aspirin, non-steroidal anti-inflammatory drugs – NSAIDs will suggest *peptic ulceration.*

3. The haematemesis of a *Mallory-Weiss tear* will classically be preceded by a dry retch or non-bloodstained vomit. The bright blood seen is a result of the mucosal tearing of forced eructation.

4. Symptoms of *oesophageal reflux* need to be sought, as does any dysphagia. It is very common indeed for elderly patients lying supine to present with a small-volume haematemesis because of gastro-oesophageal reflux.

5. Any history of *nosebleeds* or spitting bright blood needs to be considered when the problem is one of small volumes of bright blood being vomited.

6. A past history of *aortic aneurysm* repair should immediately raise the possibility of *aorto-duodenal fistula,* especially if there were any infective complications post-operatively.

7. Any past history of liver trauma or liver biopsies may suggest the rare possibility of *haematobilia* secondary to fistula formation within the liver substance.

MANAGEMENT OF GASTROINTESTINAL BLEEDING

Management is the combination of both investigation and treatment, which need to run in parallel. This is the case in all acutely ill patients, for investigations cannot proceed without satisfactory resuscitation measures.

The initial management of all types of gastrointestinal haemorrhage is similar, so they will be dealt with together (Figure 3.5.1). There will be a separate figure where the two paths diverge (Figure 3.5.2).

Once the patient has been resuscitated, an accurate diagnosis can be made at endoscopy in 90–95% of cases. This then allows for focused treatment to follow. Fortunately, the majority of causes are self-limiting or only require simple medical treatment.

Peptic ulcer disease is by far the most common cause of upper gastrointestinal bleeding (60%), and at endoscopy there are some findings that influence treatment. Active bleeding clearly needs to be arrested, but in addition there are several 'stigmata of a recent bleed' which are important because they indicate the likelihood of rebleeding. These are adherent clot in the ulcer base and a visible vessel in the ulcer base (especially if sited over a named artery). It is in this setting that endoscopic therapy may be feasible either to stop the bleeding or to prevent a rebleed. Injection around the bleeding vessel with 1:10 000 adrenalin, hypertonic saline or absolute alcohol has been shown to be effective. Similarly, coagulation of the bleeding vessel can be achieved by using a heat probe or a low-wattage neodymium:YAG laser probe. Endoscopic haemostatic methods have reduced the overall mortality of bleeding duodenal ulcers from 10% to 5%.

Occasionally the initial endoscopic treatment may have failed, or the bleeding at initial endoscopy is found to be occurring at such a rate that any endoscopic treatment is either impossible or ineffective. It is in this set-ting that surgery is indicated. As these patients are usually frail, elderly and suffering from other medical conditions, surgery is kept simple in most instances by under-running the bleeding vessel in a duodenal ulcer or excising a gastric ulcer. Once such an operation has been performed, definitive medical treatment of the ulcer is then indicated (see below). Occasionally ulcer scarring or the presence of possible malignancy may necessitate a partial or total gastrectomy, which is major surgery in a patient who may be haemodynamically compromised.

Helicobacter pylori (H. pylori)

The discovery and definition of *H. pylori* is one of the major advances in the management of peptic ulcer disease during the last decade, and as a result has not yet received mention in a number of standard surgical texts. This short-spiralled bacterium with five flagella at one end is the cause of at least 90% of duodenal ulcers and gastritis, up to 70% of gastric ulcers and probably up to 60% of gastric cancers. It is therefore important to establish whether *H. pylori* is present in a patient with bleeding peptic ulcer disease and, if present, the bacterium needs to be eradicated at some stage during the patient's treatment.

There are five techniques for diagnosing the presence of *H. pylori* (Table 3.5.2):

1. The rapid urease test – this requires a biopsy sample of the gastric antrum, which is where *H. pylori* is most prolific. *H. pylori* produces a urease which can

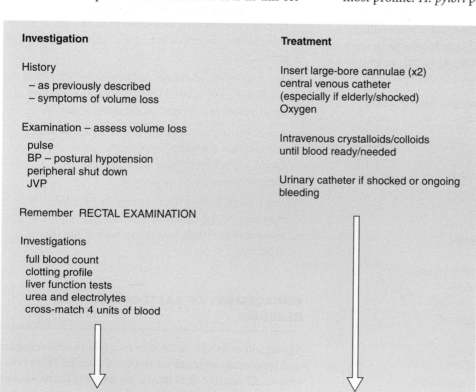

Investigation

History

  – as previously described
  – symptoms of volume loss

Examination – assess volume loss

  pulse
  BP – postural hypotension
  peripheral shut down
  JVP

Remember RECTAL EXAMINATION

Investigations

  full blood count
  clotting profile
  liver function tests
  urea and electrolytes
  cross-match 4 units of blood

Treatment

Insert large-bore cannulae (x2)
central venous catheter
(especially if elderly/shocked)
Oxygen

Intravenous crystalloids/colloids
until blood ready/needed

Urinary catheter if shocked or ongoing
bleeding

Figure 3.5.1 The management of gastrointestinal bleeding. The two streams of activity that run in parallel (Investigation and Treatment) continue in Figure 3.5.2.

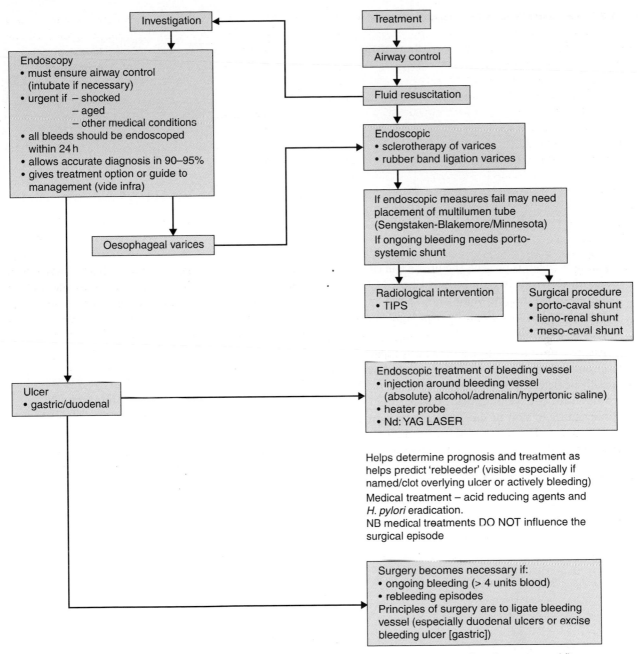

Figure 3.5.2 Ongoing management of haematemesis and melaena.

NB *Always remember* that the elderly and medically unfit do not tolerate blood loss as well as the young and fit. Therefore surgery needs to be considered at an earlier stage in this group, as does the need for insertion of a central venous catheter to monitor fluid replacement. In some circumstances a Swann-Ganz catheter to gauge left ventricular function may be helpful.

be indirectly detected by a change in the pH of the gel medium containing urea.

2. Culture – this requires endoscopic biopsy of the antrum and needs special transport media and culture techniques.

3. Microscopy – silver or Giemsa staining of an antral

biopsy will reveal the spiral organism located deep in the layer of mucus covering the gastric surface.

4. ^{13}C or ^{14}C – urea breath test (Figure 3.5.3) – this test also makes use of the urease produced by *H. pylori* by indirectly identifying its presence. Patients are given a low dose of ^{13}C- or ^{14}C-labelled urea in a test

Table 3.5.2 Current tests for *Helicobacter pylori*

Test	Sensitivity (%)	Specificity (%)	Invasive procedure
Rapid urease test	90	90–95	Yes
Culture	80	Approaching 100	Yes
Microscopy	90	90	Yes
^{13}C and ^{14}C urea breath test	95	95*	No
Serology	98	Approaching 100	No

*Note that there is a ^{14}C-associated risk for children and for women of childbearing age.

meal. If *H. pylori* is present, the urease will cleave the urea, which results in radioactively labelled CO_2 being absorbed into the blood and expired by the lungs, where it is measured (by mass spectrometer for ^{13}C and scintillation counter for ^{14}C).

5. Serology – most patients display a measurable immunological response to *H. pylori*, which can usually be detected by an enzyme-linked immunosorbent assay (ELISA). This has the disadvantage of slow or incomplete resolution after eradication of *H. pylori* and so is a screening or epidemiological tool of little use in testing for successful treatment.

Although culturing may be the 'gold standard', either the rapid urease test or a C-urea breath test are the most commonly used diagnostic tools.

Eradication of *H. pylori* has proved to be difficult and a combination of drugs is necessary for the best results. Unfortunately, a number of metronidazole-resistant strains are emerging world-wide. Drug combinations that are commonly used to achieve eradication rates of 80–90% include:

- metronidazole, ampicillin and colloidal bismuth;
- metronidazole, tetracycline and colloidal bismuth;
- metronidazole, ampicillin and proton-pump inhibitor;
- metronidazole, clarithromycin and proton-pump inhibitor.

If *H. pylori* is absent, then treatment with an H_2-blocker or proton-pump inhibitor will be indicated together with cessation of other risk factors, e.g NSAIDs and cigarette smoking.

It should be noted that acid-lowering medications have

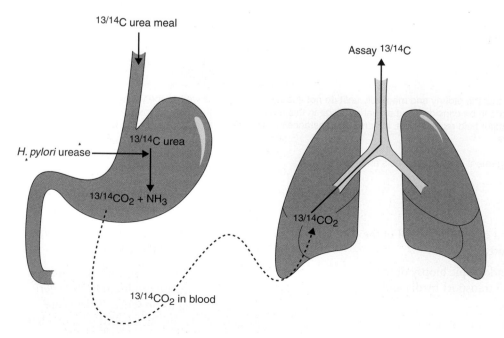

$^{13/14}$C urea meal

Assay $^{13/14}$C

H. pylori urease

$^{13/14}$C urea

$^{13/14}CO_2 + NH_3$

$^{13/14}CO_2$

$^{13/14}CO_2$ in blood

Figure 3.5.3 Urea breath test.

NOT *been shown to influence the course of active upper gastrointestinal bleeding in any way or to reduce the likelihood of rebleeding.*

Oesophageal varices

The other cause of major upper gastrointestinal bleeding is from oesophageal varices secondary to portal hypertension. It is important that endoscopy is performed even in those patients with known oesophageal varices, as 30% will be bleeding from some other cause, perhaps requiring quite a different treatment.

Having resuscitated and diagnosed bleeding oesophageal varices, the first-line treatment is usually endoscopic, involving either injection of a sclerosing agent (ethanolamine or sodium tetradecyl sulphate) or rubber-band ligation. The latter is becoming increasingly favoured as it is reputedly more effective and less likely to be associated with the uncommon complications of sepsis, oesophageal ulceration or stricture formation.

If bleeding is ongoing, the next step is to insert a Minnesota or Sengstaken-Blakemore tube. These tubes have an oesophageal balloon to tamponade the varices and a 300-mL gastric balloon to retain the tube in its correct position. Once the gastric balloon has been inflated with air or water, the oesophageal balloon is inflated with water to a pressure of 30–40 mmHg. The patient needs high-dependency-unit care to monitor vital signs and to ensure that there is no displacement of the tube, as the gastric balloon needs to be held tight against the cardia by gentle traction of about 0.5 kg on the nasal end of the catheter. Once control has been established for about 24 h, sclerotherapy or variceal ligation can again be attempted.

Continued bleeding despite tamponade is a problem. Intravenous octreotide (a synthetic somatostatin) has been demonstrated to be of benefit. Failing this, the portal hypertension must be reduced.

This is achieved by making a surgical fistula between the portal and systemic venous systems. The down-side of such a procedure is the risk of developing a hepatic encephalopathy, especially in patients with significantly impaired liver function. Such a fistula can be achieved percutaneously using radiological stenting techniques. Transjugular intrahepatic porto-systemic shunt (TIPS) involves the passing of a needle through a branch of the hepatic vein into a branch of the portal vein within the liver substance. Then, using the Seldinger technique, an expanding wire stent is positioned between the two veins to create a permanent fistula. An alternative approach is to create such a fistula surgically, usually between the portal vein and the inferior vena cava (porto-caval shunt) or between the splenic and left renal veins (lienorenal shunt).

Definition Rectal bleeding is the passage of any blood per rectum. It may be bright red, darker red, large volume, small volume, independent of stool or mixed with the stool.

Table 3.5.3 Causes of rectal bleeding

Common causes
- Haemorrhoids
- Anal fissure
- Cancer (or colonic polyps)
- Diverticular disease and angiodysplasia

Less common or rare causes
- Inflammatory bowel disease (large or small intestine)
- Infective colitis
- Ischaemic colitis
- Bleeding from upper gastrointestinal ulcer
- Small-bowel tumour, ulcer or vascular abnormality
- Rectal trauma (patients are often reticent about this possibility)
- Meckel's diverticulum (children or adolescents)
- Juvenile polyp (children or adolescents)
- Irradiation proctitis or colitis
- Carcinoma of the prostate
- Endometriosis

HISTORICAL CLUES

Frank blood (i.e. not mixed with stool)

Bright red blood:

- Small-volume and painful, seen on the toilet-paper, occasionally in the toilet bowl, and associated with defecation, is typical of an *anal fissure.*

- Small to moderate bright red blood loss, occasionally clots, seen on the toilet-paper and in the toilet bowl, but painless and associated with defecation, is usually *haemorrhoidal* in nature.

- Large-volume and painless passage of frank blood is most commonly due to *angiodysplasia* or *diverticular disease.*

Dark red blood:

- Passage of dark red blood, usually in large volumes and without pain, can be due to bleeding *diverticular disease* or *angiodysplasia*, but can also be caused by a massive bleed from the upper gastrointestinal tract (gastric/duodenal ulcer, aorto-duodenal fistula, haematobilia) or mid-gut (Meckel's diverticulum, small-bowel tumour or vascular abnormality).

- The clue for a source of bleeding proximal to the large intestine is that the patient is usually quite markedly shocked due to the large volume of blood needed to fill the intestines quickly enough to cause passage of a reddish blood per rectum.

Blood mixed with stool

- Bloody diarrhoea is much more likely to be due to a *colitis*, whether it is infective, inflammatory or ischaemic in origin.
- Small amounts of blood mixed with the stool would be suggestive of *colonic polyp* or *cancer*. *Never* ascribe this symptom to diverticular disease until proven. Both diverticular disease and colon cancer are very common in the elderly, and obviously it is a malignancy that is most likely to give rise to this symptom.

MANAGEMENT OF RECTAL BLEEDING

The major problem with rectal bleeding is to identify the bleeding point (Figure 3.5.4). Without this knowledge the most appropriate treatment may not be selected.

After taking a history, the next step is to examine the patient, paying attention to signs of shock, and seeking out a cause for bleeding. A careful abdominal and rectal examination is imperative, and this should include a *rigid sigmoidoscopy.*

Fortunately, most rectal bleeding ceases spontaneously. However, if there is clinical evidence of ongoing bleeding a technetium-labelled red-cell scan should be arranged. If the patient is actively bleeding (>0.1 mL/min) the bleeding point will show up as a 'hot spot'. An advantage of this approach is that by repeat scanning every 4 h intermittent bleeding may either show up as a hot spot or at least localize the bleeding source to one segment of the colon. Even if the bleeding ceases spontaneously (as occurs in 80% of cases), the bleeding point has been identified and, should there be a recurrence of haemorrhage, a limited resection of the involved segment of colon can be undertaken, the alternative being a subtotal colectomy in a patient who is usually a frail older person.

A mesenteric angiogram, which may require selective studies of the coeliac, superior and inferior mesenteric arteries, may help to pinpoint the precise bleeding point but, requires a greater degree of active bleeding than the technetium-labelled red-cell scan at the time of the study. Occasionally there is an abnormal vascular pattern present which may suggest – not diagnose – a site of bleeding. The combination of a mesenteric angiogram following a technetium study showing a hot spot is perhaps the most precise way of defining the site of bleeding.

If the bleeding is ongoing (>6 units of blood) then surgery is necessary. Hopefully either a technetium-labelled red-cell scan, a mesenteric angiogram or both will have identified a bleeding point which permits tailored minimal resections. If the bleeding point has not been identified, attempts to find the source of blood loss using on-table endoscopy may resolve the problem. Failing this, a bold decision has to be made to remove part or all of the colon, with the ever-present risk of perhaps leaving the bleeding point behind. Fortunately, this is an unusual situation these days.

It is well to remember that massive upper gastrointestinal bleeding can cause per rectum (PR) bleeding without haematemesis. This source of bleeding is suggested either from the history (see above) or from the observation that the patient is markedly shocked, which is unusual for someone with a colonic source. An upper gastrointestinal endoscopy can thus be indicated. Colonoscopy, while attractive in theory, is of less help in reality as blood tends to run both proximally and distally, thus easily obscuring a small focus of bleeding such as angiodysplasia or a diverticulum. However, if the episode settles, as is usually the case, a colonoscopy is essential to identify the bleeding source. It may well be possible to treat the cause of bleeding endoscopically by laser obliteration of a patch of angiodysplasia, or simple snaring of a bleeding polyp. It is worth remembering that *cancers* can also present with massive PR bleeding on occasion.

ANAEMIA/OCCULT INTESTINAL BLEEDING (FIGURE 3.5.5)

It is very important to remember that there can be a non-surgical cause of iron-deficiency anaemia, and that current faecal occult blood tests can be misleading.

The most commonly used test for faecal-occult blood detection is Haemoccult. This is a guaiac test which detects the pseudoperoxidase activity of haem. Unfortunately, this test has a false-negative rate of 60–70% for large adenomatous polyps and 20–50% for asymptomatic cancers. This is because blood loss of 1–2 mL/day is needed from a source that will often only bleed intermittently, if at all. In addition, an anti-oxidant, such as vitamin C, can produce a false-negative result. False-positives (3–5% of screened populations) can result from peroxidase activity of certain foods (e.g. broccoli, cauliflower, turnips, horseradish and melons), red meats, NSAIDs and, of course, minor anal disorders. Special dietary restrictions therefore form part of the proper use and interpretation of this test.

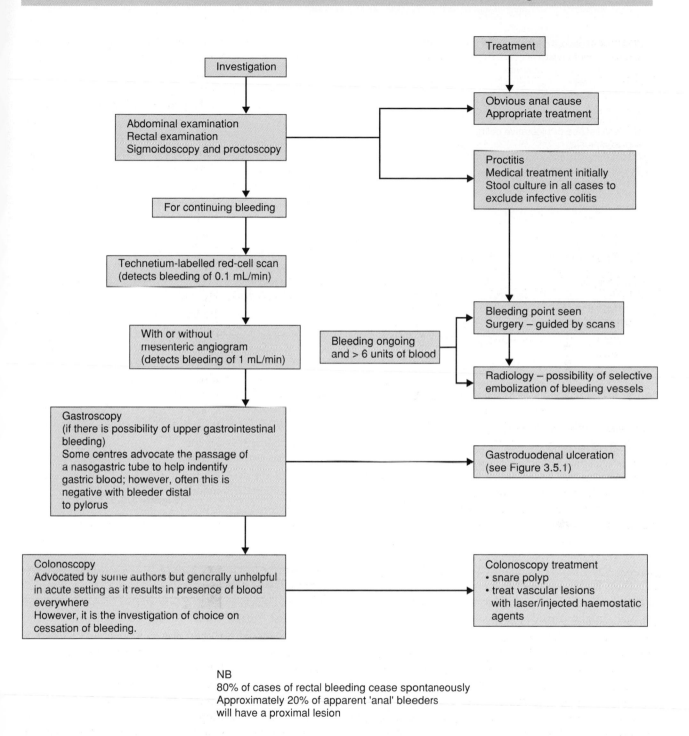

Figure 3.5.4 Ongoing management of rectal bleeding.

Several other tests for faecal-occult blood are available. One is a quantitative assay of faecal haemoglobin by fluorimetry of porphyrins derived from haem. Another assay uses immunological techniques to detect the presence of human haemoglobin.

MANAGEMENT OF ANAEMIA OR OCCULT BLOOD LOSS (FIGURE 3.5.6)

HISTORY

Again the history is important and the patient should be closely questioned regarding any possible sign of

Common intestinal causes
Colon cancer/polyps
Duodenal or gastric ulceration
Gastric cancer

Other intestinal causes
Crohn's disease or ulcerative colitis
Angiodysplasia
Vascular malformations (e.g. hereditary
   telangiectasia) anywhere in the
   gastrointestinal tract
Haemorrhoids
Puetz-Jegher syndrome

Rare intestinal causes

UPPER GI	**SMALL GUT**	**COLON AND RECTUM**
Oesophageal varices	Jejunal diverticulum	Ulcers – stercoral
Oesophagitis	Ulcers – Meckel's related	– ischaemic
Gastritis	– ischaemic	– NSAID-induced
Leiomyoma	– acquired	– infective
Anastomotic ulcer	Arteritis	
	Blind loop syndrome	
	Tumour – benign	
	– malignant	
	Polyps – Peutz-Jegher	
	Tuberculosis	

Important non-intestinal causes
Menorrhagia
Post-gastrectomy (included here because patients
often forget their gastric surgery or doctors forget
the significance of the stomach in iron absorption)
Atrophic gastritis
Inadequate diet
Thalassaemia and other haemoglobinopathies
Coeliac disease

Figure 3.5.5 Causes of occult intestinal bleeding/iron deficiency anaemia.

bleeding, and in women the specific details of their menstrual loss are vital (see Chapter 3.7). Often what a woman might consider to be 'normal' is really quite pathological. Similarly, it is essential to obtain a careful dietary history, and, as a surgical opinion is often the second or third sought, it is always important to establish what the diet was like before seeing the family doctor, as it will often have been improved since that date.

A number of vital clues can be gleaned from a past surgical history. It is important always to remember the possibility of a right-sided colon cancer – a common cause of occult blood loss that often has grumbling symptoms of intermittent subacute obstruction as well.

Before pursuing formal investigation of intestinal blood loss or anaemia, it is essential to establish that the anaemia is truly one of iron deficiency. A lot of wasteful invasive investigations can be undertaken for a macrocytic anaemia. The typical blood film shows a microcytic, hypochromic picture, while the iron studies reveal a low serum iron and serum ferritin, with decreased transferrin saturation.

INVESTIGATIONS

The first major test is for a gastroscopy and colonoscopy. This should always include a proctoscopy, as haemorrhoids are not easily seen with a colonoscope. A number of patients never observe their stool, so never have the opportunity to see rectal bleeding. If the endoscopic examination is normal, the next step would usually be a barium study of the small intestine, with perhaps even a mesenteric angiogram to follow this, although the rate of return for these two examinations is low (40%).

If the source of blood loss is still elusive, the next test to undertake is a *repeat* endoscopic examination. On many occasions a tiny vascular lesion has been found on a second inspection.

A Meckel's nuclear medicine scan is indicated in children and young adults.

If there is any doubt that the source of blood loss is in the gastrointestinal tract, a chromium-labelled red-cell nuclear medicine study can be used to document with

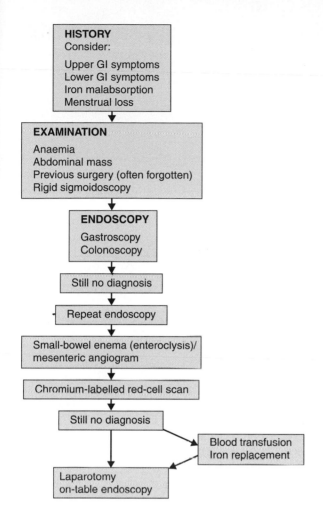

Figure 3.5.6 Investigation of anaemia (or faecal-occult blood positive).

accuracy that the gastrointestinal tract is the source of blood loss.

Occasionally, with significant and unremitting anaemia a laparotomy may become necessary, and at that time one would normally undertake an on-table endoscopic examination of the whole of the small intestine. A few specialist centres have the luxury of a thin enteroscope (an endoscope that is carried to the caecum by peristalsis, allowing the small intestine to be examined on withdrawal). However, this facility is not widely available.

Despite all of these sophisticated investigative tests,

every hospital will have on its books at least one patient with recurring anaemia from intestinal blood loss for which the source cannot be positively identified.

COMMON ERRORS

1. Not identifying the shocked or at-risk patient, and delaying resuscitation with investigation – this can cause death!

2. Not actually performing a rectal examination, and consequently spending time and money investigating the wrong end of the patient.

3. The patient aspirating and dying because of inadequate attention to the airway when combined with sedation.

4. The intern inserts a 22-G intravenous needle and is unable to run blood or resuscitate the patient adequately as a result. Venous access is increasingly difficult to obtain due to ongoing exsanguination.

5. Forgetting the possibility of *bleeding diathesis* as a cause of bleeding from any orifice. This of course includes patients taking *anticoagulants*.

6. Blaming duodenitis/gastritis for iron-deficiency anaemia, and missing the caecal carcinoma that presented later with a bowel obstruction.

7. Forgetting that *common things are common*.

FURTHER READING

Mujica VR, Barkin JP. 1996: Occult gastrointestinal bleeding. *Gastrointestinal Endoscopy Clinics of North America* **6**, 833–46.

Steele RJC, Chung SCS, Leung JWC. 1993: *Practical management of acute gastrointestinal bleeding.* Oxford: Butterworth Heinemann.

Steele RJC. 1997: The preprocedural care of the patient with gastrointestinal bleeding. *Gastrointestinal Endoscopy Clinics of North America* **7**, 551–8.

Haematuria

Alan M.F. Stapleton

Introduction

The causes of haematuria are many and varied, and no attempt will be made to list all of the possible aetiologies in this chapter. Such lists can be found in standard urological or general medical texts. Instead, this discussion will centre around the presenting features of a clinical scenario. It is frequently the history that is a key to the appropriate management of a patient who presents with haematuria, or who has haematuria noted as a sign associated with perhaps more pressing clinical concerns.

Even the common separation of haematuria into 'macroscopic' and 'microscopic', although often useful for teaching and practical purposes, can mislead one into believing that the degree of bleeding is correlated with the severity of the illness or condition. An open mind is required during the inquiry into associated clinical features when haematuria is encountered.

Urine is a very complex and dynamic product, and red cells may be concentrated or diluted simply depending on the level of hydration of the individual. Cells may also lyse in hypo-osmotic fluid, particularly if they are stored for some hours before microscopic analysis. This may be one explanation for the occasional mismatch between chemosensitive urinary dipstick analysis and formal microscopy of the urinary sediment. Similarly, one cannot rely entirely on the historical data of haematuria, since there are several foodstuffs and medications that can mimic the reddened appearance of blood in the urine. More often than not, however, the patient may have already attributed the abnormal colour of the urine to some irrelevant factor and perhaps delayed his or her presentation on that basis. Many elderly individuals assume that blood in their urine is a sign of 'cancer', and this may occasionally lead to a delay in seeking an appropriate medical opinion. A cloudy (smoky) or brackish tinge to urine is considered to be supportive of haematuria, this alteration being secondary to reduction of haemoglobin by the acidic urine.

Red blood cells can enter the urine from many different areas – from the kidney, collecting system or bladder, to the urethra and attached structures, and may even arise from a lesion on the prepuce in males or on the introitus in females – to register in the voided sample. The midstream urinalysis has stood the test of time because it reduces the risk of a false-positive result. Techniques such as bladder needle aspiration or urethral catheterization may be helpful in certain clinical situations. Red-cell morphology identified by simple light or phase-contrast microscopy can sometimes be helpful in ascribing a more likely source of bleeding (e.g. dysmorphic red cells from renal parenchymal disease). Red cells may also be added to a voided sample in order to support the aspirations of a drug-seeking individual feigning renal colic in the emergency setting.

It is certainly sensible to request that a formal microscopic urinalysis and culture be performed even when there is a history of bloodstained urine. This test identifies in the urinary sediment all cells, and occasionally casts, crystals or micro-organisms, followed by bacterial culture (and sensitivities) to diagnose bacterial infection. Analysis of urine with a multi-chemical dipstick is common practice, and ably assists in the clinic; a positive leucocyte esterase (white-cell test) or the idenitification of nitrites supports an infective aetiology. However, it is not a substitute for the more definitive laboratory analysis.

Each of the following subsections has been created to help to group common clinical presentations. They are not mutually exclusive, and this arrangement is used only as a guide.

ASYMPTOMATIC MICROSCOPIC HAEMATURIA

Painless or asymptomatic haematuria is one area that is readily subdivided into microscopic and macroscopic haematuria. Under most circumstances, microscopic haematuria in an adult is deemed worthy of investigation only in the older individual (> 40 years), once a full history and physical examination have determined the finding to be in isolation. For those individuals under 40 years of age a sinister cause or precursor lesion that will influence their health is rarely identified. Patients over 40 years of age with microscopic haematuria are much more likely to have an identifiable cause for the bleeding that requires further medical management.

The most common benign and clinically irrelevant causes of microscopic haematuria are found in young female adults, and include squamous metaplasia of the trigone (thought by many to be a normal variant) and mild abacterial cystitis. Persistent microscopic haematuria is rarely seen in younger males who do not have concomitant symptoms or signs of urological disease, e.g. urethritis, balanitis, prostatitis. Systemic disease of many types can be manifested as microscopic haematuria. A thorough general medical inquiry and physical assessment is recommended to diagnose potential clinical problems such as hypertension, vascular disease and nephritis, to mention just a few.

The fact that bleeding may be glomerular in origin is supported by the presence of dysmorphic red blood cells and urinary casts in the urinary sediment. A common accompaniment is abnormally high levels of proteinuria. The protein concentration in urine rarely exceeds 20 mg/dL under normal circumstances, although the level of hydration can influence the result. A 24-h urine collection will measure the daily loss more accurately. Bleeding secondary to a urological condition does not elevate the protein concentration in the urine into the 200–300 mg/dL range or the 2+ to 3+ range on dipstick testing.

In children and young adults with glomerular bleeding, a relatively common diagnosis is immunoglobulin A (IgA) nephropathy, often associated with a low-grade fever and an erythematous skin rash. A family history of renal impairment may suggest familial nephritis (Alport's syndrome), and haemoptysis together with haematuria suggests Goodpasture's syndrome. Individuals with a rash and arthritis may have systemic lupus erythematosus, which is more common in females than in males. A history of a recent upper respiratory tract infection or skin infection suggests post-streptococcal glomerulonephritis. Renal function is often formally evaluated in this group, and several serological tests may be required, although commonly the diagnosis is not secure until a renal biopsy has been evaluated using light, immunofluorescent and electron microscopy. Although microscopic haematuria is more often associated with these renal disorders, gross bleeding is sometimes noted during the course of the disease.

Exercise-induced haematuria has become more prevalent in recent years, and may stem from underlying renal disease, a hitherto undiagnosed renal calculus, or minor trauma from the bladder urothelium. In long-distance runners haemoglobinuria is not uncommon and is thought to be related to red-cell disruption in the peripheral circulation caused by repetitive trauma. Bleeding in these situations ought to clear quickly following cessation of the activity, and observation is recommended if, after general inquiry and physical examination, there are no suspicions of significant underlying disease.

Microscopic haematuria is not uncommon with vascular disease. Embolic phenomena in the renal arterial tree, renal vein thrombosis, and arteriovenous malformations can result in haematuria. Pertinent physical signs include moderate to severe hypertension, an abdominal bruit or atrial fibrillation. Further vascular assessment is required should the above diagnoses be entertained.

ASYMPTOMATIC MACROSCOPIC HAEMATURIA

Macroscopic bleeding almost always requires further investigation. It can be associated with bacterial infection, and in this circumstance the additional investigations may be minimal, namely repeat urinalysis following eradication of the infection. However, underlying significant illness is found in enough cases with macroscopic haematuria for routine evaluations to be recommended. The following important features are worthy of note in the history: longstanding cigarette smoking, or environmental exposure to dyes, rubber compounds, etc., increasing risk of transitional cell carcinoma (TCC) of the urinary tract; anticoagulation therapy – in itself rarely a reason not to investigate provided that the level of anticoagulation is not excessive; previous treatment of a urological condition, perhaps with the insertion of a prosthesis or ureteric stent. Physical examination may reveal signs of systemic disease or help to predict the likely source of bleeding, such as a renal mass or a palpably large or indurated prostate gland. However, more commonly the physical examination is largely unrewarding in this circumstance.

Appropriate investigation includes a peripheral blood examination (complete blood count; CBC) and an estimate of renal function (electrolytes, urea and creatinine). Whether liver function tests, prostate-specific antigen or coagulation studies, etc., are requested will depend on the findings in the history and examination.

In addition, asymptomatic macroscopic haematuria requires upper tract radiological imaging and direct lower tract visualization (cystoscopy). The choice of upper tract study may be dependent on such findings as, first, impaired renal function (e.g. creatinine >0.25 mmol/L), when intravenous contrast poorly opacifies the upper tracts and can further impair renal function; or second, pregnancy, when ionizing radiation needs to be kept to a minimum, particularly in the first trimester. In these two scenarios renal tract ultrasound as the initial test of choice would be appropriate. An intravenous pyelogram (IVP) remains the most reliable first-choice radiological investigation for frank haematuria (see algorithm in Figure 3.6.1).

Urethrocystoscopy can be safely performed in the out-patient setting using a flexible instrument with or without sedation, even in patients with severe comorbid disease. Those who are anticoagulated may undergo an initial diagnostic cystoscopy before planning definitive treatment as an in-patient under carefully controlled conditions.

The diagnosis is often apparent after these tests have been performed, although additional staging or diagnos-

tic tools may be utilized prior to therapy. For instance, a retrograde pyelogram may be indicated for a poorly filled renal calyx, and at the same time urine can be collected for cytology from the affected renal unit. It is not uncommon for a small upper tract TCC to be overlooked with renal CT, although clearly CT is used in staging to assess local and metastatic disease.

Urinary stones may be diagnosed incidently on an IVP. Typically, upper tract stones do not produce macroscopic bleeding, although microscopic haematuria is common. The finding of an upper tract stone does not obviate the need to perform a lower tract cystoscopic evaluation. A detailed description of the management of urinary stones is beyond the scope of this chapter.

HAEMATURIA IN ASSOCIATION WITH TRAUMA

Haematuria is the commonest sign of renal trauma in all large series. When present, it is suggestive of renal trauma, although its degree does not always correlate with the severity of the injury. Importantly, it is major

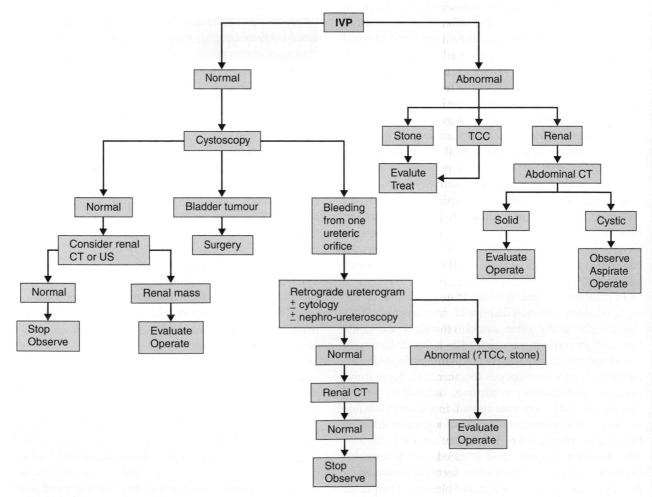

Figure 3.6.1 Evaluation of haematuria without red-cell casts or proteinuria.

renal vascular injuries that most often present with microscopic haematuria or no haematuria at all. In the latter circumstance there is typically a clue to renal injury based on the severity of the overall trauma or the mechanism of injury, e.g. a major deceleration injury or a direct blow to the flank.

The recommendation that all individuals presenting with trauma and found to have haematuria require radiological evaluation has fallen from prominence, since it would unnecessarily expose many to the discomfort, possible allergic reaction, radiation exposure and expense of a test, typically an IVP. More acceptable is an aim to identify all those in whom investigation has a low threshold of altering management, since more than 90% of individuals presenting after blunt trauma have a renal contusion only, and the yield from an IVP is low.

A clinically important renal lesion would rarely be missed if all individuals presenting with *microscopic* haematuria in association with blunt trauma and in the *absence of shock* were managed expectantly without imaging (shock in this setting is defined as a systolic blood pressure below 90 mmHg measured in the emergency department or at any time by the attendant staff prior to arrival in hospital). Conservative or expectant management is recommended. After a period of assessment (> 4 h) the individual may be discharged with simple instructions to seek medical advice if macroscopic bleeding occurs or loin pain increases such that simple (non-narcotic) pain relief is ineffective. Despite these recommendations, one must remain cognizant of the clinical picture that is more suggestive of significant renal trauma based on the mechanism of injury, and which ought to prompt radiological investigation.

The indications for imaging the renal tract in children who present with trauma and microscopic haematuria are not so well defined, since in children a normal systolic blood pressure is not as reliable an indicator of minor injury. Clinical signs of shock in children are found in less than 10% of those with significant renal injury. Furthermore, in children the kidneys are not as well protected with perinephric fat, and they are less protected by muscle and ribs. Therefore it is not unreasonable to have a lower threshold for investigation of children with suspected trauma to the kidneys, irrespective of the level of haematuria. The initial test of choice is an IVP, or if intra-abdominal pathology is suspected, then a contrast-enhanced CT scan is indicated. Of course, in the unstable patient, surgical staging of trauma may be urgently indicated, in which case knowledge of a functioning contralateral kidney ought to be obtained promptly using a 'one-shot' or infusion IVP.

Patients with macroscopic bleeding require active investigation, even if the trauma seems to be somewhat trivial compared to the amount of bleeding, since in this latter circumstance it is not uncommon to uncover a renal abnormality that predisposed the kidney to haemorrhage, e.g. a congenital abnormality or tumour. In patients who remain haemodynamically stable, an IVP is still regarded by many as the best first investigation. If renal trauma is suspected as a part of poly-trauma, and intra-abdominal imaging is required, then clearly a contrast-enhanced CT scan is appropriate in this setting. Staging of renal injury is most accurately performed with a contrast CT. However, not all patients with macroscopic haematuria require this investigation. The advantages of a CT scan include the fact that it defines the perirenal tissues and the depth of trauma to the kidney.

In the stable patient with mild to moderate renal injury, a conservative approach is recommended (Figure 3.6.2). Hospital bedrest is often required, the period of rest depending on the rapidity of clearance of macroscopic bleeding, after which there is a further period of mobilization and gradual return to normal activity over several (4 to 6) weeks. In patients with severe renal trauma, an operative approach is frequently advocated since late complications such as a urinoma or infarcted renal substance often lead to significant morbidity. However, an early operation is predictive of a higher rate of nephrectomy, and the outcome is particularly dependent on the experience of the surgeon. Clearly, those who remain haemodynamically unstable or have sustained a renal pedicle injury require prompt surgical intervention (Figure 3.6.2). Penetrating trauma also requires operative management.

In the clinical setting, haematuria in association with trauma may suggest sites other than the kidneys as the source. In particular, posterior urethral disruption may present with blood at the urethral meatus. More than 90% of cases are the result of blunt trauma, and almost all have pelvic ring disruption, many being associated with severe and often life-threatening injuries. The retrograde urethrogram is a simple, accurate and inexpensive test that can be performed early on in the assessment of trauma.

Bladder rupture is also associated with pelvic fracture in over 90% of cases, and frequently presents with gross haematuria. A cystogram is the diagnostic investigation of choice. Extraperitoneal bladder rupture may be managed conservatively, although if associated with polytrauma it is often formally closed as part of the operative management of other injuries. Intraperitoneal ruptures require surgical repair.

HAEMATURIA IN ASSOCIATION WITH IRRITATIVE SYMPTOMS

Irritative urinary symptoms include urinary frequency, urgency and urinary urge incontinence. Pain associated

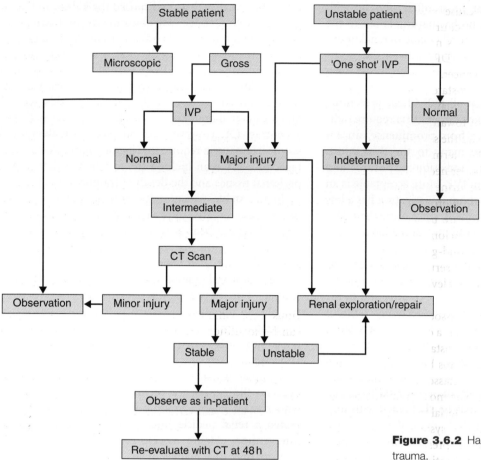

Figure 3.6.2 Haematuria associated with renal trauma.

with micturition is a common accompaniment. Haematuria in conjunction with this symptom complex necessitates further investigation. The most common cause identified is bacterial bladder infection, more commonly found in women, a finding that is partly due to the male urethra offering more resistance to ascending infection because of its length, and possibly the antibacterial properties that have been ascribed to prostatic fluid. Microscopic haematuria is common with cystitis, although gross bleeding can occur. Dipstick urinalysis is useful in the office setting, particularly if nitrites are detected. However, direct microscopy and culture with sensitivities are required. Should a bacterial infection be confirmed, then a repeat urinalysis is recommended following definitive antimicrobial therapy.

There are several other important diagnoses to consider when faced with an individual presenting with irritative voiding symptoms and haematuria. These include bladder carcinoma (particularly carcinoma *in situ*), bladder calculi, prostate cancer, an extravesical inflammatory process (e.g. sigmoid diverticular disease), urethritis and prostatitis, to mention just a few. Clearly, additional features in the history and some physical findings will assist in making these determinations.

Bladder cancer (> 90% of cases are transitional cell carcinomas in industrialized countries) has some acknowledged predisposing factors already mentioned above. Although bacterial cystitis can present concomitantly with bladder cancer, the diagnosis of a structural problem of the bladder is made more tenable when recurrent infections occur despite adequate antimicrobial therapy. Voided urine cytology can be of assistance, although well to moderately differentiated transitional cell carcinomas of the bladder do not shed malignant cells reliably. A cystoscopy is the key to the early diagnosis of bladder cancer in this setting.

Bladder calculi are commonly associated with impaired bladder emptying. In men this is frequently secondary to prostatic enlargement, and thus effective treatment involves improving the bladder outlet (e.g. transurethral prostatectomy or bladder-neck incision) as well as removing the calculi. Stranguria, or an intense pain in the bladder/urethral region at the termination of micturition, is not uncommon with infected bladder calculi, but non-infected stones can remain relatively symptom-free for years. Ultrasound is an accurate method for identifying bladder calculi, and it also has some success with exophytic bladder tumours. Despite this fact, an IVP is still recommended to evaluate the upper tracts accurately, because ultrasound will not readily identify small upper tract urothelial lesions.

An abdominal examination is never complete without a digital rectal examination (DRE), which is a useful screening tool for prostate cancer. Haematuria is not a common presenting sign of prostate cancer, which in its early stage of growth is asymptomatic. However, the timing of haematuria may point towards a prostatic source when the bleeding is initial and the stream clears as voiding continues. Occasionally, terminal haematuria is noted with lesions at the bladder neck. Also, straining to empty the last few drops of urine can cause bleeding from benign enlargement of the prostate where superficial veins are believed to rupture under the force of a Valsalva manoeuvre. The suspicion of prostate cancer may lead to transrectal ultrasound-guided needle biopsy of the prostate. Commonly, the serum prostate-specific antigen (PSA) is found to be elevated with clinically important prostate cancer.

Irritative symptoms may be associated with prostatitis, and microscopic haematuria is a common sign in this setting. Inflammation of the prostate comes in several guises, the most common perhaps being pain or a dull ache in the perineum that is unassociated with proven bacterial prostatic infection. The most dramatic form in terms of symptoms is acute bacterial prostatitis, which is often accompanied by severe systemic toxicity. An acutely tender prostate is always present with acute bacterial prostatitis, and parenteral antimicrobial treatment is indicated. Chronic prostatitis and prostatodynia often show less than satisfactory responses to conventional therapy which has centred around lengthy (4 to 6 weeks) administration of antimicrobial agents. Symptoms may be improved with anti-inflammatory preparations or sometimes by pelvic muscle relaxation techniques.

The suspicion of a perivesical cause of bleeding is often not difficult to confirm. The presence of an enterovesical fistula predisposes to pneumaturia and recurrent urinary infection. A gynaecological examination is mandatory in women presenting with irritative symptoms and haematuria, since malignancy of any of the female reproductive organs can mimic a primary urological condition. A carefully taken history is important when considering this distinction, and it ought to include questions designed to determine the presence of atypical vaginal bleeding, dyspareunia and post-coital bleeding.

HAEMATURIA IN ASSOCIATION WITH ACUTE PAIN UNRELATED TO TRAUMA

The regular appearance of patients with renal colic in the emergency departments is a situation not unfamiliar to many. The typical features include pain that stimulates movement, causing the patient to writhe about rather than lie still as with peritoneal irritation from intra-abdominal sepsis. Pain is frequently localized to the loin, but may be along the imaginary line between kidney and groin, including testicular pain in males. Systemic upset such as nausea and vomiting is common. Microscopic haematuria is common, and after initial symptomatic management, radiological assessment is required. The IVP has long been regarded as the standard investigation in the acute setting, although in recent years, a non-contrast-enhanced spiral CT scan has been advocated as a safer and more definitive investigation. Indeed, there is improved identification of small distal ureteric stones, and an assessment of stone density is readily available which correlates well with crystalline composition. However, this study gives only limited information on the function of the kidneys.

Radiological investigation usually indicates the likely cause of colic, which is typically a renal or ureteric calculus. Less commonly a blood clot or sloughed papilla can be identified, frequently secondary to upper tract malignancy in the former scenario and diabetes or analgesic nephropathy in the latter.

However, all that may initially appear to present as renal colic may not be. In particular, one needs to be vigilant in order to exclude such diagnoses as a leaking abdominal aortic aneurysm, acute porphyria or a sickle-cell crisis.

HAEMATURIA IN ASSOCIATION WITH PRIOR UROLOGICAL SURGERY

It comes as no surprise that much urological surgery is followed in the post-operative period with haematuria, gross bleeding being common after transurethral resection of a prostate (TURP) or a bladder tumour. The resected area takes several weeks to heal and, when bathed in irrigating solution in the early period, or simply in urine, cells reflective of a healing ulcer are shed from the urinary tract. To determine the presence of infection in this setting, urine culture is essential. A secondary haemorrhage following resection is not common, but can occur between 1 and 3 weeks post-operatively and is manifested by a return of gross bleeding after macroscopically clear urine for many days. Expectant management is often all that is required, although clot retention may occur if the bleeding is profuse. Frequently there is a history of rapid return to moderate or heavy physical exertion prior to the secondary bleed.

Many years after TURP, painless gross haematuria may herald the return of significant adenomatous prostatic growth. If another source is not identified, the recurrent prostatic tissue is usually resected with subsequent cessation of the intermittent bleeding. The individual concerned may or may not have experienced difficulty in voiding.

SUMMARY

Haematuria is a sign associated with a diverse range of conditions that requires careful assessment and highly specific management according to its cause. By taking a careful history the clinician is alerted to several predisposing factors that are known to cause haematuria. A thorough physical examination may also be helpful in determining the likely source. Nevertheless, radiological, surgical or pathological diagnostic tests are frequently required to diagnose the underlying condition correctly.

FURTHER READING

McAninch JW (ed.). 1996: *Traumatic and reconstructive urology*. Philadelphia, PA: W.B. Saunders.

Walsh PC, Retik AB, Vaughan ED, Wein AJ (eds). 1998: *Campbell's urology*, 7th edn. Philadelphia, PA: W.B. Saunders.

Vaginal bleeding

Hamish P. Ewing

Introduction

This is an unusual problem to arrive on the surgical doorstep, as usually women with such a symptom will be directed to a gynaecological service. The most important message for a surgeon to absorb is that abnormal bleeding from the female genital tract may:

- be a cause of iron-deficiency anaemia;
- be an obstetric cause of right iliac fossa pain;
- herald a bleeding disorder;
- be confused with rectal bleeding;
- reflect a medical disorder with surgical implications.

The answer is always to *remember to inquire about bleeding per vaginum (PV)*.

The bleeding can arise from either the uterus or the vagina, and clearly it is important to establish whether the woman is premenopausal or not. The endometrium provides a wonderful example of the effects of physiology and pathology on the triangle of hormonal interplay between pituitary, ovary and endometrium, the picture being further confused by other factors, e.g. stress, myxoedema, cirrhosis, exogenous oestrogens, etc.

There are two lists of causes of vaginal bleeding which are dependent on menopausal status.

PREMENOPAUSAL VAGINAL BLEEDING

The causes of this symptom (Table 3.7.1) can be divided into two groups, namely menstrual and other causes.

MENSTRUAL ABNORMALITIES

There are three descriptions of abnormal menstrual loss that need to be defined, as there are different causes for each of them.

Menorrhagia This is excessive bleeding in regular cycles. The usual cause is uterine fibroids, adenomyosis or faulty clotting.

Polymenorrhoea These are periods that are too frequent, and the usual cause is a disturbance of the pituitary/ovarian axis.

Polymenorrhagia These are periods that are too heavy and too frequent, usually due to a combination of any of the causes of menorrhagia and polymenorrhoea mentioned above.

In addition, there are other influences on menstrual loss.

General influences These include idiopathic thrombocytopenic purpura, aplastic anaemia, leukaemia and von Willebrand's disease.

Psychological influences For example, stress can be a significant factor.

Table 3.7.1 Causes of premenopausal bleeding

Adolescents
- Dysfunctional bleeding (due to disturbance of the balance between pituitary gland, ovary and endometrium)

Adults (20–39 years)
- Benign genital tract lesions
- Pelvic inflammatory disease
- Fibroids
- Complicated pregnancies
- Dysfunctional bleeding

Perimenopausal women (> 40 years)
- Dysfunctional bleeding
- Fibroids
- Carcinoma of the cervix
- Endometrial carcinoma

Endocrine factors Hypothyroidism can be the cause of increased menstrual loss, and in fact this symptom is found in 30% of cases of myxoedema. Pituitary disease, cirrhosis and oral contraceptives can all influence menstrual flow.

OTHER CAUSES OF VAGINAL BLEEDING

Uterine causes

With regard to (early) pregnancy, these include:

- ectopic pregnancy;

- threatened abortion;

- spontaneous abortion;

- hydatidiform mole (gestational trophoblastic disease);

- implantation haemorrhage.

It should be noted that PV bleeding occurs to some degree in up to 25% of all normal pregnancies.

Foreign bodies These can be deliberately placed, e.g. an intrauterine device (IUD), or secondary to attempted 'therapeutic' abortion.

Infection This can be seen, for example, with pelvic inflammatory disease and occasionally chronic endometriosis.

Uterine tumours These can be a simple myoma, endometrial polyps and even occasionally endometrial malignancy.

Bicornuate uterus A past history of deep venous thrombosis of the pelvic veins can lead to engorgement of the endometrium and hence bleeding.

Ovarian tumours These will only rarely cause vaginal bleeding, but a follicular cyst is a possibility.

Vaginal causes

These include the following:

- infection;

- trauma (may not be admitted to);

- cervical cancer or the after-effects of radiotherapy to treat this condition.

Any intermenstrual bleeding should raise the suspicion of malignancy.

POST-MENOPAUSAL VAGINAL BLEEDING

Post-menopausal bleeding is assumed to be due to malignancy until proven otherwise (Table 3.7.2).

Possible causes of post-menopausal bleeding include the following:

- uterine (endometrial or cervical) tumours;
- exogenous oestrogens;
- vaginal infection;
- trauma;
- irradiation.

It should be noted that in about 10–15% of cases no cause for post-menopausal bleeding can be found. Because of the high incidence of genital tract cancers in this group of women, it is very important that a careful examination of the vulva, vagina, cervix and uterus is always undertaken before more sophisticated tests are performed.

MANAGEMENT OF VAGINAL BLEEDING

This depends very much on the setting, and is largely the province of a gynaecologist.

However, the five general surgical settings listed at the beginning of this chapter will be discussed below.

Table 3.7.2 Causes of post-menopausal bleeding

- Genital malignancy (up to 25% of cases)
- Endometrial/cervical polyps
- Atrophic vagina
- Response to oestrogen therapies
- Endometrial hyperplasia
- Urethral carbuncle
- Vaginitis
- Ovarian tumour

IRON-DEFICIENCY ANAEMIA

The most important question to remember when taking the history of a woman found to have such an anaemia concerns the nature of any vaginal bleeding. It is not uncommon for a woman not to complain about her menstrual loss even though it is quite different to the norm. It is therefore necessary to ask *additional* questions concerning the length of the menstrual period, the presence of clots, excessive use of sanitary pads, etc., in order to obtain a more complete picture.

An abnormal period is one in which the duration of menstrual loss is greater than 7 days, or that is of a volume that is difficult to cope with using sanitary pads.

Having established that the anaemia may be secondary to heavy menstrual loss, a referral to a gynaecologist is indicated, as often such patients are improved by a diagnostic/therapeutic dilatation and curettage (D&C). Clearly, establishing menstrual loss as a possible cause of anaemia is *the most important clinical step*. Making a referral to the gynaecologist is the easy bit!

Menorrhagia is the commonest cause of iron deficiency in the Western world.

RIGHT ILIAC FOSSA PAIN IN ASSOCIATION WITH VAGINAL BLEEDING

As discussed elsewhere in this book (see Chapter 1.5), right iliac fossa pain can present quite a challenge to the surgeon. The possibility of an ectopic pregnancy always needs to be borne in mind. The classic story is one of right iliac fossa pain (90% of cases), amenorrhoea (80%) and vaginal bleeding (70%). Very often the bleeding is initially thought to be due to the delayed onset of the anticipated period, and can even be associated with a low-grade fever. Occasionally there is an acute rupture of the ectopic pregnancy with a collapse from massive bleeding. However, this is usually against a background of a subacute presentation. At the time of collapse there may also be some associated shoulder tip pain due to irritation of the undersurface of the diaphragm. There will be a history of sexual intercourse, although this fact will not necessarily surface if a teenager's mother is in the cubicle as well! Examination is likely to reveal lower abdominal tenderness with the presence of blood at the cervical os.

Management (Figure 3.7.1)

- Think of the possibility of an ectopic pregnancy - diagnosis made with *positive* beta human chorionic gonadotrophin (βHCG) test (99% accuracy) and ultrasound of the uterus showing absence of pregnancy.

- If the patient is in shock, resuscitate and order blood for cross-matching.

- Involve a gynaecologist early on, as this problem can often be managed laparoscopically with conservation of the Fallopian tube.

- If gynaecological assistance is not readily available, the haemorrhage is controlled by ligation and resection of the involved Fallopian tube.

The other possible cause of vaginal bleeding and some colicky lower abdominal pains is a threatened abortion. In this situation the βHCG will be positive but, on ultrasound, evidence of a uterine pregnancy is present. Of course this is not the case with an ectopic pregnancy.

VAGINAL BLEEDING HERALDING THE PRESENCE OF A BLEEDING DISORDER

The presence of abnormal vaginal bleeding in any surgical patient should suggest the possibility of a coagulopathy and flag the inherent risk for that patient during any surgery you might be contemplating. It is worth noting that 50% of patients who suffer from von Willebrand's disease and 80% of those with idiopathic thrombocytopenic purpura will experience menorrhagia.

Management

When taking the history it is important to seek evidence of easy bruising, bleeding from other orifices and any difficulties that the patient may have encountered with regard to previous operations or tooth extractions. In addition, enquire about any family history of bleeding disorders.

In order to allay concern, a coagulation profile must be ordered, possibly with a bleeding time as well. Should there be any abnormality, seek a haematologist's opinion, as the problem clearly needs to be addressed before undertaking any surgery.

VAGINAL BLEEDING CONFUSED WITH BLOOD FROM THE RECTUM

From time to time one can be misled by a patient as to which orifice is giving rise to bleeding. This confusion can work in either direction, with vaginal bleeding thought to be anal, or vice versa. This situation tends to occur more often in the elderly, who may consider it 'inconceivable' that vaginal bleeding could have started again well into the menopausal years. Surgeons need to be reminded that uterine cancer occurs in the postmenopausal age group (75% of cases are aged 55–65 years).

VAGINAL BLEEDING WITH OR WITHOUT ABDOMINAL PAIN

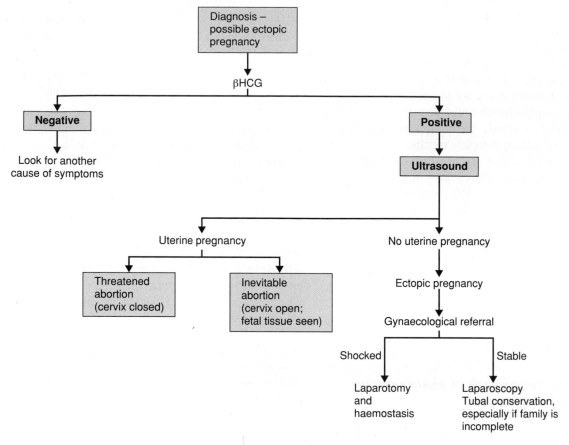

Figure 3.7.1 Management plan for vaginal bleeding.

Clearly a careful history and examination should ensure that a gynaecological cause is not missed, but if one is misled, then reaching the correct diagnosis is more challenging. The clue is provided when no cause for ano-rectal bleeding can be identified. In this setting, the genital tract must be examined by an expert. The simple measure of placing a tampon in the vagina may quickly help to pinpoint the source of bleeding.

MEDICAL DISORDERS WITH SURGICAL IMPLICATIONS

Menorrhagia has a number of causes, but it is the less common causes listed under general and endocrine factors earlier in this chapter that should perhaps be of most interest to the surgeon. For example, a missed diagnosis of *hypothyroidism* can have grave implications for any surgery undertaken, with hypotension, bradycardia and respiratory failure potentially ensuing.

Similarly, *pituitary tumours* can be manifested in a wide variety of ways, but included in this list will be vaginal bleeding.

Psychological factors, e.g. stress, can have numerous effects – menorrhagia being just one of them. How often do we spend enough time assessing and treating 'stress' in our patients? The management of irritable bowel syndrome is a prime example, but so also is the growing number of studies pointing towards the influence of the mind on the outcome of cancer treatments.

SUMMARY

Obstetric and gynaecological problems do not generally feature in surgical texts, and yet in the clinical setting this is not the case. This section should serve as a timely reminder to surgical trainees that they should always consider 'the whole patient'.

Palpitations

Leo Mahar

Introduction

Palpitations are subjective feelings of heart irregularity, and are felt as if the heart is 'missing a beat', or as thumping in the chest, an irregular pulse or even tachycardia noticed at rest.

The history is very important. It is essential to find out when the patient is aware of the palpitation, e.g. at the end of exercise or when quietly resting, or associated with a particular factor (e.g. caffeine consumption, alcohol consumption, or anxiety) and also any concurrent symptoms such as dizziness, faintness or even syncope.

USUAL CAUSES OF PALPITATIONS

Quite often in the young patient, extensive investigations will reveal that the patient is in sinus rhythm and is just very aware of their heartbeats. The most common cause of palpitations in clinical practice is ectopic beats (either atrial or ventricular ectopics; Figure 4.1). The patient is often aware of something 'missing', followed by a thump (Figure 4.2). The thump is often felt in the throat or the chest, and is caused by the more forceful post-ectopic beat. Occasionally, bursts of atrial fibrillation (Figure 4.3) will cause problems, as can bursts of supraventricular tachycardia or ventricular tachycardia (Figure 4.4). Rarely, intermittent slow heartbeats such as sino-atrial block or atrioventricular block may cause these symptoms (Figure 4.5).

As mentioned above, history-taking is vital. It is important to establish any associated precipitating factors such as coffee, tea, nicotine, alcohol or other drugs (e.g. bronchodilators), or perhaps even recreational drugs. Anxiety is a very common cause of palpitations. Overwork and missing sleep are frequently the cause (particularly in surgical registrars). It is important to obtain a history of any heart disease, hypertension, etc.

One way to determine what is going on is to ask the patient to tap out the beats or even to tap them out yourself; there is a very fast regular beat with supraventricular tachycardia (about 180 beats/min) or very fast irregular beats like 'morse code' with atrial fibrillation. Often when this is brought to the patient's attention they will be able to note more carefully what has happened the next time they have palpitations. It is important to determine any associated symptoms such as pre-syncope or syncope. Pre-syncope or syncope are particularly important if the patient indulges in dangerous leisure pursuits such as flying, scuba-diving, etc., as in such circumstances an altered state of consciousness could be life-threatening.

EXAMINATION

It is very important to examine the patient for any evidence of cardiovascular disease, such as valvular heart disease, congestive heart failure or hypertension. Although this is uncommon, it is important to look for signs of hyperthyroidism. Nevertheless, cardiovascular examination is usually normal.

INVESTIGATIONS

Resting ECG should always be taken, but is often normal. If the ectopics are very frequent, a few may show up on the rhythm strip. A resting ECG is a very unreliable sample of the patient's underlying rhythm, and other investigations will be needed. A chest X-ray is of little use. An echocardiogram is much more valuable, particularly if there is any suspicion of cardiac enlargement, cardiac hypertrophy or valvular heart disease.

Electrocardiographic monitoring is very important to

(a)
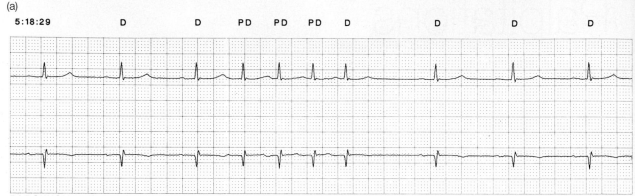
PAROXYSMAL SV TACHY. 4 Beats. Heart Rate 134. Duration 1.3 sec.

(b)
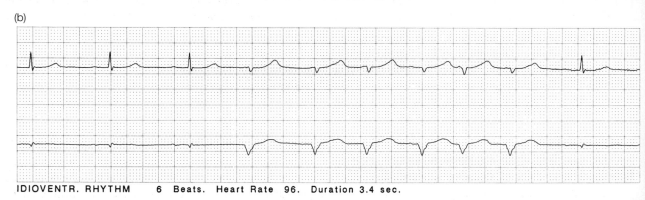
IDIOVENTR. RHYTHM   6 Beats. Heart Rate 96. Duration 3.4 sec.

Figure 4.1 Examples of palpitations from 24-h Holter recording. (a) Run of atrial ectopics. (b) Run of idioventricular rhythm (broad QRS complexes).

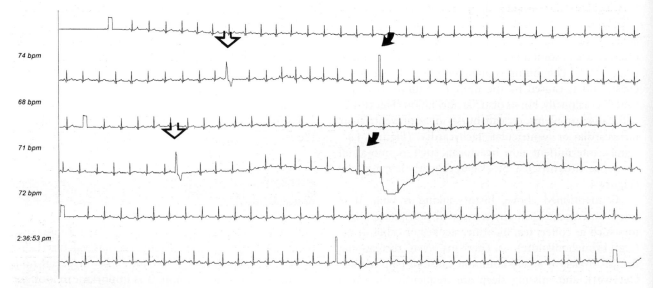

Figure 4.2 Continuous loop recording. Single premature ventricular contraction (open arrow) recorded by patient (closed arrow) as cause of symptom.

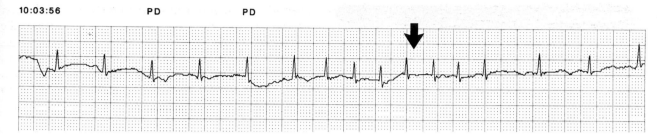

Figure 4.3 Sinus rhythm with a brief run of atrial fibrillation.

try and determine the underlying substrate of the patient's symptoms. A 24-h Holter monitor is normally very useful, but it may miss less common episodes of palpitations. In this case, an event loop recorder is useful. This continuously monitors the patient's ECG so that when the patient presses the button to mark an event that has taken place, a permanent recording of the period from 45 s before to 15 s after the event is taken. Up to five incidents can be recorded over a 6-day period. The results can be sent transtelephonically. This is particularly useful for symptoms which occur only occasionally and for patients who live some distance from the office. If the patient is very symptomatic and has had episodes of pre-syncope or syncope, it may be worth proceeding to electrophysiology studies to

attempt to resolve the problem. This is reserved for more serious arrhythmias such as suspected ventricular tachycardia, supraventricular tachycardia or even atrial fibrillation. These invasive investigations can often be performed as day-patient procedures, and may even be combined with appropriate therapy such as radiofrequency ablation of dual AV nodal pathways or abnormal atrioventricular connections (bundles of Kent).

As well as electrocardiographic monitoring investigation, the usual background blood profile and biochemical screening should be undertaken, particularly thyroid function. Often palpitations may be the presenting feature of thyrotoxicosis in the elderly. If the symptoms are related to exercise, then an exercise ECG may be appropriate.

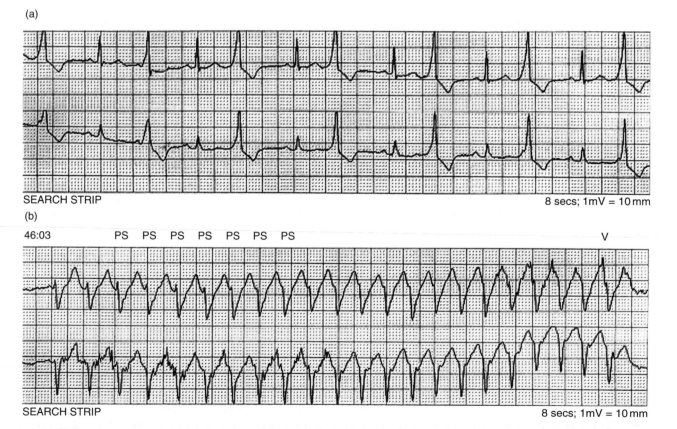

Figure 4.4 (a) Sinus rhythm with ventricular bigeminy (alternating narrow complex (QRS) preceded by P-wave and broad complex PVC). (b) Run of ventricular tachycardia.

TREATMENT

Therapy should be directed towards the underlying pathology. If the patient is hypertensive, they should be treated appropriately, preferably with agents which will damp down ectopics, such as beta-blockers or long-acting calcium antagonists, e.g. verapamil. Any thyroid malfunction should be corrected. Ischaemic heart disease may be the underlying substrate, and if symptomatic ischaemia is found, then appropriate treatment (either medical or interventional) should be given. Congestive heart failure should be treated appropriately. If an underlying rhythm is found, such as atrial fibrillation or intermittent supraventricular tachycardia, appropriate treatment (either drugs or interventional treatment) should be given.

At the end of the investigations most individuals are found to have a few ectopics. The patient should be reassured about the benign prognosis and advised on any appropriate lifestyle modifications. It is best to avoid anti-arrhythmic agents wherever possible, as they are more likely to cause harm from side-effects than to be beneficial. If the patient remains very symptomatic, then beta-blockers may be the most useful treatment if symptoms do not respond to simple measures. Any other anti-arrhythmic agents would be best managed by a consultation with a physician or cardiologist.

21:06:39

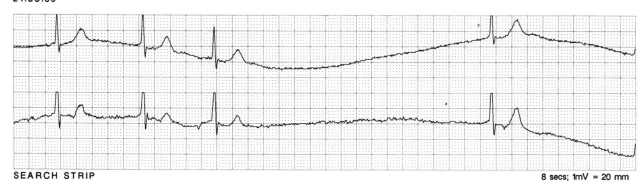

SEARCH STRIP   8 secs; 1mV = 20 mm

21:06:47

Figure 4.5 Long pause (3.6 s) with ventricular standstill and slow junctional escape rhythm.

Cyanosis

George G. Collee

Introduction

Cyanosis (from the Greek *kuanos* (adj.), meaning dark blue) is a bluish discoloration of the skin and mucous membranes, usually resulting from hypoxaemia (a deficiency of oxygen in the blood).

1. *Central cyanosis* is characterized by blue lips/tongue/mucous membranes/nailbeds, and indicates a low oxygen content in the blood.
2. *Peripheral cyanosis* is characterized by pink lips/tongue/mucous membranes but blue nailbeds and implies adequate oxygen content in the blood but slow blood flow and/or excessive oxygen uptake by tissues.

Central cyanosis is easy to miss clinically, especially in black or Asian patients or in anaemic patients. Check well-perfused mucous membranes such as the buccal mucosa, and the tongue, where the cyanosis is most readily apparent. It is the reduced haemoglobin level which gives the bluish appearance in hypoxaemia. About 3 g of reduced haemoglobin per 100 mL of blood are required to produce clinically apparent cyanosis. A patient with a haemoglobin concentration of 15 g/dL will become visibly cyanosed at a haemoglobin saturation of about 80% (i.e. 20% of 15 g/dL = 3 g/dL of reduced haemoglobin). The arterial blood gas analysis of such a patient would show a partial pressure (PaO_2) of about 7 kPa.

If the patient's haemoglobin level is only 10 g/dL, saturation must fall to 70% to produce 3 g/dL of reduced haemoglobin. The oxygen *content* of this anaemic patient is therefore very low before cyanosis becomes clinically evident at the bedside. Moreover, administering oxygen will return the saturation to normal, restore a normal PaO_2 and the patient will appear pink, even though the oxygen content of the blood remains low due to the low haemoglobin concentration.

This observation raises the concepts of oxygen content, oxygen partial pressure and percentage saturation of haemoglobin – basic scientific concepts which must be understood in order to interpret oxygen therapy.

OXYGEN CONTENT, PARTIAL PRESSURE AND SATURATION

Oxygen content This is the amount of oxygen (expressed in mL) carried by each 100 mL of blood. Fully saturated haemoglobin carries 1.3 mL of oxygen per gram of haemoglobin.

Oxygen saturation This refers to the percentage of all the available oxygen binding sites on the circulating haemoglobin (four sites per molecule) that are actually occupied by oxygen molecules. This percentage is therefore directly related to oxygen content.

Oxygen content (mL/dL blood) =
$$Hb\,(g/dL) \times 1.3\,(mL/g) \times \%\ saturation.$$

For a normal patient:
$$16 \times 1.3 \times 96\% = 19.9\,mL/dL$$

For a patient with apparent cyanosis:
$$16 \times 1.3 \times 80\% = 16.6\,mL/dL$$

For a patient with anaemia and cyanosis:
$$10 \times 1.3 \times 70\% = 9.1 \text{ mL/dL}$$

For a patient with anaemia and oxygen:
$$10 \times 1.3 \times 100\% = 13.0 \text{ mL/dL}.$$

If a normal haemoglobin level can be assumed, the percentage saturation (which can be easily measured non-invasively with a pulse oximeter) relates directly to the oxygen content of the blood. Beware of carboxy-haemoglobin in carbon monoxide poisoning. Carbon monoxide displaces oxygen from the haemoglobin molecule, but the pulse oximeter cannot distinguish between oxy- and carboxyhaemoglobin (Hb-O_2 and Hb-CO). Therefore the pulse oximeter gives a high apparent saturation in the presence of a very low oxygen content. With this important exception, percentage saturation gives an excellent indication of oxygen carriage.

Partial pressure In healthy individuals, about 20 mL of oxygen per 100 mL of blood are carried bound to haemoglobin. In addition, a very small amount of oxygen is carried in solution (0.003 mL of oxygen/mmHg or 0.02 mL of oxygen/kPa/100 mL of blood). The quantity of dissolved oxygen is virtually insignificant in most clinical settings, but it is the dissolved oxygen which is measured as the partial pressure of oxygen in blood (the PO_2 of a blood gas analysis). Knowing the affinity of haemoglobin for oxygen allows assumptions to be made whereby a partial pressure implies a certain haemoglobin saturation and oxygen content (Figure 5.1). *Blood gas analysers measure partial pressure. The clinician must interpret the PaO_2 according to the clinical setting.*

As shown in Figure 5.1, the relationship between PO_2 and oxygen content is not a straight line. The 'S'-shape of the Hb-O_2–PO_2 curve is due to the changing affinity for oxygen that the haemoglobin molecule has for each of the four oxygen molecules it can carry. The affinity of haemoglobin for oxygen is reduced by acidosis, increased PCO_2, increased temperature or increased 2,3-diphosphoglycerate (2,3-DPG). This moves the haemoglobin oxygen dissociation curve to the right so that, for a given PO_2, less oxygen is bound to haemoglobin.

Consider the interaction between dissolved oxygen and that which is bound to haemoglobin.

In the lung, oxygen passes down a concentration gradient from the alveolus into the capillary blood. By 'mopping up' dissolved oxygen as it enters the blood, haemoglobin keeps the capillary PO_2 low, thereby maintaining the gradient which facilitates oxygen transfer from the alveolus to the blood. On the Hb-O_2 dissociation curve we initially see a steep rise in oxygen content for a relatively small rise in PaO_2 as deoxygenated mixed venous blood with a PO_2 of 5.3 kPa (40 mmHg) and a saturation of 70% is oxygenated.

At the tissues, the opposite process occurs. Hb-O_2 represents a store of oxygen. As oxygen passes from the blood to the tissues, Hb-O_2 releases oxygen into solution, thereby maintaining the PaO_2. This 'props up' the gradient of PO_2 between the capillary blood and the tissues. After the initial rapid fall in PaO_2 as the saturation falls to 90%, there is a relatively small fall in PaO_2 for a relatively large fall in oxygen content as haemoglobin gives up its oxygen to the tissues. Moreover, as CO_2 enters the blood from the tissues it reduces the affinity of haemoglobin for oxygen, enhancing oxygen release (the Bohr effect).

At high PaO_2 the haemoglobin–oxygen dissociation curve is nearly flat because, once haemoglobin is fully saturated, very little additional oxygen can be carried in the blood in solution. Therefore *in anaemia, administering high inspired oxygen increases the PaO_2 but does not significantly increase oxygen content unless desaturation is also part of the clinical picture.*

OXYGEN UPTAKE

The partial pressure of oxygen in dry air at sea level is 21.2 kPa (159 mmHg). This represents the force with which oxygen molecules in the atmosphere bombard their surroundings. Within the lung, the partial pressure of oxygen falls due both to humidification of inspired gases and to the introduction of carbon dioxide. The partial pressures of water and carbon dioxide can be thought of as 'diluting' the oxygen because the sum of the partial pressures is equal to atmospheric pressure. The alveolar partial pressure of oxygen (P_AO_2) is therefore dictated by the inspired partial pressure of oxygen

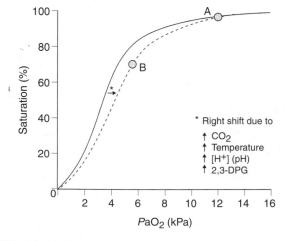

Figure 5.1 The haemoglobin–oxygen dissociation curve. The relationship between the partial pressure of oxygen and the haemoglobin saturation is shown for normal adult haemoglobin. In healthy individuals, haemoglobin operates between an arterial PaO_2 of 11.3–13.3 kPa (point A) and a venous PvO_2 of 5.3 kPa (point B).

(PiO_2), the rate of its uptake from the alveolus, and the expired partial pressure of CO_2 (P_ECO_2).

> **Key Point**
>
> Patients with decreased ventilation or increased metabolic rate require a high level of inspired oxygen.

P_AO_2 decreases when alveolar ventilation decreases, as more oxygen is taken out of the alveolus and more CO_2 is added to the alveolar gas before it is replenished from a new fresh breath. On administering oxygen, the alveolar P_AO_2 will be raised or lowered by an amount that is equal to the change in inspired gas PiO_2, provided that other factors remain constant.

Increased oxygen consumption and/or increased carbon dioxide production (e.g. in sepsis) will also cause a fall in alveolar (and thereby arterial) PO_2 and exacerbate the effect of hypoventilation.

Hypoventilation, increased oxygen consumption and increased CO_2 production lead to decreased P_AO_2 and arterial hypoxaemia, which can be corrected by the administration of oxygen. *Clinically the message is plain: patients with decreased ventilation from any cause (e.g. head injury, drugs, neuromuscular weakness) and those with increased oxygen consumption or increased CO_2 production (e.g. due to sepsis, thyrotoxicosis, shivering) require supplemental oxygen in order to maintain their arterial oxygenation.* Post-operative patients may suffer both respiratory depression (from residual anaesthetic agents and opioid analgesics) and increased oxygen consumption and CO_2 production (from sepsis or from shivering if they have become cold intra-operatively). Moreover, the alveolar oxygen is further reduced by the presence of residual anaesthetic agents. This is the reason for the routine administration of oxygen in the recovery area.

The decrease in the partial pressure of oxygen as it moves from the atmosphere to the alveolus represents the first two steps in the 'oxygen cascade'.

THE 'OXYGEN CASCADE'

A stepladder of partial pressures can be envisaged as oxygen is followed from the inspired air to the tissues (Figure 5.2). Each step is influenced by different factors. By understanding the oxygen cascade, the role of specific clinical interventions in the management of a hypoxic patient can be determined.

Partial pressure gradients in the oxygen cascade

Dry air has a PO_2 of 21.1 kPA (159 mmHg), which is 21% of atmospheric pressure ($Patm$), because air is 21% oxy-

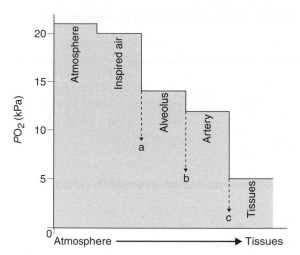

Figure 5.2 The oxygen cascade. The partial pressure of oxygen falls in steps as it moves from the atmosphere to the tissues. Each step is the consequence of specific factors. Step 'a' represents hypoxia due to hypoventilation with or without increased oxygen consumption and CO_2 production. Step 'b' is due to increased ventilation-perfusion mismatch and/or shunt. Step 'c' represents tissue hypoxia due to anaemia or low blood flow. (Modified from West JB. 1977: *Ventilation/blood flow and gas exchange*, 3rd edn, with the kind permission of Blackwell Scientific Publications, Oxford.)

gen. The partial pressure of water vapour in fully saturated air at body temperature is 6.2 kPa (47 mmHg), and therefore the partial pressure of oxygen in humidified inspired air (PiO_2) is 21% × (100 – 6.2) kPa = 19.7 kPa (149 mmHg). In the alveolus this inspired gas has CO_2 added and oxygen removed, and therefore the alveolar PO_2 (P_AO_2) falls to 13.3 kPa (100 mmHg). This is the pressure 'driving' oxygen across the alveolar membrane into the mixed venous blood. Mixed venous blood returning to the lung has a PO_2 of only 5.3 kPa (40 mmHg), so oxygen flows down a considerable concentration gradient from the alveolus to the pulmonary capillary. Equilibrium is nearly reached, so that blood leaving a pulmonary capillary from a well-ventilated area of lung has PO_2 and PCO_2 values that are very nearly equal to those within the alveolus.

Poorly ventilated over-perfused areas of the lung do not achieve equilibrium between the alveolar air and the perfusing capillary. This blood returning to the left atrium causes the partial pressure of arterial blood (PaO_2) to be less than that of the perfect pulmonary capillary. This step between alveolar PO_2 and arterial PO_2 is known as the alveolar-arterial gradient. The normal gradient is no more than 2 kPa (15 mmHg), so in healthy individuals the PaO_2 is therefore 11.3–13.3 kPa (80–100 mmHg). *Increases in the alveolar-arterial gradient are the most common cause of hypoxia in lung disease.*

Alveolar-arterial gradient (A-a gradient)

This is not a variable which is usually measured in clinical practice, but it is an important concept. The A-a gradient results from venous admixture due to *ventilation-perfusion mismatch* and *shunt*. Impaired diffusion across the alveolar/capillary membrane itself is not a significant factor. By considering the pathophysiology of a cyanosed patient, the most appropriate interventions can be selected.

Ventilation-perfusion mismatch (V/Q mismatch)

The lungs are not uniformly ventilated or perfused. Both blood flow (Q) and ventilation (V) are significantly influenced by gravity. The dependent areas of lung receive more ventilation and more perfusion than the superior areas, but the changes in blood flow and ventilation are not equal. Moving down the lung from the apex to the base there is a greater increase in perfusion than in ventilation, and therefore the upper areas are relatively over-ventilated (V/Q > 1), while the dependent areas are relatively over-perfused (V/Q < 1) (Figure 5.3).

In areas with perfect matching of ventilation and perfusion (V/Q = 1), the pulmonary capillary blood is fully saturated with oxygen and has a PCO_2 equal to that within the alveolus. In areas with a V/Q < 1 the blood is not fully saturated with oxygen, nor is it adequately cleared of CO_2. Both the under-ventilated alveoli and the blood which perfuses them have a relatively low PO_2 and relatively high PCO_2. In areas with a V/Q > 1 the over-ventilation blows off additional CO_2 but cannot achieve

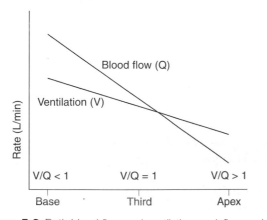

Figure 5.3 Both blood flow and ventilation are influenced by gravity. The dependent areas of lung receive more ventilation (V) and more perfusion (Q) than the superior areas. The fall in perfusion is relatively greater than the fall in ventilation moving from base to apex. This produces a range of ventilation/perfusion ratios around perfect V/Q matching at the level of the third rib. (Modified from West JB. 1977: *Ventilation/blood flow and gas exchange*, 3rd edn, with the kind permission of Blackwell Scientific Publications, Oxford.)

more than 100% saturation of blood from areas where V/Q = 1. The effects of high and low V/Q ratios on $PaCO_2$ cancel each other out. However, the effect of areas of low V/Q ratio on the PaO_2 cannot be compensated for by areas of high V/Q. V/Q mismatch therefore results in hypoxia but not hypercapnia.

Clinically, this picture is seen in pulmonary atelectasis (low V/Q in the collapsed area), bronchopneumonia, lobar pneumonia or aspiration pneumonia (low V/Q in consolidated lung). In adult respiratory distress syndrome (ARDS) the predominant defect is low V/Q and shunt in the dependent lung zones. The $PaCO_2$ often falls in the early phase of these illnesses because of the increased respiratory drive which results from collapse of lung tissue or the presence of fluid in the pulmonary interstitium. The hypoxia may be insidious in its onset. The blood flow is to some extent diverted away from under-ventilated areas of lung (so-called hypoxic pulmonary vasoconstriction). Only when this mechanism is overwhelmed does the hypoxia become severe, and therefore *cyanosis may be a late sign of respiratory distress of these aetiologies.*

Changes in the distribution of pulmonary perfusion with gravity may be clinically important. Patients with discrete areas of consolidation or collapse may have significantly poorer arterial oxygenation when they assume a posture which puts the consolidated lung in a dependent position, thereby increasing blood flow through the poorly ventilated areas. This effect is exacerbated by anaesthesia, which reduces pulmonary hypoxic vasoconstriction in the consolidated lung.

Shunt

The most extreme type of V/Q mismatch occurs when blood travels from the right side of the heart to the left side of the heart without any exposure to ventilated lung. This is called 'shunt'. In healthy individuals, shunt constitutes about 4% of cardiac output, and is accounted for by bronchial blood flow and flow though the thebesian veins. Large extrapulmonary shunts may occur in cardiac anomalies. Intrapulmonary shunt may occur in all of the situations mentioned under V/Q mismatch, but is most severe in ARDS, pneumothorax, haemothorax and one-lung ventilation.

Because shunted blood is not exposed to alveolar gas, hypoxia due to shunt does not improve with oxygen therapy. Clinical strategies must be directed instead towards re-establishing ventilation to the areas of un-ventilated lung. This involves draining the pneumo-/haemothorax, and using physiotherapy, posture and breathing exercises to help reinflate collapsed areas of lung by improving lung volumes and clearing mucus plugs. Positive end expiratory pressure (PEEP) increases the functional residual capacity and may help to recruit collapsed lung units. Post-operatively, abdominal distension, prolonged bed rest or inadequate analgesia may cause basal atelectasis with resultant shunt and/or V/Q mismatch. Anticipated changes in ventilation perfusion matching may influence the anaesthetic management considerably, especially in patients with marginal respiratory reserve.

Key Point

Patients with hypoventilation or increased V/Q mismatch require oxygen therapy. Patients with V/Q mismatch or shunt require strategies aimed at reinflating collapsed or consolidated lung.

Abnormalities of V/Q matching may have an insidious onset in the post-operative period, and it is worth considering lung volumes and how they are influenced by peri-operative events. The *functional residual capacity* (*FRC*) is the volume of gas left in the lung at the end of a quiet respiration (Figure 5.4). It represents the energy-efficient resting point at which the elastic recoil of the lung is balanced by the resting muscle tone of the diaphragm and inspiratory intercostal muscles, and by the intrinsic springiness of the rib-cage (Figure 5.5). FRC is reduced by factors which decrease muscle tone (e.g. sedation) or increase abdominal pressure (e.g. supine posture, ileus, ascites, abdominal muscle splinting).

The *closing capacity* is the volume of lung at which small airway closure occurs. At lung volumes that are persistently below closing capacity, small airway closure

results in distal atelectasis. Closing capacity increases with age. In healthy individuals, FRC is greater than closing capacity even when supine up to the age of 40 years. At 60 years of age the closing capacity exceeds FRC even when standing upright (Figure 5.6).

Consider the relevance of this clinically. An elderly obese patient undergoing abdominal surgery will have several factors contributing to a significant fall in oxygenation post-operatively. The closing volume is already greater than the FRC in this patient even in the upright

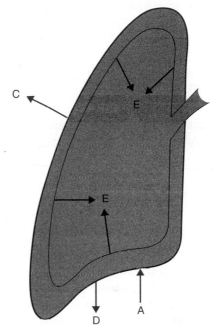

Figure 5.5 Functional residual capacity is the lung volume at which the chest wall springiness (C) and diaphragmatic muscle tone (D) are balanced by the elastic recoil of the lung (E) and the intra-abdominal pressure (A).

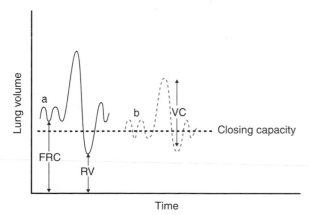

FRC = functional residual capacity

RV = residual volume

VC = vital capacity

Figure 5.4 Spirometer traces showing resting ventilation from (a) a normal FRC and (b) a reduced FRC. In post-operative patients the resting respiratory excursions may allow lung volumes to fall below closing capacity. Greater inspiratory efforts raise lung volumes above closing capacity and may reinflate atelectatic areas of lung.

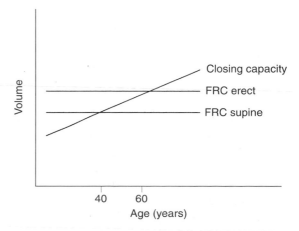

Figure 5.6 Closing capacity increases with age. At the age of 40 years closing capacity is greater than FRC when supine. By the age of 60 years, closing capacity exceeds FRC even when standing.

posture. Moreover, the FRC is compromised by increased abdominal pressure, abdominal muscle pain with poor respiratory efforts, prolonged supine posture, and the sedation which accompanies opioid analgesia. Atelectasis within the dependent lung zones is inevitable. Such patients therefore have a high incidence of post-operative hypoxia and hypostatic pneumonia.

Oxygen therapy to counter the defects in V/Q matching, early mobilization to minimize the effects of posture on FRC, adequate analgesia with minimal sedation, and physiotherapy to encourage good respiratory efforts are the mainstays of an effective post-operative strategy for the prevention of respiratory failure. Such strategies should be focused on high-risk patients in the peri-operative period. It is a grave error to reserve such interventions for patients who already show evidence of respiratory distress or hypoxia.

OXYGEN DELIVERY AND CONSUMPTION

Oxygen delivery is equal to oxygen content multiplied by cardiac output. In a normal resting adult, oxygen delivery is therefore $20\,mL/dL \times 5\,L/min = 1000\,mL/min$. Oxygen delivery to tissues depends on adequate perfusion with fully oxygenated blood. Falls in haemoglobin reduce the oxygen content of the blood. This can only be compensated for by increased flow. Because haemoglobin in arterial blood is normally nearly fully saturated with oxygen, the reduced oxygen content in anaemia cannot be compensated for by administering oxygen.

> **Key Point**
>
> Confusion or drowsiness are often the first signs of hypoxia. Do not sedate a confused patient without considering hypoxia as the cause.

Although global oxygen delivery exceeds tissue needs by a large margin, some tissues (notably myocardium and brain) have a much more critical balance between oxygen supply and demand. In hypoxia, the early clinical manifestations are most commonly seen in these organs as confusion or myocardial ischaemia. *It is a classic error of judgement to sedate a 'difficult patient' who is actually confused due to hypoxia.*
Overall oxygen consumption is approximately $250\,mL/min$ in a resting adult. It is increased by fever, pain, restlessness, shivering, convulsions or thyrotoxicosis. Increased oxygen consumption (and CO_2 production) enhances the fall in P_AO_2 for a given fall in alveolar ventilation.

OXYGEN UPTAKE BY THE TISSUES

One of the central features of hypoxia is the inability of tissues to maintain aerobic metabolism. The shift to anaerobic pathways results in inefficient metabolism and the production of lactic acid. Prolonged hypoxaemia therefore produces multiple organ dysfunction and lactic acidosis.

> **Key Point**
>
> Hypoxia requires immediate management with oxygen administration, and investigation of the cause.

In sepsis a high metabolic rate may lead to increased oxygen consumption. If this is not matched by increased tissue perfusion with adequately oxygenated blood, it will result in organ failure. The high cardiac output associated with sepsis gives less time for blood perfusing the alveoli to equilibrate with alveolar oxygen and exacerbates V/Q mismatch. Therefore supplemental oxygen should be given. In severe sepsis, ventilation perfusion mismatch and increased intrapulmonary shunt are often features of the clinical picture.

Systemic vasodilation in sepsis usually makes the patient's peripheries warm and pink with increased blood flow. However, adequate central organ oxygenation should not be assumed, as oxygen consumption may outstrip supply. Occasionally, peripheral cyanosis may also be seen in severe sepsis due to the high oxygen consumption within muscle and skin. *In practice, all patients with significant clinical evidence of sepsis should receive supplementary oxygen whether or not they appear cyanosed.*

BLOOD GAS ANALYSIS

Arterial blood gas analysis is the measurement of the partial pressures of oxygen and carbon dioxide and the pH of a sample of arterial blood. The bicarbonate (HCO_3^-) and base excess are calculated indices of acid–base balance obtained from the blood gas analyser. Consider the following three questions.

1. Is the patient hypoxaemic?
2. Is the patient hypercapnic?
3. What is the acid–base balance?

Is the patient hypoxaemic?

The normal PaO_2 is 11.3–13.3 kPa (85–100 mmHg), and the value decreases with advancing age. A PaO_2 value of $<10\,kPa$ (75 mmHg) represents significant hypoxia which requires oxygen therapy and investigation. Administer oxygen while you investigate the cause of the hypoxaemia. Chronic hypoxia is associated with a compensatory rise in haemoglobin concentration.

Is the patient hypercapnic?

The normal $PaCO_2$ is 4.8–6.0 kPa (36–44 mmHg). Elevations of the $PaCO_2$ cause acidaemia – 'respiratory acidosis'. In chronic CO_2 retention (as occurs in chronic obstructive pulmonary disease) there is a compensatory rise in bicarbonate level which reduces the severity of the respiratory acidosis (so-called compensatory metabolic alkalosis). This compensation is a gradual process taking place over days or weeks, during which the kidneys conserve bicarbonate. In acute CO_2 retention (e.g. in opiate overdose) there is no time for a compensatory metabolic alkalosis to develop, and therefore the acidosis is more severe for a given acute rise in CO_2. In acute CO_2 retention, for every 10 mmHg (1.4 kPa) rise in CO_2 there is a fall in pH of 0.08 units. In chronic CO_2 retention, the pH change is more modest, and a 4 mmol/L rise in HCO_3^- is seen for every 10 mmHg (1.4 kPa) chronic rise in CO_2.

What is the acid–base balance?

The normal pH of arterial blood is 7.36–7.44. A pH of < 7.36 represents acidosis, and a pH of > 7.44 represents alkalosis. The scale is a logarithmic representation of hydrogen ion concentration, and therefore small changes in pH represent severe derangements in acid–base balance. A pH of < 7.25 or > 7.55 represents a life-threatening degree of acid–base imbalance. The aetiology may be respiratory or metabolic, or a mixed picture with both respiratory and metabolic components. The problem may be acute or chronic, or 'acute on chronic', in which a stable chronic picture is complicated by an acute event.

In considering an arterial blood gas result, it is best to start by noting whether the overall picture is one of acidosis or alkalosis. The primary pathology is usually indicated by the direction of the pH change.

ACIDOSIS WITH HYPERCAPNIA

Is the CO_2 concentration high enough to account for all of the pH change? If so, and there is a normal bicarbonate level, the acidosis is an acute respiratory acidosis.

If the pH change is less severe than would be expected from an acute rise in CO_2, and there is a raised bicarbonate level, consider a probable chronic component with metabolic compensation. The base excess indicates the metabolic component. A positive base excess indicates conservation of bicarbonate (a compensatory metabolic alkalosis).

If the pH change is more severe than would be expected from an acute rise in CO_2, there may be a respiratory acidosis *and* a metabolic acidosis. The metabolic component is reflected in a negative base excess and a low bicarbonate level.

ACIDOSIS WITH NORMAL OR LOW CO₂ CONCENTRATION

This is a metabolic acidosis. If the CO_2 level is low it represents a respiratory compensation. The base excess will be negative, indicating a metabolic acidosis.

ALKALOSIS WITH A LOW CO₂ CONCENTRATION

Is the CO_2 level low enough to account for all of the change in pH? If so, this is an acute respiratory alkalosis (chronic respiratory alkalosis is virtually unheard of). If not, there may also be a metabolic component which will be manifested as an elevated bicarbonate level and a positive base excess.

ALKALOSIS WITH A HIGH CO₂ CONCENTRATION

This is a metabolic alkalosis with respiratory compensation. The metabolic component will be seen as an elevated bicarbonate level and a positive base excess.

OXYGEN ADMINISTRATION

Oxygen may be administered by facemask, either by a controlled-delivery facemask or by a variable-performance facemask (Figure 5.7). Controlled-delivery facemasks accurately deliver a known concentration of oxygen to the patient across a wide range of inspiratory flow rates. This is achieved using the Venturi principle. The oxygen flow to the mask passes through a narrow orifice beyond which the pressure falls in direct proportion to the flow rate through the orifice. Air is thus entrained into the mask, diluting the oxygen in a predictable ratio. These masks are especially valuable when taking arterial blood samples from patients who are receiving oxygen. Without accurate knowledge of the concentration of oxygen being inspired, it is impossible to interpret the meaning of the PaO_2 measured. Therefore, whenever an arterial blood gas sample is to be taken, the patient should be breathing a known concentration of oxygen. Masks are available to provide 24%, 28%, 35% or 60% oxygen. *Use of 24% and 28% oxygen facemasks should be reserved ONLY for patients with known chronic obstructive pulmonary disease AND chronic hypercapnia.* These patients may be dependent on their hypoxic respiratory drive. Administration of high concentrations of oxygen to such patients may lead to suppression of this hypoxic respiratory drive, with a resultant escalation of their CO_2 retention to dangerously high levels. However, it should be noted that the vast majority of hypoxic patients do *not* fall into this category. *All other hypoxic patients should receive at least 60% oxygen by facemask pending further investigation.*

Variable-performance oxygen masks (e.g. the Hudson facemask) do not utilize the Venturi principle, and the percentage of oxygen delivered varies according to the flow rate of oxygen through the mask and the peak inspiratory flow rate of the patient. When the patient's inspiratory flow rate exceeds the oxygen supply during peak inspiratory flow, air will be drawn around the sides of the mask, thus reducing the percentage of inspired oxygen. The masks can be equipped with a reservoir bag to provide enhanced oxygen concentrations. With oxygen supplied at a flow rate of 15 L/min and a reservoir bag attached, a Hudson mask can achieve 60–70% oxy-

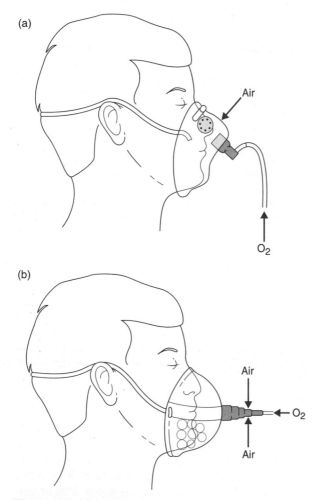

Figure 5.7 (a) A simple Hudson facemask. (b) A Venturi mask. (Reprinted from Hinds CJ, Watson D. 1996: *Intensive care: a concise textbook*, with the kind permission of W.B. Saunders Ltd, London.)

gen. Without a reservoir bag the Hudson mask provides only about 40% oxygen.

Hypoxia is difficult to detect clinically. Whenever it is suspected, oxygen should be administered pending further investigation. Oxygen toxicity is not a significant problem at inspired concentrations of 60% or less.

CLINICAL SCENARIOS

Chronic central cyanosis in a patient scheduled for elective surgery

(i.e. noticed in the out-patient department or referred to in the GP's letter)

What is the cause?
The most common cause of chronic hypoxia in adults is chronic bronchitis and emphysema, but the diagnosis must be properly established from the history and examination.

What is the severity?
Has the patient had hospital admissions with this problem? Is the patient breathless at rest? What is his or her exercise tolerance? Is there a compensatory rise in haemoglobin level? Is the patient on domiciliary oxygen?

Investigations
Early discussion with the anaesthetist is essential. Selected patients should have pulmonary function tests and arterial blood gas analysis, especially if abdominal or thoracic surgery is planned. A forced vital capacity in 1 s (FEV_1) of less than 1 L represents severe compromise with very little respiratory reserve. On arterial blood gas analysis it is important to identify baseline values while breathing room air at rest, and to identify those patients who have chronic hypoxia and hypercapnia.

Pre-operative preparation
Consider the need for peri-operative oxygen therapy, and physiotherapy with or without antibiotics and/or bronchodilators. Oxygen should be warmed and humidified to aid mucociliary clearance of bronchial secretions. Early mobilization is important, and incentive spirometry may play a role. Special techniques of analgesia should be considered (e.g. epidural infusion), and post-operative monitoring of the respiratory rate and haemoglobin saturation (with pulse oximetry) may be appropriate. Selected patients will require admission to a high-dependency unit or intensive-care unit for close respiratory monitoring and serial blood gas analysis.

Post-operative central cyanosis developing gradually on the ward

Management should be based on a knowledge of the underlying pathophysiology.

Decreased FRC occurs post-operatively due to reduced muscle tone, increased intra-abdominal pressure, supine posture and sedation leading to decreased compliance and increased work of breathing, abnormalities of V/Q matching, and atelectasis in dependent regions of the lung.

Post-operatively there is a fall in FEV_1 and FVC, and the cough reflex becomes depressed and weakened due to pain, muscle weakness and sedation. Compromised laryngeal reflexes and reduced mucociliary clearance due to intra-operative exposure to dry anaesthetic gases and the effects of intubation may lead to mucus plugging and contribute to the risk of post-operative pneumonia. Aspiration of small quantities of stomach contents may occur without clinical signs ('silent aspiration') in the immediate post-operative period, especially in the elderly and in patients with hiatus hernia or gastric stasis. Decreased respiratory drive secondary to opioid analgesia further reduces lung volumes and may reduce alveolar oxygen tension.

The post-operative abnormalities of lung function are at their most severe over the first 2 or 3 days post-operatively, returning to normal over the following 2 to 3 weeks. The changes are particularly severe following upper abdominal surgery or thoracic surgery, and are exacerbated by prolonged surgery, age, obesity, muscle weakness, poor nutritional status and cigarette smoking. It is therefore possible to identify a high-risk population who are most likely to benefit from prophylactic measures to improve their peri-operative lung function.

Key Point

Factors associated with an increased risk of post-operative hypoxia:

- Thoracic/upper abdominal surgery
- Prolonged surgery (more than 3 h in duration)
- Age > 60 years
- Chronic obstructive pulmonary disease
- Cigarette smoking
- Muscle weakness
- Poor nutritional status
- Increased abdominal pressure
- Obesity
- Symptomatic lung disease

Post-operative sudden-onset central cyanosis

Consider airway obstruction, acute respiratory depression, acute ventilatory failure and cardiovascular collapse. Immediate attention must be given to the 'ABCs' (airway, breathing and circulation) of resuscitation. Establish and maintain a clear airway, and rapidly assess the ventilation. Ensure that there is adequate bilateral air entry to both lungs and administer oxygen (by Hudson mask and reservoir bag for spontaneously breathing patients, or by the bag-valve-mask technique for apnoeic patients). Call for help!

Acute airway obstruction in the post-operative period is most commonly due to residual anaesthetic, injudicious use of opioids, or inhalation of a blood clot or foreign body. In head and neck surgery consider tracheal compression from an expanding haematoma.

Ventilatory failure may be due to central respiratory depression (e.g. neurosurgical complication, head injury, drugs), pneumothorax (especially in asthma, following positive pressure ventilation and/or placement of central venous cannulae), haemothorax (following trauma/thoracic surgery), muscle weakness (e.g. myasthenia gravis, drugs) or aspiration of stomach contents (especially in patients with hiatus hernia or reduced gastric emptying). Careful examination of the respiratory rate and the pattern of respiration is needed. Palpate the trachea (is it central?) and the rib-cage (does it move symmetrically?). Auscultate both lungs while looking for normal bilateral air entry throughout the lungs.

Cardiac events may present as acute cyanosis and/or pallor. Establish intravenous access and examine the patient for evidence of circulatory shock. Consider hypovolaemic shock and cardiogenic shock (myocardial infarction, massive pulmonary embolism). Acute pulmonary oedema may result from cardiac failure, acid aspiration, raised intracranial pressure or forced attempts at inspiration during a period of acute airway obstruction.

SUMMARY

A sound knowledge of the physiological principles of oxygen transport and pulmonary function allows the clinician to identify those patients who are most at risk in the peri-operative period, and to apply effective strategies for the prevention and treatment of hypoxia.

FURTHER READING

Hinds CJ, Watson D. 1996: *Intensive care: a concise textbook*, 2nd edn. London: W.B. Saunders.

Nunn JF. 1993: *Nunn's applied respiratory physiology*, 4th edn. Oxford: Butterworth-Heinemann Ltd.

Nunn JF, Milledge JS, Chen D, Dore C. 1988: Respiratory criteria of fitness for surgery and anaesthesia. *Anaesthesia* **43**, 543–51.

West JB. 1977: *Ventilation/blood flow and gas exchange*, 3rd edn. Oxford: Blackwell Scientific Publications.

Chapter 6

Breathlessness

Crichton F. Ramsay and Norman Johnson

Introduction

The feeling of breathlessness (or dyspnoea) is a subjective symptom. Neither tachypnoea (breathing at a rate of $\geqslant 18$ breaths/min) nor hypoxaemia (arterial $PaO_2 \leqslant 8$ kPa) correlate well with the presence of dyspnoea, although the presence of either or both often coexists with dyspnoea.

Likewise, hypercapnoea ($PaCO_2 \geqslant 6$ kPa), whilst causing acute hyperventilation in otherwise normal subjects, may have little or no effect on dyspnoea or ventilation in subjects accustomed to a chronically elevated $PaCO_2$.

Table 6.1 Factors that contribute to the sensation of breathlessness

Factors	Causes	Examples
Increase in work of breathing	Decreased pulmonary compliance Restricted chest expansion Airflow obstruction	Pulmonary oedema, pulmonary fibrosis Obesity, ankylosing spondylitis, kyphoscoliosis Asthma, chronic obstructive pulmonary disease (COPD)
Respiratory muscle weakness	Spinal cord lesions Poliomyelitis Polyneuropathy Myasthenia gravis	
Increased pulmonary ventilation	Hypoxaemia Increased dead space Metabolic acidosis	

CAUSES OF DYSPNOEA

It is practical to classify the causes of dyspnoea according to the following main systemic causes:

1. respiratory;
2. cardiac;
3. neurological;
4. skeletal;
5. systemic;
6. trauma;
7. non-organic.

Over what time period has dyspnoea developed?

The rate at which the dyspnoea has developed is an important guide to the aetiology. Together with the severity of the dyspnoea, it provides a practical way of approaching the diagnosis and management of dyspnoea. An overview will now be given of the main causes of dyspnoea by the seven categories listed above.

RESPIRATORY

Mechanism	Rate of onset of symptoms			
	Minutes → Hours	*Hours → Days*	*Weeks*	*Months*
Airways obstruction				
Upper	Foreign body inhalation			
	Angio-oedema			
	Acute epiglottitis	→		
	Croup	→		
			Tracheal compression	→
Lower	Asthma	→	→	→
		Acute bronchitis		COPD
				Bronchiectasis
				Cystic fibrosis
Alveolar filling/loss				
	Pulmonary oedema	→		
	Pulmonary haemorrhage	→		
	Adult respiratory distress syndrome	→		
		Pneumonia	TB	→
		Extrinsic allergic alveolitis	→	→
		Atelectasis		
			Alveolar proteinosis	→
			Alveolar cell carcinoma	→
Interstitial pulmonary disorders				
			Cryptogenic fibrosing alveolitis	→
			Connective tissue diseases	→
				Pneumoconiosis
Pleural disease				
	Pneumothorax			
	Haemothorax	→		
		Pleural effusion	→	
		Empyema	→	
				Pleural fibrosis
Miscellaneous/mixed			Carcinoma	→
				Sarcoidosis

CARDIAC

	Minutes → Hours	Hours → Days	Weeks	Months
Arrhythmias	Supraventricular tachycardia			
	Ventricular tachycardia			
	Atrial fibrillation	→	→	
Impaired left ventricular function	Myocardial infarction			
	Angina/IHD	→		
	Pulmonary oedema	→		
	Cardiac tamponade	Pericardial effusion		
Other causes of impaired cardiac output	Pulmonary embolism	→	Chronic multiple pulmonary emboli	→
	Rupture of inter-ventricular septum			
	'Stuck' or ruptured valve	→		
			Cardiomyopathy	→
			Pulmonary hypertension	→
			L→R shunt	→

NEUROLOGICAL

	Minutes → Hours	Hours → Days	Weeks	Months
	Guillain-Barré	→		
	Spinal cord lesion	→	→	
			Motor neurone disease	→
			Multiple sclerosis	→

MUSCULOSKELETAL

	Minutes → Hours	Hours → Days	Weeks	Months
	Diaphragmatic rupture	→		
			Kyphoscoliosis	
			Ankylosing spondylitis	
			Thoracoplasty	

SYSTEMIC

	Minutes → Hours	Hours → Days	Weeks	Months
	Metabolic acidosis (includes renal failure and diabetes mellitus)	→		
	Shock			
			Anaemia	
				Hyper-thyroidism
				Obesity

TRAUMATIC

Minutes → Hours	Hours → Days	Weeks	Months
Pneumothorax			
Haemothorax	→		
Haemopneumothorax	→		
Haemopericardium ± tamponade	→		
Rib fracture(s) ± flail segment	→		

NON-ORGANIC

Minutes → Hours	Hours → Days	Weeks	Months
Panic attacks			
Hyper-ventilation			
	Anxiety	→	
		Depression	→

Broadly speaking, patients with dyspnoea present in two different ways, either with symptoms of chronic or gradually worsening dyspnoea, or with more acute onset of symptoms which are often severe or life-threatening.

Acute severe dyspnoea can present either in an apparently previously healthy individual or in a patient with chronic dyspnoea due to a disease which has either progressed or suffered a superimposed second pathology. A relatively minor second condition will cause much more severe compromise in the presence of an underlying pathology than it would in an otherwise healthy individual.

The rest of this chapter will therefore be divided into two sections:

1. assessment of the patient with chronic breathlessness;
2. management of the patient with acute severe dyspnoea.

ASSESSMENT OF THE PATIENT WITH CHRONIC BREATHLESSNESS

HISTORY

Under what circumstances is dyspnoea experienced?

Dyspnoea may be experienced:

1. on exertion only;
2. at rest as well as on exertion;
3. intermittently and unrelated to exertion.

1. Dyspnoea that occurs on exertion only and is proportional to exertion implies a cardiorespiratory compromise or other organic pathology. It is helpful to define exactly what degree of exertion results in dyspnoea by asking how far the patient can walk on level ground and how many stairs they can climb before having to pause for a rest.

2. Dyspnoea which is present at rest and exacerbated by exertion implies a progression of or more severe form of disease from category 1.

3. Intermittent dyspnoea may have a number of causes:

   - intermittent dyspnoea associated with palpitations suggests tachyarrhythmia as a cause;
   - dyspnoea on waking the patient from sleep may be due to pulmonary oedema or airflow obstruction in asthma (or COPD);
   - the wheeze and dyspnoea of asthma are often paroxysmal in nature with unpredictable exacerbations and remissions in addition to the known precipitants (exercise, allergens, aspirin/NSAIDs and nocturnal or early-morning exacerbations);
   - dyspnoea that is present at rest and relieved by exertion is almost certainly not of organic origin.

Are any other symptoms associated with dyspnoea?

Other investigations are necessary in order to help to diagnose the cause of the dyspnoea:

1. respiratory symptoms;
2. cardiac symptoms;
3. specific inquiries.

Respiratory symptoms

These include the following:

- cough;
- sputum;
- wheeze;
- haemoptysis;
- chest pain.

Cough

If cough occurs in association with dyspnoea, the following factors should be assessed.

1. *Is the cough of recent onset or chronic?*

2. *Is the cough productive of sputum on a regular basis?* The epidemiological definition of chronic bronchitis is that of a cough productive of sputum on a daily basis for at least 3 months of the year for 2 consecutive years. Many patients with chronic bronchitis regard a morning cough with sputum as being normal, and it is necessary to ask specifically whether or not sputum is expectorated on rising.

3. *Is sleep disturbed by cough?* The normal diurnal variation in airway calibre results in airways being at their narrowest at around 4 a.m. In patients with asthma or chronic airflow limitation this may manifest itself with nocturnal wakening with cough and/or wheeze and/or dyspnoea. Nocturnal waking with cough may be the only manifestation of asthma.

Wheeze

Wheezing is the sound produced by airflow through narrowed bronchi. Wheeze may be audible to both the patient and those around him or her. Wheezes are musical or polyphonic whistling noises, and are present predominantly (or exclusively) during expiration. It is important to clarify what the patient means by the term wheeze, as many lay people use it to describe dyspnoea or to signify its severity. In asthma the wheezing is, as with the cough, typically nocturnal and worse in the early hours of the morning or on wakening. Wheeze may be a feature of asthma, chronic obstructive airways disease, bronchiectasis, multiple pulmonary emboli and also of pulmonary oedema (cardiac asthma).

Wheeze must be distinguished from stridor. Stridor is

DIFFERENTIAL DIAGNOSIS OF COUGH

Acute
  Infection (bronchitis, tracheitis)
  Inhaled
      Foreign body
      Gas

Chronic
  Productive
      COPD
      Bronchiectasis
      Tumour
      TB
      Asthma
  Non-productive
      Asthma
      Postnasal drip
      Gastro-oesophageal reflux disease
      Inhaled foreign body
      Inflammatory lung disease
      Congestive cardiac failure
      Angiotensin-converting enzyme (ACE) inhibitor
      Psychogenic
      Tumour

---

a monophonic, predominantly inspiratory rhonchus and is of a harsh crowing nature. Stridor is due to significant obstruction of the upper airway, usually the trachea (or rarely obstruction of the left or right main bronchus, and never below this level). Stridor can often be detected without a stethoscope by listening carefully as the patient takes deep breaths through an open mouth.

The presence of stridor is a serious sign that requires urgent investigation and management before complete upper airway obstruction occurs.

Haemoptysis

Haemoptysis or the coughing up of blood may be a symptom of serious respiratory pathology, and is usually accurately reported and remembered by the patient. It may be necessary to clarify that the source of the blood is the respiratory tract and that its production results from coughing and not epistaxis (nosebleeds) or haematemesis (vomiting blood). Always ask about haemoptysis in every patient with dyspnoea and clarify the following points:

- description of the blood and amount expectorated;

- presence of any sputum and its nature;

- date of the first episode of haemoptysis and the subsequent frequency and time-course.

The differential diagnosis of haemoptysis is extensive and includes the following.

1. *Neoplasms*:
Bronchogenic carcinoma and other primary and metastatic tumours of the respiratory tract (although this cause of haemoptysis is the main concern of most patients and their doctors, it accounts for less than 3% of patients with haemoptysis).

2. *Infections*:
   - tuberculosis;
   - pneumonia;
   - lung abscess/aspergilloma;
   - acute and chronic bronchitis.

3. *Immunological*:
   - Goodpasture's syndrome;
   - connective tissue disorders.

4. *Cardiovascular causes*:
   - pulmonary thrombo-embolism;
   - mitral stenosis;
   - hypertension.

5. *Miscellaneous*:
   - bronchiectasis;
   - idiopathic pulmonary haemosiderosis.

Chest pain

Chest pain is not usually associated with dyspnoea, with the exceptions of the following:

1. inflammation of the pleura;
2. chest wall or mediastinal invasion by malignancy;
3. the pain of ischaemic heart disease;
4. chest trauma (including surgical).

Pleuritic chest pain is due to the inflamed pleural surfaces rubbing against each other. Pleuritic chest pain is usually described as being sharp or stabbing in nature, it is typically worse on inspiration or coughing, and its site is usually easily described by the patient and located to one side of the thorax. A central chest pain which is 'pleuritic' in nature and is worse on lying flat and eased by leaning forward is characteristic of pericardial rather than pleural inflammation. Pleuritic chest pain is most frequently secondary to pulmonary infection or infarction. The pain of thoracic malignancy is a more constant unremitting pain of gradually increasing severity.

Cardiac symptoms

These include the following:

1. angina;
2. orthopnoea;
3. paroxysmal nocturnal dyspnoea;
4. ankle oedema;
5. palpitations:

- intermittent or constant?
- tachyarrhythmia or bradyarrhythmia?
- regular or irregular heart rate?
- do the palpitations coincide with the presence of the dyspnoea?

A history of ischaemic heart disease with exertional angina or previous myocardial infarction would imply that impaired left ventricular function is contributing to or is the main cause of the dyspnoea.

Orthopnoea is breathlessness on lying flat, and is a common feature of left ventricular failure. Patients suffering from orthopnoea attempt to sleep propped upright on a number of pillows, and it is useful to document how many pillows the patient requires. Patients with orthopnoea will awaken during the night gasping for breath if they slip down the pillows and become recumbent; this is known as paroxysmal nocturnal dyspnoea (PND).

Although orthopnoea and paroxysmal nocturnal dyspnoea are characteristic features of left ventricular failure, they are by no means specific. Any patient with significant dyspnoea will suffer from orthopnoea, whilst nocturnal exacerbations are a feature of asthma and airflow obstruction.

Chronic pitting ankle is also a feature of heart disease with impaired right ventricular function.

Palpitations may indicate underlying heart disease, but more importantly they may be the underlying cause of the dyspnoea. Palpitations which may potentially cause dyspnoea and/or hypotension include paroxysmal atrial fibrillation, supraventricular tachycardia, sick sinus syndrome (resulting in sinus bradycardia and arrest) and ventricular tachycardia.

Further specific enquiries

The patient should be questioned about the following:

- cigarette smoking;
- exposure to pets/animals;
- industrial exposure;
- full drug history;
- allergies;
- weight loss;
- fever/night sweats;
- foreign travel;
- contact with cases of TB.

Cigarette smoking

Cigarettes are a major aetiological factor in chronic bronchitis, emphysema, lung carcinoma and ischaemic heart disease. All patients should be asked about their smoking history. Never accept the answer 'No' in response to the question 'Do you smoke?' as being the end of the smoking history; always follow up with the question 'Have you ever smoked?' (many patients will have given up smoking just a matter of weeks prior to the consultation, often because of worsening dyspnoea, and some tragically because of an episode of haemoptysis). Furthermore, do not simply record 'ex-smoker', but clarify the number of years for which the patient has smoked and the maximum number and average number of cigarettes smoked per day. The total consumption can be expressed as numbers of pack-years (20 cigarettes per day for 1 year is equal to 1 pack-year).

Exposure to pets/animals

Pet owners find it hard to accept that their pet may be aggravating their illness, but there is little doubt that cats and to a lesser extent dogs exacerbate asthma. Exposure to or ownership of birds raises the possibility of an extrinsic allergic alveolitis or *Chlamydia* infection.

Industrial exposure

Industrial exposure may lead to or aggravate underlying asthma, cause an extrinsic allergic alveolitis, and increase the risk of carcinoma and specific respiratory disorders. Always check the patient's present and past occupational exposure, and specifically enquire about asbestos exposure which, because of the long incubation period, will be a cause of increasing numbers of cases of mesothelioma for the next decade and beyond.

Drugs

Many drugs are toxic to the heart and lungs. The lung is particularly susceptible to drugs that cause fibrosis, pneumonitis, eosinophilia and a variety of other disorders, and a detailed list of all of the drugs previously ingested, the doses taken and duration of treatment is essential.

Allergies

A history of allergy may be of relevance in the development of angio-oedema or exacerbation of asthma. In the case of asthmatics, always enquire about aspirin or non-steroidal anti-inflammatory drug ingestion – approximately 10% of asthmatics will have a history of nasal polyps and deterioration of their asthma with aspirin/NSAID ingestion. This reaction to asthma is not a true allergic reaction but a dose-related phenomenon as the inhibition of the cyclo-oxygenase enzyme results in increased cysteinyl-leukotriene production. Why only a small proportion of asthmatics react in this way is unclear.

Weight loss

Recent significant weight loss occurs in:

1. tuberculosis;
2. carcinoma;
3. thyrotoxicosis.

EXAMINATION

Examination of the patient with dyspnoea naturally concentrates on the cardiorespiratory systems, where most of the causes will be found, although a general examination should also be performed to detect signs of systemic disease. Examination is covered in the section on acute severe dyspnoea below.

INVESTIGATIONS

A number of investigations aid the diagnosis, management and assessment of the severity of dyspnoea.

INVESTIGATIONS

First-line investigations include the following:

- chest X-ray
- spirometry (FEV_1, FVC, PEFR)
- pulse oximetry at rest and following exertion
- ECG
- full blood count and differential white cell count
- biochemistry, urea and electrolytes and blood sugar
- arterial blood gas analysis if SaO_2 is < 94% at rest

Further investigations include the following:

- full lung volumes and transfer factor
- flow volume loop, mouth pressures
- exercise testing
- transbronchial biopsy
- CT scan of thorax
- V/Q scan of lungs
- open lung biopsy
- echocardiography

Chest X-ray

The plain chest X-ray is an essential part of the assessment of any patient with significant dyspnoea.

The chest X-ray may:

- reveal the definitive diagnosis;
- eliminate a number of important causes of dyspnoea from the list of possibilities;
- allow a shortened list of differential diagnoses to be compiled.

An erect departmental PA chest X-ray gives the most useful information. In pregnancy, it may be tempting to omit the chest X-ray in order to reduce the radiation exposure to the developing fetus. However, unless the dyspnoea is clearly due to a mild exacerbation of a known underlying condition, the chest X-ray should be performed if there are significant symptoms. The risks of missing a new diagnosis and potential hypoxic damage to the fetus (and mother) greatly outweigh the theoretical risks of the X-ray (which should be performed with lead shielding of the fetus).

Pulmonary function tests

A simple spirometric assessment of the FEV_1 (forced expiratory volume in 1 s), FVC (forced vital capacity) and PEFR (peak expiratory flow rate) will provide much useful information. However, it is important to realize that spirometry may be misleading if incorrectly performed. In order to ensure that a maximal respiratory effort and appropriate technique is adopted either perform the spirometry yourself or have it measured by a pulmonary function technician. This is particularly important in assessing the response to treatment by comparing serial measurements. Spirometry may show:

- no abnormality;
- an obstructive ventilatory defect;
- a restrictive ventilatory defect;
- a mixed obstructive and restrictive picture.

Each of these has a clear differential list of associated diagnostic possibilities. These measurements can be made easily at the patient's bedside or in the out-patient consulting room with the aid of a simple hand-held spirometer. The only circumstance in which spirometry might not be performed is in the case of a patient thought to have open tuberculosis.

Obstructive pulmonary function

Tests

FEV_1	↓↓
FVC	↓
FEV_1/FVC (%)	↓
PEFR	↓

Causes
- asthma;

- chronic bronchitis and/or emphysema (the combination of which is interchangeably known as COAD (chronic obstructive airways disease), COPD (chronic obstructive pulmonary disease), COLD (chronic obstructive lung disease), CAL (chronic airflow limitation));

- bronchiectasis;

- cystic fibrosis;

- bronchiolitis.

If positive obstructive pulmonary function test results are noted, the patient should be given a bronchodilator and the tests repeated after 30 min. In asthma (and COPD with an 'asthmatic' component) there will be a variable amount of improvement, perhaps back to normal predicted values, following administration of a bronchodilator. In asthma, the transfer factor is usually normal, whereas in the other disorders listed above the transfer factor is reduced.

Restrictive pulmonary function

Tests

FEV_1	↓/↓↓
FVC	↓↓
FEV_1/FVC (%)	→/↑
PEFR	→/↑

Causes   Divide into pulmonary parenchymal and extra-parenchymal disorders.

Pulmonary parenchymal disorders/interstitial lung disease include the following:

- sarcoidosis;
- cryptogenic fibrosing alveolitis;
- pneumoconiosis;
- drug-induced pulmonary disease;
- radiation fibrosis.

Extra-parenchymal disorders include the following:

1. neuromuscular disorders:
   - myasthenia gravis;
   - Guillain-Barré syndrome;
   - cervical spine injury;
   - diaphragmatic weakness/paralysis;

2. chest wall disorders:
   - kyphoscoliosis;
   - obesity.

Pulse oximetry

At rest on air the usual SaO_2 is ⩾ 95%. A fall of > 4% or a fall to < 90% on exertion is considered to be significant.

If the patient has a low SaO_2, then the arterial blood gases should be checked.

ECG

The ECG may give information on ventricular hypertrophy and acute or old cardiac ischaemic and rhythm disturbances. It may also be abnormal in pulmonary emboli.

FBC

The full blood count may not only reveal anaemia, but the white cell count, if low, may raise the possibility of immunocompromise, whilst an abnormal differential white cell count (such as an eosinophilia) may raise other differential diagnoses.

Biochemistry

Check for renal and hepatic function and the presence of diabetes.

Immunology

The presence of auto-antibodies for connective tissue disorders should be looked for if appropriate.

FURTHER INVESTIGATIONS

More sophisticated pulmonary function (lung volumes, transfer factor, flow volume loops and mouth pressures) and exercise testing may be necessary in some cases to aid the diagnosis. These tests, together with trans-bronchial biopsy, open-lung biopsy and high-resolution CT scanning of the chest, would usually only be arranged by or after consultation with a chest physician.

Echocardiography is useful for assessing ventricular function and valvular heart disease.

MANAGEMENT OF THE PATIENT WITH ACUTE SEVERE DYSPNOEA

Acute severe dyspnoea can present without warning and may progress over a matter of minutes to become life-threatening. It must be managed immediately and competently if the patient is to have the greatest chance of survival.

Severe dyspnoea may present in:

1. a previously well subject;

2. a patient with chronic but previously neither severe nor life-threatening dyspnoea in whom a second pathology has occurred;

3. a post-operative subject from groups 1 and 2 above;

4. a subject with chronic dyspnoea in which the underlying disease process has progressed to the terminal stages of the illness.

In the introduction to this chapter the causes of dyspnoea were categorized by their systemic aetiology as follows:

1. respiratory;
2. cardiac;
3. neurological;
4. skeletal;
5. systemic;
6. trauma;
7. non-organic.

The vast majority of causes of acute severe dyspnoea are cardiorespiratory in aetiology (see Table 6.2).

Response to the patient with acute severe dyspnoea

1. Sit the patient upright.

2. Check vital signs:

   - pulse rate and rhythm;
   - blood pressure;
   - temperature;
   - respiratory rate;
   - peak expiratory flow rate.

3. Place on SaO_2 monitor.

4. Place on ECG monitor.

5. Obtain intravenous access.

6. Check arterial blood gases (ABGs).

7. Take a venous blood sample (urea, electrolytes, cardiac enzymes, full blood count and cross-match as appropriate).

8. Request urgent ECG.

9. Request urgent chest X-ray.

10. Obtain a history.

11. Conduct examination.

12. Administer oxygen via a Venturi mask according to the guidelines given below.

13. Give specific treatments dependent on the clinical and investigational findings.

14. If the patient is deteriorating despite appropriate management, arrange for urgent intubation and transfer him or her to an intensive-care unit. Ensure that your patient's SaO_2 is $> 70\%$ (preferably $> 80\%$) at all times.

STEPS IN MANAGEMENT

Patient upright
Vital signs

Pulse oximetry
ECG monitoring

IV access
ABGs
Venous blood samples

ECG
Chest X-ray

History
Examination

O_2 therapy
Specific treatment
Ventilatory support

ITU

ARTERIAL BLOOD GAS ANALYSIS

The arterial blood gas analysis makes only three measurements, namely the PaO_2, the $PaCO_2$ and the pH (or $[H^+]$). All other values are derived from calculations involving these measurements.

Table 6.2 Causes of acute severe dyspnoea

Aetiology	Signs/Investigations	Associated risk in surgical patients
Respiratory causes:		
Airflow obstruction		Post-operative
Upper airway		
● Croup		
● Acute epiglottitis		
● Anglo-oedema	Stridor	
● Inhaled foreign body		
● Pharyngeal abscess		
Lower airways		
● Asthma	Wheeze	↑ If brittle or poor control
● COPD	Wheeze	↑ (smokers)
Pleural space disease		
● Pneumothorax	Chest X-ray (and signs) diagnostic	
● Haemothorax		
Alveolar filling/loss		
● Pulmonary oedema	Chest X-ray for all causes of alveolar	Fluid overload
● Pneumonia	filling is the same, with 'air-space'	↑ Smokers + COPD
● Pulmonary haemorrhage	shadowing and air bronchograms	
● Collapse/atelectasis		↑ Pain/excess sputum
Cardiac causes:		
Pulmonary embolism		
● Thrombus	V/Q/spiral CT scan, pulmonary angiography	↑↑
● Fat		↑ Multiple trauma
● Amniotic fluid		↑ Postpartum
Arrhythmia		
● Supraventricular tachycardia	ECG and monitor	↑ Risk
● Fast atrial flutter/fibrillation	± IV adenosine	if underlying
● Ventricular tachycardia	diagnostic	heart disease
Myocardial disease		
● Myocardial infarction	ECG, cardiac enzymes diagnostic	
● Pulmonary oedema		
● Rupture of interventricular septum		
Valvular heart disease	Requires	
● Acute valve rupture	urgent	
Pericardial disease	echocardiography	
● Cardiac tamponade		↑ In cardiothoracic surgery or chest trauma
Other causes:		
● Guillain-Barré syndrome	Watch FEV$_1$ and FVC	
● Metabolic acidosis ± shock	ABGs diagnostic	

1. *In air*:

Normal PaO_2	$PaO_2 \geqslant 12$ kPa
Normal $PaCO_2$	$4.5 \leqslant$ kPa $PaCO_2 \leqslant 6$ kPa
Normal pH	$7.35 \leqslant$ pH $\leqslant 7.45$ ($\equiv 45 \geqslant [H^+] \geqslant 35$)

2. *Type 1 respiratory failure*: $PaO_2 \leqslant 8$ kPa (hypoxia) with a normal or low $PaCO_2$

   $PaO_2 \quad \downarrow$
   $PaCO_2 \quad \downarrow/\rightarrow$

3. *Type 2 respiratory failure*: $PaO_2 \leqslant 8$ kPa (hypoxia) with a $PaCO_2 \geqslant 6$ kPa

   $PaO_2 \quad \downarrow$
   $PaCO_2 \quad \uparrow.$

If in the presence of hypercapnoea the pH is normal, this indicates that there has been sufficient time for a compensatory metabolic alkalosis to occur to balance the respiratory acidosis. A normal pH therefore implies a degree of chronicity (and stability) of the hypercapnoea. Conversely, an acidosis in association with hypercapnoea suggests an acute decompensation. The pH is therefore crucial to interpreting the blood gas results, with a respiratory acidosis being a more serious sign of severity than the absolute $PaCO_2$ value. An acidosis in the presence of a normal or low $PaCO_2$ value is of metabolic origin.

Note that most cardiac and pulmonary diseases will initially cause type 1 rather than type 2 respiratory failure. The main exceptions to this are COPD and central respiratory depression, both of which cause type 2 respiratory failure. A disease which normally causes type 1 respiratory failure that is progressing to or presenting with type 2 respiratory failure has reached a very severe (often terminal) stage of the disease process.

CHEST X-RAY

It is impractical to go into details about chest X-ray interpretation here. However, apart from the many causes of chronic diseases and abnormalities which may be present, you should be alert to the following patterns of acute change.

Check for the following.

1. *Pneumothorax* – identify by:

   - visceral pleural margin, manifested as a crisp fine line, usually parallel to the chest wall;
   - absence of lung markings peripheral to the pleural margin;
   - if there is tracheal and mediastinal deviation away from the pneumothorax, this indicates that it is a tension pneumothorax.

2. *Alveolar/air-space shadowing*:

   - lobar/segmental pattern $\Rightarrow$ pneumonia;
   - bilateral perihilar haziness or diffuse ground-glass shadowing $\Rightarrow$ *Pneumocystis carinii* pneumonia (PCP);
   - bilateral perihilar or bibasal with septal lines $\Rightarrow$ pulmonary oedema.

3. *Pulmonary collapse*:

   - if this affects the whole lung, there is a 'white-out' of one hemi-thorax with mediastinal shift *towards* the opacification (a 'white-out' of one hemi-thorax with mediastinal shift away from the opacification is due to a large effusion of haemothorax);
   - signs of lobar collapse are more subtle and rarely sufficient on their own to cause acute severe dyspnoea.

4. *Bilateral small pleural effusions* occur in the presence of multiple pulmonary emboli and cardiac failure.

5. *Bilateral multiple small areas of plate atelectasis*:

   - may occur in multiple pulmonary emboli and occasionally in the presence of retained secretions.

EXAMINATION OF THE PATIENT WITH DYSPNOEA

General examination

Table 6.3

Sign	Implication
Kussmaul's respiration	Metabolic acidosis
↓ Conscious level	$\Rightarrow$ severe hypoxia or $\Rightarrow CO_2$ narcosis or $\Rightarrow$ impending cardiorespiratory arrest or $\Rightarrow$ all of the above
Inability to speak in sentences	$\Rightarrow$ Severity
Unilateral calf swelling	$\Rightarrow$ DVT
Signs of chest trauma/ thoracic surgery	Consider haemo-/ pneumothorax

Also check briefly for signs of systemic diseases associated with pulmonary pathology, such as rheumatoid arthritis, systemic lupus erythematosus, systemic sclerosis, etc.

Upper limb

Finger clubbing is associated with:

- bronchogenic carcinoma;
- bronchiectasis;
- cryptogenic fibrosing alveolitis;
- endocarditis;
- non-cardiopulmonary causes, including inflammatory bowel disease, hepatic disorders and congenital causes.

Muscle wasting is associated with;

- motor neurone disease (fasciculation may also be present);
- multiple sclerosis;
- carcinoma.

Bounding pulse and 'flap' on wrist extension are associated with CO_2 retention.

Splinter haemorrhages are associated with:

- infective endocarditis;
- vasculitis;
- connective tissue disorders.

Head and neck

Bulbar palsy is associated with:

- motor neurone disease;
- multiple sclerosis;
- cerebrovascular accident.

The presence of bulbar palsy raises the possibility of an aspiration pneumonia as a cause of or factor contributing to the dyspnoea.

Pallor is associated with anaemia.

Lymphadenopathy is associated with:

- carcinoma;
- tuberculosis;
- lymphoma.

RESPIRATORY EXAMINATION

Inspection

Signs of *chronic airflow obstruction* include:

- ↓ crico-sternal distance and tracheal tug;
- hyperinflated barrel-shaped chest;
- use of accessory muscles of respiration (also seen in any acute severe dyspnoea).

Also look for signs of previous thoracoplasty and kyphoscoliosis.

Table 6.4 Implications of respiratory signs

Sign		Implication
Respiratory rate	↑	∝ Severity
	↓	Impending respiratory arrest
Chest wall movement		
Unilateral ↓		Chest expansion is decreased over the area of pathology
Symmetrical ↓		Bilateral disease

Palpation

Subcutaneous emphysema is due to the presence of air in the soft tissues, and gives an odd crackling sensation on palpation. It is due to a leak of air from a pneumothorax or, more rarely, from oesophageal rupture.

Subcutaneous emphysema ⇒ Pneumothorax (more rarely oesophageal rupture)

Tracheal position

The trachea should be in the midline. It is pulled towards an area of collapse/atelectasis and pushed away from an effusion or pneumothorax. Consolidation without collapse will not move the mediastinum, and pathology that affects both lungs does not usually cause any mediastinal movement.

Tracheal deviation: Away from ⇒ Tension pneumothorax
Large effusion
Emphysematous bullae

Towards ⇒ Collapse/atelectasis

Percussion

Usually the only asymmetry in chest percussion is the small area of dullness over the heart. An increase in size of the area of cardiac dullness and any other asymmetry should be considered abnormal. When asymmetry is present, it may be difficult to be certain whether or not one area is abnormally dull or another is abnormally resonant. However, integration with the other clinical findings should clarify the situation. Most pathology, such as consolidation, collapse, effusion, fibrosis and pleural disease, will lead to abnormal dullness on percussion, the few exceptions being pneumothorax and bullous emphysema, which both cause hyper-resonance.

| Unilateral hyper-resonance | Pneumothorax/ emphysematous bullae |
| Unilateral dullness | Consolidation/pleural thickening |

Bibasal dullness	Pulmonary oedema
Stony dullness	Pleural effusion

Auscultation

Stridor	Upper airway narrowing
Wheeze	Narrowing of the lower airways

Crackles

Crackles on auscultation occur in infection, fibrosis and pulmonary oedema. Always check that the crackles persist after coughing (those which do not do so are not significant).

Showers of fine-end inspiratory crackles predominating at the bases are due to pulmonary fibrosis.

The crackles due to a pneumonia may be both fine and coarse, present both in inspiration and expiration, and are localized over the area of pathology. The crackles of bronchiectasis are similar, but may be difficult to distinguish from those of fibrosis or oedema.

The crackles of pulmonary oedema start off as fine inspiratory and bibasal crackles, but gradually become coarser and extend up the chest with increasing severity.

Bronchial breathing:	High pitch	Consolidation
	Low pitch	Fibrosis

It is also heard over the meniscus of pleural effusion.

CARDIAC EXAMINATION

Inspection

Jugular venous pressure (JVP)	↑	⇒ ↑ Intravascular volume/fluid excess
		or ⇒ Right heart failure
	Fixed and ↑	⇒ SVC obstruction
	↓	⇒ Shock
	Kussmaul's sign	⇒ Cardiac tamponade

Kussmaul's sign is an abnormal rise in the JVP when the patient breathes in (it is normal for the JVP to fall on inspiration). It occurs in cardiac tamponade.

Peripheral oedema	⇒ Right heart failure/ fluid overload
Cyanosis	
Peripheral alone	May imply poor circulation
Peripheral and central	Poor oxygenation and ∝ severity
	Right → left shunt

Palpation

Pulse rate

Check for arrhythmias. A sinus tachycardia is a physiological response to cardiorespiratory compromise, and is not an arrhythmia.

Pulse rate	↑	Severity
	≥ 140/min irregular	⇒ Tachyarrhythmia Atrial fibrillation
Pulse volume	↑	⇒ Aortic regurgitation or hyperdynamic circulation (fever or thyrotoxicosis)
	Slow rising and ↓	⇒ Aortic stenosis

Blood pressure

- Hypotension is not specific to any particular cause of dyspnoea.

- Hypotension may occur in any cause of 'shock', and in combination with acute severe dyspnoea may indicate an acute cardiac cause of the dyspnoea, but may also occur in a number of the respiratory causes of dyspnoea.

- Hypotension in the presence of an arrhythmia indicates the need for urgent cardioversion.

- Hypertension may occur in the presence of an acute severe cardiorespiratory insult, and usually resolves with treatment of the underlying cause. Rarely, hypertension may be the precipitant of cardiac failure and require specific treatment.

- Pulsus paradoxus is a fall in the pulse pressure during inspiration. In practical terms, pulsus paradoxus is noted as a fall in systolic pressure during inspiration and, unless specifically looked for, it may be missed or the blood pressure misread. Pulsus paradoxus may be present in acute severe asthma, acute severe airflow obstruction, cardiac tamponade, restrictive cardiomyopathy and large pulmonary emboli.

Blood pressure	↑	Usually elevated and not discriminating
	↓	Think of causes of 'shock'
	Pulsus paradoxus	⇒ Airflow obstruction (asthma/COPD)
		or ⇒ Cardiac tamponade
		or ⇒ Large pulmonary emboli

Left parasternal heave	$\Rightarrow$ Right ventricular hypertrophy
Apex beat	
Displaced laterally and inferiorly	$\Rightarrow$ Cardiomegaly
Displaced laterally	$\Rightarrow$ Mediastinal shift

Percussion

Percussion is relatively unhelpful in cardiac examination. It may reveal an increased area of cardiac dullness in cardiomegaly.

Auscultation

Gallop rhythm	$\Rightarrow$ Heart failure
Murmurs associated with dyspnoea	
Pan-systolic	Ruptured interventricular septum/mitral regurgitation
Ejection systolic	Aortic stenosis
Early diastolic	Aortic regurgitation
Absence of prosthetic sounds (in patient with prosthetic valve)	'Stuck' valve

GUIDELINES FOR OXYGEN THERAPY IN THE MANAGEMENT OF ACUTE SEVERE DYSPNOEA

Appropriate oxygen therapy is extremely important in the acutely dyspnoeic patient. The following guidelines cover most eventualities.

1. In most conditions that cause acute severe dyspnoea, high-flow oxygen (60% via a Venturi mask) should be administered. Likewise, most patients requiring nebulized bronchodilator treatment should be nebulized with high-flow oxygen.

2. Only patients with chronic type 2 respiratory failure (hypoxia and hypercapnoea) are at significant risk from high-flow oxygen therapy. If the blood pH is normal or near normal in the presence of hypercapnoea, this indicates that the hypercapnoea is chronic. Only very occasionally will patients with chronic type 1 respiratory failure (hypoxia without hypercapnoea) develop CO_2 retention with high-flow oxygen administration.

3. In patients with acute respiratory failure from any cause, a severe respiratory acidosis (a low pH = $\uparrow [H^+]$) is a sign of impending cardiorespiratory arrest, and the treatment is urgent intubation and transfer to an ITU.

4. In most patients with acute severe dyspnoea you should be aiming to maintain their $SaO_2 > 90\% = PaO_2 > 8$ kPa, and an inability to do so in the absence of pre-existing lung disease is an ominous sign.

5. In patients with chronic type 2 respiratory failure you should aim to keep the SaO_2 between 80% and 90% (and indeed an SaO_2 of $> 90\%$ will probably aggravate the hypercapnoea and cause a respiratory acidosis).

6. In patients with chronic type 2 respiratory failure, controlled oxygen supplementation initially at 24% or 28% should be given via a Venturi mask.

7. In patients with chronic type 2 respiratory failure requiring nebulized bronchodilators, the nebulizer should be driven by air at > 8 L/min and the FiO_2 supplemented by oxygen through nasal cannulae for the duration of the nebulized treatment only, after which they should immediately return to oxygen administered via a Venturi mask.

8. A Venturi mask is the safest and most controllable way to give controlled oxygen supplementation. Other masks and nasal cannulae may give erratic FiO_2 concentrations which may change with the rate and depth of the patient's respiration. In particular, if the patient develops worsening CO_2 retention on the oxygen supplementation, the subsequent hypoventilation will cause the FiO_2 to increase, thus perpetuating the problem if oxygen is not administered by Venturi mask.

9. Nasal cannulae are preferred by some patients, and may be acceptable only if the patient is stable and closely monitored. For each 1 L/min of oxygen delivered via nasal cannulae, the FiO_2 rises by approximately 4%. Therefore 1 L/min of oxygen administered via nasal cannulae approximates to an FiO_2 of 24%, 2 L/min to 28% and 4 L/min to 35%. However, nasal cannulae have no role in the management of acute severe dyspnoea except as temporary oxygen supplementation for patients who are being given nebulized bronchodilators on air.

10. Arterial blood gases should be rechecked 20–60 min following a change in the oxygen prescription of an acutely unwell patient.

11. Any patient (even one with chronic type 1 or type 2 respiratory failure) will be in mortal danger from hypoxia with a PaO_2 much below 6 kPa ($SaO_2 = 70\%$). If the oxygen saturations are inexorably falling below 80% and certainly below 70%, then crash-call an anaesthetist and arrange urgent intubation and transfer to an ITU. Pending

intubation you may need to administer high-flow oxygen to maintain an SaO_2 of $> 70\%$.

12. If a patient with chronic type 2 respiratory failure receives an excessively high FiO_2 and develops CO_2 narcosis and respiratory acidosis, whilst reducing the FiO_2 may result in improvement, if they have progressed to a degree of severe hypoventilation then reducing the FiO_2 may result in a dangerous level of hypoxia, and in this circumstance intubation and ventilation is the only option. Again, give whatever FiO_2 is necessary to maintain an SaO_2 of $\geqslant 70\%$ pending intubation.

Remember that severe hypoxia is more life-threatening than hypercapnoea (severe hypoxia may kill in minutes, hypercapnoea in hours and acidosis in days). Do not allow your patient to die of hypoxia.

RESPONSE TO FINDINGS

By now you will have as much information as you require, or can reasonably expect to obtain in the acute situation, in order for specific action to be taken. Each finding listed below requires a specific response. Patients often have a number of components to their dyspnoea, and you should not limit your therapy to only one category. In listing the appropriate responses to each finding, it is assumed that the management procedures for acute severe dyspnoea, including appropriate oxygen therapy, will already have been followed.

STRIDOR

This is a sign of significant obstruction to the upper airway. Presenting in the chronically dyspnoeic patient, stridor is often due to a tumour of the trachea or main bronchi, and the most appropriate investigation is bronchoscopy. However, when presenting with acute severe dyspnoea, stridor must be assumed to be due to critical airway narrowing above the vocal cords. It is a serious sign and, irrespective of any other clinical finding, it requires emergency management. Acute stridor is an 'Ear, Nose and Throat' problem, and you must obtain the assistance of a senior ENT surgeon, and the patient must be admitted to a hospital with an intensive-care facility. Do not in any circumstances attempt to examine the throat, as you may precipitate complete airway obstruction. While awaiting an ENT opinion or transfer you should:

- give broad-spectrum IV antibiotics (augmentin or cefuroxime);
- give 200 mg IV hydrocortisone and 60 mg oral prednisolone;

- give 2 mg nebulized budesonide;
- if the patient is deteriorating, give nebulized racemic adrenalin.

Equipment for an emergency cricothyrotomy and intubation should be close at hand.

WHEEZE

Wheezing or polyphonic rhonchi indicates narrowing of the small- and medium-sized airways and is likely to be due to asthma, COPD or bronchiectasis, and may also occur with pulmonary oedema (cardiac asthma). Whatever the cause, the treatment is the same and it will be accompanied by low peak expiratory flow rates (PEFRs).

The treatment is as follows:

- 5 mg nebulized salbutamol;
- 500 µg nebulized ipratropium;
- 200 mg IV hydrocortisone and 60 mg oral prednisolone.

If the patient improves, commence treatment with the following:

- prednisolone 40 mg daily;
- salbutamol nebulized 2.5–5 mg 4-hourly;
- ± ipratropium 250–500 µg nebulized 6-hourly.

If the patient fails to improve:

- repeat the salbutamol, and if necessary nebulize continuously with salbutamol;
- give IV aminophylline. If the patient is already taking theophylline orally, check a level urgently and give a maintenance infusion of 0.5 mg/kg/h. If the patient is not taking aminophylline or the levels are low, give 5 mg/kg in 100 mL 5% dextrose by infusion over 20 min, followed by a maintenance infusion.

If the patient still fails to improve, then an infusion of salbutamol may be tried, but in practice intubation and ventilation will almost certainly be needed, and time should not be wasted in delaying this action.

INFECTION

An infective cause of the patient's dyspnoea is likely to take one of three forms:

1. a pneumonia (signs of focal and/or segmental consolidation on chest X-ray). Treatment is with intravenous amoxycillin and clarithromycin;

2. an infective exacerbation of established COPD or upper respiratory tract infection (URTI)

precipitating worsening asthma. Treatment is with intravenous amoxicillin;

3. infective exacerbation of bronchiectasis. Treatment is with intravenous cover for known pathogens for the individual patient (almost always *Pseudomonas*, and often *Staphylococcus*).

PULMONARY OEDEMA

Treatment is as follows:

1. IV diamorphine 2.5–10 mg (not in the presence of hypercapnoea);

2. intravenous frusemide 40–80 mg;

3. intravenous infusion of nitrate (glyceryl trinitrate (GTN) or isosorbide dinitrate);

4. repeat steps 1 and 2 after 20 min if there is no improvement;

5. if the patient still fails to improve, intravenous aminophylline may be tried. Do not delay a decision to intubate while waiting for the aminophylline to work.

PULMONARY THROMBO-EMBOLISM (PTE)

A high index of suspicion is often required in order not to miss the diagnosis of pulmonary thrombo-embolism. Post-operative patients are at high risk of PTE. The clinical findings are often non-specific or even normal. PTE should be suspected if there is pleuritic chest pain, haemoptysis or unexplained dyspnoea (either acute or chronic). The chest X-ray may show a variety of pictures. It is commonly normal or shows small bilateral effusions or bilateral basal areas of plate atelectasis. Wedge-shaped areas of oligaemia or infarcts are relatively rarely seen on chest X-ray. The ECG may also demonstrate a number of different patterns; most commonly all that is seen is a sinus tachycardia. Other patterns of ECG abnormality include right axis deviation, right bundle branch block or an $S_1Q_3T_3$ pattern. The arterial blood gas analysis in PTE shows type 1 respiratory failure. In the absence of underlying lung disease, a V/Q scan is a useful investigation. A spiral CT scan is also helpful for detecting medium-sized or larger pulmonary emboli, and may also demonstrate the presence of chronic emboli whilst an echocardiogram may show right heart strain and chamber dilatation or even thrombus. Thrombus may be demonstrated in the leg veins by venography, or in the thigh and pelvis veins alone by Doppler ultrasonography.

If the patient is not severely unwell, then anticoagulate with intravenous heparin (either unfractionated or low molecular weight) initially, and subsequently with warfarin.

Heparinization with unfractionated heparin should be carried out as follows:

- IV bolus heparin 5000–10 000 units (80 U/kg);
- IV heparin 18 U/kg (up to 1600 U/h);
- check that activated partial thrombin time (APTT) is therapeutic after 6 h and adjust the dose of infusion accordingly, aiming for a ratio of 2 to 3 times the control.

Alternatively, the newer low-molecular-weight heparins may be given provided that the patient is not too unwell.

If the patient appears to have had a massive PTE, and is haemodynamically unstable, then consideration should be given to either thrombolytic agents or surgical embolectomy. There are no well-controlled studies comparing these two options, and the decision should be made after consultation with your local cardiothoracic surgeons. If there is likely to be any delay in obtaining a decision for an embolectomy, then give intravenous thrombolysis via a peripheral cannula. Streptokinase is given as a loading bolus of 250 000 units over 30 min followed by 100 000 units/h for 24–72 h. Alternatively, alteplase may be given as a single infusion of 100 mg over 2 h, followed by full heparinization.

PNEUMOTHORAX

The chest X-ray is diagnostic in pneumothorax. Occasionally a large emphysematous bulla may resemble a pneumothorax with some pleural tethering, and it is important not to attempt to insert a drain into a bulla. Very rarely there may be bilateral pneumothoraces. In patients with significant COPD or other pulmonary disease, even a small pneumothorax may cause severe dyspnoea and should be drained. Drainage of a pneumothorax should be through the second intercostal space in the mid-clavicular line or the fifth intercostal space in the mid-axillary line by the method described in Chapter 8.6. A tension pneumothorax may be life-threatening, but it is very rarely necessary to attempt drainage prior to seeing an X-ray. If the patient is on the point of cardiorespiratory arrest and there are signs strongly suggestive of a tension pneumothorax (tracheal deviation away from the side of the chest demonstrating hyper-resonance to percussion and decreased breath sounds and perhaps subcutaneous emphysema), insert a small-bore cannula into the second intercostal space in the mid-clavicular line, and if there is a rush of air escaping then insert a larger drain.

TACHYARRHYTHMIAS

A sinus tachycardia is a normal physiological response, and should not be regarded as an arrhythmia. The only way to correct a sinus tachycardia is to treat the underlying condition. However, a number of tachyarrythmias may occur in association with breathlessness and hypoxia. These tachyarrythmias may be the primary cause of the breathlessness, or they may be secondary to the underlying cardiorespiratory cause of hypoxia. However, whether primary or secondary, correction of the arrhythmia will result in clinical improvement.

MANAGEMENT OF TACHYARRHYTHMIAS

1. Check that serum K^+ and Mg^{++} are normal, and correct levels if they are abnormal.

2. If the tachyarrhythmia is causing severe cardiorespiratory compromise, then urgent correction by direct current (DC) cardioversion is required.

3. If there is difficulty in distinguishing a supraventricular from a ventricular tachycardia, give a fast bolus of intravenous adenosine (6 mg initially and then, if there is no response, 12 mg) with ECG monitoring. Adenosine will slow and may even terminate a supraventricular arrhythmia, but will have no effect on the ventricular arrhythmia.

Fast atrial flutter or fibrillation

Rate control may be achieved by intravenous or oral digoxin, and unless contraindicated the patient should be anticoagulated with heparin whilst their rhythm is unstable.

Alternatively, intravenous amiodarone may achieve cardioversion to sinus rhythm.

Supraventricular tachycardia

Treatment is as follows:

1. intravenous verapamil (not if the patient is on a beta-blocker) slowly in 2.5- to 5-mg aliquots;

2. if verapamil fails, give intravenous amiodarone;

3. if amiodarone fails, then DC cardioversion. Beta-blockers are also useful for supraventricular tachycardia, but unless the tachycardia is the sole cause of the dyspnoea they could aggravate the dyspnoea (via increased airflow obstruction and/or pulmonary oedema).

Ventricular tachycardia

Treatment is as follows:

1. intravenous lignocaine, 100 mg by IV bolus, followed by rapidly reducing maintenance infusion;

2. if lignocaine treatment fails, DC cardioversion or intravenous amiodarone.

Pericardial effusion/tamponade, ruptured interventricular septum and cardiac valvular problems

In all of these conditions, while treatment of any pulmonary oedema and arrhythmia is needed, the most important management is to obtain an urgent echocardiogram and expert cardiac intervention.

RESPIRATORY FAILURE AND VENTILATORY SUPPORT

Additional measures for treatment of refractory respiratory failure include the following.

Type 1 respiratory failure ($\downarrow PaO_2$ with $\downarrow/\rightarrow PaCO_2$)

As described above, the patient should be on high-flow oxygen and have received specific treatment(s) for the underlying cause(s).

If the respiratory failure remains severe ($PaO_2 < 8kPa = SaO_2 < 90\%$) despite these measures, consider using continuous positive airways pressure (CPAP) with the high-flow oxygen.

CPAP is *not* appropriate for:

- asthma;
- bronchiectasis;
- type 2 respiratory failure.

However, CPAP may improve oxygenation in some patients with type 1 respiratory failure (such as patients with pulmonary oedema or pneumonia) who do not require intubation at that time.

It is not possible to administer CPAP in all patients, as the closed mask and sensation of increased airways pressure may be too distressing, particularly in the presence of severe dyspnoea. In practice, patients whose condition is severe enough to require CPAP should be treated in a respiratory high-dependency unit or an intensive-care unit. If it is not possible to maintain an adequate SaO_2 with the CPAP, or the patient is unsuitable for CPAP, then the treatment is intubation and ventilation on ITU.

Type 2 respiratory failure ($\downarrow PaO_2$ with $\uparrow PaCO_2$)

The patient should be receiving appropriate oxygen therapy and have been given appropriate specific treatment(s) as described above.

Acute on chronic type 2 respiratory failure

Patients with chronic type 2 respiratory failure will be accustomed to hypercapnoea and, when stable, will have a normal arterial blood pH despite the high $PaCO_2$ because a compensatory metabolic alkalosis occurs. The respiratory centre in such patients is desensitized to the effects of hypercapnoea, and they therefore rely on a degree of chronic hypoxia to maintain their respiratory drive. Administering a high FiO_2 to such patients removes the remaining hypoxic drive and the ventilatory rate falls, resulting in worsening hypercapnoea and an uncompensated respiratory acidosis. Therefore patients with chronic type 2 respiratory failure should in the first instance be given controlled oxygen supplementation via a Venturi mask at no more than 28%. As described above in the oxygen therapy guidelines, you should aim to keep the SaO_2 in these patients between 80% and 90%, and in fact raising the SaO_2 significantly above 90% may result in a loss of the patient's hypoxic drive.

Additional measures for the treatment of acute on chronic type 2 respiratory failure include the following.

Doxapram infusion Doxapram stimulates the respiratory centre and increases the rate and depth of respiration, and is of benefit in controlling worsening hypercapnoea.

A doxapram infusion is indicated for the treatment of type 2 respiratory failure associated with a respiratory acidosis (pH $<$ 7.25/$[H^+] >$ 55 mmol/L) where there is decreased respiratory rate or depth.

Doxapram is not indicated:

- in the absence of a significant respiratory acidosis;
- in the presence of normal or increased respiratory drive.

Bi-level positive airways pressure (BiPAP) non-invasive ventilatory support BiPAP non-invasive ventilatory support may be of benefit in acute on chronic type 2 respiratory failure, where it may avoid the need for intubation and ventilation. It should, however, not be used for:

- type 1 respiratory failure (where CPAP is more appropriate);
- in the presence of a pneumothorax.

Acute type 2 respiratory failure in a patient who has not previously demonstrated hypercapnoea

In a patient who has not previously demonstrated CO_2 retention, hypercapnoea is a serious sign and the arterial blood gas analysis will show an acidosis ($\downarrow$ pH /$\uparrow$ $[H^+]$). Acute-onset hypercapnoea may occur:

- in a patient with chronic type 1 respiratory failure whose illness has progressed to the terminal stages of the disease;
- in a patient with chronic type 1 respiratory failure with a new second pathology;
- in a patient with chronic type 1 respiratory failure and which has now progressed to a more severe stage requiring ventilation.

When type 2 respiratory failure develops in these situations, intubation and ventilation on ITU are necessary.

In these patients the hypercapnoea is due to the severity of the underlying disease and not to loss of hypoxic drive. Therefore high-flow oxygen is not contraindicated, and will be necessary to maintain adequate SaO_2 while intubation and ventilation are awaited. BiPAP, CPAP and doxapram are unlikely to be of benefit in these patients, and trials of such therapies should not delay their transfer to ITU.

INDICATIONS FOR INTUBATION AND MECHANICAL VENTILATION

The development of any of the following, irrespective of any other factors, is an indication for immediate intubation and ventilation:

- failure to maintain an adequate SaO_2;
- a rising $PaCO_2$ (i.e. worsening respiratory acidosis) that is refractory to treatment;
- patient exhaustion;
- worsening upper airway obstruction.

OPERATIVE PATIENTS

Post-operative respiratory complications can be minimized by:

- optimizing lung function and the treatment of established lung disorders pre-operatively. In patients with known respiratory disease a pre-operative assessment by a chest physician is helpful;
- prophylactic heparin peri-operatively in patients at risk of deep venous thrombosis;
- intra-operative procedures for preventing DVT in high-risk patients;
- persuading smokers to stop $\geqslant$ 6 weeks before elective surgery;
- avoiding non-emergency operations within 6 months of a myocardial infarction;
- ensuring adequate analgesia post-operatively, particularly after abdominal surgery;
- arranging post-operative chest physiotherapy for patients with underlying chest disease or undergoing abdominal surgery.

The diagnosis or anticipation of post-operative respiratory problems is greatly facilitated if pre-operative assessments have been made of:

- chest X-ray and ECG (in all patients over 40 years of age or with a known cardiac or respiratory disorder);
- SaO_2 on air;
- FEV_1, FVC and PEFR.

Most common causes of post-operative dyspnoea

Those that manifest within the first few hours include:

- myocardial infarction ± pulmonary oedema;
- cardiac arrhythmia;
- ARDS;
- shock/hypovolaemia;
- pneumothorax or haemothorax (in thoracic surgical cases);
- cardiac tamponade (in cardiac surgical cases).

Those that manifest within the first few days include:

- pulmonary thromboembolism;
- pneumonia;
- lobar or segmental collapse.

FURTHER READING

British Thoracic Society Guidelines for the management of chronic obstructive airways disease: December 1997. *Thorax* **52**(**suppl**).

British Thoracic Society: Guidelines on the management of asthma: March 1993. *Thorax* **48**(**suppl**).

Suspected acute pulmonary embolism, a practical approach: October 1997. *Thorax* **52**(**suppl**).

The British guidelines on asthma management; 1995 Review and Position Statement: February 1997. *Thorax* **52**(**suppl**).

Dysphonia

Bren Dorman

Introduction

'The human voice is very important, as it is the main instrument through which we communicate, influence our colleagues and project our personality' (Sataloff RT. 1997). The management of voice disorders is complex and requires a detailed knowledge of the anatomy, physiology and psychology of voice production.

There are three primary laryngeal functions, namely airway, airway protection and voice. Conditions that restrict or obstruct the airway may result in stridor, whereas if the protective function is altered, then cough, aspiration and subsequent chest problems may result.

There are several different ways in which voice problems present. The commonest symptoms are hoarseness, breathiness and loss of voice, but there are many others, including altered vocal range, pitch breaks, tremor, voice strain and changes in resonance. Any abnormality of phonation or voicing is called dysphonia. The signs of voice problems are perceptual, and include changes in pitch of the voice, variation in loudness and changes in voice quality.

In addition to these symptoms and signs, laryngeal abnormalities can result in pain, dysphagia, diplophonia, odynophagia, haemoptysis or even a swelling in the neck.

EPIDEMIOLOGY

Disease in any region can be considered under abnormalities of structure and abnormalities of function, and there is usually some interactive effect between them. In the larynx, abnormalities of structure include inflammation, neoplasia and degenerative changes. Abnormalities of function include neurological dysfunction (either centrally or peripherally), muscle tension dysphonia or spasmodic dysphonia.

In children, respiratory difficulty and stridor are more common than vocal changes, whereas in adults dysphonia is more common than airway obstruction. This is due to the smaller size of the larynx in children and the softer less mature cartilage. Hoarseness results whenever there is any irregularity of the vocal folds or vocal fold dysfunction resulting in incomplete approximation of the vocal folds. It usually indicates a significant abnormality in the larynx.

Acute hoarseness arises suddenly, from minutes to hours or even days, and is usually traumatic or infective in origin. Acute laryngitis may be associated with sore throat, difficulty in swallowing and even generalized symptoms of malaise and infection. External laryngeal trauma and intralaryngeal trauma e.g. endotracheal intubation, voice abuse or misuse, vomiting, inhaling irritating fumes or gases, ingesting caustic substances, and allergy can all result in the sudden onset of hoarseness.

Chronic hoarseness is defined as persistent hoarseness lasting longer than 4 weeks. The most important concern of the medical practitioner is to rule out carcinoma of the larynx. Some other causes include chronic laryngitis, contact ulcers, vocal cord polyps, benign laryngeal neoplasms such as papillomas, specific infections such as syphilis, HIV or TB, vocal fold paralysis and vocal fold nodules. The latter problem is really a localized form of chronic laryngitis at the junction of the anterior third and the posterior two-thirds of the vocal folds due to repeated trauma. It is reasonably common in young schoolchildren (especially boys) and individuals who tend to use their voice a lot in their job, such as teachers, singers, clergymen and sales personnel.

> Note: Hoarseness persisting for more than 4 weeks requires specialist otolaryngological referral for direct or indirect laryngeal examination to rule out malignancy.

ANATOMY

The structure of the larynx consists of a cartilaginous framework, intrinsic and extrinsic muscles, mucosal surfaces, nerves, blood vessels and lymphatics (Figure 7.1).

The cartilages include the thyroid cartilage, the cricoid cartilage and the two arytenoid cartilages, with the thyroarytenoid muscle extending from the arytenoid cartilage on each side to the internal surface of the thyroid cartilage. The medial aspect of this muscle forms the bulk of the vocal fold. The cartilages have complex attachments and ranges of movement. The mucosal surfaces are also complex in shape and structure, forming a multilayered covering over the internal aspects of the laryngeal skeleton. The vocal fold consists of the thyroarytenoid muscle and the overlying mucosa. In the area of contact between the vocal folds, the epithelium is

stratified squamous epithelium, whereas in the rest of the larynx it is ciliated columnar epithelium.

There are three specific areas within the larynx, namely the supraglottis, the glottis and the subglottis. The supraglottis is the area that lies above the vocal folds, the glottis is the area that lies between the vocal folds and the subglottis is the area that extends inferiorly from 1 cm below the free margin of the vocal folds to the lower border of the cricoid cartilage (Figure 7.2).

There are several intrinsic laryngeal muscles, but the most important ones are the thyroarytenoid, the cricothyroid and the posterior and lateral cricoarytenoid muscles. The extrinsic laryngeal muscles stabilize the laryngeal skeleton in the neck and lie below or above the hyoid bone. The infrahyoid group includes the thyrohyoid, sternothyroid, sternohyoid and omohyoid. The suprahyoid group includes the digastric, mylohyoid, geniohyoid and stylohyoid.

Figure 7.3 shows the relationship between the cartilages and the vocal folds and ligaments.

The nerve distribution to the larynx is via the vagus nerve. The recurrent laryngeal nerve is the motor supply to all of the muscles of the larynx except the cricothyroid muscle, which is supplied by the external branch of the superior laryngeal nerve. The sensory nerve supply to the mucosa above the vocal fold (the supraglottis) is via the internal branch of the superior laryngeal nerve. The glottis and subglottis are supplied by the recurrent laryngeal nerve. The recurrent laryngeal nerve runs a longer course on the left side of the body where it enters the thorax to loop around the aortic arch and ascends in the tracheo-oesophageal groove before entering the larynx. It is more likely to be involved in disease processes and trauma than the nerve on the right. On the right, it may run directly into the larynx as a non-recurrent recurrent

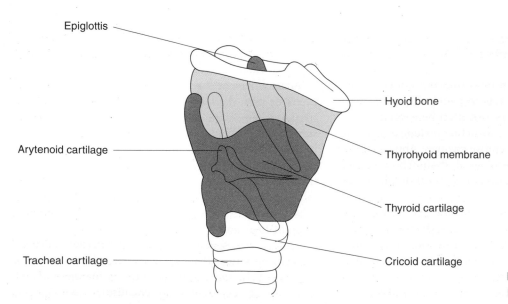

Figure 7.1 Lateral view of larynx.

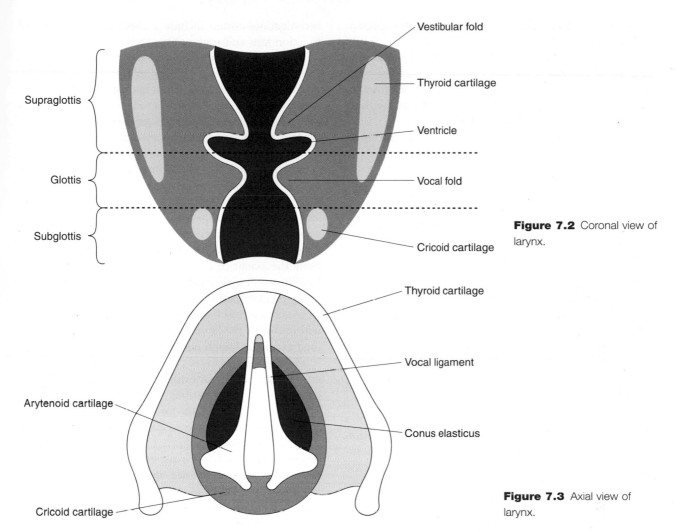

Supraglottis

Glottis

Subglottis

Vestibular fold

Thyroid cartilage

Ventricle

Vocal fold

Figure 7.2 Coronal view of larynx.

Cricoid cartilage

Thyroid cartilage

Vocal ligament

Arytenoid cartilage

Conus elasticus

Figure 7.3 Axial view of larynx.

Cricoid cartilage

laryngeal nerve, but it usually loops around the brachy-cephalic artery to ascend to the larynx.

The blood supply is from branches of the external carotid artery superiorly and from the subclavian artery inferiorly.

The lymphatic drainage of the larynx is divided into the supraglottic and subglottic areas, but the vocal folds themselves are poorly supplied with lymphatics. The supraglottic area drains to the deep cervical nodes at the level of the carotid bifurcation, and the subglottic area drains to the upper tracheal, the deep cervical and the superior mediastinal lymph nodes.

There are various regions or compartments in the larynx that may help to explain the routes of spread of laryngeal cancer. In the supraglottis there are two lateral paraglottic spaces separated by the pre-epiglottic space anteriorly. The paraglottic spaces are limited anteriorly by the thyroid cartilage, posteriorly by the piriform sinuses, medially by the quadrangular membrane and the ventricle and inferiorly by the vocalis. The pre-epiglottic space is closed inferiorly by the attachment of the epiglottis to the thyroid cartilage. It is bounded anteriorly by the upper part of the thyroid cartilage, the

thyrohyoid membrane and the hyoid bone, posteriorly by the epiglottis and superiorly by the hyoepiglottic ligament. It contains adipose tissue, lymphatics, blood vessels and mucous glands.

ESTABLISHING A DIAGNOSIS

Clinical evaluation of a patient with a voice disorder involves taking an adequate history and performing a thorough examination that requires special equipment and techniques. The equipment consists of a headlight, mirrors, flexible endoscopes and rigid endoscopes. The technique of examination varies depending on the equipment. Examination and evaluation of the larynx and the upper airways have improved greatly with flexible fibre-optic laryngoscopy and videostroboscopy. Rigid laryngoscopes with either 70- or 90-degree angulation give very detailed images of the larynx and vocal folds in particular. Voice analysis is usually conducted by the speech and language therapist both directly and with a variety of computer programs. Other investigations include electroglottography, electromyography, spectrography and air-flow analysis.

Investigations are directed towards the likely cause of the vocal symptoms once a provisional diagnosis has been made based on the history and clinical examination findings. They are tailored to help to confirm the diagnosis and direct the treatment planning.

Three common presentations will be considered here.

SOLITARY LESION ON THE VOCAL FOLD

A solitary lesion on the vocal fold in an adult may well represent a neoplastic process! It may be large and partially obstructing the airway, giving stridor, or it may be quite small, resulting only in hoarseness and perhaps some irritation in the throat. The history and examination direct the clinician to the most useful lines of investigation.

If the history is of chronic hoarseness in a moderately heavy smoker and the findings are of an irregular lesion on the vocal fold, then the provisional diagnosis is carcinoma of the larynx until proven otherwise. Squamous-cell carcinoma is the commonest malignant neoplasm of the larynx.

Hoarseness is the commonest initial symptom of a glottic or supraglottic tumour. Clinical examination would include evaluation of the rest of the upper aerodigestive tract (oral cavity, pharynx and nose) as well as the chest and neck. Second primaries can occur in up to 15% of patients with a carcinoma in the upper aerodigestive tract, and in patients with a laryngeal cancer about 5% have another primary, usually in the lung. This is the rationale for a complete endoscopic evaluation of the upper aerodigestive tract (pharyngo-oesophagoscopy, laryngoscopy and tracheo-bronchoscopy) and examination of the nasopharynx.

Patients with glottic tumours tend to develop cervical metastases later than patients with tumours in the piriform fossae, so lymph nodes may not necessarily be palpable at the time of presentation. Patients with small glottic carcinomas (T1 and T2) have an incidence of cervical metastases of 2–5%, whereas with larger tumours (T3 and T4) this rises to 20–30%. Large tumours of the supraglottis may have nodal spread in up to 60% of patients.

The most important investigation is an adequate biopsy of the lesion for histological analysis. This is usually conducted under general anaesthesia using specialized laryngoscopes and an operating microscope. The importance of obtaining a satisfactory histological specimen should not be underestimated because there is very different management if the result is a carcinoma or other malignant tumour, compared to dysplasia or carcinoma *in situ* or even a non-neoplastic process. Other

investigations would include a chest X-ray, respiratory function tests and routine blood tests.

Videostroboscopy is a useful technique for assessing the mucosal wave over the vocal fold, and the wave characterstics change with different pathology. If the stroboscopic images reveal an adynamic segment, then it is possible that the lesion is invading the deeper structures of the fold, which may influence subsequent management.

If the patient also experiences difficulty or pain with swallowing then the endoscopy may be extended to include examination of the oesophagus, the trachea and the main bronchi. Contrast studies such as a barium swallow or videofluoroscopy may be performed if evaluation of the dynamics of swallowing function is required. CT or MRI scanning have both been used to try to determine the extent of the primary lesion, the presence of local invasion into adjacent structures and the presence of lymphadenopathy in the neck. Carcinoma of the glottis tends to spread locally and is often contained initially within one of the laryngeal compartments before seeding to regional lymph nodes.

Once the diagnosis of carcinoma has been confirmed and all appropriate investigations carried out, then the tumour is staged according to the TNM classification system. This is important for treatment planning, estimation of prognosis, and to allow better comparison of different treatment regimens for similarly staged tumours. Risk factors for patients with head and neck cancer include male gender, age, smoking history, alcohol intake, previous radiotherapy to the head and neck region, the presence of other tumours, and whether the patient is immunocompromised.

If the lesion on the vocal fold seems to be smooth, rounded, polypoid or even submucosal, then although the diagnosis of a malignant neoplasm is less likely, microlaryngoscopy and excisional biopsy are still required.

VOCAL FOLD LESIONS IN A CHILD

In a child, if the history is of hoarseness and the findings on flexible endoscopy are of small irregular lesions on the vocal folds, then although one possible diagnosis is vocal fold nodules, one must exclude respiratory papillomatosis. Vocal fold nodules are usually solitary lesions present on each vocal fold at the junction of the anterior third and the middle third. A complete history will identify the child with vocal fold nodules, as they are typically 'shouters' or 'screamers' both at school and at home. No further specific investigations are required if nodules are diagnosed.

Papillomatosis is found in both the upper and lower respiratory tract, the sites in order of decreasing frequency being the glottis, the supraglottis, the subglottis and the trachea. It is the commonest benign tumour of the larynx. It is usually seen as a multifocal irregular exophytic mass, varying in colour from red to white depending on whether the mucosa is keratinizing or non-keratinizing. The presenting symptoms depend on the site and size of the papillomas. Large lesions in the glottis or subglottis can cause marked airway compromise, whereas small lesions on the free margin of the vocal fold will often only result in dysphonia. The causative agent is human papilloma virus (types 6 and 11), so eradication of the condition depends on the immune response of the patient. There appear to be two clinical pathways of respiratory papillomatosis, namely juvenile onset and adult onset. The former is more common, more aggressive, has more frequent recurrences and has an unpredictable clinical course. If papillomatosis is suspected, then a microlaryngoscopy and biopsy should be performed to confirm the diagnosis. Because the lower respiratory tract can be involved, a chest X-ray is important for helping to define the extent of the disease.

UNILATERAL VOCAL FOLD PALSY

In a patient with unilateral vocal fold palsy, the commonest and often the only symptom is hoarseness, although other voice symptoms could be loss of power and range, poor projection, altered vocal pitch and diplophonia. With the incomplete closure of the vocal folds, escape of air during phonation is common and the air flow becomes turbulent so that the voice is husky and often breathy. The rapid escape of air in a relatively uncontrolled manner results in vocal fatigue. This poor breath control and sometimes cough may result in aspiration when eating or drinking. If bilateral vocal fold palsy has occurred, then stridor and some degree of airway obstruction are usually noted. The latter situation may necessitate urgent airway access such as intubation or tracheostomy.

If the history is of relatively sudden onset of hoarseness and the findings are of an immobile vocal fold in an otherwise normal larynx, then the diagnosis is most likely to be neurological, although fixation of the cricoarytenoid joint is a possibility. Dysfunction of the vagus nerve or the recurrent laryngeal nerve will result in abnormal vocal fold movement and thus altered laryngeal function. The site of the lesion in the vagus nerve pathway may be central (supranuclear or bulbar) or peripheral (vagus nerve and its branches, the recurrent laryngeal nerve and the superior laryngeal nerve). There may also be abnormalities in muscle function within the larynx. Neurological conditions such as focal stroke, motor neurone disease, bulbar palsy, multiple sclerosis, intracranial trauma, amyotrophic lateral sclerosis or intracranial tumours are all considered to be supra-

nuclear or bulbar sites of lesion. With most of these conditions there are associated symptoms and signs which help to clarify the diagnosis. The patients with more central abnormalities in the pathway seem to have more severe effects.

In the peripheral part of the vagus nerve there are many possible causes of dysfunction, including inflammatory, degenerative, neoplastic, metabolic, traumatic and idiopathic causes. Pathology at the skull base usually affects cranial nerves IX and XI in addition to X, resulting in loss of sensation in the larynx and pharynx as well as pharyngeal paralysis, which often leads to aspiration.

The nerve most commonly affected is the recurrent laryngeal nerve, the left more commonly than the right, resulting in the vocal fold lying immobile in a paramedian position. The left nerve runs a longer course, looping down into the chest around the arch of the aorta, and as such it may be involved with chest pathology, perhaps apical tuberculosis or a lung carcinoma. A chest X-ray is often performed to help to exclude these possibilities.

The commonest causes of recurrent laryngeal nerve palsy are idiopathic, malignant disease (usually in the lung but also in the oesophagus or the thyroid), and surgical trauma, following either thyroid surgery or cardiothoracic surgery (Table 7.1). Other causes include inflammatory disorders, neck injuries and carotid aneurysms. In some patients no cause for the palsy will be identified, and in these cases it is assumed that a neuropathy has occurred, perhaps secondary to a viral neuritis.

It may be necessary to perform a microlaryngoscopy and manipulate the arytenoid cartilages to determine whether fixation or dislocation is present. Cricoarytenoid fixation can occur in patients with rheumatoid arthritis, but is more likely to be seen after endotracheal intubation or direct external laryngeal trauma. Laryngeal electromyography can be used to determine whether there is electrical activity in the muscles of the vocal folds, but it requires particular skill to place the electrodes and interpret the recordings.

Table 7.1 Causes of recurrent laryngeal nerve palsy (in decreasing order of frequency)

Idiopathic
Malignant disease:
lung, oesophagus or thyroid
Surgical trauma:
thyroid, cardiothoracic, neck or spinal
Inflammatory disorders
Neck injuries
Carotid aneurysms
Miscellaneous:
metabolic

A CT or MRI scan tracing the course of the vagus nerve and then the recurrent laryngeal nerve from the base of the skull to the larynx can be performed. This enables assessment of areas such as the base of the skull, the nasopharynx, the carotid sheath and its contents, the cervical lymph nodes and the thyroid gland. In the absence of any other clinical signs there is debate as to how cost-effective a CT or MRI scan is in these situations. If the thyroid is suspected, then a thyroid ultrasound or scintiscan may also be indicated.

MANAGEMENT STRATEGIES

The management of patients with dysphonia depends on the specific diagnosis. In some cases this may only involve the surgeon, but in most cases a team approach is required. For benign and non-neoplastic processes, close liaison between the otolaryngologist and the speech and language therapist is essential. For malignant disease, the team includes head and neck surgeons, radiotherapists, speech and language therapists, reconstructive surgeons and medical oncologists.

MALIGNANT DISEASE

Management of malignant disease of the larynx is best carried out in a multidisciplinary manner in a Head and Neck clinic which permits better discussion of each individual case and optimal use of specialized clinical time. Treatment protocols vary from one centre to another and with the specific pathology. Surgery and radiotherapy are the mainstays of treatment, although other forms of therapy, such as chemotherapy and immunotherapy, are also used.

Most large carcinomas of the larynx (T3 or T4), whether they are glottic, supraglottic or transglottic, are treated with surgery or combined surgery and radiotherapy. This surgery is usually a total laryngectomy, but may be extended to include a partial or complete pharyngectomy and, if indicated, a neck dissection. Some centres advocate various extensions of partial laryngectomy, but these procedures are reserved for highly selected cases. Histological analysis of the specimen is important, as it may indicate the need for post-operative radiotherapy. Such a situation may arise in cases where there are positive margins, cartilage invasion, perineural or vascular invasion, extranodal spread and multiple metastatic lymph nodes. The cure rates for larger tumours are lower than those for smaller tumours.

There is more controversy about the management of the smaller carcinomas (T1 and T2) of the larynx. Some advocate radiotherapy, as this modality of therapy has a similar control rate to surgery for the disease, but it preserves the voice better. T1 glottic lesions treated by radiotherapy or surgery both have 5-year cure rates of 80–95%. For supraglottic T1 and T2 lesions the cure rate is about 70% for both surgery and radiotherapy, but in these cases the neck may need to be irradiated as well, as there is a higher incidence of spread of disease to the regional lymph nodes. Others treat these smaller tumours by microlaryngoscopy and excision either directly or with the use of the CO_2 laser. Surgery may involve a cordectomy, a partial or hemi-laryngectomy, a supraglottic laryngectomy or even a near-total laryngectomy depending on the size of the lesion and the availability of other modalities of therapy. Some procedures require reconstruction to help to prevent aspiration as well as adjunctive procedures to help to improve voicing. The incidence of aspiration from supraglottic laryngectomies is 4%, and the cause is considered to be failure of elevation of the larynx at the time of swallowing. Patients in whom radiotherapy has not controlled the primary or nodal disease need salvage surgery if there are no contraindications to treatment.

In situations where the histology has revealed carcinoma *in situ* or dysplasia only, then local excision with or without the use of the CO_2 laser is usually carried out, although some centres irradiate these patients. Close follow-up is essential in patients with carcinoma *in situ* or severe dysplasia, as nearly half of these patients will progress to invasive carcinoma within 2 years.

Management of patients with malignant disease in the larynx also involves elimination of any predisposing factors such as smoking and alcohol, and regular clinical evaluation to detect any recurrence.

BENIGN DISEASE

The important benign conditions in the larynx include papilloma, adenoma, chondroma and various miscellaneous tumours such as lipoma, haemangioma and neurofibroma. These are usually removed completely at the time of biopsy, although some, like the papilloma, may recur and require several surgical excisions.

Squamous papillomas are caused by viral invasion of the mucosa with human papilloma virus types 6 and 11, so the elimination of the disease depends on the immune response of the patient. Surgery is performed to debulk the papillomas if the airway is compromised, and to reduce the irregularity on the margin of the vocal fold if voicing is a problem. At microlaryngoscopy, the CO_2 laser or the microdebrider can be used effectively to treat the disease without significant damage to adjacent normal structures. Tracheostomy has been required in some patients to secure a safe airway. The recurrent nature of this condition can result in extended and often quite difficult management.

NON-NEOPLASTIC CONDITIONS

There are many non-neoplastic conditions which involve the larynx, including vocal fold polyp, retention cyst, contact ulcer, vocal fold nodules, chronic laryngitis, vocal fold paralysis, specific infections (TB and syphilis), functional dysphonia, muscle tension dysphonia and post-radiotherapy effects.

The treatment for each of these conditions is variable, but a good working relationship between the speech and language therapist and the otolaryngologist is essential for optimal management. In most conditions treatment is usually symptomatic once the diagnosis has been made, but may consist of voice rest, modified voice protection, inhalations, inhaled bronchodilators, antibiotics, anti-allergy medication (antihistamines), steroids and other therapy depending on the aetiology.

In a child with solitary paired vocal fold lesions, the commonest diagnosis would be vocal fold nodules. The treatment consists of voice therapy that is aimed at modifying the abnormal vocal habits and thus allowing the nodules to resolve. Involvement of the family and the schoolteacher is important, so that at all times voicing is being monitored and control reinforced. Excision of the nodules is not indicated unless the underlying voice use has been modified successfully. If the nodules are considered to be fibrous and have not resolved with extended conservative measures, then microlaryngoscopy and careful excision with the CO_2 laser can be carried out.

Treatment for vocal fold paralysis depends on the symptoms that each patient experiences and how much they affect the patient in his or her work, socially and with recreational activities. There may be associated symptoms which identify the cause as being at a central site (either bulbar or supranuclear), and if this is confirmed by the appropriate investigations, treatment would be directed here.

If the vocal fold paralysis is bilateral and the patient has significant stridor, then securing the airway is of prime importance. This may require intubation or tracheostomy to relieve the airway obstruction. Other procedures may be needed to improve the airway on a long-term basis. These include lateralization of the vocal fold, arytenoidectomy (endoscopically or externally via a laryngofissure) and various other laryngeal procedures.

If the vocal folds are paralysed in a lateral position, aspiration can become a problem. Management for this is more complex, often involving more extensive surgical procedures and other adjunctive measures. This may also involve tracheostomy to protect the lower airway and reduce the incidence of aspiration pneumonia. Other procedures may include medialization as well as cricopharyngeal myotomy, partial laryngectomy or even total laryngectomy.

For unilateral vocal fold paralysis the commonest cause is dysfunction to the peripheral nerve supply, either the vagus nerve or the recurrent laryngeal nerve (Figure 7.4).

Most patients wish to improve their voice, so involvement of the speech and language therapist is important. Voice therapy is usually carried out in all patients. It is

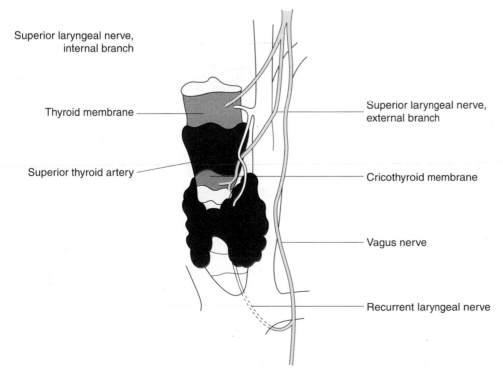

Superior laryngeal nerve, internal branch

Thyroid membrane

Superior thyroid artery

Superior laryngeal nerve, external branch

Cricothyroid membrane

Vagus nerve

Recurrent laryngeal nerve

Figure 7.4 Neurovascular supply to the larynx.

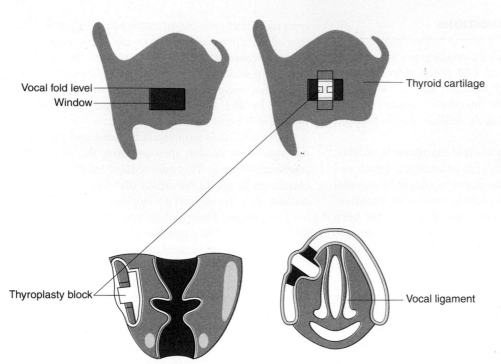

Vocal fold level

Window

Thyroid cartilage

Thyroplasty block

Vocal ligament

Figure 7.5 Thyroplasty – type I.

given early and is useful even if the paralysis is not permanent. It is aimed at achieving compensation from the uninvolved functioning vocal fold, which is then able to approximate to the paralysed side, giving clearer and stronger voicing.

The observed paralysis may not be permanent, so in cases where no obvious cause has been found, a 12-month observation period usually precedes surgical intervention. If the cause is known, perhaps carcinoma of the lung or following division of the recurrent laryngeal nerve during a thyroidectomy, then surgery is not delayed. The type of procedure varies significantly, ranging from vocal fold augmentation to thyroplasty and other complicated laryngeal framework surgery.

Vocal fold augmentation involves injecting a material into the paralysed vocal fold to create more bulk, thus allowing the non-paralysed side to make better contact with the paralysed side. The materials used include autologous fat, gelfoam, collagen, silicone, teflon, goretex and even cartilage. Autologous fat has excellent biocompatability but is only temporary, with resorption of about 50% within 12 months. Teflon is permanent, but it may migrate to a different area within the larynx or cause a granuloma formation. In some centres, fat augmentation is performed early to give immediate

voice improvement and help to reduce the likelihood of developing abnormal compensatory movements within the larynx.

Thyroplasty may be carried out under local or general anaesthetic so that the medialization of the paralysed vocal fold can be adjusted to give optimal voicing. In this procedure a small silicone or ceramic block is placed in a window carefully cut out of the lamina of the thyroid cartilage (Figure 7.5). It may be coupled with other surgical manoeuvres to adduct the arytenoid cartilage. Gortex has also been used as an implant material.

FURTHER READING

Cummings CW. (ed.) 1993: *Otolaryngology – head and neck surgery*. St Louis, MO: Mosby Publishing.

Fried MP. 1995: *The larynx – a multidisciplinary approach*. St Louis, MO: Mosby Publishing.

Sataloff RT. 1997: *Professional voice – the science and art of clinical care*. San Diego, CA: Singular Publishing.

Smee R, Bridger GP. 1994: *Laryngeal cancer*. Amsterdam: Elsevier Science.

Swelling

Robin G. Woolfson

Introduction

Symptoms of fluid retention may be local or generalized.

Local swelling may affect a single upper or lower limb, head and neck, or abdomen, with regional symptoms dependent on the site. Swelling is worse if the affected area is dependent and is improved by elevation.

Generalized fluid retention characteristically causes transient facial swelling on rising from bed in the morning, and the subsequent appearance of increasing pedal oedema during the course of the day. Additional symptoms which patients may not recognize as being due to fluid retention include tight rings on fingers, swollen fingers, a preference for wearing loose shoes, and indentations on the ankles caused by sock elastic.

THE DEMONSTRATION OF OEDEMA

Oedema is best demonstrated by the exertion of firm digital pressure on the affected area for up to 60 s, which will leave an indentation or pit. When oedema is generalized, extravascular fluid localizes to all dependent areas, with the distribution depending on the patient's posture. Typically, the face is swollen in the morning, the feet swell when sitting or ambulant, and the sacrum becomes oedematous in the bedbound. In contrast, when oedema is localized to the head or a limb, this gravitational distribution is not present.

The overlying skin appears tight and shiny if the oedema is of acute onset, whereas it is more brawny and indurated when oedema is chronic. In either case, skin lacerations result in the leakage of tissue fluid. The early identification and treatment of oedema is important, particularly in the hospitalized patient, since it predisposes to immobility, the development of bedsores, local infection and poor wound healing.

PATHOLOGY

Oedema is due to increased formation of extravascular fluid. Collection of this fluid depends on the balance between capillary extravasation of fluid and its removal by lymphatic drainage. The amount of capillary extravasation is determined by the balance between the relevant Starling forces. On one side, capillary hydrostatic pressure and tissue oncotic (colloid osmotic) pressure favour extravasation, whereas on the other, tissue hydrostatic pressure and intravascular oncotic pressure resist the formation of extravascular fluid (see Figure 8.1.1). Physiologically, there is net capillary extravasation, but homeostasis is maintained and the formation of oedema prevented by lymphatic drainage. Oedema will occur either if the volume of extravasation increases to exceed the capacity of lymphatic drainage, or if the normal lymphatic drainage is reduced (lymphoedema).

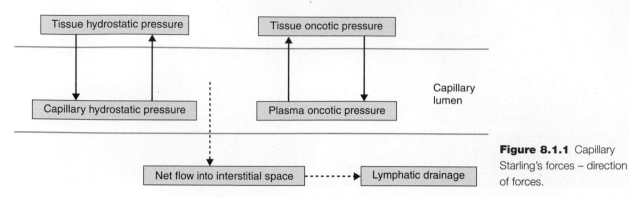

Figure 8.1.1 Capillary Starling's forces – direction of forces.

OEDEMA: IS IT LOCAL OR GENERALIZED?

Local oedema forms when local venous or lymphatic drainage is impaired. Hence this may affect an arm if axillary or subclavian vein or regional lymphatic drainage is obstructed, the head and neck if there is superior vena cava obstruction, both legs if there is inferior vena cava obstruction, and one leg if there is iliac or femoral vein or regional lymphatic obstruction. Local oedema can also result from increased capillary permeability (e.g. as a result of local infection or allergy).

The presence of generalized oedema reflects a systemic defect such as cardiac failure, hepatic failure, renal failure, nephrotic syndrome or a generalized capillary leak. The laxity of skin around the ankles, legs, sacrum and face results in low tissue hydrostatic pressure, and favours these sites as destinations for extravasated fluid. In contrast, the soles of the feet and palms of the hand, with their tightly adherent fascia, are unlikely sites. The localization of fluid is gravitational and depends on the patient's posture and mobility. In mild oedema, clinical findings need not be symmetrical, and unilateral ankle oedema is a common finding in mild congestive cardiac failure.

Conditions responsible for formation of localized oedema

Veins Oedema forms in response to impaired local venous drainage as a result of thrombophlebitis, venous incompetence due to varicose veins, or external venous compression by lymph nodes, tumours or pregnancy.

Lymphatics Local oedema can result from impaired lymphatic drainage (which may be congenital or acquired, post-infectious, malignant infiltration, post-surgical or post-radiotherapy).

Increased capillary permeability Local capillary permeability may be increased by local infection or allergy.

Conditions responsible for formation of generalized oedema

Generalized oedema is the consequence of raised capillary hydrostatic pressure, reduced intravascular colloid osmotic pressure, abnormal capillary permeability or, commonly, a combination of these factors (Figure 8.1.2).

CAUSES OF VOLUME OVERLOAD

The excessive retention of salt and water by the kidneys occurs in response to hyperaldosteronism, acute or chronic renal failure or increased secretion of anti-diuretic hormone (ADH). This circulating volume overload raises capillary hydrostatic pressure and promotes extravasation. (In contrast, arterial hypertension does not promote oedema formation, since arterial pressure is not transmitted past the pre-capillary arterioles into the capillary circulation.)

CARDIAC FAILURE

Peripheral oedema formation may complicate either solitary right heart failure or congestive (i.e. biventricular) cardiac failure, but is not a complication of isolated left ventricular failure. Common causes of solitary right heart failure include chronic lung disease, pulmonary hypertension, acute and chronic pulmonary embolism, tricuspid and pulmonary valve disease and inferior myocardial infarction. Biventricular heart failure may be due to coronary artery disease, cardiomyopathy (e.g. caused by alcohol, thyroid disease, drugs, pyridoxine deficiency), severe valvular disease, pericardial effusion (tuberculosis, malignancy, connective tissue disease) and severe anaemia.

In either clinical situation, oedema forms as a result of increased capillary hydrostatic pressure, reduced cardiac output (which leads to activation of the renin–angiotensin–aldosterone and sympathetic nervous systems, with increased ADH production resulting in retention of both salt and water) and finally hepatic congestion leading to impaired protein synthesis.

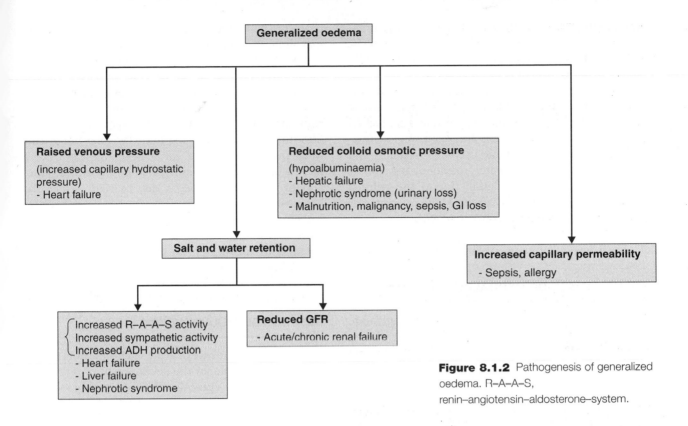

Figure 8.1.2 Pathogenesis of generalized oedema. R–A–A–S, renin–angiotensin–aldosterone–system.

ACUTE/CHRONIC RENAL FAILURE

In patients with both acute and chronic renal failure, the formation of oedema is due to circulating volume overload which reflects the impaired capacity of the kidneys to excrete sodium due to the reduced glomerular filtration rate.

ADDITIONAL CAUSES OF VOLUME OVERLOAD

Increased levels of aldosterone increase the circulating volume and may lead to oedema formation. This may be primary (Conn's syndrome) or secondary to cardiac failure, liver failure, nephrotic syndrome and recent cessation of diuretic therapy. Hypothyroidism and non-steroidal anti-inflammatory drugs impair the kidney's ability to excrete salt and water.

CAUSES OF REDUCED PLASMA COLLOID OSMOTIC PRESSURE

Reduced plasma colloid osmotic pressure, secondary to either inadequate protein and albumin synthesis or increased loss, can lead to oedema formation.

LIVER DISEASE

There is considerable overlap in the causes of both acute and chronic hepatic disease, including viral infection, drugs, alcohol, autoimmune disease and pregnancy. In general, the loss of hepatic synthetic function reflects the severity of the underlying lesion.

In acute and chronic liver disease, hepatic synthesis of albumin and protein is impaired and the reduced colloid osmotic pressure leads to oedema formation. Reduction of the circulating volume activates the renin–angiotensin–aldosterone and sympathetic nervous systems, with increased ADH production which results in renal salt and water conservation. Other humoral factors (e.g. endothelin and leukotrienes) accumulate in liver failure and affect the ability of the kidneys to excrete salt and water. Ascites is formed in response to volume overload, hypoalbuminaemia and altered splanchnic haemodynamics (with raised intrahepatic pressure and portal hypertension).

NEPHROTIC SYNDROME

Nephrotic syndrome is defined as proteinuria which exceeds 3 g per day, hypoalbuminaemia (< 30 g/ dL) and oedema. There is always an underlying glomerulonephritis, which may be primary (e.g. minimal change, membranous) or secondary to a systemic disease, such as systemic lupus erythematosus (SLE), diabetes mellitus, myeloma or amyloidosis.

The dramatic urinary loss of protein exceeds the capacity of even the normal liver to compensate, and results in reduced plasma oncotic pressure. A reduction in circulating volume activates the renin–angiotensin–aldosterone and sympathetic nervous systems and results in renal salt and water retention, but this is rapidly lost from the circulation due to the reduced plasma oncotic pressure. Occasionally, the intravascular volume has been found to be increased when the combination of low oncotic pressure and increased capillary hydrostatic pressure favours oedema formation.

OTHER CAUSES OF HYPOALBUMINAEMIA

Hypoalbuminaemia can result from malnutrition, chronic diarrhoeal states (including inflammatory bowel disease) and catabolic states (including sepsis, chronic inflammation and malignancy).

CAUSES OF GENERALIZED CAPILLARY LEAK SYNDROME

The development of oedema may reflect a generalized increase in capillary permeability, and this is seen in patients with systemic sepsis, multi-organ failure and anaphylaxis.

CLINICAL EXAMINATION

The distribution and extent of the oedema should be determined. If oedema is generalized, the extent of the oedema should be assessed by finding how far it extends proximally. If the patient is bedbound, then the sacrum should be inspected for oedema. In patients with localized oedema, evidence of regional lymphadenopathy, local infection (such as cellulitis) and venous obstruction should be sought. The condition of the overlying skin with regard to shininess, induration and integrity should be noted.

A full examination of the patient must be made to look for pyrexia, pallor, jaundice, pigmentation, spider naevi, palmar erythema, asterixis, anaemia, cyanosis, lymphadenopathy and organomegaly.

CARDIAC EXAMINATION

Evidence of increased circulating volume or heart failure should be sought. The pulse must be examined for rate, character and rhythm. The presence of hypertension may indicate volume overload, whereas hypotension may be due to circulating hypovolaemia or heart failure. Elevation of the jugular venous pulse provides evidence of raised right atrial pressure and right heart dysfunction, with prominent V-waves indicating tricuspid regurgitation. Displacement of the apex beat from the fifth intercostal space in the mid-clavicular line occurs when the left ventricular cavity is enlarged, but not if there is just left ventricular hypertrophy. The presence of a right ventricular heave is due to right ventricular hypertrophy, and usually suggests chronic pulmonary pathology. Auscultation of the heart may reveal murmurs indicative of valvular stenosis or regurgitation with the presence of a third heart sound (either left or right) suggesting elevation of the respective atrial pressure and ipsilateral ventricular dysfunction.

RESPIRATORY EXAMINATION

This may reveal evidence of acute or chronic lung disease which is responsible for the development of right heart failure. Clubbing, cyanosis, plethora, tachypnoea, reduced chest movements and evidence of pleural effusions, pleural thickening or pulmonary fibrosis should be sought.

ABDOMINAL EXAMINATION

Examination of the abdomen may reveal intra-abdominal fluid (ascites), hepatomegaly with a tender pulsatile liver in cases of tricuspid regurgitation, splenomegaly and masses. The presence of shifting dullness is a sign of ascites. Portal hypertension is suggested by splenomegaly, peri-umbilical veins with blood flow away from the umbilicus and haemorrhoids. Prominent veins on the anterior abdominal wall draining upwards may be due to occlusion of the inferior vena cava. In patients with renal insufficiency, lower tract obstruction may lead to chronic retention with a palpable bladder and enlarged prostate on rectal examination.

GENERAL INVESTIGATIONS

Full blood count will identify anaemia, with a high haemoglobin level reflecting either haemoconcentration or polycythaemia. A raised neutrophil count may provide evidence of a response to infection, and a blood film can usually exclude both acute and chronic leukaemias. In cases of infection, blood, urine and wound swabs should be sent for microbial culture and antibiotic sensitivity.

INVESTIGATIONS OF LIVER FUNCTION

Hepatic synthetic function is assessed by the measurement of plasma albumin and prothrombin time. Raised transaminases provide evidence of hepatitis, and an elevated alkaline phosphatase may be due to intra- or extra-hepatic cholestasis. Hepatitis serology (hepatitis A virus (HAV), hepatitis B virus (HBV), hepatitis C virus (HCV), Epstein-Barr virus (EBV) and cytomegalovirus (CMV)) and autoimmune screen (antinuclear antibodies (ANA), anti-DNA antibodies) should be sent. The liver, biliary tree and spleen should be examined by ultrasound, which can also be used to confirm the presence of ascites.

CARDIAC INVESTIGATIONS

An electrocardiogram will define the cardiac rhythm and can show evidence of new or old myocardial infarcts. Cardiomegaly and pericardial effusions may be identified on chest X-ray, as may lung disease, pleural effusions and mediastinal lymphadenopathy. In patients with clinical evidence of impaired cardiac function, an echocardiogram provides useful information about cardiac function, and also excludes valvular disease and pericardial effusion.

RENAL INVESTIGATIONS

A routine biochemical screen for urea, electrolytes and creatinine should be sent. Dipstick examination of the urine will identify the presence of protein, although false-negative results occur in patients with substantial Bence Jones proteinuria. Proteinuria should be measured more definitively either by sending a 24-h urine specimen for analysis of protein and creatinine content, or more simply by sending a spot morning urine sample for measurement of the protein/creatinine ratio. Urinary sodium is low in patients with hyperaldosteronism who are retaining salt and water, and also in patients with renal hypoperfusion, although this is not the case if diuretics have recently been administered. Ultrasound of the renal tract will determine kidney size (which is reduced in chronic renal failure) and echogenicity (which is increased in gross proteinuria) and exclude obstruction.

INVESTIGATIONS OF CAUSES OF LOCAL OEDEMA

Investigations of the cause for local venous and/or lymphatic obstruction depend on the site. Doppler ultrasound has largely replaced venography in the demonstration of peripheral venous thrombosis or occlusion. Abdominal lymphadenopathy can be demonstrated by ultrasound or CT scan depending on the patient's habitus. Within the mediastinum, lymphadenopathy can usually be seen on chest X-ray or CT scan. Occasionally, lymphangiography may be required to demonstrate congenital or acquired deficiencies of lymphatic drainage.

GENERAL MANAGEMENT

In patients with localized oedema, where possible the affected site should be elevated to encourage local drainage. Treatment of the cause depends on the diagnosis, but may involve anticoagulation for thrombosis and radiotherapy, chemotherapy or surgery for tumours and lymphadenopathy.

Based on the clinical and laboratory findings as detailed above, the cause for oedema should be identified. In the surgical patient, oedema is usually secondary to multiple pathologies, including malnutrition, sepsis and impaired cardiac and renal function. In such patients the clinical assessment of volume status (see above) is particularly important.

In all patients, a detailed fluid-balance chart itemizing hourly input and output should be kept together with daily measurement of weight, preferably performed at the same time each day. The amounts of intravenous fluid prescribed and their composition should be reviewed. The drug chart must be checked and drugs which reduce renal function (such as non-steriodal anti-inflammatory drugs and ACE inhibitors) identified and, if appropriate, stopped.

In patients with oedema, bedrest and compression stockings will help to mobilize extravascular fluid and improve cardiac output in patients with heart failure. The daily intake of water (including intravenous fluids) should be restricted to 1–1.5 L/day. The dietary intake of protein, carbohydrate and salt should be reviewed by the dietitian.

In patients with generalized oedema, a negative fluid balance resulting in a weight loss of 0.5–1.0 kg per day is the aim. Diuretics are often necessary to ensure this negative fluid balance. Thiazides may be given, although there is a risk of hyponatraemia, particularly in the elderly. Aldosterone antagonists take up to 48 h to work, and may cause unacceptable hyperkalaemia in patients with renal failure. Loop diuretics are generally effective, or a combination of loop and thiazide diuretics (e.g. metolazone) can be used in resistant cases. If the patient is grossly oedematous, then enteral absorption may be reduced and intravenous therapy is necessary. In bed-bound and severely hypoalbuminaemic patients, the prescription of regular subcutaneous heparin or low-molecular-weight heparin should be considered, particularly in those with cardiac failure and nephrotic syndrome.

SPECIFIC MANAGEMENT OF OEDEMA IN NEPHROTIC SYNDROME

Some patients (particularly children) with nephrotic syndrome are very hypovolaemic, and diuretic therapy should be introduced with great care in order not to precipitate acute renal failure. For this reason, aldosterone antagonists are commonly used. In profoundly nephrotic patients, dopamine may help to overcome renal salt and water retention, and in others the infusion of concentrated 20% albumin solution with loop diuretics may be required to initiate a diuresis.

SPECIFIC MANAGEMENT OF OEDEMA IN HEART FAILURE

In the oedematous heart failure patient, therapy should be directed towards improving cardiac function by the reduction of pre-load and after-load using a combination of diuretics, oral or intravenous nitrates, ACE inhibitors and possibly digoxin. In patients with severe myocardial dysfunction, intravenous dopamine or dobutamine may be required to improve cardiac output and thus increase renal perfusion and thereby promote a diuresis.

SPECIFIC MANAGEMENT OF OEDEMA IN LIVER FAILURE

Many patients with liver failure are significantly hypovolaemic, and diuretic therapy should be introduced carefully in order not to precipitate acute renal failure. For this reason, aldosterone antagonists are commonly used. In patients with severe hepatic failure and hepatorenal syndrome, loop diuretics are required and dopamine is frequently used, as are infusions of concentrated albumin and the re-infusion of ascitic fluid.

SPECIFIC MANAGEMENT IN ACUTE/CHRONIC RENAL FAILURE

In severe renal failure, the kidney responds poorly to diuretics even at high doses, and the combination of a loop diuretic with a thiazide diuretic, such as metolazone, may be required. In general, potassium-sparing diuretics (e.g. spironolactone, amiloride and triamterene) should be avoided.

Chapter 8.2

Swollen limbs

Tom W.G. Carrell and Kevin G. Burnand

Introduction

Limb swelling is a condition that commonly presents in the surgical out-patient clinic. It is usually caused by oedema, i.e. the accumulation of excessive interstitial fluid, but other causes such as gigantism, arteriovenous fistulae and excessive deposition of fat must be considered. The swelling may itself cause significant disability, or it may indicate other serious pathology.

It is essential to understand the basic mechanisms that cause oedema in order to make an accurate diagnosis of the underlying disease. Unilateral oedema suggests a venous or lymphatic cause, while patients who present with bilateral oedema must have a cardiac, renal or hypoproteinaemic cause of the swelling excluded (see Chapter 8.1).

PHYSIOLOGY

There is normally a balance between the inflow and outflow of extracellular fluid. Starling first drew attention to this equilibrium in his hypothesis of capillary fluid exchange. The capillary and interstitial hydrostatic pressures are opposed by an oncotic gradient that is determined by the different protein concentrations of the interstitial and intravascular fluid compartments. About 90% of the fluid that leaks from the capillaries is estimated to return into the post-capillary venules, while the remaining 10% enters the lymphatic system. Between 2 and 4 L of extracellular fluid and proteins are collected by lymphatic vessels (also known as lymphangioles) and channelled by lymphatic ducts into the venous system.

Oedema can be caused by changes in the capillary and venular hydrostatic pressure, capillary permeability, reduced protein concentrations or defective lymphatic function. The most common cause of limb swelling is inadequate venous drainage, which results in increased venular and capillary transmural pressure, consequently

decreasing the reabsorption of exuded extracellular fluid.

Veins have thin walls containing much less elastic tissue and muscle than their corresponding arteries, which provides a high capacitance, enabling them to distend easily with large volumes of blood (Figure 8.2.1). Two-thirds or more of the circulating volume is in the venous system at any time. Its relative distribution, determined by factors such as posture and venous tone, is controlled by both local and systemic reflexes through the sympathetic nervous system. The direction of blood flow in the venous system is controlled by valves, which are numerous in the veins of the lower limb, although they are scarce in the great veins.

In the supine position, the veins in the lower limb are collapsed and most of the blood volume is in the great veins of the abdomen and thorax. Change to an upright posture causes a large shift in distribution to the veins of the lower limb. The resting venous pressure is normally reduced by the calf muscle pump (Figure 8.2.2), but valvular incompetence renders its mechanism ineffective, causing a rise in hydrostatic pressure and resulting oedema. Oedema is much more common in the lower limbs than the upper limbs because of the higher hydrostatic pressure from the effects of gravity, the higher incidence of lower limb deep vein thrombosis, and the relatively good collateral venous drainage of the upper limb.

The volume of the calf is normally in the range 1500–2000 mL, and about 60–70 mL of this is venous blood. At rest in the upright position, the hydrostatic pressure in the veins of the leg is approximately 100 mmHg, but it can rise to 200–300 mmHg with a strong calf contraction. This increase in pressure can force up to 40 mL of blood out of the calf in a sustained contraction.

ANATOMY

Blood from the lower limbs is drained by the valveless common iliac veins and inferior vena cava to the right atrium, while the upper limbs are drained by the subclavian and brachiocephalic veins into the superior vena cava. Lymph from the lower limbs is collected in the cisterna chyli, which is in turn drained into the left internal jugular vein by the thoracic duct (Figure 8.2.3), which runs superiorly on the left side of the mediastinum. Oedema can be caused by obstruction to the venous or lymphatic drainage within the limb, or by a more proximal obstruction along the course of the intra-abdominal or intrathoracic drainage. The extent and distribution of oedema and the appearance of collateral veins often give an indication of the level and site of venous or lymphatic obstruction.

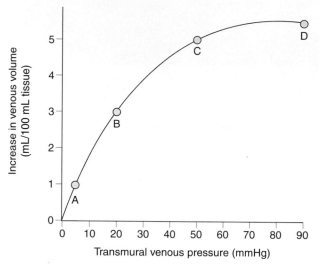

Figure 8.2.1 Venous capacitance. The pressure–volume curve of the veins in the lower limb: between points A and B an increase in volume of 0.5 mL/100 mL of tissue causes an increase in pressure of 4 mmHg; between points C and D, the same volume increases the pressure by 50 mmHg. (Reproduced with permission from Browse NL *et al.* 1988: *Diseases of the veins*. London: Edward Arnold).

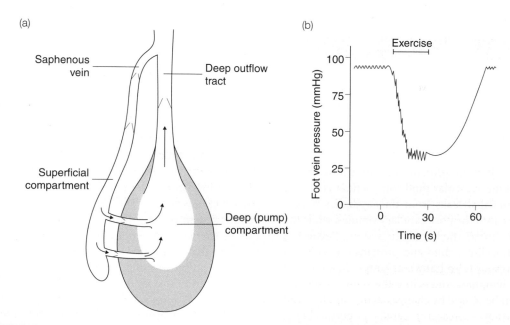

Figure 8.2.2 Calf pump mechanism. (a) Normal function of the calf pump relies on a patent deep venous system and competent venous valves. (b) The changes in foot vein pressure during a heel-raising exercise. In a normal limb, the pressure drops by 60–80% and takes 15–25 s to return to resting levels after exercise. (Reproduced with permission from Browse NL *et al.* 1988: *Diseases of the veins*. London: Edward Arnold.)

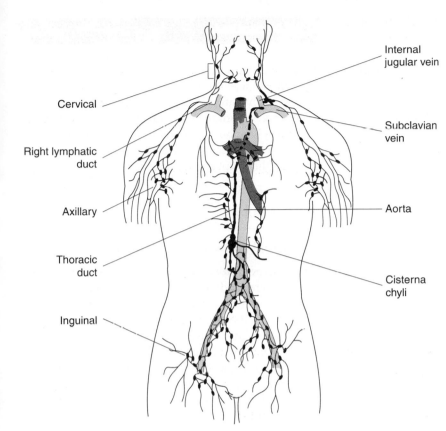

Cervical

Right lymphatic
duct

Axillary

Thoracic
duct

Inguinal

Internal
jugular vein

Subclavian
vein

Aorta

Cisterna
chyli

Figure 8.2.3 Anatomy of the lymphatic
system. Lymph from the lower limbs
collects in the cisterna chyli and is
drained by the thoracic duct into the left
internal jugular vein. The right upper limb
is drained by a separate lymphatic duct
into the right subclavian vein.

VENOUS CAUSES

ACUTE VENOUS INSUFFICIENCY

This is usually the result of an acute thrombosis occluding the deep veins draining the limb. The clinical picture depends on the site of the occlusion, the rapidity of onset and the degree of collateral venous drainage. The limb typically becomes oedematous and dilated superficial veins develop. Occasionally, massive acute thrombosis can cause sufficient venous congestion to obstruct arteriolar inflow and produce venous gangrene.

Even if the venous occlusion is relieved (e.g. by thrombolysis), fasciotomies may be necessary to avoid subsequent nerve damage and ischaemic contractures. Traumatic disruption and iatrogenic ligation are other rare causes of acute venous insufficiency.

CHRONIC VENOUS INSUFFICIENCY

Chronic venous insufficiency is the most common cause of unilateral leg oedema. Post-thrombotic damage, venous wall weakness and congenital valvular dysplasia can lead to valvular incompetence in the deep, superficial and communicating veins of the lower limb and cause oedema. Luminal occlusion of the deep veins may

be caused by fibrosis following the organization of deep vein thrombosis or congenital aplasia. Extrinsic obstruction may be caused by compression of the iliac veins by pelvic tumours, or by left iliac vein compression by the iliac artery (May-Cockett syndrome).

There is usually a long history of leg swelling, lipodermatosclerosis and even ulceration in patients with chronic venous insufficiency. There may be a history of proven or suspected deep venous thrombosis suggested by previous fractures, major injuries or past surgery. The patient may report the presence of varicose veins, or have had them operated on.

Symptoms include varicose veins, distended venules in the skin around the ankle (ankle flares), pigmentation, induration and inflammation of the skin in the classic 'gaiter' distribution (lipodermatosclerosis), eczema and ulceration. Iliac vein compression and caval occlusion may cause few signs of venous occlusion in the lower limb other than oedema, although examination of the anterior abdominal wall usually confirms dilated collateral veins. Venous oedema of the upper limb often follows axillary vein thrombosis, and sudden onset of painful swelling of the arm should be investigated by venography.

Investigation of chronic venous insufficiency

Duplex ultrasonography demonstrates reflux in the saphenous, perforating and deep veins. Ascending venography demonstrates occlusion, irregularity, filling defects, synaechiae, obstruction and collateral pathways when there has been previous thrombosis (Figure 8.2.4).

Foot volumetry and air plethysmography are techniques used for measuring the function of the calf pump.

Treatment of chronic venous insufficiency

A well-fitted and applied graduated compression stocking reduces the transmural venous pressure and is usually sufficient to reduce the oedema of chronic venous insufficiency. The stocking should be applied in the morning before any oedema has accumulated. An alternative is the regular application of compression hosiery or bandaging by a district nurse if the patient is unable to apply compression stockings because of some other disability. Surgery on the saphenous and perforating veins may reduce oedema if the deep veins are normal.

Venous collateral formation improves the oedema that follows occlusion of a major axial vein, but occasionally surgery is valuable to bypass an identified site of venous obstruction. Surgical attempts to repair or replace the damaged valves have generally been disappointing, but research on these techniques continues. Axillary vein thrombosis should be treated by fibrinolysis followed by surgical decompression of the thoracic inlet or excision of a cervical rib.

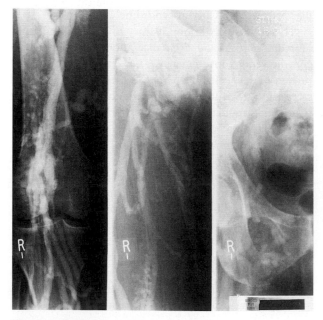

Figure 8.2.4 Post-thrombotic venous damage. The venogram demonstrates deep venous occlusions, irregularities, filling defects and collateral venous drainage following previous deep vein thrombosis.

LYMPHOEDEMA

Lymphoedema is the excessive accumulation of interstitial fluid in the extravascular compartment as a result of defective lymphatic function. The cause of primary lymphoedema is unknown, and it occurs only rarely. Secondary lymphoedema occurs more commonly, and is the result of a recognized pathological process which damages the lymphatic vessels.

PRIMARY LYMPHOEDEMA

Congenital primary lymphoedema

True congenital familial lymphoedema, or 'Milroy's disease', is a rare condition that accounts for less than 5% of all cases of primary lymphoedema and affects approximately 1 in 33 000 members of the population. The condition occurs more frequently in males than in females, and there is often a family history of swollen limbs. Limb swelling usually presents within 1 year of birth and other congenital abnormalities may coexist.

Lymphatic hyperplasia and *megalymphatics* are other rare causes of congenital primary lymphoedema. Lymphangiography shows numerous incompetent or dilated lymphatics (Figure 8.2.5).

Late-onset primary lymphoedema

In the majority of patients, primary lymphoedema is not apparent at birth and limb swelling only becomes obvious at puberty or in early adulthood. The patient may relate the limb swelling to a history of minor trauma, such as a sprained ankle or an insect bite. The resulting inflammation is thought to overwhelm a lymphatic system with little, if any, reserve function and cause oedema. Fluid retention around the time of the menarche is another common trigger factor in the presentation of late-onset primary lymphoedema. Late-onset primary lymphoedema is classified according to the lymphangiographic appearance (Figure 8.2.5).

Distal obliterative lymphoedema is the most common cause of primary lymphoedema, accounting for about 90% of cases. It usually affects women at the time of puberty. The lymphoedema is normally bilateral and rarely extends above the knee.

Proximal obliterative lymphoedema may present at any age and affects males twice as frequently as females. The lymphoedema usually starts in the thigh, but eventually it progresses to involve the whole limb, although the foot may be spared. Lymphangiography shows sparse or absent inguinal and pelvic lymphatic vessels. Occasionally, these patients are suitable for lymphatic bypass surgery.

Obliterative/hypoplastic disease

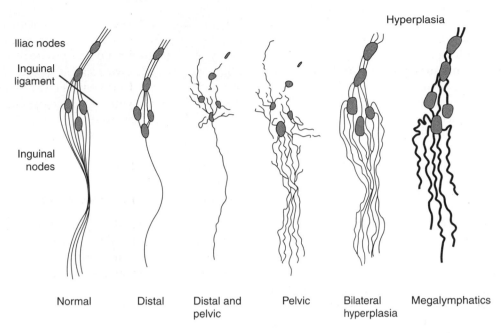

Hyperplasia

Iliac nodes

Inguinal ligament

Inguinal nodes

Normal   Distal   Distal and pelvic   Pelvic   Bilateral hyperplasia   Megalymphatics

Figure 8.2.5 Lymphangiographic appearances of primary lymphoedema. Lymphoedema may be classified according to the presence of normal, obliterated (or hypoplastic) or hyperplastic lymphatic vessels on lymphangiography. (Reproduced with permission from Burnand KG, Young AE (eds). 1997: *New Airds companion in surgical studies*. Edinburgh: Churchill Livingstone.)

SECONDARY LYMPHOEDEMA

Lymphoedema is defined as secondary if a probable pathological cause is identified. In Europe and North America, the majority of cases of secondary lymphoedema occur as a result of iatrogenic damage as part of the treatment of malignancy.

Malignancy, such as lymphomas, malignant melanomas and seminomas, can occasionally obstruct the lymphatic drainage of a limb and cause lymphoedema, but the latter is far more frequently seen after treatment of malignancy by surgical block dissection or radiotherapy.

Surgical excision and block dissection of lymph nodes often causes lymphoedema. The risk of lymphoedema following axillary node dissection is in the order of 5%, but may be over 50% after inguinal block dissection for lower limb cutaneous malignancies. These risks are greatly increased if adjuvant radiotherapy is used. Occasionally, iatrogenic disruption of the femoral lymphatics may occur during groin exploration for recurrent varicose veins, when the risk of subsequent lymphoedema is estimated to be 0.5%.

Radiotherapy, either on its own or in combination with surgery, can cause lymphoedema.

Filariasis, i.e. infection by filarial worms, is the most common cause of lymphoedema world-wide, and is seen in endemic areas of West Africa, India and South America. Filarial helminths such as *Wuchereria bancrofti*, *Brugia malayi* and *Brugia timori* are transmitted to humans by insect bites, migrate up lymphatic vessels and induce fibrosis in the local lymph nodes. This fibrosis causes lymphatic obstuction and consequent lymphoedema. The term 'elephantiasis' describes the gross deformity of severe lymphoedema that results.

Non-filarial elephantiasis has been reported in tribesmen in parts of East Africa and Ethiopia where the soil has a high silica content. It is thought that silica particles are absorbed through the bare feet and migrate to inguinal lymph nodes, and that consequent fibrosis leads to lymphoedema.

Trauma to a limb may cause secondary lymphoedema, particularly if extensive degloving has occurred.

Infection with recurrent cellulitis occasionally obliterates sufficient lymphatic vessels in a limb to cause lymphoedema. A minimal amount of further damage by cellulitis may trigger lymphoedema in a limb with preexisting lymphatic hypoplasia. In limbs with chronic lymphoedema, skin fissuring and coexistent fungal infections increase the susceptibility to cellulitis and further lymphatic destruction.

Severe chronic eczema and rheumatoid arthritis or psoriatic arthritis may cause lymphoedema, but the mechanism of the lymphatic damage is not fully understood.

Self-induced disuse of a limb can produce an oedema that is mistaken for lymphoedema. This may be a feature of psychological disturbance, such as Munchausen's syndrome, or it may be associated with prolonged inactivity after injury. A small number of patients produce oedema (lymphoedema artefacta) in response to the application of a tourniquet around a limb. Lymphoedema artefacta and disuse oedema can be distinguished by finding normal or increased lymphatic drainage on isotope lymphography.

CLINICAL FEATURES OF LYMPHOEDEMA

Patients with lymphoedema usually present with unilateral or bilateral lower limb swelling, although the arms can be affected. The history may suggest a cause in cases of secondary lymphoedema, or there may be a family history of limb swelling suggestive of primary lymphoedema. As the lymphoedema worsens and the bulk of the limb increases, the normal activities of the patient may be affected and the degree of disability is important in determining therapy.

In patients with lymphoedema, some cutaneous pitting can always be induced by firm finger pressure, and a failure to achieve this makes another diagnosis likely. The site and extent of the swelling should be noted. In distal obliterative primary lymphoedema, it is usually maximal on the dorsum of the foot and lower limb, but in proximal obliterative disease the greatest swelling is often in the thigh and buttock, and the foot may be spared. In chronic lymphoedema, warty excrescences and verrucous skin changes are often apparent. Patients with megalymphatics may develop vesicles and leak clear or milky fluid from lymphocutaneous fistulae.

INVESTIGATION OF LYMPHOEDEMA

Radioisotope lymphography determines the uptake of a technetium-labelled colloid in local and regional lymph nodes following subcutaneous injection. In lymphoedema, the uptake is markedly reduced (less than 0.3% of the injected dose), and it provides a useful diagnostic test (Figure 8.2.6).

In contrast lymphangiography, lipiodol is injected into a lymphatic vessel and radiographs provide more detailed imaging of the lymphatic vessels and nodes. The number and size of lymphatic vessels are demonstrated, and obstruction is indicated by failure of the lipiodol to advance. This is still a useful test when the isotope lymphography is equivocal, or if surgery is contemplated.

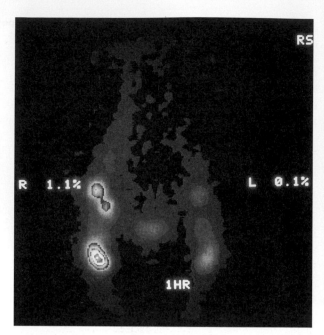

Figure 8.2.6 Radioisotope lymphogram showing decreased uptake of technetium in the left inguinal lymph nodes compared to the right, demonstrating left lymphatic dysfunction and confirming the clinical diagnosis of lymphoedema.

TREATMENT OF LYMPHOEDEMA

Physical methods

Physical methods to reduce lymphoedema provide the simplest form of treatment. Limb elevation is very effective, but impracticable for long periods in an otherwise independent patient, although the importance of elevation during the evening and at night should be stressed. Many patients benefit from regular massage to reduce limb swelling, but this is often poorly sustained unless accompanied by obsessive application of bandages. Pneumatic compression devices, either single or sequential chamber, produce a similar effect to massage in reducing oedema, and are particularly useful pre-operatively to reduce swelling, or they can be used on a regular basis at night for long-term oedema control. Correctly fitted and applied graduated compression stockings can maintain limb size and give good symptomatic relief if worn regularly. Lymphoedema of the arm can be treated by a compression gauntlet. Weight reduction is invariably beneficial in obese patients with lymphoedema.

Drug therapy

Diuretics are ineffective as they do not selectively remove fluid from the interstitial space.

Treatment of tinea pedis with terbinafine is essential to reduce the portal of entry for recurrent infection.

Appropriate antibiotics (e.g. penicillin) should be pre-scribed if cellulitis does develop to cover the likely organisms, particularly streptococci. The patient should be given a course of antibiotics to take at the first indication of an attack, when there are recurrent infections, and low-dose long-term prophylactic antibiotics may be necessary if the attacks are disabling.

Surgical treatment

Surgery is indicated in patients whose mobility is reduced by gross limb swelling.

Reduction operations

In *Homans' operation*, skin flaps are raised from the subcutaneous fat, the lymphoedematous subcutaneous tissue is excised down to the deep fascia, and the skin flaps are replaced and sutured. The operation is appropriate if the skin is in good condition.

In *Charles's operation*, all of the skin and subcutaneous tissue around the calf is excised down to the deep fascia, and split skin grafts from an unaffected donor site are applied to the denuded area. The operation produces a more radical reduction than Homans' operation, but the cosmetic result of the split skin grafts may be poor, and it is difficult to avoid a pantaloon effect.

Lymphatic bypass

Many operations have been developed over the years in an attempt to connect obstructed lymphatics to the venous system. Few of them have been successful and shown a long-term improvement in limb size. Two operations which remain in occasional use today are lymphovenous anastomosis and the mesenteric bridge bypass. Lymphovenous anastomosis of lymphatic vessels to the venous system, using an operating microscope, has been attempted in various forms to drain lymphoedematous limbs, but overall the results are disappointing. In the enteromesenteric bridge bypass, obstructed lower limb lymphatics are anastomosed to the submucosal lymphatic plexus of an isolated pedicled loop of ileum. The operation can only be attempted in a small number of patients with proximal obstruction (about 1–2% of all patients with lymphoedema), and it may only be effective in just over half of the patients in whom it is attempted.

COMPLICATIONS OF LYMPHOEDEMA

Malignancy

Lymphangiosarcoma is a rare complication of chronic lymphoedema, and is known as Stewart-Treves syndrome when it occurs following axillary node clearance and radiotherapy for breast carcinoma.

OTHER CAUSES OF LIMB SWELLING

CONGESTIVE CARDIAC FAILURE

This is the most common cause of bilateral lower limb oedema. It should be apparent from the history and clinical examination, which usually confirms a raised jugular venous pressure. A large heart, gallop rhythm, cardiac murmurs and bilateral fine crepitations are supportive of the diagnosis, and electrocardiography, chest radiography and echocardiography can be used to confirm the diagnosis.

HYPOPROTEINAEMIA

Serum albumin is responsible for most of the oncotic gradient between the interstitial and intravascular spaces. Hypoalbuminaemia causes a generalized oedema, but is more apparent in regions of increased hydrostatic pressure, especially gravity-dependent limbs. Ascites and pleural effusions can also occur. Common causes of hypoproteinaemia include chronic renal failure, malnutrition, malabsorption, burns and liver failure. The diagnosis should be suspected from the history and the generalized distribution of oedema. Serum urea, electrolytes, creatinine and albumin are diagnostic.

ARTERIOVENOUS MALFORMATIONS

Either single or multiple (Parkes-Weber syndrome) arteriovenous malformations are a cause of limb hypertrophy. The term 'Robertson's giant limb' is used to describe the condition. The limb is generally enlarged, and a 'machinery' murmur may be audible throughout diastole and systole. Tourniquet occlusion of the arterial inflow to the affected limb may cause a relative bradycardia (Branham/Nicoladoni sign), suggesting that the arteriovenous shunts are causing haemodynamic compromise and may lead to high-output cardiac failure. The diagnosis can be confirmed by flow studies or arteriography.

KLIPPEL-TRENAUNAY SYNDROME

This is the association of primitive axial veins with bony and soft-tissue abnormalities and increased limb length. Capillary naevi, abnormal or absent deep veins and lower limb oedema are frequently present. More than half of these patients have an associated abnormality of the lymphatics.

LIPODYSTROPHY (OR LIPOEDEMA)

This predominantly affects women, and is often associated with gross obesity. Abnormal deposition of subcutaneous fat is seen bilaterally in the lower limbs. Although it may have a similarity in distribution to lymphoedema, the swelling does not pit and there is no venous or lymphatic dysfunction. Gross obesity may occasionally lead to deposition of fat within lymph nodes, causing a true 'secondary' lymphoedema.

HEREDITARY ANGIO-OEDEMA

This presents as recurrent attacks of facial and peripheral oedema. It is caused by autosomal dominant deficiency of C1–esterase inhibitor. The oedema usually resolves spontaneously within 48 to 72 h, but there is significant mortality from asphyxia if it is left untreated.

IDIOPATHIC CYCLIC OEDEMA

This occurs in women of childbearing age, and typically causes mild bilateral lower limb oedema. The diagnosis should be obvious from the cyclical nature of the oedema (which is usually worse in the premenstrual week).

ERYTHROCYANOSIS FRIGIDA

This is a condition of young, often heavily built women who have cold and blotchy discoloured shins. It is the result of slow cutaneous circulation and is almost always symmetrical.

GIGANTISM

This usually affects the whole body, but it may affect one limb. It is caused by hypertrophy of the bone and soft tissues, and the buttocks or breast of the affected side may be larger.

CONCLUSIONS

The correct diagnosis of oedema is based on an understanding of the physiological mechanisms of interstitial fluid exchange. Most unilateral limb swelling is the result of venous or lymphatic dysfunction. Bilateral oedema is more often caused by congestive cardiac failure and hypoproteinaemia. Less often, limb hypertrophy presents as limb swelling, and a knowledge of the rarer causes of limb enlargement is required.

FURTHER READING

Browse NL, Burnand KG, Lea Thomas M. 1988: *Diseases of the veins.* London: Edward Arnold.

Kinmonth JB. 1982: *The lymphatics. Diseases, lymphography and surgery,* 2nd edn. London: Edward Arnold.

Reed RK, McHale NG, Bert JL, Winlove CP, Laine GA. 1995: *Interstitium, connective tissue and lymphatics.* London: Portland Press Proceedings.

The swollen abdomen: ascites

Gabriella I. Slapak

Introduction

The swollen abdomen, of which ascites is one cause, may be the first presentation of systemic illness to bring the patient to the clinic. Ascites is the collection of excess fluid in the peritoneal space. It is important to determine the cause, since the treatment and approach to the patient is usually determined by it.

CAUSES

In over 80% of cases, ascites is secondary to cirrhosis of the liver, and 80% of cirrhotics will have ascites during the course of their presentation (Table 8.3.1).

Table 8.3.1 Causes of ascites

Common causes	Others – 5%
Cirrhosis (80%)	Meigs' syndrom Familial Mediterranean fever
Malignancy (10%)	Acute alcoholic hepatitis Acute liver failure (Budd- Chiari syndrome)
Heart failure (3%)	Tuberculosis Nephrotic syndrome
Pancreatic disease (1%)	Chylous ascites Hepatoma
Dialysis (1%)	Biliary ascites Filariasis Ovarian hyperstimulation syndrome

CLINICAL HISTORY

A detailed clinical history must be taken in all cases. Frequently the patient will present with abdominal distension and discomfort. Ascites is often the first presentation of underlying disease, and may mask true weight loss. Ankle oedema is relatively rare and usually secondary to other causes, or is a late presenting feature. Dyspnoea will be present if the volume of ascites is sufficient to splint the diaphragm. In complicated ascites, such as is found in spontaneous bacterial peritonitis (SBP), there may have been deepening jaundice, gastrointestinal haemorrhage or hepatic encephalopathy as the only symptoms. Fever is frequently absent. Pain may be present with large volume ascites but it is only present in 15–20% of patients with SBP.

PHYSICAL EXAMINATION

Abdominal distension is clearly apparent, and this will be caused both by fluid and by dilated intestines. The patient is frequently thin and wasted. Although shifting dullness should be sought, this sign may not be present in large-volume tense ascites. There will be increased abdominal pressure, and congenital and incisional hernias are frequently present. Scrotal oedema is common, whilst ankle oedema is relatively rare. The abdominal wall veins may be visible, and if portal hypertension is present, caput medusea may be seen.

There may be associated poor lung expansion with elevation of the diaphragm in large-volume ascites, and pleural effusions are common and may be bilateral. The neck veins are usually distended as a result of raised right atrial pressure.

INVESTIGATIONS

The most important investigation is a *diagnostic aspirate* of the fluid. This should be obtained as soon as possible and tested for protein concentration, a cell count, Gram stain and microbial culture, including tuberculosis. Cytological examination should be performed in all cases. This can be safely achieved by aspirating 50–100 mL under aseptic conditions. Ascitic fluid should be inoculated into blood-culture bottles, which gives a much better diagnostic yield than leaving it in universal tubes overnight. It is best to use a standard complete blood count (CBC) tube (EDTA) to measure the white cell count (and red cells), as it can be assayed quickly on a 'Coulter counter'. Total protein with albumin concentration should also be requested. Glucose estimations are less useful. If the ascites is not obvious on clinical examination, aspiration can be safely performed with ultrasound guidance. A diagnostic ascitic tap should be done in all new presentations, as well as in patients with known ascites who are admitted to hospital. It is also indicated when there is clinical deterioration, particularly fever.

Probably the single most important test on ascites is the ascitic white cell count, since it provides information about possible infection which could be life-threatening. A count of $250/\text{mm}^3$ or more is assumed to be diagnostic of infection (0.25×10^9 in the Coulter counter). Ideally the neutrophil count is used, and here the count is greater than $200/\text{mm}^3$. Antibiotic therapy should be empirical (see section below on spontaneous bacterial peritonitis).

Specific culture for TB should be requested in all cases where there is uncertainty about the cause of ascites, and it should be mandatory in alcoholics, who have a higher than normal incidence compared to the normal population.

Total protein concentration has traditionally been used to differentiate between transudates and exudates. Ascites with a protein concentration of $> 2.5\,\text{g/dL}$ is termed an *exudate,* whereas a *transudate* has a protein concentration of $< 2.5\,\text{g/dL}$. This definition is not particularly helpful as a diagnostic tool, as in spontaneous bacterial peritonitis (SBP) it is usually low. In Budd-Chiari syndrome (hepatic venous outflow block), the ascitic protein concentration is frequently $> 2.5\,\text{g/dL}$. Although the serum-ascites albumin gradient (SAAG) can be used to determine the presence of portal hypertension (a value of $> 1.1\,\text{g/dL}$ suggests portal hypertension and a value of $< 1.1\,\text{g/dL}$ signifies normal portal pressures), modern ultrasonography techniques and portal wedge pressure measurement provide more useful and specific information.

Ultrasound examination of the abdomen, including Doppler examination of the vessels feeding the liver, is extremely helpful – especially in liver disease, where it is important to know whether or not there is occlusion or damped or reverse flow in the portal vein. The patency of the vena cava and the hepatic veins is thus also determined, and masses can be examined. It should be stressed that where the diagnosis is unclear from the history and examination, an ultrasound scan of the pelvis for ovarian tumours is mandatory.

An elevated serum alpha-fetoprotein (α-FP) can be useful in raising suspicion of hepatocellular carcinoma in unexpected decompensation of a cirrhotic patient (see Figure 8.3.1).

THE FORMATION OF ASCITES

The indisputable immediate cause of ascites is increased sodium and water retention. However, the precise cause of this is unclear. There are three main postulates advanced.

Underfill theory

Due to a number of known factors which include portal hypertension, peripheral vasodilatation and hypoalbuminaemia, the volume of plasma reaching the kidney (the circulating plasma volume) is low. The kidney reacts by retaining sodium and water, thus leading to ascites.

Overfill theory

The underlying cause is inappropriate sodium retention causing overfilling of the vascular system. Subsequently there is leakage into interstitial spaces and the peritoneum, resulting in oedema and ascites. As a result, reduced renal plasma volume leads to yet more sodium and water retention.

Cirrhosis

The cause here is the cirrhotic liver itself, which directly or indirectly produces vasodilatory substances. These

- 50–100 mL diagnostic aspirate
  standard culture
  cell count
  protein (albumin) conc.
  TB culture
  cytology
- Ultrasound and Doppler examination of liver vessels
- CT scan
- Renal function
- Liver function tests
- Urinary electrolytes
- Serum αFP
- Full blood count

Figure 8.3.1
Investigations in patients with ascites.

result in peripheral vasodilatation, increasing cardiac output and arteriovenous fistulae, as well as constriction of the intrarenal vasculature. Again the renal response is sodium and water retention. There are a number of observed biochemical findings which have led to the therapeutic approaches described below:

1. activation of the renin–angiotensin II system with raised aldosterone;

2. activation of the sympathetic nervous system with elevated levels of noradrenalin;

3. effects on cardiac output are thought to be partially mediated by changes in atrial naturetic peptide, as well as changes in nitric oxide levels.

Figure 8.3.2 is a diagrammatic representation of the contribution of the factors described above.

TREATMENT OF CIRRHOTIC ASCITES

The aim is to reduce the ascites and prevent its recurrence. Dietary sodium restriction of < 80 mEq/day is useful. Free water restriction is not usually required in patients with a serum sodium level of > 120 mmol/L, but abstinence from alcohol is important (Figure 8.3.3).

For mild ascites which is not causing any degree of discomfort or respiratory embarrassment, diuretic treatment may be considered as a temporary measure. It should be remembered that it is dangerous in the presence of renal failure or significant hyponatraemia. In acute alcoholic hepatitis and acute deteriorations complicated by infection, the presence of ascites may be short-lived and tends to resolve with stabilization of the patient.

DIURETICS

Spironolactone This is the mainstay of diuretic treatment, and should be started at a low dose of 50 mg/day and built up slowly to 400 mg/day in a single dose. Spironolactone acts on the distal tubule, and is an aldosterone antagonist. It binds to an aldosterone receptor on the distal tubule and prevents the forma-

tion of a protein important in sodium transport. It also interferes with testosterone synthesis and increases the peripheral conversion of testosterone to oestradiol. The onset of action is 48–72 h, so it will be important to wait at least 48 h before the effect of dose changes can be seen. Patients can be weighed three times weekly as an initial monitoring mechanism.

Amiloride This is an alternative to spironolactone (and is usually used when gynaecomastia is a problem). The starting dose is 5 mg, and 10 mg should be the maximum dose. This drug not only inhibits the sodium retention caused by aldosterone, but it also inhibits basal sodium reabsorption. Its onset of action is much shorter (2 h, with a peak effect at 6–10 h).

Frusemide and bumetanide These are loop diuretics which act at a different part of the nephron. They are usually added to a potassium-sparing agent such as spironolactone or amiloride when these agents are ineffective alone. The starting dose of frusemide is 20 mg, increasing to a maximum of 120 mg a day.

Side-effects

All diuretics should be stopped if the creatinine concentration rises above 120 µmol/L or the serum sodium level falls below 130 µmol/L. They are less effective when the serum albumin is low, i.e. < 25 g/dL. Gynaecomastia (the incidence of which depends on both dose and duration of spironolactone treatment) may lead to the withdrawal of spironolactone and its replacement with an alternative diuretic, such as amiloride.

COMPLICATIONS

Renal failure and hyponatraemia are common, and may be difficult to avoid. Regular monitoring of weight, renal function, serum sodium and albumin will allow the diuretics to be reduced and stopped when necessary. A check of urinary electrolytes may be helpful in determining whether or not hepatorenal syndrome is present when the urinary sodium falls below 10 µmol/L.

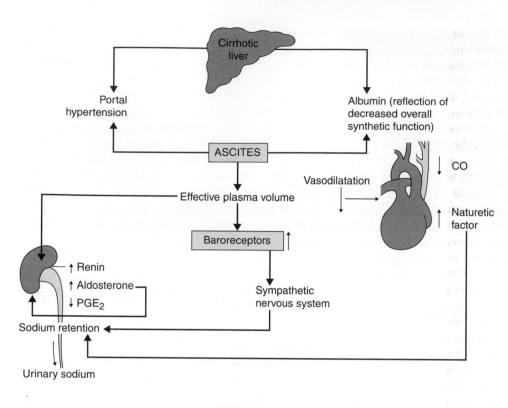

Figure 8.3.2 Diagrammatic representation of the factors involved in the formation of ascites.

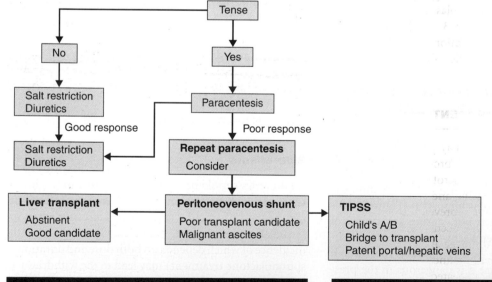

Figure 8.3.3 Treatment strategy for cirrhotic ascites.

TREATMENT FOR LARGE-VOLUME OR REFRACTORY ASCITES

Refractory ascites will occur in up to 10% of patients with cirrhosis, and is usually fatal if left untreated. A number of approaches can be taken. The ultimate treatment choice usually depends on whether or not the patient is going to be considered for liver transplantation. Intractable ascites is one of the indications for liver transplantation.

PARACENTESIS

When there is a large volume of ascites, the administration of diuretics is ineffective. The patient's comfort and respiratory function are primary indications in using paracentesis. Paracentesis may also be helpful in inducing a diuresis, since tense ascites may be the cause of renal vein compression and consequent impairment of renal function. Bed rest during paracentesis has been shown to reduce renin/angiotensin levels and to lower the speed of recurrence of ascites.

Large-volume paracentesis can be performed safely. The procedure must be performed with strict asepsis, the area being cleaned with iodine or an alternative skin antiseptic. The infra-umbilical midline region may be chosen, since it is relatively avascular and thus the risks of puncturing a vessel or varix are minimized. Alternatively, either lateral aspect of the abdomen may be approached, thus avoiding the inferior epigastric vessels. Standard IV cannulae can be used to drain the fluid under low suction into a chest-tube bottle resting on the floor. Alternatively, supra-pubic catheters can also be used. About 8–10 L of ascites can be safely removed in one session and with replacement of the lost protein (approximately 10 g/L) with intravenous salt-poor (20%) albumin. In the absence of studies examining the effects of removal of a larger volume, customary practice is to limit removal to 10 L at any one time. Each 3 L of ascites drained is replaced by 200 mL of 20% albumin intravenously. At the end of the procedure the catheter must be removed because its continued presence predisposes to a high risk of infection which may be fatal. In diuretic-resistant ascites, paracentesis may be the only treatment option whilst the patient is considered for portocaval shunting or liver transplantation. In these circumstances, it is usually needed at 2- to 3-weekly intervals. In cases where there is a coagulopathy, the INR should be corrected with fresh plasma and vitamin K administration (10 mg/day over 3 days). After large-volume paracentesis, reaccumulation of fluid can often be prevented by the administration of diuretics if these have not yet been tried.

COMPLICATIONS OF PARACENTESIS

The paracentesis needle track may provide a path for continual drainage, which may proceed externally or into the surrounding tissues and scrotum. A purse-string suture with an occlusive dressing and the use of narrow drainage catheters are helpful in preventing this complication. Bleeding is a hazard that occurs more commonly when suboptimal sites for drainage are used. The lateral abdominal approach may cause puncture of varices, and is best avoided if possible. Repeated paracentesis may also result in both hyponatraemia due to further stimulation of antidiuretic hormone (ADH) and hypo-albuminaemia. Careful replacement by the concomitant administration of intravenous albumin is helpful in this context.

TRANSJUGULAR INTRAHEPATIC/PORTOSYSTEMIC SHUNTS (TIPSS)

This is a relatively new technique available in a few specialized liver transplant centres. It involves the percutaneous placement of a stent between the intrahepatic venous and portal system via the internal jugular vein. There is a reduction in the portal pressure and ascites production. Few clinical trials have been performed, and the complication rate is high, especially in inexperienced hands. It should be considered as a bridge to transplantation. One of the complications of this procedure, namely occlusion of the portal vein and its tributaries, may make transplantation difficult if not impossible, particularly when the superior mesenteric vein is extensively involved. Only patients with Child's A and B cirrhosis should be considered, since increased hepatic encephalopathy is as common a side-effect as with standard portocaval shunts.

ORTHOTOPIC LIVER TRANSPLANTATION

Transplantation must be considered in patients with cirrhosis who have diuretic-resistant ascites. Survival rates in the best centres now exceed 75% at 1 year and 70% at 5 years. Long-term survival is usual, and is determined by disease recurrence and immunosuppressive complications, since chronic rejection is now relatively rare.

SPONTANEOUS BACTERIAL PERITONITIS (SBP)

SBP develops in approximately 10% of cirrhotics. It is particularly prevalent in decompensated cirrhosis (poor synthetic function as evidenced by prolonged prothrombin time and low serum albumin levels). Frequently clinical features are absent and the white count is normal. Ascitic protein levels are usually low, and cultures are usually monomicrobial and in 80% of cases Gram-negative. In 20% of cases non-enteric organisms are found. A broad-spectrum antibiotic such as cefotaxime or ceftizoxime is effective in 85% of cases, or alternatively ciprofloxacin and amoxycillin may be as effective. The aminoglycosides are less effective and potentially more toxic. Treatment should last for 5–7 days. If after 3 days no clinical benefit is seen, meripenem can be substituted. Treatment should be influenced by sensitivities after culture results have been obtained. Renal function and serum electrolytes should be monitored daily. In acute liver failure, antifungal cover must be empirical, beginning with fluconazole and changing to liposomal amphotericin if there is no clinical improvement.

The mortality is high, and approximately 40–50% of patients will die even with treatment. Recurrence of SBP occurs in over 60% of cases. For this reason, rapidly instituted treatment in the emergency department is vital. Since recurrence is common, prophylaxis with long-term low-dose norfloxacin is often helpful. The prognosis depends on a number of factors, including the presence of associated gastrointestinal bleeding, renal failure and the level of hepatic synthetic function, as well as the severity of infection and speed of presentation and treatment.

OTHER CAUSES OF ASCITES AND THEIR TREATMENT

MALIGNANT ASCITES

Approximately two-thirds of patients with malignant ascites have peritoneal carcinomatosis, and the remaining one-third have ascites secondary to massive liver metastasis or primary hepatoma (often having a variety of causes in cirrhotics). Chylous ascites may be found if there is lymphatic involvement. The prognosis in carcinomatosis is extremely poor, the median survival being less than 20 weeks. Physical examination of the abdomen may provide a clue as to the location of the primary and metastatic disease, since most of the tumours are adenocarcinomas. Examination of at least 1 L of ascitic fluid is important. The serum-ascites albumin gradient (SAAG) is usually $< 1.1\,g/L$ and cytology is positive in 50–80% of cases with carcinomatosis. Other tests such as cholesterol, fibronectin, α_1-antitrypsin and carcino-embryonic antigen can also be used to differentiate between malignant and benign ascites. A cholesterol level of $>$ $45\,mg/dL$ will yield $> 80\%$ positive cytology, and most cytology is negative with cholesterol levels of $< 45\,g/dL$. If ultrasound scan (USS) and examination of ascites do not give a diagnosis, then laparoscopic examination may be helpful and a tissue biopsy can be obtained. Peritoneal seedlings are frequently difficult to detect on CT scans.

Treatment should be aimed at relief of symptoms and improvement of quality of life. Paracentesis is often short-lived. However, peritoneovenous shunting may be successful in palliating 70% of patients. Complications of shunts seem to be less common than in cirrhosis, but shunts should be avoided in bloody ascites and in patients with *Pseudomyxoma peritonei*. Symptomatic palliation is the aim in malignant ascites, and there is no role for diuretics and salt/water restriction unless accompanying portal hypertension is present.

PERITONEOVENOUS SHUNTING

This is a technique in which the ascites is drained through a tube connecting the peritoneal space with the superior vena cava. Electrolyte loss and subsequent renal impairment are thus avoided. However, complication rates are relatively high due to shunt blockage, infection, disseminated intravascular coagulation or a reduced fibrinogen survival. Use of the technique in cirrhotic ascites is now decreasing, and this technique should only be considered in patients in whom liver transplantation cannot be considered. Nevertheless, either the Le Veen or the Denver shunt may provide excellent palliation in malignant ascites (Figure 8.3.4).

CHYLOUS ASCITES

This is the accumulation of lipid (chylomicron)-rich ascites, and is usually secondary to lymphatic obstruction or leakage. Patients are usually also malnourished. Diarrhoea is common, and may be associated with a protein-losing enteropathy or steatorrhoea as a result of blocked small-bowel lymphatics. In paediatric practice the majority of cases are secondary to congenital lymphatic anomalies, and neoplasms are rare in this

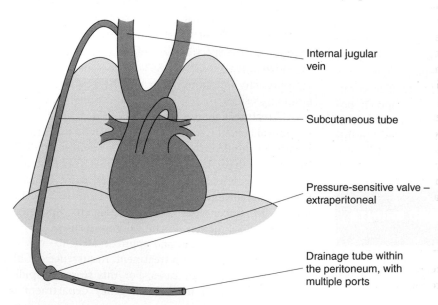

Internal jugular vein

Subcutaneous tube

Pressure-sensitive valve – extraperitoneal

Drainage tube within the peritoneum, with multiple ports

Figure 8.3.4 Peritoneovenous shunts: Le Veen shunt.

group. Surgical trauma is a relatively rare cause; in this instance, lymphangiography may sometimes be helpful in determining a site of leakage that is amenable to surgical repair. CT scanning should be undertaken to identify the site of the primary tumour, and laparotomy may be necessary to aid diagnosis. The prognosis depends on the underlying diagnosis. The survival rate is > 85% in children, but < 25% in adults.

TUBERCULOUS ASCITES

Abdominal involvement is rare in the non-immunocompromised individual, but must be seriously considered in the latter group. Onset of disease is usually insidious with intra-abdominal organ involvement (small bowel, ovary, kidney, liver). There is an increased incidence in cirrhotics in whom alcohol is the cause. There may be anorexia, weight loss, fevers and abdominal pain in over 75% of patients. Acid-fast bacilli (AFB) smears are positive in only 5% of patients, and cultures in 20%. Laparoscopy has a diagnostic yield of > 85%. With the increase in multi-drug resistance, sensitivities are important. This is a potentially lethal but treatable disease, and there should be no delay in starting empirical antituberculous chemotherapy guided by local microbiological advice. Concurrent sputum, bronchioalveolar lavage, gastric aspirate and early-morning urine samples should also be taken. Many laboratories now offer mycobacterial polymerase chain reaction (PCR) as a further diagnostic test.

PANCREATIC AND BILIARY ASCITES

Patients with chronic pancreatitis may present with massive ascites caused by rupture of a pseudocyst or disruption of a pancreatic duct. Other features of chronic pancreatitis, such as steatorrhoea, diabetes and pancreatic calcification are variably present. Pain is usually absent. Endoscopic retrograde cholangiopancreatography (ERCP) is important in defining pancreatic duct leaks, and can demonstrate abnormal ducts in patients in whom the cause of the pancreatitis is unknown. Bile leaks may be either primary (rare) or post-operative (especially after laparoscopy and liver transplantation), and can cause marked peritonitis, fever and pain. Ascitic fluid examination is usually diagnostic, with raised levels of amylase and occasionally bile-stained fluid. Management will involve a combination of endoscopy (ERCP), cholangiography and surgical approaches.

OTHER CAUSES OF ASCITES

Hypothyroidism may be both suspected clinically and diagnosed biochemically with standard measurements of thyroid-stimulating hormone (TSH), T_4 and T_3. Treatment is aimed at biochemical correction with thyroxine administration, and other approaches do not work. Peritonitis is not an infrequent complication of chronic ambulatory dialysis (CAPD), leading to increased abdominal distension and hypoalbuminaemia. Mortality is significant, and the causative bacteria, which are usually Gram-positive, differ from SBP. Intraperitoneal antibiotics are used in mild cases, but intravenous antibiotics will be required when there are signs of systemic sepsis. Peritonitis and ascites may also occur in patients who are undergoing haemodialysis, and are treated like SBP, but renal transplantation is the only definitive solution. Meigs' syndrome (ascites and pleural effusions associated with ovarian cystadenomas or fibromas) is rare, as is ascites with struma ovarii (teratoma of the ovary containing thyroid tissue). Treatment is by removal of the primary cause, usually surgically. Starch peritonitis from surgical gloves is rare, and is prevented by using starch-free gloves and thorough glove washing. A new cause of ascites is the use of ovarian stimulatory drugs for *in-vitro* fertilization (IVF) treatment, the so-called ovarian hyperstimulation syndrome. Treatment involves ascitic aspiration via the vaginal route with concomitant intravenous colloid replacement.

Ascites is a condition in which early diagnosis of the underlying cause and appropriate treatment may not only be life-saving, but is also highly effective in allowing patients a better quality of life.

FURTHER READING

Aboulghar MA, Mansour RT, Serour GI, Sattar MA, Amin YM, Elattar I. 1993: Management of severe ovarian hyperstimulation syndrome by ascitic fluid aspiration and intensive intravenous fluid therapy. *Obstetrics and Gynecology* **81**, 108–11.

Gines P, Arrovo V, Rodés J. 1992: Pharmacotherapy of ascites associated with cirrhosis. *Drugs* **43**, 316–32.

Inturri P, Graziotto A, Rossaro L. 1996: Treatment of ascites: old and new remedies. *Digestive Diseases* **14**, 145–56.

Martinet JP, Fenyves D, Legault L, *et al.* 1997: Treatment of refractory ascites using transjugular intrahepatic portosystemic shunt (TIPS): a caution. *Digestive Diseases and Sciences* **42**, 161–6.

Runyon BA. 1994: Malignancy-related ascites and ascitic fluid 'humoral tests of malignancy'. *Journal of Clinical Gastroenterology* **18**, 94–8.

Sherlock S, Dooley J. 1997: *Diseases of the liver and biliary system*, 10th edn. Oxford: Blackwell Science.

Slapak GI, Saxena R, Portmann B *et al.* 1997: Graft and systemic disease in long-term survivors of liver transplantation. *Hepatology* **25**, 195–202.

Stanley AJ, Redhead DN, Hayes PC. 1997: Review article: update on the role of transjugular intrahepatic portosystemic stent-shunt (TIPSS) in the management of complications of portal hypertension. *Alimentary Pharmacology and Therapeutics* **11**, 261–72.

Taylor MB (ed.). 1997: *Gastrointestinal emergencies*, 2nd edn. Baltimore, MD: Williams and Wilkins.

Scrotal swellings

Anthony R. Mundy

Introduction

Generations of medical students and surgical trainees have had their clinical skills assessed in various examinations by their ability to distinguish between a hernia, an epididymal cyst and a hydrocele, and have therefore been brought up to believe that the ability to distinguish a hydrocele from an epididymal cyst is important. It is not. For the same reason, the same individuals have been taught the importance of examining their patients standing up. This, too, is a fallacy except when preliminary examination suggests that the patient has either a hernia or a varicocele. The single most important point in examining the scrotum in a patient with a scrotal swelling (or any other local symptom) is to feel the testis carefully and ensure that there is no lump within the testis itself. Everything else is trivial by comparison, and the best way of palpating the testis is with the patient lying down in warm and comfortable surroundings. Likewise, the examiner should have a warm and comfortable approach and warm and comfortable hands.

The situation can be summarized as follows. As a general rule, a lump in the testis itself *is* a tumour and is serious, whereas a lump outside the testis is not a tumour and is not serious.

Other than hernias, which will not be considered further here, and skin swellings such as sebaceous cysts, there are essentially three types of scrotal swellings:

1. lumps within the testis itself – tumours;

2. cystic swellings of the scrotal contents - hydroceles and epididymal cysts;

3. swellings of the testis *and* epididymis (generally acute and painful) - torsion and epididymo-orchitis.

There are one or two conditions that do not fit neatly into this classification, such as varicocele and idiopathic scrotal oedema in children, but it does not take too much imagination to fit variocele into category 2 and idiopathic scrotal oedema into category 3 (together with trauma).

RELEVANT ANATOMY

The testicle is suspended within the scrotum from the spermatic cord. From its head the numerous efferent ductules run into the epididymis, which then runs down a narrow strip of the posterior aspect of the testis to the tail of the epididymis at the lower pole of the testis, where the epididymis makes a 'U'-turn to form the vas, and then runs back up to the neck of the scrotum and on to the inguinal canal. Other than along the attachment of the epididymis, the majority of the circumference of the testis is surrounded by the tunica vaginalis. The latter can fill with fluid to form a hydrocele, and the important point here is that this will be on the antero-inferior aspect of the scrotum and will obscure the testis itself, but will not involve the epididymis. The other important point to note is that there are 'lumpy bits' on top of the testis, at the bottom of the testis and posteriorly, and when a patient performs 'self-examination' as advocated by *Readers Digest, Men's Health* and other 'male literature', and thinks he has a lump, then it will commonly be these testicular appendages that he has actually identified.

The ducts from the testis emerge from the head of the testis to form the so-called caput epididymis. Because of this, most epididymal cysts form at the head of the testis. Apart from the vas, the spermatic cord contains the testicular artery and the testicular venous drainage known as the pampiniform plexus. Varicose dilatation of this venous plexus is known as a varicocele.

The testis and cord are surrounded by layers of spermatic fascia derived from the abdominal wall layers during the embryological descent of the testis through the inguinal canal to lie in the scrotum. These fascial layers contain the fibres of the cremaster muscle, which make the cold and anxious scrotum contract and which therefore make the cold and anxious scrotal contents difficult to examine.

Around the spermatic fascia are the skin and subcutaneous tissue of the scrotum. The subcutaneous tissue is remarkably devoid of fat and contains its own muscular layer – the dartos – which is equally prone to contract in cold and anxious states. There is a central plane of cleavage between the two halves of the scrotum, and each testis and its surroundings remains distinct. It is not possible to push one testicle into the other side of the scrotum.

The dartos and cremaster are both particularly active in young children, and reflex contraction may cause the infantile testis to disappear from the scrotum altogether. This should be anticipated in young children and steps should be taken to avoid it (see below). During early and middle adult life both reflexes become much less marked, and in general the cremasteric reflex is lost before the dartos reflex.

Anyone reading this chapter who is unaware that the testis produces both sperm and androgens might as well give up now, but it should perhaps be pointed out to the remaining readers that before continuing with the local examination of the scrotum itself, at least cursory attention should be paid to the patient's fertility and general hormonal status, although abnormalities of either of these are rarely associated with a scrotal swelling. They are far more commonly associated with the 'empty scrotum'.

THE EXAMINATION TECHNIQUE

The patient should lie comfortably on a couch or bed in a warm room. Most adults prefer to lie at a slope of 45° rather than completely flat. Young children may prefer to sit in a similar position on their mother's lap. They should not be crying, and if they are you should wait until they have stopped. Your own hands should be warm. A history of pain or tenderness, or a red angry appearance of the scrotum should lead you to be particularly gentle, but no male likes to have someone make a grab at his genitals, so a relaxed approach is important. It is equally important to start from the top of the inguinal canal and work down, particularly in young children, to prevent the retractile testis from retracting.

Each testis should be examined in turn, starting with the normal side, assuming that only one side is affected. It should be stressed that the main point is to examine the testis itself, except in the acute situation where trauma, infection or torsion may make the testis and its appendages indistinguishable. Having examined the testis for size and consistency, attention should then be given to the epididymis, then to the cord and then, in the case of an adult, the patient should be asked to stand up to allow palpation for either a varicocele or a hernia, although a hernia will usually have been suspected from the initial examination of the inguinal canal.

If the clinical examination is inconclusive, then the patient should be referred for ultrasound examination as a next step. It is often extremely difficult to examine a fat, anxious or very young patient, and it should not be regarded as a sign of incompetence to ask for a scrotal ultrasound examination, particularly in difficult or acute cases.

TESTICULAR TUMOURS

Testicular tumours only account for 1–2% of malignant tumours in men, but they are the commonest tumours in men aged 25–35 years. There is a link between undescended testes and testicular tumours, even if the testicle was treated by orchidopexy at an early age. This is by far the commonest risk factor. The majority of testicular tumours arise from germ cells. Two types exist, namely seminoma and teratoma (which in the USA is known as non-seminomatous germ cell tumour or NSGCT). Teratoma is commoner in the 20–30 years age group and seminoma in the 30–40 years age group. Each accounts for about 40% of tumours, and the other 20% of tumours consist of all the other unusual types pooled together. The tumour usually presents as a swelling in or of the testis, but occasionally it presents as a painful lump, particularly with pain occurring after mild trauma that is generally sexual in origin. It should be noted that relatively acute symptoms might obscure the diagnosis initially.

It is *extremely important* for this reason to ensure in any clinical examination that the testicle is carefully felt, and if there is any suspicion of a testicular swelling then it should be treated as a tumour until proven otherwise. Likewise, if any diagnostic confusion or uncertainty exists, the patient should be sent for an ultrasound scan immediately.

Testicular tumours of certain types can spread rapidly, and for this reason patients should be investigated and treated urgently. The testis should be explored through a groin incision within the next 24–48 h after taking blood for the two important serum markers, namely alpha-fetoprotein and beta-human chorionic gonadotrophin. It is important to explore the testis through the inguinal canal in order to avoid interfering with the superficial lymphatics of the scrotum, which drain to the inguinal lymph nodes, whereas the testicular lymph nodes are para-aortic.

Further investigation and treatment follow an accurate histological diagnosis.

CYSTIC SCROTAL SWELLINGS

The two commonest types are hydrocele and epididymal cysts. The third – not strictly speaking cystic – type is a varicocele.

HYDROCELE

A hydrocele is a collection of fluid in the tunica vaginalis. Congenital hydroceles do occur, but most are acquired. Most hydroceles are symptomless, but some cause a dragging discomfort, particularly when large. Some are tense and make it impossible to examine the testis within. If this is the case, the testis must be examined by ultrasound, as a hydrocele may mask a testicular tumour. The testis may be palpable through the hydrocele if the latter is lax. Hydroceles (and epididymal cysts) transilluminate.

No further investigation is required and the vast majority do not require treatment unless their size is causing a significant problem.

EPIDIDYMAL CYSTS

These are diverticula of the vasa efferentia, and are typically thin-walled and slowly enlarging. They might be multi-locular and are generally multiple. If there is still communication with the vasa efferentia, sperm cells may be present within the cyst, causing it to be cloudy. These are then referred to as spermatoceles. Epididymal cysts are situated above and behind the testis, rather than below and surrounding the front as with a hydrocele. Their presentation is the same as that for a hydrocele, and similarly most require no further investigation or treatment.

VARICOCELE

A varicocele is a varicosity of the veins of the pampiniform plexus which provides venous drainage for the testis. About 10% of normal males have one, almost always on the left-hand side because the left testicular vein drains into the left renal vein, whereas the right testicular vein drains into the inferior vena cava. Right-sided varicoceles are supposed to be indicative of an underlying renal tumour on that side. Varicoceles are occasionally thought to be a cause of infertility, but this is controversial.

As with other 'cystic' swellings, varicoceles are usually asymptomatic but may cause discomfort, which is the only indication for treatment.

ACUTE SCROTAL SWELLINGS

A history of trauma is usually obvious, and severe trauma may make examination impossible, which is an indication for testicular ultrasound. Further treatment depends on the finding.

TORSION OF THE TESTIS

Torsion means twisting. Twisting of the testis occurs around its longitudinal axis and occurs when there is an abnormal investment of the testis *and* epididymis by the tunica vaginalis which extends up on to the cord. This allows the testis to rotate within the tunica vaginalis. Occasionally the testis twists on a long mesentery between the epididymis and itself, but this is unusual. Even more uncommonly, and only in neonates, the spermatic cord above the testis twists. Either way it causes pain and swelling which is exacerbated by subsequent oedema and venous obstruction. This leads on to haemorrhage within the testis, arterial occlusion, and eventually infarction and necrosis of the testis. Typically a boy or young man complains of a sudden severe pain in the scrotum, often accompanied by nausea. A history of a previous incident of lesser degree that improved spontaneously is common.

The patient is usually afebrile, and the overlying scrotal skin is usually red. The whole of the testis is tender to touch, and the spermatic cord feels thickened and tender above.

This diagnosis should be suspected in any patient, particularly a boy or young man with acute scrotal pain and testicular swelling. This is the diagnosis that must be assumed until proven otherwise, because urgent exploration is required to untwist the testis, fix it in place and thereby ensure its survival, unless it is irretrievably damaged, in which case orchidectomy is necessary.

Occasionally, one of the rare testicular appendages of embryological origin twists, in which case symptoms may be severe but far more localized. It is usually necessary to explore the scrotum and excise the twisted appendage, not just to relieve pain but to exclude torsion of the testis itself.

EPIDIDYMO-ORCHITIS

This is rare before puberty, but increasingly common thereafter. The exception is in so-called idiopathic scrotal oedema in young children, in which the whole of the scrotum is red and swollen on both sides. Thus with unilateral testicular pain, swelling and redness under the age of 20 years, a torsion is more likely but a fever is usually absent, whereas over the age of 20 years epididymo-orchitis is increasingly more likely, particularly when a fever is present.

Infection reaches the epididymis either via the bloodstream or via retrograde spread from the prostatic urethra, and usually follows either a urinary tract infection or a sexually transmitted disease – occasionally following urethral instrumentation.

The onset is usually sudden, and pain is rapidly progressive, with swelling and redness of the scrotum. There is usually fever and rigors, and often a history suggestive of urinary tract infection or sexually transmitted disease. A secondary hydrocele commonly develops. The problem originally develops in the epididymis, but may then spread to the testis – hence the transition from epididymitis to epididymo-orchitis. Once this is established it may be impossible to exclude torsion clinically.

Investigation is by microscopy and culture of the urine and subsequent investigation of the urinary tract.

Occasionally an acute inflammation becomes chronic and, more rarely in this country but much more commonly in the tropics, tuberculosis may be the cause. In either case there may be a chronic fibrosis and 'lumpiness' of both the testis and the epididymis. Such a mass may be confused with a tumour, but tumours rarely spread through the testis to involve the epididymis, so if both are affected chronic inflammation is by far the most likely cause. A discharging fistula through to the skin virtually confirms the diagnosis. Viral orchitis does occur, particularly after mumps. It is usually only found in adult mumps, and is rare in pre-pubertal children.

SUMMARY

1. Remember that the main point of examining the scrotum is to satisfy yourself that the testis is normal. All other scrotal swellings are trivial by comparison.

2. Remember that if there is a lump in the testis, it is a tumour and serious. If there is a lump outside the testis, it is rarely serious unless it is acute.

3. Remember that boys get torsion and men get epididymitis.

4. Remember if you are ever unsure after a clinical examination, arrange an ultrasound examination of the scrotum to resolve the issue.

Chapter 8.5

Swollen joints

Jennifer G. Worrall

Introduction

There are 187 synovial joints in the normal human body, and any may be affected by inflammatory and degenerative change. Many joints are of course also susceptible to trauma. All synovial joints have the same basic structure, and they all respond in a similar way to insults. The cardinal sign of synovial joint pathology is *swelling*.

WHAT CAUSES JOINT SWELLING?

When a patient presents with a swollen joint, the first question to ask concerns the nature of the swelling (Table 8.5.1).

If the history is chronic, then the swelling may arise from bone or soft tissue or be due to fluid within the joint space. Bony swelling is easily identified by palpa-

Table 8.5.1 Causes of joint swelling

Sites of swelling within the joint
- Bone
- Synovium and capsule
- Fluid within the joint, i.e. synovial fluid, pus, blood

Sites of swelling around the joint
- Tendon and tendon sheath
- Bursa
- Fat
- Blood vessel
- Lymph node
- Subcutaneous tissue (oedema)

---

tion, but it can be difficult to distinguish clinically between soft-tissue swelling, arising from the synovium or capsule, and fluid. If the swelling is acute, then it is almost certainly due to fluid (synovial fluid, pus or blood) within the joint.

It is important to beware the swelling of *periarticular structures* masquerading as joint swelling. Examples are ganglia and tenosynovitis (especially around the wrist), bursitis (especially of the olecranon bursa and the anserine bursa on the medial aspect of the upper tibia) and, of course, oedema of the subcutaneous tissue (for example, dur to heart failure, disuse, cellulitis or venous thrombosis). In the knee, the infra-patellar fat pads may be prominent, but are normal structures, and swelling of popliteal structures, such as the popliteal artery and lymph nodes, may also mislead the unwary.

However, with a basic knowledge of local anatomy and careful examination you should be able to avoid these pitfalls. The following account will concentrate on swelling of the true joint, and periarticular structures will not be further considered.

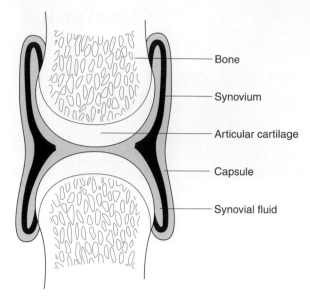

Figure 8.5.1 Structure of a normal synovial joint. The synovium is closely opposed to the internal joint surfaces, and the joint space is potential rather than actual.

OVERVIEW OF THE SYNOVIAL JOINT

Before considering each of the components of the joint which may give rise to swelling, let us take an overview of the basic structure and function of the normal synovial joint (Figure 8.5.1).

Synovial joints are joints which are specialized to permit a wide range of movement with low frictional drag. They contain a cavity lined by a specialized connective tissue called *synovium*. The cavity and the structures within it are coated with a thin layer of a highly viscous fluid, *synovial fluid*. Normal joints contain very small volumes of synovial fluid; even a joint as large as the knee contains only 1–2 mL. *Hyaline cartilage* covers the bone ends; unlike the other tissues within the joint, it is avascular and derives its nutrition from the synovial fluid. The whole joint is enclosed in a capsule of fibrous tissue. Synovium is attached to bone at the junction with hyaline cartilage, and is reflected off this junction to line the whole capsule. Normally, folds of synovium fill the spaces between non-congruous cartilage surfaces, and these folds slip away during movement as the point of contact between opposing cartilage surfaces shifts.

ARTICULAR CARTILAGE AND BONE

STRUCTURE AND FUNCTION OF ARTICULAR CARTILAGE

The articular cartilage covers the bone ends in the synovial joint and is a hyaline cartilage specialized for weight-bearing and shock absorbance. It functions in a similar way to the air-inflated tyres of a motor vehicle, in which the tensile strength of the tyre walls resists the expansion of the compressed air within, giving a structure which is resilient but sufficiently deformable to absorb shock.

Articular cartilage matrix contains a network of *collagen fibres* (mainly type 2 collagen) which restrain the swelling pressure of large, hydrophilic carbohydrate molecules contained within the network. The carbohydrates are *glycosaminoglycans*, which are heavily negatively charged and therefore attract water. As more and more water molecules are bound, the volume of the hydrated glycosaminoglycan molecules increases, until a further increase in volume is prevented by the constraints of the surrounding collagen network. When articular cartilage is subjected to *mechanical stress*, as, for example, in the heel-strike phase of walking, water is squeezed out and the cartilage deforms, thereby absorbing shock. As the stress is removed, water is reabsorbed and the cartilage resumes its original form.

ARTICULAR CARTILAGE DEGENERATION

Degeneration of the articular cartilage is the primary lesion in *osteoarthritis* (Figure 8.5.2), which is the commonest disease of synovial joints. The first step appears

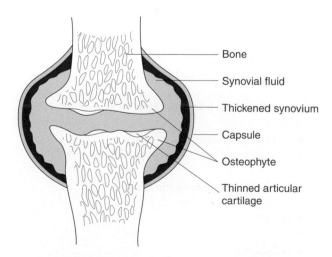

Figure 8.5.2 Osteoarthritis. There is loss of articular cartilage, and osteophytes form at the joint margins. The synovium is thickened and an effusion may be present.

to be break-up of the collagen network. This leads to loss of glycosaminoglycan molecules from the tissue, swelling pressure is reduced, and the tissue becomes less resilient and less able to withstand mechanical stress. The surface of the cartilage, which is normally smooth and glassy, becomes roughened or '*fibrillated*' (visible arthroscopically). Pieces of cartilage may break free, become coated in fibrin and form loose bodies within the joint. Mechanical irritation of the synovium by these loose bodies, and also by trapping of the synovium between roughened cartilage surfaces, may lead to mild inflammation and an effusion of synovial fluid (see below).

A number of factors predispose to osteoarthritis (see Table 8.5.2).

BONY SWELLING

Bony swelling has a number of causes (Table 8.5.3), but the commonest is the osteophytosis of osteoarthritis.

The degenerate cartilage of osteoarthritis functions poorly as a shock absorber, with the result that periarticular bone is subjected to increased mechanical stress. Bone cells respond to this stress by remodelling the bone matrix. Periarticular bone becomes more dense, or *sclerotic* (visible radiologically), and bony overgrowth, in the form of *osteophytes*, occurs at the joint margins. It is not known what precise function osteophytes serve, but they

Table 8.5.2 Factors predisposing to osteoarthritis

Abnormal cartilage
- Inherited collagen defects
- Metabolic diseases, e.g. hypercalcaemia haemachromatosis

Abnormal mechanical stress
- Professional athletes
- Obesity
- Structurally abnormal joints, e.g. developmental, post-trauma

Abnormal bone
- Paget's disease
- Osteopetrosis

Table 8.5.3 Causes of bony swelling

- Osteophytes
- Joint subluxation (chronic)
- Joint dislocation (acute, traumatic)
- Developmental abnormalities
- Tumours

may help to redistribute load-bearing, and they may also reduce the range of movement of the joint.

Osteophytes may grow to a large size, and frequently present as joint swelling. Common sites of clinically apparent osteophytes are the distal interphalangeal joints (where they are known as Heberden's nodes), the first metatarsophalangeal joint, the first carpometacarpal joint and the knee. Obviously, being bony, the swellings are fixed and hard to palpation, and they may also be slightly tender.

Another fairly common cause of bony swelling is the chronic joint *subluxation* associated with rheumatoid arthritis. Of course, the bone itself is not swollen – the swelling is only apparent and is due to malalignment. Subluxation is particularly common at the metacarpophalangeal and metatarsophalangeal joints, the wrist, the elbow and the sub-talar joints.

Other much rarer forms of bony swelling that cause joint swelling are developmental abnormalities and tumours.

SYNOVIUM

As we have seen, the synovial space is *potential* rather than actual, as it is largely filled by folds of synovium. However, the potential space is very large, and a joint such as the knee is capable of holding in excess of 150 mL of fluid.

The function of synovium is to produce synovial fluid, which it does by a combination of ultrafiltration of plasma and active secretion of large molecules, such as hyaluronan (see below).

INFLAMMATION

Before considering synovial inflammation specifically, let us briefly review the inflammatory process in general.

Inflammation constitutes the response of living tissue to injury. The clinical signs are *pain, swelling, erythema* and *heat*. The process serves to remove damaged tissue and initiate repair. The first stages of inflammation are vasodilatation and exudation of fluid into the tissue. Polymorphonuclear leucocytes migrate through blood-vessel walls into the tissue, followed by monocytes which rapidly mature into macrophages. These phagocytic cells remove debris and secrete vasodilator prostaglandins, chemotactic leukotrienes, cytokines and degradative enzymes. Endothelial cells are stimulated to form new blood vessels, and tissue repair, which occurs by a combination of regeneration and fibrosis, is effected by fibroblasts.

If the inflammation is immune-mediated, lymphocytes infiltrate the tissue in large numbers. B-lymphocytes mature into antibody-secreting cells and T-lymphocytes mature into cells specialized for cell-killing or cytokine secretion. Immune processes are triggered by antigen which must be presented to the immune cells in a way that they will recognize. Several cell types are able to present antigen, but the specialized antigen-presenting cell, or dendritic cell, is the most efficient.

If the primary insult persists, then chronic inflammation ensues. The affected tissue is disrupted, resident cells are outnumbered many times over by infiltrating cells, the matrix becomes disorganized and fibrotic and marked angiogenesis is present.

SYNOVIAL INFLAMMATION

Inflammation of synovium may be due to *mechanical, chemical, infective* or *immune-mediated* factors (Table 8.5.4)

When synovium is inflamed, it becomes swollen and secretes fluid. All types of inflammation may be associated with large synovial effusions, but immune-mediated inflammation, as in *rheumatoid arthritis*, is notable for also giving rise to gross hypertrophy of the synovial tissue itself. The surface of the synovium may be thrown into folds, or *villi*, that can be seen arthroscopically and which have the appearance of seaweed or the tentacles of a sea-anemone. On clinical examination, the grossly thickened synovium may be palpated as soft, boggy swelling. Most often, it is cool and only moderately tender but, if the disease is very active, the joint swelling may be warm, erythematous and very tender, and oedema of the overlying subcutaneous tissue may even be present.

Any chronic or recurrent inflammatory process within the joint may lead to permanent joint damage. Articular cartilage is damaged and may be completely destroyed. This process is particularly rapid in untreated septic arthritis. If bone becomes exposed, then this is also destroyed. In rheumatoid arthritis, areas of bone destruction, or *erosions*, form specifically at the site of attachment of the synovium. Radiologically, the first sign of inflammatory arthritis is increased radiolucency of the bone near the affected joint (*periarticular osteopenia*). A later sign is joint space narrowing, due to loss of articular cartilage. Bone erosions are a sign of advanced, permanent damage (Figure 8.5.3).

FLUID WITHIN THE JOINT

Fluid within a swollen joint is most commonly synovial fluid, but it may be pus or blood. We shall first consider synovial fluid.

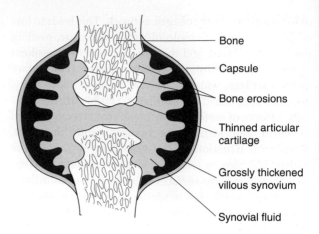

Figure 8.5.3 Rheumatoid arthritis. There is loss of articular cartilage and erosion of bone, beginning at the joint margins. The synovium is grossly thickened with a villous surface, and a large effusion may be present.

Table 8.5.4 Causes of synovial inflammation

Mechanical   e.g. cartilage fragments in osteoarthritis
Chemical   e.g. gout, pseudogout
Infective   septic arthritis, most commonly due to *Staphylococcus aureus*
Of unknown origin but immune-mediated   e.g. rheumatoid arthritis

NORMAL AND INFLAMMATORY SYNOVIAL FLUID

Normal joints contain a small volume of highly viscous synovial fluid. The fluid contains a high concentration of *hyaluronan*. Each molecule of hyaluronan is an enormous glycosaminoglycan chain with an average molecular weight in excess of 6×10^6 kDa. It is the entanglement of these large molecules which gives normal synovial fluid its viscosity. Inflammatory synovial fluid has a low viscosity because the enzymes and free radicals associated with inflammation break down these large molecules, and the smaller fragments are able to move freely without entanglement. Normal synovial fluid contains very few cells and is optically clear but inflammatory fluid contains large numbers of polymorphonuclear leucocytes, lymphocytes and macrophages, and is opalescent or even opaque.

BLOOD AND PUS WITHIN THE JOINT

Significant trauma to a normal joint may cause a *haemarthrosis*. Minor trauma to a chronically inflamed joint, in which the synovium is thickened, friable and hypervascular, may also cause intra-articular bleeding. Spontaneous bleeding may occur in haemophilia, but this is much less of a clinical problem since the advent of patient-administered clotting factor. Blood is highly irritant to the joint and, if frank blood is obtained on aspiration, the joint should be washed out.

Intra-articular pus is of course a feature of septic arthritis, but non-infective inflammation, as discussed above, may be associated with joint fluid which is opaque and visually indistinguishable from infected fluid.

THE IMPORTANCE OF JOINT ASPIRATION

The commonest causes of an acutely swollen joint, in the absence of a history of trauma, are *gout, pseudogout, infection* and an *immune-mediated inflammatory arthritis*, such as rheumatoid arthritis or reactive arthritis. An acutely swollen joint *must* be aspirated, mainly to exclude infection which can rapidly destroy the joint and lead to life-threatening septicaemia. It can be difficult to distinguish infection clinically as all of the above may give rise to a hot, red, swollen joint in association with pyrexia and leucocytosis.

Inspect the aspirated fluid for its clarity or opacity, which is a guide to the cell content. Test the viscosity by emptying the syringe; viscous fluid will form a long string, while fluid of low viscosity will drip from the syringe like water. Light microscopy and culture should be performed to detect infection. Polarizing light microscopy should be performed to detect crystals of uric acid and calcium pyrophosphate, which are pathognomonic of gout and pseudogout, respectively.

FURTHER READING

Akil M, Amos RS. 1995: ABC of rheumatology: rheumatoid arthritis. I. Clinical features and diagnosis. *British Medical Journal* **310**, 587–90.

Frankel VH. 1994: Biomechanics. In Klippel JH, Dieppe PA (eds), *Rheumatology*. London: Times Mirror International Publishers Ltd, 4.1–4.8.

Hasselbacher P. 1994: Joint physiology. In Klippel JH, Dieppe PA (eds), *Rheumatology*. London: Times Mirror International Publishers Ltd, 3.1–3.6.

Simpkin PA. 1994: The musculoskeletal system. In Klippel JH, Dieppe PA (eds), *Rheumatology*. London: Times Mirror International Publishers Ltd, 2.1–2.10.

Pleural effusion

Norman Johnson and Crichton F. Ramsay

Introduction

The surgeon or physician is frequently presented with patients who have problems related to their pleural cavity. In the majority of these cases the presenting feature is increasing breathlessness which may be associated with a cough. Chest pain is common with pneumothoraces, but rarer with pleural effusions unless there is associated pleurisy, pulmonary infarction or malignant invasion of the parietal pleura lining the chest wall.

Features in the history which aid diagnosis include the following:

- age – spontaneous pneumothorax is usually found in men in their late teens and early twenties, TB effusion is found in the same age group, while effusions in individuals over the age of 50 years are frequently malignant (if exudates);

- occupation – mesothelioma is linked to asbestos exposure years previously;

- race – recent immigrants are more likely to suffer from TB;

- trauma – pneumothorax or haemothorax or much more rarely chylothorax may complicate blunt or penetrating chest injuries;

- preceding health – pneumothorax usually occurs before a sudden event of breathlessness and pain, pleural effusions usually have a more insidious onset. If pain persists for several weeks or months, suspect a mesothelioma.

ANATOMY AND PHYSIOLOGY

The inner lining of the chest wall comprises the visceral pleura, and the parietal pleura covers the outer surface of each lung. The function of the pleura is to shape the lungs and to enable them to move as freely and with as low friction as possible across each other during inspiration and expiration. In health there is a potential rather than real space between the two layers of pleura. Movement between the two is assisted by boundary lubrication, there being a layer of surfactant absorbed on to the pleural surfaces rather than, as was previously supposed, intervening pleural fluid. There is pleural fluid in small pockets which also provide hydrodynamic lubrication.

Both layers of pleura consist of single layers of mesothelial cells with numerous microvilli which act to increase the surface area and hence aid absorption of surfactant and pleural fluid. These mesothelial cells partake in fluid and electrolyte transport and also have other functions, such as fibrinolysis and phagocytosis.

A practical point to remember is that it may be very difficult for the cytopathologist to differentiate activated mesothelial cells from malignant cells. This limits the usefulness of cytology of pleural fluid. There are stomata in the pleura via which the pleural cavity is connected to subpleural lymphatics. Hence the two mechanisms concerned with transfer of fluid across the pleural membrane are:

1. transcapillary exchange; and
2. lymphatic drainage.

At full expiration (function residual capacity, FRC) there is a negative pressure of 3–4 mmHg within the pleural space which is generated by the inward elastic recoil of the lung and the pull of the chest wall outwards. The difference between the partial pressures of gases in alveolar air and arterial blood (approximately 101 kPa or 760 mmHg) is greater than that in venous blood (94 kPa or 706 mmHg) minus 56 mmHg because this difference is in excess of the negative pressure within the pleural space minus 3–4 mmHg. The net effect is one of gaseous absorption from the pleural space. If a patient breathes oxygen, the arterial-venous blood pressure will be increased, thereby bringing about greater gaseous absorption (this is useful for treating pneumothorax).

With regard to fluid flux, firstly Starling's law can be applied to the pleural space (see Figure 8.6.1). Overall, the net drying effect is around 7 mmHg or 0.9 kPa. Secondly, there is drainage via the pleural stomata and subpleural lymphatics.

Taking into consideration these basic scientific principles, it is obvious that even in health the pleural space is an area of intense activity with constant secretion and

absorption of fluid. Even in disease with pleural effusions, it is important to recognize that there is a constant turnover of fluid, sometimes at the rate of 30% per hour.

HAEMOTHORAX

Common causes of haemothorax include:

- rupture of pleural adhesions at the time of a pneumothorax – these are usually small volume;
- rib fracture;
- a penetrating injury, e.g. a knife wound.

Therapy

A small haemothorax with merely blunting of the costophrenic angle on chest X-ray can be left, but should be monitored with daily chest X-ray to check that it is not increasing in size. If the volume is increasing, a chest drain should be inserted (well above the diaphragm). More active intervention such as thoracotomy is indicated for continued bleeding and hypovolaemic shock which is not responding to blood replacement.

Indications

These include the following:

- more than 1 L of blood aspirated immediately after insertion of a chest drain;
- continuous loss through the chest drain of 200 mL/h for more than 3 h.

Unstable patients with evidence of massive intrathoracic haemorrhage require urgent thoracotomy. Stable patients may be managed by intercostal drainage. If management of the haemothorax has been delayed by 7–10 days, the blood within the pleural cavity tends to clot and cannot be managed by intercostal drainage. In these circumstances, thoracotomy and surgical removal of the haematoma are necessary.

PLEURAL EFFUSION

Pleural effusion is the term used to describe a collection of fluid in the pleural space (cavity). Following inflammation, infection, invasion by cancer or blockage of local lymphatics, there is exudation of fluid with a high protein content (protein > 30 g/L). If fluid accumulates in the pleural space more rapidly than the normal rate of reabsorption, a pleural effusion develops. In these circumstances the volume of fluid can be very large. In order for fluid to be seen at all on a chest X-ray a volume of around 500 mL is needed. In extreme cases there can be complete obscuration of one lung on the chest X-ray

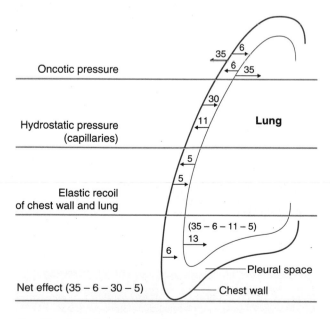

Overall result = drying effect from pleural spaces = 13 − 6 = 7 mmHg

Figure 8.6.1 Diagrammatic representation of fluid flux in the pleural space, the overall effects of which in health result in a drying effect of 7 mmHg so that fluid does not accumulate in the pleural space.

('a white-out'). In such extreme cases 3 L or more of fluid may have collected. In contrast, in conditions where the primary pathology is elevation of the venous pressure, fluid retention or a low serum albumin level, there is transudation of fluid with a low protein content (protein < 30 g/L) into the pleural cavity.

Causes of transudation (protein < 30 g/L)

Transudates (protein < 30 g/L) are usually bilateral, although they may appear on one side before the other. They are usually caused by systemic conditions which alter the hydrostatic or osmotic forces across the pleural membrane (Table 8.6.1).

Table 8.6.1 Causes of transudation

Common causes
● left ventricular failure (heart failure)
● fluid overload – excess IV fluids, or renal failure
Rarer causes
● hypoproteinaemia – cirrhosis of the liver
● failure of albumin synthesis – malnutrition
● kidney disease – excess albumin excretion, e.g. nephrotic syndrome
● constrictive pericarditis
● pulmonary emboli
● myxoedema
● peritoneal dialysis fluid leaking through the diaphragm

Clinical points

These include the following:

● cardiac failure – look for cardiomegaly and a history of cardiac problems;

● cirrhosis – look for coexisting ascites, usually right-sided (as with cardiac failure), and a history of liver disease and possible alcohol abuse. There is a poor correlation between plasma protein levels and protein in the effusion. Fluid quite often passes directly through the diaphragm via lymphatics or smaller defects;

● nephrotic syndrome – look for effusion (because of decreased plasma osmotic pressure), proteinuria and severe peripheral oedema.

Causes of exudation (protein > 30 g/L)

Exudates are usually due to local diseases causing increased capillary permeability or lymphatic obstruc-

tion (Table 8.6.2). Increased permeability is caused by inflammatory mediators such as cytokines. Lymphatic blockage is caused by obstruction of pleural lymphatics. Exudates are usually unilateral.

Table 8.6.2 Causes of exudation

Common causes
● post infective (pneumonia), usually small volume
● pulmonary infarction (pulmonary embolism), usually small volume and bloodstained
● malignancy (usually in patients over 50 years of age), either direct spread or metastases from lung cancer or spread from cancer of other sites, such as breast, ovary or lymphoma – often large volume and bloodstained
● tuberculosis – large volume, clear
Rarer causes
● subphrenic or liver abscess
● connective tissue disorders, e.g. rheumatoid arthritis or systemic lupus erythematosus
● drugs
● mesothelioma – primary malignancy of the pleura associated with asbestos exposure
● Wegener's granulomatosis
● pancreatitis
● ruptured oesophagus
● chylothorax
● trauma – haemothorax
● Dressler's syndrome
● familial Mediterranean fever
● drug induced
● Meigs' syndrome
● yellow nail syndrome
● sarcoidosis
● radiotherapy

EMPYEMA – THE COLLECTION OF PUS IN THE PLEURAL CAVITY

Common causes include the following:

● bacterial pneumonia;
● tuberculosis;
● iatrogenic – chest aspiration or surgery;

- subphrenic abscess;
- ruptured oesophagus.

CHYLOTHORAX

This is a rare condition in which there is leakage of lymph (chylomicrons) into the pleural space from an interruption, blockage or rupture of the thoracic duct which drains lymph back into the superior vena cava (Table 8.6.3).

Table 8.6.3 The commonest causes of chylothorax

- congenital in the newborn, absence or atresia of the thoracic duct
- post-operative – trauma or traumatic operations on the aortic arch
- oesophageal resection or sympathectomy
- penetrating knife wound or, very rarely, violent coughing and vomiting
- non-traumatic – malignancy involving the mediastinum which obstructs the thoracic duct, e.g. lymphoma

The diagnosis is made by finding fluid with microscopic fat in the pleural cavity. The fat content is higher in pleural fluid than in plasma. A lymphangiogram can demonstrate the size of the leakage, and a CT of the thorax is important to demonstrate the local anatomy.

Management

A medium-chain triglyceride diet or total parenteral nutrition are needed to reduce the thoracic duct lymph flow, followed by surgery if drainage has not stopped after 3 weeks (ligation of the thoracic duct immediately above the diaphragm with pleurectomy).

CLINICAL FEATURES OF PLEURAL EFFUSIONS

Symptoms

The commonest symptoms of fluid in the pleural cavity are as follows:

- increasing breathlessness, the severity of which depends on the volume of fluid and the reserve of the rest of the lung (i.e. coexisting asthma, chronic bronchitis);
- coughing;
- pleuritic pain, particularly with infection

(pneumonic), infarction, pulmonary embolism or mesothelioma (malignancy).

Physical signs

On examination of the chest, the classical abnormalities observed on the affected side (over the pleural fluid) are as follows:

- a reduction in movement;
- dullness to percussion;
- decreased breath sounds.

Imaging of the pleural cavity

- *Postero-anterior chest X-ray* – in the upright position this shows opacification on the affected side. The height of the fluid level depends on the volume of fluid. The position of the fluid level depends on gravity.
- *Decubitus chest X-ray* – if the patient lies on their side the fluid level will be at right angles to that on the upright posterior–anterior (PA) film as the fluid moves relative to the patient with gravity.
- *Ultrasound* – in particular this can be helpful for guiding aspiration and drainage.
- *CT* – this is helpful for differentiating fluid from solid masses.

MANAGEMENT AND INVESTIGATION OF PLEURAL EFFUSIONS

If the patient is extremely breathless, relief of the breathlessness by drainage is the first priority. It is important to exclude hypoproteinaemia as a cause, as removal of the pleural fluid will merely aggravate the situation. Correction of the hypoproteinaemia is needed instead. With constrictive pericarditis, urgent surgical relief by drainage of the fluid causing the constriction is required either via needle pericardial aspiration or by surgical drainage through resecting a pericardial window.

Diagnosis of the cause of pleural effusion is essential. Management of pleural effusion is shown in Figure 8.6.2.

By following this protocol with the appropriate laboratory analysis, it is almost always possible to ascertain the cause of an effusion, but occasionally the cause remains elusive.

PLEURAL ASPIRATION AND BIOPSY

The mainstay of investigation and diagnosis of pleural effusion is fluid aspiration and pleural biopsy. The pro-

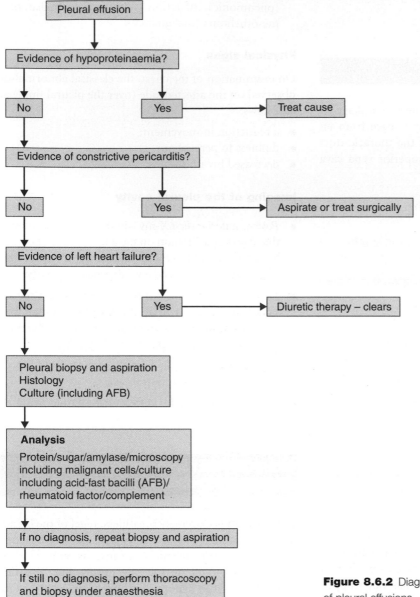

Figure 8.6.2 Diagrammatic representation of management of pleural effusions.

cedure is not without risks, and is therefore described in detail below.

- The technique is fully explained to the patient. Although some may obtain the patient's verbal consent, it is more advisable to obtain written consent for this bedside technique which is performed under local anaesthetic.

- The patient sits comfortably over the side of the bed leaning on to a bedside table, after having received a premedication of IM pethidine 100 mg (as analgesic) and atropine 0.6 mg (to prevent pleural shock).

- The chest X-ray is checked so that the operation is performed on the correct side.

- Under sterile conditions the patient's back is cleaned

and the area of maximum dullness chosen by percussion (do not go lower than the seventh intercostal space).

- The chest wall is infiltrated down to the pleura using 10 mL of 1% plain lignocaine as local anaesthetic. The approach is made over the top of a rib in order to avoid the neurovascular bundles (intercostal nerve, artery and vein) which run in a groove underneath each rib. Using this needle and syringe it is possible to check that the correct site has been chosen by aspirating 5 mL of pleural fluid into the syringe. This ensures that the approach has been neither above the level of the fluid nor below the level of the diaphragm (in the latter case there could be damage to the sub-diaphragmatic organs, such as the liver or spleen).

- After waiting for 3–4 min for the local anaesthetic to work, a small skin incision is made with a scalpel.

- An Abram's pleural biopsy needle is advanced and two or three biopsies of pleura are taken using this needle, avoiding taking a biopsy in the headwards direction, i.e. avoiding injuring the neurovascular bundle running above the needle (under the ribs). The needle is like a crochet hook with sharp jaws which are opened and closed in order to trap a piece of tissue for histological analysis. Classically biopsies are taken at 3, 6 and 9 o'clock, but not at 12 o'clock.

- Pleural fluid is then aspirated through the needle using a 50-mL syringe and three-way tap, and is collected into a bag.

- The most important factor in successfully obtaining a sample is to ensure that the patient and doctor are both comfortable. If the patient becomes uncomfortable for any reason, such as increasing pain, shortness of breath or coughing, the procedure should be discontinued.

- The fluid may be drained more rapidly by the insertion of an intercostal tube such as is used for drainage of air from the pleural space – the fluid being drained via an underwater seal by the bedside. The disadvantage of this approach is that if a large tube is being used the introduction is more hazardous and it tends to be left in the patient for a longer period of time, therefore restricting their mobility. However, with large volumes of fluid the advantage of an intercostal tube is that when all of the fluid has been drained (which is never possible with simple needle aspiration) and if it is known to be malignant, drugs such as tetracycline or other irritants such as talc can be inserted into the pleural space in order to obtain a pleurodesis, i.e. to cause a chemical irritation which will stick the two layers of pleura together, thereby abolishing the pleural space and preventing possible fluid reaccumulation. This procedure, which is commonly used for malignant pleural effusions, has a success rate of 60% and is well worth performing. A variety of irritants can be used, three commonly used agents being tetracycline, bleomycin and talc.

- A chest X-ray should be taken following aspiration to exclude hydropneumothorax and to check whether any fluid is left.

PLEURAL FLUID ANALYSIS

Once aspirated, the pleural fluid is sent to the laboratory for analysis of the following:

- appearance – transudates are usually clear, whereas exudates are often turbid, purulent or bloody;

- protein estimation – in exudate is > 30 g/L, whereas in transudate is < 30 g/L
  (*Note*: 10% of transudates have a higher protein content);

- glucose estimation – this is low in tuberculosis, rheumatoid arthritis, empyema or malignant effusions;

- amylase – this is elevated in pancreatic effusions (with high pH);

- differential cell count – increased lymphocytes > 50% indicates longstanding effusion, TB or malignancy. Polymorph leucocytes are increased in infection. Eosinophils are increased in hypersensitivity (allergic reaction), parasitic infection or malignancy;

- cytology to look for malignant cells, but many malignant effusions cannot be diagnosed solely on the basis of pleural aspirate;

- bacteriology – culture and sensitivity and tuberculosis studies. Direct smears for TB are rarely positive, but cultures are more commonly positive. PCR studies are becoming more widely available.

MEDICAL TREATMENT

Once the cause of the effusion has been found, the primary treatment is that of the underlying condition. Transudates are usually caused by heart failure or fluid overload, and thus the commonest avenue of therapy is one of careful fluid balance and diuretic therapy. The effusions are rarely large enough to warrant drainage to dryness, and drug therapy of the underlying cause is usually adequate.

However, exudates are often larger and cause more respiratory embarrassment, and their underlying causes may also prove more resistant to therapy. It is therefore probable that in many cases of exudate a pleural aspiration to relieve breathlessness will be necessary.

Treatment for the common causes of transudates are for the underlying condition:

- post pneumonia – treat the pneumonia with suitable antibiotics such as amoxycillin and clarithromycin. The effusion usually only needs to be drained if the patient is very breathless or there is an empyema (continuing fever and pus on simple aspiration);

- pulmonary embolism/infarction – anticoagulate effusion does not require draining;

- tuberculosis – treat with conventional antituberculous therapy (rifampicin, isoniazid, pyrazinamide and ethambutol). Drain the effusion if it is large and causing symptoms, and consider the use of oral steroids to prevent pleural fibrosis;

- malignant – once a diagnosis has been made, drain the effusion and refer the patient to an oncologist for treatment of the underlying cause, but consider early pleurodesis to prevent recurrence of the effusion.

COMPLICATIONS OF PLEURAL EFFUSIONS AND DRAINAGE

Hydropneumothorax This is caused by penetration of the underlying lung by the sharp needle during the aspiration of pleural fluid. It is rarely large enough to require separate drainage. A post-aspiration chest X-ray is always recommended. Increased breathlessness would be an indication for tube drainage.

Empyema This may occur either before or as a consequence of aspiration, and is recognized by the presence of swinging pyrexia. In all cases empyema needs rapid and adequate drainage through an intercostal tube with administration of appropriate systemic antibiotics. The tube needs to be of an adequate size to establish continuous drainage. If the empyema fails to drain, then check that the intercostal drain is in the correct position and perform an ultrasound scan of the chest to demonstrate that there is still fluid present and that the chest X-ray shadowing is not simply pleural thickening. If the empyema fluid persists but is not draining, it must be assumed to be loculated, and intrapleural streptokinase should be instilled. Note that streptokinase should not be instilled in the presence of a bronchopleural fistula, and caution should be exercised if tumour is present (although this is no longer considered to be an absolute contraindication). A total of 250 000 units of streptokinase should be instilled in 100 mL of saline and the tube clamped for 4 h and then allowed to drain freely. The streptokinase can be repeated daily for up to 1 week without significant risk of adverse reactions. If thrombolysis fails to clear the empyema, the patient should be referred to a thoracic surgeon for decortication.

Pleural shock This should be preventable by premedication with atropine, but if it occurs during aspiration, lie the patient flat and administer further intravenous atropine immediately.

Air embolism and pulmonary oedema These are both extremely rare complications. The patient requires full resuscitation. Neither of these two rare complications are avoidable.

SURGERY

If simple aspiration and Abram's needle biopsy do not provide the diagnosis, the patient should be referred to the thoracic surgeon for thoracoscopy. This is an operation performed under general anaesthetic in which a telescopic instrument is inserted through the chest wall into the pleural cavity so that the pleural surfaces can be directly inspected and biopsies taken. If the pleural fluid is known to be malignant, surgical pleuradhesis or pleurectomy may be performed.

PNEUMOTHORAX

Pneumothorax is the term given to the situation in which the lung has 'burst' and has collapsed down with air escaping into the pleural space. These cases are termed 'spontaneous' when there is spontaneous escape of air from the lung as a result of abnormality of the visceral pleura (usually a ruptured bulla or bleb at the apex of a lung), or 'traumatic' when they result from chest wall injury with rib fractures leading to damage and puncture of the underlying lung (Table 8.6.4).

Clinical features

Pneumothoraces are common, particularly in young men in their twenties, and are frequent causes for referral to accident and emergency departments.

Symptoms

The features of pneumothorax usually include the following:

- acute chest pain on the affected side;

- breathlessness – the severity of which depends on the size of the pneumothorax and the residual lung functions.

Physical signs

These include the following:

- diminished movement on the affected side;

- hyper-resonance on the affected side;

- diminished breath sounds on the affected side.

As there may often be difficulty in interpreting the physical signs, particularly in patients with chest disease such as asthma, a chest X-ray is essential if the diagnosis is considered.

Investigations

A chest X-ray is diagnostic. An expiratory film shows the pneumothorax as larger than on the inspiratory film

Table 8.6.4 The commonest causes of pneumothorax

- ruptured pleural bleb or bulla – common in young male adults, who are often tall and thin (they may be recurrent and bilateral, and there may be a family history)
- trauma – surgery, stabbing, fractured rib (e.g. during cardiopulmonary resuscitation (CPR) or car crash)
- ruptured emphysematous bulla in chronic obstructive pulmonary disease
- lung biopsies (either percutaneous needle or transbronchial biopsies)
- pleural aspiration
- insertion of subclavian and other central venous catheters
- rupture of cavities into the pleural space staphylococcal abscesses, cavitating tuberculosis or carcinoma
- external cardiac massage and resuscitation in adults
- artificial ventilation
- asthma
- connective tissue disorders
- cystic fibrosis
- Marfan's syndrome

because the positive intrathoracic pressure during expiration compresses the lung.

TENSION PNEUMOTHORAX

This is the term applied to the situation which develops when air continues to accumulate in the pleural space faster than it can be reabsorbed. This may occur if a ruptured bleb acts as a one-way flap valve. A tension pneumothorax constitutes a potentially life-threatening emergency which may complicate a traumatic or spontaneous pneumothorax, and it needs urgent attention.

Tension pneumothorax is recognized by the following symptoms:

- increasing shortness of breath;
- a shift of the mediastinum to the opposite side, i.e. the trachea and apex beat of the heart are displaced to the right with a left tension pneumothorax;
- increasing tachycardia;
- increasing distress.

Management

The British Thoracic Society has published guidelines for the management of spontaneous pneumothorax which also contain guidance on the management of intercostal drains (Miller AC, Harvey JE. 1993: Guidelines for the management of spontaneous pneumothorax. Standards of Care Committee, British Thoracic Society. *British Medical Journal* **307**, 114–16).

- All pneumothoraces should be managed with adequate analgesia.
- Small pneumothoraces will reabsorb spontaneously.
- In slightly larger pneumothoraces the air should be aspirated.
- For very large pneumothoraces an intercostal tube should be inserted.
- Any pneumothorax which is large enough to cause distressing shortness of breath, sweating, hypoxia or cyanosis must be drained immediately.

Drainage techniques used

Several techniques of air aspiration are used.

Simple air aspiration

- A needle covered by a plastic sheath is inserted into the second anterior intercostal space after infiltration with local anaesthetic (1% plain lignocaine).
- The needle is withdrawn and a three-way tap and 60-mL syringe are connected to the plastic sheath.
- The air is aspirated into the syringe with the patient reclining at 30°.
- The process is repeated to allow the lung to re-expand slowly.
- When no more air may be withdrawn despite repositioning of the patient, the plastic cannula is withdrawn.
- Occasionally the lung collapses again, but usually this therapy is adequate.

Intercostal tube drainage

If it is decided that an intercostal tube is needed (because of very large pneumothoraces or distress), this is carried out in a similar manner to the procedure described for pleural fluid drainage.

- Written consent is preferable.
- The drain must be performed under full sterile conditions with the patient being given a premedication (pethidine and atropine).
- The skin and intercostal space are infiltrated with 1% plain lignocaine.
- The site of insertion should be over the upper edge

of the rib in the fourth or fifth intercostal space just behind the anterior axillary line.

- The alternative site, namely the second intercostal space anteriorly (although well documented) may lead to problematic scars, particularly in young women.

- A scalpel is used to cut a hole through the chest wall skin large enough to insert the intercostal tube using blunt dissection with scissors or Spencer Wells forceps down to the pleura.

- A hole large enough for insertion of the tube is made.

- The tube is then placed gently through this preformed hole and then stitched in place with a purse-string suture.

- The tube is connected to a bottle containing 500 mL of 0.9% saline forming an underwater seal.

- Clamps are left by the bedside so that the tube can be clamped off in an emergency.

- The patient is then asked to cough to reinflate the lung.

- The tube is left in place for 24 h after it has stopped bubbling, and is then removed.

- The chest wall wound is sealed by tying the purse-string suture.

- If the lung fails to reinflate and the tube continues to bubble, this indicates a continuing air leak through the pleura (bronchopleural fistula). Gentle suction using a pump is then applied, and after several days or even weeks the bubbling usually ceases.

- Very rarely, thoracotomy is needed to seal an emphysematous bulla or to divide pleural adhesions in the case of ongoing bronchopleural fistula.

Tension pneumothorax is an acute medical emergency and a chest drain should be inserted immediately. If such a drain is unavailable, the largest available needle should be inserted into the side of the pneumothorax to relieve the tension. Even though this will not inflate the rest of the lung, it will prevent the pneumothorax from increasing in size.

COMPLICATIONS OF PNEUMOTHORAX

These include the following:

- surgical emphysema – skin crepitus due to air leaking along the drainage tube into subcutaneous tissue. This requires no therapy except in the very rare cases where the air may track up into and around the larynx, causing airway obstruction. In these cases skin incisions in the neck should be made

to allow air to escape, and in extreme cases tracheostomy may be life-saving;

- tension pneumothorax (see above);

- haemopneumothorax – this requires drainage through a large basal tube, and is usually caused by damage to the intercostal vein or artery at the original injury, or by the insertion of the drainage tube itself. In rare cases urgent referral to a thoracic surgeon for ligation of the bleeding vessel is necessary;

- re-expansion pulmonary oedema. If the lung has been collapsed for a long time and reinflates rapidly, there is a possibility that fluid will accumulate within the lung (pulmonary oedema). The patient becomes very breathless and has difficulty with gas exchange. There is little that can be done to avoid this situation, other than to stop the procedure if vigorous coughing occurs. Oxygen therapy is needed, and if pulmonary oedema occurs then artificial ventilation may be required.

Air aspiration vs. tube drainage

In general, air aspiration of pneumothoraces is recommended because it involves less trauma and a shorter stay in hospital. However, it is not suitable for very large pneumothoraces or bronchopleural fistula, or for life-threatening situations in which rapid air evacuation is essential.

Prognosis and indications for further surgery

A quarter to one-third of patients with spontaneous pneumothoraces have a recurrence. After the second recurrence, i.e. the third pneumothorax, consideration should be given to permanent elimination of the pleural space by referral to a thoracic surgeon for a pleuradhesis in which the pleural surfaces are roughened either medically with drugs or talc, or surgically by abrasion. Alternatively, pleurectomy is performed under a general anaesthetic, in which the layers of pleura on the inside of the chest wall are stripped off, and the lung then heals by sticking to the chest wall, thus obliterating any potential pleural space.

Prevention

There are certain situations in which pneumothorax is more likely to occur, and these are not always totally preventable. Special care needs to be taken with the following:

- resuscitation of the newborn;

- positive pressure ventilation, especially in emphysematous patients;

- insertion of subclavian or other central venous

pressure lines (it is particularly important to avoid bilateral approaches);

- percutaneous or transbronchial lung biopsies;
- chest aspiration;
- external cardiac massage.

ASBESTOS AND THE PLEURA

Exposure to asbestos may result in the development of a number of respiratory diseases, including the following:

- benign pleural plaques;
- fibrosis (asbestosis);
- benign pleural thickening;
- bilateral diffuse pleural thickening;
- diffuse malignant mesothelioma;
- asbestos-related lung cancer.

Asbestos is a general term covering a number of fibrous silicates. Although there are six varieties, only three have been in general use, namely chrysotile (white asbestos), amosite (brown asbestos) and crocidolite (blue asbestos). Chrysotile represents 90% of asbestos production world-wide. The use of crocidolite has been greatly restricted in the UK since 1970.

Importation has now ceased because of the association of asbestos with malignant mesothelioma. Asbestos is fire-retarding and resistant up to 800–900°C, giving it good properties as an acoustic and thermal insulator. Its use is decreasing as alternatives are found.

Occupations that are at risk include the following:

- loading and unloading asbestos sacks from boats;
- mixing asbestos for industrial purposes, particularly spraying;
- removing old lagging material in a confined space;
- lagging and textile material;
- cutting and sawing asbestos cement products;
- exposure by living close to factories.

Small straight fibres less than 3 µm in diameter are those most likely to cause harm because they are able to penetrate furthest into the lungs and thereby irritate the pleura.

Asbestos bodies are asbestos fibres coated with iron-containing protein with a bulbous end which can be found in sputum or bronchoalveolar lavage. These are an indication of past exposure and do not constitute a marker of the presence of disease.

Pleural plaques from asbestos exposure are not compensatable, as they do not cause respiratory disablement. *Diffuse pleural fibrosis* can be caused by asbestos exposure. This may occur in the absence of lung fibrosis, and can cause a restrictive functional impairment and disablement. Diffuse pleural thickening in asbestos workers is usually bilateral.

X-RAY

Chest X-ray shows widespread pleural thickening which classically obliterates the costophrenic angles on posterior–anterior (PA) chest X-ray and thins towards the apex of the lung. Diffuse thickening over the upper zone should suggest causes other than asbestos. It is likely that thickening of more than 5 mm affecting more than a quarter of the height of the chest wall is significant enough to cause symptoms.

A PA chest X-ray with oblique 45° and CT scanning are all helpful in the diagnosis. There may be difficulty in differentiating between benign pleural thickening and mesothelioma or indeed subpleural fat. A biopsy is essential for diagnosis, but not for compensation purposes alone.

Lung function tests show restrictive defect (reduced forced vital capacity) but preserved gas transfer.

MALIGNANT MESOTHELIOMA

This is a primary neoplasm of the pleura, the pericardium or the peritoneum. In 85–90% of individuals there is significant previous asbestos exposure. Crocidolite is the main form of asbestos implicated, but not the only one. There is an average delay of 20 years between exposure and development of tumour. There is usually a substantial exposure, but sometimes it is only limited.

Presentation

This is as follows:

- pleural effusion associated with an irregular pleural mass seen on chest X-ray;
- chest wall pain due to local invasion by tumour – local metastasis is common, while distant metastasis is rare but may occur;
- a definitive diagnosis (biopsy) usually needs to be made from either thoracotomy or thoracoscopy. Histology is not necessary for special medical boards to consider the diagnosis.

Prognosis

The mean expectation of life is from a year to 18 months. Surgery may be attempted for small early tumours with removal of part of the chest wall, but this is only possible in a minority of cases. Malignant mesothelioma tends to be resistant to radiotherapy and chemotherapy.

Brain swelling

James D. Palmer

Introduction

The brain responds to injury in a very similar way to any other part of the body. If you hit your thumb with a hammer it swells, and that process can be at its worst a day or two after the injury. The brain is no different, and if it is injured swelling occurs which can be maximal 48–72 h after the injury. The processes of injury of the brain show some peculiarities compared to other tissues. Injury can result from laceration of brain tissue, bruising (contusion), ischaemia, re-perfusion and release of free radicals, lack of glucose, or a sequence of events leading to excitotoxic injury.

Brain swelling is the term used to describe an increase in brain volume due to an increase in one of the compartments of the brain. This may be due to an increase in the cerebral blood volume (CBV), a mass lesion or an increase in intra- or extracellular water. The blood–brain barrier (BBB) consists of tight junctions between endothelial cells,

and water only crosses this barrier when there are differences in the osmolarity gradient. *Brain oedema* is most commonly due to disruption of the BBB following trauma or inflammation that allows plasma or a filtrate to enter the extracellular space (*vasogenic oedema*). Cellular metabolism can become disrupted following ischaemia, and certain types of drug intoxication (e.g. Reye's syndrome) leading to intracellular water retention (*cytotoxic oedema*). If an unfavourable osmotic gradient operates across the BBB, such as in water intoxication, water is retained within the brain (*osmotic oedema*). In acute renal hypertension the elevated capillary pressure can lead to capillary vasodilatation and a *hydrostatic oedema* induced by a protein-free capillary transudate. Acute hydrocephalus can lead to water extravasation into the periventricular areas (*interstitial oedema*).

BRAIN INJURY

After traumatic brain injury (TBI) the events have classically been divided into *primary* and *secondary* injury. Primary injury is that which occurs as a result of impact and leads to contusion, laceration and axonal damage which treatment cannot modify. Thereafter the injury is susceptible to further (secondary) damage due to the effects of a mass lesion, hypotension, hypoxia and metabolic disruption. The extent of the neuronal injury is determined by the consequences of a cascade of neurochemical and pathophysiological processes that are set in

motion by the initial insult. There is evidence that these events can be contained by pharmaceutical means in spinal injury with high-dose methylprednisolone, but as yet a drug of clear benefit in brain injury has not been found.

The communication between neurones in the brain is primarily through the release of the neurotransmitter glutamate. Transmission of axonal depolarization occurs following the interaction with receptors on the postsynaptic membrane. In normal circumstances small aliquots of the neurotransmitter are released. However, in brain injury the dying neurones release all of their neurotransmitters at once, and the resulting over-activation of neighbouring post-synaptic membranes results in cell death of the nearby neurones (*excitotoxic injury*), and a cascade of extending injury is triggered. Brain injury is followed by a response that includes recruitment of inflammatory cells which adhere to the endothelium, and contraction of endothelial cells with the formation of intercellular gaps. The BBB is disrupted and there is a transvascular movement of the inflammatory cells and fluid.

A free radical is an atom or molecule that possesses an unpaired electron in its outer orbit. Free radicals can be formed after ischaemia and re-perfusion of brain tissue, and they may attempt to extract an electron from nucleic acids (e.g. DNA or RNA). A primary target for these radicals is the polyunsaturated fatty acids of cell membrane phospholipids, resulting in destruction and cell lysis. It is the excitotoxic injury that leads to cell death, prostaglandin synthase activity, free-radical production and lactic acidosis, resulting in grey matter ischaemia and disruption of cell membranes. Ultimately this process spreads to the white matter, with damage to microvascular structures, ischaemia and axonal damage resulting in a neurological deficit.

CAUSES

TRAUMATIC BRAIN INJURY

One million people attend an Emergency Department each year for TBI. Of those that attend, 150 000 individuals are admitted to hospital. The severity of injury is determined by the Glasgow Coma Score after resuscitation (see Table 8.7.1). Causes of brain swelling from a 'mass lesion' may include an extradural haematoma, which is essentially a complication of a skull fracture, and subdural and intraparenchymal haematoma (contusion), which are complications of brain injury. Damage to the axons occurs as a result of the shearing or tearing of the brain in acceleration/deceleration injuries even in relatively minor head injury. Diffuse axonal injury (DAI) is a more widespread pattern of damage in the white matter, the corpus callosum, brainstem and cerebellum. DAI is responsible for coma in patients without mass lesions.

Table 8.7.1 Severity of traumatic brain injury

Glasgow Coma Score	Severity
3–8	Severe
9–12	Moderate
13–15	Mild

VASCULAR BRAIN INJURY

Vascular injury to the brain can be ischaemic or haemorrhagic. Ischaemia can result from embolism, occlusion of cerebral vessels (vasospasm, dissection and penetrating injury) or it can be caused by hypoxia, hypotension and watershed injury. Spontaneous haemorrhage may occur from a ruptured intracranial aneurysm or arteriovenous malformation. After the initial insult of a subarachnoid haemorrhage, 20–25% of patients have further ischaemic brain injury termed 'delayed ischaemic deficit' (DID) in the first 2 weeks.

TUMOURS

These have mass effects on brain tissue, and certain tumour types have a propensity to induce swelling in the substance of the brain around the lesion. Metastatic tumours (e.g. melanoma, breast carcinoma) and meningioma most commonly cause swelling.

INFECTION

The swelling of the brain in response to infection may be florid. A lesion on a brain scan with extensive surrounding oedema raises the suspicion of a cerebral abscess. Encephalitis most commonly causes oedema in the medial part of the temporal lobe.

INTRACRANIAL PRESSURE

The normal intracranial pressure (ICP) is in the range 10–15 mmHg. The Monro-Kellie doctrine is that the volume of the craniospinal compartment which is composed of blood, CSF and brain will remain constant. When the pressure rises in one compartment of the head a pressure differential can occur. The first effect is *volume compensation*, in which CSF moves to a different compartment (e.g. the lumbar thecal sac) and CSF absorption increases. Once the compensatory mechanisms are exhausted, *volume buffering* occurs, which is usually accompanied by a neurological deterioration. In a supratentorial mass lesion the shift forces the brain under the falx (*subfalcine herniation*), and then later through the opening in the tentorium (*transtentorial herniation*). The medial part of the temporal lobe of the brain (*uncal herniation*) can cause pressure on the third cranial nerve, leading to a dilated pupil on the side of the mass lesion.

Herniation of the cerebellar tonsils (*tonsillar herniation*) through the foramen magnum causes brainstem compression and respiratory arrest. The Cushing response of bradycardia and hypertension is usually a signal of irreversible brainstem damage.

Intracranial pressure is pulsatile with regard to both the cardiac and respiratory cycles. Measurement is now routinely available. The most common methods employ a fibre-optic device or a miniaturized pressure transducer implanted into the tissue of the frontal lobe. A waveform can then be recorded. When there is a critical lack of brain *compliance*, a plateau wave (A-wave) may be the first indication, where the intracranial pressure rises – usually to over 40 mmHg – for about 20 min and then falls to a subnormal level before gradually returning to the baseline pressure.

CEREBRAL PERFUSION PRESSURE

The maintenance of an adequate cerebral perfusion pressure (CPP) is the mainstay of the management of brain swelling. The CPP is calculated by subtracting the ICP from the mean arterial blood pressure (MABP). In the normal brain the CPP must fall to lower than 50 mmHg before ischaemia develops. Within certain limits, the normal brain is able to maintain a constant cerebral

blood flow (CBF) by dilating resistance vessels (*cerebral autoregulation*). An injured brain has a markedly reduced capacity to cope with periods of low CPP, and a pressure lower than 70 mmHg can lead to ischaemia and further brain injury due to loss of autoregulation. The measurement of CPP is only possible if the ICP is recorded. The importance of maintaining the MABP is therefore the most significant factor in the management of brain swelling. For example, following a moderate head injury the ICP is often 30 mmHg, and to maintain an adequate CPP the MABP must be kept above 100 mmHg. In a neurosurgical intensive-care setting, management is directed more to the CPP than to the values of the ICP.

CEREBRAL BLOOD FLOW AND CEREBRAL BLOOD VOLUME

The cerebral blood volume (CBV) is approximately 150 mL and the cerebral blood flow is 50 mL/100 g brain/min, representing 20% of cardiac output. An increase in CBV results in an increase in the intracranial pressure (ICP). When the CBF is reduced to less than

Table 8.7.2 Management modalities in brain swelling

Procedure	Indications	Physiological rationale
Airway management	The first action. Should be regularly reassessed	An obstructed airway increases the $PaCO_2$, which leads to dilatation of the cerebral blood vessels, and increases the CBV and hence the ICP. With prolonged obstruction the PaO_2 falls, increasing the risks of ischaemia
Sedation, intubation and ventilation	Should be urgently considered when the patient's Glasgow Coma Score is 8 or less. It needs to be instigated by an anaesthetist who is aware of the effects of the anaesthetic agents on the ICP	A patient in coma is more likely to obstruct their airway. Sedation reduces the brain's requirement for oxygen and glucose – CMR. As there is metabolic coupling between the CMR and CBF, if the CMR is reduced the CBF is reduced. In turn, CBV is reduced and ICP is reduced
Correction of hypoxia and hypotension	The PaO_2 in a self-ventilating patient should be > 9 kPa on air or 12 kPa on oxygen. The mean blood pressure should be greater than 100 mmHg	Hypoxia and hypotension in the resuscitation phase after a brain injury are the largest contributors to poor outcome. When brain swelling is suspected, assume the ICP is at least 30 mmHg; to maintain the CPP above 70 mmHg, the mean arterial blood pressure should be greater than 100 mmHg
Avoid constriction of the neck veins	Make sure that the head and neck are straight. Discard stiff collars as soon as possible, and use a head strap and sandbags in preference. Loosen all clothing and strapping around the neck	Constriction of the neck veins increases the venous pressure and hence the ICP
Head-up position	Avoid any head-down tilt even for central venous cannulation; 30° of head-up tilt is ideal	Head-up tilt reduces the pressure in the jugular bulb and hence reduces the CBV. The neck veins collapse when the pressure is lower than 0, so further elevation greater than 30° will not help to reduce CBV further

Table 8.7.2 (Continued)

Avoid hyperthermia	Cool with ice applied to groin, axilla and neck. Aim to keep the temperature just below normal	With each 1°C rise in body temperature the CMR rises by 6–7%. The rise in CMR leads to an increase in CBF, CBV and hence ICP
Maintain PaO_2	Monitor SaO_2 and arterial blood gases. Give oxygen and ventilation as required	A low PaO_2 will lead to ischaemia
Elective mild hyperventilation	Achieved in the ventilated patient	The cerebral vessel diameter is exquisitely sensitive to changes in CO_2 concentration. Hyperventilation lowers the CO_2 level and causes the vessels to constrict, lowering the CBV and ICP. The localized blood flow is also reduced and hyperventilation below a $PaCO_2$ of 4.0 kPa is harmful, and below 4.5 kPa should be avoided. In some circumstances hyperventilation can be used in a neurosurgical intensive-care setting when the impact on cerebral circulation can be measured by jugular venous oximetry
Steroids	Useful for brain swelling related to brain tumours. The use in cerebral abscess is more controversial as steroids limit the formation of a capsule around the abscess. They are not indicated for TBI or for VBI. They may be helpful in delayed swelling that sometimes accompanies an intracerebral haemorrhage	Steroids have a complicated effect on the brain. Within a short time of administration the ICP is reduced and swelling can be effectively controlled. They decrease CSF production and tumour capillary endothelial permeability, and have a free-radical scavenging effect. Steroids can have an oncolytic effect mainly in cerebral lymphoma. The doses required have major side-effects when given over a prolonged period, such as Cushing's syndrome, skin changes, psychoses and necrosis of the femoral head
Mannitol	Use only on the instruction of a neurosurgeon	Much harm can be done with mannitol, but timely administration can be life-saving. The function of mannitol needs an intact BBB to reduce cerebral swelling. The drug itself given in repeated doses opens the barrier. In brain injury, particularly TBI, in the damaged parts of the brain the BBB is open and mannitol will accumulate in these areas
Evacuation of mass lesions	A mass lesion taking up more than 25 mL of space in the head should be evacuated. Indicators of the need for an emergency operation include effacement of the basal cisterns, midline shift and dilatation of the contralateral temporal horn of the lateral ventricle	It is very difficult to achieve a 25-mL reduction in CBV by medical means, and therefore intraparenchymal mass lesions should be evacuated if they are polar (frontal, temporal, occipital). Brain contusion after TBI develops during the first few days after injury, and repeated scanning will identify delayed lesions which might benefit from surgery
Hydrocephalus management	Neurosurgical management with an external ventricular drain	Swelling of the cerebellum from TCI, VBI or tumour can obliterate the aqueduct leading to an obstructive, non-communicating hydrocephalus. Blood in the ventricular system may occlude the arachnoid villae, reduce the rate of absorption of CSF and lead to a communicating hydrocephalus. Ventricular drainage diverts the fluid until normal physiology is restored

BBB, blood–brain barrier; CBF, cerebral blood flow; CBV, cerebral blood volume; CMR, cerebral metabolic rate; CPP, cerebral perfusion pressure; CSF, cerebrospinal fluid; ICP, intacranial pressure; TBI, traumatic brain injury; VBI, vascular brain injury.

25–30 mL/100 g/min mental confusion develops, the EEG becomes absent at 15 mL/100 g/min and there is severe cellular disruption below 8 mL/100 g/min. The CBV is increased if there is an increase in venous pressure or a dilatation of the cerebral vessels. The venous return from the head is most commonly reduced by compression of the veins in the neck. A rotated neck in an unconscious patient is enough to compromise the venous return, increase the CBV, increase the ICP and reduce the CPP. Useful bedside methods for direct measurement of cerebral blood flow have not been established. The most useful indirect method is jugular bulb oximetry, which measures the arteriovenous difference in oxygen across the brain ($AVDO_2$) and, using the Fick principle, CBF is proportional to $AVDO_2$.

MANAGEMENT

In a similar way to the methods of the Advanced Training Life Support (ATLS) system, the establishment of the diagnosis of brain swelling should not delay the onset of management (Table 8.7.2). The aims of the management of brain swelling are to maintain the CPP by optimizing the MABP and reducing the ICP. These are the principles of resuscitation of any patient. When a patient is in coma (Glasgow Coma Score of ≤ 8) the management of brain swelling should be guided by the monitoring of ICP to measure the CPP.

FURTHER READING

Jennett B, Galbraith S. 1983: *An introduction to neurosurgery.* London: William Heinemann.

Lindsay KW, Bone I, Callander R. 1986: *Neurology and neurosurgery illustrated.* London: Churchill Livingstone.

Palmer JD. 1996: *Neurosurgery '96 manual of neurosurgery.* London: Churchill Livingstone.

Chapter 9

Change in weight

Kenneth C.H. Fearon

Introduction

It is a wonder of physiological regulation that despite variable daily food intake and expenditure, adult human beings tend to remain weight stable. Against this background, a loss of weight is frequently one of the main symptoms that brings a patient to their doctor in the belief that something is seriously wrong. Equally, a change in weight may be detected during the history or physical examination of a patient and alert the clinician to a serious underlying problem that might otherwise have been overlooked. Outside deliberate 'dieting' it is seldom that weight loss can be disregarded as of 'no significance', and hence the importance of this chapter. In contrast, progressive weight gain is commonplace in our consumer society, especially for those in middle age! None the less, the consequences of obesity in terms of excess morbidity and mortality cannot be ignored.

HUMAN BODY COMPOSITION

A knowledge of body composition is fundamental to an understanding of the significance of a change in a patient's weight. The normal 70-kg adult male (Table 9.1) consists of 60% water, 18% fat, 16% protein and 5% minerals. Changes in weight in the acute setting generally reflect alterations in hydration, whereas longer-term changes reflect an alteration in energy or protein balance. It is noteworthy that there are virtually no carbohydrate stores in the body apart from minor deposits of glycogen in the liver and skeletal muscle (and these are readily depleted within 24 h of the onset of starvation). In contrast, the major energy reserve is in the form of triglycerides, which have a high calorific value of 9 kcal/g. Thus a patient needs to be in a prolonged and severe negative energy balance in order to lose significant quantities of adipose tissue.

Fat is the most variable component of human body composition, and may vary from the negligible to the excessive! It should be noted that females in general have a higher proportion of fat than males. The presence of adipose tissue is essential if a human is to withstand a period of partial or complete starvation. However, not all tissues are immediately able to use triglycerides as their sole energy source, and thus other tissues must be auto-cannibalized. The main labile protein reserve in the body is skeletal muscle. However, recent research has drawn attention to amino-acid reserves in the gut and the concept that the physiological atrophy of the latter (with concomitant dysfunction of the gut barrier) may be of fundamental importance to the outcome of the critically injured patient. None the less, during periods of starvation it is muscle that provides the main labile pool of amino-acid precursors for hepatic gluconeogenesis to meet cerebral energy requirements (about 100 g of glucose per day). For each gram of nitrogen that is excreted as a result of amino-acid oxidation, 6.25 g of protein are lost, which is equivalent to 30–35 g in wet weight of skeletal muscle. To put this in context, during the early phase of starvation or acute injury, a patient with a

Table 9.1 Body composition

	Male (70 kg) Percentage of body weight	kg	Female (60 kg) Percentage of body weight	kg
Water	60	42	53	32
Fat	18	13	26	15.5
Protein	16	11.2	16	9.5
Carbohydrate	0.7	0.5	0.5	0.3
Minerals	5.2	3.5	4.5	2.8
Vitamins	Trace	Trace	Trace	Trace

negative nitrogen balance of 15 g N/day will be losing about 0.5 kg of skeletal muscle per day.

However, during prolonged starvation a variety of adaptations occur, including the production by the liver of ketone bodies from triglycerides. The former can substitute for glucose for cerebral energy requirements, and thus after 10–14 days of complete starvation a normal individual may only be losing 2–3 g N/day in the urine, and can thus withstand much longer periods of starvation than if this adaptation had not occurred.

NUTRITIONAL REQUIREMENTS

The normal diet has eight basic components, namely water, carbohydrate, fat, protein, minerals, vitamins, trace elements and fibre. These diverse components can be considered under three general headings – fluid and electrolytes, macronutrients and micronutrients. Fluid and electrolyte balance is covered elsewhere and will not be addressed further in this chapter.

Macronutrient (energy and protein) requirements can vary according to whether an individual needs to maintain, lose or gain weight. Requirements will also vary according to the individual's weight, age, sex, activity and clinical status. Weight is probably the most important variable, and requirements are usually expressed per kg total body weight (Table 9.2). It is important to realize that a variety of the factors mentioned above can act in concert such that the energy requirements of a 40-year-old, male, healthy, lumberjack weighing 85 kg may be two or three times that of a 40-kg, 85-year-old, female, bedridden stroke patient (3500 kcal/day vs. 1200 kcal/day).

When considering the prescription of macronutrients, it is important to appreciate that, in general, energy requirements parallel protein requirements. Moreover, in a mixed balanced diet, these elements cannot be separated from one another. Thus for most enteral or par-

Table 9.2 Estimation of energy and protein requirements in adult surgical patients

	Uncomplicated	Complicated/ stressed
Energy (kcal/kg/day)	30	35–40
Protein (g/kg/day)	1.0	1.3–2.0

enteral solutions the ratio of energy to protein is fixed (e.g. 150 kcal/1 g N) and the overall macronutrient requirements are based primarily on the energy content rather than the protein content of the feed/food.

With regard to the proportion of carbohydrate to fat in the diet, again this is relatively fixed. Current UK Government health guidelines would suggest lowering the average percentage of food energy derived from fat from current levels of 40% to no more than 35%. While this is ideal, frequently the fat content of artificial feeds exceeds these guidelines (principally to reduce the osmolality of the solution), and for short-term nutritional support this is of little consequence. A relatively high fat content is also justified in stress states where fat may be the preferred oxidative fuel, and where too much carbohydrate may lead to hyperglycaemia.

With regard to micronutrients, vitamins are generally regarded as either water soluble (the B group and vitamin C) or fat soluble (vitamins A, D, E and K), and in acute stress the requirements for the former tend to increase more than those for the latter. When refeeding a chronically starved person, it is important to recognize that as a result of anabolism there will be uptake of potassium and phosphate into cells, and that without added supplementation this can result in severe hypokalaemia and hypophosphataemia. The precise requirements for trace elements are not clearly established at present, but clinical deficiency is rare except in patients who have received long-term parenteral nutrition without a trace element supplement.

REGULATION OF ENERGY BALANCE

A change in weight is generally the result of an alteration in food intake, a change in energy expenditure, or a combination of the two. In most human disease states a reduction in food intake is the dominant cause of a negative energy balance. Resting energy expenditure can increase, especially during acute injury/inflammation, but the rise is seldom more than 20% above baseline. Many factors influence food intake, including financial or social circumstances, the presence of a functional gastrointestinal tract, and the normal psychological and physiological inputs to the hypothalamic appetite or satiety centres. It has long been recognized that various components of the diet (e.g. glucose and amino acids) as well as the classical neurohormones (e.g. insulin) may influence appetite. Recently, however, a new mediator has been described, namely leptin. This protein is produced in adipose tissue and causes suppression of the appetite centre, perhaps by altering the ratio of corticotrophin-releasing hormone (inhibitory) to neuropeptide-Y (stimulating) in the hypothalamic appetite centre. The amount of leptin in the circulation varies with dietary intake, but is also influenced by the mass of adipose tissue in the body. Thus leptin is a leading candidate for the mechanism that allows adults to remain weight stable for long periods of their lives. It is also important to recognize that it is at the level of the hypothalamus that inflammatory mediators, such as interleukin-1 or tumour necrosis factor (TNF), are thought to cause suppression of appetite.

CLINICAL ASSESSMENT OF WEIGHT CHANGE

Apart from the amount of weight change, it is important to know how rapidly the change has occurred. Clearly, the more rapid it is, the more likely it is to be due to organic disease. An overall assessment of a patient's weight status can be gleaned by calculating the body mass index (BMI) (weight (kg)/[height (m)]^2). A BMI of 20–25 is considered to be normal. A BMI of < 16 is suggestive of gross malnutrition, and a BMI of 30 indicates significant obesity. Further detailed evaluation of a patient's nutritional status can be achieved using a so-called 'subjective global assessment' (Table 9.3). This six-point scale includes evaluation of weight, appetite, gastrointestinal symptoms, performance status, stress factors and clinical features of malnutrition, and has

Table 9.3 Clinical assessment of malnutrition (subjective global assessment)

Weight change: in past 6 months; in past 2 weeks
Dietary intake: no change; suboptimal; starvation
Gastrointestinal symptoms: anorexia; nausea; vomiting; diarrhoea
Functional capacity: normal; suboptimal work; ambulatory; bedridden
Stress: nil; minimal; high
Physical signs: loss of fat/muscle; oedema; mucosal lesions

been shown to be equivalent to even the most sophisticated forms of body composition analysis or biochemical assessment of nutritional status.

In the evaluation of weight change, one of the most important variables is appetite. In a patient with weight loss there may be an obvious cause to explain a reduction in appetite, but sometimes it is difficult to gauge intake precisely without recourse to detailed in-patient dietary studies. For example, in anorexia nervosa, patients may be deliberately misleading about their intake. In a contrasting group of patients, the striking feature is the presence of a good or increased appetite in the face of weight loss. In such patients the diagnosis is often obvious (e.g. diabetes mellitus or thyrotoxicosis), but may be more obscure (e.g. steatorrhoea in pancreatic insufficiency). Finally, there is perhaps the largest group of patients in whom there is some change in appetite, but weight change seems to be in excess of that which might be expected. In such patients there may be another group of symptoms or signs that clearly leads to the diagnosis. If no other symptom or sign is apparent in the presenting complaint, then systematic questioning and careful clinical examination needs to be undertaken before organizing appropriate investigation. In the syndrome of severe weight loss known as cachexia (from the Greek words *kakos* and *hexis* meaning poor condition) careful note should be taken of associated features such as early satiety (feeling 'full' quickly), aesthenia, anaemia and oedema. It is important to realize that in addition to advanced cancer and AIDS, other conditions such as severe cardiac disease, emphysema, TB, chronic renal or liver failure and rheumatoid arthritis can also lead to a cachectic state.

IMPORTANT CAUSES OF WEIGHT LOSS

MALIGNANT DISEASE

Weight loss is frequently part of the presenting complaint, particularly in lung or gastrointestinal malignancy. Patients with oesophageal or gastric cancer may have associated dysphagia, vomiting or early satiety. The majority of patients with pancreatic cancer will usually have lost considerable weight by the time they present with painless obstructive jaundice. Patients with colorectal cancer usually present with rectal bleeding or anaemia, but may have lost weight due to symptoms of subacute intestinal obstruction. However, marked weight loss is relatively uncommon and only becomes apparent with advanced hepatic metastasis. The development of malignant ascites may mask weight loss, and this is especially important in patients with advanced ovarian carcinoma, who again may have problems with subacute intestinal obstruction. Classical 'B' symptoms of lymphoma include sweats, fever and weight loss. A similar picture can occur in renal adenocarcinoma, and both cases point to a common metabolic component of weight loss in cancer which is thought to be driven in part by pro-inflammatory cytokines.

ENDOCRINE DISORDERS

The diabetic patient who presents with weight loss will generally have associated polyuria and polydipsia and be type I or insulin-dependent. Simple urinalysis for glycosuria is a good screening diagnostic test. Very occasionally a picture of glycosuria and weight loss may occur with phaeochromocytoma, the latter being associated with attacks of pallor or palpitations with or without hypertension. Patients with thyrotoxicosis frequently present with weight loss (despite a hearty appetite), and associated sweating, heat intolerance, diarrhoea, anxiety or palpitations should aid the diagnosis. In adrenal insufficiency weight loss can be a feature. Pigmentation may be the single most helpful diagnostic clue among a variety of ill-defined features such as tiredness, nausea and postural hypotension.

GASTROINTESTINAL CAUSES

Persistent vomiting or diarrhoea will inevitably lead to progressive weight loss. In patients with vomiting, clearly an obstructive malignancy, especially of the upper gastrointestinal tract, needs to be excluded. The age of the patient, the presence of an epigastric mass or the detection of supraclavicular lymphadenopathy or hepatic enlargement may give clues to the diagnosis.

Gastric outlet obstruction due to recurrent peptic ulceration is relatively rare nowadays, but the classical features of vomiting of recognizable old food and the presence of a succussion splash aid in the diagnosis. Patients who have undergone a previous partial or total gastrectomy are prone to early satiety, dumping and malabsorption and often do not regain their usual 'fighting' weight.

Any cause of chronic diarrhoea is likely to give rise to weight loss, especially if the small bowel is involved, e.g. Crohn's disease. Malabsorption due to small-bowel problems such as coeliac disease may be associated with weight loss and steatorrhoea. Often, however, the classical features of steatorrhoea are absent, and this may give rise to confusion. In contrast, for patients suffering from pancreatic insufficiency (e.g. chronic pancreatitis) the features of steatorrhoea are often a clear part of the patient's presenting complaint.

CHRONIC INFECTIONS

In the modern era it is always important to be aware of the possibility of HIV, especially in the 'at-risk' population (IV drug abusers or homosexuals). The presence of weight loss, widespread lymphadenopathy and development of opportunistic infections heralds the development of full-blown AIDS. However, it should be remembered that the principal cause of weight loss in such patients is the development of opportunistic infections (particularly of the gut), and that adequate treatment of the latter will frequently lead to an improved appetite and restoration of normal nutritional status.

A major and increasing world-wide infectious process commonly associated with weight loss and cachexia is TB. The presence of respiratory symptoms and an abnormal chest X-ray are important clues to the diagnosis. However, miliary TB can still be a difficult diagnosis, but rarely presents with weight loss alone.

PSYCHIATRIC CAUSES

Anorexia nervosa is an increasingly recognized problem in young women, but about 10% of cases are in men. Patients have an altered image of their body habitus, and frequently it is their relatives rather than themselves who are concerned about severe weight loss. Treatment is difficult, and is often made more so by the lengths to which patients will go to hide food and deny their problem.

Weight loss is a common feature of both anxiety and depressive states. Thyroid function tests should be checked if there is any doubt about the aetiology of weight loss in a patient with anxiety. In patients with depression, other somatic symptoms such as early waking and constipation may aid the diagnosis.

IMPORTANT CAUSES OF WEIGHT GAIN

For the vast majority of the population, weight gain or the attainment of obesity is simply a reflection of over-eating and lack of physical exercise. The importance of simple obesity and its almost epidemic proportions should not be underestimated. Morbidly obese patients have a substantial excess mortality as a result of cardiovascular disease, hypertension and diabetes. Occasionally specific endocrine syndromes may account for weight gain. In hypothyroidism, associated features such as low mentation, cold intolerance, constipation and a croaking voice should alert the astute clinician. Patients with Cushing's syndrome may show specific alterations with a moon face, truncal obesity, buffalo hump, striae and hirsutism. The presence of complicating features such as hypertension or diabetes should be actively pursued. Alternatively, patients may gain weight due to fluid retention (e.g. progressive cardiac failure), but usually the underlying cause is clinically obvious.

TREATMENT OF WEIGHT LOSS

For patients with weight loss it is essential to make a clear diagnosis and treat the underlying condition. In some instances this will result in a spontaneous return of appetite and restoration of health. However, it is a sobering statistic that in a recent survey of malnutrition in hospitals in the UK, one-third of patients entered hospital in a malnourished state and two-thirds left hospital in a malnourished state! Thus one certainly cannot assume that patients will improve spontaneously, especially given the poor quality of food for in-patients and the lack of nursing time to ensure that elderly or debilitated patients are able to consume their food.

One of the main principles of nutritional support is to administer the latter via the gastrointestinal tract. Compared to intravenous nutrition, this route is safe, cheap and physiologically advantageous. As mentioned above, the first cornerstone in getting patients to put on weight is the provision of regular, warm, appetizing meals, together with the means to consume the food. For patients with early satiety, the provision of calorie-dense, high-protein, milk-based oral supplements to consume between meals can be a useful adjunct. Patient fatigue, together with a limited range of flavours and the tendency to replace the intake of normal food with such supplements, can undermine their benefit.

For patients with severe anorexia or problems with swallowing, the provision of fine-bore nasogastric feeding is a useful therapeutic manoeuvre. Longer-term feeding may require siting of a percutaneous gastrostomy (which can often be inserted endoscopically). The advice of the unit dietitian should be sought about the practical aspects of such enteral feeding.

Finally, if there is failure of the gastrointestinal tract then there should be no hesitation in the use of intravenous feeding. However, this frequently requires provision of a central venous catheter and may be fraught with a variety of mechanical, septic or metabolic complications if not carefully supervised by a dedicated hospital nutrition team. Overall, it should be remembered that regardless of the route of nutritional support, the benefits of the latter depend on the patient actually receiving what has been prescribed (rather than frequent interruptions to enteral or parenteral feeding for investigations or drug administration), and on the presence of a normal metabolic milieu in the patient. For those with chronic inflammation or cancer, there is an apparent partial block to the accretion of lean tissue. The use of specific nutrients (e.g. glutamine), endocrine manipulations (e.g. exogenous insulin or growth hormone administration) or anti-inflammatory strategies (e.g. non-steroidal drugs, fish oil) in combination with conventional nutritional support offers the best hope for the future nutritional care of such patients, but this remains an area of active research rather than an established mode of therapy.

FURTHER READING

Garrow J. 1994: Starvation in hospital. *British Medical Journal* **308**, 934.

Kinney JM, Jeejeebhoy KN, Hill GL, Owen OE. 1988: *Nutrition and metabolism in patient care.* London: W.B. Saunders.

Working Party on Enteral and Parenteral Feeding in Hospital and at Home. 1992: *A positive approach to nutrition as treatment. Report of a working party chaired by J.E. Lennard-Jones on the role of enteral and parenteral feeding in hospital and at home.* London: King's Fund Centre.

Fever

Åke Andrén-Sandberg

Introduction

Normal body temperature values are distributed in a Gaussian manner and are subject to circadian variation. Therefore, the normal body temperature of 37°C is better replaced by an upper limit of 37.1°C in the morning (6 a.m.) and 37.4°C in the afternoon (4 p.m.). The range for 95% of healthy individuals is about 1.2°C, which suggests that, for example, a temperature of 36.0°C in the early morning should be regarded as normal. Women have a body temperature about 0.2°C higher than that of men. The body temperature is raised after exercise (a marathon runner has a temperature of 40°C or more at the end of a race, even if it is cold outside) and is also subject to other physiological variations. For example, the body temperature is increased at the time of ovulation and throughout pregnancy, and it is also increased in response to psychological stress.

The temperature is usually 0.6°C higher in the rectum than in the oral cavity, where it is in turn 0.6°C higher than in the axilla. The ear-drum temperature is usually about 0.1°C higher than that in the axilla. If an increased temperature is being sought, all of these methods of measuring body temperature are adequate if applied according to the thermometer manufacturer's instructions. However, it is important to keep to one measurement modality, as it is usually the changes in temperature rather than the absolute temperature that are of interest in clinical medicine. In a cold or hot environment, rectal measurements are preferable. When diagnosing hypothermia, only a rectal measurement is sufficiently accurate, and in hospital an oesophageal measurement is recommended.

Body tissues are poor heat conductors, and the body has a high heat capacity, resulting in a long lag in body temperature change on exposure to very cold or very warm environments. Clinically, the temperature around the patient is of importance only under two circumstances: first, when the patient is outside in cold weather and cannot protect him- or herself from the cold for several hours (especially if intoxicated), and secondly when he or she is ill. The latter situation could be exemplified by the conditions that prevail in an operating theatre, where the patient can lose so much heat that the body temperature falls so low that it influences the reactions to hypoxia (a rise in chemoreceptor activity) and to the anaesthetic agents, and it also could impair the blood-clotting system. In addition, the anaesthetist needs to be aware that barbiturates and steroids selectively block the autonomic pathways for temperature control.

The temperature is raised in response to disease, this condition being known as fever (or pyrexia). Fever develops when cytokines (e.g. interleukins 1, 2 and 6, interferons and tumour necrosis factor-alpha) are released as a response (inflammation) of the body to tissue damage. Although the cytokines do not pass the blood–brain barrier, they increase the thermostatic 'set point' in the hypothalamus by inducing prostaglandins in the cells lining the brain ventricles, which in turn results in increased heat production and decreased heat dissipation. The highest and most constant fevers occur in infectious diseases, but fever is also associated with collagen disease and some neoplasms, thrombosis, ischaemia, brainstem disease and drug reactions.

The term 'hyperthermia' should be used when the thermostatic set point is normal but the heat control mechanisms fails.

There are individual differences not only in normal temperature regulation, but also in response to infection and inflammation. However, each person reacts in a fairly consistent manner, i.e. an individual who reacts with a high fever to a particular infection once will probably react in the same way the next time. In the elderly (>75 years) the fever reaction commonly declines.

FEVER – FRIEND OR FOE?

Fever is seen in most animals as a response to stress, irrespective of the cause, although the most common cause of fever is infection. Animals that cannot regulate their body temperature, such as fishes and reptiles, react to an infection by looking for warmer conditions, which might be regarded as an induced fever. This indicates that fever is in some way beneficial to those with infectious desease.

Fever may up regulate some host defence mechanisms. The increased body temperature also inhibits growth of bacteria under specified conditions, and in Gram-negative sepsis there is a positive correlation between survival and the maximum temperature. Induced fever has been used as a treatment for infectious diseases in the past. In animal experiments it has been shown that after a bacterial infection there is a higher survival rate among animals housed under the warmest conditions compared to those housed in a normal heated environment.

On the negative side, the heart rate is increased by about 9 beats/min and oxygen consumption is increased by about 7% per 1°C rise in temperature. The increased heart rate and oxygen consumption reflect a higher metabolism, which in the short term is probably relatively harmless, but which if prolonged demands so much energy that healthy tissue, i.e. skeletal muscle, is also broken down. There is also a concomitant increased water loss (300–500 mL/m^2/day per 1°C), but despite this there is an anaemia, which is part of the acute-phase reaction. High temperature is accompanied by alveolar hyperventilation which leads to alkalosis.

Therefore the question of whether fever is a friend or a foe depends on the clinical circumstances. Antipyretic pharmacological treatment should not be administered routinely. In the case of pure hyperthermia, e.g. as a result of brain damage in stroke, physical cooling is appropriate, but in the case of acute abdomen, the evolution of the untreated fever reaction might be of great value in making the right diagnosis.

FEVER MEANS DIFFERENT THINGS IN DIFFERENT CLINICAL SETTINGS

From a surgical perspective, fever should be viewed differently, for example, if seen in the emergency room in a patient with a known or unknown disease, and if it appears post-operatively. The cause of pyrexia is usually obvious after a limited investigation in most cases that present to a surgeon. In surgical practice common acute infections are also seen most often. They are not associated with diseases that should be treated surgically, but they may appear concomitantly. Usually these benign diseases have run their course within a few days to a week, and the fever has a characteristic pattern of onset, duration and lysis. Moreover, in cases of acute abdomen the fever usually follows a characteristic course, although in these cases less attention should be paid to the fever than to the localizing abdominal symptoms.

If fever is seen in the emergency room in a patient with a known surgical disease, all efforts should be made to treat the underlying disease. It is not uncommon for the fever to develop as a result of a secondary disease, but even then it is important to treat the primary disease in the most effective manner possible before looking for other causes. For example, in cases of pneumonia, which is not uncommon in patients with acute or chronic abdominal diseases, and which causes malaise, the patient should be rested and the ventilation increased to reduce atelectasis. In these patients, fever and pneumonia should always be regarded as secondary events until proven otherwise. Post-operative urinary tract infections should also be regarded as a complication of a secondary disease (e.g. outflow problems from the bladder). Under these circumstances antibiotic treatment may only form part of the management strategy.

If fever is one of the presenting symptoms that brings the patient to the doctor, the raised temperature should be regarded as a general reaction of the body, just like an increased leucocyte blood count, C-reactive protein (CRP) or erythrocyte sedimentation rate (ESR). This implies that localized symptoms from specific organs (e.g. lungs, urinary tract, appendix, gall bladder, liver, pancreas, etc.) should be looked for before the fever itself is treated.

In 1961, 'fever of unknown origin' was defined as illness of more than 3 weeks' duration, fever higher than 38.3°C on several occasions, and uncertain diagnosis after 1 week of study. However, a diagnosis is eventually made in 90% of such cases through careful and repeated history, examination and investigation. In most studies about 50% of the patients are found to have an infective source, 20% a collagen disease and 20% a neoplasm. The diagnosis is usually one of a common condition presenting in an unusual manner, rather than a rare disease.

Fever in the post-operative period greatly aids the detection of complications, and every raised temperature should be taken seriously. Around 95 % of all post-operative fevers are caused by four types of complication, namely deep or superficial wound infection, pneumonia, lower urinary tract infection or deep vein thrombosis.

DIAGNOSIS

Diagnosis involves pattern recognition. This approach may be difficult when the clinical features are few, subtle or insufficient to characterize the fever. There are no really good algorithms and few clues that reliably suggest or exclude a certain cause of fever. The diagnostic approach to fever is therefore not uniform, but must always include a thorough history and a careful physical examination. In specific situations relatively simple laboratory tests and radiographic studies are of value.

A thorough history is important, and in surgical patients should include information about previous operations and symptoms arising from the gastointestinal tract and the thorax. All aspects of pain may be important, including its characteristics, debut, duration, etc. Previous inflammatory conditions in the abdomen (e.g. Crohn's disease, cholecystitis, diverticulitis and gynaecological disorders) should always be asked for. Unfortunately, localized complaints are not always present even in these diseases. In a series in which the cause of fever was unknown for a long period, only about 50% of the febrile patients with abdominal disease had abdominal complaints. Moreover, enquires should be made about alcohol intake, smoking, medications, occupational exposure, pets, overseas travel, familial disorders and previous illnesses.

A patient in the emergency room with fever of unknown origin will probably already have had their history taken on a number of occasions. Great skill is then required to obtain previously unknown information, but enquires must always be made about new symptoms. Every organ system must be investigated by detailed questioning, and even trivial symptoms or slight incidents in the history must be fully assessed. With regard to drug history, remember to consider both prescribed medications and non-prescriptive drugs, which may have been bought over the counter for minor ailments, as well as recreational drugs and any injections.

In the physical examination, note the pulse, blood pressure and respiratory rate. In some cases it is appropriate to check the temperature while watching to ensure that the patient is not interfering with the reading. A temperature chart indicates the level and characteristics of the fever. A spiky record suggests the presence of pus, while night fever may be associated with tuberculosis. The general appearance of the patient is important, e.g. whether they look unwell despite being pyrexial, whether they are pale or jaundiced, and whether there is obvious weight loss as a sign of chronic disease.

FEVER IN THE ACUTE ABDOMEN

Hidden and unsuspected causes of fever are commonly found in the abdomen. It is important to examine for superficial, deep and rebound tenderness, and to palpate for masses and viscera, especially hepatosplenomegaly and perinephric masses. Abnormalities along the large bowel – such as malignancy or pericolic abscesses – may be palpable. Check hernial orifices to ensure that they do not contain ischaemic bowel or omentum. Pelvic examination is a very important assessment, including rectal and gynaecological digital and instrumental examination. Pus or tumour may be present in the pouch of Douglas, and tube or ovarian disease may be detected.

According to Zachary Cope:

(*About acute appendicitis*)

For lymph soon forms outside the appendix
and to parietes adjacent sticks;
Then toxins are absorbed with greater ease
So fever comes – just two or three degrees

(*About acute cholecystitis*)

There will be fever and some constipation
Which may be taken in consideration

(from Cope Z. *The acute abdomen in rhyme*, 5th edn. London: Lewis)

With regard to acute abdomen, the first and most important point to understand is that the vital signs, such as temperature, pulse rate and respiration rate, may help to differentiate those cases that have an abdominal disease which should be treated by surgeons from those who could be looked after outside hospital. On the other hand, these signs, including fever, do not often help greatly to distinguish between different 'surgical' diagnoses, and do not distinguish patients who should undergo surgery from the others. For example, the fever pattern is similar in appendicitis and non-specific abdominal pain.

Patients with bacterial diseases such as appendicitis and diverticulitis typically show a gradual increase in temperature. When the patient comes to hospital they usually have a temperature of 37.8°C or 38.2°C, rather than 39°C or 40°C. There are seldom spikes in the fever as in the septic state, and even when there is a local peritonitis, the fever is seldom more than 38.5°C. If the appendix perforates or there is diverticulitis, often a small decrease in fever is observed, accompanied by an overall increase in well-being, but if the disease progresses to a diffuse peritonitis the fever increases again, and after a further 24 h the patient may be septic with spikes of fever over 40°C.

In cholecystitis, hepatitis and pancreatitis the body temperature is often only slightly increased, if at all, on admission to hospital, even though the patient is in considerable pain and is experiencing severe malaise. It may be several days before the temperature is raised to 39°C or more, and the fever is then probably due to a secondary infection in the severely inflamed or necrotic tissues.

There are also cases with pain in the upper right part of the abdomen in which a fever above 39.5°C is the most prominent feature. This is probably a sign of a primary bacterial infection, as in cholangitis – even though the cholangitis is secondary to some obstruction to outflow of the bile (e.g. stone, stricture, neoplasm) – which is now rarely fatal, but if untreated is still very dangerous. If correctly treated, the fever is usually normalized within 24 h in such cases.

After perforation of the stomach, duodenum or colon there is also a raised body temperature. However, the other symptoms of peritonitis (pain, hypotension and tachycardia) are much more alarming in these cases. Even in severely ill patients the fever in such cases is of rather low grade. Both children and the elderly not uncommonly seek help for abdominal symptoms that turn out to be 'only' constipation. In these cases fever of around 38°C is also usually seen.

decline in rheumatic fever in the developed world and the wide availability of accurate testing for SLE that permits early diagnosis. Infective endocarditis has decreased in frequency, but may reappear under new circumstances, e.g. after longstanding intravenous treatment or nutrition.

Certain viruses, such as infective mononucleosis, hepatitis and cytomegalovirus, may have a prolonged course, as do diseases caused by granuloma-producing organisms such as tuberculosis, actinomycosis, toxoplasmosis, histoplasmosis and candidiasis. A number of endemic infectious diseases must be considered in their chosen habitat and in visitors from these areas, e.g. malaria, schistosomiasis, amoebiasis and trypanosomiasis.

Recognition that the causes of unexplained fever in patients with impaired immunity may differ from those in other febrile disorders has prompted special subgrouping in neoplastic diseases, HIV infections, etc.

The inflammatory response produces pyrexia in non-infective disorders, particularly immunological conditions, including the collagen diseases, rheumatoid arthritis, systemic lupus erythematosus, polyarteritis nodosa, temporal arteritis and polymyalgia. Some tumours characteristically have a fever, including hypernephroma, leukaemia, lymphoma and, occasionally, pancreatic carcinoma, liver metastases and sarcomas. Other less common causes include venous thrombosis, pulmonary embolism, cirrhosis and sarcoidosis.

Intracranial disease and associated surgery can interfere with hypothalamic control of temperature, producing marked pyrexia, which may be difficult to control. Almost any drug can produce a febrile reaction, but of note are those linked with sulphonamides, penicillin and barbiturates.

A fictitious pyrexia is occasionally encountered, the patient having placed the thermometer in hot water (tea or coffee) or exchanged thermometers. Watching the patient during a sublingual measurement can provide an accurate result. Suspicion is raised if the pyrexia is not accompanied by an equivalent rise in pulse rate.

FEVER OF UNKNOWN ORIGIN IN THE EMERGENCY ROOM

The proportions of cases of fever of unknown origin grouped in specific disease categories have changed little over the years. Infection accounts for about one-third of cases, followed by neoplasia and collagen vascular disease. The role of certain individual diseases has changed considerably. For example, rheumatic fever and systemic lupus erythematosus (SLE) were common in the first half of this century, probably because of the sharp

POST-OPERATIVE FEVER

Post-operatively there are four causes of fever that should always be considered first:

- deep or superficial wound infection;
- pulmonary infection;
- venous thrombosis;
- urinary tract infection.

All types of surgery may have infectious complications (Figure 10.1), and the more extensive the surgery the higher the risk. Acute operations carry a higher risk than

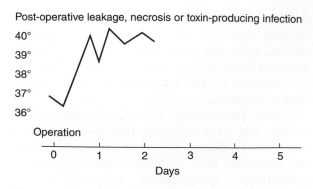
Post-operative leakage, necrosis or toxin-producing infection

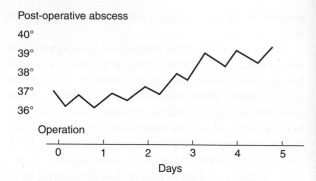
Post-operative abscess

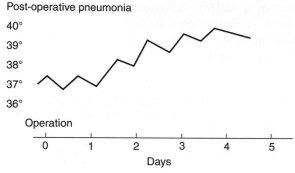
Post-operative pneumonia

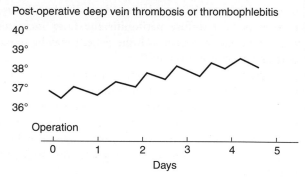
Post-operative deep vein thrombosis or thrombophlebitis

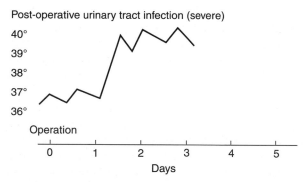
Post-operative urinary tract infection (severe)

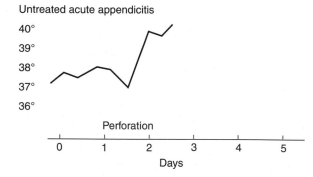
Untreated acute appendicitis

Figure 10.1 Typical fever patterns.

elective ones. The sooner the fever appears after an operation, the more serious is the complication. Patients who present with high fever on the first or second day after an abdominal or thoracic operation almost certainly have a leak in an anastomosis, a major necrosis, or an infection of toxin-producing bacteria, such as *Clostridium*. These complications have a high mortality rate and should be treated with the greatest expertise available, preferably in an intensive-care unit. Vigorous diagnostic efforts should be made to check all anastomoses, and if it cannot be established with certainty that these are intact, a laparotomy or thoracotomy must be considered. A negative result on opening of the surgical wound can also be important in these cases, and is rarely dangerous for the patient. Peroperatively cultures should be taken not only from the blood but also from any fluid collections that are found, including retroperitoneal and mediastinum sources.

Retention of blood or secretion gives low-grade and constant fever up to about 38°C, but if pus is present the

temperature will gradually increase more, and will usually be more spiky in nature.

If the fever appears later it can still be due to an insufficient anastomosis, but will not then form a diffuse peritonitis but rather a localized phlegmon or abscess, and it is then less dangerous. A rectal examination should always be performed after any abdominal surgery if there is a suspicion of infection. Localized abdominal infections should also be treated surgically, but if the leaking anastomosis appears very late, a drainage procedure (broad drains also evacuating thick pus) combined with antibiotic treatment may be sufficient for healing in some cases. Typically the fever in such cases appears as a sudden rise from normal to 38.5°C or 40°C, at which temperature it stays until the pus is evacuated.

The fever reaction is the same whether the postoperative infection is superficial (subcutaneous or intramuscular) or deep in the abdomen or thorax, but the pain pattern is different. The more superficial the infection, the more distinctly the patient can localize the throbbing pain, whereas pain due to deeper-seated infection is more difficult to pinpoint.

Post-operative pneumonia can appear at any stage of rehabilitation until the patient is fully mobilized and the bowel is functioning. Atelectasis and decreased cough efforts increase the risk considerably. The fever is rarely as high as 40°C, and may reach different levels on different days. The general state of the patient is often not so strongly influenced as with an abscess, and the diagnosis is easily made with auscultation of the lungs (the extent can be verified by X-ray).

The fever accompanying post-operative thrombosis is commonly of low grade but slowly and steadily increasing. It is not possible to draw conclusions from the fever pattern as to whether the fever is due to a low-risk superficial thrombophlebitis or whether it is due to a potentially fatal deep vein thrombosis.

Post-operative urinary tract infections are seen after the use of indwelling urethral catheters, and in older men with hyperplasia of the prostate. There is usually pain on palpation over the urinary bladder in these cases, and also over the kidneys in severe infections. The external genitalia should also be inspected, as urethritis may give an oedema at the orifice of the urethra, and in men epidydimitis always causes a swollen scrotum. These infections are more common in elderly than in young patients, in women than in men, and after more extensive surgery. The higher the temperature, the more local symptomatology arises from the lower or upper urinary tract, and the more dangerous is the infection. A sudden increase in body temperature to 40°C combined with localized symptoms indicates urinary tract sepsis, which may be fatal in old or debilitated patients if not treated promptly with intravenous fluid, antibiotics and relief of the urinary outflow obstruction.

Post-operative fever may also be due to unrelated 'common' infections. Therefore the tonsils and the pharynx should always be inspected. Drug reactions may also produce fever, which can reach 40°C without the concomitant pulse increase noted in infectious fever.

MANAGEMENT OF FEVER

The treatment methods for fever can be classified as symptomatic cooling and treating the cause. The first approach involves acceleration of heat loss by the use of external cooling processes, namely nursing the patient nude, tepid water sponging, and the use of fans and ice packs. Internal cooling by stomach or intraperitoneal lavage can be an effective way of removing heat, and has the advantage of avoiding reflex cutaneous vasoconstriction, but practically this approach is only used in severely ill patients.

The most widely used pharmacological agents include paracetamol, which in fever acts by increasing heat dissipation in normal skin by sweating and increasing peripheral blood flow secondary to internal resetting of the central thermostat back to normal levels. Occasionally the careful use of vasodilators to overcome vasoconstriction may also be necessary.

Of course, it is always preferable to treat the underlying disease that is causing fever. In surgical diseases this almost always means removing the inflammation by excision, or at least by drainage of pus. However, there is always also a place for 'one shot' of antibiotics, or alternatively a few days of treatment (not infrequently surgeons give expensive antibiotics for far too long), as a complement to the invasive procedures.

HYPOTHERMIA

Cold injury can be classified as local or systemic hypothermia.

SYSTEMIC HYPOTHERMIA

Systemic hypothermia is usually defined as a reduction in core temperature to below 35°C. In the absence of concomitant traumatic injury, the condition is classified as mild if above 32°C and severe if below 30°C. Below 28°C, lethal cardiac arrythmias may occur. The elderly are particularly susceptible to hypothermia because of their impaired ability to increase heat production and decrease heat loss by vasoconstriction. Children are also more susceptible because of their relatively large body surface area (in relation to volume) and limited energy sources.

Clinically, the hypothermic individual becomes drowsy, gradually deteriorating to unconsciousness. Intense widespread vasoconstriction produces a relative increase in circulatory volume, with hypertension and cold diuresis, the latter probably accounting for much of the weight loss observed on cold exposure. There may also be pulmonary hypertension and right heart failure ('Eskimo lung'). The blood viscosity and packed cell volume are increased, and there may be thrombosis of peripheral vessels. Low temperatures reduce nerve conduction, with reduced sensation and motor power. There is a loss of dexterity, which is also limited by stiffness of the joints due to the increased viscosity of the synovial fluid. Muscles stiffen and can rupture.

Vital signs, including pulse rate, respiratory rate and blood pressure, are all variable, and the absence of respiratory or cardiac activity is not uncommon in patients who eventually recover. Signs of respiratory and cardiac activity are easily missed unless a careful assessment is conducted.

Cardiac output falls in proportion to the degree of hypothermia. Ventricular fibrillation becomes increasingly common as the temperature falls below 25°C. Cardiac drugs and defibrillation should be reserved until the patient is warmed to 28°C. Dopamine is the only inotrope that has any utility in hypothermic patients. 'Uncorrected' blood gases, i.e. determined without warming the sample to 37°C, should be used as a guide to bicarbonate administration. Patients should be given 100% oxygen during the rewarming process. Rewarming attempts should not delay transfer to a critical-care setting.

Hypothermia alters mental function, with loss of insight, poor judgement, unnatural acts (e.g. paradoxical undressing, and attempts to kill companions) and hallucinations, deteriorating to coma.

Trauma patients are susceptible to hypothermia, and any degree of hypothermia in the trauma patient may be detrimental. In these patients hypothermia is considered to be any core temperature below 36°C, and severe hypothermia any core temperature below 32°C.

The determination of death in the hypothermic patient is difficult. It is not possible to declare a patient dead until they are warm. The exception to this axiom is the hypothermic patient who suffers an anoxic event while normothermic, is pulseless and without spontaneous respiration, and has a serum potassium level of 10 mmol/L. Death must not be diagnosed until the core temperature has returned to normal.

LOCAL HYPOTHERMIA

Local pathological responses to cold include frost nip and superficial and deep frostbite. Frost nip is a blanching of the skin, with sensory loss (numbness) and pain, but the tissue remains pliable. There is rewarming and painful hyperaemia, and there may be minor superficial skin desquamation. Tissue loss is seen only with repeated exposure. In superficial frostbite there is superficial skin death, and rewarming of the white blanched skin is accompanied by blotchy, purplish discoloration and blistering. This is gradually converted to a black carapace, which takes many weeks to separate, but a thin, new epithelial layer is in place when it falls off. Deep frostbite is accompanied by crystal formation of interstitial fluid, with cell death and associated thrombosis of small vessels. The tissues are rigid and the extent of tissue loss is difficult to determine. The gangrenous area shrivels and the inflammatory response of the adjacent viable tissue eventually forms a line of demarcation.

HYPOTHERMIA OF OPERATIVE SURGICAL PROCEDURES

There is ample evidence that substantial decreases in core temperature occur during surgical procedures under general anaesthesia, and that during recovery patients exhibit untoward skin vasoconstriction and shivering reactions. Since it is well known that hypothermia impairs coagulation and induces shivering, this requires careful management.

The cause of recovery hypothermia mainly relates to heat loss during surgery. However, it is further impaired by the immobile state of the patient, the exposure of the body to surveillance of the vital signs, and infusion of cool solutions intravenously. In addition, pharmacological agents which disturb both central and peripheral temperature-regulating mechanisms are used (e.g. atropine, general anaesthetics and skeletal muscle relaxants). The effects are more marked in infants (because of their large surface area/volume ratio and small body heat content) and in the elderly (because of their lower levels of heat production at rest, and possibly the greater susceptibility of their central temperature-controlling mechanisms to the effects of pharmacological agents).

FURTHER READING

Britt LD, Dascombe WH, Rodriguez A. 1991: New horizons in management of hypothermia and frostbite injury. *Surgical Clinics of North America* **71**, 345–70.

Jurkovich G, Greiser W, Luterman A *et al.* 1987: Hypothermia in trauma victims: an ominous predictor of survival. *Journal of Trauma* **27**, 1019–24.

Mills WJ. 1993: Summary of treatment of the cold-injured patient: frostbite. *Alaska Medicine* **35**, 61–6.

Moss J. 1986: Accidental severe hypothermia. *Surgical Gynecology and Obstetrics* **162**, 501–13.

Chapter 11

Dysphagia

Mervyn G. Neely

Introduction

Literally translated, dysphagia means a difficulty (*dys*) in eating (*phagein*). The usual presentation by a patient is a complaint of food sticking after swallowing or a sensation of slowness of the passage of food into the stomach. Most causes of dysphagia relate to oesophageal diseases, although problems in the mouth and pharynx, such as a cancer of the tongue or acute tonsillitis, must also be considered. These diseases can readily be diagnosed with the aid of a torch and spatula.

Related symptoms may be odynophagia (pain on swallowing) and regurgitation (an effortless passage of stomach or oesophageal contents into the mouth). Stomach contents usually have a sour bitter taste, while oesophageal contents are bland.

Swallowing is normally a voluntary act, but may be initiated by stimulation of the mouth or pharynx. When swallowing occurs, the tongue helps to propel the bolus into the pharynx. Entry of the food into the nose and airways is prevented by closure of the soft palate and the glottis. A peristaltic wave starts in the pharynx and rapidly propels the bolus through the upper oesophageal sphincter, which opens for about 2 s. All of this muscular activity is short-lived and high-pressure because it involves striated muscle. The peristaltic wave progresses on down the oesophagus and through the lower oesophageal sphincter that has also opened. The transit time of the peristaltic wave in the oesophagus is 8–10 s, which is slower, and the pressures are also lower, because it involves smooth muscle (Figure 11.1).

If there is any dysfunction in this normal sequence of events the patient experiences dysphagia.

The innervation of the pharynx, oesophagus and its upper and lower sphincters is from the ninth and tenth cranial nerves, also with a sympathetic supply.

If there are lesions in the brainstem or the above cranial nerves, food may not leave the oropharynx and enter the

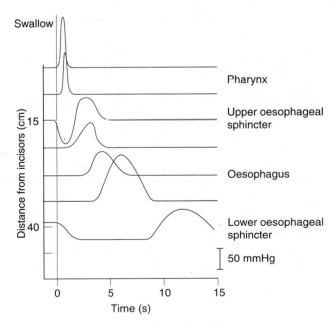

Figure 11.1 Normal oesophageal motility.

oesophagus. This may be a sequel to a head injury or a neurosurgical operation with bulbar palsy, or due to poliomyelitis, diphtheria, botulism, tetanus, lead poisoning or pseudobulbar palsy. With neuromuscular paralysis, liquids and foods may be regurgitated into the nose if the soft palate is affected, or be aspirated into the airways if there is dysfunction of the glottis.

The oesophagus starts in the neck at the level of C6, and passes through the posterior mediastinum in close relation to the aorta, thoracic duct and left atrium. It then passes through the oesophageal hiatus of the diaphragm at the level of T10 to join the stomach a few centimetres below the diaphragm in the upper abdomen. Throughout its length the left and right vagal nerves are intimately related, forming the anterior and posterior vagi as the oesophagus passes through the hiatus. Its blood supply is segmental. The oesophagus has an outer longitudinal layer and an inner circular layer of smooth muscle. There are striped muscle fibres in the uppermost few centimetres continuing caudally from the pharynx.

CASE HISTORY

Mrs DC, a 57-year-old woman, was referred with a diagnosis of achalasia by her general practitioner.

On questioning she gave a history of losing 6.4 kg in weight over the last 5 months. For the last 2 months she had experienced progressive dysphagia, regurgitation, vomiting and retrosternal pain. The vomitus usually consisted of undigested food, but on occasion consisted of thick stringy clear fluid. She had never been a smoker, and was a moderate consumer of alcohol. A peptic ulcer had been diagnosed some 4 years previously, but she was not sure whether this had been duodenal or gastric. For this she had had a 1-month course of cimetidine which had relieved her symptoms.

Examination revealed a rather thin woman who did not appear dehydrated or anaemic. No lymph nodes were palpable in her neck. Her abdomen revealed the scars of an appendicectomy as a child and tubal ligation some 30 years previously. There was no tenderness or palpable masses.

HISTORY

When taking a history from a patient with dysphagia and/or vomiting, the following key points need to be determined.

- Does the food leave the oropharynx and enter the oesophagus without difficulty?
- Does swallowing produce a swelling in the neck associated with gurgling and some regurgitation?
- Is the duration long or short?
- Has it been progressive or static?
- Is it intermittent?
- Is it mild or severe?

- Is it for both liquids and solids?
- Are there specific foods that produce it?
- Is there any accompanying pain?
- What is the perceived level of the obstruction?
- Is it accompanied by weight loss?
- What is the nature of the regurgitated or vomited material?
- Is there aspiration with concomitant cough and/or recurring chest infection?
- Is it accompanied by constipation?
- Is there a history of heartburn?
- Are there any other accompanying symptoms?

From the history and examination, this patient could have one of several diagnoses. Dysphagia may be caused by a neuromuscular disorder, such as achalasia, or by narrowing of the oesophagus by external compression, an intrinsic tumour or stricturing from reflux oesophagitis or swallowing corrosives. In this case the history of dysphagia is relatively short (2 months).

CLINICAL FEATURES

Achalasia usually has a prolonged insidious onset with plateauing of the symptoms, as the patient learns to cope with their disability. Invariably there is initial weight loss, with stabilization at a lower weight. Clinical examination does not reveal any abnormality.

Scleroderma, where there is an absence of peristalsis in the oesophagus, may be hinted at by the presence of Raynaud's phenomenon, which produces blanched fingers with atrophy of the tips (see Plate 11.1 in the colour plate section).

External compression might be caused by a mediastinal tumour such as a primary bronchial neoplasm or a mass of enlarged lymph nodes (either metastatic or primary), as in lymphoma. Here the history would be progressive and relentless. A lung neoplasm may be associated with a long history of smoking and a cough. Examination might reveal other evidence of the primary disease, such as other involved nodes or finger clubbing (see Plate 11.2 in the colour plate section).

Malignant tumours of the oesophagus are more common than benign tumours such as leiomyomas. Again the dysphagia is progressive. Clinical examination may be unrewarding, or with advanced lesions Virchow's node in the left supraclavicular fossa may be palpable or on rare occasions even visible (see Plate 11.3 in the colour plate section).

Benign oesophageal strictures are most commonly due to reflux oesophagitis. Usually there is a long history of heartburn and regurgitation preceding the formation of the stricture.

Corrosive swallowing is rare in adults but regrettably it is still occurring in young children. In the case reported here there was no history of swallowing corrosives or of heartburn, although there was a history of peptic ulceration.

INVESTIGATIONS

Investigations are essential for the correct diagnosis of dysphagia and vomiting.

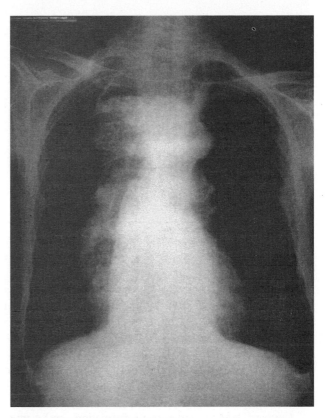

Figure 11.3 Achalasia PA fluid level.

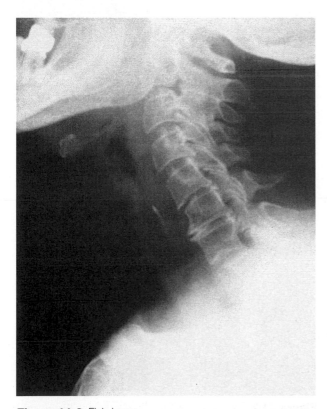

Figure 11.2 Fish-bone.

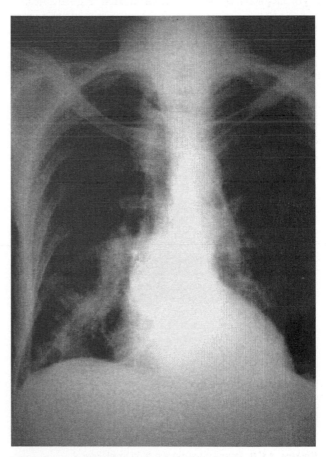

Figure 11.4 Pharyngeal pouch fluid level: PA.

BLOOD TESTS

Mrs DC had a normal haemoglobin, white count and sedimentation rate. Her biochemistry was also completely normal apart from a slightly lowered albumin level of 32 g/L. This is a reflection of reduced food intake from the dysphagia, and is not specific for any of the conditions.

RADIOLOGY

Radiological studies may yield a diagnosis. A plain X-ray of the neck may show a *foreign body* (e.g. a fish-bone) stuck there (Figure 11.2).

A chest X-ray may show an enormous oesophagus with a visible fluid level from longstanding *achalasia* (Figure 11.3).

Occasionally a large *pharyngeal pouch* may also be visible on a *plain X-ray* as an air-containing cavity at the base of the neck with a fluid level. Evidence of chronic aspiration may be seen in the right lower lobe (Figures 11.4 and 11.5).

Contrast X-rays yield more information, and a pharyngeal pouch can be clearly delineated (Figure 11.6).

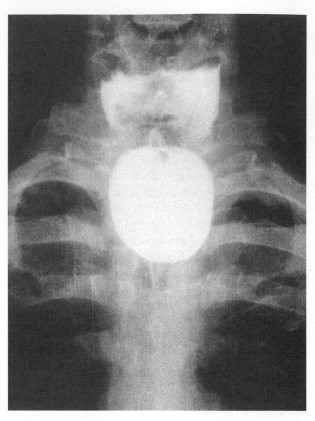

Figure 11.6 Pouch barium: AP.

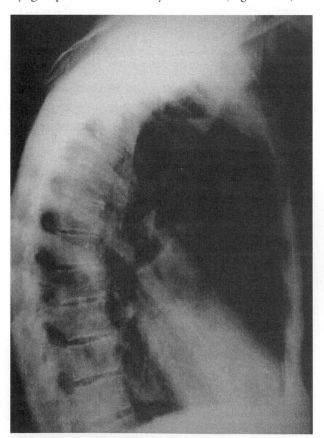

Figure 11.5 Pharyngeal pouch fluid level: lateral.

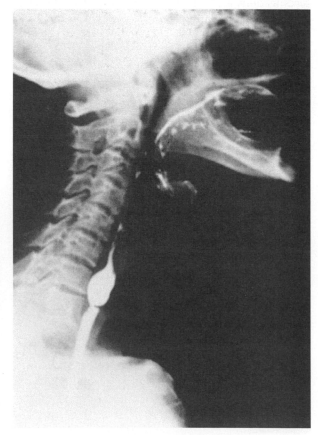

Figure 11.7 Post-cricoid web.

The pouch (*Zenker's diverticulum*) is formed by a protrusion of the mucosa through Killian's dehiscence (the triangular defect formed by the oblique fibres of the inferior constrictor of the pharynx and the horizontal fibres of the cricopharyngeus). Premature closure of the cricopharyngeus causes a sudden rise in intraluminal pressure resulting in the pulsion diverticulum. The dysphagia is high, with food entering the pouch rather than the oesophagus and usually regurgitating, either spontaneously or with pressure on the neck. This produces a characteristic gurgling sound.

A *post-cricoid web* in the Plummer-Vinson syndrome may be shown (Figure 11.7). This is a flimsy membrane of unknown aetiology that is usually ruptured (and not seen) during endoscopy.

Another web that causes dysphagia is the ring described by the radiologist Schatzki at the lower end of the oesophagus (Figure 11.8). It may be the cause of impaction of a food bolus in an otherwise normal

oesophagus. Its true nature is still unclear, but it is probably related to muscular contraction, as it is rarely seen on endoscopy.

A barium swallow may reveal external compression. The dysphagia is usually for solids. A retrotracheal thyroid nodule (see Plate 11.4 in the colour plate section) caused the displaced compressed oesophagus shown in Figure 11.9.

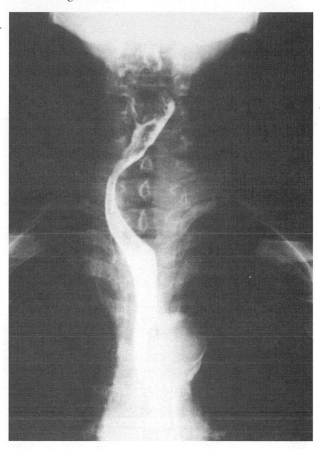

Figure 11.9 Thyroid displacement.

Congenital abnormalities of the great vessels in the superior mediastinum may also compress the oesophagus in what is known as *dysphagia lusoria* (Figure 11.10). In the patient shown in Figure 11.10 the compression was caused by the right subclavian artery with an abnormal origin crossing the oesophagus.

Malignant tumours of the oesophagus, if not detected early, are usually seen as a filling defect or an irregular stricture. They can occur at any level in the oesophagus, and can be squamous-cell carcinomas or adenocarcinomas.

A marked increase in adenocarcinomas arising in Barrett's oesophagus has been reported, and it has become the commonest carcinoma in some centres. Chronic gastro-oesophageal reflux leads to metaplasia of the squamous epithelium to columnar epithelium and intestinal glands (see Plate 11.5 in the colour plate

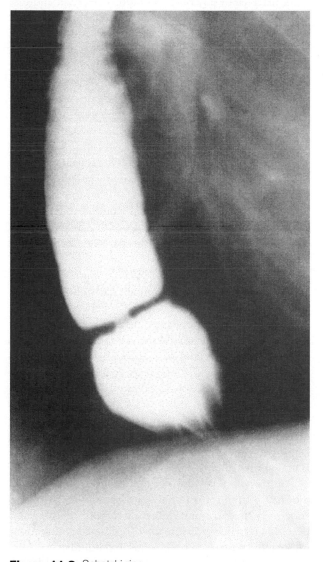

Figure 11.8 Schatzki ring.

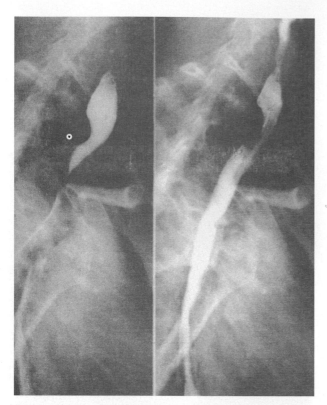

Figure 11.10 Dysphagia lusoria.

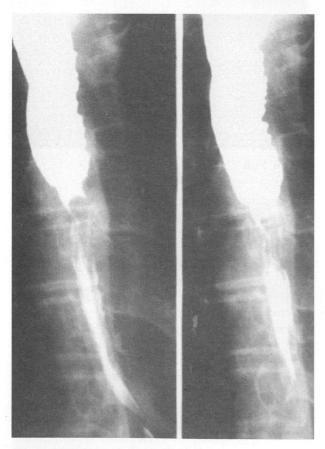

Figure 11.11 Obstructing carcinoma.

section). Ongoing inflammation leads to dysplasia, which may be mild at first, but can progress through severe dysplasia to carcinoma *in situ* and invasive carcinoma (see Plate 11.6 in the colour plate section).

It is important that ongoing surveillance of patients with Barrett's oesophagus is undertaken with endoscopies and biopsies to detect the onset of severe dysplasia, carcinoma *in situ* or early invasive carcinoma (see Plate 11.7 in the colour plate section). Resectional intervention may result in cure, which is otherwise rare in oesophageal malignancy, with 5-year survival rates of around 10%.

With an advanced malignant stricture of longer duration there may be dilatation of the oesophagus proximal to the lesion (Figure 11.11; see Plate 11.8 in the colour section).

Motility disorders can be shown with contrast studies. With video recording and slow-motion playback it may be possible to see dysmotility that cannot be demonstrated by any other method. The classic motility disorder producing dysphagia is *achalasia*, first described by Thomas Willis in 1674 without any investigations. It has an incidence of 1 in 100 000 and can occur at any age. It has an insidious onset and is often difficult to diagnose in its early stages. Dysphagia is progressive for both liquids and solids. Central severe chest pain may be a feature. Weight is slowly lost, levelling off at a lower value. Regurgitation and vomiting are common. Motility tests are essential for early diagnosis.

The aetiology is uncertain, but it appears to be a defect in the myenteric plexus where ganglia may be diminished in number rather than absent as in Hirschprung's disease. A similar condition is seen in Chagas' disease, which occurs in South America, where the ganglia are destroyed by the parasite *Trypanosoma cruzi*.

For food to enter the stomach, the resistance of the closed lower oesophageal sphincter has to be overcome. The resting pressure is usually between 20 and 30 mmHg. As the oesophagus fills in the erect position, hydrostatic pressure forces the sphincter open briefly, and spurts of contents pass through to the stomach. Patients often spontaneously learn to force food through by increasing intrathoracic pressure with the Valsalva manoeuvre.

In the advanced case shown in Figure 11.12 there is gross dilatation of the oesophagus with lengthening leading to the sigmoid appearance. The narrowed cardia is also shown.

Another motility disorder that produces intermittent dysphagia and retrosternal pain is *diffuse spasm,* as shown in the X-ray in Figure 11.13, with a corkscrew oesophagus. High-pressure unco-ordinated contractions impede the passage of both solids and liquids.

Strictures are readily shown and their site and length

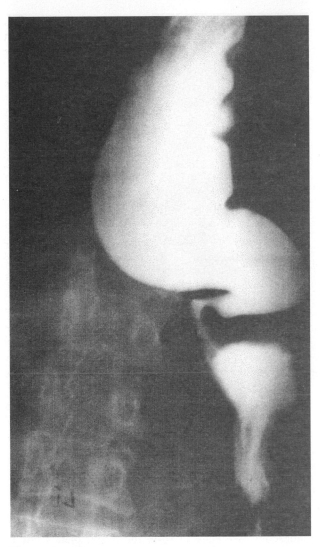

Figure 11.12 Achalasia.

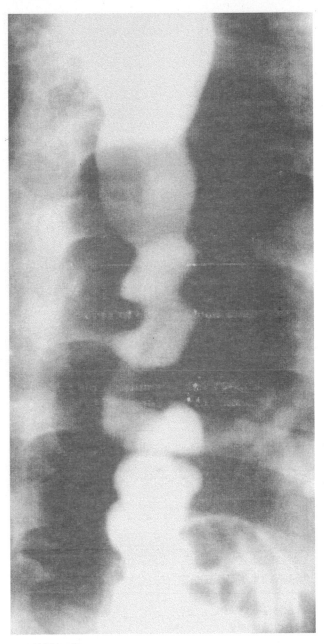

Figure 11.13 Diffuse spasm.

determined. The X-ray in Figure 11.14 shows a typical peptic stricture associated with gastro-oesophageal reflux above a hiatus hernia. The ongoing inflammation of the reflux oesophagitis results in fibrosis, which contracts to form the stricture. Reflux is very common in our society, but the incidence of strictures is not high as gastric acid suppression with drugs, or effective antireflux operations heal the oesophagitis before significant fibrosis occurs. Many patients with gastro-oesophageal reflux complain of a high dysphagia in the absence of any stricturing.

The stricture shown in Figure 11.14 is very narrow, obstructing solids and only allowing the passage of fluids. It is short and smooth.

Figure 11.15 shows an X-ray of a woman who had previously swallowed caustic soda. The corrosive agent had destroyed the whole of her oesophagus, which shows extensive irregular narrowing, and in the specimen loss of mucosa and gross fibrous replacement of

Mrs DC's barium study (Figure 11.16) showed a markedly dilated oesophagus with hold-up at a narrowed cardia.

This appearance was certainly compatible with her GP's diagnosis of achalasia, but does not exclude a cancer.

the muscle. Initially the patient could not swallow any solids, and progressively liquids could only be swallowed with great difficulty. When dilatation failed, oesophagectomy was performed.

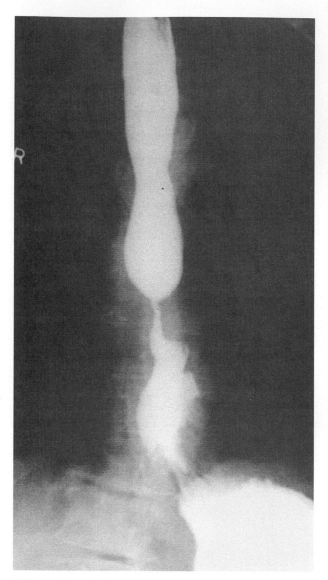

Figure 11.14 Peptic stricture above hiatus hernia.

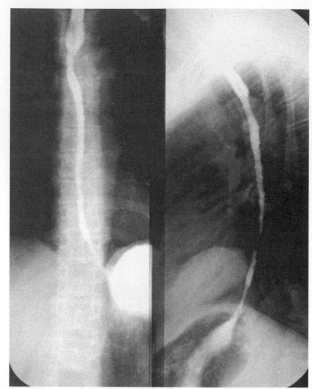

Figure 11.15 Corrosive stricture.

ENDOSCOPY

Upper gastrointestinal endoscopy should be performed in all cases of dysphagia. It may be the only way to detect early oesophageal cancers, and has the great advantage of being able to obtain a biopsy of any visualized lesion. It has the disadvantages of not being able to see beyond a stricture and hence not being able to determine its length, and being unable to see outside the lumen to determine the cause of external compression. It is necessarily an invasive procedure, and is not without associated morbidity and mortality from perforation.

Obstructing *foreign bodies* can be seen and usually removed endoscopically. Obviously the onset is acute and, depending on the size of the object, the blockage may be complete. This is often associated with profuse salivation, which exacerbates the symptoms and the dis-

comfort of the patient. The objects swallowed are many and varied, and swallowing may be intentional or accidental. The coin shown in Plate 11.9 in the colour plate section was deliberately swallowed.

Infections such as candidiasis are readily seen at endoscopy (see Plate 11.10 in the colour plate section) and the diagnosis is confirmed by biopsy and culture/histology.

Strictures are easily seen, and the visual appearance usually allows one to distinguish between malignant and benign lesions. Biopsies should be taken in every case, and the stricture may be dilated at the same time.

Plate 11.11 in the colour plate section shows a *benign stricture* in an area of oesophagitis with Barrett's oesophagus.

A *malignant stricture* is irregular and its exophytic nature is readily seen (see Plate 11.12 in the colour plate section).

MOTILITY STUDIES

Motility of the oesophagus can be assessed by inserting a pressure-measuring probe into its lumen. This is usually done through the nose and is the equivalent of passing a nasogastric tube. The patient needs to be awake and co-operative. There are two main types of probe, one of which has a series of built-in miniature transducers,

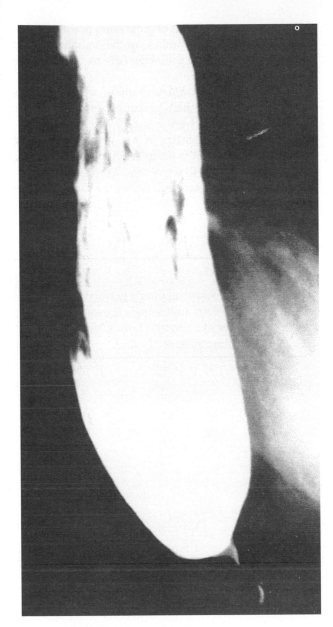

Figure 11.16 Carcinoma of cardia.

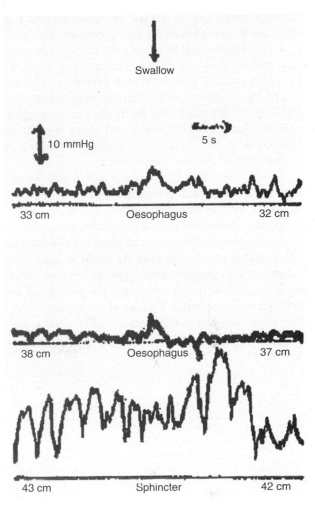

Figure 11.17 Achalasia motility.

Endoscopy in Mrs DC showed a dilated baggy oesophagus with marked narrowing at the cardia. The endoscope could not be passed through the cardia, which seemed to be quite rigid. This is not the usual finding in achalasia, where there is usually a little resistance encountered but the scope can be easily passed into the stomach.

The mucosa appeared normal and smooth. Biopsies were taken, which were reported to be normal stratified squamous epithelium. Because of the rigid nature of the stricture, malignancy was suspected, so a further endoscopy, dilatation of the stricture and biopsy were performed. On this occasion the report was of adenocarcinoma.

while the other has multiple lumens in the tube, which connect to side openings. Each of the lumens connects with an external transducer and a pump, which perfuses it with water at a constant slow rate. Variations of these tubes exist, including the Dent sleeve, which has a type of balloon over a few centimetres at the distal end and is useful for delineating the lower sphincter. Usually the miniature transducers or side openings are situated at 5-cm intervals and there are at least three of them. However, any number is possible, and the interval

The motility study for Mrs DC showed synchronous contractions in the oesophagus on swallowing. It was not possible to pass the probe through the lower oesophageal sphincter to assess the lower sphincter. The synchronous contractions (common channel phenomenon) are produced in dilated tubes containing fluid. These synchronous contractions are also seen in the early stages of achalasia.

between them can be varied. In some probes a pH electrode is incorporated for the assessment of reflux.

A test is performed by passing the tube into the stomach initially and withdrawing it in 1-cm steps. The patient is asked to swallow at each centimetre. The timing of the swallows can be marked using signals from EMG electrodes placed on the neck. The investigation enables a profile of the lower and upper oesophageal sphincters to be obtained, as well as indicating the contractility of the oesophagus itself.

In patients with a *pharyngeal pouch*, if the oesophagus can be intubated, premature closure of the upper sphincter may be demonstrated.

In *scleroderma* there is an absence of peristalsis and the lower oesophageal sphincter does not function and has a resting pressure of zero. As eating is usually performed in the upright position, gravity coupled with the *vis à tergo* from the pharynx aids the passage of food through the oesophagus. Because of the incompetence of the lower oesophageal sphincter, reflux occurs which may lead to oesophagitis and subsequent stricture formation.

In *achalasia* there is loss of progressive peristaltic contractions in the smooth muscle of the oesophagus, and the lower oesophageal sphincter fails to relax (Figure 11.17).

Motility studies in *diffuse spasm* of the oesophagus show unco-ordinated high-pressure contractions. The progressive peristaltic wave is lost.

Oesophageal manometry is not necessary in most cases of dysphagia, but in disorders of motility it may be the only investigation to reveal the diagnosis. This is particularly true in early achalasia before the barium studies are conclusive.

MANAGEMENT

Mrs DC had an oesophagectomy performed. The specimen showed an infiltrating adenocarcinoma of the cardia rather like a linitis plastica (see Plate 11.13 in the colour plate section).

Chapter 12

Constipation and diarrhoea

John P.V. Collins

Introduction

Constipation and diarrhoea are common symptoms, each of which may mean different things to different people. Constipation, which literally means 'crowding together', is defined as irregularity or difficulty in defecation, whereas diarrhoea is a condition of frequent and loose bowel movements. In clinical practice, constipation is defined as the passage of two stools per week and diarrhoea as an increase in liquid stool with a daily weight greater than 200 g, usually associated with three or more motions per day. It is difficult to define what is normal because the frequency of defecation varies so widely. A desire to defecate normally follows the ingestion of food or distension of the rectum with faeces, but habits and cultural factors play an important role in determining when defecation takes place. This explains why it may be normal for one individual to produce one stool every 2 days, while another may produce one or even three stools each day. For these reasons it is important to establish a person's normal bowel habit and stool consistency before regarding these as abnormal.

In this chapter the important background principles are first outlined, followed by a description of the aetiological factors. Diagnostic evaluation is then discussed using a problem-based approach to the history, clinical examination and investigations.

IMPORTANT BACKGROUND PRINCIPLES

Changes in bowel habits may occur through an alteration either in the normal transit time of ingested food to the rectum and its subsequent evacuation, or in the fluid movements which occur across the gastrointestinal tract.

Ingested food enters the stomach and 3–4 h later (Figure 12.1) passes through the pylorus into the duodenum and small intestine, arriving at the caecum 4–6 h later. This is followed by a slow transit time of 12–18 h through the colon to the rectum.

Distension of the rectum by faecal material initiates reflex contractions of its musculature and the desire to defecate. At the same time, nerve impulses travel to the internal sphincter via its parasympathetic nerve supply, causing it to relax. The external sphincter which receives its nerve supply via the pudendal nerve remains in tonic contraction and only relaxes when defecation is initiated.

About 8.5 L of fluid are secreted into the gastrointestinal tract each day, being composed of approximately 1.5 L saliva, 3.0 L gastric juice, 1.0 L bile, 1.0 L pancreatic juice and 2.0 L small intestine secretion (Figure 12.1). In addition to this, 1.5 L of fluid are ingested with food. Of this total volume of 10 L, 85–90% is absorbed in the small intestine, 1 L is absorbed in the colon, leaving about 0.1 L to be excreted in the faeces.

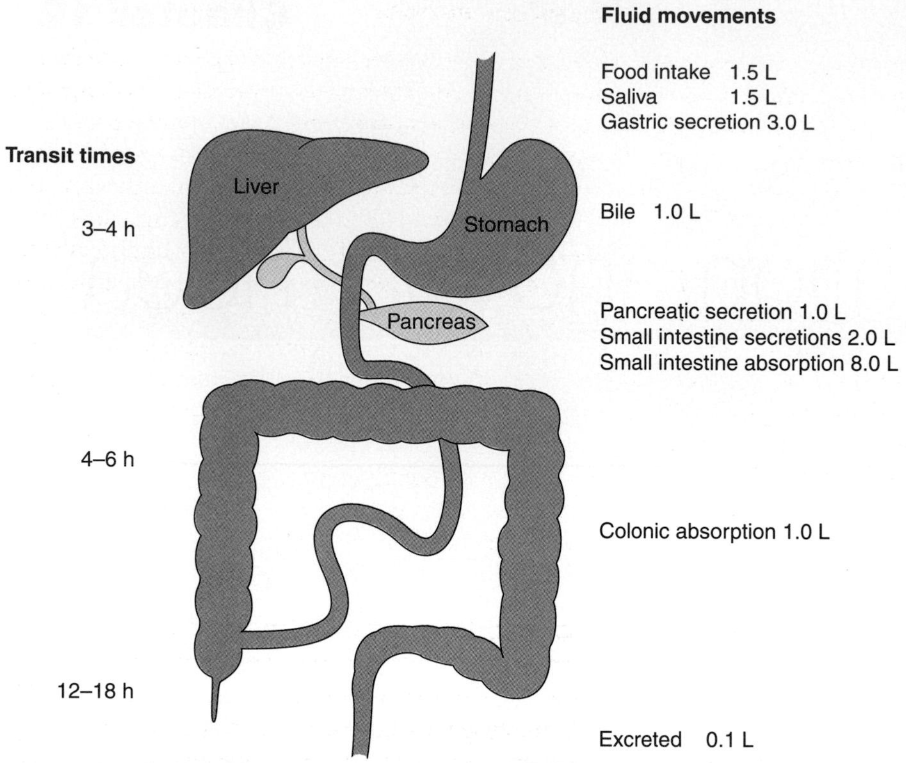

Fluid movements

Food intake 1.5 L
Saliva 1.5 L
Gastric secretion 3.0 L

Transit times

Liver

Stomach

Bile 1.0 L

3–4 h

Pancreas

Pancreatic secretion 1.0 L
Small intestine secretions 2.0 L
Small intestine absorption 8.0 L

4–6 h

Colonic absorption 1.0 L

12–18 h

Excreted 0.1 L

Figure 12.1 Transit times and fluid movements in the gastrointestinal tract.

CONSTIPATION

Constipation may be due to general causes (Table 12.1) or to a local cause in the colon, rectum or anus (Table 12.2). Exclusion of these causes leads to a diagnosis of idiopathic constipation.

GENERAL CAUSES

The following account describes the different general causes of constipation, although in an individual case several of these may be working together.

Table 12.1 General causes of constipation

Dietary	Psychogenic	Endocrine	Neurological	Metabolic	Drugs/poisons
Low fibre	Stress	Hypothyroidism	Autonomic	Hypokalaemia	Opiates
	Anxiety	Hyperparathyroidism	neuropathy	Uraemia	Anticholinergics
	Depression	Hypopituitarism	Multiple sclerosis	Porphyria	Phenothiazines
	Obsessional personality	Diabetes	Tabes dorsalis	Amyloid	Iron
					Lead/mercury/arsenic

Table 12.2 Local causes of constipation

Obstructive bowel disorders	Painful anorectal conditions	Colorectal and anal dysfunction
Benign stricture	Anal fissure	Anorectal anomalies
Carcinoma	Thrombosed haemorrhoids	Absence of ganglia
Polyps	Perianal infection	Post-pelvic operations
Volvulus		
Hernia		
Adhesions		
Rectal prolapse/intussusception		

Dietary causes

The intake of dietary fibre is closely related to the water content of the stool, which in turn influences stool bulk, weight and transit time. The use of convenience foods and other foods lacking in dietary fibre is a common cause of constipation.

Psychogenic causes

Stress in relation to toilet training or the use of inadequate toilet facilities at school – particularly lack of privacy – may lead to constipation in children. Constipation may occur as part of an unhappy childhood for whatever reason. It is also a prominent feature in those of any age with depression, especially in the elderly, where cerebral deterioration and blunted awareness may be a feature. A low-fibre diet may be part of this background, particularly in the elderly. Anxiety states and an obsessional personality may also be associated with constipation.

Endocrine causes

Constipation may be associated with hypothyroidism and hypercalcaemia due to either hyperparathyroidism or milk alkali syndrome. There is some evidence that constipation in the reproductive age group may be associated with a reduction in certain steroid hormones. Diabetic patients with autonomic neuropathy may suffer from constipation, although incontinence may be a more major symptom.

Neurological causes

The congenital absence of parasympathetic ganglion cells in the anal canal, rectum or distal colon (Hirschsprung's disease) may lead to acute constipation within a few days after birth, but may occasionally persist undiagnosed into adult life. The diseased segment which is constricted varies in length, and most commonly terminates 1–2 cm above the dentate line. Proximal to this the bowel is dilated with hypertrophy of its wall.

Damage to the myenteric nerves may occur in diabetes, amyloid disease, scleroderma, Chagas' disease, advanced malignancy, Crohn's disease or with certain medications. Constipation may also be a feature of the demyelinating disorder multiple sclerosis, or of posterior column degeneration from tabes dorsalis.

Metabolic causes

Constipation may occur in hypokalaemia, uraemia or porphyria as a result of altered muscle contraction, and in amyloid disease due to local nerve damage.

Drugs and poisons

Several medications that are prescribed for headache and menorrhagia contain opiates, particularly codeine, and may account for constipation. As mentioned previously, patients with depression may suffer from constipation, and this may be made worse by certain antidepressant medications. These include tricyclic compounds, phenothiazines and monoamine oxidase inhibitors, and may cause constipation through damage to the myenteric nerves. Iron supplements, medications that cause hypokalaemia, such as diuretics, ganglion-blocking drugs and drugs used to treat Parkinson's disease may also cause constipation. An important drug-induced cause of constipation is the chronic use of laxatives, which leads to damage to the myenteric plexus of the colon. Lead, mercury and arsenic poisoning may cause chronic constipation.

LOCAL CAUSES OF CONSTIPATION

These may be subdivided into three categories (Table 12.2), namely those which cause obstruction of the large bowel, painful anorectal conditions and dysfunction of the anus, rectum and colon.

Obstructive bowel disorders

Benign strictures due to diverticular disease, endometriosis or following ischaemic colitis may lead to constipation, and neoplastic strictures due to carcinoma or large polyps may similarly affect intestinal transit. Volvulus, adhesions and hernia may lead to chronic constipation. Mucosal prolapse or intussusception may also be associated with constipation.

Painful anorectal conditions

Some painful conditions of the anus may be accompanied by fear of defecation and lead to constipation which may then become chronic. Examples of such conditions include anal fissure, thrombosed haemorrhoids and perianal infections.

Colorectal and anal dysfunction

Minor anorectal anomalies such as an anteriorly placed anus or stenosis of the anal canal may explain constipation in infants. Congenital absence of ganglia in the myenteric plexus, as in Hirschsprung's disease or acquired autonomic neuropathy, as discussed earlier, may lead to constipation. Constipation is also a feature of irritable bowel syndrome. Some pelvic operations, including hysterectomy, ovarian cystectomy, rectopexy and cystectomy, may be complicated by constipation and this may be due to local autonomic damage.

IDIOPATHIC CONSTIPATION

This diagnosis is made after exclusion of all previously mentioned causes. Physiological studies of these individuals suggest three subgroups, namely those with colonic inertia, those with defecation problems and those with irritable bowel syndrome. Clearly more than one mechanism may coexist in any one patient.

Colonic inertia delays transit time either through the entire colon and rectum or through a segment, depending on the extent of altered motility. Disorder of the mechanism of defecation may result from inappropriate contraction of the pelvic floor and external sphincter, both of which should relax during defecation. Constipation is a prominent symptom in individuals with irritable bowel syndrome.

DIARRHOEA

Diarrhoea may occur through any one of four mechanisms (Table 12.3), or a combination of these. The presence of non-absorbable solutes in the intestine may result in osmotic diarrhoea by attracting fluid and electrolytes into the small bowel. Simple laxatives and those used in bowel preparation, such as mannitol or magnesium salts, act in this way. Lactase deficiency leads to malabsorption of carbohydrate, which may cause diarrhoea for a similar reason.

Stimulation of gut secretion may occur with certain hormone-secreting tumours or as a result of bacterial toxins produced by *Escherichia coli*, *Clostridium difficile* and *Vibrio cholera* or *Shigellosis*.

In inflammatory bowel disease, mucosal damage leads to increased capillary permeability and exudative diarrhoea. Mucosal damage may also result from bacterial infection. Exudative diarrhoea may also occur in association with villous adenoma, large-bowel cancer or radiation colitis.

Intermittent diarrhoea may occur in disorders of intestinal motility, such as irritable bowel syndrome and the blind loop syndrome. Malabsorption may lead to increased faecal bulk and diarrhoea. This may result from a lack of digestive enzymes or bile salts, loss of absorptive area following massive bowel resection, or in coeliac disease which involves damage to the epithelium of the small intestine.

DIAGNOSTIC EVALUATION

A problem-orientated approach to the history, physical examination and investigations must be undertaken in order to determine the pathological basis of the predominant symptom. It is essential to clarify at the outset what the patient really means by either constipation or diarrhoea.

A PROBLEM-ORIENTATED HISTORY IN CONSTIPATION

A general history should enquire about occupation and social and family background. Specific questions should address the duration and pattern of the complaint, and the presence or absence of systemic symptoms. Dietary and medication history should be clarified, and any accompanying symptoms such as rectal bleeding or the passage of pus should be sought.

The age of the patient is an important predictor of the most likely diagnosis. The *onset of constipation in childhood* may have a simple explanation. Changes of environment or diet or periods of inactivity may be the cause, especially if the symptoms have a more acute onset. The passage of normal stools at abnormal times or in abnormal places suggests psychogenic causes. While it may be difficult to unravel the factors responsible, evidence of an unhappy childhood should be enquired for. The duration of constipation must be clarified, and if it dates back to birth or infancy, the possibility of Hirschsprung's disease must be considered. A history of pain on defecation should be enquired about and, if present, the diagnosis of anal fissure becomes likely, particularly with constipation of a more acute onset. Fresh blood on the toilet-paper after defecation may be further evidence of an anal fissure.

In *older patients with constipation*, obstructive causes are more likely. If a person with previously normal bowel

Table 12.3 Mechanisms of diarrhoea

Osmotic	Secretory	Exudative	Motility disorder
Laxatives	Hormone-producing tumours	Inflammatory bowel disease	Irritable bowel syndrome
Lactase deficiency	Bacterial enterotoxins	Gastroenteritis	Blind loop syndrome
		Villous adenoma	
		Colorectal cancer	
		Radiation colitis	

habits develops constipation, the diagnosis of large bowel cancer must be considered. The likelihood of this diagnosis is increased in individuals with rectal bleeding or a family history of bowel cancer. Specific details of the bleeding should be sought, particularly its colour, as dark blood supports the diagnosis of a malignancy. A history of incomplete emptying of the rectum after defecation or straining at stool suggests rectal cancer, especially in a person with increasing constipation and rectal bleeding. Occasionally the blood loss in rectal cancer may be bright red and accompanied by mucus. Abdominal pain should be enquired about. It may be a feature of constipation from any cause, but if it is of short duration and increasing severity, obstructive causes are more likely. The site of the pain is important, generalized pain occurring in large bowel obstruction. Pain confined to the left iliac fossa occurs in diverticular disease. This diagnosis is supported if a patient passes small fragments of hard stool. Questions should be asked about tiredness and weight loss. A history of tiredness may reflect the anaemia which occurs in bowel cancer, and weight loss may occur following spread of this disease.

In those patients without these major symptoms, more simple causes of constipation are likely. Inadequate intake of fibre, lack of exercise and chronic use of laxatives may be significant aetiological factors. A history of depression should be sought and, if present, may be accompanied by inactivity and laxative abuse. Painful anorectal conditions such as anal fissure will present in adults as in children. Only after common causes have been excluded should idiopathic constipation be considered.

A PROBLEM-ORIENTATED HISTORY IN DIARRHOEA

The age of the patient is again paramount in determining the most likely diagnosis. Diarrhoea at any age, especially with an acute onset, is most often due to gastroenteritis; this is particularly so in children. A history of eating suspect food or of diarrhoea in siblings, family or friends, or diarrhoea following recent overseas travel, should be sought as it supports the diagnosis.

A history of bloody diarrhoea may still be due to gastroenteritis, particularly with *Campylobacter* infection. The passage of pus in the stool is a further feature of infective diarrhoea. Bloodstained diarrhoea may be due to inflammatory bowel disease, particularly ulcerative colitis. Further support for this diagnosis may be obtained on enquiring about the duration and pattern of the diarrhoea. Previous episodes of remissions and relapses are typical of ulcerative colitis. Diarrhoea in a patient who has recently been on antibiotics may be due to *Clostridium difficile* infection.

Urgency or even incontinence may occur, particularly in inflammatory bowel disease, but may also be found in malignancy or rectal prolapse. Symptoms of extracolonic manifestations of ulcerative colitis should be enquired about and may relate to joints, the eye, the skin or the liver. Weight loss may occur in severe diarrhoea from any cause, and is a marker of severity rather than aetiology.

Less commonly, diarrhoea may be due to chronic laxative abuse, and it may be difficult to obtain this from the history. Faecal material which floats in the toilet pan or is difficult to flush away suggests malabsorption. In those who have previously been treated for a sexually transmitted disease or who are involved in homosexual activity, diarrhoea may be due to a variety of intestinal infections, parasites or, more rarely, AIDS-related proctitis.

Mucus loss with diarrhoea may occur with villous adenoma, solitary rectal ulcer or rectal prolapse. In patients with a history of previous abdominal surgery, diarrhoea may occur following gastrectomy or intestinal resection.

On completion of the history a list of possible differential diagnoses – in order of probability – should be recorded. The clinical examination then attempts to establish whether confirmatory or other signs are present. The absence of abnormal physical findings is in itself an important consideration.

PROBLEM-ORIENTATED CLINICAL EXAMINATION

Physical examination must include a general examination followed by assessment of the abdomen, anus and rectum. Evidence of weight loss, anaemia, dehydration and sepsis should be sought. Extracolonic manifestations of inflammatory bowel disease, particularly arthritis and skin lesions, should be looked for where appropriate. Examination of the abdomen may demonstrate an abdominal mass, distension or signs of peritonism. Examination of the perianal area and of the anus may reveal the cause of the symptoms.

The possible diagnoses suggested by the history should be looked for. Abdominal distension and palpable faeces in the colon may be a feature of chronic constipation. Faecal soiling of the perianal area may be present in children in whom psychogenic constipation is suspected. In these children the anus will be normal but faecal impaction is likely. A painful anal fissure may be present which precludes digital rectal examination. Faecal impaction may be found in the elderly, particularly in chronic laxative abusers and in those with depression.

An abdominal mass in the older patient suggests cancer, but this finding may be obscured in the presence of abdominal distension. Rectal examination may demonstrate a palpable tumour in a patient with constipation and rectal bleeding.

In acute gastroenteritis, signs of dehydration and abdominal tenderness should be looked for. Signs of anaemia and acute blood loss may be present in ulcerative colitis. These findings, together with a tender distended abdomen, raise the possibility of impending megacolon. Occasionally no physical findings can be elicited, and this raises the possibility of rarer causes of diarrhoea, such as hormone-producing tumours.

PROBLEM-BASED APPROACH TO INVESTIGATIONS

Basic investigations should include a full blood count, liver function tests, urea and electrolytes. A sigmoidoscopy is indicated in all patients with significant symptoms, and a biopsy of any abnormality should be performed for histological analysis. In a patient with bloody diarrhoea the finding of a normal rectum on sigmoidoscopy is suggestive of an infective cause rather than ulcerative colitis. In those patients with suspected *Clostridium difficile* infection, a typical membrane may be seen on the rectal mucosa and this should be biopsied. Biopsy of the rectum in inflammatory bowel disease is important both for establishing the diagnosis and for differentiating ulcerative colitis from Crohn's disease.

Stool examination for bacteria and parasites may establish the cause of diarrhoea. If malabsorption is a possible diagnosis, excess faecal fat may be demonstrated by the Sudan stain. Daily stool volumes should be measured in diarrhoea, and an output of more than 1 L per day suggests a significant disorder.

If Hirschsprung's disease is being considered, a full-thickness rectal biopsy, involving removal of a longitudinal strip of mucosa and muscle over a distance of 3–6 cm from the anal verge, will be required.

Anal manometry, rectal sensation and compliance (ability to distend) may each play a part in the diagnosis of some patients with idiopathic constipation. Colonic motility studies using administered radio-opaque markers and daily abdominal radiographs for 1 week may help to establish the site of impaired motility. Electromyography of the puborectalis and external sphincter may help to identify the cause of defecation problems. Balloon proctography has been used to assess pelvic floor function during defecation, but it has now been superseded by video proctography in the identification of treatable causes of outlet obstruction.

FURTHER READING

Ganong WF. 1997: *Review of medical physiology.* London: Prentice-Hall International.

Keighley MRB, Williams NS. 1993: *Surgery of the anus, rectum and colon.* London: W.B. Saunders.

Chapter 13

Jaundice

Robert M. Jones

Introduction

Management of a patient with the yellow-black pigmentation of jaundice remains a diagnostic challenge. Hyperbilirubinaemia has multiple causes and is rarely a benign condition.

The normal plasma bilirubin level is 5–15 μmol/L.

Hyperbilirubinaemia occurs when the plasma bilirubin is above the upper range of normal, which for most laboratories is around 17 μmol/L. Clinical jaundice occurs when the pigment can be observed in the skin or sclera, usually at around 40 to 50 μmol/L.

BIOCHEMISTRY

Bilirubin is an endogenous, insoluble, negatively charged molecule. Several isomeric forms can be detected in the serum, but the IXα pigment predominates. Although bilirubin IXα is a linear structure of linked carbon rings and should be soluble, it is folded with six intramolecular hydrogen bonds, and as a result the molecule is insoluble (Figure 13.1).

Light energy of the correct wavelength can disrupt the hydrogen bonds, producing soluble photoisomers that can be excreted in the urine. This is the basis of 'phototherapy' for neonatal jaundice.

PRODUCTION

An adult produces 500 μmol of bilirubin daily, of which 400 μmol are derived from the reticulo-endothelial system breakdown of the haem component of haemoglobin. As 1 g of haemoglobin yields 61 μmol of bilirubin, appoximately 6 g of haemoglobin are catabolized daily. The remaining bilirubin is derived from the metabolism

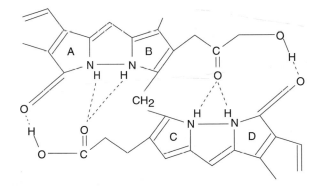

Figure 13.1 Billrubin IXα. Note the intramolecular hydrogen bonds between the propionic acid and nitrogen of the opposite pyrrole groups. (Reproduced with permission from Sherlock S. 1985: *Diseases of the liver and biliary system.* Oxford: Blackwell Scientific Publications, p. 200.)

of other haem-containing proteins such as myoglobin and the cytochrome P450 enzyme system.

The administration of radiolabelled haem shows an initial peak of biliary excretion within a few hours, due to incorporation of haem into the rapid-turnover cytochrome P450 enzymes. A second peak in a few days is due to abnormal haemoglobin production and early red-cell destruction, and most of the radiolabelled haem is excreted at around 120 days, reflecting the average lifespan of the red blood cells.

Porphyrin is converted to biliverdin IXα by the microsomal enzyme haemoxygenase, which oxidizes the closed methane bridge, producing a linear tetrapyrrole molecule. This produces one molecule of carbon monoxide, which can be measured in order to estimate haem metabolism. Biliverdin is then reduced to bilirubin IXα by the cytosolic enzyme biliverdin reductase. These two enzymes are concentrated in the liver and spleen but can be induced in other tissues if haem production is increased (Figure 13.2).

The enzyme haemoxygenase is localized to the endoplasmic reticulum and works in conjunction with the NADPH cytochrome P450 enzyme system. Haemoxygenase is also the pathway for the degradation of the cytochrome P450 enzymes and hence indirectly influences the biotransformation of many drugs.

Haemoxygenase is the rate-limiting step of bili-rubin production from protoporphyrins. Tin and zinc protoporphyrins are potent inhibitors of haemoxygenase and may prevent kernicterus in neonatal hyperbilirubinaemia.

PLASMA TRANSPORT

The majority of bilirubin derived from hepatic metabolism passes directly into the biliary canaliculus and does not enter the plasma. Plasma bilirubin is derived from splenic and reticulo-endothelial system breakdown of red blood cells, together with a smaller proportion of the pigment derived from hepatic haem metabolism. This water-insoluble unconjugated bilirubin is transported almost entirely bound to albumin with only a minute unbound fraction remaining free.

Albumin has a high binding affinity for bilirubin. Two binding sites have been described, namely a high-affinity site binding up to 350 μmol/L and a second site of lower affinity binding up to 650 μmol/L. Above this level the concentration of free bilirubin increases rapidly.

Other anions such as sulphonamides, salicylates and

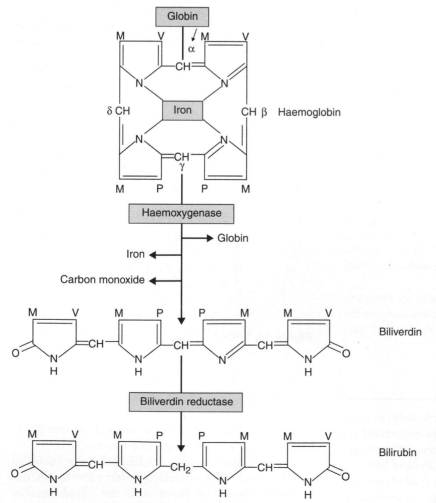

Biliverdin

Bilirubin

Figure 13.2 Metabolism of haemoglobin to bilirubin IXα. (Reproduced with permission from Billing BH. 1978: Twenty-five years of progress in bilirubin metabolism (1952–1977). *Gut* **19**, 481–91.)

radiological contrast media can compete and displace unconjugated bilirubin into the serum. In chronic liver disease some bilirubin becomes irreversibly bound to albumin (delta-bilirubin) and the half-life of this pigment is then that of the metabolism of albumin at 15–20 days.

Exchange transfusion with albumin replacement can remove bilirubin from tissues, and is used as a temporizing measure to lower severe hyperbilirubinaemia and prevent kernicterus.

HEPATIC METABOLISM

Free unconjugated bilirubin is lipid soluble and can traverse cell membranes and enter cells, where it is toxic. However unconjugated bilirubin does not enter cells and is almost exclusively metabolized by the liver. Albumin gives up bilirubin selectively to the liver by an active, membrane-linked transport mechanism. Bilirubin is bound to intracellular hepatocyte proteins which prevent its return to the plasma. Reflux is also prevented by the continued excretion of bilirubin into the bile, maintaining a concentration gradient across the cell.

Bilirubin IXα is made water soluble by the hepatic enzyme UDP-glucuronosyltransferase (UGT), which disrupts the hydrogen bonds by conjugating a sugar at two sites on the bilirubin molecule. This is the natural equivalent of the alcohol solvent used to measure the unconjugated fraction. Most bilirubin in bile is in the diconjugate form with glucuronic acid, but small amounts of bilirubin are conjugated with other sugars.

UGT consists of a group of isoenzymes within the endoplasmic reticulum of the hepatocyte, which have glucuronidase action on many compounds, including morphine, steroids and other drugs.

A small amount of conjugated bilirubin refluxes back into the sinusoids and systemic circulation, but this represents less than 5% of the total circulating bilirubin.

EXCRETION

Excretion of bilirubin into the biliary canaliculus is mediated by an energy-dependent carrier mechanism that secretes conjugated bilirubin across a concentration gradient. The secretion can be saturated (T_{max}) and competitively inhibited by drugs such as indocyanin green and tetrabromosulfopthalein (BSP) which do not require glucuronidation.

The secretion of bilirubin is independent of bile acid secretion and operates by a different carrier system. Conjugation of bilirubin rather than canalicular transport is the rate-limiting step.

Bilirubin within the bile is mostly conjugated and incorporated into mixed micelles with cholesterol and bile salts. A small unconjugated fraction remains solubilized in bile micelles. Some bilirubin is deconjugated within the intestine and can be reabsorbed for reconjugation in the liver and resecretion into the bile. However, most bilirubin is reduced by bacteria to colourless stercobilinogen which is excreted unchanged in the faeces. Some stercobilinogen is oxidized to urobilinogen, which is a mixture of isomers that contribute to the brown pigment of stool colour.

Urobilinogen forms part of the enterohepatic circulation of bilirubin. Absorption occurs in the terminal ileum, but this and the enterohepatic circulation of substances formed in the colon are of little surgical significance. However, some enters the circulation, and this explains the presence of urobilinogen in the urine and its increased levels in patients with haemolytic disease or liver disease, and its reduction in patients with complete biliary obstruction. This is in contrast to the surgically important enterohepatic circulation of bile salts, where approximately 90% of bile salts are reabsorbed via the terminal ileum.

SYMPTOMS OF JAUNDICE

The level of hyperbilirubinaemia is quite variable within each disease. Even with complete bile duct occlusion, serum bilirubin levels may range between 200 and 600 µmol/L. The final level depends on the amount produced and excretion by the kidney, which is limited. Skin discoloration varies from yellow to green-black in chronic jaundice, due to the variable amount of biliverdin in the skin. Water-soluble conjugated bilirubin penetrates tissue and produces a more intense discoloration than jaundice derived from unconjugated bilirubin.

The tissue bilirubin concentration varies and is dependent on protein binding. An exudate with a high protein level will contain more bilirubin than a low-protein transudate. Bilirubin binds readily to elastic tissue in the skin, which may remain deeply pigmented despite falling serum levels.

Patients with isolated hyperbilirubinaemia may be completely normal apart from marked jaundice. This is typified by Crigler-Najjar syndrome, where patients with a bilirubin level of greater than 300 µmol/L lead normal lives.

It is debatable whether bilirubin itself is toxic, but it probably is at high levels, particularly to the kidneys and brain.

Most surgical patients will be jaundiced due to extrahepatic biliary obstruction. The resulting jaundice is usually accompanied by some degree of discomfort or epigastric pain, weight loss and hepatosplenomegaly. In these patients hyperbilirubinaemia will be associated with cholestasis, and most of the symptoms will be caused by the reduction in bile flow. The clinical features commonly associated with jaundice, namely steatorrhoea, pruritis and malabsorption of fat-soluble vitamins and calcium, are due to the reduction in bile salt flow and bile salts retained within the circulation.

TESTING

Bilirubin is measured using a diazo colour dye, originally described by van den Bergh in 1913. The level of bilirubin present is proportional to the depth of colour change. Water-soluble, 'conjugated' bilirubin reacts 'directly' with the diazo reagent, while insoluble, 'unconjugated' bilirubin requires solvent extraction to be measured – hence the term 'indirect'. Solvent-treated plasma measures both conjugated and unconjugated bilirubin, giving the total bilirubin. The difference between the total, solvent-extracted 'indirect' bilirubin and the direct reaction is assumed to represent the unconjugated fraction.

The reaction depends on the time, temperature and concentration of the solvent, and this may produce considerable inter-laboratory variation. Bilirubin is degraded by light, and this may affect the level if the samples are left exposed to the light.

At high levels of bilirubin ($> 400\,\mu\text{mol/L}$) the accuracy of the diazo method decreases and there may be considerable day-to-day variation. It is the trend over several days that is important.

Accurate estimate of the bilirubin fractions requires high-performance liquid chromatography (HPLC), but this not practicable for day-to-day use.

KERNICTERUS

During the first few weeks of life the blood–brain barrier is immature, and unconjugated bilirubin can cross, causing kernicterus. This results in diffuse brain damage with cortical, cerebellar and basal ganglia signs. Kernicterus is rare in adults with an intact blood–brain barrier, but can occur in the presence of very high levels of bilirubin if the blood–brain barrier is disrupted by sepsis, acidosis, surgery or osmolality changes.

CHOLESTASIS

In cholestasis bile flow is reduced or absent. Obstruction to bile flow can occur anywhere from the hepatocyte to the ampullary sphincter. Cholestasis can occur without hyperbilirubinaemia, as bile flow and bilirubin excretion are independent. However, most surgical patients will present with jaundice in association with cholestasis.

Most of the symptoms associated with 'jaundice' are due to the cholestatic reduction of bile flow, i.e. pruritus, xanthomas, hepatic osteodystrophy, bone pain, joint pain, neuropathy, steatorrhoea and malabsorption of the fat-soluble vitamins K, D, A and E.

The common causes of cholestasis without marked jaundice are the liver diseases primary biliary cirrhosis (PBC) and primary sclerosing cholangitis (PSC), cholestasis of pregnancy and some myeloid leukaemias, particularly lymphomas, leukaemia and myeloma.

CIRRHOSIS

Cirrhosis is the manifestation of the end-stage of a multiplicity of liver diseases. Although the diagnosis of cirrhosis can be established clinically, it is characterized by the histological appearance of interlobular bridging fibrosis. This may be impossible to see on a fine-needle biopsy, and a large sample may be needed before the pathologist can be confident of the diagnosis. The liver may respond to injury with discrete areas of nodular regeneration that can mimic hepatoma.

Cirrhotic patients may present with no history to indicate the cause of the underlying liver disease. While jaundice may be the presenting symptom of cirrhosis, most cirrhotic patients are not jaundiced until the end-stage of their disease.

Most of the diseases listed in Table 13.1 can result in cirrhosis, which is a term describing the liver architecture with little aetiological connotation.

CLASSIFICATION

Jaundice is due to:

1. excess production of bilirubin;

2. a defect in hepatocellular transport or conjugation; or

3. extrahepatic biliary obstruction.

However, this classification groups diverse pathologies that have little in common. A more logical classification based on the main biochemical abnormality is suggested in Table 13.1. This classification is also the basis for the investigation and diagnosis of the jaundiced patient. A surgeon may encounter children who survive to adult life, and the table includes the major causes of paediatric hyperbilirubinaemia.

Jaundice can be classified into two biochemical categories. In the first the plasma increase is predominantly unconjugated, and in the second it is mostly conjugated or mixed. Conjugated bilirubin should always be less than 5% of the circulating total bilirubin, in normal adults and children. Jaundice due to unconjugated or

Table 13.1 Basic classification used for investigation and diagnosis of the jaundiced patient

Bilirubin type	Site of defect	Disease	
Unconjugated	Increased production	Spherocytosis	Thalassaemia
		Sickle-cell disease	Enzyme deficiencies
		Haemoglobinopathies	Haemolytic uraemic syndrome (HUS)
	Intracellular/Transport defect	Gilbert's syndrome	
		Crigler-Najjar syndrome	
		Acquired sepsis, drugs	
Conjugated/mixed	Extrahepatic	Stone obstruction	Benign stricture
		Congenital	Iatrogenic
		Biliary atresia	Post-inflammatory
		Allagile's syndrome	Trauma
		Choledochal cysts	Malignant stricture
		Infective	Recurrent jaundice of pregnancy
		Cholangitis	
		Parasitic	
	Intrahepatic	Viral	Cholestatic
		Alcohol	Primary biliary cirrhosis
		Drug	Primary sclerosing cholangitis
		Oestrogen	Malignancy
		Anabolic steroids	Primary/secondary
		Sepsis	Diffuse
			Fatty liver of pregnancy
			Paediatric causes

conjugated hyperbilirubinaemia can be easily differentiated on blood test.

UNCONJUGATED HYPERBILIRUBINAEMIA

Patients with unconjugated hyperbilirubinaemia will have increased production of bilirubin, a defect in transportation or hepatic bilirubin uptake. These conditions are common and remain surgically relevant.

Unconjugated hyperbilirubinaemia can be divided into the haemolytic disorders and familial non-haemolytic hyperbilirubinaemia (Gilbert's syndrome, Crigler-Najjar syndrome). In these disorders no bilirubin passes into the urine – hence the term *acholuric jaundice.*

The normal liver has considerable excess capacity to excrete bilirubin, and red-cell turnover must increase significantly before unconjugated bilirubin accumulates in the blood. With a normal liver, excess production of bilirubin will not raise the serum bilirubin above 100 µmol/L.

Increased red-cell turnover is usually due to a haemolytic disorder associated with abnormal red cells. In haemolytic disorders, both unconjugated and conju-

gated bilirubin levels increase, but the unconjugated form predominates.

FAMILIAL NON-HAEMOLYTIC UNCONJUGATED HYPERBILIRUBINAEMIA

These include Gilbert's syndrome and Crigler-Najjar syndrome. The other congenital syndromes, namely Dubin-Johnson and Rotor syndromes, are extremely rare and interestingly result in jaundice due to conjugated bilirubin. These will not be discussed.

Gilbert's syndrome may affect up to 5% of the population. It affects males predominantly, and in some patients is familial. The elevated unconjugated bilirubin level is probably due to an impaired intracellular ability to conjugate bilirubin. Gilbert's syndrome is usually detected serendipitously by noting hyperbilirubinaemia which fluctuates around the upper limit of normal and rarely exceeds 40–50 µmol/L. Rapid increases can be precipitated by fasting, alcohol, surgery and other illness. Gilbert's syndrome appears to be benign, and only rarely causes symptoms.

The diagnosis is made by finding an increase in the unconjugated fraction of bilirubin with otherwise normal liver function tests (LFTs). Fasting the patient should increase the bilirubin level. Other hepatic investigations, including liver biopsy and PTC, are not needed, and patients do not require treatment.

Crigler-Najjar syndrome is characterized by high levels of unconjugated bilirubin. It is due to a deficiency of the hepatic enzyme UDP-glucuronosyltransferase (UGT).

Type 1 Crigler-Najjar syndrome is an autosomal recessive condition that presents soon after birth. There is no UGT activity on liver biopsy and no bilirubin in the bile. Children will develop kernicterus unless the condition is treated aggressively with long daily sessions of phototherapy or plasmapheresis.

The definitive treatment for type 1 Crigler-Najjar syndrome is liver transplantation. Allograft transplantation of intraportal isolated hepatocytes is under investigation, and may preserve the native liver for subsequent gene therapy.

Type 2 Crigler-Najjar syndrome is less severe, as there is some UGT activity, and it may not become apparent for months or years. Because of this, kernicterus is less of a problem. UGT is reduced on biopsy and bilirubin is present within the bile. Phenobarbitone can induce transferase activity and lower the bilirubin levels. Most children can lead normal lives, although they are permanently jaundiced with bilirubin levels up to 300 μmol/L. Type 2 Crigler-Najjar children may need plasmaphereses to lower bilirubin levels prior to major surgery, to prevent kernicterus.

Most children with Crigler-Najjar syndrome have a defect in the *UGT1* gene on chromosome 2, and this may be amenable to gene-transfer therapy in the future.

HAEMOLYTIC ANAEMIAS

These are characterized by an accelerated destruction of the red blood cells. Haemolytic anaemias can be congenital or acquired.

HEREDITARY SPHEROCYTOSIS

Hereditary spherocytosis is an autosomal dominant condition in which the red blood cell (RBC) membrane is defective. The RBCs have a spherical shape with increased fragility, and the cells have difficulty passing through the microcirculation. Hereditary spherocytosis is characterized by anaemia, jaundice, increased reticular cell count and splenomegaly. Jaundice is not severe, but cholelithiasis may occur in 50% of patients. Splenectomy is the accepted therapy and it is recommended that this be performed in middle childhood. If gallstones are present, the gall bladder should be removed.

HEREDITARY ENZYME DEFICIENCY

Glucose-6-phosphate dehydrogenase (G6PD) deficiency affects the hexosemonophosphate shunt. The RBCs are fragile and prone to haemolysis. However, the spleen is rarely enlarged. The affected patients, although anaemic, are usually asymptomatic and do not require therapy. Diagnosis is based on a G6PD assay. Splenectomy is not indicated for this disease.

THALASSAEMIA

Thalassaemia is inherited as an autosomal dominant defect in haemoglobin synthesis, and is more common in individuals of Mediterranean origin.

Homozygous thalassaemia (thalassaemia major) is a severe condition that presents in the first year of life with jaundice and growth retardation. Gallstones are common.

Heterozygous thalassaemia (thalassaemia minor) may be relatively minor and not detected until a routine blood examination is performed. Affected patients have a mild anaemia, mild jaundice and splenomegaly.

Thalassaemia is usually diagnosed on blood film which reveals the abnormally shaped red cells with a hypochromic microcytic anaemia. Patients require repeated transfusions, but may occasionally benefit from splenectomy.

SICKLE-CELL DISEASE

In this autosomal dominant condition, normal haemoglobin is replaced by an abnormal form (HbS) which undergoes a configurational change under reduced oxygen tension, altering the shape of the red blood cell. This increases blood viscosity, leading to tissue thrombosis, ischaemia and necrosis.

Sickle-cell trait is present in up to 10% of the black African population, and can present a significant clinical problem for surgeons. In Australia the condition is rare, but a detailed knowledge of its management is important.

Patients have a mild anaemia with characteristic sickle cells on blood film. There is a mild to moderate elevation of serum bilirubin levels and gallstones are common. Patients typically complain of joint and bone pains, haematuria, neurological problems or limb ulceration. Abdominal pain is common, and may simulate an acute abdomen. Multiple splenic infarcts are common, as is eventual fibrosis and atrophy of the spleen. Splenectomy is only indicated for splenic pain or abscess.

Patients may present with a sickle-cell crisis with severe abdominal pain, which does not require surgery if the diagnosis is known.

IDIOPATHIC AUTOIMMUNE HAEMOLYTIC ANAEMIA

In this condition warm or cold haemoagglutination antibodies react with red cells which are phagocytosed by the reticulo-endothelial system, particularly in the spleen. Gamma-globulins bind to the red cell membrane and precipitate macrophage destruction. The condition is common in middle age and in females. Jaundice is usual, and splenomegaly and gallstones are common. Affected patients are mildly anaemic with an elevated reticulocyte count and mild elevation of bilirubin. A direct Coomb's test will reveal antibody on the surface of the red cells.

Autoimmune haemolytic anaemia is usually benign. Steroids may be needed to treat patients who are severely affected, and splenectomy may be required for patients who fail to respond. Radiolabelled red blood cells (CR51) may indicate splenic sequestration and be a useful predictor for the ultimate success of splenectomy in treatment.

HAEMOLYTIC URAEMIC SYNDROME (HUS)

This rare condition has surgical significance, as affected patients typically present with abdominal pain. It is due to severe haemolytic destruction of the red cells, and has been associated with bacterial infection, particularly *E. coli*.

The patients are usually young and well, and present with a severe febrile illness and abdominal pain. Renal function may be only marginally elevated on presentation, but progresses to complete anuria within hours. This rapid progression of acute renal failure is the key to the diagnosis.

Treatment is supportive with antibiotics and dialysis, and surgery is not needed.

CONJUGATED/MIXED HYPERBILIRUBINAEMIA

Patients with a conjugated or mixed conjugated and unconjugated hyperbilirubinaemia can be classified according to whether the site of the problem is extrahepatic or intrahepatic.

Table 13.1 lists the major surgical causes of extrahepatic jaundice. The majority of surgical patients will have mechanical obstruction of the large extrahepatic bile ducts. However, the surgeon must be aware of the major causes of intrahepatic or parenchymal liver disease that result in jaundice.

It is common for jaundice to have more than one presenting cause. For example, a patient with a traumatic or benign bile duct stricture may become infected and present with ascending cholangitis, the patient whose primary disease is parasitic infection of the bile ducts may present with benign or malignant strictures, and a patient with a congenital choledochal cyst may present with malignant obstruction and ascending cholangitis, which are known risks with this pre-malignant condition.

The exact intracellular consequences following large duct obstruction are unknown. Typically the liver will be enlarged with a dark green pigmentation due to the accumulation of bilirubin.

Mechanical obstruction of the bile duct will result in an increase in luminal pressure. The intra-luminal bile duct pressure is dependent on the sphincter of Oddi, which has a resting pressure of 15 to 25 mmHg. Transient ampullary contractions can raise the luminal pressure to 200 mmHg in normal patients, and it is likely that pressures within the obstructed bile duct rise toward this level. As a consequence of this, the extra- and intra-hepatic bile duct dilate. Duct dilatation may not occur in the cirrhotic or fibrotic liver.

Biliary secretion into the canaliculus is carrier-mediated and energy-dependent, and is limited by the increasing pressure and concentration of luminal bilirubin. The carrier mechanism may also be poisoned by other accumulating substances such as bile salts.

The portal tracts become oedematous and inflamed with proliferation of bile ductules that can fill the portal tracts. Extravasated bile may be seen in the tracts, and inflammation may result in an inter-lobular fibrosis, which can progress rapidly to a secondary biliary cirrhosis. Nodular regeneration may occur.

It is common for the obstructed bile to become infected, and bacteria and endotoxins can reflux across the hepatic sinusoids into the hepatic veins and into the systemic circulation. This can be demonstrated in patients who become septicaemic within minutes of biliary manipulation.

Bile-duct enzymes reflux into the blood in the presence of obstruction. The typical pattern is a marked elevation of alkaline phosphatase (ALP) and gamma-glutamyl transpeptidase (γGT) and mild elevation of alanine aminotransferase (ALT) or aspartate aminotransferase (AST).

GALLSTONES

It is of interest that hyperbilirubinaemia from the haemolytic disorders may result in the formation of gallstones in one patient, while gallstones may be the cause of jaundice in another.

It is estimated that 10% of the population (1.8 million Australians) will have gallstones at any one time. The incidence is higher in females and may reach 20–30% in older age groups. The female:male ratio is 5:1 in patients with cholesterol stones, but is approximately 1:1 for pigment stones. The gallstone risk is increased by obesity, disease in a first-degree relative, Crohn's disease or ileal resection, which reduces the bile salt pool.

Cholesterol predominates in 70–80% of gallstones and bile pigment in the remainder. A cholesterol-saturated bile is essential for the formation of cholesterol stones, but gall bladder motility is frequently abnormal with delayed or poor emptying, and this may contribute to stone formation.

Pigment stones may be brown or black. Black stones are typically formed in patients with increased bilirubin production, while brown stones are associated with infection within the biliary system. It has been suggested that a glucuronidase produced by the bacteria reacts with the soluble bilirubin within bile to produce insoluble free bilirubin glucuronic acid, which combines with other salts such as calcium to form stones.

Gallstones may cause jaundice by causing infection or by obstruction of the biliary tree. Acute cholecystitis due to impaction of a stone within the cystic duct or Hartmann's pouch may cause a mild jaundice. This is likely to be due to a low-grade ascending cholangitis, but alterations in the hepatocyte handling of bilirubin secondary to sepsis may be a contributing factor.

, Patients who present with jaundice due to acute cholecystitis may be indistinguishable from those who present with choledocholithiasis and cholangitis.

The hepatic or common bile duct can be obstructed by the distended gall bladder, compressing the ductal system and causing jaundice (Mirizzi syndrome).

At operation, around 10% of patients with gallstones have choledocholithiasis. These patients typically have smaller-diameter gallstones and larger-diameter cystic ducts, which allow passage of stones into the common bile duct. Stones within the common bile duct may impact within the narrow ampullary region and precipitate jaundice with or without cholangitis. Choledocholithiasis is usually associated with elevation of ALP and GGT.

Patients with common bile duct stones or common hepatic stones should have them removed in order to alleviate symptoms and jaundice.

Jaundiced patients with choledocholithiasis may present with acute pancreatitis due to the passage of stones through the ampulla.

Investigations with ultrasound, CT and liver function tests, and clinical examination usually allow differential diagnosis between these entities. Endoscopic retrograde cholangiopancreatography (ERCP) will usually clarify bile duct pathology, and sphincterotomy may allow stones to be removed or an obstructed duct stented. Magnetic resonance cholangiopancreatography (MRCP) is becoming the investigation of choice in patients who are unlikely to require therapeutic intervention.

While liver function tests (LFTs) are usually abnormal with choledocholithiasis, they are normal in patients with uncomplicated gallstones.

CONGENITAL DILATATION OF THE BILIARY TRACT

Choledochal cysts or congenital dilatation of the biliary tract are rare, and the cause is unknown.

Cystic dilatation can occur at different sites in the biliary tree, and is classified according to these criteria. Caroli's disease with multiple intrahepatic dilated cysts is now classified as a type 5 choledochal cyst (Figure 13.3).

Cysts are thick-walled with a high incidence of gallstones. The epithelium of the cysts is abnormal and there is a high risk of malignant degeneration over a 20 to 30-year period. Choledochal cysts are associated with an anomalous pancreaticobiliary duct junction above the ampullary sphincter, and this allows free reflux of pancreatic juice into the cyst. This may be a factor in the malignant change.

Although cysts are usually detected in childhood, patients may present in middle age with a combination of jaundice from obstruction, abdominal pain, cholangitis or a palpable mass. The development of a malignant stricture may precipitate jaundice or cholangitis.

The diagnosis can be made by a combination of CT, ultrasound and ERCP. Choledochal cysts must be differentiated from proximal dilatation of the biliary tree secondary to a low stricture.

Because of the malignant potential, all patients

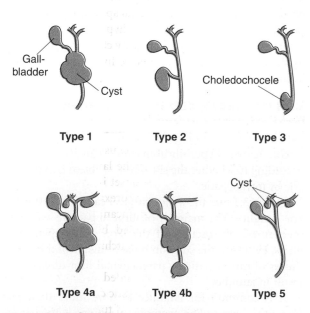

Figure 13.3 Classification of choledochal cysts. (Reproduced with permission from Morris PJ, Malt RA (eds) 1994: *Oxford textbook of surgery*. Oxford: Oxford University Press, p. 1217.)

should undergo surgical excision of the dilated cystic component of the extrahepatic ducts.

BILIARY ATRESIA

Biliary atresia affects approximately one child in every 15 000 live births. Originally thought to be a congenital defect, it was not until 1970 that a characteristic inflammatory process which obliterates the intra- and extrahepatic bile ducts was recognized. Biliary atresia is classified according to the predominant site of extrahepatic duct atresia. The smaller intrahepatic bile ducts are less involved with this sclerotic process and may allow the drainage of bile if the extrahepatic ductal tissue is excised.

Babies with biliary atresia are otherwise normal, but rapidly develop neonatal jaundice which does not resolve.

The prognosis depends on the severity of the destructive process and the delay to definitive surgical drainage. Early excision of the extrahepatic bile ducts and anastomosis of a Roux loop to the hilum of the liver may provide successful drainage in up to 50% of patients (the Kasai procedure). However, the remainder will become progressively cirrhotic and will die without liver transplantation, usually before 5 years of age.

ALLAGILE SYNDROME

Children with this rare, congenital condition have anomalies which include hypoplasia of the biliary tree, small stature, a characteristic facial appearance and complex vascular anomalies such as hypoplasia of the pulmonary arteries. Despite this, many children will survive to the age of 5 to 10 years before liver transplantation becomes necessary.

MALIGNANT STRICTURES

Jaundice due to obstruction is the usual presenting feature of malignant strictures of the large bile ducts and the head of the pancreas. The onset is usually insidious and accompanied by malaise, anorexia and weight loss, and only rarely is there significant pain. Bile duct obstruction will be accompanied by cholestasis and many patients will complain of itching. Cholangitis is rare.

The gall bladder may be distended and palpable with distal obstruction and a patent cystic duct (Courvoisier's sign), but it may not be palpable if tumour involves the gall bladder, cystic duct or proximal bile ducts.

Extrahepatic bile duct tumours can be classified as primary gall bladder, primary bile duct or head of pan-

creas. Tumours of the extrahepatic bile ducts, including the gall bladder, may be scirrhous, polypoidal or nodular.

Tumours spread by direct extension into the surrounding structures such as the duodenum, gall bladder and liver, or by nodal involvement into the pericystic and periduodenal lymph nodes and coeliac axis. Perineural invasion is common and has a poor prognosis.

Radical surgery usually requires resection of the bile ducts accompanied by occasional hepatectomy and a *Roux-en-Y* choledochojejunostomy reconstruction.

Despite aggressive surgery, the overall 5-year mortality rate for malignant strictures causing jaundice is poor at around 1–5%. Non-resectable patients may be palliated by percutaneous or endoscopic stenting.

Experimental combinations of surgery and combined chemoradiation are currently being tried, but their role is not well defined.

Metastatic tumour from colon, breast or other primary sites may occlude the liver hilum by growth in hilar lymph nodes and result in jaundice.

TOTAL PARENTERAL NUTRITION

Hyperbilirubinaemia may occur in up to 25% of patients who receive parenteral nutrition. This typically occurs after 8 to 12 days, and may be accompanied by elevations of ALT and ALP.

Liver biopsies show areas of fatty infiltration. It is likely that this change is due to the hepatotoxic effect of metabolic products of the parenteral solutions.

BENIGN BILE DUCT STRICTURE

Hyperbilirubinaemia is the usual presenting symptom of a benign bile duct stricture, often in association with cholangitis. Benign bile duct strictures are typically postinflammatory, and may follow episodes of cholangitis, parasitic infection, cholecystitis, pancreatitis, radiotherapy or trauma. A significant number will be due to injury sustained during cholecystectomy, or will follow endoscopic or percutaneous biliary manipulation.

Benign bile duct strictures are classified according to the site and extent of bile duct damage.

Benign strictures must be treated aggressively as recurrence is common and may lead to a secondary biliary cirrhosis.

INTRAHEPATIC CONJUGATED HYPERBILIRUBINAEMIA

The multiple causes of intrahepatic hyperbilirubinaemia are linked only by the fact that they are due to a defect in hepatocyte metabolism and excretion of bilirubin. Any agent that is toxic to the hepatocytes may result in elevation of the bilirubin. However, this does not occur in isolation and other hepatocyte functions are usually disturbed, particularly the manufacture of export proteins such as albumin and clotting factors.

VIRAL HEPATITIS

Viral hepatitis is a common precipitant of jaundice within the Australian population, and it typically affects younger patients.

Hepatitis A is an RNA virus belonging to the enterovirus subgroup. It is limited to humans, and no chronic carrier state exists. After an incubation period of 3 weeks, patients become jaundiced. Virus excretion in the stools remains for a week or so, and transmission is by the faecal oral route.

Vaccination is available for hepatitis A, and excellent short-term protection can be obtained from passive immunization with anti-HA antisera.

The hepatitis B virus is a DNA virus belonging to the hepadnavirus group. Transmission occurs at birth or via body fluids. Most affected children are infected at birth, and chronic infection may occur in up to 10% of patients. The virus has a predilection for the liver and secretes large quantities of surface antigen (HbSAg) into the blood. The HbSAg and the E antigen which arises from the core component of the virus are usually detected within a few weeks of infection. Clinical illness will follow infection within days or a few weeks. The virus may be cleared and be followed by the appearance of anticore antibodies. The viral genome can become incorporated into the hepatocyte genome, and this is thought to be necessary for the subsequent development of hepatitis B-associated hepatoma.

Administration of vaccine containing synthesized hepatitis B surface antigen provides good immunity.

Hepatitis D is caused by an RNA delta virus. It is unique in that it can only infect patients who are already infected with hepatitis B, which it requires for replication.

Hepatitis C has recently been identified as the cause of a significant percentage of the patients previously labelled as non-A non-B hepatitis (NANB). Infection is usually transmitted by blood or body fluid contamination, and it remains a significant surgical risk. Most infected patients will develop antibodies 2–6 months after the onset, which are used to screen for the disease. Plasma viral RNA can be quantified and used as a marker of the severity of infection. Although infection may be occult, up to 50% of the patients will develop ongoing chronic infection that cannot be cleared. Early treatment with interferon may limit the progression to a carrier

state. Cirrhosis may occur after an average of 20 years, and is a significant risk for the development of hepatoma.

INVESTIGATION OF THE JAUNDICED PATIENT

Figure 13.4 shows a simple method of investigating the jaundiced adult patient. It is based on the principal biochemical abnormality and follows the classification of jaundice previously described. Determination of the type of hyperbilirubinaemia combined with ultrasound should allow a rapid determination of the likely diagnosis. A patient with hyperbilirubinaemia that is predominantly conjugated and who has non-dilated ducts is likely to have an intrahepatic and non-surgical cause of jaundice.

The conjugated/unconjugated fraction of bilirubin should be estimated, and can be used as a marker to follow the progress of the disease or treatment. Although the hepatic enzymes do show characteristic patterns of change with specific diseases, there is great variability, and the tests are rarely diagnostic.

Gamma-glutamyl transpeptidase (γGT) is membrane bound and occurs at high levels in the biliary secretory

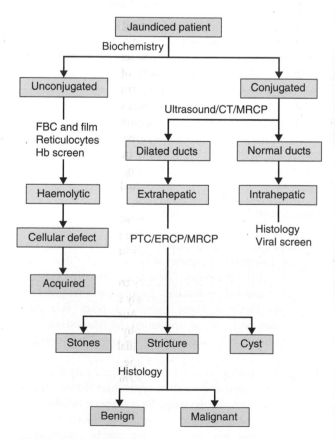

Figure 13.4 Schematic diagram of the investigation of the jaundiced patient.

epithelium. The level of GGT in the bile is 100 times that in the serum. Although GGT is a sensitive marker of liver disease it is not specific. ALP is also secreted by biliary canalicular epithelium and refluxes back into the circulation with biliary obstruction. Together, ALP and GGT are useful markers of biliary obstruction or cholestasis, especially if the levels are more than four or five times higher than normal.

AST is not a useful marker of liver disease, because it is present in many tissues, including heart, liver and muscle, and its origin cannot be determined. ALT exists only in the cytosol of the hepatocyte, and its level is a specific marker of the severity of hepatocyte damage, which releases ALT into the circulation. Marked elevation of ALT (1000 IU/L) usually indicates hepatocellular damage (hepatitis), which is rarely higher than two or three times normal with obstruction or cholestasis.

Ultrasound examination requires no preparation and is non-invasive. It is sensitive and specific in determining dilatation within the biliary tree, and it may demonstrate the site of obstruction, e.g. dilatation of the common bile duct indicates distal obstruction. Although ultrasound may show air, stones and debris within the bile ducts, it is not sensitive or specific in determining the cause of obstruction in most patients. If the liver is fibrotic or cirrhotic the biliary tree may not dilate even in the presence of distal obstruction.

Magnetic resonance cholangiopancreatography (MRCP) is rapidly becoming the investigation of choice for visualizing the biliary tree. The sensitivity and specificity of MRCP approaches that of ERCP in skilled hands. The examination is performed on the newer, faster magnets that allow rapid data collection during a short breath hold. MRCP is non-invasive and requires no contrast media, as the biliary tree is visualized by its water content alone. The digital information can be reconstructed in any plane, allowing three-dimensional rotation of the biliary tree and visualization of its relationship to other hepatic structures.

CT scanning is used as an adjunct to ultrasound. It will demonstrate dilated ducts or the presence of stones, and may show a gall-bladder, periductal or pancreatic mass that is not otherwise evident.

The patient with a dilated biliary tree will require further imaging to determine accurately the site of obstruction and causative pathology. In Australia, endoscopic retrograde cholangiopancreatography (ERCP) has been the initial choice, as it is widely available and may allow therapeutic intervention at the same sitting. ERCP can be performed successfully in over 90% of patients, and is sensitive and specific in determining the site and cause of obstruction in most patients. However, separating malignant from benign strictures remains difficult, and the diagnosis will depend on the age and history of the patient as well as the appearance of the stricture. Bile and brushings for cytology can be taken at ERCP, but have poor sensitivity, and bile-duct malignancy may require percutaneous fine-needle aspiration cytology, core biopsy or surgery to obtain a histological diagnosis.

A sphincterotomy dividing a short segment of the intraluminal ampullary sphincter will open the lower end of the common bile duct and improve drainage. Baskets can be passed up the duct and stones crushed or retrieved. Impacted stones or strictures can be palliated by the passage of one or more biliary stents that traverse the stricture or stone proximally and drain into the duodenum. This can provide short-term palliation, and it may be the definitive 'treatment' in older patients with malignant strictures.

If the obstruction is complete, ERCP will only outline the lower, non-obstructed duct. The dilated biliary tree above the site of obstruction will require injection of contrast into the upper ductal system in order to be visualized. Percutaneous transhepatic cholangiography (PTC) is performed under radiological screening by passing a fine needle into the liver, with simultaneous injection of water-soluble contrast to detect duct puncture. PTC also allows decompression of the proximal biliary tree by the passage of a drain into the ductal system, and it may enable a stricture to be stented or dilated.

PTC and ERCP may be needed in the same patient to diagnose or treat strictures.

Laparoscopy may provide an accurate assessment of the liver and hepatic hilum and contribute to staging of malignant disease. In addition, it may allow fine-needle biopsy of the periductal and gall-bladder area.

FURTHER READING

McIntyre N, Benhamou J-P, Bircher J, Rizetto M, Rodes J. 1991: *Oxford textbook of clinical hepatology.* Oxford: Oxford University Press.

Morris PJ, Malt RA. (eds) 1994: *Oxford textbook of surgery.* Oxford: Oxford University Press.

Sherlock S. 1985: *Diseases of the liver and biliary system.* Oxford: Blackwell Scientific Publications.

Terblanche J. (ed.) 1994: *Hepatobiliary malignancy.* London: Edward Arnold.

Chapter 14

Coma, confusion and convulsions

Nigel R. Jones

Introduction

What is consciousness? It can be described as a state in which one is aware of one's surroundings and one's own being. Disturbances of consciousness may follow focal damage to the reticular formation which extends from the rostral midbrain to the caudal medulla. It receives input from all sensory pathways and projects widely to the cerebral cortex and limbic system. Focal cortical lesions do not affect conscious level, but coma may be produced by general depression of the cerebral cortex.

Although coma is the opposite of consciousness, it is not quite as clear-cut as, for example, being pregnant or not pregnant. Consciousness is a continuum, and we therefore speak of levels of consciousness.

For various reasons it can be useful to define levels of consciousness. This allows us to compare groups of patients at different times, or to follow an individual patient's progress over time. The use of purely descriptive methods is fraught with difficulties. One observer's idea of

somnolent is another's idea of drowsy. When is a person stuporose and when are they obtunded? What is a semi-conscious state, and when does a clouded conscious state become coma? These terms are like describing the weather. What is warm to an Eskimo may well be cold to a Queenslander. Some sort of objective scale is required, but there is no equivalent of a thermometer to give us a numerical measure of conscious level. What we use instead is the Glasgow Coma Scale. This scale was developed as a simple and reproducible measure of conscious level. It has both inter-observer and intra-observer consistency, allowing it to be used as a measure of a patient's progress, despite recordings being made by many different staff members. It can also be used as a research tool to compare results in different centres.

The Glasgow Coma Scale has three components. These are assessed separately and charted to give a visual representation of a patient's progress over time (Figure 14.1).

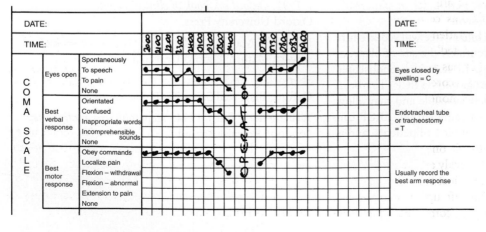

Figure 14.1 A Glasgow Coma Chart showing recording made at frequent intervals in a patient who developed an extradural haematoma. The patient's decline is illustrated graphically, followed by an operation and subsequent recovery.

It is important to note that it is the *best* score that is recorded. The reason for this is obvious if one considers what we are trying to assess. This is a measure of conscious state, not focal deficit. Someone who had a stroke many years ago may have abnormal flexion in their affected arm even though they are wide awake and will obey commands with their good arm. As they are fully conscious, their best motor score ('obeys commands') is much more appropriate than their worst motor score ('abnormal flexion'). The best score also implies the best of all four limbs, and although assessment of the lower limbs is more difficult, it may be relevant in patients with bilateral upper limb fractures or other injuries.

Each response on the GCS is given a number – up to 4 for eyes, 5 for speech and 6 for motor response. Note that these start from 1, not 0, so a patient scores 3 points just for attending, even if they have already expired!

The total is 15, and a score can be given out of this total, e.g. 6/15. This is more meaningful if it is divided into its component parts, e.g. E1, V2, M3, 6/15.

It is not necessary to remember these numbers as they will be on the charts, and provided that the correct assessment is made the numbers can be easily derived.

GLASGOW COMA SCALE

Eye opening

This is quite straightforward. If the patient's eyes are open, 'spontaneous' is recorded. If the eyes are closed initially, say the patient's name or ask them to open their eyes. If they do, record 'to speech'. If the eyes remain closed, apply a painful stimulus (a rub to the chest or pressure over the supra-orbital margin). If the eyes open, record 'to pain', otherwise record 'none'.

If the eyes are too swollen to open, record 'C' for closed. This part of the scale then becomes invalid.

Best verbal response

Each level on the verbal response section represents an increased level of complexity in communication. Starting at the bottom is 'none', which should not cause too many difficulties. Next is 'incomprehensible sounds', which means groans or other noises which do not constitute a word. One level higher is 'inappropriate words', which are usually of the four-letter variety. Putting words together to make sentences comes next. If these sentences are incorrect (e.g. Where are you? At the supermarket), the patient is recorded as 'confused', whereas if the answers are correct and the patient knows where they are, they are recorded as 'orientated'.

If the patient is intubated or has a tracheostomy they will be unable to talk and are recorded as 'T' for tube. They should not be recorded as 'none'.

Best motor response

This section is the most difficult one, but with a little practice it can be completed quickly and reproducibly.

'Obeying commands' means just that. The patient is asked to perform a task (e.g. lift up their arm). It is important to be wary of using the command 'squeeze my fingers', as this may be confused with a grasp reflex. One needs to be confident that the patient has understood the command, processed it and then produced the appropriate response.

'Localizes pain' implies that the upper limb is brought up above shoulder level when a stimulus is applied to the supra-orbital margin. If a stimulus is applied to a nailbed on one hand and the other hand comes across to push it away, this is also localizing. A stimulus applied to the sternum will not usually distinguish between 'localizing' and 'normal flexion'.

'Normal flexion (withdrawal)' implies that the upper limb is flexed when a stimulus is applied to the supra-orbital area but it does not go above shoulder level. A similar response can be produced using nailbed pressure, but it is important to try supra-orbital stimulation first to distinguish localization.

'Abnormal flexion' is more of a primitive reflex response. It can be distinguished from normal flexion by the presence of initial extension followed by flexion or any two of the following:

1. stereotyped flexion posture;
2. extreme wrist flexion;
3. abduction of the upper arm;
4. flexion of the fingers over the thumb.

'Extension' is easily recognized and is accompanied by pronation of the forearm and flexion of the wrist.

'None' implies no response at all to painful stimuli, which should include a stimulus in a cranial nerve territory in case of spinal cord injury.

Using the Glasgow Coma Score we can define coma as not speaking words, not obeying commands and not opening the eyes. Using this definition, most patients with a GCS of 9 and all patients with a GCS of 8 or less are unconscious (in coma).

The GCS is also used to categorize head injury as mild (14–15), moderate (9–13) or severe (3–8).

ASSESSMENT OF THE UNCONSCIOUS TRAUMA PATIENT

The surgical resident will be confronted with unconscious trauma victims in the Emergency Department in most surgical rotations. It is frequently a source of great anxiety, but does not need to be so. Little needs to be done beyond standard trauma management (ABCs, etc.) and history and examination. As part of the primary survey, the pupillary size and reactions are noted and the GCS assessed. This is the extent of the neurological examination at that stage, as other areas have a higher priority. Even though an open head wound may appear dramatic, it is much more important to secure the airway and maintain adequate oxygenation and perfusion than to be concerned about a CT head scan. While the ambulance officers are available an assessment of the GCS at the earliest possible time after the injury should be obtained. The main value of charting the GCS is to provide a record of conscious level over time. The relevance of a GCS of 9 now would be quite different if it was 3 an hour ago than if it was 15 an hour ago.

Once the primary survey is complete, the secondary survey should include a more thorough neurological examination, as well as an examination of the head, face and neck. The neurological examination will be limited because of the lack of co-operation by the patient, but it should still be possible to determine whether there are lateralizing signs such as a hemiparesis or a third cranial nerve palsy. The head and face should be examined for fractures and the nose and ears inspected for CSF leaks. If there is CSF rhinorrhoea or otorrhoea, a basal skull fracture is present (regardless of whether or not it can be seen on radiographs).

Patients who are unconscious (GCS < 9) as a result of a head injury should be intubated and ventilated, as they will be unable to protect their airway or maintain ideal oxygen and carbon dioxide levels. Table 14.1 details the indications for CT head scan in head injury and Table 14.2 lists the indications for neurosurgical referral.

Table 14.1 Indications for CT scan in head injury

GCS < 9 after resuscitation
Neurological deterioration (2 GCS points)
Drowsiness or confusion (GCS 9–13 for > 2 h)
Persistent headache, vomiting
Focal signs
Fracture
Penetrating injury
Age (over 50 years)

Table 14.2 Indications for neurosurgical consultation in head injury

Skull fracture with GCS < 15 or signs
GCS < 9 after resuscitation
Deterioration (2 GCS points, fits, new signs)
GCS 9–13 > 2 h, no fracture
Compound depressed skull fracture
Skull base fracture
Penetrating injury
Abnormal CT scan

ASSESSMENT OF THE PATIENT WITH SUBARACHNOID HAEMORRHAGE

Patients with subarachnoid haemorrhage (SAH) are among the most difficult to diagnose and treat. When seen in the Emergency Department they will usually give a history of sudden onset of severe headache, but they may present with sudden collapse and loss of consciousness. Clues to the diagnosis are neck stiffness, subhyaloid haemorrhages and a history of a preceding 'warning leak'.

The difficulties for the surgical resident increase during the days following a subarachnoid haemorrhage. These patients can develop a wide range of complications, which can often be difficult to distinguish from each other. Close observation is critical to detect these complications, which can occur many days after the haemorrhage. Increasing confusion, decreasing conscious level, epilepsy and the development of focal neurological deficits frequently occur following SAH. When called to see a patient who has deteriorated following SAH, the following conditions should be considered.

Rebleed

This should be considered if the aneurysm has not been clipped and the deterioration is fairly sudden. Increased neck stiffness or new subhyaloid haemorrhages may occur, but the diagnosis will usually rest on the demonstration of new subarachnoid blood on CT. The risk of rebleeding is greatest soon after the first SAH, and decreases with time. The mortality rate of a second SAH is 60%.

Vasospasm

This is a common, serious and poorly understood complication of SAH. It can occur up to 3 weeks after haemorrhage, but is most common after 4 to 10 days. Many prophylactic treatments have been tried in the past, and currently calcium-channel antagonists (nimodipine) are used. Vasospasm is more common in patients with large amounts of subarachnoid blood on the initial CT, and can produce confusion, drowsiness and any combination of neurological deficits which are not necessarily confined to the distribution of the artery harbouring the ruptured aneurysm. Transcranial Doppler ultrasonography is used routinely in many centres to predict the onset of vasospasm, but definitive diagnosis usually rests with angiography, during which vasodilatory treatment may be instituted. Vasospasm is a common cause of both neurological deficit and death in patients with SAH, and it needs to be treated aggressively. Apart from controversial invasive measures such as angioplasty and intra-arterial papaverine, hypertensive, hypervolaemic and haemodilution (HHH) therapy is frequently used in patients whose aneurysms have been clipped. Patients with unclipped aneurysms are more difficult to treat, since measures aimed at reducing vasospasm may increase the risk of rebleeding.

Hydrocephalus

SAH may cause acute hydrocephalus by blocking the normal CSF flow with massive intraventricular haemorrhage, but it more commonly produces a block to the reabsorption of CSF, which is usually transitory. This can cause raised intracranial pressure and require ventricular drainage or permanent ventricular shunting.

Electrolyte disturbance

Patients with SAH are particularly prone to syndrome of inappropriate antidiuretic hormone (SIADH) and consequent hyponatraemia. Low sodium levels can produce confusion, drowsiness and epilepsy.

Hypoxia

Hypoxia can be due to respiratory depression from impaired conscious level, but SAH may also cause neurogenic pulmonary oedema which can be severe enough to require ventilation.

ASSESSMENT OF POST-OPERATIVE CONFUSION OR COMA

One should first obtain a history of the onset of coma or confusion. Abrupt onset suggests causes such as haemorrhage, stroke or epilepsy, while a more gradual onset suggests metabolic causes. The most common causes of post-operative confusion are hypoxia, drugs and alcohol withdrawal. Hypoxia may be due to pain inhibition of respiration, sedative drugs, pneumonia, pulmonary oedema or pulmonary embolism. All confused patients should have arterial blood gases taken and be given supplemental oxygen.

Hyponatraemia can develop insidiously in the post-operative period due to SIADH, and requires determination of serum and urinary sodium and osmolality levels. Many analgesics used in the post-operative period can produce drowsiness and confusion as well as hypoxia from respiratory depression. If narcotics are thought to be the cause, they can be reversed with naloxone.

Alcohol withdrawal should always be considered, even without a history of alcoholism. Physical signs of liver failure and abnormal liver enzymes support the diagnosis. Other causes of liver failure or renal failure may also cause post-operative confusion.

Diabetes may produce confusion and coma through hypoglycaemia or hyperglycaemia. As with status epilepticus, it is worth giving a dose of intravenous glucose in an unconscious patient without a diagnosis, after taking blood for analysis.

Epilepsy may occur without being noticed by staff, and the post-ictal state is often characterized by drowsiness and confusion.

Cerebrovascular accidents may occur in the perioperative period, and should be considered especially in patients who have been on cardiac bypass or anticoagulants, or who have undergone carotid or intracranial surgery.

When called to the post-operative neurosurgical patient, there are even more possibilities to consider. The causes of deterioration in the SAH patient have been covered above. Any patient who has had intracranial surgery may develop epilepsy, and this is dealt with below. Haemorrhage also needs to be considered. This may be intracerebral, subdural or extradural. Intracranial infection usually causes significant neurological deficit, and seizures occur frequently. Hydrocephalus may also develop following neurosurgical procedures, particularly in patients with a ventriculo-peritoneal shunt which may become blocked or infected. It is also important to consider shunt malfunction in a patient who has had abdominal surgery or infection. Brain swelling is particularly common following surgery for gliomas, but may also occur after other intracranial procedures.

These intracranial causes of confusion or coma are best diagnosed with a CT scan, but the general conditions described above should not be ignored. The author has woken up more than one patient on the CT table with intravenous glucose.

EPILEPSY

The study of epilepsy is a complicated field, but for our purposes epilepsy may be regarded as generalized or partial, with partial seizures including focal motor, focal sensory and temporal lobe seizures. All may be seen in neurosurgical patients, but generalized seizures are predominant in other surgical patients. Table 14.3 outlines the major causes of symptomatic fits (i.e. excluding idiopathic epilepsy, which is the most common category overall).

Complications such as hypoglycaemia, hyponatraemia or meningitis can all occur in post-operative or trauma patients, and must not be overlooked.

POST-TRAUMATIC EPILEPSY

Post-traumatic epilepsy (PTE) is categorized as early (within the first week) or late (after the first week). The incidence of each type is approximately 5%. The rare immediate seizure occurring within moments of injury is different and does not predispose to late epilepsy. Approximately one-third of early seizures occur within the first hour, one-third within the next day and one-third within the following 6 days. Half are focal, especially focal motor. The risks for an individual can be predicted to some extent, with features such as intracerebral or subdural haematoma, missile wounds, compound depressed fracture, infection and

Table 14.3 Causes of symptomatic fits

1. Metabolic causes
Hyponatraemia
Hypoglycaemia
Hypocalcaemia
Uraemia
Hyperthyroidism
Drug withdrawal (especially alcohol)
Porphyria
Hypoxia
Hypertensive encephalopathy
Hyperthermia, especially in children

2. Infection

3. Trauma (including post-craniotomy)

4. Cerebrovascular causes
Rare with thrombosis except venous thrombosis
25% early seizures with SAH
Focal seizures after embolic stroke

5. Tumours

6. Congenital causes
Tuberous sclerosis
Neurofibromatosis
Inborn errors of metabolism

early epilepsy all being associated with significantly higher risks of late epilepsy.

Anticonvulsant prophylaxis has undergone changes over the last few years. Whereas most patients with severe head injury used to be given prophylactic anticonvulsants for 2 years, this is now mostly restricted to higher-risk patients and for much shorter periods (often only 1 week). Patients who develop early post-traumatic epilepsy have a risk of late epilepsy of at least 25%, and will usually be treated with anticonvulsants. Phenytoin is often the initial drug of choice, as it can be given intravenously, starting with a loading dose and then regular once-daily doses with blood levels checked after a steady state has been reached in about 5 days. Carbamazepine can also be used in patients who are able to take oral medication.

Epilepsy occurring in the post-operative neurosurgical patient should be treated in a similar manner. It is important to exclude one of the general underlying causes described in Table 14.3 before accepting the surgery as the sole cause.

STATUS EPILEPTICUS

Status epilepticus refers to two or more tonic-clonic seizures occurring without an intervening return of consciousness. It is a medical emergency, as prolonged status can cause permanent neurological deficit or death. Treatment begins with attention to airway, breathing and circulation. Blood should be withdrawn for analysis of glucose, electrolytes (particularly sodium and calcium), creatinine/urea, osmolality and anticonvulsant levels if appropriate. This should be followed immediately by 50 mL of 50% glucose and 100 mg thiamine intravenously. Seizures can usually be controlled with diazepam 3–10 mg intravenously. This should be followed by a loading dose of phenytoin (500–1000 mg IV slowly at 50 mg/min). If diazepam does not control the seizures, clonazepam 0.5–1 mg IV may be used. If this is unsuccessful, barbiturates or general anaesthesia may be required. The above doses are for adults and care must be taken when using these sedating drugs in children.

Attention should also be given to identifying and treating underlying causes. Examination should include inspection for evidence of head trauma, needle marks, neck stiffness, signs of renal or hepatic failure and fundoscopy for evidence of subarachnoid haemorrhage (subhyaloid haemorrhages). Urine should be collected for a drug screen, arterial blood gases should be obtained and hypoxia corrected, body temperature should be returned to normal, and acid–base and electrolyte disturbances should be corrected. More specific tests such as CSF analysis, blood culture, thyroid and liver function tests may also be required.

TETANY

PARATHYROID TETANY

This is an uncommon complication of thyroidectomy, due to hypoparathyroidism when two or more parathyroid glands have been removed. Symptoms of tingling and numbness of the lips and extremities occur between 1 and 5 days after surgery. This is followed by painful cramps throughout the body, but particularly in the hands and feet (carpopedal spasm). Clinical signs of tetany rely on hyperexcitability of the nerves and their susceptibility to ischaemia.

Chvostek-Weiss sign Tapping the facial nerve just in front of the ear produces a muscular twitch on the ipsilateral side of the face.

Trousseau's sign A sphygmomanometer cuff is placed on the arm and inflated to 200 mmHg. If tetany is present, typical contractions of the hand will occur within 5 min. The fingers flex at the metacarpophalangeal (MCP) joints and extend at the interphalangeal joints. The thumb is strongly adducted (obstetrician's hand).

TETANUS

Tetanus is caused by the exotoxin of *Clostridium tetani*. Despite immunization programmes, tetanus still occurs in non-immunized or partially immunized individuals. Although it is rare in Australia, cases are reported every year and mortality rates are very high.

The spores of *C. tetani* are found in the soil, and dirty, contaminated wounds are therefore most at risk. However, tetanus may follow elective surgery and burns. A recent case of tetanus following elective surgery in Australia led to criticism of the surgeon by the court for not checking the patient's tetanus immunization status pre-operatively.

The incubation period is between 2 and 56 days, with most cases occurring within 14 days. Early, non-specific symptoms are soon replaced by muscle stiffness, followed by rigidity. Trismus is usually seen early, and facial muscle contractions produce the typical *risus sardonicus*. More widespread spasms follow, including laryngeal and respiratory muscles.

The best treatment is prevention with active immunization. Contaminated wounds should be cleaned and thoroughly debrided. Immunization status should be determined. Full immunization involves three injections of adsorbed toxoid, with a further dose every 10 years. If a patient is considered to be fully immunized and has a tetanus-prone wound, they should be given a further 0.5 mL of adsorbed toxoid if more than 5 years have elapsed since the last dose. For a non-immunized individual suffering a tetanus-prone wound, both active and passive immunization should be given. This involves 0.5 mL adsorbed toxoid and 250 units of human tetanus immunoglobulin (TIG). These should be given using different syringes and administered to different sites.

FURTHER READING

American College of Surgeons Committee on Trauma. 1969: Prophylaxis against tetanus in wound management. *Ohio State Medical Journal* **65**, 506–7.

Jennett B. 1975: *Epilepsy after non-missile head injuries*, 2nd edn. London: Heinemann.

Neurosurgical Society of Australasia and Royal Australasian College of Surgeons. 1992: *The management of acute neurotrauma in rural and remote locations. A set of guidelines for the care of head and spinal injuries.* Melbourne: Joint publication of The Neurosurgical Society of Australasia and the Royal Australasian College of Surgeons.

Plum F, Posner JB. 1980: *The diagnosis of stupor and coma*, 3rd edn. Philadelphia, PA: F.A. Davis Company.

Chapter 15

Paresis and paraesthesia

Gordon G. Stuart

Introduction

Paresis refers to a weakness of muscles and is usually taken to mean a partial paralysis.

Paralysis refers to loss of voluntary movement due to interruption of the motor pathway at any point from the cerebrum to the muscle fibre (Table 15.1).

Monoparesis is weakness of one limb, whereas *monoplegia* is complete paralysis of one limb. Hemiparesis (incomplete) and *hemiplegia* (complete) refer to weakness of one side, i.e. the leg, arm or lower portion of the face. The upper face is spared due to the bilateral cortical supply to the cranial motor neurones. *Paraparesis* or *paraplegia* refers to weakness or paralysis of the lower limbs. *Paresis* is divided into *upper motor neurone* or *spastic paralysis* and *lower motor neurone* or *flaccid paralysis*.

Paraesthesia is defined as altered or diminished sensation. Lesions that produce paraesthesia will involve the peripheral nerves, posterior root ganglia, dorsal roots or rootlets, dorsal white columns of the spinal cord and brainstem (medial lemniscus), corona radiata or the post-central gyrus of the cerebral cortex.

A lesion of a *peripheral nerve* produces sensory loss in the cutaneous distribution, whereas lesions of *posterior root ganglia, roots or segments of the spinal cord* produce a dermatomal sensory loss which gives an accurate segmental level of the lesion, the so-called *sensory level*, e.g. C4 – shoulder tip, T4 – nipple, T10 – umbilicus, L1 – groin, L3 – knee.

MANAGEMENT OF A PATIENT WITH PARESIS AND/OR PARAESTHESIA

As in all forms of clinical practice, the most important factor which forms the basis for diagnosis, management and treatment is the history of the symptomatology.

Essential points in history taking are the age of the patient, family and occupational history and duration of symptoms. Also important is the speed of onset of symptoms (rapid in stroke and slow in benign tumours), and the progression of the disease, which improves after a stroke, is relentlessly progressive in tumours, rapidly progressive in CSF obstruction and fluctuating in chronic subdural haematoma (the great mimic of stroke and tumour). A past history of hypertension, blood dyscrasias, trauma, embolic source, cardiac arrhythmia or primary malignancy should be sought, as should associated or accompanying features of paranasal, mastoid or middle-ear infection. The presence of pain, such as headache, spinal pain or root pain, is highly relevant.

PHYSICAL EXAMINATION

An accurate physical examination should enable anatomical diagnosis of the site of pathology.

1. *Lower motor neurone* lesion features place the lesion at the spinal cord nerve root, peripheral nerve or muscle.

Table 15.1 Upper and lower motor neurone paralysis: distinguishing features

	Upper motor neurone paralysis	Lower motor neurone paralysis
Muscle tone	Increased (spasticity)	Decreased (flaccidity)
Deep tendon reflexes	Hyperactive	Absent
Plantar response	Extensor	Flexor or absent
Muscle wasting	Minimal	Pronounced
EMG changes	Minimal	Marked
Site of lesion	Pyramidal cells or axones (corticospinal tract)	Anterior horn cells or axones (peripheral nerve)

2. *Upper motor neurone* lesion features place the lesion at the spinal cord brainstem, internal capsule, corona radiata or motor cortex opposite to the side of the paresis.

3. *Cauda equina* lesions classically produce saddle or perineal anaesthesia and sphincter loss.

4. *Mixed peripheral nerve* lesions typically produce lower motor neurone weakness, sensory impairment, autonomic loss (absence of sweating) and trophic changes (wasting and neuropathic ulcers).

IMAGING INVESTIGATIONS

These will confirm or possibly alter the clinical hypothesis of the anatomical site of the lesion.

SUSPECTED SPINAL PATHOLOGY

Plain X-ray shows spinal collapse, destruction of vertebral bodies or pedicles, narrowed disc spaces, intraspinal calcification and spinal canal stenosis.

CT scan shows disc protrusions or extrusions and, if combined with intrathecal contrast injection (myelography), shows cord or nerve root compression or displacement.

MRI has become the main imaging investigation for spinal pathology. It will show all of the information of CT myelography, as well as altered signal characteristics of the spinal cord, as in myelopathy, intramedullary haemorrhage or tumour.

SUSPECTED INTRACRANIAL PATHOLOGY

CT scan without and with IV contrast is the first line of investigation. If a haemorrhage is found, further investigation with CT angiography, digital angiography or MRI angiography may be indicated.

STROKE

Stroke is defined as a sudden neurological deficit of vascular aetiology lasting more than 24 h. A transient ischaemic attack (TIA) is a transient neurological deficit of vascular origin lasting less than 24 h.

Stroke is the third commonest cause of death in most countries, and the most important cause of chronic neurological disability. It may be due to cerebral haemorrhage (20%) or cerebral ischaemia (80%). The incidence of strokes has declined in recent decades due to better management of the following risk factors:

- hypertension;
- smoking;
- cardiac disease, including arrhythmias;
- diabetes;
- hyperlipidaemia;
- excessive alcohol consumption.

However, the incidence of subarachnoid haemorrhage due to ruptured cerebral aneurysm has remained constant at 12 per 100 000 members of the population annually.

Ruptured cerebral aneurysm is the commonest cause of non-traumatic subarachnoid haemorrhage, which typically occurs in patients over 40 years, as aneurysms take years to develop. It is a myth that berry aneurysms are congenital.

Ruptured berry aneurysm is a lethal condition with a mortality rate of at least 50%. Rebleeding, hydrocephalus and progressive cerebral ischaemia are significant complications which add to both morbidity and mortality.

Anatomy

Aneurysms occur at bifurcations of the circle of Willis, which lies in the subarachnoid space at the base of the brain. Figure 15.1 illustrates the common aneurysm sites.

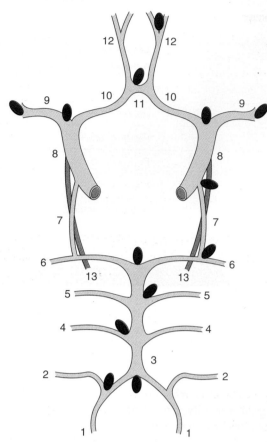

Figure 15.1 Diagram of circle of Willis and common aneurysm sites. 1, vertebral artery; 2, posterior inferior cerebellar artery; 3, basilar artery; 4, anterior inferior cerebellar artery; 5, superior cerebellar artery; 6, posterior cerebral artery; 7, posterior communicating artery; 8, internal carotid artery; 9, middle cerebral artery; 10, proximal anterior cerebral artery; 11, anterior communicating artery; 12, distal anterior cerebral artery; 13, oculomotor nerve.

Management

For details of diagnosis, see Chapter 1.2 on headache.

Premonitory headaches or warning leaks are present in 40% of aneurysmal haemorrhages, and are frequently misdiagnosed by patients, local medical officers and hospital staff as migraine, tension headache or influenza. If the diagnosis is made at this stage and appropriate investigations and surgical management carried out, a good outcome can be expected in 80–85% of patients. Missed diagnosis may result in a second haemorrhage with high morbidity and a mortality rate of at least 50%. The most important safeguard is to enquire about the mode of onset in any patient with a severe headache. The cardinal feature of subarachnoid haemorrhage is *sudden headache,* often described as being like a blow on the head or an explosion inside the head.

The definitive diagnosis of cerebral aneurysm is made by digital subtraction angiography.

Treatment of ruptured aneurysms involves:

1. prevention of rebleeding by excluding the aneurysm from the circulation by direct microvascular surgery or endovascular coiling.

2. prevention of cerebral ischaemia by promoting adequate hydration, avoiding hypotension and 'anti-vasospastic' drugs such as nimodipine.

Transient ischaemic attacks (TIAs)

These are brief and reversible episodes of cerebral or retinal vascular dysfunction lasting less than 24 h.

The risk of stroke after a TIA is approximately 5–10% per year, compared to about 1% in an age-matched control population.

Carotid territory TIAs produce transient monocular blindness or hemisensory disturbance, hemiparesis or dysphasia.

Vertebrobasilar TIAs are often more complex, with a variety of symptoms which may include vertigo, amnesia or occasionally loss of consciousness (described as 'drop attacks').

Investigation with a CT head scan will demonstrate lesions such as chronic subdural haematoma, cerebral tumour or abscess, which may all mimic TIAs. Duplex scanning and/or digital subtraction angiography will demonstrate extracranial atherosclerosis, which often occurs at the common carotid bifurcation in the neck. Atheromatous plaques at this site may ulcerate and produce platelet thrombi and micro-embolism. Cardiac investigation, including echocardiography, should be undertaken, particularly if the patient is in auricular fibrillation, which may produce embolism from the cardiac site.

Treatment

If TIAs are found to be due to carotid disease, the following options are available:

1. medical – antiplatelet aggregation drugs, aspirin or ticlopidine;

2. percutaneous transluminal angioplasty;

3. carotid endarterectomy.

Cardiogenic thrombo-embolism

Auricular fibrillation is associated with a fivefold increase in stroke incidence, which can be reduced by up to 70% with warfarin therapy.

Intracerebral haemorrhage (non-aneurysmal haemorrhagic stroke)

Non-traumatic intracerebral haemorrhage is most commonly due to hypertension, which causes rupture of small vessels in the putamen, thalamus, central white matter, brainstem and cerebellum.

Diagnosis is readily confirmed on CT scan, which will show the mass-effect site and allow estimation of volume.

Surgical treatment

Evacuation of intracerebral haematomas by surgical methods is of value if the patient is suffering from the mass effect of the haematoma. Patients who are comatose with haematomas of volume greater than 75 mL as estimated on a CT scan are unlikely to benefit from surgery.

Patients with cerebellar haematomas are at risk of sudden deterioration due to hydrocephalus and/or brainstem compression. They often do well with surgical evacuation of the haematoma.

Arteriovenous malformation (AVM)

Arteriovenous malformation is a true congenital lesion which is thought to be due to persistence of fetal-type circulation. Classically the lesions are wedge-shaped, with the base presenting on the brain surface and the apex pointing towards the ventricle. They commonly occur at sites of fusion, such as the Sylvian fissure, Rolandic fissure and the great fissure of the cerebellum.

The effects produced may include rupture of the thin-walled vessels, with resultant subarachnoid and/or intracerebral haemorrhage, and arteriovenous shunting through fistulae in the malformation with resultant steal phenomena such as epilepsy or neurological deficit.

AVM is the commonest cause of subarachnoid haemorrhage in the first two decades of life, accounting for 60% of subarachnoid haemorrhages in children. About 70% of AVMs that are destined to bleed have done so by the age of 40 years. The mortality rate from bleeding AVMs (about 10%) is much lower than that from cerebral aneurysms and the risk of rebleeding is estimated to be 2–3% per year. Small lesions are thought to be more prone to rupture than large ones.

Investigation

1. CT scanning will detect many unruptured AVMs with contrast enhancement of the lesion.

2. A ruptured AVM shows as a haemorrhage on CT.

3. MRI angiography will demonstrate ruptured and unruptured AVMs.

4. If treatment is being considered, digital subtraction angiography is essential.

Management

Microsurgical excision to prevent haemorrhages is the method of choice for small lesions in a young person if a significant increase in neurological deficit is unlikely, i.e. the lesion is not in an eloquent site. Pre-operative embolization by endovascular techniques may make surgery easier and safer.

Small lesions in an eloquent site, e.g. left parietal lobe or brainstem, may be treated by focused radiotherapy to the nidus of the AVM, aiming to produce endarteritis and thrombosis of the lesion. This affords protection against haemorrhage after a lag period of 2 to 3 years.

SPINAL INJURIES

Approximately 5 in 100 000 members of the population per year suffer spinal column injuries, and young adult males are most commonly affected. The spinal cord is injured in 1 in 200 000 members of the population annually.

ANATOMY OF THE CORD

The spinal cord extends from the craniocervical junction to the conus medullaris at level L1–L2.

BLOOD SUPPLY TO THE SPINAL CORD (SEE FIGURE 15.2)

The arterial supply is by anterior and posterior spinal arteries which run longitudinally from the foramen magnum and anastomose inferiorly at the conus medullaris in the cruciate anastomosis. Segmental reinforcements occur by anastomotic arteries entering along spinal nerve roots. The largest of these occur at the spinal cord enlargements of T1 and T11, and are known as the arteries of Adamkiewicz.

The *anterior spinal artery* is the dominant arterial supply of the cord, supplying the anterior grey columns and anterior and lateral white columns. Thus the *anterior spinal artery syndrome* causes loss of motor function due to involvement of the ventral horns and corticospinal tracts, loss of pain and temperature due to lateral spinothalamic tract involvement, but preservation of touch, vibration and joint position sense, due to intact posterior columns. The anterior spinal artery is formed by the union of one branch from each vertebral artery.

The *posterior spinal arteries* consist of one or two vessels on each side which branch from the posterior inferior cerebellar or vertebral arteries. They supply the posterior grey and white columns only.

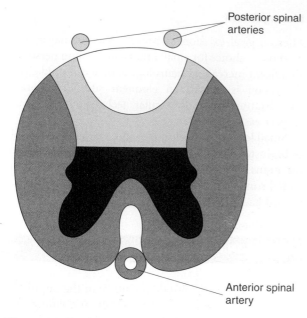

Posterior spinal arteries

Anterior spinal artery

Figure 15.2 Blood supply to spinal cord.

MECHANISM OF INJURY

Most undisplaced fractures of the spine are not associated with spinal cord injury, although fracture dislocations usually cause cord damage and neurological dysfunction.

The spinal cord may be damaged by direct mechanical compression (as in fracture dislocations), traction (as in hyperextension and flexion injuries) or there may be vascular damage producing ischaemia, particularly with damage to the anterior spinal artery which supplies the anterior columns, lateral columns and anterior grey matter.

Injuries to the spinal column may include flexion and flexion rotation, compression, hyperextension and penetrating injuries. Flexion and flexion rotation are often associated with posterior ligamentous damage and instability. Compression injuries are usually stable, as are hyperextension and penetrating injuries from gunshot wounds or stab injuries.

CLINICAL FEATURES

Initially there is an immediate flaccid paralysis and sensory loss below the level of the lesion, with loss of vasomotor control and resultant hypotension, loss of temperature control, and sphincteric loss with impairment of bladder and bowel control. This is referred to as spinal shock, and it usually lasts from 3 days to 3 weeks. Priapism in males during this early stage usually indicates spinal cord injury.

When spinal shock wears off, a spastic paralysis appears with hyper-reflexia and extension plantar responses.

PREHOSPITAL MANAGEMENT

Remember that airway care is always the first priority.

1. Always consider spinal injury, especially injury to the cervical spine or thoracolumbar junction in the *unconscious patient.*

2. Rapid clinical assessment:
   - respiratory pattern (is the breathing only diaphragmatic?);
   - voluntary movement and sensation in limbs;
   - muscle tone and reflexes.

3. Extrication from a vehicle:
   - maintain spinal alignment, especially avoiding flexion or rotation;
   - avoid movements which increase pain;
   - if cervical injury is suspected, apply a cervical collar or substitute (e.g. rolled up jacket).

4. Transport to primary hospital:
   - if the patient is conscious, place them in the supine position. If respiratory distress is aggravated, place them in the head-up position (unless hypotensive);
   - if the patient is unconscious, clear and control the airway. Place them in the lateral position with neck support. Protect the airway from obstruction and/or inhalation;
   - arrange an appropriate lifting device and transport;
   - give supplemental oxygen.

PRIMARY HOSPITAL MANAGEMENT

1. Emergency resuscitation – cardiopulmonary support with possible treatment for surgical shock (beware spinal shock) – see below.

2. Always consider spinal injury:
   - history (mechanism of injury) and symptoms;
   - clinical examination will assess vital signs, especially bradycardia and hypotension, respiratory pattern (e.g. diaphragmatic in high cord injury), neurological signs (e.g. motor response in all limbs; paralysis is usually flaccid in spinal shock), sensory level to pain, joint position and response to touch. In particular, check perineal sensation, sweat level or altered triple response in the unconscious, plantar responses, priapism (an uncommon but characteristic sign of a usually 'complete' lesion), hyperelevated

shoulders in cervical injury, sphincter tone (flaccid in cauda equina lesion and reduced in cord lesion) and urinary retention.

3. Suspect other injuries, such as head injury, haemopneumothorax or ruptured aorta with thoracic spinal injury, ruptured abdominal viscus with thoracolumbar injury. In particular beware of the retroperitoneal injury (especially duodenum) with lap-type seatbelt injuries. Symptoms and signs of such injuries may be masked in a patient with a complete spinal cord lesion.

4. Management of 'spinal shock' due to acute 'shutdown' of spinal cord function below the injury level, which may last for several days:

   - intravenous fluids, taking care not to overtransfuse – the blood pressure may be 'normal' at 80/50 mmHg with bradycardia in a high cord injury (but beware surgical shock which may also be present from other injuries, e.g. splenic tear or ruptured aorta);

   - steroids may be helpful, but their value is not proven;

   - insert a large-bore nasogastric tube;

   - insert a urinary catheter and monitor urinary output;

   - avoid hypoxia, monitor vital capacity and beware respiratory failure from sputum retention or fatigue;

   - a careful lift or log roll is needed every 2 h to avoid trophic skin ulceration;

   - maintain normothermia.

INVESTIGATION OF SUSPECTED SPINAL INJURY

Once primary triage of airway, breathing and circulation has been performed and their functioning optimized, an assessment of the spinal column and cord can be made.

In order to prevent further damage to the spinal cord, any movement or transfer of patients with a possible spinal injury should be made with caution, with adequate help and expertise available. Unconscious patients should have a protective cervical collar applied initially, until adequate imaging of the spine has been performed. Plain X-rays to include the whole cervical spine C1–C7 with lateral view should be performed on all unconscious patients following trauma to the head and neck region, and on conscious patients who have symptoms or signs of neck or spinal cord injury. CT scan of the spine may be indicated to assess bone injuries more effectively.

MRI of the spine will show cord ligament and soft-tissue abnormalities.

If plain X-ray and CT do not demonstrate an abnormality, but cervical injury is suspected, then flexion and extension views of the cervical spine under careful medical supervision may be required to exclude instability due to ligamentous injury.

Suspicion of thoracic or lumbar spinal injury (e.g. widened posterior mediastinum on chest X-ray) will indicate X-ray and CT of the appropriate spinal segments.

MANAGEMENT

Initial management

During spinal shock, secondary insult to the already damaged spinal cord must be prevented by correction of hypoxia (administration of oxygen, or assisted ventilation if necessary) and correction of hypotension. Use of a pressure mattress prevents pressure areas and secondary infection. Prevention and treatment of infection can be achieved by sterile bladder catheterization and regular culture of urine samples to detect subclinical infection. Deep vein thrombosis and pulmonary embolus may be prevented by administration of low-dose heparin and compression stockings. Nasogastric tube decompression of the stomach is used to prevent vomiting and diaphragm splinting due to ileus.

SPINAL REDUCTION AND STABILIZATION

Once the patient's general condition has been stabilized, a reduction of dislocations by traction manipulation or open surgical techniques may be indicated.

Immobilization by spinal bed nursing, traction, internal or external fixation techniques is then maintained until bone and ligamentous healing has occurred.

INDICATIONS FOR SURGICAL TREATMENT

Damage to the spinal cord occurs at the time of injury, and there is little evidence to show improved neurological outcome as a result of acute surgical decompression procedures.

Indications for surgical intervention are limited to the following:

1. progressive neurological deterioration if a compressive lesion such as a bone disc or haematoma is shown on imaging;

2. incomplete cord lesions where there is failure to improve and a compressive lesion is demonstrated;

3. in cases of penetrating injury (e.g. gunshot wound,

knife or blade wound, or spear) removal of foreign bodies, debridement and dural repair are indicated;

4. operative stabilization and fixation to avoid prolonged traction or bedrest.

GENERAL CARE OF SPINAL CORD INJURY

This involves the following:

1. metabolic care – fluid, electrolyte and calorie balance need to be maintained;

2. skin care – careful regular turns and care of the anaesthetic skin are needed to prevent pressure sores and infection;

3. bladder care – maintain bladder drainage to prevent dilatation of the upper urinary tract. This involves indwelling catheters initially, with careful antisepsis and bladder training or drainage later. Regular urine examination for infection is needed so that appropriate treatment of infection can be instituted.

4. limb care – passive limb movements should be regularly made to prevent joint stiffness and muscle contractures as muscle tone returns and spasticity develops;

5. rehabilitation – this commences early after injury. It involves emotional, financial and physical support for the patient and their family, and requires a multidisciplinary approach.

PERIPHERAL NERVES

ANATOMY

Nerves may be injured acutely by physical trauma (traction or laceration) or chronically by entrapment or compression (Figure 15.3).

Acute nerve injuries are classified as neuropraxia, axonotmesis or neuronotmesis.

Neuropraxia

This is the mildest form of injury, where the nerve remains in continuity and recovery usually occurs within days or weeks.

Axonotmesis

In this form of injury there is interruption of axons and their myelin sheaths, but the encapsulating epineurium and perineurium remain in continuity. These sheaths guide regenerating fibres to their distal connections, and complete functional recovery is likely. Regeneration occurs at the rate of 1 mm/day.

Neurotmesis

This involves complete disruption of the nerve, and Wallerian degeneration occurs distally. Regeneration is unlikely unless the nerve is repaired surgically. If surgical repair can be achieved, regeneration occurs at the rate of 1 mm/day, but complete functional recovery is imperfect.

Wallerian degeneration

When a peripheral nerve is transected, changes occur central and peripheral to the transection.

Peripheral to the transection there is proliferation of the Schwann cells, myelin breaks down and the myelin debris is phagocytosed by the Schwann cells. Complete phagocytosis may take 1 to 3 months. Endoneural tubes (the basal lamina of the Schwann cells) now collapse because of phagocytosis of the myelin and axons.

Central to the transection similar changes occur, which occasionally result in death of the cell body.

Regeneration

Axons sprout into regenerating units within 1 to 2 days of injury. Initially all of the fibres are non-myelinated, but with time some of them become myelinated as the Schwanncells forming the endoneural tubules regenerate.

When these regenerating fibres reach the distal nerve and receptors, function may return. If the regenerating fibres are unable to enter distal tubules because of inadequate repair (due to various factors), then a neuroma develops. Functional recovery requires alignment of correct fascicle to fascicle, particularly in mixed nerves.

Examination of peripheral nerves

This implies an accurate and detailed knowledge of anatomy.

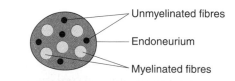

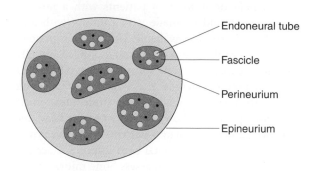

Figure 15.3 Anatomy of peripheral nerves.

A **SMART** practitioner will examine for:

- Sensory changes – light touch, pin-prick, detection of hot and cold;
- Motor changes – power;
- Autonomic changes – sweating, skin colour;
- Reflex changes – deep tendon jerks;
- Trophic changes – wasting of muscles, ulcers.

FURTHER READING

Adams RD, Victor M, Ropper AH. 1997: *Principles of neurology*, 6th edn. London: McGraw-Hill.

Kaye AH. 1997: Subarachnoid haemorrhage. In Kaye AH (ed.). *Essential neurosurgery*, 2nd edn. New York: Churchill Livingstone, 179–98.

Kaye AH. 1997: Stroke. In Kaye AH (ed.). *Essential neurosurgery*, 2nd edn. New York: Churchill Livingstone, 199–229.

Kaye AH. 1997: Spinal injuries. In Kaye AH (ed.). *Essential neurosurgery*, 2nd edn. New York: Churchill Livingstone, 329–39.

Newcombe R, Merry G. 1999: The management of acute neurotrauma in rural and remote locations. *Journal of Clinical Neuroscience* 6, 85–93.

Van Gijn J. 1992: Subarachnoid haemorrhage. *Lancet* **339**, 653–5.

Chapter 16

Deafness, vertigo and tinnitus

Joseph L. Hegarty and Scott M. Graham

Introduction

The diagnosis of diseases of the ear and associated structures may often require rigorous history-taking, examination extending beyond visualization of the tympanic membrane and thoughtful interpretation of specific tests. This chapter reviews the anatomy and physiology of hearing and balance, with a subsequent clinically directed examination of the sometimes disabling disorders of these systems.

DEAFNESS

ANATOMY AND PHYSIOLOGY OF HEARING

The ear is physically separated into external, middle and inner ear components (Figure 16.1). The external ear consists of the auricle and external auditory canal. The middle ear is separated from the external ear canal by the tympanic membrane, and contains the ossicles (malleus, incus and stapes) and an air-containing cavity continuous with the mastoid air cells. The inner ear consists of the bony otic capsule, which encompasses the organs of hearing and balance. The cochlea (Latin, snail shell, from Greek *kokhlias*) makes 2.75 turns and is separated into three fluid-filled chambers (Figure 16.2). The two outer chambers, namely the scala vestibuli and scala tympani, contain perilymph which has an ionic composition similar to that of extracellular fluid. The middle cochlear chamber, the scala media, is a separate space maintained within the perilymphatic compartments which contains endolymph. The composition of endolymph is similar to that of intracellular fluid, with a very high potassium content.

The ability to hear depends on the transduction of mechanical energy (sound) into neural impulses and the interpretation of those impulses by the central nervous system. We perceive this mechanical energy (sound) as variations in loudness (intensity) and pitch (frequency). Loudness of sound is measured in decibels (dB), whereas the pitch of sound is measured in Hertz (Hz). The human ear is able to perceive frequencies in the range 20–20 000 Hz, although the range 500–4000 Hz is most important for understanding speech. Sound waves travel from their source through the external auditory canal, causing the tympanic membrane and the underlying ossicular chain to vibrate. The role of the middle ear is to transmit vibrations of air into vibrations of fluid within the inner ear, taking into account the difference in impedance (resistance to vibration) between air and water. The middle ear compensates for this impedance mismatch through the lever action of the ossicles and the difference in the vibratory surface areas of the tympanic membrane and oval window. The magnitude of sound pressure amplification is approximately 22-fold, which is equivalent to *c.* 25 dB in acoustic amplification. Once past the oval window, perilymphatic fluid waves in the common fluid space between the cochlea and labyrinth, known as the vestibule, are transmitted to the cochlea. This fluid disturbance, called the travelling wave, enters

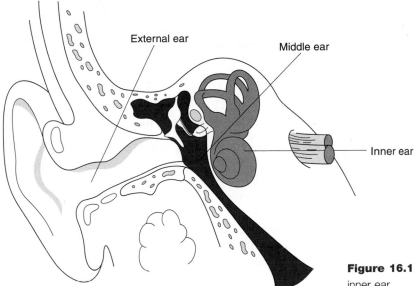

Figure 16.1 Anatomy of the external, middle and inner ear.

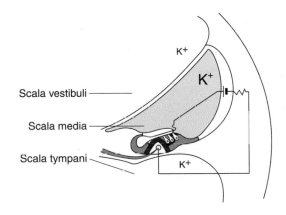

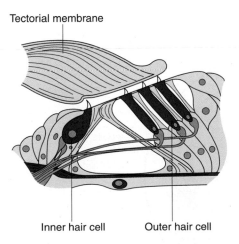

Figure 16.2 Cross-section of the cochlea. The endolymph is separated from the perilymph within the scala media. The high potassium concentration in the endolymph produces a large electrochemical gradient across the hair cells, similar to that of a battery.

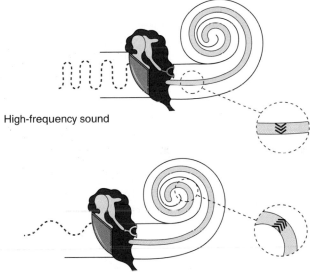

Figure 16.3 The travelling wave within the cochlea. High-frequency sounds have maximum resonance at the base of the cochlea, whereas low-frequency sounds have maximal vibration at the cochlear apex. This accounts for the tonotopic organization of the cochlea.

the cochlea at its base and courses the length of the cochlea, displacing the basilar membrane at precise locations based on the frequency of fluid vibration (Figure 16.3). Basilar membrane motion results in deflection of the hair cells, which are specialized mechanical transducers that respond to basilar membrane displacement with a change in membrane potential. The inner hair cells (numbering only 3000 per cochlea) are the critical elements in sound transduction, converting mechanical energy into bioelectrical energy. They are the only cells that actually provide acoustic input to the auditory cortex. The outer hair cells (numbering approximately 12 000 per cochlea) enhance the function of the inner hair cells by sharpening sound input, and do not have any significant cortical input. The unique ability of the outer hair cells to amplify acoustic input is dependent on their contractility in response to hair cell deflection. The inner hair cells do not have the ability to contract. Stereociliar deflection at the apical surface of the hair cell allows either opening or closing of elastically gated, mechanosensitive transduction channels, causing either depolarization or hyperpolarization of the hair cell. Larger deflections of the hair cell stereocilia result in stronger depolarization and more frequent action potentials, which are interpreted as a louder sound. The unique ability of the cochlea to code for varying sound frequency is based on its tonotopic organization within the auditory cortex. Fluid vibrations at the base of the cochlea are perceived as high-frequency sound in the central auditory system, whereas vibrations at the apex of the cochlea are interpreted as low-frequency sound. If an individual suffers a loss of sensory or neural function at the base of the cochlea, as occurs for instance in noise-induced hearing loss, high-frequency sound perception is lost.

CAUSES OF HEARING LOSS

The causes of hearing loss are classified as *sensorineural*, *conductive* or *mixed*. Sensorineural hearing loss is due to a dysfunction of the sensory (hair cells) or neural elements (acoustic nerve and central connections) of the auditory system. Conductive hearing loss is due to an obstruction of the acoustic signal at the level of the external canal, tympanic membrane or middle ear space. Mixed hearing loss describes a combination of sensorineural and conductive hearing losses. Proper identification of the type of hearing loss is critical to successful treatment of the patient.

Sensorineural hearing loss

Sensorineural hearing loss (Table 16.1) is most commonly the result of age-related, cochlear degeneration and is commonly referred to as presbycusis (from the Greek *presbys*, meaning old, and *akouein*, meaning to hear). Approximately 30% of the population over 70 years of age have a debilitating, bilateral hearing loss due to the effects of presbycusis. Schuknecht has described four patterns of audiometric loss attributed to presbycusis, namely sensory, neural, metabolic and mechanical (Figure 16.4). Sensory presbycusis is the most common type, and most often represents loss of hair cells at the basal turn of the cochlea. Neural presbycusis represents

Table 16.1 Common causes of sensorineural hearing loss

Presbycusis
Acoustic trauma
Hereditary causes
Infectious causes
Ototoxic medications
Syphilis
Trauma/perilymphatic fistula
Tumours
Sudden hearing loss

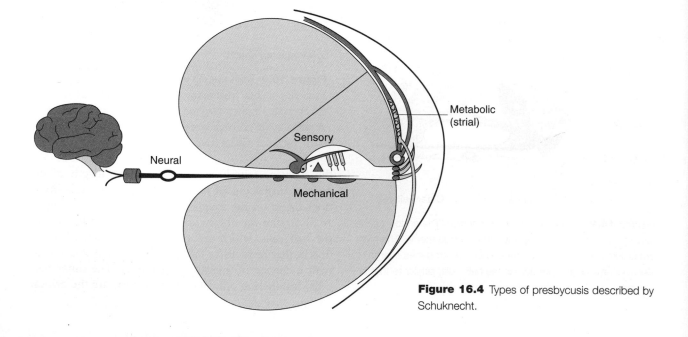

Figure 16.4 Types of presbycusis described by Schuknecht.

degeneration of first-order cochlear neurones of the auditory nerve. Metabolic presbycusis represents atrophy and dysfunction of the stria vascularis. Mechanical presbycusis represents stiffness at the level of the basilar membrane or hair cells. Noise exposure is a common form of sensorineural hearing loss in industrialized societies. Hair cell damage at the basal turn of the cochlea results from the acoustic trauma, and is seen audiometrically as a 'notched' loss at 4 kHz following a single exposure to loud noise. Alternatively, a gradual, downsloping pattern in the high frequencies may result from prolonged exposure to less intense sound. Current US standards mandate limiting continuous noise exposure to less than 90 decibels during an 8-h working day. Sensorineural hearing loss can often be genetically determined. The estimated incidence of severe to profound hereditary hearing loss is approximately 1 in every 1000 live births in the USA, and a further 6 in every 1000 live births can have a mild to moderate sensorineural hearing loss. Dominant inheritance (25%) is typically seen in those cases manifesting after birth, and is progressive, whereas recessive inheritance (75%) is typically congenital and non-progressive. Although dysmorphic features are often found with sensorineural hearing loss, at least 50% of all heritable deafness is not associated with other organ defects. Because the first 10 months of life are thought to be critical for language development, the majority of US hospitals have adapted universal newborn hearing screening. Congenital hearing loss is not always inherited. Perinatal insults to the auditory system are well documented as a consequence of rubella, measles, mumps, ototoxic drugs, anoxia, hyperbilirubinaemia and bacterial meningitis. Deafness is a permanent sequela in about 20% of cases of bacterial meningitis. Ototoxicity following intravenous gentamicin or cisplatin chemotherapy is also often seen in acquired deafness, and is usually dependent on the cumulative dose of the medication. Sudden sensorineural hearing loss is seen in 1 in 10 000 individuals, and although the exact pathogenesis is obscure, most believe that it has a viral or ischaemic aetiology. The large vestibular aqueduct syndrome (LVAS) is an increasingly recognized disorder, characterized by a stepwise, progressive sensorineural hearing loss associated with isolated enlargement of the vestibular aqueduct. LVAS is typically found in children, and is associated with intermittent balance disturbance. Although rare, tumours of the cerebellopontine angle (such as acoustic neuromas and meningiomas) will often present with hearing loss. These tumours are symptomatic in 1 in 100 000 individuals and should be considered in any patient with a significant asymmetry in pure tone hearing or speech discrimination or significantly asymmetrical tinnitus.

Conductive hearing loss

Conductive hearing loss (Table 16.2) is caused by the disruption of acoustic transmittance at the level of the external or middle ear. External canal obstruction may be due to cerumen accumulation, a foreign body, exostoses, oedema or a neoplasm. Abnormalities of the tympanic membrane that cause conductive hearing loss include perforation and tympanosclerosis. Tympanosclerosis results from hyaline and calcium deposition within the tympanic membrane and middle ear. Conductive hearing loss can also be caused by disorders of the middle ear, including effusions, ossicular fixation and ossicular discontinuity. Serous otitis media is the most common cause of conductive hearing loss in children, often producing a 20–40 decibel hearing loss. If serous otitis media is found in adults, evaluation of the nasopharynx is indicated to rule out a neoplasm obstructing the Eustachian tube orifice. Otosclerosis is the most common form of conductive hearing loss in adults, with a 1% prevalence in the Caucasian population. In otosclerosis, hearing loss is the result of abnormal bone growth at the joint between the stapes and the vestibule of the cochlea, rendering the stapes immobile. Occasionally, malleus fixation occurs within the middle ear space, usually as a result of fibrous tissue or bony growth following chronic inflammation. Ossicular discontinuity often occurs with trauma or necrosis of the long process of the incus, resulting in a significant con-

Table 16.2 Common causes of conductive hearing loss

External ear	Tympanic membrane	Middle ear
Cerumen	Myringosclerosis	Otitis media
Foreign body	Perforation	Haemotympanum
Oedema	Retraction	Otosclerosis
Stenosis/atresia		Tympanosclerosis
Exostosis		Cholesteatoma
Osteoma		Ossicular discontinuity
Tumours		Tumours
Cysts		

ductive hearing loss, up to 60 decibels. Cholesteatoma is an ingrowth of tympanic membrane squamous epithelium into the middle ear and mastoid cavity, and should be sought in any patient with a draining ear and hearing loss. Ossicular mass effect with progressive ossicular erosion from the cholesteatoma results in a conductive hearing loss.

TREATMENT OF HEARING LOSS

Conductive hearing loss is often amenable to surgical correction. Surgery will address the source of acoustic block, either in the external canal or in the middle ear. External auditory meatal stenosis is dealt with using a canalplasty, a perforated eardrum is addressed with a myringoplasty, ossicular discontinuity is re-established with an ossiculoplasty, and an immobile stapes footplate is corrected with a stapedectomy. Patients who elect to have non-surgical treatment or in whom surgery fails can be helped with the use of a hearing-aid.

The progressive loss of the outer hair cells results in the loss of the cochlear amplifier. This amplifier can often be supplanted using external acoustic amplification by way of a hearing-aid. However, progressive loss of the inner hair cells leads to poor word understanding despite adequate amplification. Intracochlear electrical stimulation through a cochlear implant allows stimulation of the remaining spiral ganglion neurones and is a successful method of achieving usable hearing following the loss of inner hair cells. This is especially important for children deafened by bacterial meningitis and adults suffering a rapid onset of hearing loss prior to the loss of spiral ganglion neurones.

VERTIGO

ANATOMY AND PHYSIOLOGY OF BALANCE

The inner ear not only contains the sensory organ for hearing, but also five sensory organs of balance, namely three semicircular canals, the utricle and the saccule (Figure 16.5). These organs are responsible for both stabilization of gaze during head movement and postural control. To function appropriately, labyrinthine input must be coupled with visual, proprioceptive, auditory and other sensory cues so that eye and body movements occur in a co-ordinated fashion. Like the auditory system, the basic sensory cell in the vestibular system is the hair cell. Within the three orthogonally positioned semicircular canals, named lateral, posterior and superior for their location within the temporal bone, hair cells are arranged along the crista ampullaris with their cilia

embedded in a gelatinous cupula. The cupula is a neutrally buoyant structure that spans the height and width of the ampulla, allowing detection of head movements in the plane of that particular canal. Cupular displacement causes deflection of the hair cell bundle, resulting in a change in hair cell membrane potential. The arrangement of the semicircular canals in opposite ears is such that the input in the ipsilateral canal has opposite effects to that in the contralateral canal. The lateral semicircular canals lie in roughly the same plane in both ears, whereas the superior canal lies in the same plane as the contralateral posterior canal. These reciprocally acting canals are exquisitely sensitive to head movement. A particular head movement will stimulate the ipsilateral canal and inhibit the contralateral, complementary canal. For instance, turning one's head to the left will stimulate the left lateral canal and inhibit the right lateral canal. Taken together, this 'push-pull' mechanism amplifies the asymmetrical neural input to the brainstem that results in the perception of head movement to the left.

The otolith organs, the utricle and saccule, are primarily responsible for detection of linear acceleration, including that due to gravity. Otolith hair cell cilia are embedded in the gelatin layer of the otolithic membrane, which is covered by calcium carbonate crystals, namely the otoconia. The otoconia have a higher specific gravity than the surrounding endolymph, making static head tilt or acceleration in the vertical or horizontal plane detectable through the otolith organs. Although each organ is capable of multidirectional sensitivity, the utricle has receptor cells predominantly in a horizontal plane, whereas the saccule has receptor cells predominantly in the vertical plane. Vestibular input arrives in the vestibular ganglion, located just outside the otic capsule, and proceeds to synapse in the vestibular nucleus of the brainstem. Vestibular nuclei likewise receive input from the cerebellum, the spinal cord and the contralateral vestibular nuclei, and integrate information about posture, movement, tilt and co-ordinated eye and head movements.

EVALUATION OF VERTIGO

Balance disorders are an important health care concern, significantly interfering with the life of about 5% of the American population over the age of 65 years. Vertigo (from the Latin *verto*, to turn) is defined as a sensation of rotation in any plane, and is often imprecisely used as a general term to describe dizziness (a term that should be reserved for light-headedness or unsteadiness). Vertigo and balance disorders can often be categorized into central (originating from the brainstem or brain), peripheral (originating from the vestibular labyrinth) and metabolic aetiologies (Table 16.3).

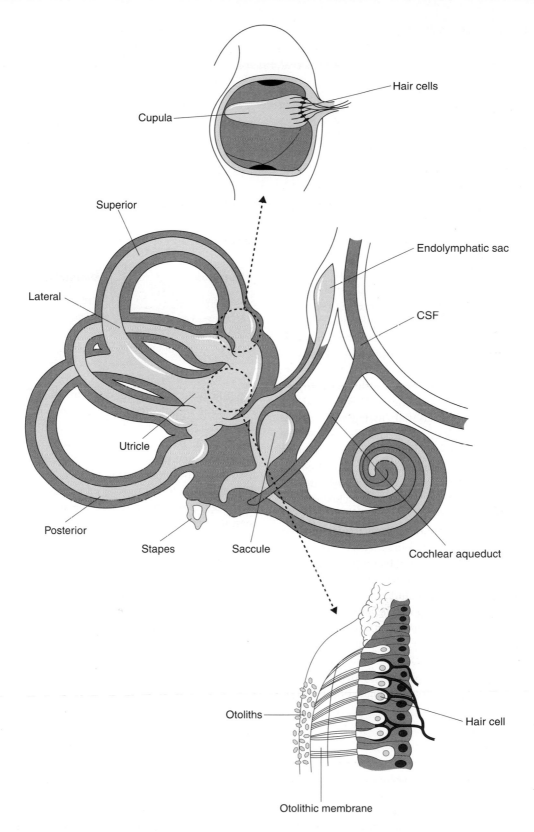

Figure 16.5 Anatomy of the vestibular system. The ampullae of the three semicircular canals detect angular acceleration. Movements of the otolithic membranes of the utricle and saccule detect linear acceleration.

Table 16.3 Possible causes of vertigo

Central causes	Peripheral causes	Metabolic causes
Vertebrobasilar insufficiency	BPPV	Diabetes
TIA, stroke	Ménière's disease	Thyroid disease
Multiple sclerosis	Vestibular neuronitis	Syphilis
Acoustic neuroma	Labyrinthitis	Cogan's syndrome
Arnold-Chiari malformation	Autoimmune inner ear disease	Anaemia
CNS tumours	Perilymph fistula	Autoimmune diseases
Cervical vertigo	Otosclerosis	
Vascular loops	Labyrinthine concussion	

When evaluating patients with balance complaints, a detailed history, physical examination and laboratory testing are all important for establishing an accurate diagnosis. A detailed history is crucial, and should include the character, duration and triggering factors of the vertiginous spells. However, one of the most important questions to ask is '*How long* do your dizzy spells last?' The answer to this question is often helpful in making a diagnosis.

The physical examination should include a comprehensive evaluation of the cranial nerves, cerebellar function, spontaneous or positional nystagmus, vision, hearing and proprioception. A Dix-Hallpike manoeuvre should also be performed to elicit evidence of benign paroxysmal positional vertigo (see below). Supplemental tests that are helpful in establishing a diagnosis include an audiogram and electronystagmogram (ENG). The ENG allows electronic evaluation of the visual tracking system and responses of the lateral semicircular canal to caloric irrigation and positional manoeuvres. The ENG is very helpful for differentiating between peripheral and central vestibular lesions. Laboratory testing is helpful in some patients, and will often include a haemoglobin test (for anaemia), fluorescent treponemal antibody absorption test (FTA-Abs, for tertiary syphilis) and a heat-shock protein-70 (HSP-70) Western blot (for autoimmune inner ear disease). Gadolinium-enhanced magnetic resonance imaging is often performed to rule out a lesion of the cerebellopontine angle, brainstem or brain.

CAUSES OF VERTIGO

Benign paroxysmal positional vertigo (BPPV) is the most common cause of vertigo, accounting for nearly 20% of all vestibular complaints. Patients will typically relate brief episodes of some seconds of vertigo precipitated by rolling over in bed or looking upward (Table 16.4). BPPV can be seen after head trauma, vestibular neuronitis or Ménière's disease, although most commonly there is no identifiable antecedent event. A Dix-

Table 16.4 Duration of common vestibulopathies

Duration	Diagnosis
Seconds	BPPV
Minutes	Vertebrobasilar insufficiency
Hours	Ménière's disease
Days	Vestibular neuronitis

Hallpike head positioning confirms this clinical diagnosis, placing the affected posterior semicircular canal into a dependent position (i.e. lying down with the head turned). A pathognomonic response reveals a brief (1–5 s) latency prior to the onset of geotropic, rotary nystagmus (beating toward the floor), a limited duration of symptoms (10–30 s), reversal nystagmus on resuming an upright position, and a fatigable response on repeated manoeuvres. There are two proposed pathophysiological mechanisms, namely canalithiasis (free-floating otoconial particles in the posterior canal) and cupulolithiasis (otoconial particles adherent to the posterior canal cupula). Displaced otoconia from the superiorly positioned utricle are believed to gravitate to a more dependent part of the inner ear, the posterior canal (Figure 16.6). With provocative head positioning, the posterior canal cupula is believed to be excessively stimulated, producing brief symptoms of vertigo. A canalith-repositioning manoeuvre has proved to be very helpful in dramatically shortening the length of symptoms. This manoeuvre theoretically rotates free otolithic particles out of the affected canal and back into the utricle, where they remain asymptomatic. This manoeuvre resolves symptoms in over 90% of patients in just one or two treatments. Although BPPV is usually self-limiting, resolving within weeks to months without treatment, intermittent and chronic forms exist that result in long-term symptoms. Patients with persistent symptoms can pursue surgical treatment, which includes a singular neurectomy (i.e. nerve section of the posterior canal) or a posterior semicircular canal occlusion (i.e. plugging of the canal with fascia or bone wax).

Menière's disease is one of the most commonly diagnosed aetiologies of vertigo, affecting 1 in 5000 individuals in the USA, and 1 in 1000 in the UK. Menière's disease is characterized by spells of ear full-

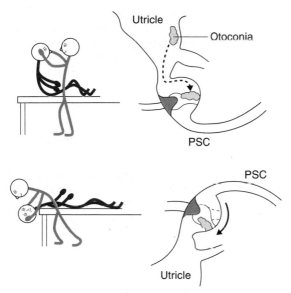

Figure 16.6 A Dix-Hallpike manoeuvre demonstrates evidence of benign paroxysmal positional vertigo. Otoconia from the utricle dislodge and attach to the posterior semicircular canal (PSC) cupula, giving the patient a sense of exaggerated movement with the head in a dependent position.

ness, decreased hearing and roaring tinnitus, followed by severe, rotatory vertigo lasting at least 20 min (typically 2–4 h), but not more than 24 h. A definitive diagnosis requires that the patient should have at least two or more of these episodes with an audiometrically documented sensorineural hearing loss (usually low-tone loss) that eventually returns to baseline. Histopathologically, every patient with Menière's disease shows evidence of an enlarged endolymphatic fluid compartment, or endolymphatic hydrops. This is presumably due to an overproduction or under-resorption of endolymph. This increased endolymphatic pressure is thought to cause ear fullness and distorted hearing. However, the 'membranous rupture' theory proposed by Schuknecht is helpful for understanding the pathophysiology of episodic vertigo and transient hearing loss. This theory argues that continued expansion of the endolymphatic space ultimately results in a membranous rupture, spilling the potassium-rich endolymph into the perilymph (Figure 16.7). This disturbs the tonic discharge of the sensory hair cells and ultimately the neural ganglion cells, resulting in a transient neural 'short-circuit'. Since the central vestibular system is dependent on balanced input from both ears, this acute loss of unilateral input results in a sensation of vertigo. In most cases, the ruptures affect both the cochlear and vestibular systems. If the rupture involves only the cochlea, only transient hearing loss and aural fullness occur. If the rupture is

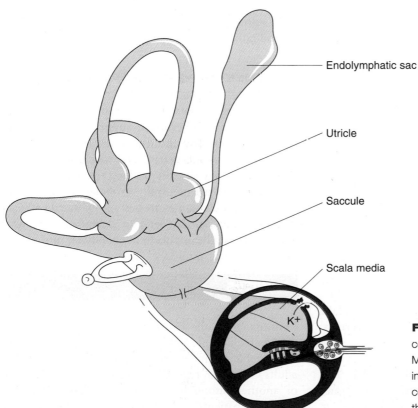

Figure 16.7 Enlarged endolymphatic fluid compartment of Menière's disease. Membranous rupture with potassium intoxication of the sensory and neural compartments of the cochlea may explain the pathophysiology of this disease.

confined to the labyrinth, only episodic vertigo occurs. This incomplete symptomatology will often lead to the diagnosis of atypical Menière's disease, i.e. cochlear Menière's or vestibular Menière's disease. There are still many poorly characterized biochemical alterations in the hydropic inner ear, including excessive glycoprotein accumulation and a perturbed ionic composition, which are all likely to contribute to the cochlear and vestibular symptoms of this disease. Fortunately, the vertiginous episodes of Menière's disease are controllable. Approximately 80% of patients can be managed medically with a low sodium diet (1500–2000 mg/day). A sodium-wasting diuretic (hydrochlorothiazide with or without triamterene to spare potassium wasting) can also be used if diet alone does not give satisfactory control of vertigo. For those who fail successful management on medical therapy, multiple surgical options exist. For patients with good hearing, an endolymphatic shunt or a vestibular nerve section have met with considerable success. For those with poor hearing, intratympanic gentamicin or a labyrinthectomy are potential options. However, despite medical or surgical therapy, aural fullness, tinnitus and fluctuating hearing persist until the disease eventually becomes inactive or 'burned out.'

Other disorders can often give rise to atypical vestibular symptoms, and can initially be erroneously diagnosed as Menière's disease. These less common neurotological diagnoses include acoustic neuroma, autoimmune inner ear disease, chronic labyrinthitis, perilymph fistula, vertebrobasilar insufficiency, multiple sclerosis, ototoxicity and syphilis. A detailed patient history will often help to ensure a proper diagnosis. Unilateral tinnitus, asymmetrical sensorineural hearing loss, decreased speech discrimination and disequilibrium often characterize the symptoms of an acoustic neuroma. Vertigo is not a predominant symptom of this benign neoplasm. Autoimmune inner ear disease (AIIED) is typically a bilateral, rapidly progressive, non-fluctuating sensorineural hearing loss. Only 25–50% of patients will have episodic vertigo and aural fullness, and 30% will have a pre-existing systemic autoimmune disease. Although up to 50% of Menière's patients will have some evidence of bilateral symptoms, only a small percentage of patients will show bilateral symptoms at presentation. Chronic labyrinthitis should be suspected in a patient with a history of ear surgery, ear pain or drainage. A perilymph fistula is typically seen following straining or barotrauma, and is usually associated with a sudden, severe sensorineural hearing loss. Patients will usually complain of disequilibrium, although some report vertigo. Vertebrobasilar insufficiency is characterized by a sudden loss of balance without a loss of consciousness, due to transient ischaemia of the vestibular nuclei. The symptoms are often accompanied by nausea and vomiting, and are occasionally precipitated by neck flexion or extension. Vertigo occurs in over one-third of patients with multiple sclerosis, presumably due to focal demyelinization of the middle cerebellar peduncle, but occasionally as a result of plaques in the cochlear or vestibular nuclei of the brainstem. Ototoxicity is usually seen during a course of ototoxic medication, such as gentamicin or cisplatin, although patients will typically complain of oscillopsia (bouncing of the visual field with walking) and ataxia, rather than true vertigo. Tertiary syphilis (syphilitic labyrinthitis) is often referred to as the 'great imitator' because of its protean cochleovestibular symptoms. Although less common today than in the past, the spread of HIV has increased the incidence of syphilitic infections during the past decade. Any bilateral sensorineural hearing loss with associated balance complaints warrants a FTA-Abs to rule out syphilis, as this disease can be effectively treated with penicillin and oral steroids.

In addition to BPPV and Menière's disease, vestibular neuronitis is one of the most common causes of vertigo seen in general practice. This disorder occurs as long as 2–3 weeks after an upper respiratory infection, and is thought to be due to a viral infection of Scarpa's (vestibular) ganglion. The vertigo is usually sudden and severe, lasting for many days and gradually improving over the next few weeks. Hearing is typically not affected, although high-frequency sensorineural hearing loss may be observed. Histopathologically, there is loss of vestibular nerve fibres with subsequent fibrosis. Spontaneous recovery of balance is generally obtained following central vestibular compensation. Otherwise, vestibular rehabilitation exercises can greatly facilitate recovery.

TREATMENT OF VESTIBULOPATHIES

Pharmacological treatment of an acute vestibular crisis is most effective with vestibular suppressants, most commonly diazepam and antihistamines. However, vestibular suppressants are detrimental to chronic vestibular disorders, as they actually prolong the balance disturbance by delaying central vestibular compensation. Chronic vestibulopathies are best rehabilitated with daily vestibular exercises that serve to strengthen the sensory and proprioceptive inputs to the vestibular nucleus.

TINNITUS

Tinnitus (from the Latin *tinniere*, to ring) refers to a non-hallucinogenic auditory perception that is not attributable to an external source. About 30% of all adults in the USA report having had tinnitus at one time or another, although its presence is reported in over 80% of patients with sensorineural hearing loss.

Approximately 6% of the US population report their tinnitus to be severe or disabling. Tinnitus can be located in the ear (tinnitus aurium) or in the head (tinnitus cranii), and may be perceived unilaterally or bilaterally. Subjective tinnitus can be heard only by the patient, affecting 95% of tinnitus sufferers. Objective tinnitus is also heard by others, and affects less than 5% of tinnitus sufferers.

Subjective idiopathic tinnitus (SIT) is commonly encountered in clinical practice and is often a diagnosis of exclusion. SIT is most often attributable to a sensorineural hearing loss, although the hearing loss may not always be detectable with standard audiological testing. The precise pathophysiology and site of origin of the event causing tinnitus are also unclear, but many theories exist. The hair cell 'decoupling' theory is helpful for understanding one aspect of tinnitus. The stereocilia tips of the outer hair cells insert into the undersurface of the tectorial membrane, bending as the travelling wave displaces the underlying basilar membrane (see Figure 16.2). One consequence of noise exposure and ototoxic drugs is the alteration of the stereocilia microstructure, leading to their separation from the tectorial membrane. This decoupling leads to 'leaking' of potassium-rich endolymph into the hair cell, resulting in an increase in the basal neural firing rate from that portion of the damaged cochlea. High-frequency noise damage, typically occurring at the base of the cochlea, results in a high-pitched tinnitus. Narrow-band tinnitus is often described in patients with discrete lesions of the inner ear. Although initiated in the ear, this chronic signal is thought to lead to central auditory changes that often continue to trouble the patient even after surgical ablation of the cochlea.

SUBJECTIVE TINNITUS

Subjective tinnitus (Table 16.5) is often a symptom of an underlying disease, and correction of the underlying problem often ameliorates the tinnitus. Tinnitus is commonly reported in patients with anaemia, blood dyscrasias, hypertension, hyperlipidaemia, thyroid dysfunction, diabetes, migraine, syphilis, multiple sclerosis, Menière's disease, brain/brainstem tumours, perilymph fistulae, Paget's disease or exposure to ototoxic drugs. Prescription and non-prescription drugs are frequent contributors to tinnitus, specifically aspirin, non-steroidal anti-inflammatory drugs (NSAIDs), quinine, heart medications (quinidine, beta-blockers, loop diuretics), antibiotics (aminoglycosides, doxycycline, ciprofloxin) and chemotherapeutic medications (cisplatin). Conductive hearing loss (e.g. from a cerumen impaction, middle ear effusion or otosclerosis), is a potentially treatable cause of tinnitus that should be sought. Important aspects of the history should involve questions about loudness, pitch, temporal characteristics, localization, psychological influences, effects of environmental noise and, most importantly, severity. Tinnitus, like pain, is subjective, and two patients may have identical loudness and pitch matches on testing, yet may rate the severity very differently.

OBJECTIVE TINNITUS

Objective tinnitus (Table 16.6) can be heard by the examiner, and can be further categorized into pulsatile and non-pulsatile tinnitus. Common causes of pulsatile tinnitus are glomus tumours (paraganglioma of the temporal bone), vascular malformations (e.g. dural arteriovenous fistula, cavernous-carotid fistula, dehiscent jugular bulb, aberrant carotid artery, persistent stapedial artery) and transmitted bruits (e.g. hypertension, atherosclerotic carotid artery, pseudotumour cerebri, heart murmur). Common causes of non-pulsatile, objective tinnitus are patulous Eustachian tubes, palatal myoclonus and temporomandibular joint (TMJ) disorders.

The physical examination of patients with tinnitus should include a thorough evaluation of the tympanic membrane, specifically seeking evidence of a vascular, retrotympanic mass (glomus tumour). Examination of the soft palate for contractions (palatal myoclonus) should be performed together with visualization of the nasopharynx for Eustachian tube abnormalities. A detailed cranial nerve examination is important, especially with regard to the lower cranial nerves exiting

Table 16.5 Common causes of subjective tinnitus

Sensorineural hearing loss
Drugs, ototoxins
Systemic diseases (hypertension, hyperlipidaemia, anaemia, diabetes, thyroid disease, multiple sclerosis)
Acoustic neuroma
Menière's disease
Perilymph fistula
Conductive hearing loss (otosclerosis)
Paget's disease
Syphilis

Table 16.6 Common causes of objective tinnitus

Pulsatile	Non-pulsatile
Glomus tumours	Patulous Eustachian tubes
Vascular malformations	Palatal myoclonus
Transmitted bruits	TMJ disorders

the jugular foramina. An audiogram will evaluate evidence of sensorineural or conductive hearing loss. Pitch and loudness matching should be documented prior to initiation of treatment. Although not routinely used, additional testing with otoacoustic emissions (OE), evoked auditory brainstem response (EABR) testing and electrocochleography (ECoG) can be obtained. Enhanced magnetic resonance imaging of the brain and brainstem is performed in nearly all patients with unilateral tinnitus, as subjective tinnitus is present in over 80% of acoustic neuromas.

MANAGEMENT OF TINNITUS

Treatment goals for tinnitus should be directed at identifying and treating the underlying disorder that is producing the symptom of tinnitus. In most cases, however, the underlying problem is neither identifiable nor treatable. Hearing loss is most frequently identified, and should be treated with hearing-aids. Hearing-aids alone are probably the most frequently used devices for treatment of tinnitus, because they not only improve hearing but also provide tinnitus masking. External sound stimulation in the affected ear is thought to inhibit or alter the production of tinnitus, giving at least partial relief to a substantial number of patients. Patients will often have found an effective masking device prior to physician consultation, usually an FM radio tuned between stations. Tinnitus maskers without amplification are also available for patients without significant hearing loss. Biofeedback with behavioural therapy often helps to alleviate bothersome tinnitus in individuals who are refractory to traditional methods of relief. Avoidance of certain foods, such as caffeine, red wine, aged cheeses and food additives such as salt and monosodium glutamate, may also help to reduce tinnitus substantially. There is currently no drug therapy that gives long-term tinnitus relief without significant side-effects. Reassurance is probably the most important 'treatment' that physicians can give tinnitus sufferers. Despite the lack of effective treatments for tinnitus, the tinnitus sufferer must not be told to 'learn to live with it'. Like patients with any chronic disease with multiple treatment options, those with tinnitus need to be involved in their choice of treatment. Importantly, they must not feel abandoned by the medical community. Investigational treatments, such as electrical stimulation of the cochlea and cortex, are currently being investigated and offer future hope for the tinnitus sufferer.

FURTHER READING

Becker W, Naumann HH, Pfaltz CR. 1989: *Ear, nose and throat diseases.* New York: Thieme Medical Publishers.

Hughes GB, Pensak ML. 1997: *Clinical otology,* 2nd edn. New York: Thieme Medical Publishers.

Northern JL. 1996: *Hearing disorders.* Needham Heights, MA: Simon & Schuster.

Vernon JA, Moller AR. 1995: *Mechanisms of tinnitus.* Needham Heights, MA: Simon & Schuster.

Wilson WR, Nadol JB. 1983: *Quick reference to ear, nose and throat disorders.* Philadelphia, PA: J.B. Lippincott Co.

Dysuria

Brian R. Landers

Introduction

While many practitioners think of dysuria only as a urethral burning discomfort associated with voiding, the broader definition of dysuria is pain or difficulty on urination, and this implies that a wider range of potential causes needs to be considered. Many conditions that affect the lower urinary tract in men and women, or the vagina and introitus in women, may produce dysuria (Figures 17.1.1 and 17.1.2). Patients may complain of pain with a full bladder which is diminished by voiding, suprapubic or urethral pain during voiding, or pain at the end of voiding. Pain may be referred from the bladder or prostate to the glans penis in men, occasionally to such an extent that the patient is convinced that the pathology is located submeatally. Similarly, bladder pain may be referred to the distal urethra or perineum in women.

In this chapter I shall give an overview of the more common causes of dysuria in clinical practice, and I shall describe an approach to the investigation of this symptom. I have not attempted to create an exhaustive list of possibilities, but I would direct the reader to the references for further details and also for information about treatment.

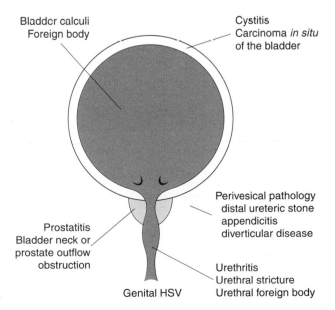

Figure 17.1.1 Causes of dysuria. Prostatic causes obviously only occur in men. The remaining causes may occur in either men or women.

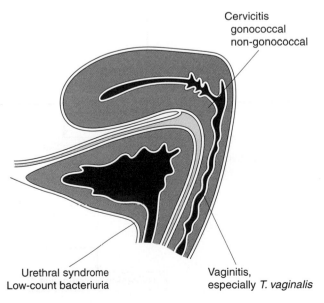

Figure 17.1.2 Additional causes of dysuria in women.

DYSURIA IN CLINICAL PRACTICE

There are four broad patterns of dysuria which may be recognized in clinical practice. First, conditions which widely affect the bladder wall, such as cystitis or carcinoma *in situ* of the bladder (Figures 17.1.1 and 17.1.3), may produce a suprapubic ache or pain which is increased when the bladder is full and the bladder wall is stretched. This ache is diminished to some extent by voiding. Such conditions may also produce a functional or fixed reduction in the bladder capacity and thereby cause nocturia, increased daytime frequency and diminished voided volumes. Uncommonly, similar symptoms may occur when perivesical pathology is present (Figure 17.1.1), although the symptoms and signs of the primary pathology usually then predominate over the bladder symptoms.

Secondly, patients with bladder pathology may also describe a suprapubic or urethral pain at the end of voiding (strangury). Some men report a similar symptom for a period following transurethral resection of the prostate or a bladder neck incision, and this symptom is then presumably caused by considerable inflammation at the bladder neck. Bladder calculi or foreign bodies (ureteric stents or self-inserted foreign bodies) may also be associated with bladder irritability or strangury.

A third pattern of dysuria may be recognized when there is obstruction to the free flow of urine from the bladder, and this is more commonly diagnosed in men. It may be due to obstruction at the level of the bladder neck or prostate or, less frequently, caused by urethral strictures or neuropathic conditions. Acute urinary retention is painful, but chronic urinary retention may be merely a little uncomfortable or even painless. Patients with a lesser degree of obstruction to the flow of urine may describe urinary hesitancy and a poor or stop–start flow together with variable degrees of nocturia, frequency, urgency or incontinence. Some patients also describe a suprapubic or urethral ache which begins immediately before the flow, and this is caused by the bladder contracting strongly on the urine in the bladder to overcome the outflow resistance and produce the flow. Finally, pain which occurs only during the flow suggests urethral pathology (Figure 17.1.1).

CYSTITIS

The common causes of cystitis are shown in Figure 17.1.3.

The most common cause of dysuria is acute bacterial cystitis. There may be pain when the bladder is full and stretched, a urethral burning discomfort during voiding, or terminal strangury. Acute bacterial cystitis may be accompanied by urinary urgency or haematuria. General malaise, fever and rigors are not symptoms of cystitis in adults, and these symptoms imply the development of acute pyelonephritis, acute bacterial prostatitis or acute epididymo-orchitis.

Candidal cystitis occurs sporadically, usually in patients with an indwelling urinary catheter. It is more common in patients with diabetes mellitus or immunosuppression, or in those receiving antibiotics or steroids. It is often asymptomatic as a bladder infection.

Mycobacterial cystitis is uncommon. Tuberculous

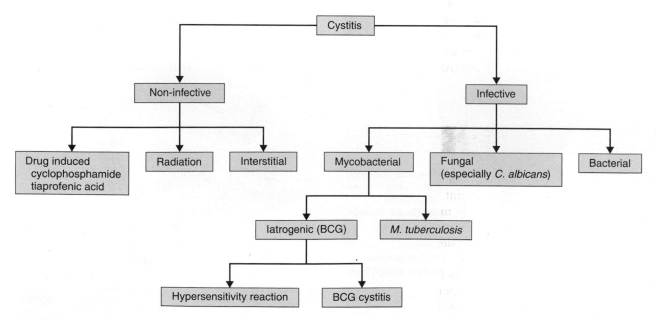

Figure 17.1.3 Common causes of cystitis.

infection begins in the kidney and spreads via the ureter to the bladder, where symptoms develop more slowly than in acute bacterial cystitis. Patients may develop urinary frequency and nocturia, but urinary urgency is less common. Macroscopic haematuria occurs in 10% of cases, but most patients will have pyuria or microscopic haematuria, and 20% of them will have a superimposed bacterial infection. The intravenous pyelogram (IVP) will be abnormal and show changes characteristic of renal and ureteric involvement. If a diagnosis of mycobacterial cystitis is suspected, then 3 to 5 early-morning urine samples should be collected and sent for mycobacterial culture. Mycobacterial cystitis can also occur sporadically in patients treated with intravesical installations of bacille Calmette-Guérin (BCG) for carcinoma *in situ* of the bladder. Non-infective hypersensitivity reactions to intravesical BCG include bladder irritability, dysuria, haematuria, fever and malaise, and these are more common than BCG infection. There will be a history of recent administration in all of these patients. Alternatively, the BCG is instilled via a urethral catheter, and the patient may therefore have an acute bacterial urinary infection.

The aetiology of interstitial cystitis is uncertain. It is an uncommon condition which occurs in at least 1.8 per 10 000 women, and it occurs up to 11 times more frequently in women than in men. In common with the other causes of bladder wall inflammation, it may produce suprapubic discomfort or pain with a full bladder, which diminishes with voiding, together with a reduced bladder capacity, nocturia, frequency and reduced voided volumes. Previous pelvic radiotherapy may produce similar symptoms.

Among medications, cyclophosphamide can produce haemorrhagic cystitis, and there are a number of reports of dysuria, haematuria or urinary frequency associated with the use of the non-steroidal anti-inflammatory agent tiaprofenic acid (Australian Adverse Drug Reactions Advisory Committee (ADRAC), personal communication).

BLADDER CANCER

Pain is not a presenting feature of papillary bladder tumours in the absence of significant haematuria causing clot urinary retention. Similarly, most invasive bladder cancers do not present with pain unless this is caused by ureteric obstruction, invasion of surrounding structures or clot urinary retention.

Transitional-cell carcinoma *in situ* (CIS) of the bladder is a high-grade, superficial carcinoma which usually appears endoscopically like a red rash. In contrast to the other forms of transitional-cell carcinoma (TCC) noted above, widespread CIS involves the bladder more diffusely. It may produce unexplained nocturia, frequency or urgency, and a suprapubic ache with a full bladder or strangury similar to other inflammatory conditions of the bladder wall, and this diagnosis should be suspected in cases where such symptoms are otherwise unexplained. Urine microscopy usually shows microscopic haematuria and sterile pyuria. Voided urine cytology is positive for malignant cells in up to 95% of patients with CIS where three urine samples are submitted on separate days, and the diagnosis is then confirmed by cystoscopy, bladder biopsy and histopathological analysis. CIS or TCC can also occur in the upper urinary tracts or prostate, and it is important to exclude these sites by appropriate investigation. Importantly, voided urine cytology is much less reliable in the detection of low-grade papillary TCC.

URETHRITIS, VAGINITIS AND SEXUALLY TRANSMITTED DISEASES

Gonococcal (GU) or non-gonococcal urethritis (NGU) in men usually presents with a urethral burning discomfort during voiding, and a urethral discharge, each being due to the urethral inflammation. The discharge may be absent, and some men complain only of a urethral itch. There is usually no other pain or disturbance of the voiding pattern. Women do not usually have a urethral discharge, and only about 20% will report burning during voiding. A large proportion of women may therefore be asymptomatic of similar infections.

Symptoms due to isolated urethritis in women are uncommon, and most symptoms are due to the coexistence of cystitis or vaginitis. The most important cause of non-gonococcal infection in men and women is *Chlamydia trachomatis. Trichomonas vaginalis* infection in women can produce dysuria together with the symptoms of vaginitis, and genital herpes simplex virus infection (HSV) may produce dysuria in 44% of men and 83% of women.

Most women with *Neisseria gonorrhoeae, C. trachomatis* or *T. vaginalis* infection will show polymorphonuclear leucocytes on a urethral smear, and it is uncommon to find these organisms if leucocytes are absent. A midstream urine may show sterile pyuria. Vaginitis should be suspected if there is a vaginal discharge or itch associated with the dysuria, and endocervical and vaginal swabs should be taken when indicated. Fluid from suspicious vesicles should be cultured for HSV in either sex. The urinary polymerase chain reaction testing for *C. trachomatis* on a voided urine sample is positive in up to 85% of women and almost 100% of men with this infection.

Prostatitis can be divided into four subgroups. Acute bacterial prostatitis is a severe acute febrile illness with retropubic or perineal pain and the possibility of outflow obstruction, including sudden urinary retention, superimposed on the symptoms of acute bacterial cystitis. The prostate is tender to rectal examination, but prostatic massage should be avoided. The renal areas and scrotum are usually normal at examination, unless there is coincident acute pyelonephritis or acute epididymoorchitis. Urine microscopy and culture confirm a urinary tract infection (UTI), and patients with a febrile UTI should undergo an early urinary ultrasound examination to exclude upper urinary tract obstruction.

By comparison, chronic bacterial prostatitis (CBP), non-bacterial prostatitis (NBP) and prostatodynia (PD) produce similar symptoms to one another, including bladder irritability, cystitis-like pain, urethral discomfort during voiding, perineal, pelvic or scrotal discomfort, and sometimes pain with ejaculation. CBP produces recurrent bacterial cystitis caused by the same organism, and the causative focus for the UTIs may be localized to the prostate by segmented cultures of the lower urinary tract. NBP and PD produce prostatitis-like symptoms in the absence of positive bacterial cultures. Microscopy of expressed prostatic secretions (EPS) shows an increased number of white blood cells in NBP but no abnormality in PD. The underlying cause of NBP or PD is uncertain.

Oestrogen deficiency in women may produce atrophic changes in the urethral mucosa, vagina and vulva, and some women may report a urethral or perineal burning discomfort during voiding. Other diagnoses must be excluded, but these atrophic changes and the associated symptoms usually respond to local oestrogen therapy.

ASSESSMENT OF DYSURIA

A broad outline for the assessment of dysuria is shown in Figure 17.1.4. The cause of dysuria can be largely determined by a careful history, especially with regard to the age and sex of the patient, the site and timing of the pain, and the presence or absence of any associated symptoms or significant past history, as discussed above. Pneumaturia or dyspareunia should be noted when present. The drug history should include an enquiry about antibiotic use, steroids, immunosuppression, chemotherapy or the recent intake of tiaprofenic acid. Bladder cancer is more common when there has been a history of smoking. The range of common causes of dysuria (Figures 17.1.1, 17.1.2 and 17.1.3) should be kept in mind, together with an understanding of the conditions as outlined in the text above. A careful physical examination may confirm the tentative diagnosis or suggest an alternative (Table 17.1.1).

All patients should have a carefully collected midstream urine sample (MSSU) assessed by microscopy and culture. Men should retract the foreskin and women should separate the labia. Despite this manoeuvre, the

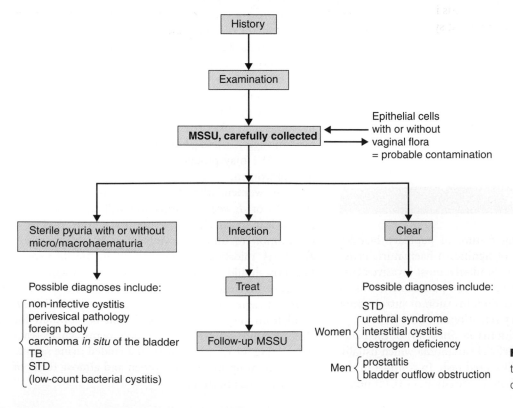

Figure 17.1.4 Flow chart to aid the assessment of dysuria.

Table 17.1.1 Examination related to dysuria

General
  Pallor, jaundice, weight loss, neck nodes

Abdomen
  Bladder (palpable?), kidneys (palpable or tender?),
  masses, tenderness

Male external genitalia
  Testes, epididymes (swollen or tender?), urethral
  palpation (tender?), external urethral meatus
  (discharge?), penis and glans (lesions?)

Digital rectal examination in men
  Prostate (tender or irregular?)
  Rectal lesion
  Pelvic mass or tenderness

**Female external genitalia, vaginal and rectal
examinations (as necessary)**
  Atrophy, lesions, vaginal discharge, cervicitis
  Mass or tenderness on vaginal or rectal examination

collection of a midstream urine sample is more difficult for women, and the sample may be contaminated by epithelial cells and vaginal flora. When such contamination occurs, apparent pyuria or microscopic haematuria may be entirely due to the contamination. Importantly, some women with symptomatic urinary tract infections (UTIs) have fewer than 100 000 organisms/mL, and any organism which is cultured should be reported if a diagnosis of low-count bacterial cystitis is postulated (Figure 17.1.2). Women with the urethral syndrome have cystitis-like symptoms but negative midstream urine microscopy and culture results and no other evidence of local disease. The cause of the symptoms in these patients is unclear.

If the diagnosis is unclear from the history and examination, and if the urine culture has excluded infection, then further assessment is required (Figure 17.1.4). With clinical experience, the differential diagnosis is usually limited to two or three possibilities. Appropriate further investigation may then include an assessment of plasma biochemistry, glucose and creatinine levels, voided urine cytology, early-morning urine samples for mycobacterial culture, investigations to exclude a sexually transmitted disease (STD), an intravenous pyelogram or urinary ultrasound, voiding flow rate analysis, urodynamic assessment or cystoscopy to establish the diagnosis.

FURTHER READING

Lamm DL. (ed.) 1992: Superficial bladder cancer. *Urologic Clinics of North America* **19**(3).

Mellinger BC, Smith AD. (eds) 1992: Sexually transmitted diseases and other lesions of the external genitalia. *Urologic Clinics of North America* **19**(1).

Schaeffer AJ. (ed.) 1986: Urinary tract infections. *Urologic Clinics of North America* **13**(4).

Walsh PC, Retik AB, Stamey TA, Vaughan ED. (eds) 1992: *Campbell's urology*. Philadelphia, PA: W.B. Saunders.

Oliguria/anuria

Robin G. Woolfson

Introduction

Oliguria is the passage of less than 400 mL urine per day, which need not necessarily imply renal pathology. When a patient is sweating profusely and is receiving little fluid intake, a low urine output may be entirely appropriate. However, in other situations, oliguria may be due to renal parenchymal injury affecting glomeruli, tubules, or both, or it may result from an obstruction to the free flow of urine. In either case, elevation of the plasma creatinine levels indicates that there is a significant reduction of glomerular filtration rate, that the capacity of the kidneys to purify the blood is reduced, and that intervention is required.

Anuria is the passage of less than 100 mL urine per day, and is rare in clinical practice. It usually reflects surgical pathology such as severe obstruction or a vascular catastrophe which has affected the arterial supply of both kidneys (if present).

SYMPTOMS

Most patients are not aware of a reduction in urine output, and the symptoms resulting from oliguria and anuria reflect the volume status of the patient. In patients with a depleted circulating volume, the patient may complain of thirst, dry mucous membranes, cool peripheries and symptomatic postural hypotension. In contrast, the patient with fluid overload will complain of peripheral oedema as well as dyspnoea and orthopnoea due to pulmonary congestion.

AETIOLOGY

Hypovolaemia

In the surgical patient, the most common cause of oliguria/anuria is the response to renal hypoperfusion. Most commonly, this 'pre-renal' problem is the result of a reduced circulating volume secondary to loss from haemorrhage, burns, diarrhoea and polyuria (including inappropriate diuretic administration). Alternatively, under-replacement of fluids can occur due to inadequate prescription, inaccuracies in fluid balance measurements, and the failure to correct insensible loss, particularly in pyrexial patients on air beds. Fluid may extravasate from the circulation (but is not lost from the body) as a result of systemic sepsis, pancreatitis, peritonitis or severe soft-tissue injury. The renal consequences of hypovolaemia are exacerbated by injudicious treatment with diuretics, inadequately monitored aminoglycosides, the prescription of non-steroidal anti-inflammatory drugs (NSAIDs) or angiotensin converting enzyme (ACE) inhibition and the use of radiocontrast medium.

Heart failure

Renal hypoperfusion may follow loss of cardiac function as a result of acute cardiac arrhythmias (either bradycardia or tachycardia), acute myocardial infarction, acute ventricular septal rupture or acute cardiac valve leak due to myocardial infarction or endocarditis.

Circulatory failure

Systemic vasodilatation with loss of blood pressure due to sepsis or vasodilatory drugs can cause renal hypoperfusion and oliguria.

PATHOLOGY

Severe renal hypoperfusion may lead to the development of acute tubular necrosis (ATN), which is a histological diagnosis. The same pattern of injury may occur following exposure to nephrotoxic drugs, such as radiocontrast medium, aminoglycosides and NSAIDs, and indeed renal injury is commonly due to a combination of both hypovolaemia and nephrotoxic medication. The patients most likely to develop ATN under these circumstances are those with coincident sepsis, diabetes mellitus or congestive cardiac failure. Since diagnostic renal biopsy is seldom undertaken in this situation, the diagnosis of ATN is mostly presumptive rather than proven. Therefore the differential diagnosis (see below) must be considered, and other diagnoses (which require different management) excluded.

The renal response to hypoperfusion is graded and reflects the evolution of progressive tubular epithelial dysfunction and injury. At first there is intense and appropriate urinary sodium and water conservation, as well as the preservation of excretory function. Urinary sodium levels are characteristically less than 20 mmol/L (unless there has been recent diuretic administration), urine osmolality is greater than 500 mOsm/kg H_2O, and the ratio of urine creatinine (U_{Cr}) to plasma creatinine (P_{Cr}) exceeds 40. The development of tubular dysfunction is suggested by a rising urinary sodium level and the production of isothenuric urine, which indicates the loss of medullary concentrating power. Finally, as more severe tubular epithelial cell injury occurs, oliguria or anuria develops.

This sequence of events reflects the underlying pathophysiology. As the renal perfusion pressure falls, there is *autoregulation* of the renal circulation, which leads to vasodilatation of the afferent arteriole and proximal renal circulation together with increased (angiotensin II -mediated) efferent arteriolar tone. The net result of these reflexes is to maintain renal blood flow and glomerular capillary hydrostatic pressure, and thereby to preserve glomerular filtration in the face of falling perfusion pressure. Increased aldosterone and ADH production, in response to changes in renal and systemic haemodynamics, leads to the formation of highly concentrated urine with a low sodium content.

However, if hypoperfusion persists, autoregulation

progressively fails and the renal microvasculature constricts under the influence of vasoconstricting factors, including the sympathetic innervation, angiotensin II, endothelin, constrictor prostaglandins, ADH and the loss of endogenous vasodilators. Failure of the proximal tubule to reabsorb filtered sodium and water increases the delivery of tubular fluid to the macula densa. This excess delivery stimulates reflex afferent arteriolar vasoconstriction, which results in a reduction in glomerular filtration, presumably in order to conserve the circulating volume and reduce tubular work (tubuloglomerular feedback). However, as renal blood flow decreases, the metabolically active tubular epithelium becomes ischaemic, and its capacity to conserve sodium and water is lost. The urine becomes isothenuric, with urinary sodium exceeding 40 mmol/L. The medulla is particularly sensitive to ischaemia and hypoperfusion. Even under physiological conditions, the ambient medullary PO_2 (20 mmHg) borders on hypoxia. This situation reflects the limited blood supply, countercurrent transport of O_2 out of the medulla and the high rate of local metabolic (ATP consumptive) activity. As a result, reduction of medullary blood flow results in injury/necrosis of the tubular epithelium, with the severity of injury reflecting the degree and duration of the insult. As vasoconstriction develops, the reduction in glomerular filtration rate is disproportionately greater than that of the total renal blood flow. This reflects not just the loss of glomerular hydrostatic pressure, but also tubular obstruction by casts, back-leakage of tubular filtrate through abnormally permeable tubules, and perhaps mesangial contraction, which leads to a reduction

Table 17.2.1 Factors responsible for reduction in renal blood flow and glomerular filtration rate

Renal vasoconstriction is mediated by:
- increased sympathetic activity
- activation of the renin–angiotensin system
- catecholamines
- endothelin
- prostanoids
- adenosine
- loss of endogenous vasodilatory factors (nitric oxide, prostaglandins)
- tubuloglomerular feedback

Factors responsible for loss of glomerular filtration:
- vasoconstriction (tubuloglomerular feedback)
- tubular obstruction by casts and epithelial cell debris
- back-leakage of urinary filtrate across damaged tubular basement membrane
- mesangial contraction

in filtration area. The net result is the development of oliguria.

CLINICAL CORRELATES

This sequence of pathological events has clinical correlates which allow for the identification of diagnostic groups that reflect the extent of tubular dysfunction and injury, and the prospects for recovery.

Pre-renal

Recent-onset renal hypoperfusion is associated with oliguria. Characteristically, urine has a low sodium content (less than 20 mmol/L) and a raised osmolality (greater than 500 mOsm/kg H$_2$O), although recent administration of diuretics may give misleading results. The plasma urea may be disproportionately elevated, reflecting circulating volume contraction in the context of preserved glomerular filtration rate (GFR). Correction of hypovolaemia will lead to the rapid recovery of urine output and biochemical abnormalities.

Persistent medullary hypoperfusion

More persistent hypoperfusion may be associated with the loss of urinary concentration, which is a medullary function. This intermediate state is also seen in patients with NSAID toxicity, cyclosporin toxicity and burns, and in these circumstances urinary sodium is low, which implies preserved proximal tubular function. However, GFR and urine osmolality are reduced, and renal recovery does not immediately follow the correction of hypovolaemia, but may take several days.

Acute tubular necrosis (medullary ischaemia)

Prolonged hypoperfusion will result in ATN. This is characterized by isothenuria with urinary sodium which characteristically exceeds 40 mmol/L and urine osmolality comparable to that of plasma. The GFR is reduced significantly (to 5 mL/min or less). The time to recovery following resuscitation is prolonged and a period of renal replacement is often required.

CLINICAL ASSESSMENT

This begins with an assessment of the oliguric patient's circulating volume and cardiac status.

VOLUME STATUS

Hypovolaemia

The nurses' charts and notes are generally very informative, and may reveal a falling blood pressure and rising pulse over the preceding hours or days. These sources should be closely scrutinized for evidence of negative balance, usually associated with inadequate fluid replacement (either prescribed or delivered), inappropriate diuretic usage, large gastrointestinal aspirates, diarrhoea, excessive wound drainage and frequent dressing changes due to haemorrhage. The significance of a negative fluid balance can be confirmed by the daily weight charts. Intra-operative and post-operative charts should be examined to identify periods of hypotension, intravenous fluid regime including blood, and the recent prescription of nephrotoxic drugs, such as NSAIDs and aminoglycoside antibiotics, as well as other drugs, including ACE inhibitors, angiotensin II receptor antagonists and diuretics.

Hypovolaemia is suggested by symptoms of thirst, dry mouth, cold peripheries and orthostatic hypotension. The presence of normotension does not exclude hypovolaemia, so evidence of postural hypotension should be sought. Under normal circumstances, the fall in systolic blood pressure when moving from the supine to the erect position should not exceed 10 mmHg, and the associated increase in pulse rate should be less than 10 beats/min. Many older patients are hypertensive, and therefore an apparently normal pressure may actually be low for them.

The jugular venous pulse (JVP) must be identified even if the patient has to lie flat or even head down. This sign provides vital information about volume status, right atrial pressure (right heart function) and venous tone. Examine the peripheral veins on the dorsum of the

Table 17.2.2 Biochemical analysis of the urine helps to discriminate between different severities of hypoperfusion injury

	Urine sodium (mmol/L)	Urine osmolality (mOsm/kg H$_2$O)
Pre-renal	< 20	> 500
Medullary hypoperfusion	< 20	< 350
ATN	> 40	< 350

feet and the backs of the hands. In a euvolaemic individual, these are visible and not guttered. Finally, the hands and feet should be warm; if the toes are cold, then move proximally and check whether the feet, ankles, shins, knees or thighs are warm.

The patient should be examined for evidence of third spacing, which is suggested by the presence of ascites, pleural effusions, oedema or soft-tissue injury.

Hypervolaemia

This may be suggested by symptomatic breathlessness, othopnoea and peripheral oedema. Examination may reveal a dyspnoeic and cyanosed patient with tachycardia, hypertension, a raised JVP and the presence of a left ventricular third heart sound. Chest examination may reveal bibasal inspiratory crackles suggestive of pulmonary oedema or dullness due to pleural effusions. Venous congestion and right heart failure can give rise to tender hepatomegaly, peripheral oedema in dependent sites and ascites.

Investigations

The decision regarding the volume status of the patient is a clinical one. Demonstration of upper lobe blood diversion (pulmonary venous congestion), pulmonary oedema (Kerley B lines), fluid in the horizontal fissure, pleural effusions (loss of costophrenic angle) and cardiomegaly on chest X-ray support the diagnosis of volume overload. Conversely, the presence of pulmonary oligaemia and reduced heart size are not reliable indicators of hypovolaemia, which is best confirmed by fluid challenge.

Management: the fluid challenge

A total of 250 mL of colloid or normal saline are infused intravenously over 10 min and the JVP, central venous pressure, blood pressure or pulmonary artery wedge capillary pressure is measured before and afterwards to monitor the response. In the hypovolaemic patient, a reduced value will be corrected *transiently* before falling back to a value close to the previous measurement within 20–30 min. In contrast, in a euvolaemic or overfilled patient the rise in pressure will be sustained.

Hypovolaemia should be corrected as rapidly and accurately as possible using salt-containing fluid, such as a synthetic colloid or normal saline. Excessive replacement in elderly patients with poorly compliant circulations will lead to volume overload, hypertension and pulmonary oedema. In such patients, who tend to have high sympathetic tone, judicious use of low-dose intravenous nitrate may help to promote vasodilatation and allow space for further filling.

When hypovolaemia has been corrected, many doctors give a dose of frusemide, or mannitol, or start renal-dose dopamine infusion to initiate a diuresis. However, there is no evidence of efficacy for these interventions and they are certainly not substitutes for the rapid and effective correction of hypovolaemia.

CARDIAC STATUS

The presence of impaired cardiac function may be suggested by the patient's premorbid symptoms or medical history. The pulse should be examined for its strength, rate and rhythm. A raised JVP reflects right or biventricular heart failure, a displaced apex beat reflects a dilated left ventricle with dyskinesis due to an aneurysmal segment, and auscultation may reveal new murmurs. The presence of bilateral inspiratory crackles can be due to pulmonary oedema or basal atelectasis, and dull bases due to pleural effusions should be sought.

Investigations

The ECG may provide evidence of a rhythm disturbance or recent myocardial infarction. The chest X-ray may demonstrate signs of heart failure with cardiomegaly, pericardial effusion, upper lobe blood diversion, pulmonary oedema and pleural effusion. In some patients an echocardiogram may be required to confirm impaired myocardial function and to exclude important valve pathology. Cardiac enzymes should be measured if there is a suggestion of recent myocardial infarction.

Management

Optimization of cardiac output may require invasive cardiac monitoring and the judicious use of fluids, inotropes, vasodilators and anti-arrhythmics, with the aim of maximizing systemic perfusion. These interventions are best undertaken by an experienced physician.

EVIDENCE OF SEPSIS

The patient should be examined for evidence of sepsis suggested by a history of chills, pyrexia and the presence of warm, bounding peripheries due to systemic vasodilatation. Systemic sepsis may derive from a post-operative chest infection, surgical wound, venous cannulae, infectious diarrhoea or urinary infection.

Investigations

Urine, blood, sputum and stool specimens should be sent for culture, wounds should be swabbed, and venous cannulae should be removed if the puncture site is erythematous and the catheter tips sent for culture.

Microbiology records should be reviewed for relevant results.

Management

Advice regarding antibiotic therapy should be sought from the microbiology team. If the patient is haemodynamically affected, then invasive monitoring and the use of vasoconstrictors and inotropes should be considered.

OTHER MISCELLANEOUS FACTORS WHICH SHOULD BE CONSIDERED IN THE OLIGURIC PATIENT

The patient's notes should be examined for evidence of recent studies or procedures involving radiocontrast medium. Acute pigment-induced nephropathy should be considered in patients who have undergone revascularization (rhabdomyolysis), prolonged surgery or who could have received a mismatched blood transfusion. Finally, the possibility of an obstructed bladder catheter should be excluded.

ESTABLISHING THE CAUSE OF OLIGURIA

In addition to the clinical approach detailed above, only four tests are required to diagnose the cause of the patient's oliguria or impaired renal function. These are:

1. plasma creatinine (test of renal function);

2. urinary sodium (for evidence of renal hypoperfusion and appropriate oliguria);

3. urinalysis and microscopy (for evidence of primary renal disease rather than hypoperfusion injury, see below);

4. renal imaging – ultrasound to measure renal size and cortical thickness, diagnose nephrolithiasis, exclude obstruction and demonstrate perfusion using Doppler.

MANAGEMENT (SEE FIGURE 17.2.1)

Following scrutiny of the charts and examination of the patient, a list of the probable causes and relevant comorbidities should be made. Hypovolaemia should be corrected as rapidly as possible and cardiac function optimized. All nephrotoxic drugs should be stopped. If assessment of circulating volume and cardiac status provide no clue to the cause of oliguria, then the differential diagnosis should be considered and a referral to a physician or nephrologist (if available) made.

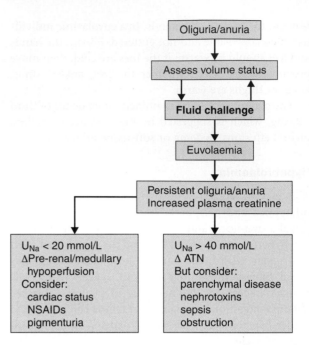

Figure 17.2.1 Algorithm for the management and diagnosis of the oliguric patient.

Additional causes of ARF

The free flow of urine may be obstructed by the presence of bilateral calculi, clot or tumour in the renal pelvicalyceal systems, bilateral extrinsic ureteric compression due to primary or secondary (malignancy, inflammatory aortitis, drugs) retroperitoneal fibrosis or lymph nodes, the presence of tumour, stones or clot in the bladder, or urethral obstruction by prostate or stricture. The diagnosis of obstruction is suggested by the presence of dilated upper tracts on ultrasound, but renography may be required to confirm this. Management requires specialist advice, and a nephrologist or urologist should be contacted.

Urine microscopy is mandatory if primary renal parenchymal disease is suspected. The presence of coarse granular casts suggests parenchymal disease, and dysmorphic red cells and red cell casts are pathognomonic of glomerular bleeding due to acute glomerulonephritis (e.g. post-infectious, systemic lupus erythematosus (SLE), microscopic polyarteritis, Goodpasture's syndrome, Henoch-Schönlein purpura). Deeply pigmented casts are found in patients with acute pigment nephropathy, due to mismatched blood transfusion or intra-operative limb ischaemia leading to rhabdomyolysis. Interstitial nephritis due to infection, drugs, myeloma or systemic disease is suggested by eosinophiluria, pyuria and white cell casts, and the presence of copious urinary crystals may reflect tumour lysis (urate) or ethylene glycol (oxalate) poisoning. Renal infiltration by malignancy, myeloma, sarcoid or amyloid may also require exclusion. All of these conditions require specialized management by a nephrologist.

Acute catastrophic renovascular insufficiency may complicate abdominal aortic aneurysm rupture, aortic dissection, renal artery thrombosis and renal vein thrombosis. Although the diagnosis may be apparent on Doppler ultrasound, a dynamic renogram should be performed to confirm the diagnosis when the patient is stable. Oliguria may be due to acute microvascular disease caused by renal cholesterol embolization following interventional vascular radiology or surgery, haemolytic uraemic syndrome, malignant hypertension or pre-eclampsia. All of these conditions require specialized management by a nephrologist.

Prognosis

The prognosis of the oliguric patient depends on the cause. About 95% of patients with established ATN will recover renal function within 6 weeks, although some of these will subsequently develop chronic and even end-stage renal failure. Even after 12 months, patients who appear to have made a complete recovery will show defects in urinary acidification and concentration, and will remain more vulnerable to further episodes of ATN.

The development of ATN may complicate up to 5% of hospital admissions, and commonly the aetiology is multifactorial, involving both renal hypoperfusion and nephrotoxins. A significant proportion of these cases are potentially avoidable. In general, the mortality is twice as high in patients with cardiac insufficiency as in those in whom ATN is due to nephrotoxins alone. Nevertheless, the overall mortality of acute renal failure remains about 50%.

Prophylaxis

A variety of strategies have been proposed to protect the kidney against insult. These are based on attempts to reduce metabolic activity in the face of hypoperfusion, i.e. to reduce mismatch between the energy demand of tubular epithelium and blood supply. The Na^+/K^+-ATPase in the distal segment of the proximal tubule and the thin ascending limb of the loop of Henlé are the most metabolically active segments of the nephron, and are therefore the most vulnerable to hypoperfusion. Theoretically, inhibition of active (ATP-dependent) pumps (by frusemide, dopamine or cardiac glycosides) should reduce the vulnerability of these nephron segments to hypoperfusion. However, there are few clinical data which provide clinical evidence of efficacy. It seems likely that the only benefit of these interventions is to cause a diuresis and facilitate fluid balance, rather than to improve renal function.

Effective prophylaxis against ATN depends on the early recognition of the high-risk patient, who may have cardiac failure, diabetes mellitus, chronic renal failure, a recent episode of acute renal failure, hypertension or systemic atherosclerosis. In all patients, hypovolaemia should be rapidly identified and treated. In patients who are to be starved prior to a procedure, or who are to receive radiocontrast medium, intravenous fluids (normal or half-normal saline to prevent sodium overload) should be infused for at least 12 h prior to the intervention. There is no proven renal protection from pretreatment with mannitol, frusemide or dopamine. Finally, in the post-operative period, adequate intravenous fluids must be administered, NSAIDs avoided and aminoglycoside levels carefully monitored.

Erectile dysfunction and ejaculatory disorders

David Ralph

ERECTILE DYSFUNCTION

'Erectile dysfunction' has now replaced the term 'impotence', and is defined as the inability to initiate and maintain an erection of sufficient rigidity for sexual intercourse. It is a common disorder, varying in severity, with persistent erectile dysfunction occurring in 5% of 40-year-olds and increasing to 15% of 70-year-olds.

ANATOMY

The penile erectile tissue consists of two corpora cavernosa (Figure 18.1). Each corpus cavernosum is attached by its crus to the pubic rami and joins in the midline forming the pendulous part of the penis. Each corpus cavernosum consists of smooth muscle lining the vascular sinusoidal spaces supplied by branches of the central cavernous artery. This erectile mechanism is encased within the tough tunica albuginea of the penis, which in the midline forms the septum of the penis. The urethra is surrounded by the corpus spongiosum, which terminates by forming the glans penis. The cavernous artery within the corpus cavernosum and the dorsal artery supplying the glans penis are branches of the internal pudendal artery. Venous drainage is via the emissary veins which pass through the tunica albuginea into the circumflex veins and into the deep dorsal vein of the penis. The erectile mechanism is innervated by the autonomic nervous system. The sympathetic fibres (T10 to L2) via the hypogastric nerves and parasympathetic fibre (S2 to 4) enter the pelvic plexus. The cavernous nerves, containing both autonomic pathways, exit the pelvic

plexus, travel posterolateral to the prostate and membranous urethra, and enter the corpus cavernosum to innervate the smooth muscle (Figure 18.2). Penile sensation occurs via the dorsal nerve of the penis and the internal pudendal nerve.

MECHANISM OF ERECTION

In the flaccid penis (Figure 18.3), vasoconstriction of the helicine arteries and contraction of the cavernous

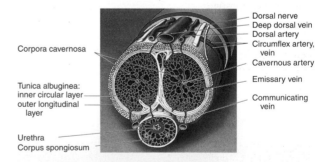

Corpora cavernosa

Tunica albuginea:
inner circular layer
outer longitudinal
layer

Urethra
Corpus spongiosum

Dorsal nerve
Deep dorsal vein
Dorsal artery
Circumflex artery,
vein
Cavernous artery

Emissary vein

Communicating
vein

Figure 18.1 Cross-section of the penis.

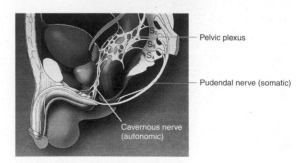

Pelvic plexus

Pudendal nerve (somatic)

Cavernous nerve
(autonomic)

Figure 18.2 Innervation of the penis.

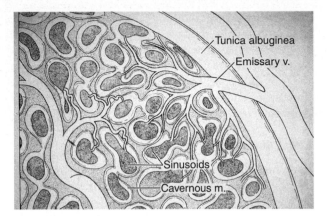

Figure 18.3 Mechanism of erection: flaccidity.

smooth muscle are mediated via the sympathetic nervous system. The sinusoidal spaces therefore contain a minimal amount of blood, the intracorporeal pressure is low, and blood is allowed to drain out of the corpora cavernosa via the emissary veins into the circumflex and deep dorsal vein.

During erection, the most important feature is relaxation of the cavernous smooth muscle. Together with the vasodilatation that occurs, this allows the sinusoidal spaces to be filled with blood with an increase in intracavernosal pressure (Figure 18.4). This increased intracavernosal pressure allows for compression of the subtunical venous plexus and occlusion of the emissary veins by the expanding tunica albuginea. There is therefore an increased arterial inflow and also a reduced venous drainage from within the corpus cavernosum. The whole erectile event is mediated by the autonomic nervous system in that there is a reduction in sympathetic tone and an increased parasympathetic inflow. The major neurotransmitter is nitric oxide synthesized locally within the nerves and endothelium, but other neurotransmitters (prostaglandin E_1, vasoactive intestinal polypeptide and acetylcholine) also contribute.

At the time of ejaculation there is a huge sympathetic outflow, thereby causing arterial vasoconstriction and smooth muscle contraction, and the penis will therefore revert to the flaccid state.

AETIOLOGY

A classification of erectile dysfunction is given in Box 18.1.

BOX 18.1 CLASSIFICATION OF CAUSES OF ERECTILE DYSFUNCTION

Psychogenic
Vasculogenic
    Arteriogenic
    Venogenic
Neurogenic
Endocrine
Local diseases of the penis
    Peyronie's disease
    Fibrosis
Drug induced

Psychogenic causes

Erectile dysfunction may be a symptom of many psychiatric disorders, as well as being the initial cause. Performance anxiety or the fear of failure are the commonest psychogenic causes of erectile dysfunction (Figure 18.5). In this situation there is a high sympathetic outflow, resulting in vasoconstriction and corporal cavernous smooth muscle contraction. Consequently, when this occurs either the patient cannot obtain an erection, or the erection cannot be maintained during sexual intercourse.

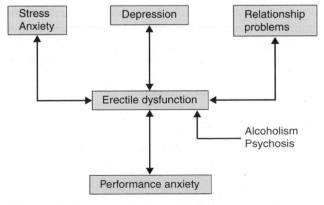

Figure 18.4 Mechanism of erection: rigidity.

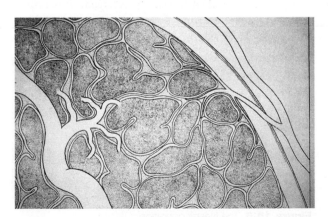

Figure 18.5 Cause and effect of psychogenic erectile dysfunction.

Vasculogenic causes

The risk factors for vasculogenic erectile dysfunction are as follows:

- diabetes;
- hypertension;
- smoking;
- cardiac disease;
- peripheral vascular disease;
- hyperlipidaemia;
- trauma.

Arteriogenic causes

An increased arterial inflow is necessary during erection. Patients with generalized vascular disease or vascular risk factors are therefore at risk of being unable to meet the increased arterial demand necessary for erection. Arterial trauma can result from a direct injury to the cavernous artery in the perineum following a fall-astride injury or an injury to the internal pudendal artery in association with a fractured pelvis, as it travels in Alcock's canal. It is important to identify isolated arterial injuries, as patients may benefit from revascularization.

Venogenic causes

Veno-occlusive dysfunction or venous leakage is said to occur when there is a normal arterial input but the blood cannot be maintained within the penis. Patients usually have similar vasculogenic risk factors, but it is thought that there may well be an abnormality of the cavernous smooth muscle.

Neurogenic causes

The most common causes of neurogenic erectile dysfunction are as follows:

- trauma (spinal or pelvic);
- multiple sclerosis;
- diabetes;
- pelvic surgery.

Other central nervous system disorders can result in erectile dysfunction. Injury to the cavernous nerves commonly occurs following radical prostatectomy, cystectomy and abdominoperineal (AP) resection of the rectum. Injury to the pelvic plexus can also occur during anterior resection of the rectum. Ejaculatory dysfunction is often present in these patients.

Endocrine causes

The endocrinological causes of erectile dysfunction are as follows:

- hypogonadism;
- hyperprolactinaemia;
- thyroid disease.

Testosterone is important for cavernous smooth muscle relaxation and the ability to have an erection. Associated symptoms of hair loss, gynaecomastia and loss of libido, together with small-sized testicles, should alert one to the possibility of hypogonadism. Treatment of the underlying endocrine abnormality usually successfully cures any erectile dysfunction.

Local diseases of the penis

Peyronie's disease

This is a disease of unknown aetiology that is common in men aged 40–60 years. In the early stages there is inflammation of the tunica albuginea, which heals by forming a 'plaque' which is often palpable. The plaque is usually situated on the dorsal surface of the penis and results in a dorsal penile deformity on erection. Erectile dysfunction due to Peyronie's disease can be psychogenic in nature, due to embarrassment about the shape of the penis, the deformity itself may prevent sexual intercourse, or in extensive disease there may be involvement of erectile tissue and an impaired erection. Medical therapy is often unhelpful, and approximately 20% of patients finally have a surgical intervention. This is an operation to straighten the penis either by excision of an ellipse of tunica albuginea opposite the apex of the deformity – the Nesbit operation (Figure 18.6 and see Plates 18.1 and 18.2 in the colour plate section) – or by an incision of the plaque and insertion of a vein graft to lengthen the shorter side. Patients who also have impaired erectile capacity usually need to have a penile prosthesis inserted.

Penile fibrosis

Fibrosis of the cavernous muscle can occur following trauma (either direct or iatrogenic), and is also commonly found at the injection site of patients who are on a self-injection treatment programme.

The commonest reason for penile fibrosis is priapism (a painful persistent erection lasting more than 6 h), for which there are many causes (Box 18.2), the commonest being self-injection with a vasoactive agent. It is important to take the erection down as soon as possible, as

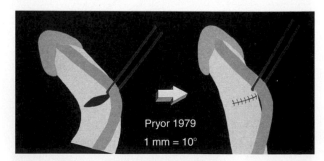

Pryor 1979
1 mm = 10°

Figure 18.6 The Nesbit operation.

with time the cavernous smooth muscle becomes anoxic and eventually necrotic, with subsequent healing by fibrosis. Conservative treatment includes exercise and an attempt to ejaculate. If this is unsuccessful, aspiration of the anoxic blood and instillation of a vasoconstrictor (e.g. phenylephrine) into the penis should be cautiously administered. Patients who do not respond to this regimen usually develop severe penile fibrosis with complete erectile failure, and require the insertion of a penile prosthesis (see Plate 18.3 in the colour plate section). For other causes of priapism the underlying condition should be treated first, and the erection then usually settles.

BOX 18.2 CAUSES OF PRIAPISM

Injection of vasoactive drug
Sickle-cell disease
Haematological malignancy
Antipsychotic medication
Idiopathic causes
Trauma

Drugs associated with erectile dysfunction

These are listed in Table 18.1.

ASSESSMENT

Clinical history

A good clinical history forms the basis of assessment, with the physician attempting to decipher whether the cause is psychogenic or organic in nature. It is important to establish the nature of the erectile problem and to distinguish it from other forms of sexual dysfunction, such as penile curvature or premature ejaculation. Patients who experience normal waking erections, normal erections in certain situations, and who have no risk factors and give a short history are likely to have psychogenic erectile dysfunction. It is important for the clinician to distinguish between psychogenic and organic erectile dysfunction, as treatment pathways may differ (Table 18.2).

The clinical history should include a description of the nature of the erectile dysfunction, the relevant current medical history, with known risk factors for erectile

Table 18.1 Drugs related to erectile dysfunction

Major tranquillizers	Antidepressants	Antihypertensives	Miscellaneous
Haloperidol	Amitriptyline	Beta-blockers	Anti-androgens
Thioridazine	Imipramine	Vasodilators	Cimetidine
Carbamazepine	Fluoxetine	Diuretics	Clofibrate
Fluphenazine	Monoamine-oxidase inhibitors	ACE inhibitors	Digoxin
			Indomethacin

Table 18.2 Factors suggesting aetiology of erectile dysfunction

Organic factors	Psychogenic factors
Gradual onset	Sudden onset
Constant dysfunction	Situational
Obvious cause (spinal injury, pelvic surgery)	Relationship problems
Absent erections at all times	Normal waking/self-stimulated erections
Age > 60 years	Young men
Ejaculation normal except in specific diseases	Premature/absent ejaculation
Risk factors present	No risk factors

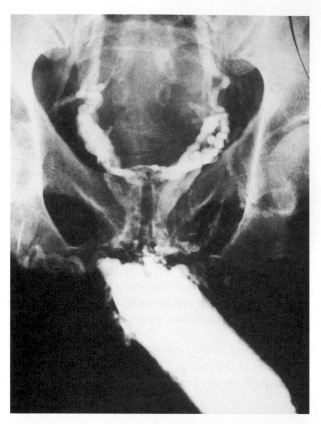

Figure 18.7 Cavernosography demonstrating venous leakage to the prostatic plexus.

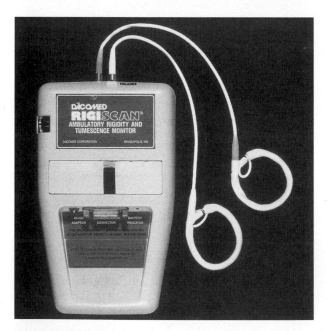

Figure 18.8 A Rigiscan used to monitor nocturnal penile tumescence.

dysfunction, and any relevant past medical history of systemic illness or surgical procedures. A full sexual and relationship history with a list of the medications used should also be taken.

Clinical examination

A physical examination of the patient is important in order to reassure him that due attention has been given to organic factors. The penis should be examined to exclude Peyronie's plaques or areas of penile fibrosis, and the size of the testicles assessed to exclude hypogonadism. Rectal examination should be performed to exclude prostate carcinoma, together with measurement of the blood pressure, peripheral pulses and a brief neurological examination.

Investigations

It is always important to rule out unsuspected diabetes mellitus, and ideally a random blood glucose test should be performed together with a serum testosterone level. The majority of patients do not require further investigations (see Plate 18.4 in the colour plate section, and Figures 18.7 and 18.8) unless specifically indicated as outlined in Table 18.3. It is important to refer any specific endocrine, neurological or psychiatric abnormality to the appropriate speciality.

MANAGEMENT

Patients should be advised to reduce smoking and alcohol consumption, and possibly there should be a change of drug regimen. Patients with purely psychogenic erectile dysfunction should be referred for psychosexual counselling with or without medical therapy to improve the outcome. Patients with organic disease will also be affected psychologically, and will benefit from some form of sexual counselling, although medical therapy is usually instigated in this group.

Testosterone replacement therapy should only be administered for confirmed isolated testosterone deficiencies and in cases where digital rectal examination and prostate-specific antigen tests have been normal.

Treatment options (Box 18.3) should preferably start with the least invasive oral therapy, graduating through to surgical therapy in patients in whom all other treatments have failed. An outline protocol for management is shown in Figure 18.9.

BOX 18.3 TREATMENT OPTIONS

Oral therapy
Intra-urethral injections
Intracavernosal injections
Vacuum device
Penile prosthesis
Other surgical options

Table 18.3 Further investigations

Investigation	Rationale	Indication
Prolactin	To exclude pituitary adenoma	Low testosterone levels
LH/FSH	To assess cause of hypogonadism	Low testosterone levels
Free testosterone		
Colour Doppler ultrasound	Assesses vascular integrity	Young patient being considered for surgical intervention
Phalloarteriography	To clarify vascular abnormality	Arterial abnormality found on Doppler ultrasound
Cavernosometry/ cavernosography	Assess venous occlusive mechanism	When primary venous leakage is suspected in a young man
Nocturnal penile tumescence	Assesses nocturnal erections when smooth muscle is relaxed. Reduces false-positive investigation rate	When other investigations are inconclusive, or prior to surgery

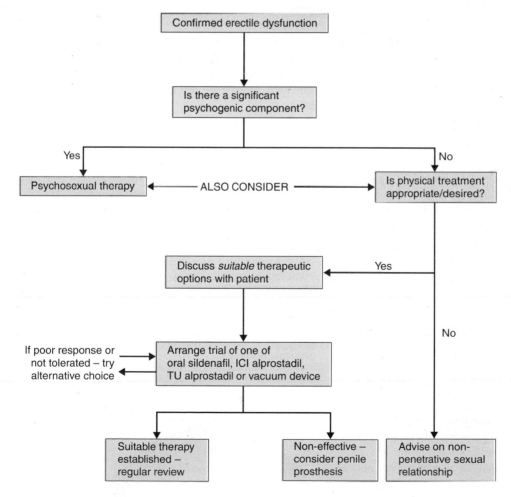

Figure 18.9 Suggested plan for the treatment of erectile dysfunction.

Pharmacological agents

Mechanism of action

The fundamental event that occurs during erection is relaxation of the corporal smooth muscle. This is brought about by the second messengers cAMP and cGMP, and drugs act to influence their concentrations within the penis. The main neurotransmitter for erection is nitric oxide, which stimulates guanylate cyclase to produce cGMP. This is subsequently broken down by the enzyme phosphodiesterase 5, which is specifically inhibited by sildenafil (Viagra). It is important to note that nitric oxide

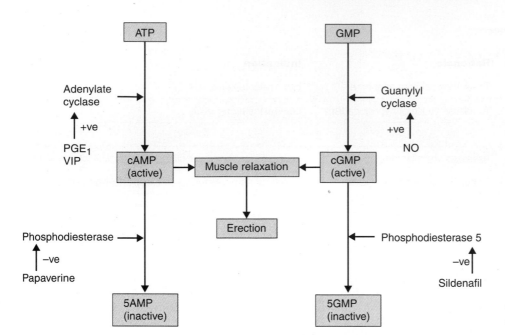

Figure 18.10 Mechanism of action of pharmacological agents.

is formed only on demand following sexual arousal, and therefore sildenafil is ineffective for patients who are not sexually aroused. Injection therapy with prostaglandin E_1 (PGE_1) and vasoactive intestinal polypeptide (VIP) stimulates adenylate cyclase to produce cAMP and smooth muscle relaxation. The breakdown of cAMP is inhibited by papaverine's effect on phosphodiesterase (Figure 18.10).

Oral medication

Sildenafil is available in doses of 25, 50 or 100 mg, and is taken 1 h prior to sexual intercourse. It is well tolerated, and is effective in 40–80% of men, but should not be taken by those already on nitrate therapy, due to the risk of severe hypotension.

Transurethral therapy

Diffusion of prostaglandin E_1 (alprostadil) can occur when it is administered into the urethra. The chemical will diffuse through the corpus spongiosus and into the corpus cavernosus within 15 min, thereby producing an erection. It is a minimally invasive technique which is well accepted by patients, although the efficacy is not as good as intracavernosal injection therapy (see Plate 18.5 in the colour plate section).

Intracavernosal injection therapy

The injection of a vasoactive agent into the penis to cause an erection was first performed in 1982, and has since revolutionized the treatment of erectile dysfunction (Figure 18.11). The following drugs are currently available for intracavernosal injection:

- alprostadil (prostaglandin E_1);
- VIP/phentolamine;
- papaverine (unlicensed).

An erection will occur within 5 min of injection and should ideally last for approximately 30 min. The drugs are effective in 80% of patients, and complications include penile pain on injection, priapism and penile fibrosis at the injection site. Side-effects are more prevalent with papaverine, which was one of the first agents used.

Vacuum devices

The penis is inserted into the vacuum device (see Plate 18.6 in the colour plate section) and a vacuum is created, thereby drawing venous blood into the penis. Once it is erect, a band is slipped off the plastic cylinder around the base of the penis to maintain the erection. These devices are potentially effective in all patients, although they are cumbersome to use. The penis feels cold due to being filled with venous blood, and ejaculation is usually blocked by the compression band at the base. Vacuum devices are particularly useful in older men in stable relationships when other treatment options are ineffective, and can sometimes be used in combination with pharmacotherapy.

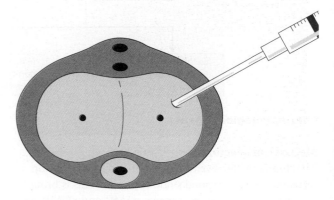

Figure 18.11 Intracavernosal injection of a vasoactive drug.

Penile prostheses

In general, penile prostheses should be considered in patients who have an organic cause for their impotence, or who are unwilling to consider or have failed to respond to medical therapy or external devices. They are particularly useful in patients who have an impaired erection due to Peyronie's disease or post-injection penile fibrosis. There are basically two types of prosthesis. The semi-rigid malleable prosthesis is easy to insert through a penoscrotal incision, and complications are minimal (see Plates 18.7 and 18.8 in the colour plate section). However, the penis has the same rigidity at all times, and therefore concealment may be a problem. If concealment is desired, a more natural erection that allows both flaccidity and rigidity can be obtained by the use of inflatable penile prostheses. The cylinders of such prostheses are inserted into the corpora cavernosa on each side, a scrotal pump is placed and a reservoir is inserted into the retropubic space (Figure 18.12). Mechanical problems with these devices are reported to occur at the rate of 5% per year, and they are now highly reliable. The cost of the inflatable models is high, and infection and erosion rates of approximately 2% can be expected.

Other surgical options

Penile revascularization

This operation involves harvesting of the epigastric artery and anastomosing it to the dorsal vein of the penis to increase arterial inflow to the corporal bodies. It is particularly useful in patients who have an isolated arterial lesion, usually due to trauma, which has been diagnosed on a selective arteriogram. These patients are young and have no other risk factors, and with careful selection can achieve a 65% success rate.

Surgery for veno-occlusive dysfunction (venous leakage)

Venous ligation procedures for this condition have previously been widely used, although success rates have been poor. Ligation of the dorsal venous complex should now be reserved for patients with primary veno-occlusive dysfunction who are likely to have congenital focal abnormalities which are diagnosed by cavernosography.

EJACULATORY DISORDERS

The main disorders of ejaculation are as follows:

- premature;
- anejaculation;
- retrograde;
- low volume.

PHYSIOLOGY

The average ejaculated volume is 2–5 mL, 95% of this being formed from secretions of the seminal vesicles and prostate, and is highly androgen dependent. The mechanism of ejaculation is mediated through the sympathetic

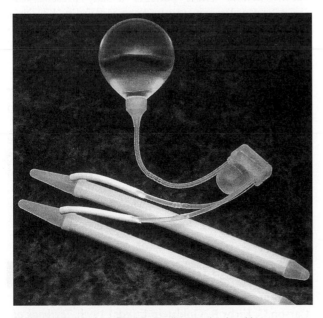

Figure 18.12 An inflatable penile prosthesis with two cylinders, a scrotal pump and a reservoir.

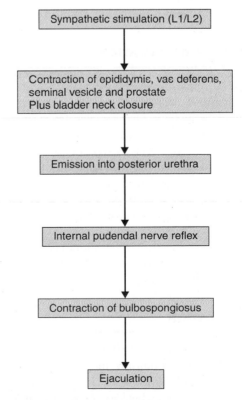

Figure 18.13 Mechanism of ejaculation.

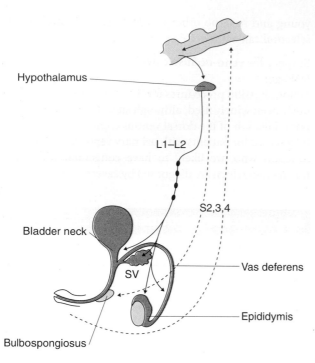

Figure 18.14 Mechanism of ejaculation.

nervous system (L1/L2), fibres of which run in the hypogastric nerves to supply the epididymis, vas deferens, seminal vesicles, prostate and bladder neck. Expulsion of the ejaculate from the posterior urethra is mediated by a reflex within the internal pudendal nerve to cause contraction of the striated muscle, in particular the bulbosponsiosus (Figures 18.13 and 18.14).

PREMATURE EJACULATION

Excessive stimulation of the ejaculatory centre in the hypothalamus is usually of cortical origin due to over-excitement or anxiety. Occasionally deformities of the penis or inflammatory lesions causing pain may precipitate this condition. Previous treatments, including the application of local anaesthetic jellies to the glans penis to reduce sensitivity, have been unsuccessful. Surgical remedies such as division of the dorsal nerve of the penis should be discouraged. Favourable results have been obtained using selective serotonin reuptake inhibitors (e.g. fluoxetine – Prozac), which should be taken 2 to 3 h prior to intercourse. Psychosexual counselling is the preferred treatment option.

ANEJACULATION

This term refers to patients who fail to ejaculate and are anorgasmic. This condition may be psychogenic in nature, particularly when there is no history of nerve injury or disease and when nocturnal emissions occur,

which would therefore suggest that the normal ejaculatory pathways are intact. Causes of an organic nature include spinal injury and surgical injury to the hypogastric nerves. This is particularly relevant in patients having retroperitoneal lymph node dissections for germ cell tumours, aorto-iliac surgery and rectal excision where the hypogastric nerves can be damaged as they traverse the pelvic brim. Patients with autonomic neuropathy, usually due to diabetes, may also present with anejaculation due to loss of contraction of the epididymis, vas and seminal vesicles.

Treatments for organic disease in the group of patients with spinal injury include vibratory stimulation with high lesions and electro-ejaculation with a rectal probe for the remainder.

RETROGRADE EJACULATION

This condition presents with anejaculation, but orgasm is maintained. It is due to failure of the bladder neck to close during ejaculation, and could be either congenital in nature or acquired. Acquired causes include excision of the bladder neck during transurethral resection of the prostate (TURP) and a diabetic autonomic neuropathy. Damage to the sympathetic nerves during pelvic surgery may also present with an isolated incompetent bladder neck. The diagnosis can be made by observing the presence of sperm in a post-ejaculatory urine sample, as well as a transrectal ultrasound examination revealing an incompetent bladder neck. Treatment with the sympathomimetic agents desipramine and imipramine is occasionally successful, as is major bladder neck reconstruction. These patients usually present with infertility, and sperm can be harvested from the urine, washed and used for assisted conception.

LOW VOLUME

A low-volume ejaculate (less than 1 mL) may be due to reduced production, an obstruction, or partial retrograde ejaculation. Serum testosterone levels should be measured as seminal vesicle and prostatic fluid production is testosterone dependent. A transrectal ultrasound examination will exclude ejaculatory duct obstruction, which can be treated by a transurethral incision of the ejaculatory duct.

FURTHER READING

Carson C, Kirby R, Goldstein I. (eds) 1999: *Textbook of erectile dysfunction.* Oxford: Isis Medical Media.

Feldman HA, Goldstein I, Hatzichristou DG. 1994: Impotence and psychosocial correlates: results of the Massachusetts male ageing study. *Journal of Urology* **151**, 54–61.

Goldstein I, Krane RJ. 1997: Diagnosis and therapy of erectile dysfunction. In Walsh PC, Retik AB, Stamey TA, Vaughan ED (eds), *Campbell's urology*. Philadelphia, PA: W.B. Saunders, 3033–72.

Morales A. (ed.) 1998: *Erectile dysfunction: issues in current pharmacotherapy*. London: Martin Dunitz.

Chapter 19

Vaginal discharge

Friedericke Eben

Introduction

Although women with vaginal discharge, odour, pruritis and pain are usually seen by general practitioners and gynaecologists, they may also be seen by surgeons, especially if other symptoms are present. Doctors often have a poor understanding of the condition, and so treat it ineffectively. Clinical examination, together with microscopic examination and culture where appropriate, are essential to make a diagnosis.

The causes of vaginal discharge may be bacterial, parasitic, viral, atrophic, cancerous or traumatic, and are associated with cervical or vulval lesions. Referral to a sexual health clinic and treatment of the sexual partner must always be considered. Vaginal discharge may also be due to a vesicovaginal or rectovaginal fistula.

PHYSIOLOGY

Vaginal secretions consist of cervical mucus, endometrial and oviductal fluids, and vulval secretions from sebaceous, Bartholin's and Skene's glands. Secretion varies with the stage of the menstrual cycle, and is affected by the concentrations of oestrogen and progesterone.

Vaginal fluid is acidic (pH 4–5) and contains high levels (2–3%) of lactic acid resulting from the conversion of glycogen by Doderlin bacilli (*Lactobacillus*) under the influence of oestrogens. The low pH is bactericidal and helps to maintain a healthy vaginal environment. Vaginal levels of glycogen are high at birth and during ovulation, but very low during childhood and after the menopause, which accounts for the differences in vaginal flora during a woman's life.

VAGINAL DISCHARGE DUE TO INFECTION

Case 19.1 A recently divorced woman, aged 25 years, with two children, had just entered into a new sexual relationship. She had had an intrauterine contraceptive device fitted 1 year previously and presented to an Emergency Department with an increased vaginal discharge over the last 2 weeks.

The clinical assessment is illustrated by the following case presentation.

What questions would you ask?

Q. *Is the discharge thick and cheesy and associated with vaginal or vulval pruritis (suggesting vaginal* candidiasis), or is it malodorous (suggesting bacterial vaginosis)?

A. Yes it smells.

Q. *Has the patient noticed any dysuria, or symptoms of endometritis, such as pelvic pain or intermenstrual bleeding (suggesting chlamydial infection or more rarely gonorrhoea)?*

A. Yes, she had noticed mild, intermittent pelvic ache, but no pain on micturition.

Q. *Has she noticed any tender spots on her vulva (possibly suggesting a genital herpes infection)?*

A. No.

Q. *Has her partner noticed any dysuria or urethral discharge (suggesting urethritis)?*

A. Not that she was aware of.

Q. *Are the patient and her partner using condoms?*

A. No.

Which specific examinations would you perform?

- Check the patient's temperature.
- Perform an abdominal examination to elicit any pelvic tenderness and exclude obvious pelvic masses.
- Perform a speculum examination of the vagina. This will allow you to assess the colour, smell and consistency of the vaginal discharge and to check the cervix for any abnormality.
- Perform a bimanual examination to assess cervical excitation suggestive of pelvic infection, or pelvic masses in association with a pelvic abscess.

Which tests would you perform?

- High vaginal swab (HVS) for Gram staining or amine test to diagnose bacterial vaginosis, HVS for culture to diagnose candidal or streptococcal infection and trichomoniasis.
- Separate endocervical swabs for chlamydial and gonococcal culture.
- Ultrasonography if a pelvic mass is suspected.
- Midstream urine culture.
- Consider assessment of the patient's partner.

Subsequent treatment

The patient had a positive amine test and was treated with a course of metronidazole for suspected bacterial vaginosis after the attending doctor had taken high vaginal and endocervical swabs to exclude coinfection with other organisms. The endocervical swab proved positive for chlamydia for which the patient was treated with doxycycline. Although he was asymptomatic, her partner was found to have chlamydial urethritis.

BACTERIAL VAGINOSIS

Nearly one-third of women with symptomatic vaginal discharge will have bacterial vaginosis, which results from replacement of the normal lactobacilli-predominant flora with a mixed flora containing mainly anaerobic bacterial species, including *Gardnerella vaginalis*, *Bacteroides* and *Mycoplasma hominis*. Whether the condition is sexually transmitted is uncertain.

Clinical features

The commonest presenting symptom is excessive vaginal discharge with a fishy smell, particularly after unprotected sexual intercourse. This is due to the release of amines by alkaline semen.

Diagnosis

The most accurate diagnostic test is microscopy of vaginal secretions. Its Gram-stain appearance shows the normal vaginal flora replaced by organisms such as *Gardnerella*. The amine test, which involves the addition of two drops of potassium hydroxide solution to a sample of the vaginal secretions on a slide or a swab, has a sensitivity of 80–90%. The sudden release of a fishy odour represents a 'positive' result. The appearance of the discharge to the naked eye, high vaginal swab culture and a raised vaginal pH are poor diagnostic markers.

Treatment

Oral metronidazole is very effective, with 2% clindamycin cream administered intravaginally for 3 to 7 days as a useful alternative for patients who cannot tolerate metronidazole. Recurrence is common, and may be treated with short monthly courses of oral metronidazole or vaginal clindamycin cream. Treating the male sexual partner has not proved helpful in preventing the recurrence of bacterial vaginosis.

VAGINAL CANDIDIASIS

This common infection is usually caused by the yeast *Candida albicans*. It grows by producing budding yeast cells (spores) and hyphal filaments (mycelia).

Colonization with *Candida albicans* is widespread, with a prevalence of 15–20% in asymptomatic healthy women. It is not considered to be a sexually transmitted disease.

Predisposing factors

These include the following:

- pregnancy;
- oral contraception;

- broad-spectrum antibiotics;
- clothing and detergents;
- diabetes mellitus;
- immunosuppression.

Clinical features

The vaginal discharge is thick and white with a cheesy appearance, and vaginal examination may be painful. In symptomatic women there is often associated intense vaginal and vulval irritation. The vulval skin may appear red and inflamed, and these appearances may spread to the anus and the region around the thighs.

Diagnosis

High vaginal swabs should be taken, as the organism grows easily in culture. Gram stains and examination of wet preparations may also be performed, but are not as sensitive as culture.

Treatment

Asymptomatic candidal infection does not usually require treatment. The acute episode is best treated with intravaginal tablets or pessaries and topical cream for the vulva using imidazole derivatives such as clotrimazole. Oral therapy with fluconazole or itraconazole has been promoted as an alternative to intravaginal treatment, and may produce lower long-term recurrence rates.

Recurrent candidiasis may be associated with:

- persisting predisposing factors;
- reinfection from an intestinal reservoir;
- reinfection from an untreated sexual partner.

Treating recurrent candidal infections

Various prophylactic regimes reduce recurrence rates. These include a 100-mg miconazole pessary weekly over a period of 6 months, or a single clotrimazole vaginal tablet after each period. Some success has been reported with the use of intravaginal yogurt or yeast-free diets.

TRICHOMONIASIS

Trichomonas vaginalis is a motile flagellated protozoon with a diameter of 10–20 μm (slightly larger than a pus cell). Trichomoniasis is usually transmitted sexually, but may be acquired from towels and toilet seats. *Trichomonas vaginalis* attaches itself to the vaginal mucosa and, after multiplication, depletes the number of lactobacilli by depriving them of glycogen.

Clinical features

About 50% of infected patients have a profuse, yellow, frothy discharge which may smell offensive, and about 20% of women have an associated vulvovaginal pruritis. However, many women have little discharge or are asymptomatic.

In addition to the discharge, vaginal examination may reveal inflamed vaginal walls and numerous minute punctate ulcers on the cervix ('strawberry spots').

Diagnosis

The condition is diagnosed by identifying motile trichomonads on a wet mount of the discharge. Culture of a high vaginal swab and staining of a fixed preparation with Papanicolaou are other diagnostic methods.

Treatment

Metronidazole cures up to 98% of patients. A single dose of 2 g metronidazole is as effective as multidose regimens.

The organism is difficult to detect in men, and whether asymptomatic partners without detectable infection need to be treated is the subject of controversy. Nevertheless, women and their partners should be fully screened for sexually transmitted diseases, as *Trichomonas* often coexists with other infections, especially gonorrhoea and chlamydial infections.

GONORRHOEA

Neisseria gonorrhoea is a Gram-negative intracellular diplococcus which is sexually transmitted and has an incubation period of around 1–14 days. Squamous epithelium such as that lining the vagina is resistant to infection by the gonococcus. The site of infection is commonly the glandular epithelium of the urethra, Bartholin's gland and the endocervix. The buccal and anal mucosa may also be involved.

Clinical features

Infected women are frequently symptomless. Initial complaints may include dysuria, urinary frequency and vaginal discharge. Bartholin's abscess is associated with gonococcal infection, and complications include endometritis and pelvic inflammatory disease. Disseminated gonococcal infection complicates 1% of genital infections, and is characterized by fever, pleomorphic skin lesions and swollen, painful joints which in some cases dominate the picture.

Most men develop a purulent discharge and dysuria within 2 to 3 days of acquiring the infection, and then seek treatment. However, about 10% of men are asymptomatic and therefore act as a reservoir of disease.

Diagnosis

Accurate diagnosis is dependent on correct swab-taking. A positive swab is most likely to be obtained from the cervix (89%), the rectum or urethra. A high vaginal swab will miss the infection.

If facilities for direct microscopy are available, an immediate diagnosis can successfully be made by examination of a Gram-stained smear in 50% of cases. Alternatively, specimens should be sent for culture in transport media such as Stuart's or Amies.

Treatment

Patients who are not allergic to penicillin should be given 3 g amoxycillin and 1 g probenecid orally. Patients who are allergic to penicillin may be treated with 250 mg ciprofloxacin or 2 g spectinomycin IM. This regime may also be used for penicillin-resistant strains.

CHLAMYDIA

Chlamydia trachomatis is a Gram-negative intracellular bacterium that causes genital and eye infections. It is transmitted sexually and may lead to pelvic inflammatory disease, ectopic pregnancy and subfertility. As the infection may be asymptomatic in both men and women, it may be present in couples who have been in a stable relationship for months or years. Thus, in contrast to gonococcal infection, its presence does not necessarily indicate recent infidelity.

Clinical features

Most women with symptomatic chlamydial infection will complain of pelvic ache, which is usually bilateral. There may be associated deep dysparunia, intermenstrual or postcoital bleeding, and (rarely) urethritis. Vaginal speculum examination may show a mucopurulent endocervical exudate with cervicitis. In symptomatic women, bimanual examination reveals cervical excitation with uterine and adnexal tenderness.

Some women may present with right upper quadrant pain rather than pelvic symptoms. This is due to chlamydia perihepatitis (Fitz Hugh Curtis syndrome).

Diagnosis

Swabs should be taken from the endocervix and urethra. Urine may also be tested for *Chlamydia trachomatis* infection.

Previously, the standard diagnostic test was isolation of *Chlamydia* from tissue culture. However, at best this detected only 90% of positive specimens. Nucleic acid amplification techniques, including the polymerase and ligase chain reactions, have recently been introduced and increase the test's sensitivity. Women with suspected pelvic inflammatory disease may benefit from a laparoscopy, which when supplemented with a careful microbiological and histological examination of the gen-

ital tract, and inspection of the liver, makes an important contribution to the effective management of their disease.

Treatment

Clinical trials have shown that 1 g azithromycin administered orally in a single dose is as effective as 100 mg doxycycline given orally twice a day for 7 days. Sexual partners should be traced, tested and treated, and patients should abstain from sexual intercourse until both partners have completed treatment.

ATROPHIC VAGINITIS

In postmenopausal women, lack of oestrogens causes thinning of the vaginal epithelium. In addition, there is a progressive fall in the vascularity of the underlying tissue and a gradual loss of elastin and collagen. The vaginal skin becomes pale and fragile, with an increased predisposition to infection, and the pH of the vaginal wall and urethra falls.

Clinical features

Vaginal symptoms include discharge (sometimes blood-stained), dryness and pruritus. There may be urinary symptoms such as dysuria, frequency and urgency. On examination, the vaginal walls appear inflamed and may bleed on contact.

Diagnosis

If there is significant vaginal discharge, high vaginal and endocervical swabs should be taken to exclude infection. Bloodstained discharge must be investigated with a hysteroscopy and endometrial biopsy to exclude endometrial carcinoma.

Treatment

Topical oestradiol creams, pessaries or an oestradiol ring are very successful in reversing the atrophic changes without endometrial stimulation, if used correctly. Some women may prefer systemic hormone replacement therapy.

FISTULAE CAUSING VAGINAL DISCHARGE

VESICOVAGINAL FISTULA

Introduction

Vesicovaginal fistulae have obstetric, surgical, malignant, radiation and miscellaneous other causes. In the developing world most fistulae are due to obstetric causes, whereas in developed countries previous surgery is responsible for most cases.

Case 19.2 A 39-year-old woman presented to the Emergency Department with a 5-day history of increasing lower abdominal pain and a profuse watery vaginal discharge, which smelled like urine.

What questions would you ask?

Q. *What is the patient's obstetric history? (A prolonged labour and instrumental delivery suggests possible cephalopelvic disproportion and obstetric vesicovaginal fistula.)*

A. The patient's last child was born by Caesarean section 5 years ago.

Q. *Has she had any abnormal cervical smear? (Carcinoma of the cervix can invade the bladder and cause a malignant vesicovaginal fistula.)*

A. Her cervical smear 6 months ago was normal.

Q. *Has she recently undergone pelvic surgery, such as an abdominal hysterectomy? (This raises the possibility of a surgical vesicovaginal fistula.)*

A. Yes, she underwent a hysterectomy for fibroids 2 weeks ago.

What specific examinations would you perform?

- Abdominal examination to exclude any large pelvic masses.
- Speculum examination to assess the cervix, particularly if cervical carcinoma is suspected.
- Examination with a Sims speculum may allow visualization of the site where the vesicovaginal fistula lies in the anterior vaginal wall.
- Bimanual examination may reveal a fixed pelvic mass of an invading cervical carcinoma.

Which tests would you perform?

- A midstream urine culture to exclude urinary tract infection in association with the vesicovaginal fistula.
- An intravenous urogram.
- If the fistula is small, injection of methylene blue into the bladder after placing a swab in the vagina may show the level of the fistula in the vagina after withdrawal of the swab.
- An examination under anaesthetic, and cystoscopy.

Subsequent treatment

A vesicovaginal fistula had formed near the vault, which was related to the patient's earlier hysterectomy. This had been difficult, because the bladder had been stuck to the lower segment of the uterus due to her previous Caesarean section, and an anterior uterine wall fibroid had distorted the anatomy. Dissection of the bladder from the uterus had compromised the blood supply to the bladder, which had led to subsequent tissue necrosis. The vesicovaginal fistula was successfully repaired using a vaginal approach.

Obstetric injury

The commonest cause of vesicovaginal fistula is obstructed labour. Prolonged compression of the anterior vaginal wall, the bladder base and the urethra between the fetal head and the posterior surface of the pubis leads to devitalization of the intervening tissues by ischaemia. A few days after the delivery, the bladder base sloughs and a fistula develops.

Other obstetric causes of vesicovaginal fistulae include accidental injury at the time of Caesarean section, forceps delivery, craniotomy or symphysiotomy.

Surgical injury

Vesicovaginal fistulae are more common after abdominal or vaginal hysterectomy and colporrhaphy if the following are present:

- anatomical distortion within the pelvis by an ovarian tumour or fibroid;
- abnormal adhesion between the bladder and uterus or cervix following previous surgery, such as Caesarean section or cone biopsy;
- previous sepsis, endometriosis or pre-operative radiotherapy.

Malignancy or radiation

These are most commonly associated with carcinoma of the cervix, but occasionally carcinoma of the endometrium or vagina may invade the bladder and cause a fistula. Bladder cancer invading the vagina is a rare cause of fistula.

Fistulae may be caused by vaginal application of caesium or other radioactive elements.

Prevention and management of vesicovaginal fistulae

- Fistula formation is mostly avoidable by adopting a high standard of obstetric care.
- The surgical management of fistulae is best undertaken by surgeons with a special interest in this problem.
- The surgical closure of a vesicovaginal fistulae entails either an abdominal combined transperitoneal and transvesical or a vaginal approach.

COLOVAGINAL, RECTOVAGINAL AND ANOVAGINAL FISTULAE

Introduction

Fistulae into the vagina may arise from the colon due to inflammatory bowel disease or, more rarely, from the sigmoid colon, due to diverticular disease. Recto and anovaginal fistulae most commonly follow obstetric trauma. Fistulae may also develop in association with neoplastic disease or post radiation.

> **Case 19.3** A 26-year-old woman was referred by her gynaecologist to the surgical out-patient clinic with a 6-month history of recurrent vaginitis and a more recent history of passing flatus and faeces through her vagina. This happened only during bouts of diarrhoea. Initially she thought that she was suffering from faecal incontinence, and was too embarassed to consult her general practitioner.

What questions would you ask?

Q. *Has the patient recently suffered from increasing episodes of diarrhoea and abdominal pain (suggestive of a fistula due to inflammatory bowel disease)?*

A. No, her recent bout of diarrhoea was associated with food poisoning.

Q. *Has she lost any weight or passed any blood in her stool (suggesting a malignant rectovaginal fistula)?*

A. No, there has been no weight loss or bloody stools.

Q. *Has she undergone any gynaecological vaginal surgery (suggesting surgical injury as a possible cause)?*

A. No, but her perineum was badly torn during the birth of her first child 7 months ago.

The history thus pointed towards a fistula due to obstetric injury.

Which specific examinations would you perform?

- Rectal and vaginal examination and proctoscopy should be performed to exclude any tumours or abscesses.
- Inspection of the posterior vaginal wall will usually identify the fistula.
- Smaller fistulae may be demonstrated by using a probe.

Which tests would you perform?

- Higher colovaginal fistulae may be demonstrated on a barium enema.
- If the fistula is difficult to locate, inserting a tampon into the vagina and methylene blue into the anus can be helpful. The presence of blue coloration on the tampon after 15 to 20 min shows the presence and level of the fistula.
- An examination under general anaesthetic may be useful.
- Anal endosonography.

Subsequent management

On examination this woman's perineum appeared deficient, and careful examination of her posterior vaginal wall showed a small rectovaginal fistula.

As the delivery was more than 6 months ago and the fistula had not healed spontaneously, it was repaired using a vaginal approach.

Colovaginal fistula

This is uncommon, but may result from the rupture of a pericolic abscess into the posterior fornix of the vagina due to acute diverticulitis. More commonly, a diverticular sigmoidovaginal fistula may perforate the vaginal vault some years after a total hysterectomy, and this should be considered as a cause of foul-smelling vaginal discharge in women over 50 years of age.

Rectovaginal fistula

Rectovaginal fistula is a rare complication of vaginal delivery (0.1% of cases). Other causes include infection, trauma, inflammatory bowel disease, radiation and malignancy.

The success rate of surgical repair in a series of non-inflammatory rectovaginal fistulae was very good. The management of rectovaginal fistula depends on size, location, cause and anal sphincter function. Surgical techniques include an endorectal advancement flap, perineoproctotomy, and a transperineal or vaginal repair. A temporary stoma may be used during the time of the repair.

Anovaginal fistula

Anovaginal fistulae may be congenital or acquired. Most acquired cases are due to obstetric injury. Tears in the perineal body and anal canal during vaginal delivery, including those secondary to episiotomies and forceps use, are often responsible. The fistula may develop immediately after delivery, but more commonly it presents 7 to 10 days later with dissolution of the suture material and infection. Necrosis of the rectovaginal septum from prolonged compression by the fetus is another cause of anovaginal fistula, and is mainly a problem in developing countries.

Surgical procedures involving the perineal body, or operations such as coloanal anastomoses for low rectal cancers, may also cause anovaginal fistula.

Crohn's disease with transmural inflammation leads to anovaginal fistulae in some cases. Fistulae may also arise as a result of perineal infections, in particular abscesses of Bartholin's gland, and more rarely tuberculous abscesses, diverticulitis and endometriosis.

Anal carcinomas, vaginal tumours and haematological malignancies such as leukaemia can cause fistulae, as may radiotherapy for malignant disease.

Finally, violent trauma from a foreign body or forceful sexual intercourse may be responsible for a fistula.

FURTHER READING

Anonymous. 1998: Guidelines for treatment of sexually transmitted diseases. *Morbidity and Mortality Weekly* 47, 1–111.

Bevan CD. 1997: The role of laparoscopy in the diagnosis and management of women with pelvic infection. In O'Brien S (ed.), *The yearbook of obstetrics and gynaecology*, Vol. 5. London: RCOG Press, 93–101.

Goldaber KG, Wendel, PJ, McIntyre DD, Wendel GD Jr. 1993: Postpartum perineal morbidity after fourth-degree perineal repair. *American Journal of Obstetrics and Gynecology* 168, 489–93.

Ison C. 1996: Antimicrobial agents and gonorrhoea: therapeutic choice, resistance and susceptibility. *Genitourinary Medicine* 72, 253–7.

LeBar W. 1996: Keeping up with new technology: new approaches to diagnosis of *Chlamydia* infection. *Clinical Chemistry* 42, 809–12.

Tsand C, Rothenberger D. 1997: Rectovaginal fistula. Therapeutic options. *Surgical Clinics of North America* 77, 95–114.

Venkatesh K, Ramanujam P, Larson D, Haywood, M. 1989: Anorectal complications of vaginal delivery. *Diseases of the Colon and Rectum* 32, 1093–41.

Watson S, Phillips R. 1995: Non-inflammatory rectovaginal fistulae. *British Journal of Surgery* 82, 1641–3.

Overview of clinical approach to lumps

Jonathan W. Serpell

Introduction

A great deal of the practice of surgery is concerned with the patient who has a lump or tumour. A lump is a form of focal lesion with which surgeons are concerned. Much of surgery concerns the management of focal lesions such as tumours, defects (e.g. hernia) and deformities (both congenital and acquired).

The word 'tumour' in its broader sense should be considered equivalent to the word 'lump'. Often, however, 'tumour' is considered to be synonymous with 'neoplasm'. Lumps are best classified on a pathological and aetiological basis. A number of examples are listed in Table 20.1.1. For example, lumps may be traumatic in origin (e.g. fat necrosis), vascular in origin (e.g. an aneurysm), inflammatory (e.g. a phlegmon), or neoplastic (both benign and malignant).

Whenever a patient presents with a lump, such a classification of possible differential diagnoses should be considered. The possibilities are extremely varied, but are dictated to a considerable extent by the anatomical features of the local region involved. In practical terms, therefore, a number of lumps are extremely characteristic, such as sebaceous cysts on the scalp and scrotum, pleomorphic adenoma of the parotid gland in the pre-auricular region, supraclavicular lymph nodes in the supraclavicular fossa, and an olecranon bursa on the elbow.

However, many lumps are common to multiple sites because the structures from which they arise are common to all regions, e.g. boils, lipomas, sebaceous cysts, haematomas and neurofibromas.

CLINICAL APPROACH TO LUMPS

To determine the pathological basis of a lump in a particular region, a problem-orientated history and examination are undertaken. The onset of the lump and its duration are important. A lump that has been present for several years suggests a congenital lesion, whereas a lump which has been present for several months to perhaps several years is likely to be benign, a lump which has been present for weeks to months may be malignant, and a lump which has been present for only days is likely to be inflammatory. A lump which is increasing in size suggests a neoplastic growth. Pain suggests inflammation, but may signify malignancy. Intermittency and fluctuation in size of the lump suggest benign processes such as obstruction and inflammation. A discharge may signify an inflammatory process, but malignant masses if neglected will often ulcerate and discharge. A mass which is reducing in size suggests resolution of an inflammatory process or a cystic lesion, e.g. a cyst in the breast or thyroid gland. Ulceration and bleeding of a lump suggest underlying malignancy. Multiplicity of lumps is not uncommon, and suggests that the lump in question may be an abnormal lymph node, a lipoma, a sebaceous cyst or a neurofibroma.

General questioning is important and should include the patient's occupation, a complete past history, a

Table 20.1.1 Pathological classification of lumps with examples

Pathological category	Examples
Congenital	Hamartoma
	Naevi
	Defect → hernia
	AV malformation of liver
Developmental	Branchial cyst
	Inclusion dermoid
	Thyroglossal cyst
Traumatic	Haematoma
	Seroma
	Fat necrosis
	Oil cyst
	Fracture callus
	Implantation dermoid
	Muscle tear → pseudotumour
Inflammatory	
Acute	Phlegmon – appendiceal
	– cholecystitis
	Abscess – boil, carbuncle
Chronic	Granuloma
Vascular	
Arterial	Aneurysms
	Infarction, e.g.
	1. Omentum
	2. Torsion testis
	3. Volvulus small bowel → mass
Venous	Saphena varix
	Varicocele
Arterial and venous	Arteriovenous fistula, traumatic, iatrogenic, and therapeutic for dialysis
Neoplastic	
Benign	Lipoma
	Neurofibroma
Malignant	Primary, secondary. Carcinoma, melanoma, lymphoma, sarcoma
Hyperplasia	Keratoacanthoma
	Hyperplasia of the breast
Degenerative and reactive	Baker's cyst, olecranon bursa
	Ganglia
	Heberden's nodes
	Foreign body granuloma, e.g. silicone
Metabolic	Gouty tophi
Autoimmune	Rheumatoid nodules
Iatrogenic, drug-induced	Lipodystrophy secondary to insulin
Cysts	Sebaceous cyst
	Infective – hydatid
	Inflammatory – pseudocyst pancreas
Obstruction	Calculus – submandibular duct
	Hydronephrosis
	Mucocele gall bladder
	Pharyngeal pouch

history of medications and also a general enquiry about systemic features of malignancy such as weight loss, anorexia, back pain, dyspnoea and headache.

This should be followed by a detailed problem-orientated examination. In summary, there are four essential elements to such an examination. First, all of the general clinical features of any lump are noted. These are listed in Table 20.1.2. Secondly, any special regional features of the suspected lump and its pathology are noted. For example, the facial nerve must always be tested for a lump in the pre-auricular region. Thirdly, an examination of the regional draining lymph nodes is mandatory for any focal lesion. Finally, a complete general examination is always essential.

The site of the lump is critical, and the region will often dictate possible diagnoses. The depth and plane of the lump in a particular focal site are also important. For example, a mass within a limb may be in the skin, the subcutaneous tissue, the deep fascia, the muscle or the bone. The size of any lesion should be determined in three dimensions, and the shape of the lesion should be described as regular or irregular. The surface and contour of the region may be bosselated (e.g. a pleomorphic adenoma of the parotid) or lobulated with an associated slipping sign (e.g. a lipoma). Consistency can really only reliably be subdivided into soft, firm and hard. Fixation should be determined both superficially and to deeper structures. Distal neurovascular function will be specific to the site of the particular lump in the region under examination.

In many cases a detailed clinical examination of a lump will allow a precise clinical diagnosis which dictates subsequent management.

In the following chapters on lumps in the breast, the head and neck, the limbs (bones, muscles and joints), abdominal lumps and inguinoscrotal lumps, a detailed problem-orientated clinical approach to regional lumps is adopted.

As a general principle it must be emphasized that the clinical impression of any lump is of at least equal importance to any investigational diagnosis of a lump, such as imaging or biopsy. Therefore if there is clinical suspicion about a lump in the breast or the thyroid or a lipoma, that clinical suspicion should outweigh and overrule any apparently benign result obtained from an imaging process or biopsy. Lipomas are a good example of this. They are extremely common, and clearly it would be neither reasonable nor practicable to remove all lipomas from every patient. The indications for removal of lipomas are therefore cases where there is clinical suspicion that the lipoma may be a liposarcoma. This would be indicated, for example, if the tumour is more than 5 cm in diameter, deep to the deep fascia, or increasing in size. Other indications for removal would be cases where a lipoma is painful or causing pressure, or where a malignant cytological or histological core-biopsy specimen has been obtained.

Table 20.1.2 General examination of any lump

Site – region, plane or depth
Size – three dimensions
Shape – regular or irregular
Surface and contour – bosselated or lobulated
Edge
Consistency – soft, firm or hard
Compressibility
Emptying
Cough impulse
Reducibility
Tenderness
Temperature
Fluctuation
Indentable
Transilluminable
Bruit
Thrill
Percussion
Changes in the overlying skin
Fixation – superficial or deep
Distal neurovascular function – specific to region
Regional lymph node examination
General examination

Lumps of bones/joints and nerves

Andrew M. Ellis

Introduction

When considering a problem-solving approach to 'lumps' or discrete swellings in the limb, it is important to recognize the potential tissue of origin from which such a lesion might arise. The application of anatomical knowledge, particularly of surface anatomy, is critical to this end. In this chapter a brief overview will be provided of lesions arising from bone, joint or nerve that might present with swelling. The general principles that characterize a lump, both in history and in physical examination, have already been stated. Specifically excluded from this chapter is a discussion of joint swelling, which is dealt with elsewhere. The management of these conditions will be dealt with by general overview, and only common examples will be highlighted.

LESIONS OF BONE PRESENTING AS A LUMP

The best way to approach any lesion of bone is with a healthy suspicion for potential malignancy, and an understanding of the patterns of the various pathological entities, which are generally well described and recognizable. A helpful approach is to consider lesions of bone as either benign or malignant neoplasms or 'tumour-like' conditions. Malignant lesions of bone may be primary, secondary or locally aggressive. 'Tumour-like' conditions of bone are often associated with metabolic disease or an underlying hamartomatous change. 'Tumour-like' conditions of bone are encountered from time to time, and may mimic more serious pathology. Usually a collaborative approach to diagnosis is required in which the surgeon, radiologist and histopathologist combine to consider the diagnosis. This multidisciplinary approach is critical, and in most states of Australia is managed via state-based Bone Tumour Registries or regular diagnostic meetings at a few centres in each capital city, where such work is concentrated.

HISTORY AND PHYSICAL EXAMINATION

Swelling and tumours of bones should be considered along the general lines which are established for any growth. One critical factor is the *age* of the patient, because most tumorous and tumour-like lesions of bone have particular peaks at various stages of life (see Table 20.2.1). The *duration* of symptoms is also important, together with rapidity of growth to help in initially discriminating benign from malignant lesions. *Swelling* is a common complaint especially in the appendicular skeleton. Within the axial skeleton, pelvic lesions in particular may grow to a large size and bulk before being noticed by the patient (Figure 20.2.1). Always consider *local pressure effects* from tumour, especially on peripheral nerves. Compressive neuropathies from both benign and malignant lesions are not uncommon. Nerves are

Table 20.2.1 Age predilection for skeletal tumours

	1–5 years	6–18 years	18–40 years	>40 years
Tumour-like condition	Osteomyelitis	Osteomyelitis Fibrous dysplasia	Brown tumour (renal osteodystrophy)	
Malignant neoplasm	Metastatic disease Neuroblastoma Leukaemia	Ewing's sarcoma Osteosarcoma	Ewing's sarcoma Osteosarcoma (rare)	Metastatic disease Chondrosarcoma Fibrosarcoma/malignant fibrous histiocytoma

Benign neoplasm	Eosinophilic
	    granuloma
	Unicameral bone
	    cyst (rare)
		Unicameral bone
		    cyst
		Aneurysmal bone
		    cyst
		Non-ossifying fibroma
		Enchondroma
		Chondroblastoma
		Chondromyxoid fibroma
		Osteoblastoma
			Giant-cell tumour	

always vulnerable to compression where they pass through narrow spaces (e.g. the spinal foramen or the carpal tunnel) or around bony prominences (e.g. the head of the fibula). For example, the lumbar sacral plexus may be compressed by pelvic tumour mimicking symptoms of a prolapsed inter-vertebral disc, or the common peroneal nerve at the knee by diaphysial aclasia, leading to foot drop.

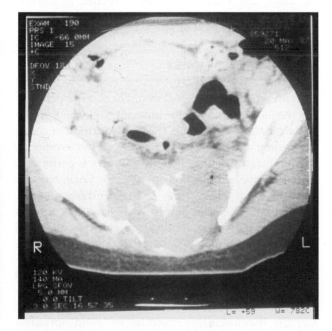

Figure 20.2.1 A large chordoma of sacrum (malignant) with extensive destruction at the time of presentation. This illustrates the size to which pelvic tumours might grow before presentation.

Pain is a variable symptom, and lesions may develop without pain. Pain at rest or night pain are thought to be characteristic of aggressive benign or malignant lesions of bone. Pain may be non-specific and vague initially, although there are several exceptions to this. *Referred* pain is a particular feature of musculoskeletal pathology, especially around joints. This reflects Hilton's law and may lead to pain being experienced at a site distant from the lesion. For example, there are well-documented reports of patients with osteosarcoma of the femur undergoing knee arthroscopy for the investigation of knee pain. Similarly, as mentioned above, pressure effects from compressive neuropathy may lead to radicular pain and signs of nerve root irritation. A pathological *fracture* may develop in association with weakening caused by any lesion in which bone is replaced, removed or destroyed. Such a fracture occurs when normal force is applied to abnormal bone. It is characterized by the usual signs of fracture, including local pain, loss of function, abnormal mobility, and sometimes deformity.

Patients may complain of other symptoms. A history of injury is not uncommon. This probably does not reflect an aetiological process, but rather a time which for the patient first represents symptoms due to tumour mass or microfracture. Gait disturbance and limp, especially in lesions of the lower limb, are not uncommon.

By far the most common tumour encountered in surgical practice is metastatic carcinoma. Usually, but not always, the diagnosis is obvious. Among the primary malignant lesions of bone, myeloma is the most common, followed by osteosarcoma, chondrosarcoma and small-cell sarcoma (e.g. Ewing's sarcoma). Benign tumours of bone occur more frequently than primary malignancy, and their radiological features are usually unique. The most common of these are osteochondroma and non-ossifying fibroma. Less common are osteoid osteoma, enchondroma and giant-cell tumour (which may be locally aggressive, and in which metastases have been described). Figure 20.2.2 shows a giant-cell tumour of the sacrum.

Lesions that are likely to represent primary malignancy include those that are large or deep, as well as bone lesions that are suspected on the basis of their radiographic appearance of being potentially malignant.

APPROACH TO DIAGNOSIS

Biopsy of potentially malignant lesions of bone is not necessarily a simple process. Because of the hardness of bone, closed biopsy may not be possible. Specific risks include causing a pathological fracture, spreading tumour, and contamination of tissue planes and limb compartments. Limb salvage surgery is well advanced, and wherever possible this will be performed rather than amputation. Combination (neoadjuvant and adjuvant) chemotherapy in combination with surgery has significantly improved survival in both osteosarcoma and Ewing's sarcoma. Improved survival and advances in prosthetic implants make such surgery highly specialized. Without appropriate planning and preparation, biopsy may lead to an adverse outcome in terms of prognosis and treatment options for malignant neoplasia in particular.

Prior to biopsy of the lesion, adequate diagnostic tests must have been performed. These include appropriate blood tests (including full biochemical analysis, full blood count, sedimentation rate, prostate-specific antigen, and serum and urine protein electrophoresis) and radiological investigations to characterize the lesion (plain radiographs, CT scans and MRI). The radiological appearance of the lesion is often characteristic. Malignant lesions will often have an ill-defined edge, with permeative or 'moth-eaten' infiltration of adjacent bone. A vigorous periosteal reaction is seen with surface lesions. This so-called Codman's triangle is characteristic of osteosarcoma. Extra-osseous extension and associated soft-tissue mass are typical of malignancy. Benign lesions often have a longstanding host reaction (sclerosis and remodelling), a clearly defined border, and lack the aggressive destruction of a malignancy.

Staging of the suspected tumour must be performed, and the important question of the existence of metastatic disease must be answered. Chest radiographs and a CT scan should be performed to exclude metastatic disease, together with a CT scan of the abdomen if a soft-tissue sarcoma is suspected. Technetium nucleotide bone scanning has a role in determining whether polyosteotic disease is present, but has limited usefulness in characterizing lesions. In multiple myeloma the bone scan may be 'cold', and a skeletal survey is needed to confirm polyosteotic disease.

PRINCIPLES OF BIOPSY

Certain principles are recognized. The surgeon performing the biopsy should be the same surgeon who will ultimately manage the patient. The biopsy incision or needle entry should be placed so as to allow *en bloc* excision of scar and tract when the definitive surgery is performed. Careful consideration of flaps used in reconstruction must be given at this time. If an open biopsy is performed, an incisional biopsy is preferred, as tumour spillage can then be minimized. The biopsy should include the interface of the pseudocapsule. Biopsy should be taken away from the zone of periosteal reaction (Codman's triangle). Care must be taken to avoid the creation of a pathological fracture by careful technique and avoiding the creation of stress risers in bone. Careful haemostasis is essential to avoid spreading tumour together with haematoma. If a drain is used, its exit point should be near the incision, and should be able to be included in the *en bloc* excision at the time of definitive surgery.

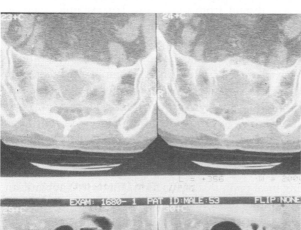
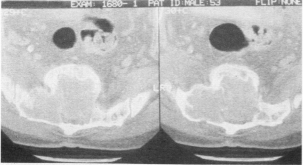

Figure 20.2.2 Giant-cell tumour of sacrum, expanding into the pelvis. Characteristically it is a solitary lytic lesion.

CLASSIFICATION OF SURGICAL PROCEDURES

Surgical removal has been the traditional means of managing skeletal neoplasia, according to site and surgical access. Methods have included curettage, resection and amputation. In recent times limb-sparing procedures have been developed, based on the concept of *limb compartment*, in which fascia or bone acts as a border with regard to local spread. The following surgical procedures based on this concept have been recognized:

1. *intralesional* – an intralesional procedure passes through the pseudocapsule and directly into the lesion. Macroscopic tumour is left, and the entire operative field is potentially contaminated;

2. *marginal* – a marginal procedure is one in which the entire lesion is removed in one piece. The plane of dissection passes through the pseudocapsule or reactive zone around the lesion. When performed for a sarcoma, it leaves macroscopic disease;

3. *wide (intracompartmental)* – this is commonly called *en bloc* resection. A wide excision includes the entire tumour, the reactive zone and a cuff of normal tissue;

4. *radical (extracompartmental)* – the entire tumour and the structure of origin of the lesion are removed. The plane of dissection is beyond the limiting fascial or bony borders.

Malignant tumours require a wide or radical procedure, and benign lesions may be adequately treated by an intralesional or marginal procedure. The local anatomy and the extent of the lesion determine how a margin can be obtained – hence the value of pre-operative staging. It is important to recognize that an amputation may not necessarily provide the wide margin required for a malignant lesion.

BENIGN BONE TUMOURS

Solitary and multiple osteochondromas (diaphyseal aclasis)

Osteochondromas are the most common benign tumour, occurring in any bone formed by enchondral ossification. They may be sessile or pedunculated, and they may be regarded as a form of developmental dysplasia.

When they occur multiply they may represent diaphyseal aclasia (hereditary multiple exostosis), as shown in Figure 20.2.3. Individuals with this disorder are often of short stature, and have skeletal deformity and premature osteoarthritis. Inheritance is autosomal dominant. The risk of malignant transformation is less than 1%, and may be indicated by a thick cartilage cap

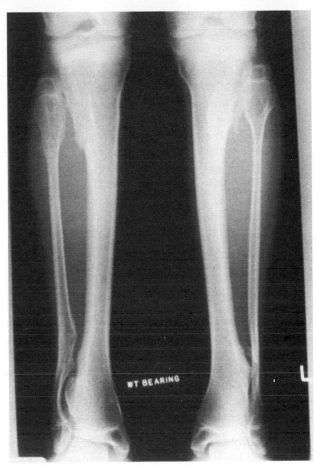

Figure 20.2.3 Diaphyseal aclasis (hereditary multiple osteochondroma). Typical benign-looking radiological appearance. Multiple well-corticated lesions in the metaphysis with trabeculae entering the osteochondroma. Absence of bone destruction.

(> 2 cm), increasing pain or an associated soft-tissue mass.

Unicameral bone cyst

This is typically present in children as a metaphyseal cyst, often in the proximal humerus and femur. If treatment is required, intralesional steroid injection or curettage and bone grafting have been described. The natural history is of involution with growth, and occasionally the presentation is precipitated by pathological fracture.

Giant-cell tumour

This is often a lesion of adulthood, and is characterized by a solitary, lytic lesion of long bone seen in close proximity to the articular surface of joints (e.g. the knee). Giant-cell tumours of the sacrum are problematic and may be locally aggressive. Intralesional curettage, combined with grafting and local adjuvant cryotherapy, is the preferred treatment.

MALIGNANT TUMOURS

Osteosarcoma (OS)

This is typically an aggressive neoplasm of adolescence and young adulthood. There is a second peak of incidence in later life due to secondary osteosarcoma in relation to disease such as Paget's disease or previous radiotherapy. The classic lesion develops in the metaphysis near the knee or proximal humerus, arising from mesenchymal soma (spindle cells) which produce osteoid. The most common sarcoma of bone has a number of subtypes that vary in aggression. High-grade lesions are treated with neoadjuvant chemotherapy, wide resection with limb salvage and adjuvant (postoperative) chemotherapy. The 5-year survival rate is about 50%.

Chondrosarcoma

This malignant tumour arises from the cartilage line and affects a slightly older age group than OS. The tumour is usually slow-growing and often of histological low grade. Surgery is the mainstay of treatment, as chondrosarcoma responds poorly to chemotherapy and radiotherapy.

Ewing's sarcoma

Ewing's sarcoma is a small-cell undifferentiated sarcoma of children and young adults. Extra-osseous (soft-tissue) Ewing's sarcoma is a well-recognized variant. The pelvis and lower limb are most commonly affected. The tumour is potentially curable by a combination of chemotherapy and surgery. Radiotherapy is reserved for inaccessible sites (e.g. pelvis) or incomplete resection.

Malignant fibrous histiocytoma

This occurs in an older age group than OS, and the lesion has its cell of origin in fibrous cells. It has a skeletal distribution similar to that of OS. Radiologically, it has a lytic and destructive appearance without osteoid formation. The 5-year survival rate is poor.

LESIONS OF JOINTS PRESENTING AS A LUMP

GANGLION

The most common swelling around joints is a ganglion, which is a fibrous-walled cyst filled with clear mucinous fluid and usually lacking a recognizable lining. Ganglia occur in the soft tissue, often dissecting between tendon planes. They are commonly seen around the hands, feet and knees (Figure 20.2.4). Ganglia may arise either

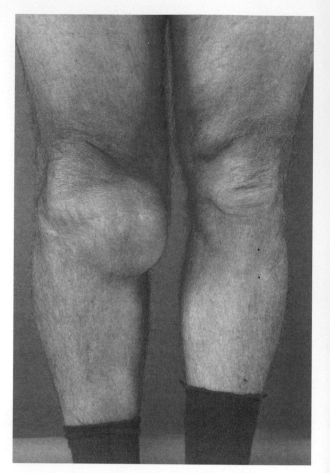

Figure 20.2.4 A large ganglion cyst of the knee.

(rarely) as herniations of the synovium or (more commonly) from cystic degeneration within dense fibrous connective tissue. Only rarely do they communicate with the joint. They may develop into very large lesions, especially around the knee, and they may be symptomatic due to local tissue pressure. Treatment of a ganglion is by simple excision, but recurrence is possible.

Cysts of the knee-joint meniscus are special examples of ganglion cysts. They occur more commonly in the lateral meniscus, and are often seen in association with horizontal cleavage tears. Treatment is by arthroscopic menisectomy with drainage of the cyst into the joint. Occasionally a pseudocyst of the meniscus is seen. Associated with a meniscal tear, the patient will describe a hard lump at the joint line (usually medial) caused by prolapse of the torn meniscus.

Around 50–70% of soft-tissue tumours in the hand and wrist are ganglion tumours. These occur in two anatomical sites in particular. Dorsal carpal ganglion cysts, often from the scapholunate ligament, are the most common type. Volar carpal ganglia are commonly seen at the volar wrist crease between the flexor carpi radialis and abductor pollicus longus, and may relate to the scaphotrapezoid joint capsule. Transillumination should confirm the nature of the ganglion, differentiating it from solid lesions that may occur in close proximity.

BURSAE

Inflammation of synovial-lined soft-tissue bursae can lead to marked swelling around joints. Soft-tissue bursae typically occur in close proximity to joints to allow the wide range of soft-tissue excursion required, especially at the knee, elbow and hip. Inflammation and enlargement of such bursae can occur through over-use (e.g. pre-patellar bursitis, caused by kneeling), or in association with crystal deposition or inflammatory arthritis (e.g. gout and olecranon bursitis) or infection. Synovial cysts are distended bursae. The popliteal cyst (Baker's cyst) may dissect into the gastrocnemius muscle of the posterior calf compartment. Painful rupture with swelling can occur, mimicking the symptoms of an acute deep venous thrombosis.

The diagnosis of bursitis will usually be obvious from the history and careful physical examination. Ultrasound examination has an important role in separating cystic from solid lesions, especially in the diagnosis of a Baker's cyst.

Primary malignant tumours of bone are rare. However, when they do occur they often arise from the metaphysis near joints. For example, osteosarcoma more commonly arises from the distal femur and proximal tibia or humerus. In these cases presentation may occur as a lump or swelling near the joint, and due consideration must be given to possible malignant potential.

LESIONS OF NERVES PRESENTING AS A LUMP

NEUROFIBROMA

Neurofibromas are benign tumours of mixed origin (neural and fibrous tissue). When they are multiple, familial and congenital they may represent neurofibromatosis (or Von Recklinghausen's disease). Neurofibromatosis type 1 (NF1) is the common form, occurring in 1 in 3000 individuals. The diagnosis is based on the presence of two or more of the following:

1. six or more *café-au lait* macules, the greatest diameter of which is more than 5 mm in prepubertal patients and more than 15 mm in post-pubertal patients;

2. two or more neurofibromas of any type, or one plexiform neurofibroma;

3. freckling in the axillary or groin region;

4. two or more Lisch nodules (dome-shaped elevations on the surface of the iris, seen with a split lamp);

5. a distinctive osseous lesion such as sphenoid dysplasia or pseudoarthrosis;

6. a first-degree relative with NF1 according to the preceding criteria.

The importance of this disorder is that it is multi-system and inherited in an autosomal-dominant pattern with a 50% risk of transmission to offspring. The gene is on chromosome 17 (17g11.2). About 50% of cases are sporadic and due to new mutations, and about 50% of people with the disorder will be only mildly affected and may not know that they have it. Management is best conducted through multidisciplinary clinics with screening of first-degree relatives and appropriate genetic counselling of affected individuals.

NEUROFIBROSARCOMA (MALIGNANT SCHWANNOMA)

Malignant tumours arising from peripheral nerves are exceedingly rare, representing about 10% of all sarcomas. A large percentage of neurofibrosarcomas (NFSs) arise in association with NF1, but the lifetime risk for such a patient developing malignancy is 5% higher than the risk for the general population.

A limb mass associated with neurological symptoms must be considered potentially malignant. The approach to management is similar to that for other suspected soft-tissue sarcomas of the limb, with appropriate staging performed before biopsy and definitive treatment. Wide (compartmental) excision and neoadjuvant chemotherapy is the treatment of choice.

FURTHER READING

Kasser JR (ed.) 1995: *Orthopaedic knowledge update 5.* Rosemont IL: American Academy of Orthopaedic Surgery.

Simon MA, Biermann JS. 1993: Biopsy of bone and soft-tissue lesions. *Journal of Bone and Joint Surgery* **75**, 616–21.

Simon MA, Finn HA. 1993: Diagnostic strategy for bone and soft-tissue lesions. *Journal of Bone and Joint Surgery* **75**, 622–31.

Head and neck lumps

Jonathan W. Serpell

Introduction

This chapter aims to provide the clinician with a problem-orientated clinical approach to establishing the diagnosis of a patient who presents with a lump in the head or neck. Because head and neck lumps are heterogeneous, the first point to establish is the region in which the lump is located, and then a problem-orientated regional approach to the suspected lump can be implemented. The regions are dictated anatomically, and lumps in the pre-auricular region, the thyroid or the supraclavicular fossa will have different problem-orientated algorithms to establish diagnosis.

Head and neck lumps are diverse and numerous. However, there are four groups of common lumps:

1. thyroid swellings (goitre);

2. salivary gland swellings;

3. lymph node swellings;

4. skin and subcutaneous lesions, which are cornmon but not specific to the head and neck, and are usually superficial to the deep cervical fascia.

Each of these four groups is subclassified, and the first three groups will be considered in more detail. The less common lumps (Box 20.3.1) are in general developmental cysts and will be considered briefly. Specifically excluded from this discussion of head and neck lumps are carcinoma of the lip, tongue and floor of the mouth, and many of the conditions of oral medicine, such as mouth ulcers and gum swellings.

CLASSIFICATION OF HEAD AND NECK LUMPS

As well as classification by frequency of occurrence, head and neck lumps may be classified by region, and naturally fall into midline lumps (Figure 20.3.1) and lateral lumps (Figure 20.3.2). In general, midline lumps arise from unpaired structures, whereas lateral lumps arise from paired structures.

Once the region of the patient's swelling has been established, a much more defined problem-orientated approach can then be used.

GENERAL PROBLEM-ORIENTATED HISTORY

A number of points are applicable to all lumps in the head and neck. First, age will give an indication of aetiology. Congenital lesions are more common in patients under 25 years of age, and neoplastic lesions are more common in those aged over 45 years.

How the lump was noted, who noted it, the history of the lump and its duration are all important factors. A lump which has been present for many years and is unchanging is unlikely to be malignant, whereas a lump which has been present for weeks to months and is rapidly enlarging is suggestive of malignancy. A lump

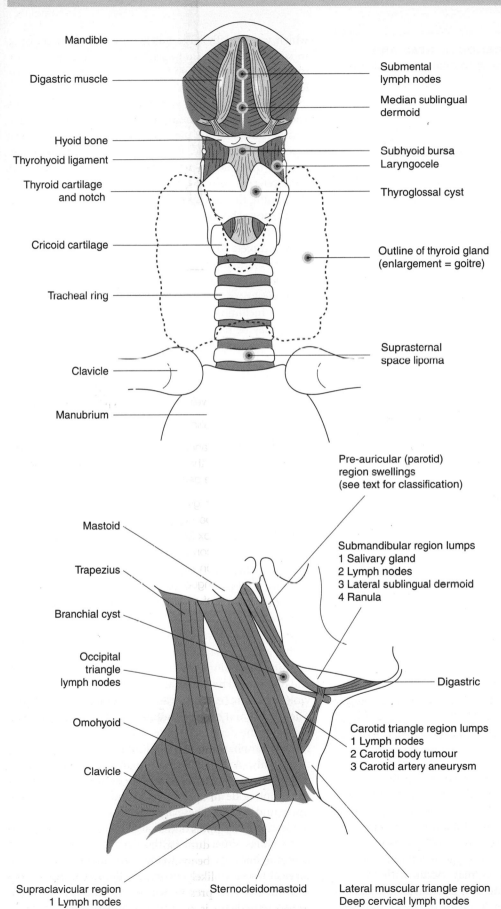

Mandible

Digastric muscle

Hyoid bone

Thyrohyoid ligament

Thyroid cartilage
and notch

Cricoid cartilage

Tracheal ring

Clavicle

Manubrium

Submental
lymph nodes

Median sublingual
dermoid

Subhyoid bursa
Laryngocele

Thyroglossal cyst

Outline of thyroid gland
(enlargement = goitre)

Suprasternal
space lipoma

Figure 20.3.1 Midline
neck lumps. Schematic
diagram after removal of
the strap muscles.

Pre-auricular (parotid)
region swellings
(see text for classification)

Mastoid

Trapezius

Branchial cyst

Occipital
triangle
lymph nodes

Omohyoid

Clavicle

Submandibular region lumps
1 Salivary gland
2 Lymph nodes
3 Lateral sublingual dermoid
4 Ranula

Digastric

Carotid triangle region lumps
1 Lymph nodes
2 Carotid body tumour
3 Carotid artery aneurysm

Supraclavicular region
1 Lymph nodes
2 Cervical rib

Sternocleidomastoid

Lateral muscular triangle region
Deep cervical lymph nodes

Figure 20.3.2 Lateral
neck lumps.

<table>
<tr><td>

BOX 20.3.1 CLASSIFICATION OF HEAD AND NECK LUMPS BY FREQUENCY OF OCCURRENCE

Common head and neck lumps

1. Thyroid swellings (goitre)
2. Salivary gland swellings
3. Lymph node swellings
4. Skin and subcutaneous lesions
   - BCC
   - SCC
   - Benign naevi
   - Keratotic horns
   - Melanoma
   - Lipoma
   - Sebaceous cyst
   - Boils
   - Carbuncles
   - Neurofibroma
   - Fibroma
   - Papilloma
   - Pilomatricoma
   - Dermatofibroma

Less common head and neck lumps

1. Thyroglossal cyst
2. Branchial cyst
3. Ranula
4. Cystic hygroma (cavernous lymphangioma)

Rare head and neck lumps

1. Pharyngeal pouch
2. Dermoids – sublingual (median and lateral)
3. Carotid body tumour (chemodectoma)
4. Soft-tissue sarcomas
5. Aneurysms and arteriovenous fistulae
6. Ludwig's angina
7. Laryngoceles
8. Parathyroid carcinoma
9. Subhyoid bursa
10. Ectopic thyroid
11. Cervical rib
12. Clavicular tumours
13. Sternomastoid tumour/torticollis
14. Pre-auricular sinus
15. Deep cervical and spinal abscesses

</td></tr>
</table>

which has appeared suddenly and is painful suggests haemorrhage or cystic formation, and may occur in the thyroid and parotid regions. Alternatively, a rapid onset of a painful mass may signify inflammation. The progression of the lump over time may indicate its nature. A lump which fluctuates in size suggests inflammation or intermittent obstruction, as may occur with salivary gland duct obstruction due to a calculus or inflammation of a salivary gland. A lump in the head and neck which was initially large but is progressively decreasing in size suggests a lesion such as cystic degeneration or inflammation which is in the process of resolution. Such lesions are not uncommon.

Pain is an important symptom, and in general benign and inflammatory conditions are painful whereas neoplastic conditions are painless. However, there are many exceptions to this rule, and a rapidly enlarging thyroid or parotid malignancy may be painful. In the head and neck, referred pain to the ear from lesions in the floor of the mouth, the tongue and the thyroid is important, and such lesions should be specifically looked for in patients with ear pain.

A complete history must be taken and, in particular, enquiry made about symptoms of generalized metastatic malignancy such as loss of appetite, loss of weight, bone pain, weakness, dyspnoea and chest pain. The previous history, including surgery and a full history of medications, may be relevant. Social circumstances and family support are important for any patient diagnosed with cancer, but may also be a significant factor in determining a treatment policy for head and neck cancer where major ablative resections may be required.

GENERAL EXAMINATION OF THE HEAD AND NECK

For all patients with a head and neck lump a general systematic and thorough examination based on all anatomical regions is essential. There are specific features for regional examination of thyroid, salivary and lymph node swellings which will be described separately under those sections. The patient must be adequately exposed, and free of clothing to the waist. Adequate illumination and equipment to examine all orifices, including a tongue depressor and gloves, must be available. A headlight is useful, as are a magnifying glass and a dermatoscope to examine skin lesions. The state of the patient's skin, scalp and hair should be noted, and evidence of excessive ultraviolet exposure (e.g. solar elastoses and keratoses) sought. The state of oral hygiene should always be assessed, and a record of the dentition made. All cavities, especially the mouth, oropharynx, nose and ears, must be examined thoroughly. A full examination of each cranial nerve should be undertaken. A complete examination of all of the lymph node areas in the head and neck must be routinely undertaken. These are described in more detail in the section on lymph node enlargement.

Swellings superficial to the deep cervical fascia are common but not specific to the head and neck. The deep cervical fascia splits to encompass the sternocleidomastoid muscle. Therefore by tensing the muscle, the fascia is also tensed, thus enabling a distinction to be made between a lump which is superficial and one which is deep to the fascia. A superficial lump will be more prominent and a deep lump less prominent when the fascia is tensed.

Recognition of normal structures which may be confused with abnormal head and neck lumps is essential. It must be appreciated that lymph nodes are normal structures in the head and neck, and that up to 200 of these are normally present. Normal nodes are palpated as soft, small, indistinct subcutaneous nodules. In children in particular, lymph nodes may be slightly enlarged, and any lymph node may be up to 1 cm in diameter and still be within normal limits. The jugulo-digastric or tonsillar lymph node is often palpable in normal patients. Firm nodes that are more than 1 cm in diameter are almost always abnormal. However, nodes of < 1 cm in diameter can on occasion still be pathological. The carotid artery may be tortuous in the elderly and mistaken for a lymph node. The lateral mass of the atlas, the transverse process of the C6 vertebra and the greater cornu of the hyoid bone may be mistaken for abnormal lymph nodes. In the elderly, increasing flexion deformity of the neck is common, and results in ptosis of the submandibular gland and the thyroid gland. Ptotic submandibular glands are often mistaken for abnormal neck lumps. The normal mobility of the larynx on the underlying pharynx, which usually produces a palpable clicking sensation, should be assessed. A problem-orientated examination is then undertaken for each region, and the lesion must be described accurately both in writing and also in detailed diagrams in several views. Clearly, therefore, a detailed knowledge of the anatomy of the head and neck is essential. A full general examination of the patient is always important both to look for systemic signs of disease and to assess the general medical condition.

INVESTIGATION OF A HEAD AND NECK LUMP

Triple assessment of any lump in the head and neck should be undertaken, and this involves clinical examination including endoscopy, imaging and biopsy, usually with fine-needle aspiration cytology.

Flexible panendoscopy may be performed as an outpatient procedure, and is useful for defining a tumour, excluding a second tumour and obtaining a biopsy.

The most appropriate imaging for a head and neck lump will depend on its likely suspected nature, but may include ultrasound, CT scanning, sialography, nuclear medicine scanning and magnetic resonance imaging. Magnetic resonance imaging is increasingly being used to assess the extent of squamous-cell carcinoma of the head and neck, particularly in the larynx, and to assess the involvement of cranial nerves by infiltration of tumour at the base of the skull and the carotid sheath. A chest X-ray is essential for patients with head and neck lesions, as associated primary and secondary diseases are common.

Fine-needle aspiration cytology is of great value in the head and neck because of the multiple accessible organs and the heterogeneous pathology encountered. It has an accuracy of at least 90%, but it is important to appreciate that it provides a cytological rather than a histological diagnosis. Thus while it can diagnose lymphoma, it is unable to diagnose subtypes of lymphoma. None the less, it will usually establish the tissue of the organ of origin, and also in many cases the tumour type. It has a 2% false-negative rate, and therefore any suspicious lump should still be explored or otherwise investigated, even if the cytology is negative. As with breast lesions, ultrasound-guided fine-needle aspiration cytology is often useful for small lesions in the thyroid, but most lumps in the head and neck are readily accessible to aspiration using a free-hand technique. The technique used is exactly the same as for breast lumps. There are no reports of seeding with fine-needle aspiration cytology of the track with head and neck tumours, including parotid tumours. Fine-needle aspiration cytology will usually enable a pre-operative diagnosis and facilitate one-stage surgery for patients. Importantly, cytology will usually avoid the need for an open biopsy for conditions such as a lymph node deposit of squamous-cell carcinoma in the neck, which is contraindicated.

THYROID SWELLINGS

THYROID PRACTICAL ANATOMY

The thyroid gland is bilobed in the shape of a shield, and is located in the midline visceral compartment of the neck, invested by pretracheal fascia. The upper pole is related to the inferior constrictor and cricopharyngeus, and the lower areas of the lobe are related to the trachea and oesophagus. The two lobes are joined by an isthmus, usually crossing the second to fourth tracheal rings. The pyramidal lobe is a variable tongue of thyroid tissue derived from the thyroglossal duct remnant. The thyroid is covered by two layers of strap muscles anteriorly (the sternothyroid and sternohyoid), each with its own layer of fascia, the more superficial of which is the investing layer of deep cervical fascia. These two layers cover the pretracheal fascia. Thus during thyroidectomy, after elevation of the subplatysmal flaps, three layers of fascia are divided longitudinally to separate the strap muscles before the thyroid gland itself is reached.

The superior thyroid artery runs in close proximity to the external branch of the superior laryngeal nerve (the external laryngeal nerve). At thyroidectomy, this structure is at risk during mass ligation of the superior pedicle, and therefore the branches of the superior thyroid artery should be individually ligated at the level of the thyroid gland capsule after identification of the external laryngeal nerve. Damage to this nerve may not be recognized by either the clinician or the patient. However, it will be apparent to patients who sing.

The inferior thyroid artery supplies both parathyroid glands before passing across the recurrent laryngeal nerve (more usually anteriorly, especially on the left side) to divide into tertiary branches within the capsule of the thyroid gland.

The recurrent laryngeal nerve is at risk during thyroidectomy, particularly in its upper portion in the 1–2 cm prior to entry into the larynx. In this region it is closely applied to the posterolateral margin of the thyroid, invested by Berry's ligament, and at this level has often divided into anterior and posterior branches. Berry's ligament is a condensation of pretracheal fascia, and attaches the upper deep surface of the thyroid gland to the cricoid and upper trachea. As well as its surgical importance in preservation of the recurrent laryngeal nerve, it is responsible for elevation of the thyroid gland with the larynx when swallowing. The recurrent laryngeal nerve has a variable relationship to the inferior thyroid artery, and anatomically there is more variation on the right side than the left. Non-recurrent laryngeal nerves also occur on the right side in 0.5% of cases.

DEFINITION OF A GOITRE

The term 'goitre' derives from the Latin word '*guttur*' meaning 'throat'. A goitre is best regarded as a non-specific enlargement of the thyroid gland due to any aetiology.

PROBLEM-ORIENTATED HISTORY FOR PATIENTS WITH SUSPECTED THYROID PATHOLOGY

Age is important, and the risk of malignancy increases with age, but is also increasingly common in children with solitary nodules.

A history of irradiation to the neck should be enquired for. It is well established that patients with irradiation to the neck are at increased risk of thyroid malignancy. Irradiation was previously used to treat acne, tonsillitis, thymic enlargement and facial hair.

A family history of thyroid disease should be enquired for and, in particular, note taken of the possibility of multiple endocrine neoplasia type II (Sipple's

syndrome). This is divided into two subgroups: multiple endocrine neoplasia (MEN) type IIA (hyperparathyroidism, medullary carcinoma of the thyroid and phaeochromocytoma) and MEN type IIB (medullary carcinoma thyroid, mucosal neuromas and phaeochromocytoma).

Enquiry should be made for geographical origin, as endemic goitres were previously more common in iodine-deficient areas such as South Wales in the UK, areas of Gippsland in Victoria, and Tasmania in Australia.

A history of the goitre itself, indicating how it was found, whether it is painful, how long it has been present and whether it is fluctuating or increasing in size rapidly, is important. In the thyroid, rapid growth may signify malignancy, but equally a malignant nodule can grow slowly over a number of years before a diagnosis is made.

Specific enquiry should be made for pressure symptoms in the neck. Symptoms include dysphagia, cough, sore throat, hoarseness, breathlessness and a general feeling of pressure and fullness in the neck. Difficulty in breathing and, in particular, noisy breathing on tilting the head to one side, or while sleeping when lying on one or the other side, is not uncommon when large multinodular goitres cause pressure effects. Pain in the goitre should be noted and may signify malignant change, haemorrhage into a degenerating nodule causing distension or subacute thyroiditis.

A previous history of thyroid disease and surgery should be noted, and a specific enquiry made about associated autoimmune diseases. A full record of medications is essential.

A problem-orientated history to establish over-active thyroid function includes enquiry about increased appetite, weight loss, palpitations, altered bowel habit, temperature sensitivity, tremor, nervousness, muscle weakness, tiredness, low efficiency, anxiety, irritability and excessive sweating. A menstrual history should be taken, as thyrotoxicosis tends to be associated with oligomenorrhoea. An ophthalmic history should be taken, and note made of any deterioration in vision, pain, a sensation of grittiness and diplopia. Specific symptoms of hypothyroidism include intolerance of cold, constipation, tiredness, poor appetite, weight gain, forgetfulness, dryness of the skin and hair, a general slowing down mentally and physically, menorrhagia, symptoms of carpal tunnel syndrome and symptoms of anaemia.

PROBLEM-ORIENTATED EXAMINATION FOR PATIENTS WITH SUSPECTED THYROID DISEASE

The patient must be examined while adequately exposed, free of clothing to the waist and free of necklaces. Detailed inspection and palpation should be undertaken in the sitting position, both from in front and from behind. Previous thyroidectomy scars should be noted. The first question to be addressed is whether the swelling is in the thyroid. Movement of the swelling upwards with swallowing indicates that it is enveloped by the pretracheal fascia and that it is therefore related to the thyroid gland. The next question to be answered is whether the swelling represents a diffuse enlargement affecting both lobes of the thyroid gland, or whether it appears to be a solitary nodule within an otherwise normal thyroid gland. The next point to investigate is if it appears to involve the whole of the thyroid gland, whether it is a diffuse process, or whether the process consists of multiple nodules such as may occur in a multinodular goitre or in the nodular variant of Hashimoto's thyroiditis.

The cervical trachea should be palpated. On occasion it is not palpable because it is totally hidden by a large goitre. Its position and deviation should be noted. The outline of the goitre should be assessed both from in front and from behind the patient for both lobes. The extent of the goitre superiorly, laterally and inferiorly is noted. In assessing this, it is important to note at the same time any degree of fixed flexion deformity of the neck, which is increasingly common with age. Retrosternal extension can be assessed by asking the patient to swallow, and attempting to define the lower limit of the gland. If it is not possible to get below the gland, then retrosternal extension exists. Secondary confirmation can sometimes be obtained by percussion over the upper chest, but this is a less reliable sign. Occasionally patients will have goitres which are reversely plunging in the sense that they only appear on swallowing, and are almost totally retrosternal. Note should be made of any obvious stridor at rest, and Pemberton's sign should be performed, whereby both arms (fully extended) are placed vertically into the air, thereby narrowing the thoracic inlet and potentially increasing the pressure within it if a retrosternal goitre is present. This sign highlights the presence of pressure and obstructive symptoms. In particular, the sign detects distension of neck veins occurring with this manoeuvre (superior vena caval obstruction). Pressure on a narrowed trachea may elicit stridor. Nerves in association with the thyroid should be assessed, and recurrent laryngeal nerve function can be assessed by the ability to phonate the letter 'e', the ability to cough, and an assessment of palatal movement, as well as indirect laryngoscopic assessment of vocal cord function. All patients who may later undergo thyroidectomy should undergo pre-operative laryngoscopic assessment of vocal cord function. A detailed examination of regional lymphadenopathy should be undertaken.

If there is a solitary nodule in the thyroid, all the usual features of a lump should be assessed, including its site, size, shape, surface, edge, consistency, fluctuance and tenderness. A firm to hard lump raises the suspicion of carcinoma, but equally a cyst under tension may be very hard on palpation. A diffuse goitre is assessed for a thrill and a bruit, which suggest Graves' disease. The overall consistency of a diffuse goitre should be assessed, i.e. whether it is soft, firm or hard, and whether it is diffuse or nodular. A detailed general examination must be undertaken to look for clinical features of hyperthyroidism and hypothyroidism. In addition to the symptoms already listed above, signs of thyrotoxicosis include tachycardia, cardiac arrhythmias, cardiac failure, sweating, tremor, hyperkinetic movements, myopathy, pretibial myxoedema, thyroid acropathy, vitiligo, alopecia and ophthalmic signs. The ophthalmic signs may include lid retraction, lid lag, exophthalmos, conjunctival injection and oedema (chemosis), ophthalmoplegia, keratitis and corneal ulceration, papilloedema and decreased visual acuity. The assessment is completed by a full general examination.

INVESTIGATION OF THYROID DISEASE

Pathophysiology of investigations

A basic understanding of thyroid physiology allows interpretation of investigations. Thyroid hormones (thyroxine, T_4 and tri-iodothyronine, T_3) are synthesized in three stages in the thyroid follicle, namely iodine trapping, iodine organification by combination with tyrosine to form iodotyrosine, and coupling of iodotyrosine to form active T_4 and T_3. The hormones are released in two further stages, namely hydrolysis of thyroglobulin and passage of iodotyrosine into the circulation. Both T_4 and T_3 are transported in the blood bound mainly to thyroid-binding globulin (TBG). Only a small proportion of each of T_4 and T_3 is free in the circulation. Currently free (non-protein-bound) T_4 and T_3 are measured. Previously a correction for increases in protein-binding capacity (but with normal free T_4 and T_3 levels), as in pregnancy (which increases serum-bound levels), was made using T_3 resin uptake (T3RU) to assess the free tyroxine index (FTI).

T_3 is responsible for the principal metabolic effects of thyroid hormone. About 80% of T_3 is produced peripherally by conversion from T_4. T_3 is the more active physiological hormone, and its measurement is particularly important in T_3 toxicosis, where there is a clinical picture of thyrotoxicosis but normal serum T_4 levels.

Thyroid function is controlled by thyroid-stimulating hormone (TSH), which is secreted by the anterior pituitary. TSH secretion is controlled by both the hypothalamus (via thyroid-releasing hormone) and a negative feedback of peripheral free T_4 levels. Thyroid-stimulating hormone is a sensitive assay and is routinely measured. TSH is elevated in hypothyroidism and suppressed in thyrotoxicosis, except for some cases of mild disturbance in multinodular goitre-associated T_3 toxicosis.

Thyroid antibodies are measured by radioimmunoassay. Microsomal antibodies are the most sensitive type. Antibodies to thyroid microsomes are elevated in Graves' disease and Hashimoto's disease, and thyroglobulin antibodies are elevated in both of these diseases. Thyroglobulin is a normal constituent of colloid in the thyroid, and can therefore be used to detect residual or recurrent tumour in those patients with differentiated thyroid carcinoma who have been treated by a total thyroidectomy.

Serum calcitonin levels will be elevated in individuals with medullary carcinoma of the thyroid.

Erythrocyte sedimentation rate (ESR) is elevated in subacute thyroiditis.

Thyroid imaging

Thyroid isotope scanning with the radio-isotopes ^{123}I, ^{131}I or technetium 99^M allows classification of thyroid nodules into those which are cold (non-functioning), those which are warm (normally functioning) or those which are hot (hyper-functioning). Of all cold nodules, 20% will be malignant, and although the vast majority of hot nodules are benign, thyroid isotope scanning cannot distinguish thyroid malignancy from benign nodules. Ultrasound examination may identify nodules as small as 0.3 mm in diameter, and can distinguish solid from cystic nodules. However, ultrasound cannot distinguish between benign and malignant nodules. Cysts which are more than 4 cm in diameter may have a malignancy rate of up to 20%. Ultrasound examination is useful for guiding precise needle biopsy.

CT scanning is an increasingly useful investigation for assessing large multinodular goitres, and also for assessing the extent of malignancy, and in particular it can assess the extent of retrosternal extension and pressure and distortion of structures in the neck. CT scanning should be undertaken without intravenous contrast, as the iodine-containing contrast can precipitate thyrotoxicosis, which can subsequently be difficult to treat.

All patients with thyroid disease should have a chest X-ray to assess the thoracic inlet, and to look for evidence of metastatic disease.

Biopsy

Needle core biopsy will provide histological data and has a high diagnostic accuracy rate. It is particularly useful for very large goitres which have grown rapidly, to distinguish lymphoma from anaplastic carcinoma, and to subclassify the lymphoma. It is much less useful for smaller goitres, and should not be used for solitary nodules, as it is difficult to obtain a core safely. The risks are those of haematoma, tracheal puncture and recurrent laryngeal nerve damage.

Fine-needle aspiration cytology is highly accurate and cost-effective, with low morbidity and excellent patient compliance. In the thyroid it will accurately diagnose colloid nodules, thyroiditis, papillary carcinoma and medullary carcinoma. It may diagnose anaplastic carcinoma and lymphoma, but its major limitation is its inability to distinguish benign follicular adenomas from follicular carcinomas. This distinction can only be made histologically by the demonstration of capsular and/or vascular invasion after resection of the nodule.

Fine-needle aspiration cytology of a thyroid nodule will give one of four possible results:

1. a malignant result;

2. an entirely benign result, which should show benign follicular cells with a substantial amount of colloid, and often macrophages and blood, with no suspicious features;

3. an indeterminate or suspicious result is usually associated with a follicular neoplasm, where it is not possible to distinguish a benign cytological aspirate from a malignant one;

4. the aspirate may be inadequate or non-diagnostic.

The accuracy of fine-needle aspiration cytology may be increased by performing it under ultrasound control, and this is especially applicable to nodules which are difficult to feel clinically, and also cysts which have an associated solid component where it is desirable to sample the solid area.

In several large series, no false-positive results in thyroid cytology have been found, with false-negative rates of 0.7–2.2%. A non-diagnostic specimen will be obtained in about 15% of cases, and should not be regarded as a benign diagnosis, but rather as an indication to repeat the cytology in order to obtain a definitive diagnosis. Increasingly, patients are presenting with ultrasound-identified thyroid nodules, and naturally, because most of these are not clinically palpable, they require sampling under ultrasound guidance.

CLINICAL CLASSIFICATION OF GOITRES

Goitres are most usefully classified on the basis of clinical findings. In many instances a firm diagnosis will be established before any investigations are undertaken. The first distinction to be made is whether the whole of the gland is enlarged, or whether there is a solitary nodule within an otherwise apparently normal gland.

Enlargement of the whole thyroid gland (diffuse goitre)

Simple non-toxic goitre

Physiological goitre A smooth, diffuse, hyperplastic goitre is physiologically normal during puberty and pregnancy, and is often described as parenchymatous or colloid in nature. It is largely due to hormone changes affecting iodine uptake by the gland. Thyroxine suppression may reduce the size of the goitre. Very rarely, surgical intervention is necessary for cosmesis or pressure symptoms.

Multinodular goitre Multinodular goitre is common, and occurs in both endemic forms in iodine-deficient areas, and in sporadic forms. Like all thyroid conditions, it is more common in females. It may affect up to 5% of the population, but most of these patients are asymptomatic. Whatever the aetiological cause, the thyroid reacts in a similar manner. Inadequate thyroid hormone production causes an increased TSH level, resulting in hyperplasia and multiplication of thyroid follicles. The end result is a diffuse hyperplastic goitre. Areas of the gland may then regress in an irregular fashion, with some areas remaining hyperplastic and others becoming filled with colloid. Colloid follicles may coalesce and degenerate, forming large colloid nodules or cysts. Areas of haemorrhage into cysts, fibrosis and calcification occur, resulting in a goitre consisting of multiple nodules of varying size. The whole gland is affected by these multiple nodules, which may be macroscopic or microscopic. However, the extent of disease in the two lobes may be asymmetrical.

Indications for surgery include the following:

1. cosmesis;

2. local pressure symptoms;

3. large size that is increasing;

4. retrosternal extension because of risk of progressive airway obstruction and inaccessiblity to fine-needle aspiration cytology (FNAC);

5. a dominant nodule which is clinically or cytologically suspicious;

6. thyrotoxicosis (if there are associated pressure symptoms or retrosternal extension; or if radio-iodine is contraindicated).

Thyrotoxic goitre

Diffuse thyrotoxic goitre A diffuse hyperplastic goitre is characteristic of Graves' disease and causes 75% of cases of thyrotoxicosis. The female:male ratio is 8:1, and typically there is a moderately enlarged goitre which is soft, vascular and with an associated thrill and bruit. The clinical features of thyrotoxicosis are present. The treatment of thyrotoxicosis may require a multidisciplinary approach, with antithyroid drugs, radio-iodine (^{131}I) and surgery being the available treatment modalities.

Multinodular goitres Multinodular goitre which has become thyrotoxic (Plummers' disease) (25% of cases of thyrotoxicosis) occurs in an older age group, and is often associated with cardiac complications (arrhythmias and cardiac failure). Ophthalmic signs are unusual or absent.

The radio-iodine scan will determine the site(s) of over-activity, and will also exclude factitious thyrotoxicosis. Treatment is with radio-iodine or thyroidectomy.

A solitary toxic adenoma is a rare cause of thyrotoxicosis (1%), and is usually not palpable. It is diagnosed by thyroid scan, and may be treated by surgical excision or radio-iodine therapy.

Special goitres

Rapidly enlarging goitre There are three differential diagnoses of a rapidly enlarging goitre:

1. *sub-acute thyroiditis* – also known as De Quervain's thyroiditis, granulomatous thyroiditis, giant-cell thyroiditis and viral thyroiditis. This is a rare inflammatory condition of the thyroid often following an influenza-like illness. Thyroid antibodies are elevated and the main clinical feature is a painful, tender goitre. Fine-needle aspiration cytology shows thyroid cells, macrophages and multinodular giant cells. ESR and T_4 are elevated, and radio-iodine scanning shows a reduced uptake. The condition is self-limiting, but if necessary it will respond rapidly to oral prednisolone;

2. *anaplastic carcinoma*;

3. *lymphoma* – fine-needle aspiration cytology may distinguish lymphoma from anaplastic carcinoma, but often histological diagnosis (usually by a core biopsy) is required.

Hashimoto's thyroiditis Hashimoto's thyroiditis is more common in females, and is diagnosed by a combination of cytology and elevated antibodies. Stimulated follicular cells (Hürthle or Askanazy cells) are mixed with lymphocytes and plasma cells on cytology. Hashimoto's goitre is a diffusely enlarged firm goitre which is only occasionally nodular, and is therefore a differential diagnosis of multinodular goitre. Hypothyroidism is the usual sequel in established disease. There is an increased risk of subsequent development of lymphoma. The usual treatment is with thyroxine, but rarely – if the goitre is large and resulting in pressure symptoms – thyroidectomy is required.

Riedel's thyroiditis This condition is very rare. The thyroid gland is replaced by dense fibrous tissue which results in a firm, diffuse, painless swelling which may lead to tracheal compression.

A solitary nodule within an otherwise normal thyroid gland

This may be any of the following:

1. a dominant nodule in a multinodular goitre;

2. a degenerative cyst occurring in an adenoma or hyperplastic colloid nodule;

3. follicular adenoma;

4. thyroid carcinoma:
   - papillary;
   - follicular;
   - medullary;

5. secondary metastases, especially carcinoma of the breast, kidney and lung;

6. Hashimoto's thyroiditis with nodule formation.

The prevalence of thyroid nodules at autopsy is approximately 50%, but many of these will be less than 1 cm in diameter. Although the vast majority of thyroid nodules are benign, the clinical problem of distinguishing benign from malignant disease remains. Of all of the apparently solitary thyroid nodules, 50% will represent a dominant nodule of a multinodular goitre. A true solitary nodule which is cold has a 10–20% chance of malignancy. As already indicated, ultrasound examination and nuclear medicine scanning, whilst giving an indication of the likelihood of malignancy, cannot exclude malignancy for an individual thyroid nodule.

For a degenerative thyroid cyst, fine-needle aspiration for cytology may be both diagnostic and therapeutic. A cyst should be aspirated so that there is no residual mass, and provided that it is not bloodstained and the cytology is negative, the process can be repeated three times. However, cysts which recur more than three times should be excised. Indications for removal of a thyroid cyst are refilling after three aspirations, frank blood, positive cytology, a cyst larger than 4 cm in diameter, and previous irradiation of the neck.

Cytology cannot distinguish between benign and malignant follicular neoplasms, and therefore when cytology suggests a follicular neoplasm, surgery is always indicated.

It is likely that a dominant nodule in a multinodular goitre may have a malignancy rate similar to that of a true solitary nodule.

Clinical examination of a thyroid nodule is helpful, and a hard, firm or rapidly growing fixed nodule is likely to be malignant. However, a papillary carcinoma may be cystic and soft. Furthermore, a very hard lesion may in fact be a calcified colloid nodule. A proven recurrent laryngeal nerve palsy on the side of a nodule suggests that it is likely to be malignant.

Fine-needle aspiration cytology remains the procedure of choice for diagnosing solitary thyroid nodules. A benign aspirate should be repeated at 3 months, and provided that both aspirates are benign, the nodule can be observed. A suspicious or malignant cytological result requires thyroidectomy. Other indications for thyroidectomy for a solitary nodule are a nodule that is rapidly increasing in size, painful, associated with lymphadenopathy, greater than 4 cm in diameter, fixed, or found in the context of a positive family history or previous neck irradiation. A hard nodule associated with hoarseness, airway obstruction or pressure symptoms is an additional indication for surgery. In summary, the indications for surgery are clinical and cytological. Surgery for a solitary thyroid nodule should involve a complete thyroid lobectomy and removal of the isthmus and pyramidal lobes.

PATHOLOGY OF THYROID CANCER

Thyroid cancer is rare, and accounts for less than 1% of all malignancies and only 0.5% of all cancer deaths. Like all thyroid diseases, it is commoner in females. The relative proportions are as follows: papillary, 50%; follicular, 25%; anaplastic, 20%; medullary, 5%. Papillary, follicular and anaplastic carcinomas arise from follicular cells, whereas medullary carcinomas arise from the parafollicular cell.

Papillary carcinoma

This tumour is the commonest thyroid cancer, and it occurs in young adults as well as in children. It typically presents as a solitary thyroid nodule, with a thick fibrous capsule, but is often multifocal and associated with palpable lymph node metastases. It may occur subsequent to previous irradiation of the neck. The condition of lateral aberrant thyroid is now known to represent secondary papillary carcinoma in a lymph node from an occult primary papillary carcinoma. Whilst the primary nodule may be firm or hard, cystic change can occur and, similarly, cystic change in lymph nodes is not unusual in secondary papillary carcinoma. The lesion is often multifocal throughout the thyroid gland, due to lymphatic spread, and therefore total thyroidectomy is indicated for treatment. Metastases may occur to the lungs, but the overall 10-year survival rate is of the order of 90%.

Follicular carcinoma

Follicular carcinoma occurs in an older age group, 30–50 years, and typically has a well-defined capsule and is solitary. It invades vessels, and metastases occur to bone and lung. It is more common in individuals with endemic goitre. The overall 10-year survival rate is 50%. The diagnosis will be suggested by fine-needle cytology showing a follicular neoplasm, especially with a microfollicular pattern. However, of all follicular lesions on cytology, only 20% will subsequently be found to be malignant.

Anaplastic carcinoma

This may occur *de novo* or be superimposed on a multinodular goitre. It is a disease of the elderly, and presents with rapidly aggressive local growth with invasion. It has an extremely poor prognosis and there is no effective treatment. Diagnosis can be confirmed by fine-needle aspiration and core biopsy.

Medullary carcinoma of the thyroid

This may be inherited as part of the multiple endocrine neoplasia syndrome type II (20%), or it may occur sporadically (80% of cases). Typically it presents as a solitary thyroid nodule. It may occur bilaterally, and lymph node metastases occur in up to 50% of cases. Distant metastases are also common. The lesion arises from the parafollicular or C-cells which secrete calcitonin, which is used as a marker for the disease.

Lymphoma

This may occur as a complication of Hashimoto's disease, and is usually of the non-Hodgkin's B-cell type. It occurs in the elderly, and appears as a rapidly growing, painless, firm thyroid mass. Clinically it therefore needs to be distinguished from anaplastic carcinoma, and this may be done by fine-needle aspiration cytology, but core biopsy may be required to make the differentiation, and also to subclassify the lymphoma. The treatment is usually chemotherapy. On occasion radiotherapy is required in addition, and surgery is rarely necessary for airway obstruction.

GENERAL POLICY ON TREATMENT OF THYROID MALIGNANCIES

In general, differentiated thyroid carcinomas and medullary carcinomas should be treated by total thyroidectomy and ablation of any thyroid remnants with radio-iodine. Subsequently, scanning for residual disease is undertaken with radio-iodine, and therapeutic doses of radio-iodine can be given for any evidence of metastatic disease. The condition may also be monitored with thyroglobulin antibodies. Thyroxine replacement is required, and this should be of a sufficiently high dose to cause TSH suppression. Excision of involved lymph nodes or a modified neck dissection may be required for involved lymph nodes. In discussing treatment options for surgery with patients, the possible complications of thyroidectomy will need to be considered. Apart from the general complications, the specific complications of thyroidectomy are asphyxia due to haemorrhage, recurrent laryngeal nerve damage, external laryngeal nerve damage, hypothyroidism and hypoparathyroidism.

SALIVARY GLAND SWELLING

PAROTID SWELLINGS

Swellings in the pre-auricular region are relatively common. Their main importance lies in recognizing a parotid swelling as arising from the parotid gland, rather than mistaking it for an upper deep cervical lymph node. This distinction is important because the technique of exploration differs, and the risk of damage to the facial nerve is high if the parotid swelling is not recognized.

Applied anatomy

The parotid is a serous salivary gland located in the pre-auricular retromandibular region below the zygomatic arch, and its inferior pole is separated from the submandibular gland by the stylomandibular ligament. The parotid is covered by the investing layer of deep cervical fascia, and within the parotid fascia are up to 8 lymph nodes. Up to 12 lymph nodes are actually embedded in the glandular tissue of the parotid itself.

The facial nerve emerges from the stylomastoid foramen at the base of the skull and enters the gland posteromedially. Figure 20.3.3 illustrates the methods of identifying the facial nerve at operation. These include the tragal pointer – the facial nerve is 1 cm below and 1 cm medial to the tip of the tragal pointer. Another method involves the mastoid process – if a finger is placed on it, the facial nerve will be 1 cm in front of a line bisecting the fingernail. Finally, if the posterior belly of the digastric is followed upwards along its superior border in the angle between it and the tympanic plate, the facial nerve will be found to emerge.

The facial nerve divides into two main trunks about 1 cm after emerging from the base of the skull, namely the temporozygomatic and cervicofacial trunks. The five branches of the facial nerve, which arise from the trunks, are the temporal, zygomatic, buccal, marginal mandibular and cervical branches. It is important to realize that the marginal mandibular branch may be given off low down from what appears to be solely the cervical branch. Thus although the cervical branch may be sacrificed, this should not be done until a definite identification of the marginal mandibular nerve has been made.

The division of the parotid into superficial and deep lobes by the facial nerve is an artificial one and created only at operation by superficial parotidectomy, but it is described in many operative texts as the faciovenous

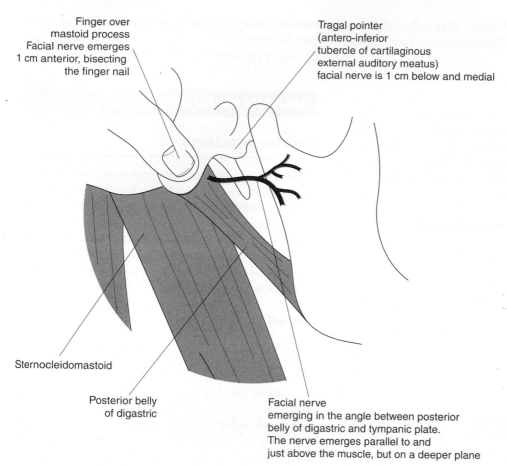

Finger over mastoid process
Facial nerve emerges 1 cm anterior, bisecting the finger nail

Tragal pointer (antero-inferior tubercle of cartilaginous external auditory meatus) facial nerve is 1 cm below and medial

Sternocleidomastoid

Posterior belly of digastric

Facial nerve emerging in the angle between posterior belly of digastric and tympanic plate. The nerve emerges parallel to and just above the muscle, but on a deeper plane

Figure 20.3.3 Facial nerve identification at superficial parotidectomy.

plane. In reality the parotid is embedded right around the facial nerve, without any true anatomical plane separating the two lobes.

Problem-orientated history

Having established that a lump is in the parotid region, it is important to obtain a history of the duration of the lump, whether it fluctuates and whether it is painful. Intermittency of the lump suggests sialectasis or calculus disease. Although pain is usually indicative of a benign process, a rapidly enlarging mass which has become painful may indicate malignancy.

Problem-orientated examination

The first question to be answered is whether the whole of the parotid gland is swollen, i.e. parotidomegaly, or whether there is a focal lump within an otherwise normal parotid gland. Secondly, it must be established whether the process is unilateral or bilateral. Once these two questions have been addressed, a classification of parotid swellings naturally arises (Box 20.3.2).

Examination includes a detailed description of all of the physical features of the lump, including site, size, shape, surface, tenderness, fixity, overlying skin changes

(including tethering, oedema and inflammation), fluctuance and transilluminability. The facial nerve must be examined in detail in all of its five peripheral branches. The parotid duct is palpated while the jaws are clenched as it passes across the masseter muscle, and its orifice is inspected on the buccal surface of the cheek opposite the crown of the second upper molar tooth. An attempt should be made to massage the parotid to see if any purulent material is discharged from the duct orifice. The oral cavity is examined and, in particular, the tonsillar region and the anterior pillar of the tonsil are examined for deep lobe extension. Bidigital palpation of this region and of the parotid duct is undertaken. A detailed examination of all lymph node areas in the neck is essential.

The characteristics of a parotid swelling are that it is in the region of the parotid gland as outlined in Figure 20.3.2, and that it leads to a fullness in the retromandibular space, often causing the ear lobe to protrude laterally. It is located anterior to the mastoid process and the upper part of the sternocleidomastoid muscle. Clinically, it may appear to be very superficial. In the region of the parotid tail, careful differentiation is required to distinguish it from an upper deep cervical lymph node.

BOX 20.3.2 CLASSIFICATION OF PAROTID ENLARGEMENT

Diffuse enlargement of whole gland – unilateral or bilateral

1. Viral – mumps
2. Acute suppurative parotitis
3. Calculus disease
4. Sialectasis
5. Sjögren's syndrome
6. Stenosis duct papilla
7. Infiltrations
   (a) Fat – alcohol, diabetes
   (b) Myxoedema
   (c) Cushing's disease
   (d) Drugs – thiouracil, oral contraceptive pill
   (e) Sarcoidosis
   (f) Tuberculosis

Discrete lump within the parotid

I. Benign tumours
   A. Epithelial
      1. Pleomorphic adenoma
      2. Monomorphic adenoma
         (a) Adenolymphoma (Warthin's tumour)
         (b) Oncocytoma (oxyphilic adenoma)
   B. Non-epithelial
      1. Haemangioma
      2. Lymphangioma
      3. Neurofibroma
      4. Benign parotid cyst
      5. Parotid lipoma
II. Malignant tumours
   A. Intermediate malignancy
      1. Muco-epidermoid tumour
      2. Acinic-cell tumour
   B. Malignant
      1. Adenoid cystic carcinoma
      2. Adenocarcinoma
      3. Malignancy in a pleomorphic adenoma
      4. Anaplastic carcinoma
      5. Squamous-cell carcinoma
      6. Lymphoma
      7. Soft-tissue sarcoma
      8. Metastases – squamous-cell carcinoma, melanoma

Swellings in the parotid region but not arising from the parotid gland

1. Lymphadenopathy within the parotid gland
2. Benign masseter hypertrophy
3. Mandibular tumours and dental cysts
4. Branchial cysts (first arch remnant)
5. Myxoma masseter
6. Aneurysm in the superficial temporal artery

Investigation of parotid swellings

Fine-needle aspiration cytology for solitary parotid swellings is appropriate and highly accurate. There is no risk of seeding of the needle track. Incisional biopsy is never appropriate, because there is a high risk of local recurrence of a pleomorphic adenoma if the capsule of the tumour is broken, and also of injury to the facial nerve.

Imaging of parotid tumours is best performed with CT scanning and the use of intravenous contrast medium, which enables the fasciovenous plane to be identified and therefore it can be established whether it is likely that there is deep lobe extension of the parotid tumour. It provides useful anatomical information for planning subsequent surgery.

Parotid calculi tend to be radiolucent and therefore, if suspected, sialography will be required to demonstrate the calculus. If sialectasis is suspected, sialography is required to confirm the diagnosis.

Salivary gland tumours

Pleomorphic adenoma
This is the commonest type of salivary gland tumour, which is slow-growing and usually occurs in the tail of the parotid, in the superficial lobe. It is usually unilateral and forms a firm swelling with a bosselated surface which feels surprisingly superficial. Male and female incidences are similar, and pleomorphic adenoma tends to occur in patients older than 40 years. It is the commonest benign tumour in the parotid gland, and accounts for 60% of salivary gland tumours overall. It never involves the facial nerve if it is benign. Its main importance is that it has a high risk of local recurrence if it is enucleated or the capsule is breached at surgery. Therefore the principle of surgery is intact removal with a cuff of normal tissue around it. This is usually best achieved by a superficial parotidectomy.

Adenolymphoma (Warthin's tumour or papillary cystadenoma lymphomatosum)
This is a neoplastic proliferation of heterotopic parotid tissue within a lymph node within the parotid. It is therefore a variety of monomorphic adenoma. It is commoner in males, and occurs in the tail of the parotid. It occurs in an older age group and is bilateral in 10% of cases. It is often fluctuant, and tends to be slow-growing. It is the second commonest benign tumour in the parotid.

Oncocytoma (oxyphilic adenoma)
This is a rare benign monomorphic adenoma which occurs in the parotid.

Haemangiomas and lymphangiomas
These tend to occur in children, and are uncommon.

Cysts of the parotid

These include retention cysts, hydatid cysts, cystic change in Warthin's tumour, branchial cysts which may occur within lymph nodes of the parotid, and HIV-related cysts. Fine-needle aspiration cytology for some of these will be diagnostic as well as therapeutic.

Muco-epidermoid tumour of the parotid

This is a form of low-grade carcinoma, and it becomes increasingly malignant as the epidermoid elements increase. It may therefore be misdiagnosed as a squamous-cell carcinoma. Pure squamous-cell carcinoma of the parotid is extremely rare.

Acinic-cell tumour

The majority of these tumours behave like pleomorphic adenomas. However, they have a slightly more aggressive malignant course.

Adenoid cystic carcinoma

The particular feature of this tumour is its tendency to neural invasion and therefore to presentation with pain.

Carcinoma arising within a pleomorphic adenoma

About 1% arise *de novo*, but most arise from a pre-existing benign pleomorphic adenoma which has usually been present for longer than 15 years.

Adenocarcinoma and pure squamous-cell carcinoma

These are both rare.

Malignant salivary gland tumours are less common than benign salivary gland tumours. One in six parotid tumours is malignant, and one in three submandibular tumours is malignant. This is in contrast to minor salivary gland tumours, where one in two is malignant. These tend to involve the hard palate in particular. Malignant parotid tumours tend to involve the retromandibular area and parapharyngeal space extending into the deep lobe, and therefore treatment by total parotidectomy is required. Among patients with malignant parotid tumours, less than 25% have a facial nerve palsy.

Detailed discussion of the treatment of parotid malignancy is beyond the scope of this chapter, but consideration should be given to total parotidectomy with or without facial nerve sacrifice. If facial nerve sacrifice is necessary, consideration should be given to facial nerve grafting. If lymph node metastases are present, radical neck dissection may be required and consideration should be given to post-operative radiotherapy.

Miscellaneous parotid conditions

Sjögren's syndrome

This is a multisystem disease characterized by xerostomia and xerophthalmia with associated connective tissue disease, usually rheumatoid arthritis. Some of these patients will subsequently develop lymphoma in the parotid gland. The diagnosis is established by biopsy of a minor salivary gland in the lip.

Sialectasis

This is a common bilateral diffuse cause of parotid gland enlargement which is intermittent and painful. The pain and distension are due to stasis, infection and dilatation of the parotid ducts. The condition is diagnosed by sialography and managed by massage and antibiotics. Surgery is not usually required.

Superficial parotidectomy

The details of surgery are beyond the scope of this chapter. However, the principles of the operation are important. Although a parotid tumour may be relatively small, the operation is a significant one as a large incision is required to enable superficial parotidectomy and full exposure of the facial nerve to be undertaken. Consequently, it is necessary to explain to patients the magnitude of the operation and the accompanying risks, which include those of anaesthesia, wound infection and haemorrhage, as well as the specific risk to the facial nerve with facial muscle weakness post-operatively. A vital part of the operation is division of the greater auricular nerve as it courses through the parotid gland, and it is necessary to warn patients pre-operatively of anaesthesia in the region of the ear lobe, which will be permanent. As the commonest reason for operating is a pleomorphic adenoma which has a significant risk of local recurrence, this should be mentioned to patients pre-operatively. Frey's syndrome is uncommon, and consists of gustatory sweating in the distribution of the auriculotemporal nerve.

SUBMANDIBULAR GLAND

Submandibular gland swellings lie in the digastric triangle, and superficially they are related to the marginal mandibular branch of the facial nerve, while on their deep surface they are related to the lingual nerve and hypoglossal nerve.

The submandibular gland is bidigitally palpable in the floor of the mouth. With increasing age the gland becomes ptotic into the neck. A stone in the duct or the orifice will be palpable, and examination should include palpation of the gland to see whether pus discharges from the duct orifice at the side of the frenulum of the tongue in the floor of the mouth.

Sialolithiasis

Intermittent painful swelling of the submandibular gland is common, and calculi are more common in the submandibular gland than in the parotid gland. Submandibular gland calculi tend to be radio-opaque, and are composed of calcium carbonate and calcium phosphate. It is usually possible to feel the calculus and to visualize it with floor-of-mouth X-ray, plain films and/or sialography. In general the stone can be removed if it is mobile and located anteriorly in the duct. However, if it is located more posteriorly and impacted at the junction of the duct and the gland, or if the condition has been allowed to become chronic (with chronic inflammation and fibrosis with a chronically enlarged gland), then removal of the submandibular gland will be necessary.

Submandibular gland swellings are most commonly due to calculus disease, but other causes, such as salivary gland tumours, simple cysts and dermoids, and all causes of enlarged lymph nodes, require consideration. These conditions are differentiated by the usual triple assessment of clinical examination, imaging and fine-needle aspiration cytology.

LYMPH NODE SWELLINGS

PRACTICAL ANATOMY

Several hundred lymph nodes are scattered throughout the head and neck, but the majority fall into well-recognized groups (Figure 20.3.4). The six groups or levels of nodes shown in Figure 20.3.4 are designed to describe lymph node groups removed during radical neck dissection.

Classically, the pre- and post-auricular and submandibular nodes are thought to drain into the upper, middle and lower deep cervical chain, as are axillary lymph nodes and posterior triangle lymph nodes. From these, jugular lymph trunks are formed which drain to the thoracic duct on the left and the internal jugular vein or brachiocephalic vein on the right. With the evolving technique of lymphoscintigraphy to enable performance of sentinel node biopsy, especially for melanoma, it is becoming apparent that the sentinel node (the first lymph node site of drainage) may not be consistent with classical anatomical descriptions. For example, a primary melanoma on the upper arm may have its sentinel node in the posterior triangle of the neck, rather than in the axilla. This highlights the importance of always undertaking a thorough general examination of a patient who presents with lymphadenopathy.

The problem is compounded by the ability of tumours to skip expected lymph node groups. Lymph

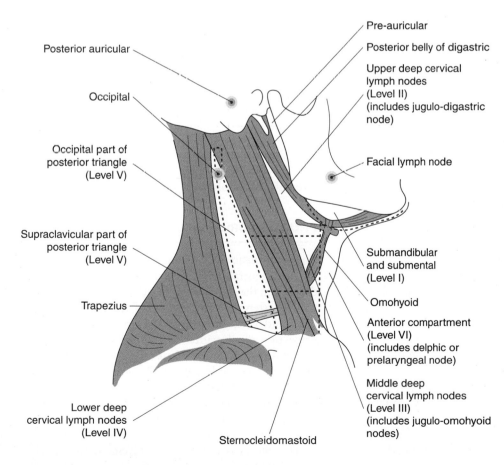

Figure 20.3.4 The lymph node regions and levels of the neck.

Pre-auricular
Posterior belly of digastric
Upper deep cervical lymph nodes (Level II) (includes jugulo-digastric node)
Facial lymph node
Submandibular and submental (Level I)
Omohyoid
Anterior compartment (Level VI) (includes delphic or prelaryngeal node)
Middle deep cervical lymph nodes (Level III) (includes jugulo-omohyoid nodes)
Sternocleidomastoid
Lower deep cervical lymph nodes (Level IV)
Trapezius
Supraclavicular part of posterior triangle (Level V)
Occipital part of posterior triangle (Level V)
Occipital
Posterior auricular

⌐ - - - - - ⌐ = outline of lymph node levels in the neck

nodes usually only become palpable when they are at least 1 cm in diameter, but they can be histologically involved while they are impalpable. Differences in children and adults are important, because children tend to have chronically enlarged non-tender palpable lymph nodes because of the frequency of recurrent upper respiratory tract infections. This type of lymphadenopathy in children has much less significance than palpable nodes in older patients, which should therefore always be investigated.

CAUSES OF CERVICAL LYMPHADENOPATHY

The causes of cervical lymphadenopathy are numerous, but are best classified into acute and chronic inflammatory conditions and malignant conditions. The malignant conditions are best subdivided into secondary squamous-cell carcinoma from the head and neck, secondary visceral carcinoma and lymphoma. Finally, there is a miscellaneous group of rare causes (Box 20.3.3).

PROBLEM-ORIENTATED HISTORY

A detailed problem-orientated history is essential for a patient with suspected cervical lymphadenopathy, and should include many of the points under the general problem-orientated history. Aetiological factors predisposing to head and neck squamous-cell carcinoma include smoking, alcohol, excess exposure to ultraviolet light and previous irradiation. A previous history of surgery and treatment for malignancy is noted, and the presence of lumps elsewhere and skin lesions is enquired for. Then follows a detailed systematic questioning about possible primary sites of inflammatory or neoplastic conditions which may result in cervical lymphadenopathy. Any skin lesion is enquired about in detail, including sun exposure, the use of sun blocks, occupation and changes in the lesion, including colour changes of increasing darkness or depigmentation, bleeding, pruritus and repeated scabbing and failure to heal. Such changes may suggest a clinical diagnosis of malignant melanoma, squamous-cell carcinoma or basal-cell carcinoma.

Ear, nose and throat symptoms must be enquired for, and these include epistaxis, oral ulceration, dental intervention, sore throat, bleeding from the mouth or gums, and details of diet and dental hygiene.

Upper aerodigestive tract symptoms may include dysphagia, hoarseness, odynophagia, dyspnoea, cough, sputum, haemoptysis, stridor and chest pain.

Abdominal symptoms include nausea, vomiting, epigastric pain, rapid satiation, back pain, steatorrhoea and jaundice.

Symptoms of lymphoma of a symptomatic nature

BOX 20.3.3 CERVICAL LYMPHADENOPATHY

A. **Acute lymphadenitis**
   1. Non-specific viral or bacterial
      (a) Infectious mononucleosis
      (b) Rubella
      (c) Chicken-pox
      (d) Pharyngitis, tonsillitis
   2. Suppuration and abscess formation

B. **Chronic lymphadenitis (> 3 weeks duration)**
   1. Non-specific
   2. Chronic skin sepsis (acne, eczema)
   3. Lymphadenopathy secondary to HIV infection
   4. Atypical mycobacterial (MAIS complex) infection
   5. Tuberculosis

C. **Malignancy**
   1. Secondary squamous-cell carcinoma of the upper aerodigestive tract
   2. Melanoma
   3. Visceral carcinoma (stomach, pancreas, breast, lung, kidney, oesophagus, testis)
   4. Lymphoma, leukaemia

D. **Other rare causes**
   1. Toxoplasmosis
   2. Cat scratch disease
   3. Brucellosis
   4. Actinomycosis
   5. Syphilis
   6. Sarcoidosis
   7. Rheumatoid arthritis

---

should be enquired for. These are termed B-symptoms, and they include anorexia, weight loss, night sweats, fever, alcohol intolerance and pruritus.

PROBLEM-ORIENTATED EXAMINATION

The examination will follow very closely the procedure for the general examination of the head and neck detailed in the early part of this chapter. It is emphasized that a systematic examination of the lump, and of all head and neck regions, for a primary site, as well as inspection of all orifices and panendoscopy, should be performed in the out-patient clinic. A complete examination of the whole patient should be undertaken for possible sites of malignancy outside the head and neck region, such as the abdomen, and melanoma in any site, and also for evidence of leukaemia and lymphoma in other lymph node groups.

The site of lymph node involvement should direct attention to various areas. For example, neoplastic upper deep cervical lymph nodes require attention to be directed to pre- and post-auricular regions, including the parotid, oral cavity, sinuses and nose. In contrast, a neoplastic node in the inferior deep cervical region, particularly on the left side (Trosier's sign, Virchow's node), should suggest a primary intrathoracic or intra-abdominal cause, such as carcinoma of the stomach, pancreas, lung, oesophagus, kidney or testis. Breast carcinoma can also cause this sign.

The number, size, consistency and discreteness of enlarged nodes are helpful in diagnosis. Inflammatory nodes are usually softer than malignant nodes, which are often multiple, discrete, hard and non-tender.

INVESTIGATION OF AN ENLARGED CERVICAL LYMPH NODE

This follows the principles outlined in the general introduction. Particularly important is the role of fine-needle aspiration cytology. It is essential that an incisional or excisional biopsy of a neoplastic cervical lymph node is not performed, as this may predispose the patient to local recurrence, cause a wound complication, and therefore interfere with the performance of the subsequent radical neck dissection, and some studies have suggested that it reduces long-term survival. Fine-needle aspiration cytology will be able to distinguish between inflammatory and neoplastic lymph nodes. In addition, fine-needle cytology will be able to establish whether the neoplasm is squamous-cell carcinoma from a primary in the head and neck, melanoma, secondary adenocarcinoma from a visceral tumour, or lymphoma. For melanoma and squamous-cell carcinoma, the subsequent steps in management would be to stage the patient prior to proceeding to radical neck dissection. In contrast, for patients with secondary carcinoma or lymphoma, a formal lymph node biopsy can then be performed to confirm the diagnosis and classify the type of lymphoma, as this will dictate treatment.

Computed tomography scanning of the head and neck is particularly useful for all head and neck tumours, and will help to define the extent and involvement of cervical lymph nodes and their relationship to major structures.

As part of the examination, investigation and staging process of a head and neck tumour, a formal examination under anaesthesia with multiple biopsies may be required.

Occasionally, special investigations such as HIV status, Paul-Bunell or monospot test for infectious mononucleosis and toxoplasma serology are required.

Specimen handling of a lymph node biopsy suspected of being lymphoma is critical to accurate diagnosis. Frozen-section examination should not be performed, and the specimen should be sent fresh to the pathologist, who has been notified in advance that it will be sent. Lymph node imprints, immunofluorescent studies and tissue culture may be undertaken in addition to routine sections. It is preferable for the lymph node to be excised intact so that the architecture can be assessed accurately.

ACUTE LYMPHADENITIS

Viral and bacterial infections of the tonsils and pharynx and dental infections are extremely common and result in lymphadenopathy. Rarely these suppurate, resulting in abscess formation which may require drainage. Occasionally the condition becomes chronic, and any chronic lymphadenitis of more than 3 weeks duration should be investigated. Often excisional biopsy will be required after fine-needle aspiration cytology has excluded secondary squamous-cell carcinoma and melanoma as the diagnosis.

Specific infections which commonly cause lymphadenopathy include infectious mononucleosis, chickenpox and rubella, most of which have specific diagnostic clinical features.

Chronic lymphadenitis

Tuberculosis and atypical tuberculosis with the MAIS (*Mycobacterium avium, intracellulare* and *scrofulaceum*) complex are rare, as are other specific chronic infections such as syphilis, actinomycosis, cat-scratch disease, toxoplasmosis and brucellosis.

NEOPLASTIC CERVICAL LYMPHADENOPATHY

Lymphomas

Patients with lymphoma frequently have bilateral, rubbery, firm, discrete cervical lymph nodes. Lymphadenopathy may be present elsewhere, and hepatosplenomegaly is also not uncommon. Cervical lymph node excisional biopsy is required after fine-needle aspiration cytology has excluded squamous-cell carcinoma and melanoma.

Secondary carcinoma

In a patient over 45 years of age with a painless lymph node swelling, the most likely diagnosis is a primary squamous-cell carcinoma of the head and neck. Possible sites include the lip, tongue, floor of the mouth, pharynx, larynx, tonsil and scalp.

If a supraclavicular node is involved, potential primary tumours in addition to those in the head and neck include carcinoma involving the lung, breast, stomach, pancreas, kidney, testis and oesophagus.

Secondary lymphadenopathy from malignant salivary

gland tumours and thyroid tumours has already been described earlier in this chapter.

The surgical details of lymph node biopsy and radical neck dissection are beyond the scope of this chapter. However, two points require emphasis. First, it is never appropriate to perform a lymph node biopsy in the neck under local anaesthetic, as the lymph node is always much deeper than is clinically appreciated. Secondly, whenever one is operating on a lymph node anywhere in the posterior triangle, the patient must be warned pre-operatively of the possibility of accessory nerve damage, as the lymph node is almost always in close proximity to the accessory nerve. Although in anatomical textbooks the posterior triangle appears to be splayed out with plenty of room in it away from the accessory nerve, in the living patient the triangle is closely packed together and dominated by the centrally situated accessory nerve.

LESS COMMON HEAD AND NECK LUMPS

BRANCHIAL CYST

The aetiology of a branchial cyst is controversial. It may either represent an embryologically derived cyst from remnants of the pharyngeal pouches, or it may derive from epithelial inclusions within upper deep cervical lymph nodes. It usually occurs in children and young adults. In middle-aged and elderly patients with an apparent branchial cyst, the diagnosis is more likely to be cystic degeneration of a secondary deposit of squamous-cell carcinoma in a lymph node. Characteristically it is situated anterior to the upper third of sternocleidomastoid muscle at the level of the carotid bifurcation, often partially covered by the muscle. The mass is soft, cystic and fluctuant, and secondary infection is common. The differential diagnosis is an enlarged upper deep cervical lymph node. Cytology shows opalescent fluid with cholesterol crystals, degenerate squamous cells and lymphocytes. Treatment by excision is recommended.

CYSTIC HYGROMA (CAVERNOUS LYMPHANGIOMA)

Typically this is a large, fluctuant, brilliantly translucent cystic swelling at the root of the neck laterally in childhood.

THYROGLOSSAL CYST

The thyroid gland develops from the median thyroid diverticulum in the floor of the pharynx, growing downwards between the first and second pharyngeal arches.

The stalk of this diverticulum elongates and forms the thyroglossal duct. The ultimobranchial bodies from the fourth pharyngeal pouch become applied to the lateral part of the thyroid gland and contribute the parafollicular C-cells.

A thyroglossal cyst may develop at any level from remnants of the thyroglossal tract, which extends from the foramen caecum in the posterior tongue, through the neck, closely related to the hyoid bone and down to the pyramidal lobe or isthmus of the thyroid gland. Most commonly situated at the hyoid bone level or below, the cyst characteristically moves upwards on swallowing and protrusion of the tongue. The cyst is usually just to one side of the midline, and usually occurs in children and young adults. Cysts are lined by columnar epithelium with islands of thyroid and lymphoid tissue. Because of the lymphoid tissue, they are prone to secondary infection. Infected cysts are best treated by aspiration and antibiotics, rather than by drainage, as incision may result in thyroglossal fistula formation. Rarely, papillary thyroid carcinoma may develop in a thyroglossal cyst.

Surgical treatment involves excision of the whole thyroglossal duct remnant and cyst, and includes resection of the central portion of the body of the hyoid bone (Sistrunk's operation).

RANULA

A ranula forms from the sublingual salivary gland, representing a mucoid degeneration, and resulting in a translucent swelling laterally in the floor of the mouth. Rarely this may extend downwards to appear in the submandibular region of the neck. Treatment is by marsupialization into the floor of the mouth.

FURTHER READING

Freid MP. 1994: The evaluation of a neck mass in an adult patient. In Morris PJ, Malt RA (eds), *Oxford textbook of surgery*. Vol. 2. New York: Oxford University Press, 2215–20.

Lynn J, Bloom SR (eds) 1993: Thyroid. In Lynn J, Bloom SR (eds), *Surgical endocrinology*. Oxford: Butterworth-Heinemann, 193–330.

Maran AGD, Gaze M, Wilson JA. 1993: *Stell and Maran's head and neck surgery*. Oxford: Butterworth-Heinemann, 269–309.

Wheeler MH. 1997: The thyroid gland. In Farndon JR (ed.), *Breast and endocrine surgery*. London: W.B. Saunders, 35–75.

Breast lumps

Jonathan W. Serpell

Introduction

This chapter contains the necessary information for the clinician to undertake a problem-orientated approach to a lump in the breast of a post-pubertal female patient. The chapter emphasizes clinical features, and includes a broad outline of treatment principles rather than specific details. Specifically excluded from this chapter are developmental abnormalities, male gynaecomastia and a detailed discussion of mastalgia. As nipple discharge may be associated with a breast lump, a short description of this is also included.

The relatively simple macroscopic and microscopic anatomy of the breast provides the framework for understanding the pathogenesis of many breast conditions, and these are indicated on the applied anatomical diagrams.

Breast lumps are common, and half the female population will at some time seek medical attention for a breast problem. It is estimated that up to 25% of the female population will undergo a breast biopsy. Of those presenting to a breast clinic, 90% will be found to have a benign breast condition, but breast cancer itself is also common. The lifetime risk for developing breast cancer is of the order of 1 in 13 in both Australia and the UK. The incidence of breast cancer is increasing. This increase has been noted since the mid-1980s, and is not completely explained by an increased detection rate through screening, or by the ageing of the population. As a consequence, breast screening is well established in many countries, including Australia and the UK, and increasingly breast conditions are initially being diagnosed by screening mammography. Breast screening with mammography has been shown to reduce the risk of death from breast cancer in screened women in the 50–65 years age group by 29%. This is because screen-detected cancers are more likely to be smaller, of lower grade, node negative, and of special histological subtypes compared to symptomatic cancers. Ductal carcinoma *in situ* (DCIS) is found in about 30% of screen-detected breast cancers, compared to less than 2% of symptomatically detected breast cancers.

HOW DOES BREAST CANCER PRESENT?

In order of decreasing frequency, breast cancer presents as:

1. a lump in the breast;

2. a screen-detected lesion;

3. a nipple change (either nipple retraction or ulceration);

4. an alteration in the contour of the breast (included in this category are skin dimpling, *peau d'orange*, distortion of the breast and asymmetry);

5. nipple discharge;

6. pain (although this is rarely the sole presentation of a breast carcinoma).

RISK FACTORS FOR DEVELOPING CARCINOMA OF THE BREAST

Risk may be defined in absolute and relative terms (Table 20.4.1). If the normal risk of development of carcinoma of the breast is expressed as 1, a low but increased risk is a relative risk of 1.1 to 1.9. A medium relative risk signifies a relative risk of 2 to 4 times, and a high level of risk signifies a relative risk greater than 4 times normal (Table 20.4.1). Absolute risk is often useful in providing explanations to patients. In the USA the risk of a 25-year-old woman developing breast cancer is 1 in 19 608. By the age of 40 years the risk is 1 in 217, by 50 years it is 1 in 60, by the age of 60 years it is 1 in 25, and by the age of 80 years, 1 in 10 women will have developed breast cancer. Therefore, if a 50-year-old woman has a risk factor that increases her relative risk twofold, then her absolute risk increases to that of a 60-year-old.

Table 20.4.1 Factors associated with increased risk of breast cancer

1.1 Relative risk increased more than four times
1. Evidence of susceptibility genes, *BRCA1, BRCA2*
2. Premenopausal breast cancer in mother and sister
3. Atypical hyperplasia
4. *In-situ* ductal or lobular carcinoma

1.2 Relative risk increased between two and four times
1. Premenopausal breast cancer in mother or sister
2. Moderate or severe hyperplasia without atypia
3. Previous breast cancer
4. Ageing Caucasian women

1.3 General markers increasing risk up to two times
1. Post-menopausal breast cancer in a first-degree relative
2. Previous ovarian or uterine cancer
3. Excess ionizing irradiation to chest wall or breast
4. High alcohol consumption
5. Higher socio-economic status
6. Obesity

1.4 Hormone-related markers increasing risk up to two times
1. Nulliparous
2. Early menarche
3. Late menopause
4. Late age at birth of first child
5. Short duration of breast-feeding
6. Prolonged use of oral contraceptives
7. Prolonged use of oestrogen replacement therapy

More minor markers are associated with up to a two-fold increase in risk, but are not consistently identified as significant in all studies.

As a corollary to this, the American College of Pathology issued a statement indicating factors which do not increase the risk of breast cancer (see Box 20.4.1).

BOX 20.4.1 PATHOLOGICAL CONDITIONS *NOT* ASSOCIATED WITH INCREASED RISK OF BREAST CANCER

Adenosis
Apocrine metaplasia
Macro- or microcysts
Duct ectasia – periductal mastitis
Mastitis
Fibrosis
Fibroadenoma
Mild hyperplasia
Squamous metaplasia

CLASSIFICATION OF BREAST LUMPS

There are many differential diagnoses of breast carcinoma. The common and important breast cancer differential diagnoses include a macroscopic cyst, a fibroadenoma, and a breast lump in association with aberrations of normal development and involution (ANDI). All other breast conditions are less common (see Box 20.4.2).

Radiologically detected abnormalities in both diagnostic mammograms and screening mammograms are increasingly the presentation of patients with breast conditions. The common radiological abnormalities detected are listed in Box 20.4.3.

APPLIED MACROSCOPIC ANATOMY OF THE BREAST

The developed female breast is a modified sweat gland situated in the subcutaneous layer of the anterior chest wall overlying the second to sixth ribs anteriorly. The axillary tail extends along the infero-lateral margin of the pectoralis major muscle. A greater proportion of the fibroglandular breast tissue is situated in the upper outer quadrant of the breast, and therefore the upper outer quadrant is the commonest site of breast cancer and pathologies associated with ANDI. The breasts are often asymmetrical, and more commonly the left breast is slightly larger than the right. The non-lactating developed breast consists of varying proportions of fibroglandular breast tissue and adipose tissue, depending on the

BOX 20.4.2 BREAST LUMPS

3.1 Common breast lumps

1. Carcinoma – invasive and *in situ* (5% of *in-situ* carcinomas will form a mass)
2. Macrocyst
3. Fibroadenoma
4. Cyclical change with mastalgia and nodularity (ANDI)

3.2 Less common breast lumps

1. Lactational mastitis and abscess
2. Periductal mastitis – ectasia, inflammatory lump
3. Hyperplasia – especially if florid and atypical
4. Fat necrosis – oil cyst
5. Haematoma
6. Intramammary lymph node
7. Galactocele
8. Granulomatous mastitis
9. Lipoma
10. Pseudolipoma
11. Giant fibroadenoma
12. Phyllodes tumour
13. Sebaceous cyst – Montgomery tubercle
14. Mondor's disease
15. Silicone granuloma
16. Papillary cystadenoma
17. Sclerosing adenosis
18. Radial scar
19. Complex sclerosing lesion

3.3 Rare breast lumps

1. Lymphoma
2. Secondary metastasis, e.g. melanoma
3. Soft-tissue sarcoma
4. Desmoid tumour
5. Nodular fasciitis
6. Tuberculosis
7. Pilonidal sinus
8. Hidradenitis suppurativa

BOX 20.4.3 COMMON MAMMOGRAPHIC ABNORMALITIES

1. Mass lesion
2. Calcification
3. Stromal distortion
4. Asymmetry
5. Stellate lesion
   (a) Carcinoma
   (b) Radial scar
   (c) Sclerosing adenosis
   (d) Complex sclerosing lesion
   (e) Fat necrosis
   (f) Hyalinized fibroadenoma

number of pregnancies and the state of involution (Figure 20.4.1). The fibroglandular tissue runs in the interlobar connective tissue planes and contains the ducts and acini of the non-lactating breast. Fat lobules are located between the fibroglandular tissue, and are often prominent and palpable. The majority of the bulk of the breast is due to the fat lobules, except during lactation. The breast is normally mobile on the underlying pectoralis major muscle with its associated deep fascia, and is connected via a layer of loose areolar tissue. The deep fascia of the pectoralis major muscle should be taken as a deep clearance plane when performing a mastectomy or wide local excision of a breast cancer. The suspensory ligaments of the breast (Astley Cooper) extend from the deep pectoral fascia and insert into the skin, and they therefore support the breast. They are more prominent in the upper part of the breast. Pathological conditions adjacent to these suspensory ligaments may cause fibrosis and shortening of the ligaments, and consequently produce a skin dimple as a marker of the underlying disease. Such conditions include inflammatory conditions (fibrosis following abscess formation and fat necrosis) and, importantly, the desmoplastic reaction associated with a typical scirrhous carcinoma. The nipple drains between 15 and 20 lobes of the breast via a lactiferous duct which has a dilatation beneath the areola, namely the lactiferous sinus. Each lactiferous duct and lobe roughly equates to a radial sector of the breast. During lactation, cracking of the nipple may allow entry of *Staphylococcus aureus*, and this may result in lactational mastitis and/or abscess formation. Consequently, the inflammatory process tends to be related to a sector or sectors of the breast. The lactiferous ducts are normally palpable as thickened cords at the peri-areolar margin, and should not be mistaken for abnormal breast masses. Traumatic fat necrosis with subsequent inflammation and fibrosis can result from trauma but may be idiopathic, and it affects one of the macroscopic fatty lobules. It may result in skin and nipple retraction and a mass identical to that of a carcinoma.

Lymphatic drainage of the breast occurs through the ipsilateral axillary lymph nodes (75%), the internal thoracic lymph nodes, and the infra- and supraclavicular lymph nodes. Contralateral drainage may also occur.

APPLIED MICROSCOPIC ANATOMY OF THE BREAST

The breast lobule is the specialized histological feature of the breast. The essential feature is the terminal duct – lobular unit, and into the terminal duct drain a number of related acini which make up a single lobule. Lobules

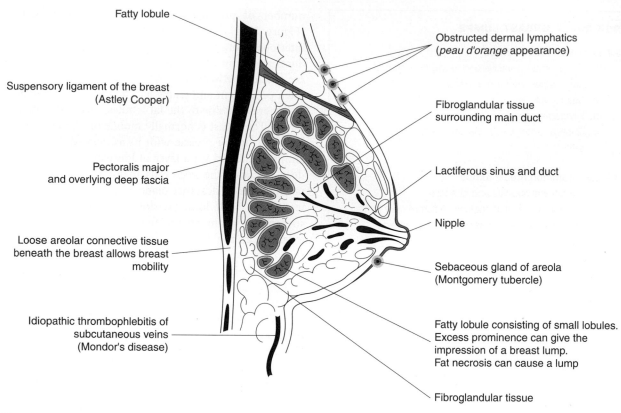

Fatty lobule

Suspensory ligament of the breast
(Astley Cooper)

Pectoralis major
and overlying deep fascia

Loose areolar connective tissue
beneath the breast allows breast
mobility

Idiopathic thrombophlebitis of
subcutaneous veins
(Mondor's disease)

Obstructed dermal lymphatics
(*peau d'orange* appearance)

Fibroglandular tissue
surrounding main duct

Lactiferous sinus and duct

Nipple

Sebaceous gland of areola
(Montgomery tubercle)

Fatty lobule consisting of small lobules.
Excess prominence can give the
impression of a breast lump.
Fat necrosis can cause a lump

Fibroglandular tissue

Figure 20.4.1 Macroscopic breast anatomy.

are located between adipose tissue and interlobular dense connective tissue, as part of the fibroglandular tissue of the breast. However, within the lobule the acini are separated by loose intralobular specialized connective tissue. The acini consist of a single layer of epithelial cells with an underlying layer of myoepithelial cells. Both the specialized intralobular connective tissue and the acini are under hormonal control.

Menstrual cyclical changes of heaviness of the breasts and associated nodularity and tenderness of the breasts are so common that they should be considered physiologically normal, but they are not associated with significant histological changes within lobules. However, histological changes do occur during breast development, pregnancy, lactation and involution of the breast. Involution of the breast is evident by the age of 35 years, and results in a reduction in the fibroglandular tissue and a relative increase in the adipose tissue of the breast. As a result, there is disappearance of the lobular epithelium and specialized lobular connective tissue, with replacement by the more usual fibrous tissue of the interlobar region. When the stroma involutes at a faster rate than the acini, these remain and form microcysts, and are so common as to be regarded as normal. Obstruction of the related efferent duct can subsequently result in a macroscopic cyst. Sclerosing adenosis is an aberration of stromal fibrosis with epithelial acini surrounded by

fibrosis. Involution of the stroma and epithelium may not occur at the same rate in all areas of the breast over the 20 years of the process, and some remaining fibroglandular specialized breast tissue may appear clinically and radiologically as asymmetrical involution, particularly in the upper outer quadrant of the breast. The histological changes of microcysts, adenosis, fibrosis, lymphocytic infiltration and apocrine change are therefore considered to be part of the normal breast involution process.

THE CONCEPT OF ABERRATIONS OF NORMAL DEVELOPMENT AND INVOLUTION (ANDI)

The essential feature of the concept of ANDI developed by Hughes and colleagues is that most benign breast conditions are due to disorders based on the normal processes of development, cyclical change and involution. These benign breast conditions show a predominance at each phase (Table 20.4.2). For each disorder there is a spectrum from normal through mild abnormality (aberration) to disease (Table 20.4.2). The concept replaces that of fibrocystic disease, and explains the common occurrence of benign histological changes with no clinical correlation. Furthermore, it replaces the

Table 20.4.2 Classification of common benign conditions: aberrations of normal development and involution

Stage	Normal process	Benign breast disorder or aberration	Benign breast disease
Development	Lobule development	Fibroadenoma	Giant fibroadenoma
	Stromal development	Adolescent hypertrophy	Severe hypertrophy
Cyclical change	Hormonal cyclical change	Mastalgia	Severe mastalgia and
		Nodularity – focal	nodularity
		– diffuse	
	Epithelial activity	Benign papilloma	
Pregnancy and lactation	Lactation	Galactocele	
Involution	Lobular involution (including microcysts, apocrine changes, adenosis, fibrosis)	Macrocysts	Extensive and recurrent cysts
		Sclerosing adenosis	
	Ductal involution	Nipple retraction	Periductal mastitis with
	Fibrosis		suppuration
	Dilatation	Duct ectasia	
	Micropapillomatosis	Simple hyperplasias	Lobular hyperplasia with atypia
			Ductal hyperplasia with atypia
			Intracystic papilloma

Reproduced with permission from Hughes LE, Mansell RE, Webster PJT. *Benign disorders and diseases of the breast.* London: Balliere-Tindall; 1989: 23.

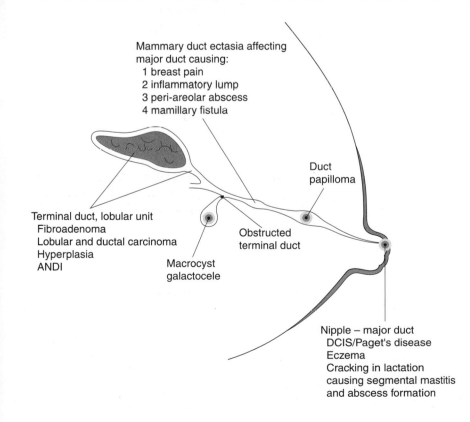

Mammary duct ectasia affecting
major duct causing:
  1 breast pain
  2 inflammatory lump
  3 peri-areolar abscess
  4 mamillary fistula

Duct
papilloma

Terminal duct, lobular unit
Fibroadenoma
Lobular and ductal carcinoma
Hyperplasia
ANDI

Obstructed
terminal duct

Macrocyst
galactocele

Nipple – major duct
DCIS/Paget's disease
Eczema
Cracking in lactation
causing segmental mastitis
and abscess formation

Figure 20.4.2 Diagrammatic outline of breast microscopic anatomy correlated with sites of pathology.

obsolete synonyms of fibrocystic disease, namely fibroadenosis, chronic cystic mastitis, mastodynia, cystic mastopathy, benign mammary dysplasia, cystic epithelial hyperplasia and Schimmelbusch's disease. Common examples are shown in Table 20.4.2, emphasizing that the concept encompasses pathogenesis, histology, clinical features and treatment principles.

The sites of pathology of various breast diseases are indicated in Figure 20.4.2 in relation to the nipple areolar complex, the major ducts and the terminal duct lobular unit.

BENIGN BREAST DISORDERS

FIBROADENOMA

This is a common condition, occurring in young women, in which there is formation of a smooth, firm, rubbery, well-circumscribed, mobile lump, usually between 1 and 2 cm in diameter. Because of its mobility it is sometimes likened to a 'breast mouse'. Although it is most commonly diagnosed in a younger age group, it may be detected for the first time as a calcified lesion by screening mammography in those over 50 years of age. It is part of the ANDI complex, and originates from the whole of a breast lobule. A spectrum exists from microscopic hyperplastic lobules which are identical to fibroadenomas through to macroscopic fibroadenomas. The lesion therefore develops from the whole lobule rather than from one cell of an acini of a lobule, and is therefore not thought to represent a true neoplasm. The fact that continued growth is unusual and that it usually ceases at between 1 and 2 cm in diameter also argues against it being a true neoplasm. Fibroadenomas tend to show hormonal dependence and exhibit lactational changes and involution in the menopause. They usually become static in size, but may also involute and disappear. They are occasionally multiple and bilateral. Clinically, fibroadenomas can usually be diagnosed with confidence. However, of all lumps thought to represent a fibroadenoma, there is a potential error rate in up to 50%. Therefore triple assessment is required to confirm a positive diagnosis of a fibroadenoma. The risk of carcinoma developing within a fibroadenoma is small (1 in 1000). Therefore a concordant triple assessment positively diagnosing a fibroadenoma enables the lump to be observed or, if the patient wishes, removed. By definition, a fibroadenoma larger than 5 cm in diameter is termed a giant fibroadenoma. This is more common in patients from African countries. However, it is to be distinguished from and is not synonymous with a phyllodes tumour.

CYSTS

Macroscopic cysts are one of the major features of ANDI, and are commonest between the ages of 38 and 53 years. Other cysts may form in the breast which are not part of the ANDI complex. These include galactoceles, oil cysts following resolution of fat necrosis, papillary cystadenomas, and necrosis in phyllodes tumours and carcinomas.

Cysts may be associated with microcalcifications on mammography. All lumps that are suspected of being cysts should be aspirated. Provided that the lump completely disappears, the fluid is not bloodstained and the cyst does not reform, the lesion can be observed. However, if the fluid is bloodstained, the cytology is positive, there is a residual mass or the cyst keeps re-filling after more than three re-aspirations, then a histological diagnosis is required. For similar reasons, if an ultrasound examination shows a solid component to the cyst, it should be investigated in the same way as a solid lump, usually by ultrasound-guided biopsy.

EPITHELIAL HYPERPLASIA

This term indicates an increased number of epithelial cells in the terminal duct lobular unit, and supersedes the previous terms 'epitheliosis' and 'papillomatosis'. Three aspects of epithelial hyperplasia are classified:

1. whether it is ductal or lobular;
2. whether the hyperplasia is mild, moderate or severe;
3. whether the hyperplasia is typical or atypical.

Atypical ductal or lobular hyperplasia is associated with a four- to fivefold increased risk of breast cancer. Mild degrees of hyperplasia are common, may be regarded as part of ANDI and, as indicated in the American College of Pathology list, should not be considered to be associated with increased risk. However, a moderate degree of hyperplasia is associated with a mildly increased risk of breast cancer. Epithelial hyperplasia is usually asymptomatic and detected as an incidental finding on a breast biopsy for some other reason. On occasion it can form a mass, especially if florid and atypical. Fine-needle aspiration for cytology of such a mass will usually show a cellular and possibly suspicious aspirate, so that excisional biopsy is indicated.

RESIDUAL BREAST TISSUE

Not infrequently different areas in the breast involute at different rates, and the resulting asymmetry may cause clinical and/or radiological confusion. Radiologically residual breast parenchyma will compress away on coned compression magnification views, in contrast to stellate lesions, which will become more obvious and prominent on magnification views.

MAMMARY DUCT ECTASIA – PERIDUCTAL MASTITIS

These conditions are common, and pathologically they involve the major ducts and may be associated with linear macroscopic calcification on mammography. They may present in four clinical ways:

1. breast pain;
2. abscess formation;
3. an inflammatory lump;
4. as a mammillary fistula.

The constellation of features of non-cyclical mastalgia, nipple discharge (which may be bloodstained), nipple retraction, peri-areolar inflammation with or without a mass, a non-lactating peri-areolar abscess and mammillary fistula are typical. Histologically, the condition involves a major duct with associated plasma cells, granulomas, ductal dilatation and periductal inflammation and fibrosis. *Bacteroides*, staphylococci, *Proteus* and streptococcal organisms have all been isolated, and antibiotic treatment is required, including anaerobic cover.

DUCT PAPILLOMA

This is a common condition that is regarded as an aberration of cyclical change rather than a true benign tumour. Usually it presents with a bloodstained or clear watery nipple discharge. A duct papilloma itself is not palpable. The treatment is excision of the involved duct or ducts.

LIPOMAS

Lipomas are relatively common within the breast, but are an important diagnosis to be distinguished from pseudolipomas. Pseudolipomas are due to underlying desmoplasia in association with a carcinoma, resulting in contraction and fibrosis of breast tissue, throwing a fatty breast lobule into prominence and thereby creating a pseudolipoma.

NIPPLE DISCHARGE

Nipple discharge is an important symptom which demands full investigation. If it is associated with a breast lump, investigation should include a complete investigation of the associated breast lump. Physiological lactation is excluded from this discussion.

The common causes of nipple discharge are mammary duct ectasia, duct papilloma, epithelial hyperplasia, galactorrhoea, ductal carcinoma *in situ* and underlying carcinoma of the breast. A problem-orientated history is essential. Is the discharge from a single or multiple duct(s)? Is the discharge unilateral or bilateral? Is the discharge spontaneous or does it occur on expression only? The ductal system of the breast is not a vacuum, and therefore in at least two-thirds of women with expression, a small amount of greenish-yellow discharge is possible, and this should be viewed as physiological. The colour of the discharge is important (whether it is milky or non-milky, bloodstained or clear and watery, and yellow serous, brown or black). The causes of bloodstained nipple discharge include epithelial hyperplasia, ductal carcinoma *in situ*, invasive carcinoma, duct ectasia and duct papilloma. On historical grounds alone, a discharge from multiple ducts that is bilateral and only occurs on expression, and is not bloodstained or clear and watery, is highly unlikely to be significant. In contradistinction, a nipple discharge from a single duct which is unilateral, occurs spontaneously and is bloodstained or clear and watery is highly significant, and is most likely to represent an underlying duct papilloma. The nipple discharge should be tested for blood with one of the commercially available biochemical dipsticks, a specimen sent for cytology and mammography undertaken. For single-duct discharge, microdochectomy is the treatment of choice, but in patients older than 50 years, and especially those in whom multiple ducts are involved, total duct excision (Adair's or Hadfield's operation) is appropriate.

DISORDERS OF INVOLUTION

These include sclerosing adenosis, radial scars and complex sclerosing lesions (formerly termed sclerosing papillomatosis or duct adenoma). These are all examples of sclerosis occurring during the period of breast involution. Each condition may present with breast pain, a breast lump, or be mammographically detected. Because they may closely mimic carcinoma, excisional biopsy is usually required.

ASSESSMENT OF A BREAST LUMP

The mainstay of assessing a breast lump is triple assessment. This includes clinical assessment, imaging assessment and microscopic assessment. A detailed clinical assessment is essential, while a problem-orientated history based on an understanding of risk factors and pathogenesis of breast diseases is essential, and will often provide the correct diagnosis. Diagnostic imaging of the breast with diagnostic mammography and on occasion special views, particularly coned compression magnification views, and ultrasound examination should form part of any breast assessment. Microscopic assessment may involve cytological or histological examination of a breast lesion. Cytology is obtained by fine-needle aspiration (either free-hand or image-controlled). Histological tissue for examination may be obtained by core biopsy (either free-hand of a palpable lump, or image-guided with ultrasound or a stereotactic mammography). Histology may also be obtained at open biopsy, which may be either incisional or, as is more usually preferred, excisional.

ACCURACY OF THE TRIPLE ASSESSMENT

The triple test will be positive in 99.6% of breast cancers. A positive triple test is defined as positive if any one of its three components is malignant or suspicious for malignancy. A negative triple test on all components indicates that cancer is unlikely (less than 1% of cases), and further investigation can be avoided for most of these women, and their lesion can be observed rather than removed. The sensitivity of the individual components of the triple assessment is as follows: clinical examination, 85%; mammography, 90%; and fine-needle aspiration cytology, 91%. Therefore any clinical lump which is suspicious must be treated as such, even though mammography will on occasion be negative.

PROBLEM-ORIENTATED HISTORY

The age of the patient is likely to give an indication of the likely pathology. The commonest type of lump in a young adult is a fibroadenoma. Macroscopic cysts are commonest in the 38–53 years age group. Carcinomas become increasingly common with age; 90% of all breast cancers occur after the age of 40 years, and they are extremely rare in women under 25 years of age. By the age of 70 years the majority of discrete breast masses will be carcinomas (Figure 20.4.3). The history of the lump itself is critical. It is most important to know when, how and by whom the lump was first noted. Did the patient feel it, and can she still feel it? Has the patient's referring doctor felt it definitely, or only suspected it? How long has the lump been present? Has it fluctuated in size or varied during the menstrual cycle? Is it associated with pain? Is there a history of trauma to the breast? Is there a previous history of benign breast disease, including cysts, fibroadenomas and hyperplasia, or is there a previous history of carcinoma of the breast? Has there been irradiation to the breast (e.g. in the treatment of

Hodgkin's disease)? A full reproductive history, including age of menarche, regularity of cycles, oral contraceptive pill usage and duration, and hormone replacement therapy usage and duration is critical. Parity, age of first birth, breast-feeding duration, mastitis and abscess formation must be recorded. The age at menopause and whether the patient has undergone hysterectomy and/or oophorectomy is important. Cyclical mastalgia should be noted. Mastalgia is cyclical in two-thirds of patients and non-cyclical in one-third. Premenstrual discomfort and nodularity are so common that they should be regarded as physiologically normal, and they affect 70% of women significantly at some stage of their life. A family history of breast cancer in particular and other carcinomas on both maternal and paternal sides of the family should be enquired for. About 95% of breast cancer is sporadic and only 5% is inherited. Breast cancer associated with *BRCA1* and *BRCA2* genes is autosomally dominantly inherited, but with 80% penetrance. Typically the characteristics of an inherited susceptibility are early age of onset and premenopausal, bilateral multifocal disease in which two or more affected first-degree relatives and the index case are noted. The family tree should be drawn and all other cancers entered as well. The presence or absence of nipple discharge and its features should be noted. General systematic questioning suggesting metastatic disease, including loss of appetite, loss of

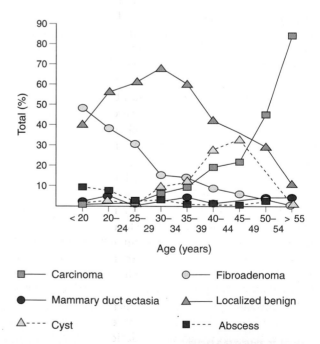

Figure 20.4.3 Percentage of patients in 5-year age groups with a discrete breast lump who have common benign conditions and breast cancer. (Reproduced from Dixon JM, Mansell RE. 1992: The breast. In Burnand KG, Young AE (eds), *The new Aird's companion in surgical studies*. Edinburgh: Churchill Livingstone, p. 813, Fig. 34.1b, with permission.)

weight, back pain and dyspnoea, should be noted. Enquiry should be made about the most recent mammograms and their results, and copies of the X-rays and reports obtained if possible.

PROBLEM-ORIENTATED EXAMINATION

The first question to be answered is whether a lump is present or not. A dominant or discrete lump is usually three-dimensional, distinct from the surrounding tissue, and may produce asymmetry. It should be distinguished from areas of thickening and nodularity which do not cause a discrete or dominant lump.

Nodularity and thickening are common, and may be diffuse or focal. They occasionally produce lumpy areas which tend to fluctuate in size, are non-discrete and often tender. These patients who clinically do not have a dominant lump are appropriately managed by ultrasonography to examine specifically for a dominant lump, and mammography if they are over 35 years of age or if there is any degree of suspicion. The patient should also be re-examined at a different phase of the menstrual cycle at either 3 or 6 weeks, and subsequently followed for at least 3 months before discharge back to the referring doctor.

Experience is required to recognize some normal features of the breast on examination. The normal nodularity, tenderness and prominence of the upper outer quadrants and axillary tails is common and often asymmetrical. Involutional change may produce a fibro-fatty ridge running across the lower half of the breast, and this is particularly a feature of older patients with ptotic breasts. Palpable fatty lobules and fibroglandular tissue and ducts are commonly felt at the areolar margin. Postoperative palpable defects of the walls of a biopsy cavity at previous excisional biopsy sites are common, and require recognition rather than misinterpretation as a new breast lump. Undue prominence of underlying costal cartilages should not be confused with a breast lump.

Occasionally, for a patient with a non-discrete lump, a fine-needle aspirate for cytology taken blindly from the general area indicated by the patient will provide further reassurance for her. Only in this circumstance can a non-diagnostic aspirate (C1) be accepted without the need for repeating the needle cytology.

The importance of a second clinical examination at a different phase of the menstrual cycle is emphasized, as on occasion it can be difficult to decide whether a dominant or discrete lump is present or not, particularly in dense younger breasts.

Greater significance should be attributed to a change noted by the patient, which is difficult to palpate, than to a change observed by the referring doctor, which the patient is unable to feel.

The clinical features of a benign breast lump are a smooth, spherical, tense or firm, tender mass, with no associated skin dimpling, and with a clear margin, which is mobile and not fixed. This is in contrast to the clinical features of a carcinoma, which tends to be an ill-defined dominant mass. The mass may have associated nipple retraction, skin dimpling, *peau d'orange*, skin discoloration and erythema. The mass will be non-tender and firm to hard, with poorly defined margins, immobility and sometimes fixity. Lesions less than 1 cm in diameter are difficult to palpate.

EXAMINATION TECHNIQUE

The patient must be adequately exposed and free of clothing to the waist. They are first examined in the sitting position and then in the supine position. It is useful to ask the patient to indicate the position of the lump.

Inspection

This is undertaken in four positions, firstly with the patient sitting straight up, secondly with the patient placing the arms above and behind the head, and thirdly with the arms above and behind the head while the patient leans forwards so that the breast should move off the chest wall. Finally, the patient is asked to place her hands on her hips, pressing in firmly and thereby contracting the pectoralis major muscle to which the suspensory ligaments of the breast are attached; this manoeuvre may make a lump more prominent. Lumps often may not be visible in the supine position, but may only be drawn into prominence with the patient sitting and with the arms above the head.

The features to note on inspection are asymmetry, scars, alteration in contour, distortion by a mass, accessory nipples, skin retraction and dimpling, *peau d'orange*, skin discoloration and nodules. Changes in the nipple such as retraction, ulceration, eczema and discharge are noted, as are prominent Montgomery's follicles. A cord-like thickening over the anterior lateral part of the chest wall and breast may signify underlying superficial vein thrombophlebitis (Mondor's disease).

Palpation

This should be undertaken on the unaffected side first to establish the normal texture and nodularity of the breast for the individual patient. It is undertaken initially in the supine position with the arm behind the head and the shoulder slightly forwards, so that the breast lies flat on the chest wall. This enables a lump to become apparent as it is palpated between the flat of the outstretched fingers and the underlying chest wall. Following full examination in the supine position on both sides, the patient is examined in a sitting position, both palpating against the chest wall and also palpating bimanually.

Palpation is undertaken with the flat of the hand using the palmar surfaces of the outstretched fingers. The whole breast, including the axillary tail and the central nipple areolar complex, must be examined. The most reliable way of examining all areas is to do this in strips both vertically and horizontally, usually divided into three strips in both directions. If the tips of the fingers are used to examine the breast, it is much easier to mistake a fatty lobule or glandular tissue for an abnormal lump, and this is a common problem in breast self-examination. If a lump is discovered, all of the usual physical characteristics of the lump should be described. Deep fixation should also be tested by contracting the pectoralis major whilst palpating. An attempt to elicit any discharge should be made and the characteristics noted.

The examination is completed by a careful examination of both axillae in the pectoral, posterior, anterior, central and apical regions, and the supraclavicular fossae. A general examination for evidence of metastatic disease should include assessment of the head and neck for anaemia and jaundice, examination for bone pain (particularly over the vertebrae), and examination of the chest and the abdomen for hepatomegaly and ascites.

The clinical assessment should be concluded by creating a detailed medical record, including a diagram such as that shown in Figure 20.4.4. Such a written record is of increasing medico-legal importance.

IMAGING OF THE BREAST

MAMMOGRAPHY

Mammography is performed by compressing the breast between two perspex paddles in both the oblique and the cranio-caudal position while X-rays are taken. It is important that all of the breast is included on the X-ray. Mammography is less useful in patients under 35 years of age because dense fibroglandular breast tissue may obscure underlying pathology. However, mammography in all age groups should be undertaken if clinical or ultrasonographic findings are suspicious or malignant. The changes of involution of increasing fat and decreasing fibroglandular tissue result in an increased resolution and accuracy of mammography with ageing. For this reason, the target population for screening by mammography is the 50–70 years age group in particular. A detailed request form should be provided to the radiologist so that the most appropriate targeted images of a suspected area of pathology can be undertaken. This is why diagnostic mammograms are considered different to screening mammograms, in which standard two-view films are taken in the first instance only. For diagnosis, coned compression magnification views of abnormalities such as asymmetrical involution tend to compress away, whereas significant underlying lesions such as stellate carcinomas become more prominent. Mammography must always be undertaken even if clinical examination shows that a carcinoma of the breast is obvious. This is to detect associated ductal carcinoma *in situ*, multifocality, a tumour in the other breast, and to serve as a baseline for follow-up examinations. Mammography underestimates the extent of DCIS, but none the less helps to plan the extent of surgery required. Mammograms should ideally be discussed with a radiologist prior to planning biopsies and surgery, and in particular it should be realized that needle localization biopsy can only be undertaken if the lesion can be seen in two views, whereas a stereotactic core biopsy can usually be undertaken if the lesion is seen in one view only.

ULTRASONOGRAPHY

Ultrasonography is especially useful for patients under 35 years of age, during pregnancy and lactation, and for women with severe mastalgia, where compression between the paddles of the mammogram machine is poorly tolerated. It is particularly useful to elucidate whether a mass is cystic or solid, and to measure accurately the size of a mass. It may be used to obtain a fine-needle aspirate for cytology or a core biopsy for histology of an ultrasound-identified lesion, and it may also be used to localize impalpable disease for needle localization biopsy. It is particularly useful for doubtful clinical lesions in determining whether or not an underlying lump is present. Ultrasound examination is not useful for diagnosing occult cancers and, as such, ultrasound is not a useful screening investigation. Furthermore, not all carcinomas will be visible clinically, mammographically or ultrasonographically, the typical example of this being a lobular carcinoma, which tends to be diagnosed late by all modalities because it does not initially form a mass. It is essential that if a known lump which is clinically present cannot be seen on mammography and ultrasound, then this should not deter the clinician from going ahead with the appropriate biopsy to establish its nature. More recent techniques of breast imaging, such as magnetic resonance imaging and PET scanning, are currently undergoing further evaluation.

BIOPSY OF THE BREAST

FINE-NEEDLE ASPIRATION CYTOLOGY

This technique is safe, simple, inexpensive, easily mastered, and increasingly widely used and available. It has a high degree of accuracy and, when combined with

CLINICAL FEATURES:

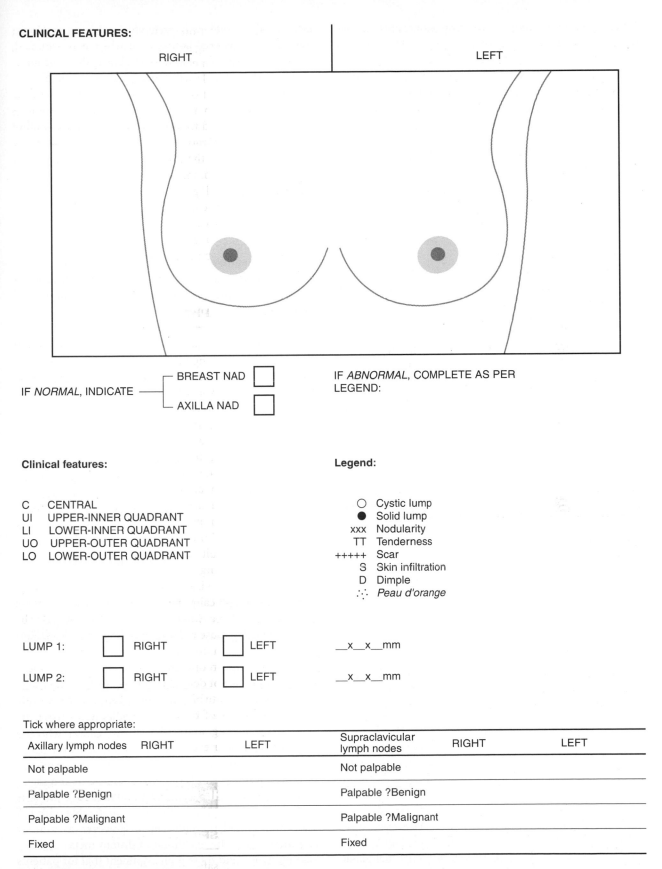

RIGHT   LEFT

IF *NORMAL*, INDICATE — ⌐ BREAST NAD ☐

⌐ AXILLA NAD ☐

IF *ABNORMAL*, COMPLETE AS PER LEGEND:

Clinical features:

C   CENTRAL
UI   UPPER-INNER QUADRANT
LI   LOWER-INNER QUADRANT
UO   UPPER-OUTER QUADRANT
LO   LOWER-OUTER QUADRANT

Legend:

○ Cystic lump
● Solid lump
xxx Nodularity
TT Tenderness
+++++ Scar
S Skin infiltration
D Dimple
∴. *Peau d'orange*

LUMP 1:   ☐ RIGHT   ☐ LEFT   __x__x__mm

LUMP 2:   ☐ RIGHT   ☐ LEFT   __x__x__mm

Tick where appropriate:

Axillary lymph nodes	RIGHT	LEFT	Supraclavicular lymph nodes	RIGHT	LEFT
Not palpable			Not palpable		
Palpable ?Benign			Palpable ?Benign		
Palpable ?Malignant			Palpable ?Malignant		
Fixed			Fixed		

Figure 20.4.4 Record of breast examination.

clinical, mammographic and ultrasonographic assessment, it has an accuracy approaching 100% for mass lesions. The result of a cytology can be classified from C1 to C5 as shown in Box 20.4.4. Fine-needle cytology may be performed on a clinically palpable lesion or on an ultrasound or mammographically detectable lesion.

BOX 20.4.4 CLASSIFICATION OF BREAST CYTOLOGY

CI Acellular aspirate or fibro-fatty tissue, but no diagnostic epithelial cells
C2 Benign ductal epithelial cells
C3 Probably benign, but some atypical features
C4 Suspicious epithelial cells
C5 Malignant epithelial cells

The technique for a clinically palpable lesion is to immobilize the lump between the index and middle fingers of the non-dominant hand. Local anaesthetic is not necessary. A 10-mL syringe and a 21-G needle are used, and after applying an alcohol skin swab to prepare the skin, the needle is inserted into the lump. Negative pressure is created on the syringe, and multiple quick stabbing passes are made with the needle through the lump whilst maintaining negative pressure. Up to 10 passes are made. Suction is released and then, prior to removing the needle from the lump, the syringe is disconnected from the needle and the needle is then removed. Air is subsequently drawn up into the syringe, and the contents within the needle are then squirted on to a glass slide and a cytological smear is prepared. One slide is air-dried (this is particularly useful for cytoplasmic detail) and one slide is fixed (this is particularly useful for nuclear detail). Complications are rare, and firm pressure should be applied following withdrawal of the needle to avoid haematoma formation.

A C1 result is satisfactory as a random sample from a thickened area, but should not be accepted as a benign diagnosis if a discrete solid lump is present. This is an indication to repeat the aspirate. A C5 diagnosis is sufficient to proceed to definitive surgery, and pre-operative triple assessment enables a definitive diagnosis of breast cancer to be made prior to surgery in most cases. This has the advantage of allowing an informed discussion and consideration of treatment options with the patient, who can be involved in decision-making and also involve others prior to surgery. It is possible to assess oestrogen and progesterone receptor status on cytological material using the immunocytochemical assay technique. However, it is important to realize that a cytological rather than a histological diagnosis is obtained. Therefore, whilst malignant cells are seen it is not possible to tell whether they are from an *in-situ* or an invasive cancer purely on the basis of the cytological aspirate. It is preferable to have a cytologist examine the material at the time when it is aspirated, whether this is performed free-hand or with image guidance to ensure that the specimen is adequate for diagnosis. This also increases the likelihood of an accurate triple assessment following one clinic visit. With the diagnosis achieved after one visit, treatment, planning and any other pre-operative investigations can be undertaken, and the open biopsy rate is reduced.

CORE BIOPSY

A core biopsy will obtain a core of tissue which allows both a histological diagnosis and assessment of invasion, as well as identifying malignant cells. It may be undertaken by a Trucut core biopsy device (which requires both hands of the operator) or by various commercial automated guns (which can be fired with one hand alone). Local anaesthetic is required for use of the technique, but this is well tolerated. It may be performed free-hand or under image guidance both by ultrasound and stereotactically mammographically. It is preferable to use a 14-G core instrument, as smaller cores tend to make diagnosis more difficult and less reliable.

OPEN BIOPSY

Occasionally, fine-needle aspirates for cytology and core biopsies will fail to establish an adequate diagnosis, and open biopsy is then required. Usually this should be excisional biopsy, but the number of patients requiring open biopsy (whether performed on a palpable lesion or needle-localized biopsy) is steadily decreasing.

PRE-OPERATIVE STAGING FOR PATIENTS WITH CARCINOMA OF THE BREAST

Routine investigation for all patients who are to undergo surgery for breast cancer includes serum urea, creatinine and electrolytes, full blood examination, a chest X-ray and liver function tests. Multiple studies have repeatedly shown that patients with early breast cancer who are asymptomatic do not benefit from bone and liver scans, as the yield from these investigations is minimal. However, if bone pain is present, a bone scan and skeletal X-ray should be undertaken, and if liver function tests are abnormal, imaging of the liver (preferably with CT scanning) should be undertaken. However, as tumour size increases so the likelihood of distant metastatic disease increases, and there is an argument that for patients with stage-3 tumours who are to undergo surgery it is reasonable to perform bone scanning and liver imaging.

PATHOLOGY

SPECIMEN HANDLING AND THE REQUEST FORM

The major factor associated with local recurrence is incomplete surgical excision or close surgical margins. Consequently, accurate assessment of surgical margins by the pathologist is essential to determine whether re-excision is necessary. This is only possible if the excised breast specimen is sent appropriately orientated and labelled with explanatory notations and a detailed request form to the pathologist, who is aware of in-house established methods of orientation. Several methods of orientating specimens are available, including the use of clips and sutures. A combination of sutures, such that a long suture is placed laterally, a short suture is placed superiorly and a medium suture is placed medially, orientates the specimen appropriately. It is then useful to suture the specimen to a sheet of sterile paper and to label this in indelible ink with a detailed notation of the site in the breast and an explanation of the specimen and the margins. The expectation is then for the pathologist to measure the margins macroscopically and microscopically in six dimensions. This specimen labelling and orientation should be performed for all complete and wide local excision specimens, for mastectomy specimens, and the axillary contents should also be labelled. It is of prognostic value to know whether the apical axillary node is involved with carcinoma, and therefore a suture applied to the apex of the axillary contents enables the pathologist to determine this. The specimen should be sent fresh to pathology. The request form should be detailed and should routinely include a request for oestrogen and progesterone receptor analysis.

All needle-localized biopsy specimens should be submitted to specimen radiography and two copies of the X-ray taken (one to be sent to the pathologist with explanatory notations, so that the correct area of the needle-localized biopsy specimen can be examined histologically). If feasible, it is ideal for all wide excisions of breast cancer specimens to undergo specimen radiography, as this is helpful in determining whether clear margins are likely to be achieved. It is not appropriate to perform a frozen section on mammographically detected impalpable lesions.

PATHOLOGY REPORT

A detailed pathology report is required to determine prognosis, and for all of the parameters discussed in this section, a positive or negative statement with regard to their presence or absence should be made. The report should include a description of the type of surgical specimen (e.g. mastectomy or a wide local excision specimen) and a macroscopic description of the specimen. The size in three dimensions in millimetres should be stated. The histological subtype and grade of the tumour according to the Elston modification of the Bloom and Richardson classification should be recorded. Grade is determined by mitoses, tubule formation and nuclear pleomorphism. Evidence of skin and nipple involvement should be noted where appropriate. The margins should be recorded in six dimensions in millimetres both macroscopically and microscopically. A separate statement should be made as to whether the margin is clear or not, and if it is not clear which of the six margins is involved. Multifocality should be recorded, and is defined as two areas of breast cancer greater than or equal to 20 mm apart. Ductal carcinoma *in situ* both within the tumour and surrounding it should be noted, together with its type and grade. It should also be noted whether extensive *in-situ* carcinoma is present, as this correlates with local recurrence. Invasion of lymphatics, vascular structures and perineural invasion should be noted. Evidence of necrosis and inflammation should also be documented. Associated pathology in the breast should be noted, particularly lobular carcinoma *in situ*, atypical ductal hyperplasia and atypical lobular hyperplasia. The presence or absence of histological evidence of calcification should be noted.

The axillary specimen should be described macroscopically, and as a minimum the total number of lymph nodes examined histologically should be noted. The number of involved lymph nodes with carcinoma should be recorded, together with the status of the apical node. The extent of the involvement should be documented, whether this is a solitary focus of subcapsular involvement or total replacement of the node, and also extranodal spread. A comment should be included in the initial report that tissue has been sent for oestrogen and progesterone receptor analysis.

BREAST CANCER HISTOLOGICAL SUBTYPES

It is difficult to determine whether the cell of origin of breast cancer is from the ductal or lobular elements of the terminal ductal lobular unit, and the classification of tumour histology indicated in Box 20.4.5 is therefore descriptive rather than histogenetic. The commonest histological type is invasive ductal carcinoma of no special type (NST) or not otherwise specified (NOS). The special subtypes collectively account for approximately 10% of all breast carcinomas, and have a better prognosis than invasive ductal carcinoma (NOS).

BOX 24.4.5 CLASSIFICATION OF HISTOLOGICAL SUBTYPES OF INVASIVE BREAST CANCER

Invasive ductal carcinoma not otherwise specified (≥ 80%) or no special type

Invasive ductal carcinoma with predominant ductal carcinoma in situ (DCIS)

Invasive lobular carcinoma

Mixed invasive ductal and lobular carcinoma

Mucoid or mucinous carcinoma

Medullary carcinoma

Well-differentiated tubular carcinoma

Cribriform carcinoma

Squamous-cell carcinoma

Adenoid cystic carcinoma

Papillary carcinoma

Secretory carcinoma

Paget's disease

STAGING OF BREAST CANCER

This is necessary in order that precise details of an individual breast cancer can be recorded and therefore comparisons made in clinical trials and treatment outcomes.

The TNM classification is detailed in Box 20.4.6, and is correlated with the Manchester staging system in Table 20.4.3.

Table 20.4.3 Correlation between TNM and Manchester staging systems

TNM staging system	Manchester staging system
T0–T2 N0	Stage I
T1, T2 N1	Stage II
T3, T4 N2, N3	Stage III
M1	Stage IV

TREATMENT OF EARLY BREAST CANCER

SURGERY

The aims of treatment of early breast cancer are to achieve local control, to stage the patient accurately and achieve a diagnosis, and therefore to enable a prognosis

BOX 20.4.6 THE UICC–TNM CLASSIFICATION OF BREAST CANCER (5TH REVISION, 1997)

Primary tumour = T

Tx Not assessable

T0 No primary tumour

TIS Carcinoma in situ

Ti < 2 cm in diameter

   T1a < 0.5 cm in diameter

   T1b 0.6–1 cm in diameter

   T1c 1.1–2 cm in diameter

T2 > 2 cm, < 5 cm in diameter

T3 > 5 cm in diameter

T4 Any size with chest wall or skin extension

   T4a Chest wall

   T4b Oedema/ulceration/nodules

   T4c Both 4a and 4b

   T4d Inflammatory cancer

Nodes = N

Nx Not assessable

N0 No nodal metastases

N1 Ipsilateral axillary, mobile

N2 Ipsilateral axillary, fixed

N3 Ipsilateral internal mammary nodes

Distant metastases = M

(includes supraclavicular nodes)

Mx Not assessable

M0 No distant metastases

M1 Distant metastases present

to be given to the patient. Decisions can then be made on the basis of this histological information about adjuvant therapy and entry into clinical trials. When breast conservation is utilized, the aim should be to achieve cosmesis, and following mastectomy the aim should be reconstruction to preserve body image. Where preoperative triple assessment establishes a pre-operative diagnosis, one-stage surgery should be the aim. For some early and/or small breast cancers, ductal carcinoma in situ and minimally invasive cancer, cure may be achieved by local treatment.

It is now well established that breast conservation is a safe option for the treatment for breast cancer, and results in equivalent survival rates to treatment of early breast cancer by mastectomy. Breast conservation is achieved by wide local excision of the tumour with clear histological margins, axillary dissection and post-operative radiotherapy to the breast. Omission of post-operative radiotherapy to the breast results in higher rates of local recurrence, and therefore it should be part of the standard treatment of breast conservation. The latter should be offered as the preferred treatment to most women with early breast cancer, and in a symptomatic population the rate of breast conservation will be of the order of 50%, while in a screened population it will be of the order of 70%.

The alternative treatment is total mastectomy and axillary clearance. This will be necessary for patients with multifocal tumours, where margins are involved despite re-excision, where the tumour is large in relationship to the size of the breast, or where it is greater than 4 cm in diameter. Extensive *in-situ* breast cancer or proven invasive breast cancer with extensive microcalcification mammographically over more than one quadrant is also a relative indication for mastectomy. A previous high dose of radiation given to the area (e.g. for Hodgkin's disease) is a relative contraindication to breast conservation. Scleroderma because of the associated vasculitis and reduced cosmesis following radiotherapy is a relative indication for mastectomy. A central tumour or a tumour involving the nipple can be treated by wide local excision, but some would also regard it as a relative contraindication to conservation. The ability to undertake radiotherapy must be established prior to breast conservation being planned, and in remote parts of Australia may influence the decision towards mastectomy. Finally, patient choice may dictate one or other treatment.

The incidence of local recurrence following breast conservation is approximately 1% per year, whereas the incidence of local recurrence following mastectomy is approximately 0.5% per year, but the survival rates are equivalent.

Axillary dissection treats potential metastatic disease in the axilla, enables a prognosis to be established, and provides the necessary information for decisions to be made about adjuvant therapy. It is performed either in continuity with a total mastectomy or through a separate transverse incision as part of breast conservation. A level-2 radical axillary dissection is usually undertaken, and this includes the nodes below and also behind the pectoralis minor. Axillary sampling is not recommended. Post-operative radiotherapy to the axilla is not recommended, as this significantly increases the risk of lymphoedema.

If mastectomy is undertaken, breast reconstruction should be offered and the advantages and disadvantages of immediate or delayed reconstruction, and the various types available, discussed in detail with the patient.

Pre-operative discussions about treatment options are preferably undertaken while a support person is present with the patient, and also with a breast nurse counsellor present. Treatment options and choices must be provided both verbally and in written form.

Treatment planning is ideally undertaken with a multidisciplinary approach, including a surgeon, radiation oncologist, medical oncologist, plastic surgeon and breast nurse counsellor to plan the most appropriate treatment for the individual tumour in the patient.

ADJUVANT CHEMOTHERAPY AND HORMONAL MANIPULATION

The current biological model of breast cancer suggests that micrometastases occur at an early stage and may lie dormant for varying periods of time, up to many years. The purpose of adjuvant chemotherapy and hormonal manipulation is to reduce the micrometastatic burden following initial treatment of the early breast cancer, and thereby to improve survival. Meta-analyses have shown that combination chemotherapy, tamoxifen or ovarian ablation (in those under 50 years of age) significantly reduce the risk of recurrence and death from breast cancer in both node-positive and node-negative breast cancer patients. Accordingly, adjuvant chemotherapy and/or hormonal manipulation should be offered routinely as a treatment option for most women with early breast cancer.

RADIOTHERAPY FOLLOWING MASTECTOMY

Radiotherapy to the chest wall flaps may be indicated following mastectomy if the tumour is large or high grade, or extensive lymphatic, vascular or neural invasion has been detected histologically.

PROGNOSTIC FACTORS FOR BREAST CANCER

The two most important prognostic factors for breast cancer are involvement of axillary lymph nodes and the size of the primary tumour. With increasing involvement of lymph nodes and increasing size of the primary tumour, the prognosis worsens. Other prognostic factors of importance include the grade, lymphovascular invasion, S-phase fraction, KI/67 staining, epidermal growth factor receptor, oestrogen receptor, progesterone receptor and histological subtype.

For an individual patient, assessment of all of these prognostic factors is often of more importance than placement within a category in the TNM or Manchester staging system.

FOLLOW-UP OF EARLY BREAST CANCER PATIENTS

Regular clinical examination and annual mammography should be undertaken for all breast cancer patients. It has been repeatedly shown that there is no survival benefit for the routine use of bone scans, chest X-rays, liver imaging or blood tests in the follow-up of asymptomatic patients. However, if patients develop specific symptoms they should be thoroughly investigated.

FURTHER READING

Anonymous. 1995: Guidelines for surgeons in the management of symptomatic breast disease in the United Kingdom. *European Journal of Surgical Oncology* **21** (Suppl. A), 1–13.

Bilimoria ML, Morrow M. 1995: The woman at increased risk for breast cancer: evaluation and management strategies. *Cancer. A Cancer Journal for Clinicians* **45**, 263–78.

Collins JP, Simpson JS. 1998: Guidelines for the surgical management of breast cancer. *Australian and New Zealand Journal of Surgery* **68** (Suppl.), 1–28.

Early Breast Cancer Trialists' Collaborative Group. 1992: Systemic treatment of breast cancer by hormonal, cytotoxic or immune therapy: 133 randomised trials involving 31 000 recurrences and 24 000 deaths among 75 000 women. *Lancet* **339**, 1–15, 71–85.

Fisher B, Anderson S, Redmond CK *et al.* 1995: Reanalysis and results after 12 years of follow-up in a randomised clinical trial comparing total mastectomy with lumpectomy with or without radiation therapy in the treatment of breast cancer. *New England Journal of Medicine* **333**, 1456–61.

Giard RW, Herman J. 1992: The value of aspiration cytologic examination of the breast. A statistical review of the medical literature. *Cancer* **69**, 2104–10.

Hughes LE, Mansel RE, Webster DJT. 1989: Aberrations of normal development and involution (ANDI): concept of benign breast disorders based on pathogenesis. In Hughes LE, Mansel RE, Webster DJT (eds). *Benign disorders and diseases of the breast: concepts and clinical management.* London: Baillière Tindall, 15–25.

International Union Against Cancer. 1997: *TNM classification of malignant tumours*, 5th edn. New York: John Wiley Inc. Publications.

National Health and Medical Research Council. 1995: *Clinical practice guidelines. The management of early breast cancer.* Eastwood, NSW: The Stone Press.

Abdominal lumps

Jonathan W. Serpell and Anthony J. Buzzard

Introduction

The presentation of an abdominal lump (mass) is a common manifestation of intra-abdominal pathology. This chapter describes the clinical features, investigation and diagnosis of a patient with an abdominal lump. However, because of the great diversity of pathologies, treatment is not considered. It is assumed that the patient is known to have an abdominal lump prior to their clinical assessment. This enables an appropriate problem-orientated clinical approach. Often, however, an abdominal mass is noted as an incidental finding on clinical examination, and the patient has been unaware of its presence. At the other end of the clinical spectrum an increasing amount of surgical practice is spent investigating vague abdominal symptoms and endeavouring to exclude significant pathology such as the presence of an abdominal mass.

HISTORY

The history of the presenting complaint must be thoroughly explored. This includes how the lump was noted, the length of time for which the lump has been present, any change in size, pain in the lump, factors producing an alteration in size of the lump, and any other features associated with it.

Even at the stage of initial exploration of the presenting complaint of an abdominal lump, the clinician will be considering the possible differential diagnoses. With increased experience he or she will become more adept at this, and at all times it is important to be mindful of the need to change or reconsider the diagnosis. It is essential that at the conclusion of the clinical assessment the clinician formulates a working diagnosis which subsequent investigations will support or refute.

Systematic questioning enables the clinician to elicit unpresented symptoms of which the patient may be unaware. For example, if the abdominal lump is an abdominal aortic aneurysm, during systematic questioning other historical features of vascular disease may be obtained. For many abdominal masses a detailed gastroenterological history is required, and it will be important to pay particular attention to appetite, weight change, indigestion, abdominal pain and its characterization, bowel habit, rectal bleeding and history of jaundice.

A past history of abdominal malignancy or other malignancies which may have spread to the abdomen causing hepatomegaly, an omental mass, or ovarian or adrenal metastases must be sought. Previous abdominal surgery may be crucial (e.g. a biliary stricture with portal hypertension resulting in splenomegaly as the underlying cause of a presenting left upper quadrant abdominal mass). A history of liver disease, or any other history of abdominal pathology, such as Crohn's disease or diverticular disease, which could, for example, produce a phlegmon or abscess, must be noted.

A family history of certain conditions (e.g. colorectal cancer, neurofibromatosis, familial polycystic kidney disease and familial adenomatous polyposis) may be of significance to an abdominal mass. A family history of haematological conditions (e.g. hereditary spherocytosis), may explain underlying splenomegaly.

A drug history may provide the clue to the underlying pathological process. Examples include chemotherapy resulting in phlegmonous caecitis and a right iliac fossa mass, and methysergide resulting in retroperitoneal fibrosis and hydronephrosis producing a renal mass.

Occupation may be of relevance, such as exposure to hydatid disease or amoebiasis, both of which may cause hepatomegaly. A further example is asbestos exposure, which can produce mesothelioma.

CLINICAL EXAMINATION OF THE PATIENT

ABDOMINAL EXAMINATION

Apart from the general examination, specific examination of the abdomen to elucidate the nature of the abdominal lump must always follow a standard pattern.

Specifically excluded from this discussion are the causes of generalized abdominal distension which are considered elsewhere under the heading of abdominal swellings. These include pregnancy, obesity, ascites, the flatus and fluid of a bowel obstruction, generalized gaseous distension of the stomach, small and large bowel (tympanites), generalized faecal loading (e.g. in megacolon) and, rarely, a massive tumour (e.g. an ovarian cyst) filling the whole abdomen. Occasionally, other intra-abdominal tumours which normally produce a localized mass may present as generalized abdominal distension due to the large size of the mass. Examples include retroperitoneal soft-tissue sarcoma, lymphoma, massive bladder distension, massive splenomegaly and fibroids.

INSPECTION

Inspection of the abdomen for abdominal scars, generalized or localized abdominal distension, dilated subcutaneous veins, visible peristalsis and abnormalities of the umbilicus is routine. The lump itself may be visible and, if so, it may be visibly pulsatile.

There may be discoloration of the abdominal wall, such as peri-umbilical bruising (Cullen's sign, an umbilical black eye, a late sign of intra-abdominal haemorrhage) or discoloration in the flank (Grey-Turner's sign, which may suggest a pancreatic phlegmon as the cause of the abdominal mass). There may be a visible umbilical secondary cancer nodule or discharge, or there may be an obvious abdominal wall lump and, if so, the patient should be asked to cough in order to assess whether it changes and therefore whether a hernia is suggested.

There may be abnormal hair distribution (e.g. loss of the male hair distribution seen in cirrhosis of the liver). The patient should always be asked to cough and raise the head from the bed to allow assessment for abdominal wall herniae, which may become apparent with this manoeuvre before palpation is undertaken.

PALPATION

Palpation of the abdomen should follow a standard pattern. Light palpation is undertaken in the first instance to ascertain whether or not there is any local or generalized tenderness and/or guarding. Deeper palpation is undertaken next to explore for masses and deep tenderness. It is usually prudent to commence abdominal palpation away from any expected area of tenderness. Palpation for specific organs and their enlargement is then undertaken, using a standard technique to ascertain whether or not these are the source of the presenting abdominal lump, or whether these organs are affected by the presenting lump. The liver, spleen and kidneys are therefore routinely palpated for.

At this stage of the clinical examination the presenting abdominal lump is specifically examined.

The clinician must be conversant with normal intra-abdominal structures which may be mistaken for intra-abdominal pathologies. These are learned by clinical experience. Examples include the caecum (particularly if it contains much faecal material) and the sigmoid colon (which in a constipated patient may contain multiple masses in the line of the colon which have the distinguishing feature of being mobile, multiple and indentable). Tendinous intersections in the rectus abdominus, particularly in the upper abdomen on the right side, may produce the apparent impression of a right upper quadrant abdominal mass. Occasionally, the lower poles of the right and left kidney are palpable, especially in aesthenic patients and if the diaphragm is ptosed. The normal liver is very rarely palpable, but is occasionally so in emphysematous patients or if it is ptosed due to a sub-diaphragmatic lesion.

The site of the lump is determined first. It can be determined whether or not it is within the abdomen or within the abdominal wall simply by tensing the abdominal wall musculature. This can be achieved by asking the patient either to lift their head from the examining couch, or to raise their legs from the examining couch while the lump is being examined. If the tensed abdominal wall musculature appears to hide the lump, it is intra-abdominal, whereas an abdominal wall lump will become more obvious with this manoeuvre. The regional site of the lump is described according to the nine anatomical regions illustrated in Figure 20.5.1. There is no precise delineation of abdominal areas.

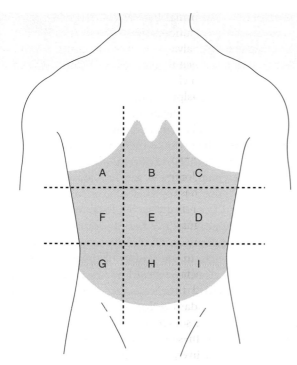

Figure 20.5.1 Anatomical regions of the abdomen. A, right hypochondrium; B, epigastrium; C, left hypochondrium; D, left flank or lumbar; E, umbilical; F, right flank or lumbar; G, right iliac fossa; H, hypogastrium or suprapubic; I, left iliac fossa.

Rather, abdominal lumps are described as being in a certain area if they best fit into that area. The region will determine the range of possible differential diagnoses of the mass.

The usual physical characteristics of any mass are then assessed. The size of the lump is measured, and the clinician must remember that the lump is being felt through the thickness of the abdominal wall, which will cause the lump to appear larger than its true size. Thus accurate measurement is clinically unreliable. For this reason, measurement in finger-breadths and hand-spans rather than centimetres is recommended. The shape of the lump may suggest its origin. For example, a fusiform lump suggests a lesion arising from a longitudinal organ, whereas a rounded lump suggests a neoplasm, cyst or inflammatory mass. Typically gall bladder, splenic and renal masses tend to feel like their native organ of origin. If the surface of the lump is craggy and irregular, this suggests a malignant tumour, in contrast to a smooth lump, which suggests a benign expanding lesion such as a cyst. The consistency is assessed. If the lump is fluctuant, this is indicative of it being fluid filled, whereas if it is indentable this is indicative of it being faecal. A hard lump suggests malignancy. If it is sufficiently large, a fluid-filled mass will have a thrill, e.g. massive enlargement of the bladder or a massive ovarian cyst. Movement

with respiration suggests a relationship with the diaphragm. Fixity, as opposed to free mobility, suggests local invasion by pathological processes. However, a number of benign masses are characteristically fixed because of their anatomical situation (see below). Expansile pulsation of a mass suggests an aneurysm, whereas transmitted pulsation may be present in many masses, but particularly in retroperitoneal masses such as those arising from the pancreas. Hepatomegaly due to congestion from cardiac failure may have venous pulsation.

PERCUSSION AND AUSCULTATION

Percussion and auscultation must always be undertaken for completeness, but are of less value than a thorough history, inspection and palpation. Clinical characteristics of various masses may be determined in part by their percussion note, but in general this is not a very reliable sign. Auscultation for the presence or absence of bowel sounds and their quality and the presence of bruits should always be undertaken for completeness. However, their contribution to the overall clinical diagnostic process is limited.

INGUINO-SCROTAL EXAMINATION

An inguino-scrotal and groin examination is a crucial and routine part of any abdominal examination. In the context of an abdominal lump, the lump may be secondary to, for example, a testicular tumour (e.g. secondary lymph node deposits presenting as an epigastric mass). An empty hemi-scrotum may suggest that an intra-abdominal mass in the right iliac fossa could be due to malignancy in an undescended testis.

RECTAL EXAMINATION

Rectal examination is an essential part of any abdominal examination. An abdominal lump may be secondary to rectal pathology, e.g. rectal cancer may be palpable and cause hepatic metastases. There may be a palpable shelf of intraperitoneal tumour (Blumer's shelf) at the rectovesical and rectovaginal peritoneal reflection, which would be an indication of intra-abdominal malignancy. When extensive and associated with a fixed malignant pelvic mass, this constitutes a frozen pelvis. An intra-abdominal or pelvic mass may only become evident during a rectal examination. For example, a carcinoma of the sigmoid colon or a diverticular mass may only be palpable when it is felt through the rectal wall in the rectovesical pouch or pouch of Douglas. There may be bloodstained faeces on the examining glove, associated with a colorectal tumour. Bimanual examination of a pelvic mass may be possible. Sigmoidoscopy may be indicated at this stage as part of the clinical examination.

GENERAL EXAMINATION AND EXTRA-ABDOMINAL MANIFESTATIONS OF ABDOMINAL DISEASE

A thorough general physical examination is mandatory, and will provide many pointers to intra-abdominal pathology. The general state of the patient is noted, particularly temperature, pulse rate, respiratory rate, blood pressure and the state of hydration. The colour of the patient may show evidence of anaemia, plethora, jaundice, cyanosis or the yellow tinge of various anaemias. These features have obvious relevance to hepatobiliary conditions and haematological conditions which may be associated with splenomegaly. Pyrexia may be due to inflammatory masses, abscesses, or paraneoplastic processes such as carcinoma of the kidney, and is also commonly seen in cirrhosis and in patients with hepatoma. Generalized skin pigmentation is not uncommon in cirrhosis, but in particular is seen in haemochromatosis and the condition of acanthosis nigricans, which may indicate abdominal malignancy. The patient may appear cushingoid, which could be due to a secretory adrenocortical carcinoma. Hypertension is most likely to be essential. However, it is of relevance to aneurysmal disease, and may be secondary to renal disease or a phaeochromocytoma.

Examination of the head and neck may reveal features such as angular stomatitis, cheilitis, mouth ulceration and leukoplakia, which may reflect general nutritional status. Left-sided supraclavicular lymphadenopathy of a malignant nature (Virchow's node, Trosier's sign) may indicate intra-abdominal malignancy. Gynaecomastia may be idiopathic, but may also be secondary to chronic liver disease, a testicular tumour or an adrenal tumour. Extra-abdominal manifestations of chronic liver disease should always be sought, and should include palmar erythema, clubbing of the fingernails, spider naevi, loss of the male hair distribution, testicular atrophy, Dupuytren's contracture, ecchymosis, parotid enlargement and gynaecomastia. Portal hypertension may be manifested by dilated abdominal wall veins and a caput medusae. Evidence of generalized lymphadenopathy should be sought. Other features of haematological disease, such as purpura, bruises and ecchymoses, should be noted. The lower limbs are examined for features such as oedema (evidence of inferior vena caval obstruction, perhaps due to a retroperitoneal sarcoma), peripheral neuritis (which may be associated with alcoholic liver disease) and vascularity (which may be of relevance to abdominal aortic aneurysmal disease).

DESCRIPTION OF CHARACTERISTIC FEATURES OF ABDOMINAL MASSES AND ORGAN ENLARGEMENTS

Enlargement of specific organs is usually characteristic and is described in detail for each organ below. In general, organ enlargement may be due to diffuse enlargement of the organ or there may be a solitary mass lesion within an otherwise normal organ. Generally this causes enlargement of the organ in a focal sense, which may or may not be appreciable compared to diffuse enlargement. Occasionally such a focal mass lesion is so large that it appears to give the impression of enlarging the whole organ (e.g. a massive carcinoma of the kidney). Throughout, the causes of organ enlargement are therefore classified according to diffuse or focal enlargement and by their degree of importance and commonness. Rare conditions are listed, but are not described in any detail. Only conditions that a practising surgeon may expect to encounter are listed, and some rarities are deliberately excluded. It is therefore important to realize that these lists of causes are not exhaustive. Within each list the causes are generally ordered according to the pathological type of classification given in the overview of clinical approaches to lumps. Many of the conditions of hepatomegaly, splenomegaly and hepatosplenomegaly would traditionally be viewed as medical, but are also important for a surgeon to recognize. For example, a patient with breast cancer who has a slightly enlarged but definitely palpable liver will require investigation. It is necessary to understand the possible differential diagnoses and the methods of investigation in order to establish whether such a patient has secondary breast cancer in the liver, or whether the problem is due to one of the other common causes of hepatomegaly.

A simple clinical examination will establish whether a mass is within or superficial to the abdominal wall, or contained within the abdominal cavity. Abdominal wall masses can be categorized as follows:

1. *skin and subcutaneous masses* – lipomas, sebaceous cysts, neurofibroma, abscess, fat necrosis and lipodystrophy secondary to insulin;

2. *hernias* – epigastric, umbilical (true umbilical and para-umbilical), incisional, inguinal, femoral, and divarication of the recti;

3. *umbilical masses* – hernia, endometrioma, secondary metastasis (Sister Joseph's nodule);

4. *rectus sheath haematoma;*

5. *rare abdominal wall conditions* – desmoid tumours, endometrioma, soft-tissue sarcoma.

Organ enlargement and masses arising within each of

the nine regions of the abdomen will now be considered sequentially, commencing in the upper abdomen and working downwards.

Right hypochondrial masses are most often due to liver and gall bladder pathology, but other rare conditions may cause a mass in the right hypochondrium. These include the following:

1. liver masses;
2. gall bladder masses;
3. others:
   - carcinoma of the colon;
   - renal masses;
   - high retrocaecal appendiceal mass;
   - high ileocaecal Crohn's disease;
   - pyloric masses;
   - choledochal cyst;
   - primary adrenal carcinoma.

Masses in the left hypochondrium may be classified according to their organ of origin in a similar way to right hypochondrial masses:

1. stomach tumours;
2. carcinoma of the distal transverse colon;
3. left lobe liver masses;
4. splenic masses;
5. renal masses;
6. gastric distension due to pyloric outlet obstruction;
7. pancreatic masses;
8. primary adrenal carcinoma.

Gastric distension due to pyloric outlet obstruction may cause a diffuse fullness in the left hypochondrium and epigastrium, with visible gastric peristalsis and a succussion splash. Pancreatic masses will usually cause a swelling in the epigastrium, but may be a cause of left upper quadrant abdominal mass when they occur predominantly in the distal body and/or tail of the pancreas. In general, stomach tumours are rarely felt because much of the stomach lies beneath the lower rib-cage and costal margin. However, on occasion some stomach tumours do become palpable in the left upper quadrant.

The characteristics of a palpable gall bladder are that it is a smooth, rounded, globular gall bladder-like mass in the right hypochondrium. Usually only the fundus is felt, which may be tender. The mass moves downwards and forwards on inspiration, and will be dull to percussion. It can be distinguished from an enlarged liver when both are palpable, (e.g. in malignant obstructive jaundice of the distal biliary tree). The mass appears from beneath the tip of the right ninth rib in the transpyloric plane. A gall bladder mass tends to be characteristic, and with experience is recognized in the same way that one recognizes a friend's voice on the telephone without needing to analyse the features of the voice. The

gall bladder greets the examining fingers with an unmistakable feel. The causes of a palpable gall bladder are as follows:

1. obstruction of the biliary tree;
2. acute cholecystitis with a phlegmon;
3. mucocele;
4. empyema;
5. pericholecystic abscess;
6. carcinoma of the gall bladder;
7. massive gallstone;
8. torsion of the gall bladder.

Box 20.5.1 details the general classification of liver and spleen enlargements.

BOX 20.5.1 GENERAL CLASSIFICATION OF HEPATIC AND SPLENIC ENLARGEMENTS

1. **Hepatomegaly**
   - **1.1** Diffuse enlargement
   - **1.2** Solitary mass in the liver
   - **1.3** Causes of massive hepatomegaly

2. **Hepatosplenomegaly**

3. **Splenomegaly**
   - **3.1** Diffuse enlargement
   - **3.2** Solitary mass in the spleen
   - **3.3** Causes of massive splenomegaly

The causes of hepatosplenomegaly include many but not all of the causes of hepatomegaly and splenomegaly individually. However, it is important to understand the common and/or important causes of hepatosplenomegaly that occur.

The main clinical feature of hepatomegaly is a mass in the right hypochondrium which may extend across into the epigastrium or left upper quadrant, or on ocassion be felt in these areas only. It is an anteriorly situated mass within the abdomen, and one cannot get above the mass under the costal margin. The mass moves down on inspiration, and tends to be smooth with a liver-like, well-defined inferior border which is felt as an edge. It is dull to percussion, and this dullness is continuous with the normal liver dullness under the lower rib-cage. A massive liver enlargement may be bimanually palpable, but it is not ballottable. Having determined that the mass is due to liver enlargement, it is then necessary to decide whether it is smooth diffuse enlargement or a nodular enlargement. The causes of diffuse hepatomegaly are listed in Box 20.5.2.

Cirrhosis of the liver is characterized in the early stages by enlargement of the liver, which may be micro- or macronodular in nature, but later because of increasing fibrosis and contracture the liver may become

---

BOX 20.5.2 CAUSES OF DIFFUSE HEPATOMEGALY

Inflammatory
Infective
 Viral Hepatitis A, B and C
    Infectious mononucleosis
    Cytomegalovirus
    HIV infection
 Bacterial Ascending cholangitis, multiple liver
    abscesses, pylephlebitis
 Protozoal Malaria
Alcohol
 Fatty infiltration
 Alcoholic hepatitis
Chronic active hepatitis
Collagen-vascular disease (e.g. systemic lupus
erythematosus)

Growth disorders
 Cirrhosis
 Multiple nodular hyperplasia

Neoplastic causes
 Secondary malignancy
  Carcinoma
  Melanoma
  Sarcoma
  Carcinoid
 Primary malignancy
  Hepatocellular carcinoma
  Cholangiocarcinoma

Bile duct obstruction
 e.g. Obstructive jaundice due to carcinoma of the head
 of the pancreas

Haematological causes
 Hodgkin's and non-Hodgkin's lymphoma
 Chronic leukaemia
  Chronic myeloid leukaemia
  Chronic lymphatic leukaemia
 Myelofibrosis
 Anaemias

Infiltrations
 Fat
  Alcohol
  Diabetes mellitus
 Others
  Amyloid
  Lipid and glycogen storage diseases

Vascular causes
 Suprahepatic portal hypertension
 Congestive cardiac failure
 Tricuspid valve disease
 Constrictive pericarditis
 Hepatic vein thrombosis, Budd-Chiari syndrome

Cystic disease
 Polycystic liver
 Multiple or single solitary large hydatid disease

---

impalpable. The causes of cirrhosis of the liver include alcohol, cryptogenic causes, primary and secondary biliary cirrhosis, cardiac cirrhosis, Wilson's disease, haemochromatosis and post-hepatitic cirrhosis, as well as rarer causes.

The causes of hepatomegaly due to a solitary mass in the liver are listed in Box 20.5.3.

Reidel's lobe is a normal anatomical variant of the liver in which the normal liver extends down as a tongue in the anterior axillary line from the right costal margin. Hepatic-cell adenoma and focal nodular hyperplasia are both usually solitary. The adenoma is a true neoplasm and may become malignant. It is associated with the oral contraceptive pill, and may spontaneously rupture and bleed. Focal nodular hyperplasia is not neoplastic, and may regress after cessation of the oral contraceptive pill. Cavernous haemangiomas are only rarely palpable, and are usually discovered incidentally at the time of operation. Because of their nature, they should not be biopsied intra-operatively. The causes of massive hepatomegaly are as follows:

1. multiple metastases;
2. alcoholic fatty infiltration;
3. hepatocellular carcinoma;
4. chronic myeloid leukaemia;
5. myelofibrosis;
6. congestive cardiac failure.

The features of splenomegaly are a mass in the left hypochondrium, emerging from beneath the costal margin in the line of the tenth rib. It is not possible to get between the mass and the costal margin. The mass is anteriorly situated in the abdomen, and whilst one can insert the examining finger behind the mass, this is not possible in a renal mass. The mass moves downwards, medially and forwards on inspiration. It has a well-defined medial border in which a notch may be felt. It is dull to percussion, and the dullness is continuous with the normal splenic dullness. It is sometimes better felt with the patient slightly rolled to the right side. Like a liver mass, it may be bimanually palpable, but it is not ballottable. It is firm, smooth and splenic-

BOX 20.5.3 CAUSES OF HEPATOMEGALY DUE TO A SOLITARY MASS IN THE LIVER

Congenital causes
Riedel's lobe

Traumatic causes
Solitary cyst

Inflammatory causes
Liver abscess
Bacterial
Amoebic
Hydatid cyst

Growth disorder
Focal nodular hyperplasia

Neoplastic causes
Benign
Hepatic cell adenoma
Haemangioma
Hamartoma, fibroma, lipoma, leiomyoma
Malignant
Primary (hepatocellular carcinoma, cholangiocarcinoma, angiosarcoma)
Secondary (solitary metastasis, especially in colon, rectum, breast or lung)

Apparent solitary nodule of a multiple nodular process
Multiple
Hepatocellular carcinoma
Secondary metastases
Multiple cysts
Polycystic disease
Multiple hydatids

BOX 20.5.4 CLASSIC CAUSES OF SPLENOMEGALY WITH COMMON EXAMPLES

Inflammatory causes
Infective
Acute
Viral
- Infectious mononucleosis
- Hepatitis A, B, C
- HIV infection
Bacterial
- Septicaemia
Chronic
Bacterial
- Subacute bacterial endocarditis
Protozoal
- Malaria
Collagen vascular disease
- Rheumatoid arthritis
- Systemic lupus erythematosus

Circulatory causes
Portal hypertension
- Suprahepatic (constrictive pericarditis)
- Hepatic (cirrhosis)
- Portal vein thrombosis

Neoplastic and haematological conditions
Anaemias
- Pernicious anaemia
- Haemoglobinopathies
- Hereditary spherocytosis
- Other haemolytic anaemias
Leukaemias
- Chronic myeloid leukaemia
- Chronic lymphatic leukaemia
Lymphoma
- Hodgkin's and non-Hodgkin's
Myeloproliferative disease
- Polycythaemia rubra vera
- Myelofibrosis

Infiltrations
Sarcoid, amyloid, storage diseases

shaped. The causes of diffuse splenomegaly are listed in Box 20.5.4.

A solitary mass within the spleen may cause splenomegaly, but it is unusual to realize that the enlargement is due to a solitary mass rather than diffuse enlargement of the spleen. The causes are listed in Box 20.5.5.

The causes of massive splenomegaly are as follows:

1. chronic myeloid leukaemia;
2. myelofibrosis;
3. lymphomas;
4. malaria.

The causes of hepatosplenomegaly are as follows:

1. acute hepatitis;
2. chronic active hepatitis;

3. alcoholic liver disease (and the other causes of cirrhosis with hepatomegaly) with associated portal hypertension;

4. neoplastic and haematological conditions – leukaemias, lymphomas, myelofibrosis and some haemolytic anaemias;

5. collagen vascular disorders;

6. infiltrations – sarcoid, amyloid and storage disorders.

BOX 20.5.5 CAUSES OF A SOLITARY MASS GIVING RISE TO SPLENOMEGALY

Congential cyst

Traumatic degenerative cyst

Inflammatory cyst
  Hydatid
  Splenic infarction
  Splenic abscess

Tumour
  Benign
    Haemangioma
    Lymphangioma
  Malignant
    Primary (excluding lymphoma and leukaemia, are very rare; an example is haemangiosarcoma)
    Secondary tumours are similarly rare; an example is melanoma

BOX 20.5.6 CLASSIFICATION OF CAUSES OF EPIGASTRIC MASSES

1. Stomach tumours
   1.1 Carcinoma
   1.2 Lymphoma
   1.3 Leiomyoma
   1.4 Leiomyosarcoma
2. Carcinoma of the transverse colon
3. Abdominal aortic aneurysm
4. Solitary liver masses
5. Pancreatic masses (see separate list)
6. Gastric outlet obstruction with gastric dilatation
7. Para-aortic lymphadenopathy
   7.1 Lymphoma
   7.2 Secondary testicular cancer (e.g. seminoma)
8. Hypertrophic pyloric stenosis with a palpable 'pyloric tumour'
9. Others (e.g. choledochal cysts, lesser sac abscess following a sealed perforated gastric ulcer)

Epigastric masses are diverse in their possible origins. The classifications of causes is shown in Box 20.5.6.

Abdominal aortic aneurysms are a common cause of an abdominal mass. The mass tends to be smooth, fusiform and located just to the left of the midline above the umbilicus. It is immobile and does not move on respiration, and characteristically has an expansile pulsation. It may or may not be tender

Pancreatic masses tend to be located in the epigastrium or central abdominal region, and have their long axis running across the abdomen. They are deeply situated posteriorly in the abdomen, and therefore are usually large if palpable. Because of their deep situation and the pathology causing them, they are usually ill-defined. They do not move on repiration because they are fixed in the retroperitoneal tissue. They may have transmitted pulsation from the aorta. They are usually firm in consistency and resonant on percussion because of the overlying stomach and/or colon. A classification of causes of pancreatic masses is shown in Box 20.5.7.

The causes of central abdominal masses (umbilical) include most of the causes of epigastric masses, but in addition they include masses arising from the small bowel and omentum. The causes are listed in Box 20.5.8.

A mesenteric cyst is a characteristic but rare abdominal swelling which tends to be mobile at 90° to the long axis of the small bowel mesentery, but not in the long axis of the mesentery. Like all cysts, it is smooth, spherical and mobile.

Retroperitoneal swellings often present late because they are posteriorly situated, and are therefore large and associated with abdominal distension when first discovered. They tend to be firm to hard and irregular, and are

BOX 20.5.7 CLASSIFICATION OF CAUSES OF PANCREATIC MASSES AND PERIPANCREATIC MASSES

1. Inflammatory causes
   1.1 Pancreatic necrosis with acute severe pancreatitis
   1.2 Pancreatic pseudocyst
   1.3 Pancreatic abscess

2. Cysts
   2.1 Multiple congential cysts (in association with cysts in the liver and kidneys)
   2.2 Retention cysts secondary to duct obstruction

3. Neoplastic causes
   3.1 Benign (cystadenoma, serous or mucinous)
   3.2 Malignant (e.g. adenocarcinoma)

usually obviously malignant on examination. They may have transmitted pulsation from the aorta, or they may produce occlusion of the inferior vena cava with gross oedema of the lower half of the body. Because of their retroperitoneal situation, these masses tend to be fixed and do not move with respiration. The causes of retroperitoneal masses include lymphomas, soft-tissue sarcomas (which may arise in any abdominal region), secondary metastases to lymph nodes (particularly testicular and ovarian cancer) and massive lipomas.

The characteristics of renal swellings are that they lie laterally and posteriorly in the flank or loin. They have a rounded lower pole and feel reniform. They move down on inspiration and are resonant to percussion because of the overlying colon. Because of their posterior situation it is not possible to insert an examining hand behind the mass and in front of the erector spinae, but on occasion it will be possible to feel above the mass. The mass will be bimanually palpable and ballottable. Unlike an enlarged liver it does not have an edge, and unlike an enlarged spleen it does not have a notch on its medial border. In distinguishing a large kidney from a large liver or spleen, percussion is useful, as a liver or spleen will be dull whereas a kidney is resonant. The term 'ballottable' refers to the ability to bounce the mass like a ball being patted between the front and the back examining hand. The causes of renal masses may be divided into those giving rise to bilateral renal masses and unilateral renal masses.

Causes of bilateral renal masses include the following:

1. polycystic kidneys;
2. bilateral hydronephrosis;
3. bilateral primary carcinoma of the kidney or nephroblastoma;
4. bilateral simple cysts;
5. horseshoe kidney.

Causes of unilateral renal masses include the following:

1. solitary cyst;
2. primary carcinoma and nephroblastoma;
3. secondary malignancy, e.g. melanoma;
4. hydronephrosis;
5. renal abscess (carbuncle);
6. pyonephrosis;
7. compensatory hypertrophy;

8. staghorn calculus;
9. acute pyelonephritis;
10. others (e.g. oncocytoma, angiomyolipoma).

Right iliac fossa masses are a common surgical problem. There are three common causes as well as other less common causes (see Box 20.5.9). In addition, there are a number of rare causes which may give rise to a mass in the right iliac fossa as well as the left iliac fossa, and these unusual masses which are common to both iliac fossae are listed in Box 20.5.10.

Causes of left iliac fossa masses include the following:

1. sigmoid colon carcinoma;
2. diverticular mass (phlegmon, abscess).

Appendiceal masses are characteristically felt low down and laterally in the right iliac fossa immediately adjacent to the anterior superior iliac spine, whereas a carcinoma of the caecum tends to be more centrally located in the right iliac fossa. A carcinoma of the caecum may have perforated locally, causing a peri-caecal abscess, and here it may be very difficult to make the distinction clinically from an appendiceal inflammatory mass. Ileo-caecal Crohn's disease tends to result in several inflamed loops, producing an elongated sausage-shaped mass which will lie transversely in the right iliac fossa.

Rectus sheath haematoma due to rupture of the inferior epigastric artery is not uncommon. Strictly speaking it is an abdominal wall mass. However, it is deep to the musculo-aponeurotic layer, and is therefore

---

BOX 20.5.10 UNUSUAL MASSES COMMON TO BOTH RIGHT AND LEFT ILIAC FOSSAE

Psoas abscess

Retroperitoneal sarcoma

Deep iliac lymph node enlargement

    Lymphoma

    Deep iliac adenitis

    Secondary tumour (e.g. squamous-cell carcinoma and melanoma)

Common iliac artery aneurysm

Renal transplant

Tumour in an undescended testis

Chondrosarcoma of the ilium

Rectus sheath haematoma

An abnormally situated kidney

Structures from other abdominal regions

    Ovarian masses

    Renal masses

    Fibroid uterus

---

often confused with a right iliac fossa mass. The haematoma is located extraperitoneally, and hence tracks beneath the musculo-aponeurotic layer of the abdominal wall.

Colonic swellings are characteristically felt in either the right or left iliac fossa. They usually have well-defined lateral borders, but tend to have poorly defined superior and inferior borders. They tend to be mobile from side to side but not superiorly and inferiorly, and they also tend not to move with respiration. They give the impression of being able to be rolled under the examining hand, and in so doing may produce a gurgling sound. They tend to be comparatively fixed, and therefore the differential diagnosis of tumour vs. inflammation is clinically difficult. Percussion is of limited value in a colonic mass.

A pelvic swelling is located in the hypogastrium, but may be eccentric and move into the right or left iliac fossa. It is not possible to reach below the swelling, and it has no lower edge. If extremely large it may cause generalized abdominal distension. It may be palpable on bimanual examination per rectum or per vaginum. When extremely large, ovarian masses will become centrally situated in the pelvis and then in the abdomen as they enlarge even further. Pelvic masses tend to have a well-defined upper border. It is essential that the bladder is demonstrably empty before an opinion is given on a mass in the hypogastrium which is thought to be arising from the pelvis. This may necessitate catherization. The bladder arises from the pelvis, is dome-shaped, immobile and dull to percussion, and direct pressure on it causes a desire to micturate. An ovarian cyst tends to be smooth, spherical and distinct, arises from the pelvis, and may have mobility from side to side. It tends to be dull to percussion, and may be eccentrically situated on the right or left side. A fibroid uterus arises out of the pelvis, is firm to hard, knobbly, and may have slight movement transversely. It tends to be dull to percussion. Other causes of hypogastric masses include the following:

1. bladder:
   - acute retention;
   - chronic retention;
   - bladder tumour;
   - bladder stone;
2. uterus:
   - pregnancy;
   - fibroids;
   - endometrial carcinoma;
   - uterine sarcoma;
3. ovary:
   - cysts;
   - tumours;
4. tubo-ovarian masses:
5. colonic:
   - carcinoma;
   - diverticular mass;
6. lymph node mass.

CLINICAL PROVISIONAL WORKING DIAGNOSIS

At this stage a provisional diagnosis and list of possible differential diagnoses should be written down. This in turn dictates subsequent investigations which will confirm or refute the diagnosis.

INVESTIGATIONS

INTRODUCTION

The assessment of any lump should be considered by applying the generality of triple assessment, similar to that used in diagnosing a breast lump. For an abdominal lump this will involve clinical assessment, history and examination, imaging or visualizing the lump (this will usually involve computed tomography (CT) scanning and/or ultrasound, and often endoscopy) and biopsy (which is usually performed percutaneously and image-guided). This generality of triple assessment has dramatically changed surgical practice with the advent and availability of ultrasound examination, CT scanning and the safety and accuracy of percutaneous biopsy and endoscopy. It has reduced the need for contrast radiology such as barium meal and barium enemas, and has also decreased the need for diagnostic laparotomy.

There is much to be said for obtaining a CT scan of the abdomen as an early investigation for the patient with an abdominal mass. Ultrasound examination can often provide important information of a complementary nature, and is also required. For example, in a patient with a pancreatic mass due to pancreatitis, CT scanning will be the best investigation to assess the mass, but the clinician will wish to know whether or not gallstones are present in the gall bladder, and here ultrasound examination is the investigation of choice. These investigations are readily available and will clarify the organ of origin of the mass and its precise anatomy. In addition, they may provide information about the underlying pathology producing the mass, and enable planning and performance of a percutaneously guided biopsy. A core biopsy obtaining histology is in general preferable to a fine needle aspiration biopsy which provides cytology only.

Direct consultation with the radiologist before and after investigations are performed is often invaluable, and may make the difference between the timely establishment of a correct diagnosis and an ongoing apparently elusive problem.

Other investigations will be discussed in this section, but all of these should be considered ancillary to a CT scan, which confirms the mass and organ of origin. Ancillary investigations will help to determine the pathological nature of the regional anatomical abnormality that the CT scan had identified. For example, in diffuse hepatomegaly, CT scanning will confirm that the liver is enlarged and diffusely affected, and a liver biopsy and other investigations will be required to determine the pathological nature of the process. Similarly, a left iliac fossa colonic mass will be confirmed by CT scanning, but colonoscopy and biopsy will be required to determine whether the mass is due to a carcinoma or diverticular disease.

COMPUTED TOMOGRAPHY SCANNING OF THE ABDOMEN

CT scanning of a mass in the abdomen may be used to establish the diagnosis, to aid percutaneously obtained biopsies, and to drain abscesses percutaneously. A CT scan of the abdomen may take images from as small a distance as 3 mm apart, and therefore in general will identify lesions larger than 1 cm in diameter. It is important that an oral contrast agent or water is given to outline the gut so that areas of local ileus can be distinguished from abscesses. Intravenous contrast is also necessary to establish the vascularity and enhance the definition of any identified lesion. In addition, it provides an indication of renal function and may show the relationship of a retroperitoneal mass to the ureters. CT scanning has increased resolution in obese patients, and conversely is somewhat reduced in very aesthenic patients.

The CT scan will determine the site of the tumour (e.g. the segment of liver involved) and the size of the lesion. Local invasion of adjacent structures can be assessed, particularly by looking at fascial planes. Involvement of regional lymph nodes and distant metastases to liver and lung should be noted. Ascites, peritoneal seedlings and omental secondaries may also be identified. Invasion of vessels (e.g. carcinoma of the kidney invading the renal vein and inferior vena cava) may be noted with a dynamic CT scan.

CT scanning will provide some information about the texture of hepatomegaly, but not as much as that provided by ultrasound examination. However, CT scanning is more sensitive in diagnosing liver metastases.

In general, CT scanning is excellent for lesions in the liver, spleen, pancreas, kidney, adrenal glands, omentum, lymph nodes and retroperitoneum. It will provide some information about the bowel, such as the level and cause of a bowel obstruction, and it will provide detailed information about the retroperitoneal lymph nodes, the aorta and the inferior vena cava. Adrenal masses less than 1 cm in diameter will often not be detected, and for this reason a number of Conn's tumours (which tend to be of the order of 1 cm or less in diameter) will not be identified by CT scanning.

CT scanning will distinguish between an inflammatory phlegmon (e.g. accompanying diverticulitis) and a peri-colic diverticular abscess. This distinction is important, as drainage will be required for the latter.

CT scanning is the modality of first choice for draining abdominal abscesses and fluid collections, because of its ability to delineate air, fat and fascial planes. These collections should first be needled with a fine-bore needle and fluid obtained by aspiration. Contrast is then injected and, if it is deemed to be suitable, a percutaneous drain can then be inserted. In addition, samples for microscopy and culture are obtained by this technique (e.g. to culture fluid from a possible infected pancreatic collection).

CT scan-guided biopsy has a major role in determining the histology of a mass lesion, although some lesions may be better seen by ultrasound examination. In general, a core biopsy is preferable to fine-needle aspiration cytology. If possible, the pathologist should be present to determine that the aspirate is satisfactory and diagnostic. Complications of these percutaneous techniques are rare. Contraindications to percutaneous core biopsies include a suspected hydatid cyst, as there is a risk of spillage of hydatid fluid with anaphylaxis and intraperitoneal seeding with hydatids. A lump associated with bowel should not be subjected to this technique, as there is a risk of perforation. Coagulation studies should be performed prior to the procedure, and any bleeding tendency is a contraindication. Vascular tumours such as cavernous haemangiomas of the liver should not be subjected to percutanous needle biopsy. Dilated intrahepatic bile ducts are a relative contra-indication to liver biopsy, as they may result in a bile leak. A phaeochromocytoma subjected to core biopsy may result in a hypertensive crisis, and should be avoided.

ULTRASOUND EXAMINATION

Ultrasound examination is the best investigation for establishing the presence of gallstones. It is useful for measuring the size of the common bile duct and for establishing flow in vessels (e.g. in the mesenteric, splenic, portal venous system and the inferior vena cava). It also provides useful information about liver texture (e.g. fatty infiltration seen in alcoholic liver disease and diabetes mellitus). It is less useful in obese patients and in individuals in whom a large amount of bowel gas is present.

When ordering an ultrasound examination, the area to be examined should be specified, whether this is the upper or lower abdomen, and whether a renal ultrasound scan is required.

Ultrasound examination measures the size of masses accurately and is therefore useful in some situations where follow-up of the size of a lesion is critical (e.g. an abdominal aortic aneurysm).

Ultrasound equipment is portable, and thus the examination can be performed at the patient's bedside if necessary.

Ultrasound-guided biopsy is often easier and quicker than a CT-guided biopsy, and percutaneous drainage can also be undertaken, if necessary at the bedside. This is particularly useful for intensive-care patients who cannot be transported to the radiology department.

Ultrasound examination is excellent for determining whether a lesion is cystic or solid, and this is of importance in many situations (e.g. space-occupying lesions in the liver and kidney).

IMAGE-GUIDED BIOPSY

Image-guided biopsy may be performed under ultra-sound or CT scan control. Abdominal paracentesis of ascitic fluid should be subjected to cytology, and may for example establish the diagnosis of an ovarian carcinoma.

ENDOSCOPY

Depending on the clinical features and the CT scan result, the suspected lesion may be subjected to endoscopy. This may involve gastroscopy, colonoscopy, cystocopy, hysteroscopy or endoscopic retrograde cholangiopancreatography (ERCP). Each of these inves-tigations may also provide biopsies for histology, and brushings and washings for cytology.

ANCILLARY INVESTIGATIONS

Haematological, biochemical and serological investigation

An endless number of possible investigations may be performed, but these are determined by the suspected diagnosis on the basis of the clinical features and CT scan or ultrasound images.

Full blood examination may show evidence of anaemia or polycythaemia (e.g. in carcinoma of the kidney and polycythaemia rubra vera). Urea, creatinine and electrolytes are essential baseline investigations, and may show evidence of renal failure. Serum amylase and lipase will be elevated in patients with phlegmons asso-ciated with acute pancreatitis and in those with pancre-atic pseudocysts. Liver function tests will give an indication of underlying liver pathology. Elevation of bilirubin, alkaline phosphatase and gamma-glutamyl transferase (γGT) may suggest a picture of obstructive jaundice, whereas elevation of the liver enzymes (aspar-tate transaminase (AST) and alanine transaminase (ALT) indicates a parenchymal process affecting the liver, such as acute viral hepatitis. The ESR and acute-phase reactants such as C-reactive protein may be elevated in many inflammatory processes and also, for example, in carcinoma of the kidney. Coagulation studies should be performed prior to percutaneous image-guided biopsy. Detailed haematological investigations may be required for patients with splenomegaly (e.g. in order to deter-mine the nature of an underlying haemoglobinopathy or haemolytic anaemia).

On occasion, serum tumour markers may be indi-cated. These include carcino-embryonic antigen (CEA), which is useful in a number of different tumours and also as a follow-up for patients with colorectal cancer, and alpha-fetoprotein (AFP), which may be elevated in patients with hepatoma and testicular tumours, as well as lactate dehydrogenase (LDH), which may be elevated in testicular tumours, CA125, which may be elevated in ovarian carcinoma, and prostate-specific antigen (PSA), which may be elevated in prostatic carcinoma and underlie the cause of urinary retention resulting in a palpable bladder. Hydatid serology will be required for patients with suspected hydatid cysts.

Patients with features suggesting acute viral hepatitis are investigated with hepatitis A IgM antibody, hepatitis B surface antigen and hepatitis C antibodies. Patients with suspected cirrhosis of the liver may be investigated with auto-antibodies (e.g. smooth muscle antibodies for patients with chronic active hepatitis and anti-mitochondrial antibodies for patients with suspected primary biliary cirrhosis). Serum and/or urinary beta human chorionic gonadotrophin may be estimated to assess pregnancy, and is also a marker of some tumours, such as testicular and ovarian carcinomas and hydatidiform moles. Adrenal tumours tend to be non-palpable, but large adrenal carcinomas may be palpable and are also quite commonly functional. Twenty-four-hour urinary cortisol measurements and a low-dose dexamethasone suppression test will detect Cushing's syndrome. Plasma renin and plasma aldosterone will detect aldosterone excess, and 24-h urinary vanillylmandelic acid (VMA) will detect catecholamine-producing tumours.

Simple investigations such as a midstream urine specimen for microscopy for cells, casts, crystals, and culture should be routinely undertaken. Faeces examination should include microscopy and culture (e.g. looking at a fresh faecal specimen for amoebae which may explain a right iliac fossa mass (amoeboma) and/or a liver abscess).

Ancillary radiological investigations

A chest X-ray and/or CT scan of the thorax is undertaken to detect the presence of possible pulmonary metastases. A CT scan of the thorax is a more sensitive investigation than a chest X-ray. A plain abdominal X-ray may show evidence of a bowel obstruction, calculi in the renal tract, and evidence of pancreatic calcification and calcification in degenerate hydatid cysts in the liver. It may also identify conditions such as staghorn calculi and a porcelain gall bladder. These represent only a few examples of specific diagnoses which may be obtained by relatively simple investigations.

Intravenous urography should be performed if the patient has haematuria, and will detect a space-occupying lesion in the kidney. The next test would be an ultrasound examination to determine whether such a lesion was cystic or solid.

A small-bowel enema is useful for small-bowel Crohn's disease, and will also help both to identify other small-bowel pathology and to determine the pathologi-cal nature of masses in the right iliac fossa. On occasion a gastrographin or barium enema will be indicated to differentiate a diverticular colonic mass from a neoplastic one.

An arteriovenous (AV) malformation in the liver is best confirmed by performing a blood pool scan. Hepatobiliary scintigraphy is useful for confirming that a right upper quadrant mass is a non-functioning gall bladder with cystic duct obstruction. On occasion a bone scan will be useful for a bone tumour arising within the pelvis and producing a right or left iliac fossa mass.

Selective angiography is also useful on occasion to determine the resectability of tumours, and also to perform pre-operative embolization to reduce their vascularity. This is occasionally indicated (e.g. in soft-tissue sarcomas in the retroperitoneum and large malignant renal masses). Contrast studies of the renal vein and inferior vena cava will be indicated to determine whether invasion and tumour thrombus are present in carcinoma of the kidney and primary adrenal carcinomas. Magnetic resonance imaging will provide useful additional information about the relationship of tumours to vessels and nerves.

LAPAROSCOPY

There is an increasing role for laparoscopy in diagnosing abdominal lesions, obtaining biopsies and assessing the resectability of lesions. A good example is a suspected hepatocellular carcinoma. At the same time the patient may be examined under anaesthetic, and for pelvic lesions a thorough bimanual examination should be performed and biopsies obtained. Diagnostic laparotomy is therefore only rarely indicated to determine the nature of an abdominal mass.

CONCLUSIONS

A very diverse range of pathological conditions may result in an abdominal mass. With a careful triple assessment – including clinical examination, imaging and/or endoscopy and biopsy and other ancillary investigations – to determine the pathological nature of a regionally identified anatomical mass, a precise diagnosis is usually achievable.

Inguino-scrotal lumps

Jonathan W. Serpell

Introduction

Inguino-scrotal lumps are common, and can usually be definitively diagnosed by careful history and examination. They provide a good example of applied anatomy dictating pathological processes, in turn producing clinical disease entities. Because of this, investigations have a smaller role than in other areas, such as breast, head and neck lumps, and in many cases no investigation at all is required after clinical assessment prior to treatment.

ANATOMY

A thorough understanding of inguino-scrotal, perineal and perianal anatomy enables a practical regional approach to lumps in the groin. A simplified schematic diagram of the anatomical regions which may give rise to groin lumps is shown in Figure 20.6.1. A systematic examination of all of these areas will be required, and in each area the range of differential diagnoses is significantly dictated by the underlying anatomy (Table 20.6.1). The regions to be considered are as follows: region A, inguino-scrotal lumps, subdivided into B (inguinal) and C (femoral) lumps; region D, spermatic cord lumps; region E, testis; region F, epididymis; region G, tunica vaginalis; region H, scrotal skin. (Femoral lumps are not strictly inguinal, but present as groin lumps and are therefore important differential diagnoses of inguinal swellings.) All of these areas (inguinal, testis, epididymis, inguinal lymph nodes, femoral artery, spermatic cord, perineum and perianal region, penis, and front and back of the scrotal skin, including inspection of Cowper's glands region) must be systematically examined. Hernias, hydroceles and epididymal cysts are common, and several different pathological conditions are often present in one patient.

The surface anatomy of the region is critical to successful examination. Students and textbooks often confuse the terms mid-inguinal point and mid-point of the inguinal ligament. The mid-inguinal point is the point midway between the anterior superior iliac spine (ASIS) and the symphysis pubis. Located at the mid-inguinal point is the femoral artery. The mid-point of the inguinal ligament is a point midway between the anterior superior iliac spine and the pubic tubercle. This point is slightly lateral to the mid-inguinal point. It is also known as the mid-Poupart point. It both marks the site of the femoral nerve and, about a centimetre above a line between the ASIS and pubic tubercle, it also marks the deep inguinal ring. When examining patients, it is useful to imagine the site of the inguinal ligament stretching between the anterior superior iliac spine and the pubic tubercle. The inguinal canal lies above the recurved inguinal ligament. Therefore inguinal hernias are manifestly above the line of the inguinal ligament. For the same reason, as the femoral canal lies below the inguinal ligament, femoral hernias are manifestly below the inguinal ligament. Much confusion arises about their relationship to the pubic tubercle. Inguinal hernias will emerge above and medial to the pubic tubercle because that is the site of the superficial inguinal ring, but both

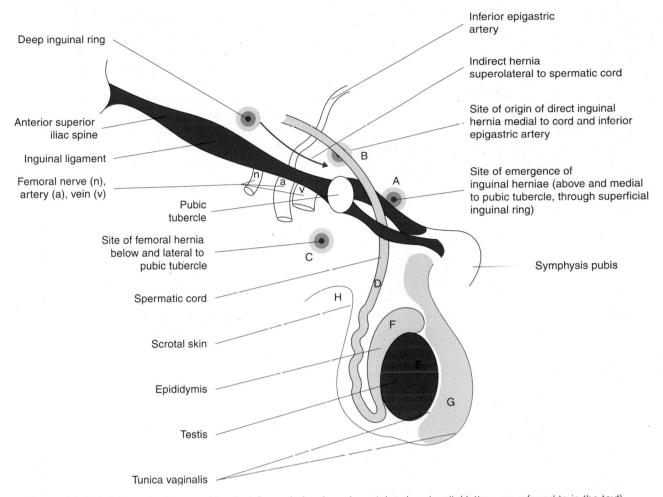

Figure 20.6.1 Schematic diagram of inguinal, femoral triangle and scrotal regions (capital letters are referred to in the text).

indirect and direct hernias occupy the inguinal canal commencing laterally to this area. Therefore the statement that inguinal hernias are above and medial to the pubic tubercle really refers to the site of emergence from the inguinal canal, and not necessarily to their full position. Femoral hernias, on the other hand, do lie below and lateral to the pubic tubercle. However, once they have emerged from the femoral canal, they tend to turn upwards over the lower part of the inguinal ligament. For this reason, femoral and inguinal hernias can on occasion be difficult to distinguish from one another.

The inguinal canal is an oblique slit-like canal 4 cm long, stretching from the internal ring to the external ring. Its posterior wall is weak laterally where it is formed by the fascia transversalis. This is divided into two areas by the inferior epigastric artery. Lateral to the inferior epigastric artery is the deep inguinal ring, whereas medial to the inferior epigastric artery is the region through which a direct inguinal hernia arises (Hesselbach's triangle). An indirect inguinal hernia arises through the deep inguinal ring, usually superolaterally to the spermatic cord, but within the three fascial coverings of the cord. Because the hernia is within the

cord and its coverings, it is directed along the line of the cord into the scrotum. It therefore passes obliquely down the inguinal canal, and is sometimes referred to as an oblique inguinal hernia. For the same reason it tends to reduce upwards, backwards and laterally. In contrast, a direct inguinal hernia emerges through the weak posterior wall medial to the inferior epigastric artery and also medial to the spermatic cord. Consequently, it is not covered by the fascial layers of the spermatic cord and is therefore rarely directed into the scrotum.

The femoral triangle is below the inguinal ligament, and contains the femoral nerve, the femoral artery and the femoral vein, and most medially the femoral canal, which is normally occupied by fat and a lymph node (Cloquet's node). The boundaries of the femoral ring are the lacunar ligament medially, the femoral vein laterally, the inguinal ligament anteriorly, and the ilio-pectineal ligament posteriorly. Superficially the femoral canal is covered by the cribriform fascia. The boundaries of the femoral ring are therefore rigid except for the lateral wall (femoral vein), which is pliable. The long saphenous vein will enter into the femoral vein in this area. The inguinal lymph nodes are arranged in superficial and deep

Table 20.6.1 Classification of inguino-scrotal lumps

Inguinal lumps

Inguinal lump

- Hernia, direct inguinal, indirect inguinal, recurrent inguinal
- Maldescended testis
- Encysted hydrocele of the cord or canal of Nuck
- Lipoma of the cord

Inguino-scrotal lump

- Indirect inguinal hernia
- Varicocele
- Congenital hydrocele
- Haematoma of the specific cord
- Miscellaneous others

Femoral triangle lump

- Femoral hernia
- Inguinal lymphadenopathy
- Saphena varix
- Lipoma
- Femoral artery aneurysm
- Psoas abscess
- Psoas bursa
- Ectopic testis

Scrotal lumps

Body of testis lumps (testicular mass)

- Tumour
- Mumps
- Others e.g. gumma

Epididymal mass

- Acute epididymo-orchitis
- Chronic epididymo-orchitis e.g. T.B.
- Others e.g. rare tumours

Para-epididymal mass

- Cyst of epididymis
- Spermatocele
- Torsion hydatid of Morgagni

Scrotal covering mass

- Squamous cell carcinoma
- Sebaceous cyst
- Idiopathic scrotal oedema

Tunica vaginalis masses

- Hydrocele – primary and secondary
- Haematocele – acute and chronic

groups. The superficial group tends to form a T-shaped arrangement along the inguinal ligament and extending in a vertical limb downwards along the saphenous vein. The deeper lymph nodes are arranged along the femoral vein and artery.

The anatomy of the spermatic cord, epididymis and testis and their coverings is relatively simple. The normal epididymis lies posterolaterally to the testis and is clearly distinguishable from it. The tunica vaginalis is a mesothelial-lined sac which covers the testis and epididymis anteriorly, medially and laterally. The region may be represented by a simple scheme as shown in Figure 20.6.1. By systematically examining each area, it should be possible at the conclusion of examination to produce a diagram so that the anatomical regional abnormality can be marked on it. In this way an accurate clinical diagnosis can be achieved.

HISTORY OF INGUINO-SCROTAL LUMPS

The history is no different to the history of any other lump but, in particular, intermittency may suggest a hernia. Pain and discomfort are common with inguinal hernias, and a history of trauma may be of importance. General symptoms of carcinoma, such as weight loss, are important.

Risk factors for development of groin hernias are important. The patient's occupation and the circumstances in which the hernia occurred or was first noted are highly significant and must be accurately documented. It is usual for such hernias to be regarded as secondary to work, and they are therefore covered under most work-care schemes. In the history, smoking and coughing, chronic bronchitis, straining, heavy lifting, constipation and altered bowel habit may all be significant. Genito-urinary symptoms must be enquired for, in particular to assess for prostatism, urethral stricture and symptoms of urinary tract infection. Urinary tract infection, a history of urethral discharge and sexually transmitted disease may all be associated with epididymo-orchitis.

INGUINO-SCROTAL EXAMINATION

There is an unfortunate but common misconception among medical students that the first thing to do when asked to examine a patient's inguino-scrotal area is to ask the patient to stand. This practice has arisen as a result of the artificial and clinically inappropriate so-called 'Short Case Surgical Examination'. In clinical practice, patients present and give their history and are then examined logically and systematically. This will include a careful

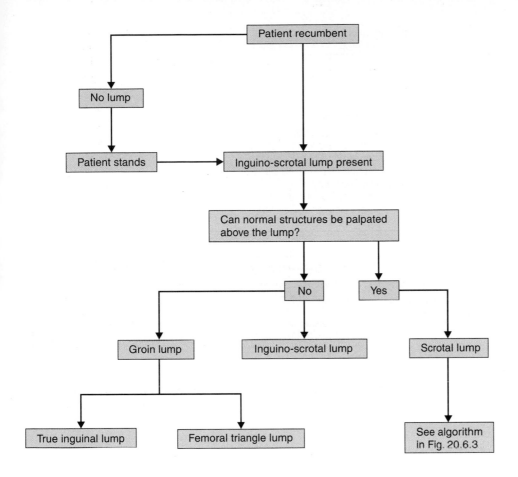

Key examination questions

1. ?Cough impluse
2. ?Reducible

Figure 20.6.2 Algorithm for diagnosis of inguino-scrotal lumps.

general examination, including the head and neck, chest, and abdomen, prior to a focused examination of the patient's problem, i.e. the inguino-scrotal mass. This is usually therefore conducted as a logical extension of the preceding examination in the lying position. Clearly, however, it is essential to examine the inguino-scrotal area in both lying and standing positions, as the two examinations are complementary. Obviously some inguinal hernias will only be manifested on standing, but, equally, much of the examination is more easily performed in terms of both patient comfort and accuracy of examination with the patient lying down. This particularly pertains to the ability to reduce an oblique indirect inguinal hernia, which reduces upwards, backwards and laterally. It always seems inappropriate for someone to be struggling to reduce such a hernia while the patient is standing, when the same manoeuvre can be achieved more elegantly and with less patient discomfort with the patient lying in comfort and the examiner actually able to see what he or she is doing. As well as conducting the examination with the patient in the lying and standing positions, it is also essential that the examination is systematic and thorough, and that it includes the inguinal

region, the femoral region, the penis, testis, scrotum, perineum and lower limbs.

Virtually all inquino-scrotal lumps can be diagnosed by following the algorithms presented in Figures 20.6.2 and 20.6.3. The algorithms are based on a detailed understanding of the regional anatomy and a problem-orientated examination to answer the following five questions.

1. Is it possible to feel normal structures above the lump? If the answer to this question is yes, the lump is scrotal; if the answer is no, then the lump is either inguinal or inguino-scrotal.

2. Is it possible to distinguish the testis from the epididymis, and if so, is the mass arising from one or other of these structures, or is it arising from another structure?

3. Is the mass tender?

4. Is the mass fluctuant?

5. Is the mass transilluminable?

It goes without saying that both sides must be examined. A lump in the inguino-scrotal region which it is not

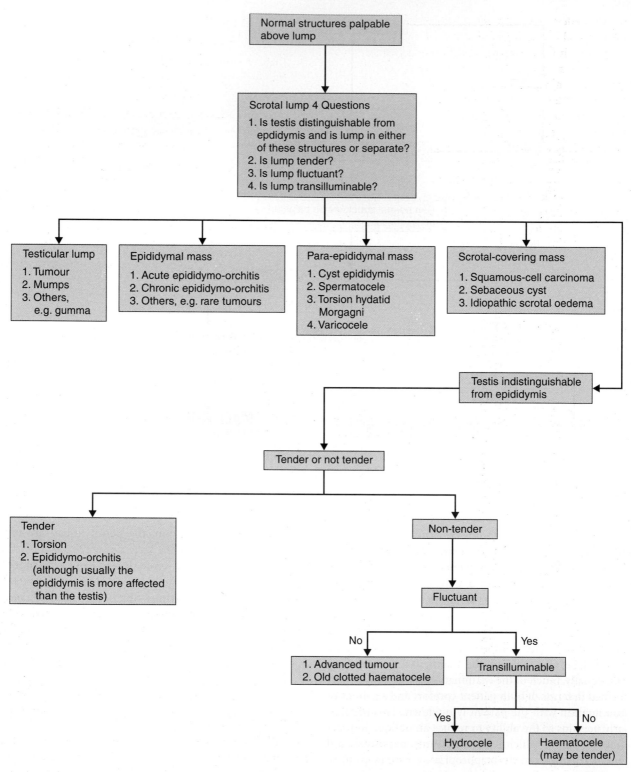

Figure 20.6.3 Algorithm for diagnosis of scrotal lumps.

possible to feel above may be either an inguinal lump, a femoral lump or an inguino-scrotal lump. As previously mentioned, students often have difficulty feeling the pubic tubercle, and therefore struggle to distinguish an indirect inguinal hernia (which is said to be above and medial to the pubic tubercle) from a femoral hernia

(which is said to be below and lateral). Two points deserve emphasis here. First, an inguinal hernia is always manifestly above the inguinal ligament and a femoral hernia is below it. Secondly, an indirect inguinal hernia emerges from the inguinal canal through the superficial inguinal ring medial to and above the pubic tubercle, but the distended inguinal canal which contains the rest of the inguinal hernia is lateral to the pubic tubercle.

An inguinal or inguino-scrotal swelling can be diagnosed by answering two further questions. First, does the mass have an expansile cough impulse? If so, this indicates that it is a hernia. Secondly, is the mass reducible? Again this indicates that it is a hernia or alternatively a varicocele or saphena varix.

Essentially all of the physical signs of any lump outlined in the general introduction to lumps should be assessed in any inguino-scrotal lump.

The particular features to be noted on any lump suspected of being a hernia include the site (inguinal, direct or indirect, and femoral). This may be determined by the relationship to the pubic tubercle and, secondly, having determined that a hernia is inguinal, an indirect inguinal hernia is controlled after reduction by pressure over the deep inguinal ring at the mid-point of the inguinal ligament, whereas a direct hernia is not. Conversely, a direct hernia will be controlled by pressure over the superficial inguinal ring, whereas an indirect inguinal hernia will not be controlled by this manoeuvre. If it descends into the scrotum, it is almost certainly an indirect inguinal hernia. The colour and temperature of the overlying skin will usually be normal, but if it is reddened and the temperature is elevated, this suggests underlying strangulation, as does the presence of pain and tenderness. The shape and surface of an inguino-scrotal lump may be characteristic. Hernias tend to be pear-shaped with a smooth surface, whereas a varicocele tends to feel like a bag of worms in the standing position, and a spermatocele characteristically feels like a third testis. The composition of a hernia may be either bowel (in which case the contents will feel soft, resonant and fluctuant), or omentum (which may be firm, rubbery and non-fluctuant). If strangulated, the contents will become much firmer and also tender. Massive inguinal hernias may have visible peristalsis, as they may contain a considerable amount of bowel. Two diagnostic features of a hernia are that it has an expansile cough impulse and that it is reducible. It should be noted that the site of the hernia refers to the site of reduction rather than its ultimate site in the body. This is because hernias, once they reach the subcutaneous plane through either the superficial inguinal ring or the femoral ring, tend to pass in the direction of least resistance. Auscultation of an inguino-scrotal lump has little role, as bowel sounds heard over a hernia may be transmitted from the abdomen rather than from the underlying mass which is being auscultated.

The features of direct inguinal herniae that distinguish them from indirect inguinal herniae are as follows:

1. Direct inguinal herniae are less common.

2. Direct inguinal herniae occur in older patients and are uncommon in children and young adults.

3. They are rare in women.

4. They do not descend into the scrotum.

5. They are not controlled by pressure over the deep inguinal ring, but are controlled by pressure over the superficial inguinal ring.

6. A direct hernia will reduce spontaneously on lying flat, whereas an indirect inguinal hernia reduces upwards, backwards and laterally.

7. A direct hernia rarely strangulates.

8. Direct hernias are often bilateral.

9. A direct hernia bulges forwards on reappearing, whereas an indirect hernia passes downwards medially and forwards in an oblique fashion.

A list of terms which may be used to describe groin herniae is given below:

1. indirect inguinal;
2. direct inguinal;
3. recurrent inguinal;
4. sliding inguinal;
5. femoral;
6. reducible or irreducible;
7. right or left;
8. unilateral or bilateral;
9. incarcerated;
10. obstructed;
11. strangulated;
12. Maydl's;
13. Littre's;
14. Richter's.

A sliding hernia is one in which bowel, usually sigmoid colon or caecum, forms one of the walls of the sac, rather than purely peritoneum. An incarcerated hernia is simply a non-reducible hernia, usually due to adhesions, although some texts claim that the term should only be applied when the hernia is irreducible due to inspissated faeces in the bowel contained within the hernia preventing its reduction. The important feature is that an incarcerated hernia is not reducible, but also not obstructed or strangulated. An obstructed hernia is tender and associated with a small-bowel obstruction, and a strangulated hernia indicates ischaemic compromise of the contents of the hernia, usually bowel in association with obstruction. For practical purposes, the terms 'obstructed' and 'strangulated' are the same, and indicate an acute complication of the hernia which requires urgent surgical intervention. Spontaneous reduction should always be followed by surgery within 24 h because of the risk of reduction *en masse* whereby the hernia is reduced but the bowel contents are still caught within the peritoneal sac. The reason for this is that the site of strangulation in most herniae is a narrowing in the peritoneal sac, rather than the rigid confines of the superficial inguinal ring, for example. In Richter's hernia a loop of small bowel is kinked off and completely obstructed, but on reduction it appears that only a portion of the circumference of the bowel has been involved in the hernia. Figure 20.6.4 explains this apparent paradox. It seems highly unlikely that the often quoted explanation of a portion of the circumference of the bowel becoming caught within a hernia could occur without causing obstruction. In Maydl's hernia there are two loops of small bowel within the hernia, and in this setting the intermediate loop is at risk of strangulation within the abdomen rather than within the hernial sac. Littre's hernia contains Meckel's diverticulum.

The differential diagnosis of any inguinal hernia includes all inguinal masses, the femoral triangle masses and inguino-scrotal masses. A congenital hydrocele occurs when the peritoneal cavity communicates with the processus vaginalis and the tunica vaginalis. This forms an inguino-scrotal lump which is not reducible, does not have a cough impulse, where the testis is not palpable and the swelling is brilliantly translucent. This is in contrast to an indirect inguinal hernia, where the testis is palpable, and the mass has a cough impulse, is reducible and is non-transilluminable. In addition, there are two emergent swellings which may pop out of the external inguinal ring. These are a maldescended testis and a hydrocele of the spermatic cord.

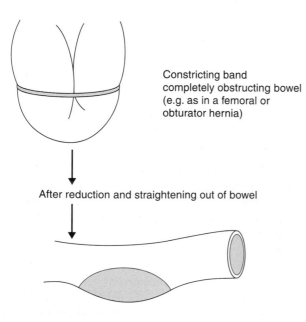

Constricting band completely obstructing bowel (e.g. as in a femoral or obturator hernia)

After reduction and straightening out of bowel

Apparent partial involvement with 'pseudo-pod' of bowel wall

Figure 20.6.4 Richter's hernia.

FEMORAL TRIANGLE LUMPS

FEMORAL HERNIA

The majority of femoral herniae occur in elderly women. However, it is important to realize that in women the commonest groin hernia is still inguinal. There is a high risk of strangulation because of the rigid walls of the femoral ring. A femoral hernia lies below and lateral to the pubic tubercle, tends to be small and firm, and is often not completely reducible. This is due to adhesions, and for the same reason there is often no cough impulse.

DIFFERENTIAL DIAGNOSES OF FEMORAL HERNIAE (FEMORAL TRIANGLE LUMPS)

Saphena varix

This is a soft, smooth, reducible swelling in the region of the cribriform fascia, which has a thrill and a bruit on coughing, and empties when the limb is elevated. It is associated with varicose veins of the long saphenous system, and tapping over the long saphenous vein transmits an impulse to the swelling.

Lymph node mass

This lies in the femoral triangle region, has no cough impulse, thrill or bruit, and is not reducible. It is shaped like a lymph node and may or may not be mobile. Its size and degree of hardness depend on the underlying pathology. It is often multiple, and it is easy to confuse it with an irreducible femoral hernia. Similarly, a strangulated femoral hernia may be confused with acute lymphadenitis. Lymph nodes in the groin drain a number of areas, and all of these must be systematically examined for any evidence of pathology. The sites to examine include the lower limb, penis, scrotum, anus and anal canal, perineum, buttock, lower back and anterior abdominal wall. It is always particularly important to examine the back of the scrotal skin, as this is the commonest site for a scrotal squamous-cell carcinoma.

Lipoma

Lipomas are ubiquitous and are usually subcutaneous, not attached to skin, and mobile to a degree with a slipping sign. Lobulation is often detectable and the mass is fluctuant. There is no cough impulse, and the mass is neither reducible nor tender.

Psoas abscess

A psoas abscess will present beneath the inguinal ligament lateral to the femoral artery. The patient will usually show systemic signs of sepsis, and may have a mass in the ipsilateral iliac fossa. The overlying skin is reddened, and the mass is fluctuant and tender, but has no cough impulse and is not reducible.

Femoral artery aneurysm

Femoral artery aneurysms are increasingly common, and may be due to atherosclerosis, but are more commonly due to traumatic punctures. A false aneurysm following procedures in interventional radiology, for example, where the femoral artery is the site normally used to access the vascular system is not an uncommon clinical entity. The site is characteristic and the mass will have an expansile impulse. It tends to be non-tender and non-reducible, and does not have a cough impulse.

Ectopic testis

Abnormalities of testicular descent may be categorized as either maldescent or incomplete descent; or ectopic or abnormal site. Incompletely descended testes are in the correct line of descent but have failed to reach the scrotum. They may therefore be abdominal, inguinal or high scrotal. They are prone to complications of trauma, torsion, malignancy, association with indirect inguinal hernia and infertility. Incompletely descended testes tend to be atrophic.

Ectopic testes are situated in abnormal sites, and the testicle is often not atrophic. The commonest site is in the superficial inguinal pouch, but they may also be located in the femoral triangle, at the base of the penis and in the perineum. For this reason, a femoral triangle ectopic testis is a differential diagnosis of a femoral hernia.

Psoas bursa

This is an uncommon mass which appears from beneath the psoas major tendon from a situation deep within the femoral triangle region. Ultrasound examination will help to distinguish the site of the mass and therefore the nature of the mass from the other differential diagnoses in the femoral triangle region.

SCROTAL LUMPS

Virtually all scrotal lumps can be diagnosed clinically according to the algorithm shown in Figure 20.6.3. Careful examination of the known anatomical structures enables a diagram to be drawn with a sketch of the pathology. In turn this usually indicates the diagnosis. A schematic representation of the common pathologies is shown in Figure 20.6.5.

HYDROCELES

Hydroceles may be primary or secondary. Secondary hydroceles tend to be small and lax, and the important underlying diagnoses are infection, trauma and neoplasia. Diagnosis is directed towards the underlying condition. Primary hydroceles tend to occur in older patients, and therefore a small lax hydrocele in a young patient should raise suspicion about the underlying diagnosis. A primary vaginal hydrocele is the commonest type in the older patient. The cord is palpable above the lesion, but because of the situation of the tunica vaginalis, the testis and epididymis are not palpable and usually the hydrocele is somewhat tense, smooth-walled and well defined. The swelling is fluctuant and brilliantly translucent. There is no cough impulse and it is not reducible. If it is extremely large, a fluid thrill may be present and, if large enough, the swelling will also be found to be dull to percussion. If a scrotal swelling can be felt separate to the testis, then the swelling manifestly cannot be a hydrocele.

EPIDIDYMAL CYSTS

These are thought to be derived from the tubules of the epididymis. An epididymal cyst by definition contains clear fluid, whereas a spermatocele contains opalescent fluid. Otherwise there is little difference between these two diagnoses, except that a spermatocele is considered by many to feel like a third testis. Epididymal cysts are often multiple, multilocular and bilateral. The testis and epididymis can be palpated separately to the mass, which is situated superolaterally to the testis. The mass is fluctuant, translucent, dull and non-reducible, and does not have a cough impulse. If multilocular, it may feel bosselated and give a Chinese-lantern effect on transillumination.

VARICOCELE

A varicocele will usually only become evident on standing or, if it is evident on lying down, will become much more prominent on standing. It consists of dilated, elongated and tortuous veins of the pampiniform plexus, almost always occurring on the left side. The reason for the left-sidedness of the pathology is unknown, and it seems overly simplistic to attribute this to the junction of the left testicular vein into the renal vein. The swelling has been described as feeling like a bag of worms. It may be associated with reduced spermatogenesis and relative infertility. Surgery may be indicated both for cosmetic reasons and in an attempt to improve fertility.

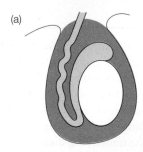

(a)

Hydrocele surrounds testis
and epididymis, neither of
which can be felt

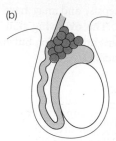

(b)

Multilocular epididymal cyst
above and lateral to epididymis

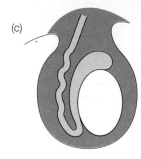

(c)

Inguino-scrotal swelling enveloping
testis and epididymis. Distinguished
from an indirect inguinal hernia by the
absence of a cough impulse and its
non-reducible nature

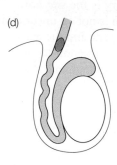

(d)

Small, translucent, mobile
mass within spermatic cord

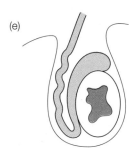

(e)

Irregular, hard mass within
the testis

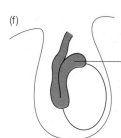

(f)

Swollen, tender epididymis
and spermatic cord

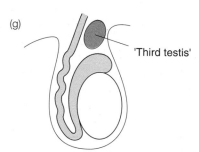

(g)

'Third testis'

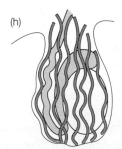

(h)

Dilated veins pampiniform
plexus giving the impression of a
'bag of worms'

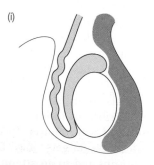

(i)

Complete or scrotal hernia,
encompasses testis.
The mass has a cough impulse, and may be reducible,
fluctuant, non-transilluminable and resonant

Figure 20.6.5 Schematic diagrams of scrotal lumps. (a) Vaginal hydrocele. (b) Cyst epididymis. (c) Congenital hydrocele. (d)
Encysted hydrocele of cord. (e) Testicular tumour. (f) Acute epididymitis. (g) Spermatocele. (h) Varicocele. (i) Indirect inguinal hernia.

HAEMATOCELE

By definition this is blood within the tunica vaginalis, and it may be due to trauma or malignancy. An acute haematocele has the same features as a vaginal hydrocele, but is not translucent and is often slightly tender. A chronic haematocele occurs when the blood of an acute haematocele has clotted and contracted, forming a small hard mass which is non-tender and non-fluctuant. Clinically this may be indistinguishable from advanced malignancy, and in this situation investigation with ultrasound examination and often ultimately inguinal exploration may be necessary.

TORSION OF THE TESTIS

This important condition is most common in patients under 25 years of age. The condition is usually due to torsion of both the testis and the epididymis because of a bell-clapper testis abnormality, in which the tunica vaginalis descends right around the testis and epididymis so that they are hanging within the scrotum like a bell-clapper within a bell, suspended by the spermatic cord. Consequently, the condition of torsion is usually torsion of the spermatic cord. As a result, as in other conditions of torsion (e.g small bowel), there is initially venous obstruction and subsequently, as venous swelling and venous infarction continue, arterial occlusion. Therefore torsion may still be present while ultrasound Doppler duplex studies show flow within the testicular artery. The condition presents acutely, but there may have been previous episodes of pain. It is unilateral, the scrotum may be reddened and the testis is elevated, tender and indistinguishable from the epididymis. The condition is a surgical emergency, and surgical exploration will be required. The differential diagnoses of the acute surgical scrotum are as follows:

1. torsion of the testis;
2. torsion of a testicular appendage (hydatid of Morgagni);
3. acute epididymo-orchitis;
4. idiopathic scrotal oedema;
5. strangulated inguinal hernia.

The abnormality predisposing to testicular torsion is almost always bilateral, and therefore if torsion is found at operation the other side should be explored and an orchidopexy performed.

ORCHITIS

Mumps is the commonest cause of orchitis, and is usually associated with a less significant secondary epididymitis.

ACUTE EPIDIDYMO-ORCHITIS

This is a common condition and must be distinguished from testicular torsion. It may be associated with *Chlamydia trachomatis*, *E. coli* or gonococcal infection. There may be a history of urinary tract infection, urinary tract instrumentation or sexually transmitted disease. Urethral discharge should be enquired for. The patient is often systemically unwell with malaise, fever and toxicity. Examination of the scrotum will reveal an acutely tender hemiscrotum. With careful palpation it is usually possible to determine whether the epididymis is distinguishable from the testis, and whether the epididymis itself is particularly swollen and is the site of maximal tenderness. There may be a small lax secondary associated hydrocele. The spermatic cord is usually thickened, and a rectal examination to assess the prostate is mandatory.

TUBERCULOUS EPIDIDYMO-ORCHITIS

This condition is rare in Western communities, but can cause a mass in the epididymis which can ulcerate through to the skin, causing a sinus to appear posteriorly in the scrotum.

TESTICULAR TUMOURS

About 95% of testicular tumours arise from germ cells, and may be classified as seminomatous, non-seminomatous (teratoma) and others. Up to 40% of testicular tumours present with tenderness and are often associated with small secondary hydroceles. Clinically there will be a solid mass within the testis which is irregular and hard, non-fluctuant, non-translucent and non-reducible. The lymphatic drainage of the testis is to the para-aortic nodes, and therefore abdominal examination is mandatory, as is examination of the neck. Differential diagnoses of a solid mass within the testis include the following:

1. testicular tumour;
2. acute and chronic epididymitis with secondary orchitis;
3. chronic haematocele;
4. gumma of the testis.

All such solid masses will require testicular exploration via an inguinal approach to exclude malignancy.

INVESTIGATIONS

As previously indicated, careful clinical assessment usually enables a specific diagnosis to be achieved in the inguino-scrotal area. Occasionally, some investigations will be required. If testicular tumour is suspected, tumour markers, beta human chorionic gonadotrophin (HCG), LDH, and alpha-fetoprotein should be assessed, as these data can subsequently be used for monitoring. Secondary spread should be looked for with chest X-ray, CT scan of the chest and CT scan of the abdomen.

Ultrasound examination of the inguinal canal, spermatic cord and scrotal contents is often helpful. Colour Doppler can show flow within vessels, and although the flow is increased in epididymo-orchitis and decreased in torsion, this distinction is not absolute, and if there is any doubt surgical exploration is mandatory. Ultrasound examination is useful for determining whether masses are present, and is often a reassuring investigation for the patient who is concerned about the possibility of testicular cancer. It is useful to docu-ment the site of a swelling as being in the epididymis, within the testis or elsewhere. It is also useful on occasion for patients who present with chronic groin pain and in whom an inguinal hernia is not clinically apparent.

MANAGEMENT

In general, all hernias require repair because of the risk of strangulation and because they are symptomatic. Only in exceptional circumstances would a conservative approach be indicated. For most other inguino-scrotal swellings, exploration and surgical removal or repair are indicated, but the specific details are beyond the scope of this chapter.

Integrity of the skin barrier to infection

Rodney D. Cooter and David Belford

Introduction

The skin is the largest organ of the human body. In an adult its area exceeds $1.5–2\,m^2$ and its mass is greater than that of any other organ. It covers the entire body in a layer of varying physical thickness, ranging from 8 mm at the soles to 1 mm over the eyelids, and it contains several appendageal structures, including sebaceous, apocrine and eccrine glands, hair and nails. Skin acts both as a barrier to the environment and as a communication with it, and its total destruction is incompatible with survival. As an organ it subserves a multitude of activities, including thermoregulation, fluid loss control, immune protection, sensory transduction, mechanical and solar protection, and infection control. While recognizing the importance and complexity of these functions, this chapter will focus on skin as a barrier to infection.

For the purpose of this chapter, infection will be regarded as the transcutaneous transfer and subsequent multiplication, growth, metabolic activities and pathophysiological effects of micro-organisms. Clinically, for bacteria this translates to $>10^5$ micro-organisms per gram of tissue, except for *Streptococcus*, which may cause clinical infection at substantially lower levels, of the order of 10^2 micro-organisms per gram of tissue. It is important to note that under normal biological conditions humans exist in equilibrium with surface micro-organisms – this equilibrium represents a balance between local and systemic host defences and action of the bacteria. Normal skin contains a resident flora of around 10^3 micro-organisms per gram, predominantly *Staphylococcus epidermidis*, Corynebacteria and Propionibacteria. Infection only occurs when this equilibrium becomes unbalanced.

During surgical intervention it is important to consider the integrity of two skin barriers, namely the patient's skin barrier against wound infections, which are predominantly bacterial, and the surgeon's skin barrier to the transmission of blood-borne viral pathogens.

Of surgical relevance, therefore, is an appreciation of the normal properties of skin as a barrier to infection, as well as an understanding of the methods that are used to enhance that barrier function in order to avert the infective consequences of a breach in skin integrity.

THE NORMAL BARRIER FUNCTION OF SKIN

Skin is composed of two layers of differing embryological origin. The most superficial layer, the epidermis, is an ectodermal derivative, while the innermost thicker layer, the dermis, is of mesenchymal origin. A subepidermal basement membrane separates the epidermis and the superficial or papillary dermis along an undulating border that results from the upward extension of numerous dermal papillae into the epidermis. The ridges of epidermal cells that interdigitate between the dermal papillae are known as rete ridges.

EPIDERMIS

The epidermis is a stratified squamous epithelium that

envelops the external surface and is continuous with the internal surfaces of the respiratory, gastrointestinal and urogenital systems. In addition, the skin appendages, namely hair, nails, sweat glands and sebaceous glands, are all derived from the epidermis. The epidermis is the primary barrier to invasion by micro-organisms and, if damaged, it has a large regenerative capacity. It contains no blood vessels, but derives nutrients by diffusion from capillaries in the superficial or papillary dermis. There are three different cell types in the epidermis, namely keratinocytes, melanocytes and dendritic cells.

Keratinocyte layer

The nomenclature of the stratified epidermal layers relates to the maturation phase of the keratinocytes, which are continuously developing from the basal layer to the anuclear horny layer.

The basal layer (also known as the stratum basale or stratum germinativum) is a single layer of columnar cells attached to the basement membrane via hemidesmosomes, a complex of transmembrane proteins which consist of bullous pemphigoid antigens 1 and 2 (also known as type XVII collagen) and the α6β4 integrin heterodimer.

Basal keratinocytes actively divide and advance from the basal layer to the skin's surface over a period of 28 days. In so doing they undergo structural and functional changes commensurate with the various epidermal strata. Immediately above the basal layer the cells form the squamous cell layer (the stratum spinosum or prickle cell layer) which is several cells thick. In this layer, intercellular bridges or desmosomes appear as prickles, and the cells become flattened and accumulate keratin filaments. Superficial to the squamous cell layer is the granular cell layer (also known as the stratum granulosum) in which the cell's cytoplasm is filled with keratohyaline granules and the nuclei shrink as the cells begin to degenerate. The granular cell layer thickness is proportional to that of the horny layer above. In areas such as the palms and soles, where the horny layer is thick, there is an identifiable zone above the granular cell layer known as the stratum lucidum (or stratum conjunctum). The outermost horny layer (the stratum corneum, or stratum disjunctum) contains flattened anuclear cell remnants and keratin. Desiccation and desquamation of surface cells shed some organisms but, more importantly, the keratin layer is indigestible by most micro-organisms, and therefore protects the deeper viable keratinocytes from surface organisms and their toxins. Equally, however, the resident surface flora helps to protect the skin from surface invasion by more virulent species, as they coexist as opportunists and compete for nutrients.

It is this insoluble, tough keratinized layer that mechanically protects the body from the environment, as epidermal tissue is subjected to more trauma than any other body tissue.

Melanocytes

About 10% of the cells in the basal layer are melanocytes, which have processes through which they transfer melanin to the basal keratinocytes. In this way each melanocyte delivers melanin to several keratinocytes, so that at any given time there is usually more melanin in the keratinocytes than in the melanocytes.

Dendritic cells

Langerhans' cells account for approximately 3% of the epidermal cells, and are found just above the basal layer of the epidermis. They are antigen-presenting cells, and have a pivotal role in the skin immune system by inducing primary immune responses. In response to skin contact by allergens, Langerhans' cells show enhanced migration, which in turn activates paracortical cells in the draining lymph nodes, and specific T-cell populations expand.

BASEMENT MEMBRANE

The dermis and epidermis are separated by a band known as the basement membrane zone, which consists of about 20 different structural proteins that serve to attach the basal keratinocytes to the underlying dermis. Electron microscopy identifies separation of the basement membrane into two zones. The upper electron-lucent lamina lucida is traversed by anchoring filaments that are thought to attach the hemidesmosomes to the underlying basement membrane complex. Recent evidence suggests that these anchoring filaments are composed of laminin 5. The underlying lamina densa contains laminin 1, type IV collagen, heparin sulphate proteoglycans and nidogen, and is secured to the underlying dermis via anchoring fibrils which consist of type VII collagen.

DERMIS

Like the epidermis, the dermis varies in thickness in different parts of the body. The connective tissue of the dermis contains collagen, predominantly of mature type 1 with smaller amounts of immature type 3 collagen and some reticulum fibres adjacent to the basement membrane. Hydrated glycosaminoglycans occupy the spaces between the structural fibres. In addition there are thin elastic fibres in the superficial dermis which become thicker in the lower portion of the dermis. The pivotal cell of all the dermis is the fibroblast, which is responsible for the production of these dermal constituents. The superficial dermis is termed the papillary layer, as it contains the above-mentioned dermal papillae that project into the undersurface of the epidermis. The deeper layer, known as the reticular dermis, contains the more robust elastic fibres that produce the skin's relaxed tension lines. The uniqueness of the skin's physical properties mainly depends on the dermal networks of collagen and elastin, and the pattern of their interwoven architecture. The dermal layer is the nutrient source for the epidermis, and is important surgically as the producer of scar tissue that confers physical strength to a wound after surgical closure. Disruption of this layer creates a portal of entry for organisms to subcutaneous tissues as they bypass the natural protective barrier mechanisms of intact skin.

ADNEXAL STRUCTURES

The basal cell layer of the epidermis gives rise to the dermal appendages, namely hair, sebaceous and eccrine sweat glands, and apocrine glands. Hair follicles are essentially down-growths of the epidermis. Sebaceous gland ducts open into the follicles and thence to the surface, while erector pili muscles insert into the follicles more deeply. Hair follicle epidermal cells are controlled by a special stromal region known as the dermal papilla. Sebaceous glands are found in all skin except the palms of the hands and soles of the feet. They are most abundant in the skin of the forehead, nose and cheeks. Their secretions are formed from the decomposition of their cells by lysosomal enzymes. Greasy sebum contains bactericidal activity, and also prevents dehydration of the epidermis. Skin secretions vary in composition at different stages of development, with some childhood fungal infections being cleared by puberty with its increased rate of sebaceous secretion.

Eccrine glands are abundant in human skin and can produce large volumes of sweat in response to heat. They have a deep coiled secretory portion with an epithelial cell-lined duct that passes upwards through the dermis and epidermis to open directly on to the skin's surface, where they secrete a colourless fluid. Like sebaceous secretions, sweat contains bactericidal and fungicidal activity that protects against pathogenic micro-organisms.

Skin secretions contain a multitude of compounds with proposed bactericidal activity, including lysozyme, sterols, amino acids, phospholipids, lactic acid and uric acid, fatty acids and triglycerides. The high concentration of salt in drying sweat is a further barrier to the survival of skin micro-organisms.

The apocrine glands are to be found in the hair-bearing axillary and genital regions, where their ducts lead directly into a pilosebaceous unit above the entry point of the sebaceous duct. Apocrine secretions are more viscous than their eccrine counterparts, and unlike the heat regulation of sweat, they are essentially scent glands that become active at puberty.

All skin gland ductal systems can act as a repository for micro-organisms. Normal skin contains a resident flora of around 10^3 micro-organisms per gram, predominantly consisting of *Staphylococcus epidermidis*, Corynebacteria and Propionibacteria.

Nails consist of compacted keratinized cells that originate in the epidermis of the nail matrix. Beneath the nail is the dermal bed, which consists of a germinal matrix (the proximal one-third) and a sterile matrix (the distal two-thirds). The soft tissue around the nail is termed perionychium, while that along the nail sides is known as the paronychium. The hyponychium is the junctional area where the sterile matrix and the fingertip skin meet. In this region there are increased numbers of leucocytes and lymphocytes.

ENHANCING THE BARRIER FUNCTION OF SKIN

INFECTION CONTROL PROTOCOLS

Although infection is uncommon with an intact skin barrier, with surgical interventions other measures must be taken to replace or reconstitute the protective barrier function of skin in order to reduce the risk of transmission of infectious agents between patient and surgeon. Enhancement of the skin's barrier function may take many forms, including physical measures (e.g. gloves, gowns, caps, masks, drapes, etc.), appropriate choice of disinfectant solutions, pharmacological measures (e.g. antibiotic prophylaxis, vaccinations, etc.), and the routine use of safe surgical techniques. To help guide this process in the surgical setting, infection control protocols have been developed.

Hand-washing

Before any invasive surgical procedure, the initial surgical 'scrub' each day should last for 5 min, with subsequent washes lasting 3 min. Prolonged vigorous pre-operative scrubbing is not necessary. Recommended hand cleansers should contain 4% (w/v) chlorhexidine or detergent-based povidone-iodine containing 0.75% available iodine.

Gloves

While resident skin flora can be significantly reduced by hand-washing, as noted above, they persist within the ductal conduits of skin glands and can readily multiply.

In addition, the distal fingertip skin beneath the fingernails is often heavily contaminated with *Staphylococcus epidermidis*, which is difficult to eradicate even with pre-operative hand scrubbing. For these reasons, sterile gloves should be worn during any procedure that physically breaches the skin, to ensure patient protection against iatrogenic inoculation.

Protective clothing

Other protective clothing and equipment include gowns, which should be impervious or fluid-resistant, and face masks; both are recommended to reduce the risk of wound contamination by desquamating epithelial cells from the surgeon and, of course, for the wearer's own protection. Surgical caps or hoods are worn to prevent hair from falling into the wound. Like surgical gowns, sterile drapes should be impervious, as wet drapes can have a wick-like effect which permits the transmission of micro-organisms from one side to the other. To enhance their barrier effect further, drapes can be secured with sterile adhesive film around the perimeter of the operative site, or alternatively across the whole operative field, and incisions can then be made through the clear film.

Disinfectants

Skin disinfectants are designed to aid the removal of the skin's bacterial flora. Those recommended for the skin are chlorhexidine (0.5–1.0%, w/v), or aqueous povidone-iodine (10%, w/v, with 1% available iodine).

Prophylaxis

Pharmacological and immunological enhancement of the infection barrier are important adjuncts to the prevention of infection. In surgical patients who are at significant risk of developing infection, either from a surgical procedure or from a presenting complaint, antibiotic prophylaxis should follow recommended guidelines. Tetanus prophylaxis for patients and surgical staff should be current, and all surgical personnel require hepatitis vaccinations. It is well known that steroid-dependent patients have a reduced wound-healing capacity and higher post-operative infection rates, but this can be corrected by a short course of peri-operative vitamin A administered orally for 2 weeks at a dosage of at least 25 000 IU/day. Vitamin A acts as a pro-inflammatory cytokine to enhance the early inflammatory phase of healing by offsetting the anti-inflammatory effect of steroids.

Debridement

Skin wound surgical techniques are designed ultimately to reconstitute the skin's layers and thereby restore its barrier function. To achieve this reliably, surgeons must pay particular attention to thorough wound debridement, employ atraumatic tissue-handling principles, close the skin with edge eversions, and avoid diathermy burns to the skin.

Local factors in the wound that promote infection include necrotic or ischaemic tissue, the presence of a foreign body, haematoma, dead space and decreased local perfusion.

WOUND CARE

Most normal skin healing will lead to scar formation that acts as a substitute barrier. The healing skin wound gains strength over a period of several months, but in the early stages may be liable to dehiscence unless it is adequately splinted, either internally by dermal sutures or externally by taping. Skin tapes or adhesive dressings help to control scarring and offer added protection for the skin by reducing the abrading effect of clothing and the risk of inadvertent scratching by fingernails. If suture lines are kept moist with antibiotic ointment, there is less local inflammation post-operatively, as the ingress along sutures by micro-organisms is impeded; suture removal is also facilitated due to a lack of crusting around the suture knots.

From the myriad of dressing technologies now available, surgeons must choose a product to match a particular wound's requirements, one of which is to maintain sterility (or at least cleanliness) of a wound by acting as a barrier to nosocomial infection. An occlusive dressing, providing this function, also creates a moist wound environment which is optimal for wound healing.

To enhance further the integrity of healing skin wounds around joints, immobility splintage may be prudent in the early post-operative phase, followed by taping measures both to control scarring and to offer longer-term support. Excessive movement of a joint before a skin scar is mature may result in dehiscence or scar fissuring, which may in turn lead to infective problems.

THE BREACHED SKIN BARRIER

THE PATIENT'S BARRIER

From the foregoing account it will be apparent that the normal barrier function of skin maintains microbial balance under normal conditions. However, during surgical procedures it is necessary to isolate the patient's skin from that of the surgeon by interposing alternative barriers. In routine elective surgical procedures the protocols are straightforward, but surgeons are often required to deal with wounds that are potentially contaminated, dirty or frankly infected as a result of breaches in the skin barrier. In addition, breaches in the skin may be secondary to other pathologies such as ulcerating skin tumours, pressure ulcers, leg ulcers, sinuses and fistulae, unstable scars or fissures at mucocutaneous junctions.

Traumatic wounds

When presenting with physical trauma, patients and their wounds should both be classified according to their infection risk. Often neglected, but of vital importance, is the documentation of a thorough history of the mechanism and environment of an injury, and an inquiry into the patient's viral exposure risk.

Open-hand injuries are at particular risk of breaching several structures in close proximity because the hand anatomy is so compact. Skin wounds over volar joint creases are very likely to have penetrated the flexor tendon sheath. Antibiotic prophylaxis is important in these cases, and should be tailored to the types of organisms expected. Obviously contaminated wounds or those caused by high-pressure industrial accidents will need aggressive debridement, even though some pressure injection injuries only breach the protective skin layer with a deceptively minor skin wound.

Another challenging concern is the burn wound, which soon becomes colonized and often infected because necrotic tissue serves as an excellent culture medium. Burn wounds must be cleansed of surface dirt and contaminants in order to reduce the likelihood of mycotic infection from fungal spores. With such a large surface barrier loss and the impending infection risk, it is now customary to debride early and replace the lost skin function with a split skin graft or an alternative skin equivalent layer. However, electrical burns, like pressure injuries, can penetrate the skin via a relatively small surface wound from which a deep zone of necrosis may extend. In these cases restoration of the integrity of the skin can be complicated by the progressively deepening necrosis.

Bite injuries physically breach the skin barrier and inoculate subcutaneous tissue or even joints and tendon sheaths with a variety of micro-organisms. A human bite can contain up to 10^8 organisms/mL of saliva. The commonest human 'bite' wound involves the fist punch injury, in which the assailant's metacarpophalangeal joints are at risk of being punctured by the victim's teeth. What appears initially to be a rather innocuous laceration on the extensor aspect of the proximal phalangeal region may quickly develop into septic arthritis as the extensor tendon hood seals the metacarpophalangeal joint as the hand adopts a normal posture on relaxation of the clenched fist. Anaerobic organisms 'injected' by human bites include *Eikenella corrodens*, which is sensitive to pencillin. Animal bites carry similar risks because

the inoculum can be injected deeply by the long slender teeth of some species. For example, cat bites are particularly prone to *Pasteurella multocida* infections, and these too are sensitive to penicillin. Antibiotics are not usually sufficient treatment in isolation, and should be combined with debridement and irrigation and, in some cases, delayed primary closure.

Occasionally leeches are used to relieve venous congestion of skin flaps or digital replants. At the point of skin attachment, the leech (*Hirudo medicinalis*) releases an anticoagulant (hirudin) locally to assist blood flow. Being a waterborne organism, the leech can also infect the host with micro-organisms such as *Aeromonas hydrophila*, so antibiotic prophylaxis should include an aminoglycoside such as gentamicin.

Hair

Hair at an operative site can be clipped in preference to shaving, because wound infection rates are significantly higher with pre-operative shaving. Organisms harboured within the ducts of the skin's adnexal glands can also lead to chronic infective problems around hair follicles, as is seen in conditions such as sycosis barbae and kerion, and treatment is effected with appropriate antibiotic and antifungal therapies, respectively. Glandular infections may develop more deeply in the condition hidradenitis suppurativa, which may be temporarily controlled with systemic antibiotics, but which may ultimately require excision of the offending glands. This usually entails excision of the affected hair-bearing areas of the groin or axilla, otherwise the problem will be perpetuated by the persistently moist and infected environment.

Moisture

While wound healing is promoted in a moist environment, excessive sweating softens the keratin layer, so inactivating the most superficial barrier and leading to infection. For example, covering the skin with a water-impermeable dressing can result in the loss of this barrier and the appearance of staphylococcal folliculitis. The higher skin infection rate in tropical environments bears testimony to the contribution of excessive sweating in weakening the keratin barrier.

Skin closure

The choice of skin-closure technique can significantly influence the post-operative infection rate. Because tapes, tissue glues and staples do not traverse the wound, they are associated with lower rates of infection than sutures that pass through all of the skin layers as well as the wound itself. Local complications of sutures, such as stitch abscesses, can cause chronic breaches in the skin barrier. If dermal apposition sutures are not buried deeply enough or not tied with the knot's ears pointing deeply, they may lead to a chronic communication with the surface and act as a nidus of infection. Higher risks of infective complications occur with multifilament sutures compared to their much less reactive monofilament counterparts. Suture composition is also relevant, catgut and silk sutures being particularly noxious if left in the skin for extended periods. A single silk suture decreases the number of staphylococci required to form a pustule by around 10 000-fold.

Foreign bodies

All foreign bodies, including dirt and debris as well as iatrogenic bodies, decrease host resistance. Consideration should be given to all other sites of skin breaching, including intravenous drip sites, intra-arterial lines, drains and '-ostomies'. Colonization of these breaches can become a nidus for infection elsewhere in the body, e.g. tracheostomy-related organisms can be transferred to craniofacial osteotomy sites and result in severe infection.

THE SURGEON'S BARRIER

While much of our surgical emphasis is on the protection or restoration of the patient's barrier function, it is becoming increasingly important to protect staff from exposure to blood-borne viruses.

Pre-existing breaches

As the integrity of the skin acts as a natural barrier to infection, any cuts or abrasions on the surgeon's hands should be covered with a sterile wound tape and then sealed with a water-resistant occlusive dressing after a normal hand 'scrub'. Double-gloving over the dressing then decreases the risk of blood exposure during the procedure.

Double-gloving

To protect the surgeon from sharp injuries and patient blood exposure, simple precautions such as double-gloving and developing safer operating techniques can decrease the exposure risk to blood and body fluids by an estimated 74%. While no double-gloving technique will prevent sharp injuries, it has been shown that in operations exceeding 2 h in duration where more than 100 mL of blood were lost, a 51% incidence of single-glove perforation and blood exposure was noted. This figure decreased to 7% with the use of double gloves. Despite such evidence, many surgeons have resisted changing their single-gloving practices as they are concerned that wearing two gloves may be cumbersome and reduce

tactile sensitivity. A comfortable method is to wear a half-size greater than normal glove as an inner glove, with a normal-size glove worn as the outer layer. Powder-free surgical gloves are recommended.

Sharps injuries

In a report of 70 sharps injuries, 67% were caused by needles, usually while suturing. The non-dominant index fingertip was the commonest site of injury, and three main mechanisms were identified: injured hand retracting tissue; injury occurring during the passage of a needle into or out of the incision; injury of the hand by sharp objects left in the operating field. To overcome these 'breaches in the barrier', it is recommended that a free hand should not be used to retract tissue, the hands of the assistant should be distanced from an incision by using longer instruments, and all sharp objects should be removed from the operating field when not in use. The transfer of needles out of the field can be made safer by clamping the sharp tip of a needle in the jaws of a needle-holder before returning it. In the case of other sharp objects, it is sensible practice to pass the instruments via an intermediate tray or receptacle to avoid hand-to-hand transfer.

Self-inflicted injuries are often the result of hand-held needles being passed through tissue that is splinted with the operator's fingers. For this reason, hand-held needles should not be used, and when passing trochars percutaneously the skin counterpressure should be provided with an instrument and the trochar then placed directly into a sharps receptacle. Kirschner wires should be covered or bent down away from the operative field, and dental wires should be left long, draped out of the mouth and splinted with a small artery clip to cover their sharp ends during the application of other wiring.

FURTHER READING

Bos JD. 1977: The skin as an organ of immunity. *Clinical and Experimental Immunology* **107** (Suppl. 1), 3–5.

Cooter RD, Lim I, Ellis D, Leitch I. 1990: Burn wound zygomycosis caused by *Apophysomyces elegans*. *Journal of Clinical Microbiology* **28**, 2151–3.

David DJ, Cooter RD. 1987: Craniofacial infection in 10 years of transcranial surgery. *Plastic and Reconstructive Surgery* **80**, 213–23.

Edlich RF, Rodenheaver GT, Thacker JG. 1995: Technical factors in the prevention of wound infections. In Howard RJ, Simmons RJ (eds), *Surgical infectious diseases*, 3rd edn. Norwalk, CT: Appleton & Lange.

Ehrlich HP, Hunt TK. 1973: Effects of vitamin A and

glucocorticoids upon inflammation and collagen synthesis. *Annals of Surgery* **177**, 222–7.

Fry DE. 1991: Blood exposure in the operating room: reducing the risk. *Bulletin of the American College of Surgeons* **76**, 17.

Fuller JC, Cutroneo KR. 1992: Pharmacological interventions. In: Cohen IK, Diegelmann RF, Lindblad WJ (eds), *Wound healing: biochemical and clinical aspects*. Philadelphia, PA: W.B. Saunders Co., 305–15.

Gardner JF, Peel MM. 1991: *Introduction to sterilization, disinfection and infection control*, 2nd edn. Melbourne: Churchill Livingstone.

Gibson T. 1990: Physical properties of skin. In McCarthy JG (ed.), *Plastic surgery. Vol. 1. General principles*. Philadelphia, PA: W.B. Saunders Co., 207–20.

Heggers JP. 1991: Systemic causes of decreased resistance. In Heggers JP, Robson MC (eds), *Quantitative bacteriology: its role in the armamentarium of the surgeon*. Boca Raton, FL: CRC Press, 35–52.

Hotcherg J, Murray GF. 1997: Principles of operative surgery. In Saliton DC (ed.), *Textbook of surgery: the biological basis of modern surgical practice*, 15th edn. Philadelphia, PA: W.B. Saunders Co., 253–6.

National Health and Medical Research Council 1996: *Infection control in the health care setting. Guidelines for the prevention of transmission of infectious diseases*.

Poon C, Morgan DJ, Pond F, Kane J, Tulloh BR. 1998:

Studies of the surgical scrub. *Australian and New Zealand Journal of Surgery* **68**, 65–7.

Quebbeman EJ, Telford GL, Wadsworth K *et al.* 1992: Double gloving: protecting surgeons from blood contamination in the operating room. *Archives of Surgery* **127**, 213–16.

Rayan GM, Flournoy DJ. 1987: Microbiologic flora of human fingernails. *Journal of Hand Surgery* **12A**, 605.

Robson MC. 1991: The equilibrium between the bacteria and the host. In Heggers JP, Robson MC (eds), *Quantitative bacteriology: its role in the armamentarium of the surgeon*. Boca Raton, FL: CRC Press, 1–8.

Royal Australasian College of Surgeons. 1998: *Infection control in surgery*. Melbourne: Policy document.

Smoot EC. 1998: Practical precautions for avoiding sharp injuries and blood exposure. *Plastic and Reconstructive Surgery* **101**, 528–34.

Wright JG, McGeer AJ, Chyatte D *et al.* 1991: Mechanisms of glove tears and sharp injuries among surgical personnel. *Journal of the American Medical Association* **266**, 1668.

Zook EG. 1990: Anatomy and physiology of the perionychium. *Hand Clinics* **6**, 1.

Zook EG, Van Beek AL, Russell RC *et al.* 1980: Anatomy and physiology of the perionychium: a review of the literature and anatomic study. *Journal of Hand Surgery* **5**, 528.

Skin ulcers

Rodney D. Cooter and David Belford

Introduction

Skin ulcers are an unpleasant burden on patients, families, clinicians and health systems world-wide. While many different clinicians are involved in their management, skin ulcers are frequently encountered in surgical practice, the most common types being leg ulcers from vascular disease and pressure ulcers from pressure around the hip girdle. This chapter deals predominantly with these two groups.

Skin ulcers can have widely varying aetiologies, but most result from tissue necrosis caused or sustained by factors such as vascular disease, prolonged pressure, trauma, infection and neuropathy (principally diabetes related). Other factors that may retard ulcer healing include steroid therapy, vitamin deficiencies, anaemia and malnutrition. Several of these factors may coexist.

As epidemiological data emerge on the prevalence and high cost to society of these chronic skin ulcers, research efforts are starting to unravel their aetiologies and pathophysiologies, and this information will help to shape clinical practice guidelines for effective prevention strategies and optimal treatment protocols. At the present time, however, despite the debilitating nature of these ulcers, there is still a disappointing lack of evidence-based information from large prospective randomized controlled trials on which to base conclusions. Until more rigorous supporting evidence becomes available, the recommendations for the management of many skin ulcers will continue to be based on small prospective non-randomized trials, retrospective studies, or even anecdotal evidence from uncontrolled trials or case reports.

LEG ULCERS

EPIDEMIOLOGY

Chronic leg ulceration is usually a non-fatal condition of predominantly elderly patients, and it can be frustratingly recalcitrant to treatment. It remains a common problem in clinical surgical practice, with an estimated point prevalence in the range of 1–2 per 1000 total population. Most studies collecting prevalence data have relied on postal questionnaires, and these results almost certainly represent an underestimate of leg ulcers in the general population. The problem is compounded further by the fact that many leg ulcers persist for several years and, even if they heal, recurrence rates are high. These prevalence and recurrence rates reflect a virtual epidemic of recurrent leg ulcers that are managed ineffectively and so persist as a burden on health resources.

AETIOLOGY

The majority of leg ulcers are due to venous disease, arterial ischaemia or neuropathy. Chronic venous insufficiency is a recognized contributor to leg ulceration in up to 80% of cases. A further 10% have arterial ischaemia, and the remainder are due to neuropathy or combined aetiologies.

Venous leg ulceration is the result of chronic venous insufficiency which leads to venous hypertension. Damage to the communicating, superficial or deep vein valves, deep vein occlusion or failure of the calf muscle pump results in 'venous insufficiency' or 'venous hypertension'. This term is something of a misnomer, and refers to the situation where venous pressure, while not actually increasing, does not drop with contraction of the calf muscle pump. Nevertheless, the link between increased pressure in the venous system and the cellular pathology of the venous ulcer has not yet been established, although several somewhat overlapping hypotheses have been suggested, as follows.

Fibrin cuff hypothesis This postulates that venous hypertension promotes leakage of plasma proteins, notably fibrinogen, from a distended capillary bed. Extravascular fibrinogen polymerizes to form a peri-capillary fibrin cuff. Recent work has shown that these cuffs also contain other serum proteins, such as α2-macroglobulin and factor XIIIa, as well as the matrix proteins laminin, fibronectin, tenascin and collagens I and III, suggesting that certain components of fibrin cuffs are actively synthesized by the surrounding connective tissue cells. These cuffs are proposed to act as a diffusion barrier to oxygen and nutrients, and to inhibit capillary sprouting. Similar peri-capillary cuffs containing fibrin, collagen, laminin and fibronectin are found in diabetic ulcers.

White-cell-trapping hypothesis It has been suggested that increased pressure in the venous system reduces the perfusion pressure and capillary flow rate, and that this results in the trapping of white blood cells in skin capillaries. The trapped leucocytes become activated and release toxic metabolites, enzymes and cytokines, damaging endothelial cells and allowing the passage of plasma proteins, including fibrinogen. In addition, the trapped leucocytes result in areas of local ischaemia. More recently it has been further proposed that the matrix proteins found in fibrin cuffs are synthesized by fibroblasts and smooth-muscle endothelial cells in response to cytokines from activated leucocytes trapped in skin capillaries.

Trap hypothesis The co-localization of growth factors and serum-binding proteins (e.g. of α2-macroglobulin and transforming growth factor-β1) in fibrin cuffs has led to the suggestion that the trapping or inactivation of growth factors essential to the wound repair process by extravasated plasma proteins inhibits the repair response.

Unifying hypothesis Recently, a unifying hypothesis has been proposed to provide a basis for wound chronicity. This hypothesis stems from a significant body of evidence showing that the fluid and tissue collected from chronic wounds contain markedly elevated levels of pro-inflammatory cytokines, proteolytic enzymes and matrix degradation products compared to acute wounds. In contrast, chronic wound fluid contains reduced levels of protease inhibitors and low growth factor activity.

According to this hypothesis, the chronic wound is locked in a pro-inflammatory cycle such that tissue injury as a result of trauma, ischaemia and bacterial infection results in the release of inflammatory stimuli, including endotoxins, platelet products and extracellular matrix fragments that promote the entry of inflammatory cells into the wound. The release of inflammatory cytokines (e.g. tissue necrosis factor-α, interleukin-1) by these cells promotes production or release of proteases by resident neutrophils, macrophages, fibroblasts and keratinocytes. High levels of these enzymes (e.g. matrix metalloproteinases and neutrophil elastase) combined with low concentrations of their inhibitors (e.g. α1-proteinase inhibitor, α2-macroglobulin, tissue inhibitor of metalloproteinase) alters the delicate balance of protein synthesis and proteolysis required for normal wound repair. Ongoing degradation of proteins vital to wound repair, including matrix proteins (e.g. fibronectin), integrin matrix receptors, growth factors and growth factor receptors, results in wound chronicity.

DIABETIC ULCERS

Diabetic ulcers result from a combination of neuropathy, vasculopathy and infection. Peripheral neuropathy affecting sensory, motor and autonomic nerves leads to a lack of sensation, deformity of the foot and dry fragile skin at risk of breakdown. This situation is compounded by the ischaemia due to distal atherosclerosis and increased susceptibility to infection. Ulceration occurs at sites of repeated trauma, such as the toes, heels and prominent metatarsal heads.

EVALUATION

In the clinical setting it is important to document the ulcer's duration and any antecedent contributing factors. Comorbidities that should be enquired about include diabetes, rheumatoid arthritis, cardiovascular disease, anaemia, vitamin deficiencies, alcohol-related problems and infections. An attempt should be made to differentiate venous from arterial insufficiency. A venous ulcer sufferer may have had a deep vein thrombosis or suffer from varicose veins, whereas an arterial ulcer patient may report ischaemic calf pain or even pain in the toes or forefoot.

Appropriate ulcer treatment strategies depend on accurate diagnosis, and clinical examination will help to guide the process. Typically a venous leg ulcer is found on the medial aspect of the lower third of the leg. In addition to the ulcer, there should be other signs of chronic venous insufficiency, namely oedema, hyper-pigmentation, lipodermatosclerosis and dermatitis. Varicose veins may be obvious.

The venous ulcer usually has granulation tissue in its base, and there is often evidence of peripheral attempts at healing, as reflected in uneven epithelial margins. Arterial ulcers are less specific and occur in any area of poor blood supply. They are painful and have pale granulations in their bases which are often covered by a dark necrotic slough. Distal pulses are absent and the foot may be cool. The edges lack evidence of epithelialization, and the ulcer base is sharply demarcated.

Care must be taken in the elderly, who commonly have concomitant venous and arterial insufficiency, and both conditions must be further investigated and treated appropriately. If typical features of vascular insufficiency or diabetes are not present, an alternative diagnosis should be considered. These include the following.

1. Tumour:
   - basal-cell carcinoma;
   - squamous-cell carcinoma (especially in transplant patients);
   - haemangiomas;
   - vascular malformations.
2. Trauma:
   - burn scars (if long-standing, consider Marjolin's ulcer);
   - foreign bodies.
3. Infection:
   - osteomyelitis with sinus;
   - tropical ulcer;
   - tuberculous lesion;
   - fungal infection;
   - syphilis;
   - leprosy.
4. Medical:
   - hypertension;
   - lymphoedema;
   - AIDS-related Kaposi sarcoma;
   - immune suppression.
5. Inflammatory:
   - pyoderma gangrenosum;
   - rheumatoid vasculitis;
   - dermatitis.

Simple investigations, such as plain radiographs to exclude osteomyelitis, serology for systemic conditions, an incisional biopsy for local conditions, or a medical review, will clarify the situation.

NON-INVASIVE INVESTIGATIONS

Doppler ultrasound

This is a simple hand-held ultrasound probe that detects blood flow using the audible Doppler principle (5 MHz for venous investigations and 8 MHz for arterial investigations). The severity of arterial disease can be evaluated by measuring the ankle brachial index (ABI). This is the ratio of ankle artery systolic pressure to brachial artery systolic pressure (measured in both arms, and using the higher brachial pressure for the calculation).

Measurement of venous flow and velocity helps to delineate venous disease. Leg vein patency is detected by spontaneous venous signals that are modified by respiration, or by compressing the distal leg. Valvular incompetency can be assessed by the retrograde flow after a Valsalva manoeuvre, or following release of calf compression.

Duplex scan

An ultrasound system can include a pulsed Doppler facility to generate blood-flow data (velocity and direction). All leg veins can be assessed for forward flow and reflux, and the competence of individual valves may be assessed.

Skin perfusion studies

Transcutaneous oxygen measurement reflects skin perfusion when the probe is preheated to 45°C for the measurement.

Plethysmography

This technique, usually limited to vascular laboratories, evaluates limb blood flow from limb volume changes.

Photoplethysmography

In this technique, infrared light is directed into the skin and a detector in the same probe measures changes in the intensity of light reflected. It is useful for assessing patients with small-vessel disease where characteristic waveforms are generated from the probe, which is attached to the ankle region, while the patient activates their calf muscle pump with ankle movements. In this way it can help to differentiate oedema of venous origin from that due to lymphoedema or cardiac or other causes.

INVASIVE INVESTIGATIONS

Arteriography

An arteriogram is a method used to display arterial anatomy by digitally recording the data from contrast medium injected into an artery. Digital subtraction angiography has the advantages over conventional angiography of increased contrast sensitivity and therefore the need for a smaller amount of contrast medium, as well as providing data that can be more easily manipulated and quantified.

Venography

Contrast medium is injected into the venous system, and postural and other manoeuvres may be required to achieve appropriate venous filling. Venography provides precise anatomical information.

Intravascular pressure measurements

By cannulating specific vessels, intra-arterial pressures can be compared on either side of stenoses, and intravenous pressures can be monitored in response to exercise, or to diagnose proximal occlusion.

NON-SURGICAL TREATMENT

Prophylaxis

As deep vein thrombosis (DVT) is implicated in chronic venous insufficiency, surgical attention to DVT prophylaxis is imperative. If patients present with early signs and symptoms of chronic venous insufficiency, then clear instructions should be given in order to avoid deterioration. Simple measures such as leg elevation, good skin care, avoiding prolonged standing and using appropriate calf compression hosiery can all help to prevent the progression of skin ulceration. Comorbidities such as cardiac failure, anaemia, diabetes, liver failure, hypoproteinaemia, alcoholism, renal impairment, obesity, poor nutrition and skin conditions need to be treated effectively, and the management plan should encompass advice on appropriate lifestyle modifications to help to sustain the effects of early treatment. The association of smoking with vascular disease is well documented, and every attempt should be made to help patients to stop smoking.

Infection

To facilitate ulcer healing, treatment should remove as many 'ulcer-promoting' factors as possible. Surface necrotic tissue needs to be debrided, as it inhibits healing by preventing epithelialization and encouraging infection. Overt infection needs to be treated with appropriate antibiotics. However, caution must be exercised when choosing such an antibiotic on the basis of topical wound swabs, as most ulcers are colonized by several organisms, but their presence does not always constitute an infection. The most accurate technique for diagnosing infection is quantitative bacteriology, where a bacterial load of $> 10^5$ organisms per gram of tissue is considered to be positive. The exception to this is the presence of β-haemolytic streptococcus, which is pathogenic at levels of 10^2 per gram of tissue.

If patients are being treated with steroids for other conditions, such as rheumatoid arthritis or asthma, consideration should be given to a short course of high-dose oral vitamin A therapy administered as a pro-inflammatory cytokine to aid the inflammatory phase of wound healing which is otherwise dampened by the steroids.

Compression strategy

To counteract venous hypertension and thereby stimulate healing, legs with venous ulceration require firm compression bandaging. However, before applying such compression it is most important to exclude arterial disease, otherwise the bandage could render the limb ischaemic. A plethora of dressings and bandaging techniques exist. These differ in their composition, method of application, level of compression, longevity of compression, interval between changes, and cost. Ideally they should provide a compression of around 40 mmHg at ankle level, with a graduated pressure profile that promotes venous return from the limb. High-compression four-layer bandaging can achieve complete ulcer healing in 69% of venous ulcers by 12 weeks, and in 83% by 24 weeks.

Pharmacological treatment

While pharmacological treatment for leg ulceration is an attractive concept, there are no universally accepted oral or topical formulations in routine use. Those investigated include fibrinolytic-enhancing drugs (e.g. stanozolol, defibrotide), inhibitors of granulocyte aggregation (e.g. oxpentifylline), vasodilators (e.g. prostaglandin derivatives) and drugs that alter vascular permeability. Platelet-derived growth factor has shown some promise.

At the time of writing, three new biological treatments have been approved for the treatment of chronic wounds.

1. *Regranex*, a gel containing human recombinant platelet-derived growth factor (hrPDGF) at a concentration of 0.01% (100 µg/g), has been approved for the treatment of diabetic neuropathic ulcers.

2. *Apligraf* is a tissue-engineered skin substitute containing both dermal and epidermal layers that has been approved for the treatment of venous leg ulcers.

3. *Dermagraft* is a dermal replacement produced by culturing dermal fibroblasts in a biosynthetic scaffold. It has been approved for the treatment of diabetic ulcers.

Several other biological treatments, including tissue-engineered skin substitutes and growth factors (e.g. TGF-β2 and TGF-β3), are currently being tested in phase II pivotal trials.

However, the early over-enthusiasm for exogenously applied growth factors has generated several results that are difficult to interpret with confidence because the trial designs lack rigour.

SURGICAL TREATMENT

Surgical treatment of leg ulcers is tailored to the specific type and its aetiology. The excision and skin grafting of venous ulcers, for example, would be futile unless the venous disease was also corrected; typically this means operative correction of varicose veins and an operation for perforator vein incompetence. In order to have lasting benefits, such procedures need strict adjunctive behavioural regimens of early leg elevation and then prolonged elastic stocking support, often for life. Ischaemic-type ulceration may be the result of large-vessel occlusion, small-vessel disease, or a combination of both. Conservative measures include cessation of smoking, sympathectomy and intravascular prostacyclin. Limbs with weak or absent pulses may require balloon angioplasty or arterial reconstruction.

For ulceration of mixed arterial and venous aetiologies, it is usual to treat the arterial lesion first. In persistent leg ulcerations that are painful, amputation may be the only option.

PRESSURE ULCERS

EPIDEMIOLOGY

Pressure ulcers result from tissue necrosis caused by compression of soft tissue against a bony prominence. The prevalence of pressure ulcers varies according to the subpopulation of patients, the clinical setting and the staging of the ulcers. The Australian studies are limited, and report an incidence range of 5–14% in acute-care settings.

An American survey of 177 hospitals reported a prevalence rate of 11.7%. Much higher rates have been recorded in acute spinal cord injuries (60%), in elderly patients with femoral fractures (66%) and in critical-care units (41%).

AETIOLOGY

Pressure ulcers are characterized by deep tissue loss, often with undermining of the wound margin. Prolonged pressure is the main causative factor, with the critical determinants being the intensity and duration of the pressure, and the soft-tissue toleration of that pressure.

Pressure necrosis occurs when the external pressure exceeds that of the venous capillary limb, resulting in increased tissue pressure, increased capillary arteriolar pressure, capillary filtration, oedema, occlusion of lymphatics and ultimately cell death. Pressure over a bony prominence leads to a cone-shaped pressure gradient with its base on the bone.

The susceptibility of underlying tissue to prevent necrosis reflects both the anatomy of the circulation and the inability of muscle and other subcutaneous tissue to withstand prolonged periods of hypoxia. In the elderly, severely ill and steroid dependent, and also after spinal cord injury, the threshold of pressure that causes capillary collapse is lower, and these groups of patients have higher rates of pressure ulceration. The duration of pressure is also important, with low pressure that is maintained over long periods being just as detrimental as high pressure sustained for short periods. Significant tissue ischaemia can result from unrelieved pressure of 70 mmHg for 2 h.

Commonly identified risk factors include immobility, diminished activity and sensory loss, particularly as a result of spinal cord injury. Surgical patients undergoing lengthy procedures are clearly at risk. Other aetiological factors include sheer stress between tissue layers that can compromise blood supply to the dermis, fricitional forces across the skin, and the presence of moisture. Body fluids, wound fluid or pooled surgical antiseptic fluid may cause skin maceration and make the skin more susceptible to pressure injury. In addition, intrinsic factors such as old age, diabetes, chronic illness, anaemia, circulatory problems and smoking have all been implicated in contributing to pressure ulceration.

EVALUATION

In an attempt to focus on preventative management, various pressure ulcer risk assessment tools have been developed. Most of these employ a numerical scoring system to weight the severity of each risk factor.

The Norton risk assessment score is based on an assessor rating five areas, namely physical condition, mental state, activity, mobility and incontinence. To each of these areas is assigned a number from 1 to 4 (e.g. for 'activity' the four choices are as follows: 1, bedfast; 2, chairbound; 3, walks with help; 4, ambulant). A total Norton risk assessment score of 16 or below identifies a patient 'at risk' of developing a pressure ulcer. This is a rather simplistic tool that is based on the care of geriatric patients, so it has been modified to reduce the subjective nature of some of the ratings.

Similar but more comprehensive risk assessment tools include the Waterlow risk assessment card and the Braden scale for predicting pressure sore risk.

Pressure ulcers are classified according to the extent of tissue damage as follows:

- stage 1 – non-blanchable erythema of intact skin;
- stage 2 – partial-thickness skin loss, e.g. a superficial ulcer;
- stage 3 – full-thickness ulceration down to but not through the underlying fascia;
- stage 4 – extensive tissue necrosis involving deep tissues, e.g. muscle, bone, tendon, joint structures. Stage 4 ulcers may have undermined edges and sinus tracts.

INVESTIGATIONS

The multifactorial contributors to pressure ulceration make a comprehensive medical overview an essential prerequisite for determining the most appropriate investigations. The latter should include an assessment of the patient's nutritional status, full blood examination, electrolyte status and diabetic control, as well as excluding other remedial causes of ulceration. If an ulcer is present and infection is in question, then quantitative bacteriology will best guide antibiotic selection.

Before embarking further on any surgical strategy to excise the ulcer, it is imperative that the patient demonstrates compliance with pressure area care to ensure that the reconstruction is not subjected to pressure post-operatively. As the post-operative 'weight-free' period is at least 6 weeks, it is prudent to check patient compliance pre-operatively, because failure to follow a strict regimen after the operation may render the procedure useless. The pre-operative test period should assess the spinal-injured patient's ability to lie in the required position with comfort, as well as checking for control of muscle spasms that may require additional prophylaxis.

Radiological investigations are often useful for defining the extent of the pressure ulcer, particularly in stage 4 lesions where bony involvement is common. Plain radiographs often suffice, but occasionally a CT scan or bone scan may be required for information on the underlying bony prominence, which may show signs of osteomyelitis. The extent of sinus tracts needs to be determined pre-operatively with a sinogram.

Fistulae may connect the pressure ulcer to nearby structures such as bladder or bowel, and relevant specialist investigations are then determined in collaboration with the appropriate team.

NON-SURGICAL TREATMENT

Attention to pressure relief is fundamental to the management both of patients at risk of developing a pressure ulcer and of those with an established pressure ulcer. Regular skin monitoring should alert the clinician to an impending or extending ulcer. Bedridden individuals should be repositioned 2-hourly, but if they are considered to be at risk of developing a pressure ulcer, then hourly repositioning may be necessary.

Surveillance of the pressure-prone bony prominences (greater trochanters, ischial tuberosities, sacrum and heels) warrants particular attention.

Skin hygiene becomes a priority for patients at risk of pressure ulceration, and body fluids should not be in contact with the skin for prolonged periods. A stable skin temperature should be maintained, as increased skin temperature results in a significant elevation of metabolic rate, with its attendant systemic demands and increased perspiration rate. This may be relevant intra-operatively during long procedures when the patients are on warming blankets.

When transferring a patient to or from an operating table, care must be taken to avoid shearing forces on the skin.

Post-operatively, patients should be encouraged to mobilize as early as is practicable, and thereafter to steadily increase their activity, perhaps with assistance from a physiotherapist.

While they are immobile, surgical patients should be provided with a support surface appropriate to their risk of developing a pressure ulcer. A standard hospital mattress with pressure-reducing properties is needed for patients at low risk; whereas pressure-relieving support surfaces, which maintain the tissue pressure below capillary-closing pressure, are required for high-risk patients.

Local treatment is appropriate for ulcers of grades 1 and 2. With dressings and pressure control, most superficial ulcers will heal within 3 weeks.

Enzymatic debriding agents may be a useful adjunct to sharp bedside debridement to clear away slough. Useful dressings include hydrocolloids, alginates and hydrogels. Deeper ulcers usually require surgical intervention.

SURGICAL TREATMENT

The principal objectives of any surgical procedure for a pressure ulcer are to remove all necrotic tissue and to resurface the area with a robust healthy flap of vascularized tissue that will remain intact. Pre-operatively, the patient's medical condition should be optimal, and consideration should be given to relief of muscular spasms, catheterization, bowel preparation or even diversion, and blood group matching.

Specific surgical principles for pressure ulcers include the following.

- General anaesthesia is preferable.

- Position the patient so that the surgical defect is exaggerated (to ensure comfortable closure).

- Delineate the ulcer externally on the skin and internally with methylene blue.

- Excise the ulcer *en bloc* as if it was a tumour.

- Avoid incisions over prominences.

- Remove by osteotomy any bony prominence beneath the ulcer.

- Plan flaps to preserve as many future reconstructions as possible.

- Secure haemostasis and use large suction drains long term.

- Carefully consider the flap tissues, as muscle is more susceptible to pressure than skin, and muscle is not usually draped across bony prominences in normal anatomy.

Examples of common flaps used for reconstructing defects after excision of pressure ulcers include the following:

- sacral pressure ulcer – gluteal rotation flap which may incorporate skin, fascia and muscle, and is based on the gluteal vessels;

- ischial pressure ulcer – biceps femoris V to Y advancement flap which transfers in a sliding fashion the posterior thigh skin with the underlying biceps femoris muscle, and relies on femoral perforating blood vessels for its viability;

- trochanteric pressure ulcer – the tensor fascia lata flap can be mobilized by freeing its distal insertion into the iliotibial tract and then turning it back to cover the trochanteric region; the lateral femoral artery supplies this flap.

FURTHER READING

Angle N, Bergan JJ. 1997: Chronic venous ulcer. *British Medical Journal* **314**, 1019–23.

Baker SR, Stacey MC. 1994: Epidemiology of chronic leg ulcers in Australia. *Australian and New Zealand Journal of Surgery* **64**, 258–61.

Fu X, Sheng Z, Cherry GW *et al.* 1998: Epidemiological study of chronic dermal ulcers in China. *Wound Repair and Regeneration* **6**, 21–7.

McGowan S, Hensley L, Maddock J. 1996: Monitoring the occurrence of pressure ulcers in a teaching hospital: a quality improvement project. *Primary Intention* **4**, 9–16.

Mast BA, Schultz GS. 1996: Interactions of cytokines, growth factors and proteases in acute and chronic wounds. *Wound Repair and Regeneration* **4**, 411–20.

Phillips TJ. 1994: Chronic cutaneous ulcers: etiology and epidemiology. *Journal of Investigative Dermatology* **102**, 28S–40S.

Waterlow J. 1985: A risk assessment card. *Nursing Times* **81**, 24–7.

Skin cancer

Miklós J. Pohl

Introduction

Skin cancer is the most common form of cancer in Caucasian populations. Of the non-melanocytic skin cancers, basal-cell carcinoma (BCC) is the commonest type and squamous-cell carcinoma (SCC) is the second commonest.

The patient presenting with skin cancer may be very anxious. Their family doctor has almost certainly used the word 'cancer' or 'tumour' when filling out their referral to a specialist. The very fact that they are now going to need an operation merely confirms their reason for feeling anxious. Even with the excellent information now available, some of it from the Internet, patients may not be able to put their 'cancer' diagnosis into perspective. *Reassuring* the patient right at the beginning of the consultation that they are not going to die and that most skin cancers are not melanoma, and are easily cured by minimally invasive techniques, is time well spent. On the other hand, a patient with a thick melanoma has to be given his or her prognosis. This may be best left to the second consultation.

Patients with skin cancer also have to be *informed* of their increased risk of developing other skin lesions, and given details about the procedure that they are about to undergo.

EPIDEMIOLOGY OF NON-MELANOCYTIC SKIN CANCER (NMSC)

INCIDENCE OF BCC AND SCC

NMSC is so common in Australia that cancer registries are unable to calculate rates for the whole population. Incidence rates for Australia are therefore based on surveys and studies.

BCC is the most common of all skin cancers. Its incidence in Queensland has been estimated to be as high as 2074/100 000 in men and 1519/100 000 in women. These rates were based on a study of treated cases in the 18–69 years age groups in Nambour, Queensland, between 1985 and 1992. Since NMSC is even more common in those aged over 70 years, the total population rates of NMSC could well be double those reported. In addition, rates have been rising rapidly in the 1990s across all age groups, so they may have doubled by 1999.

The rates in more southern regions of Australia are lower, but even in Tasmania (at latitude 40–42°) NMSC is at least twice as common as all other types of cancer combined.

MORTALITY

In contrast to the high incidence, death from NMSC is not very common. In 1994 there were 358 NMSC-related deaths (261 men and 97 women) in Australia, which represents a crude rate of 2/100 000 individuals. Deaths from NMSC are rising, and the steeply increasing rates of SCC are believed to be the reason for this. To put this death rate into perspective, in Tasmania in 1995 there were 8 deaths from NMSC, and in the same year there were 9 deaths from uterine cancer and 12 deaths from all combined forms of buccal cancer.

RISK FACTORS FOR SKIN CANCER

These are as follows:

1. ultraviolet radiation (both UVB and UVA);
2. fair skin colour;
3. skin lesions such as solar keratosis (actinic keratosis), Bowen's disease (SCC *in situ*), naevus sebaceous (naevus of Jodassohn);
4. strong family history;
5. immunosuppression;
6. albinism;
7. xeroderma pigmentosum;
8. basal-cell naevus syndrome;
9. chronic scars;
10. radiation;
11. arsenicals.

AETIOLOGY

SCC usually, but not always, affects an older age group than BCC. It mainly occurs on sun-exposed parts of the body, and is more common in the outdoor-working population (e.g. fishermen, linesmen and farmers) who have a high cumulative sun exposure. Patients with a fair complexion are also at higher risk for both types of NMSC.

Early retirement and outdoor hobbies/occupations such as gardening, bowls and sailing are putting more people into high-risk categories.

GENERAL PRINCIPLES OF TREATMENT

Histological diagnosis is essential in the treatment of all skin lesions. Lesions should be biopsied by incision, trephine or total excision whenever possible.

The width of excision depends on the type of tumour, the site of the tumour, the age of the patient and other clinical circumstances. Excision is the preferred method of treatment, as this affords confirmation of tumour-free edges, both of margins and depth of excision. Most small skin cancers can be excised under local anaesthetic and the defect closed primarily. Larger lesions require local flaps or skin grafts, either split skin grafts or, more commonly, Wolfe grafts (full-thickness grafts), especially on the face. In larger defects, free tissue transfer may be necessary.

Regional lymph nodes are only resected if they are clinically involved or shown to be involved on CT or MRI scans.

- Radiotherapy may be used as a primary mode of treatment or as an adjunct to surgery for recurrent disease, high-grade tumours and tumours exhibiting perineural invasion.
- Radiotherapy may also be employed in the elderly and in areas of the body that would require a magnitude of reconstruction that could not be tolerated by the patient.

HISTORY

A careful family history should be obtained, as well as a past history of skin cancers and skin lesions. The patient should be asked how much sun exposure they have experienced in their work and leisure activities. Enquiries should also be made about how sun conscious the patient is. Do they wear protective clothing when going out? Do they use ultraviolet blockout cream? Are they aware of the dangers of exposure to the sun between 10 a.m. to 3 p.m? This is useful to know not only for research purposes, but also in order to be able to counsel the patient appropriately.

In more general terms, the patient should be asked about medications, especially immunosuppressive drugs. Immunosuppressed patients (e.g. renal transplant patients) are more prone to developing skin cancers than the normal population.

Specific information should be obtained about the behaviour of the lesion. Has it bled? Has it been itching? Has it changed colour? Has it changed size, and if so over what period of time?

A long-standing lesion undergoing sudden change is always a cause for suspicion. A lesion that has not healed, or which has bled or remains crusty, should be considered malignant until proven otherwise by biopsy.

EXAMINATION

The size, site, shape, surface, edge, colour and induration of the lesion and its adherence to deeper structures should be noted. Regional lymph nodes need to be examined thoroughly, and the patient should be checked completely wearing only their underwear, under a good light with loupe magnification and/or a dermatoscope. Patients with numerous skin lesions, whether they be naevi or lesions acquired from sun damage, should be photomapped. A minimum of four to six photos should be taken, and a spare set may be sent to the primary-care physician for their files for future reference.

INVESTIGATIONS

In general investigations should include a biopsy of some kind. In very advanced cases, CT scans or MRI scans may delineate the extent of surrounding tissue involvement or regional gland involvement.

NON-MELANOCYTIC SKIN CANCER (NMSC)

BASAL-CELL CARCINOMA

Pathological classification

Basal-cell carcinoma (BCC) can be classified into the following categories:

- papulonodular – these may be solid or cystic (45% of cases, Figure 21.3.1);
- infiltrating (8%, Figure 21.3.2);
- multifocal (35%);
- morphoeic or sclerosing (9%; Figure 21.3.3);
- metatypical or basisquamous (1.4%);
- other – pigmented, naevoid BCC (1.6%).

Differential diagnoses include squamous-cell carcinoma, solar keratosis, kerato-acanthoma, amelanotic malignant melanoma, angiosarcoma, Merkel cell tumour, desmoplastic malignant melanoma or neurotrophic malignant melanoma, appendigeal tumours of the skin

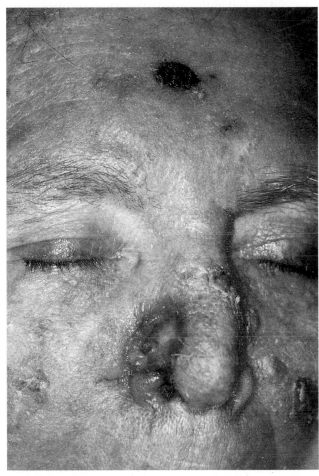

Figure 21.3.2 Infiltrating basal-cell carcinoma.

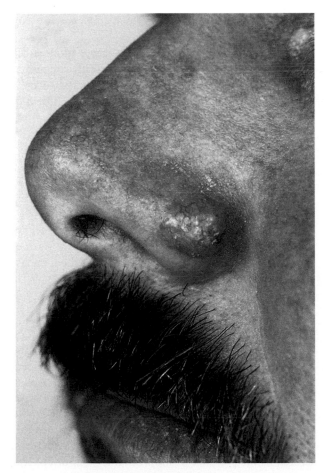

Figure 21.3.1 Nodular basal-cell carcinoma.

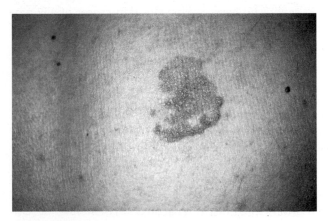

Figure 21.3.3 Morpheic basal-cell carcinoma.

(e.g. tricho-epithelioma or hydro-adenoma), dermato-fibroma, naevi, hypertrophic scar, chondrodermatitis nodularis helicis, seborrhoeic keratosis, Bowen's disease, perifolliculitis and pyogenic granuloma. Rarer tumours may also mimic BCCs, e.g. discoid lupus or atypical fibroxanthoma. Basal-cell carcinomas have a smooth, raised and waxy, often pearly, translucent appearance. They may present as a single nodule or as multiple nodules with or without a central ulcer. There are often small telangiectatic vessels running over the tumour.

Morphoeic basal-cell carcinomas are more difficult to identify, and the edges are often difficult to determine. Any basal-cell carcinoma may be ulcerated. The infiltrative type, as the name suggests, may infiltrate deeper underlying tissues. Of particular relevance are the 'danger areas', namely the nose (the base of the lateral alae), the ear (around the external auditory meatus) and the eye (around the lateral and medial canthi). Any BCC may be pigmented, and pigmentation as such is of little significance.

Surgical treatment

Surgical excision is the preferred method of treatment whenever feasible. The specimen should be marked with an orientating suture. This aids the pathologist in reporting the orientation of the tumour with regard to clear margins.

If numerous tumours are found, the patient is best managed jointly with their family practitioner, dermatologists and radiation oncologists. Following biopsy, electrocautery and curettage may be the treatment of choice, especially in cases where there are numerous lesions on the back, for example. In some instances radiotherapy may be employed alone.

Follow-up should be performed routinely, but obviously some tumours are more prone to recurrence than others. Morphoeic and infiltrative tumours are more likely to recur, as well as those in the danger areas mentioned above. These should be followed intensively at 4- to 6-month intervals initially, and annually thereafter. Patients who have developed a skin cancer of any type are at a higher risk of developing subsequent tumours.

Immunosuppressed patients, individuals who present at an early age and albinos should be followed more intensively for life.

Excision margins

Excision margins depend on the site of the tumour and the type. Nodular lesions may be excised by a narrow (0.5-mm) margin, whereas infiltrating and morphoeic lesions need a wider margin. Intra-operative frozen section reduces the likelihood of incomplete excision margins.

Moh's progressive tangential excision may be employed in very difficult, extensive or recurrent lesions.

Prognosis

The basisquamous variety can metastasize, but BCC is very rarely a cause of death. However, cases are reported of patients with advanced localized disease which defies all management strategies and which eventually results in the death of the patient. This occurs by direct invasion and destruction of full-thickness skin and deeper tissues, leading to sepsis, haemorrhage and death.

Conclusion

Basal-cell carcinoma is the commonest of all tumours. Fortunately, most patients with BCC present early, and nearly all tumours can be excised and the defect closed primarily. Recurrences are rare, but histological confirmation for diagnosis must always be obtained, as well as confirmation of tumour-free margins.

SQUAMOUS-CELL CARCINOMA

Squamous-cell carcinoma (SCC) is the second commonest malignant tumour of skin. The ratio of BCC to SCC in most studies varies between 2:1 and 3:1. The incidence of SCC increases with age, and appears to be related to cumulative rather than intermittent sun exposure.

Whereas only the basisquamous subtype of basal-cell carcinoma metastasizes, all squamous-cell carcinomas can potentially metastasize, but rarely do so – hence the need for accurate diagnosis and thorough assessment of regional lymph glands.

Pathological classification

Squamous-cell carcinomas are classified as well differentiated (76%, Figure 21.3.4), moderately differentiated (16%) and poorly differentiated or anaplastic (8%, Figure 21.3.5). Staging of the tumour is done according to TNM guidelines. By far the majority of SCCs are low-grade or well differentiated, and very few of them metastasize.

Clinical presentation

SCCs may appear anywhere on the skin surface, but are more common in the head and neck region and the upper limbs, as well as on the lower half of the lower limbs (i.e. the sun-exposed parts of the body). Squamous-cell carcinoma presents in a number of ways, as a persistently crusty or bleeding lesion that may also be itchy. At clinical examination the degree of differentiation of the tumour, its attachment to deeper structures, as well as the presence of induration are important features to note.

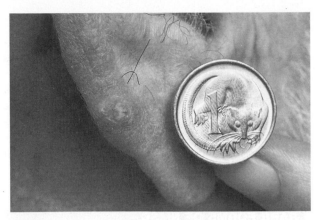

Figure 21.3.4 Well-differentiated squamous-cell carcinoma.

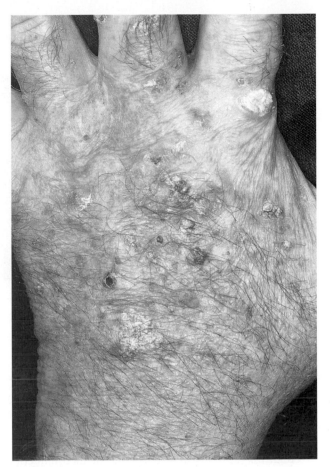

Figure 21.3.6 Solar keratosis.

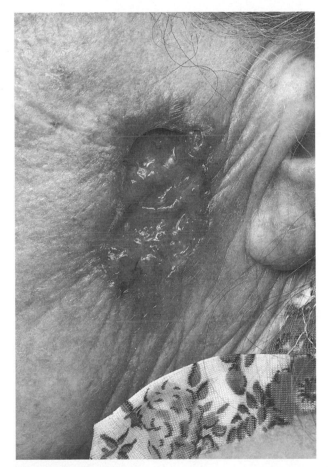

Figure 21.3.5 Undifferentiated (anaplastic) squamous-cell carcinoma.

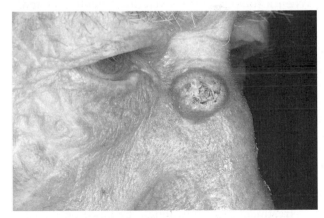

Figure 21.3.7 Kerato acanthoma.

Induration is pathognomonic of squamous-cell carcinoma, and is an important sign that can be elicited by careful palpation.

Differential diagnosis

Differential diagnoses include hyperkeratosis (Figure 21.3.6), kerato-acanthoma (Figure 21.3.7), basal-cell carcinoma, amelanotic malignant melanoma and numerous chronic dermatological conditions, as well as Bowen's disease (Figure 21.3.8).

Investigations

The tumour, if large, should be biopsied first for histological confirmation. Smaller lesions may be excised and the defect closed directly. Regional lymph nodes are examined, and if any doubt exists about their involvement, or if the tumour is aggressive, fine-needle aspiration is performed and a CT scan or MRI scan of the suspected lymph glands may also be undertaken.

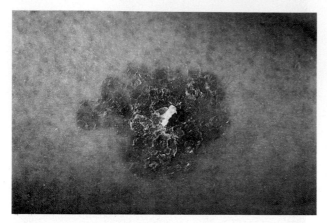

Figure 21.3.8 Bowen's disease.

Treatment of the primary tumour

If the primary tumour is small, treatment is usually by excision and primary closure. Larger tumours require a local flap or graft, and very large tumours may require reconstruction by a microvascular free flap.

Radiotherapy may be used alone or in conjunction with surgery, depending on the clinical circumstances. When a tumour shows severe local infiltration and/or perineural infiltration, radiotherapy is usually employed as an adjunct to surgery.

The aggressiveness of the tumour, its site, and the age and well-being of the patient determine the margins of excision. The width of margins may range from 0.5 to 3 cm.

Treatment of regional lymph nodes

Involved lymph nodes are treated by radical lymph-node dissection. If nodes are not demonstrated to be involved, then close clinical follow-up is all that is necessary.

Treatment guidelines should be based on the entire clinical picture, which includes the type of tumour, its stage of differentiation and site, and the well-being of the patient, as well as consideration of cosmetic outcome.

Follow-up

Most secondary lymph nodes develop within 12 months of primary treatment. However, long-term follow-up is recommended as some tumours (e.g. those involving the lower lip) may present at a much later stage. Initial close follow-up, up to 4- to 6-monthly, followed by annual review for life, is recommended.

Prognosis

Although only a small proportion of SCCs will metastasize and cause death, it is important to identify the ones that are most likely to do so.

The risk of metastasis for squamous-cell carcinoma has been reported to be as low as 0.5% overall. The tumours that metastasize are mainly anaplastic or undifferentiated and have escaped early detection and treatment. The recurrence rate for well-differentiated, small tumours is extremely low.

RARE FORMS OF NMSC

These include rare but highly malignant skin cancers such as eccrine poroma, Merkel cell tumours and dermatofibrosarcoma.

MALIGNANT MELANOMA

Cutaneous malignant melanoma (CMM) is the third commonest skin cancer in Australians, and the fifth

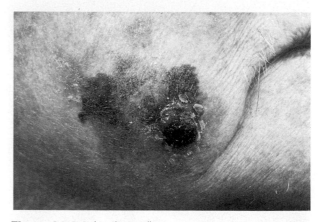

Figure 21.3.9 Lentigo maligna.

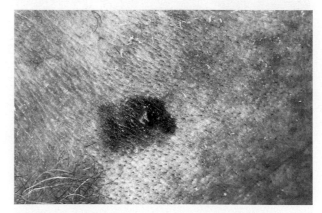

Figure 21.3.10 Superficial spreading malignant melanoma.

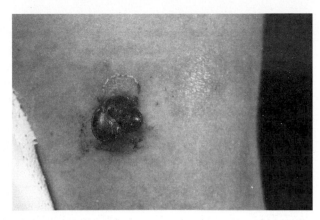

Figure 21.3.11 Nodular malignant melanoma.

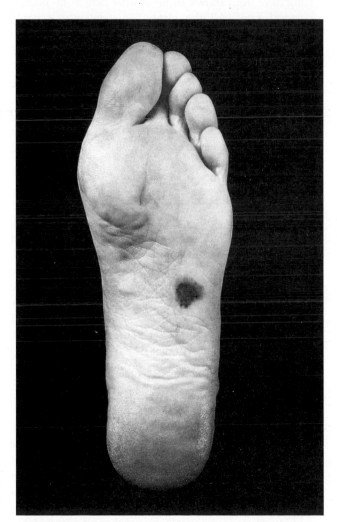

Figure 21.3.12 Acral lentigenous malignant melanoma.

commonest cancer overall in Australia. Patients are presenting much earlier than in former years, as a result of the very active publicity campaigns regarding the harmful effects of sun exposure. This has led to an increased awareness of the warning signs of skin cancer, including

malignant melanoma. None the less, the incidence of CMM is still rising, not only in Australia but also globally.

Approximately 900 people die of malignant melanoma each year in Australia. Early detection of thin lesions has raised the overall survival figures substantially. The mortality rate from CMM is approximately 10% of the incidence rate, i.e. 1 to 5/100 000. Fortunately, we now seldom see the very thick advanced melanomas with which patients used to present two decades ago. Patients are referred with either a primary, suspicious skin lesion or a biopsy-proven malignant melanoma. More often than not, the primary has been removed and the patient presents to the surgeon with a surgical scar and a pathology report. In most instances further wider local excision is required. As with all skin cancers, a thorough general physical examination should be performed, and the patient should be reassured and given information and printed material (available from Cancer Councils) about the disease.

PATHOLOGICAL CLASSIFICATION OF CUTANEOUS MALIGNANT MELANOMA

Cutaneous malignant melanoma can be classified as follows:

1. *non-invasive melanomas* – account for 25% of all CMMs. They include lentigo maligna (Figure 21.3.9, Hutchinson's melanotic freckle) and superficial spreading CMM *in situ*;

2. *invasive lesions*:

   - *superficial spreading malignant melanoma* – accounts for 57% of invasive lesions (Figure 21.3.10);

   - *nodular malignant melanoma* – accounts for 16% (Figure 21.3.11);

   - *acral lentiginous malignant melanoma* – accounts for 1% (Figure 21.3.12);

   - *desmoplastic malignant melanoma* – accounts for less than 1%.

Any of the above melanomas may be amelanotic.

Tumour thickness, as originally described by Breslow using an ocular micrometer, is the most useful guide to formulating treatment.

P	=	primary; T = tumour
PTIS	=	melanoma *in situ*
PT2	=	thickness of > 0.75–1.5 mm
PT3a	=	thickness of > 1.5–3.0 mm
PT3b	=	thickness of > 3.0–4.0 mm
PT4	=	thickness of > 4.0 mm

RISK FACTORS FOR MALIGNANT MELANOMA

Most risk factors for malignant melanoma are the same as for NMSC, namely the following:

- UVA and UVB radiation from sunlight and solariums;
- skin colour;
- genetic factors;
- naevi (dysplastic, large congenital naevus);
- immunosuppression;
- ionizing radiation;
- for CMM in particular, intermittent sun exposure associated with a history of sunburn and naevi;
- sunburn associated with an increased number of naevi in darker as well as light-skinned adolescents of Northern European descent.

INCIDENCE OF MALIGNANT MELANOMA

In Australia, the incidence of malignant melanoma is rising. In 1982 it was 18/100 000, compared to 30/100 000 in 1994. This pattern of increase has also been observed in European countries and the USA, although rates there are about one-third of those in Australia.

In Australia, Queensland (at latitude 10–27°) has the highest incidence at 50/100 000 compared to Tasmania (at latitude 40–42°), which has an incidence of 30/100 000. This is referred to as the latitudinal gradient.

DIAGNOSIS

Patients usually present either because they have noticed a recent change in a pre-existing lesion, or because a lesion has appeared *de novo*. The lesion may have become itchy, scaly or darker, or it may have bled or developed irregular edges. Less than 30% of melanomas arise from pre-existing naevi. A useful way to record change in any skin lesions is the ABCDE system where A = asymmetry, B = border, C = colour, D = diameter, E = elevation. Patients with dysplastic naevi should be carefully monitored, especially if there has been a history of malignant melanoma in a first-degree relative. Some lesions are best just observed, whereas others are best photomapped. It is useful to take two sets of photographs, one for your own files and one for the referring physician who may follow the patient at their leisure. As well as being photomapped, patients are given special charts to help them to keep a record of their lesions and complete a thorough self-examination. These charts are available from Cancer Councils.

DIFFERENTIAL DIAGNOSIS

Differential diagnoses of malignant melanoma (CMM) include compound, junctional and intradermal naevi, blue naevi, seborrhoeic keratosis, dermatofibroma and subungual haematoma. Pigmented BCCs and SCCs, as well as pyogenic granulomas, may also mimic malignant melanoma.

INVESTIGATIONS

Dermatoscopic examination of skin lesions allows a more accurate diagnosis. However, extensive investigations such as CT scanning, chest X-ray and liver scanning have been shown to be of little benefit in altering survival rates. All the same, for suspicious regional lymph glands and also in patients with thick tumours, a routine chest X-ray, liver ultrasound and possibly a CT scan may be ordered, as well as isotope bone scanning.

Scintiscanning and sentinel lymph node biopsy are employed in some of the larger units, but at this stage are best regarded as a research tool. These techniques allow highly selective sampling of lymph nodes to help to stage the disease and formulate treatment.

TREATMENT

As most lesions presenting to the clinician are small, excision biopsy is the commonest form of treatment, and a minimum margin of 5 mm is recommended. Hutchinson's melanotic freckle (lentigo maligna) may be shave excised (see below). Incision biopsy should be avoided if possible, but may be necessary in broader-based lesions. Wider margins are necessary in superficial spreading, nodular and acral lentigenous melanomas, the margin being determined by tumour thickness and site and the general well-being of the patient.

Lentigo maligna (Hutchinson's melanotic freckle, *in situ* malignant melanoma)

When an invasive focus is not evident, tangential shave biopsy may be performed. This is the treatment of choice, as it allows both full histological examination and cure of the lesion at the same time. As Hutchinson's freckles are broadly based, a full-thickness excision would inflict a cosmetically unsightly and unwarranted scar. If an area of a lentigo maligna appears to have changed, i.e. if it has become darker, developed an irregular edge, thickened or become scaly or bled, that area should be biopsied in its own right and the whole area then excised, depending on the maximum thickness of the area sampled.

Summary of recommended margins

The generally recommended excision margins for malignant melanomas are as follows:

1. melanoma *in situ* (lentigo maligna (LM), Hutchinson's melanotic freckle (HMF)) – 5 mm margin;
2. melanoma 0–1.5 mm thick – 1-cm margin;
3. melanoma 1.5–4 mm thick – 1- to 2-cm margin;
4. melanoma > 4 mm thick – 2- to 3-cm margin.

Management of regional lymph nodes

Clinically suspicious lymph nodes should be investigated by fine-needle aspiration and/or CT scanning. Elective lymph-node dissection in the case of clinically negative lymph nodes has not been demostrated to be beneficial. Therapeutic lymph-node dissection should only be performed on involved lymph nodes by surgeons trained in the procedure.

Management of visceral secondaries

It may well be worth resecting singular metastases from involved viscera. Radiotherapy, chemotherapy and immunotherapy also have a role in the management of secondaries.

Limb recurrences may be very successfully treated by isolated limb perfusion or infusion in specialized units.

FOLLOW-UP

The frequency of follow-up is determined by tumour thickness. For example, a tumour less than 1.5 mm in thickness should be followed 4- to 6- monthly for up to 2 years. Tumours that are more than 1.5 mm thick should be followed up 4-monthly for 3 years and 6- to 12-monthly thereafter. About 85% of recurrences occur within the first 3 years after excision of the primary.

At every follow-up visit, total skin surveillance should be practised. This allows detection of new primary lesions and other skin cancers. A patient who has had one melanoma has at least a 4% increased risk of having a second primary as well as developing other skin cancers.

PROGNOSIS

The prognosis for malignant melanoma is as follows:

1. melanoma *in situ* – 100% survival at 10 years;
2. melanoma 0–0.75 mm thick – 98% survival;
3. melanoma 0.75–1.05 mm thick – 91% survival;
4. melanoma 1.05–3.00 mm thick – 75% survival;
5. melanoma > 3.00 mm thick – 55% survival.

CONCLUSION

As with most cancers – and skin cancer is no exception – early detection and treatment equate to cure, or at least to good survival rates. Despite the rising incidence of all types of skin cancer, cure is usually possible because the majority of tumours are thin at the time of presentation.

FURTHER READING

Australian Cancer Network. 1997: *Guidelines for the management of cutaneous melanoma*. Epping, NSW: Stone Press.

Emmett AJJ, O'Rourke MGE. 1991: *Malignant skin tumours*. 2nd edn. Edinburgh: Churchill Livingstone.

Mandell MA (ed.). 1980: *Symposium on skin tumors*. Philadelphia, PA: WB Saunders, 289–336. (Rogers BO (ed.). Clinics in plastic surgery; vol 7(3)).

McCarthy JG (ed.). 1990: *Volume 5: Tumors of the head & neck and skin*. In Plastic surgery. Philadelphia, PA: WB Saunders, 3614–3662.

Milton GW. 1977: *Malignant melanoma of the skin and mucous membrane*. Edinburgh: Churchill Livingstone.

Limp and gait

Andrew M. Ellis

Introduction

There is no doubt that the study of limp and gait affords insight into the manner in which musculoskeletal disease affects the individual. Upright stance and bipedal gait have conferred a tremendous evolutionary advantage on hominids, our gait setting us apart from other animals. To be able to analyse limp, to break the abnormal gait cycle into discrete phases, and to observe carefully and diagnose the cause of disability, is to enter the fascinating world of Sherlock Holmes. There is so much to be learned from quiet, precise observation.

The normal pattern of bipedal gait is studied as a cycle consisting of two principal phases. As the subject participates in weight-bearing on one limb (the stance phase) the other limb advances (the swing phase), and thus forward locomotion is achieved. Normally this is smooth and rhythmic, but in disease it can be altered in subtle or more obvious ways. Disturbance of balance, weakness, shortening (or lengthening), pain or disruption of normal joint function can all impact upon gait.

NORMAL GAIT

Normal human locomotion is smooth and energy-efficient. Balance is maintained by keeping the centre of gravity over the limb that is taking weight. To allow for the opposite leg to be cleared from the ground during the swing phase, it is necessary for the pelvis to be tilted, relying on strong hip abductors and strong lateral abdominal muscles. The pelvis and trunk shift laterally about 2.5 cm and the centre of gravity oscillates approximately 5 cm about the anatomical centre. In addition to tilt and side-to-side movement, the pelvis rotates internally during the swing phase to allow further forward movement.

The width of the normal base in gait is 5–10 cm. During normal walking the step length is about 35 cm and the average cadence is about 90 to 120 steps per minute. During running, step length may increase together with cadence, thus requiring more energy expenditure.

In recent times it has been possible to make direct measurements of joint reaction forces during function. The resultant hip joint reaction force, its orientation and its moment have been measured in patients during walking and running using an instrumented hip prosthesis. These data show peak forces at the hip ranging from 2.8 to 4.8 times body weight when accelerating from slow to fast walking speed. Jogging and uncontrolled stumbling increase the forces to between 6 and 9 times body weight.

PHASES OF GAIT

A cycle of gait is defined as the movement of a single limb from heel-strike to heel-strike (Figure 22.1). The gait cycle begins with the stance phase, which represents 60% of the cycle, at initial contact with the heel

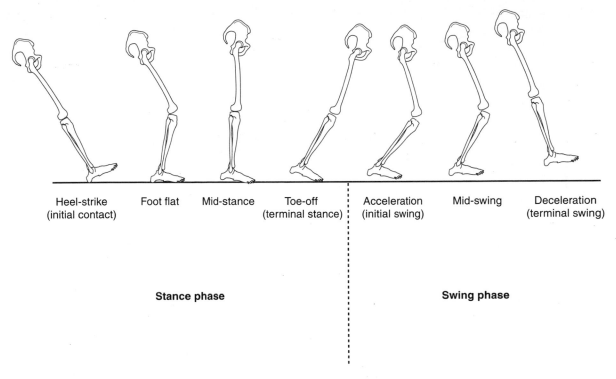

Heel-strike (initial contact)	Foot flat	Mid-stance	Toe-off (terminal stance)	Acceleration (initial swing)	Mid-swing	Deceleration (terminal swing)

Stance phase   **Swing phase**

Figure 22.1 The gait cycle, which consists of two major phases, each composed of a number of segments.

(heel-strike). The loading response occurs next, with plantar flexion occurring at the ankle, and controlled descent of the heel allowing the entire foot to be placed on the ground (foot flat). Mid-stance follows, in which body weight passes forward over the stabilized foot as the ankle dorsiflexes. Finally, the forward movement continues, the heel is lifted and body weight shifts further forward leading to the terminal phase of stance, namely toe-off. The remaining 40% of gait is spent in the swing phase, during which the limb is lifted through for ground clearance. Initially there is a period of acceleration, finally decelerating in terminal swing to allow for heel-strike, and thus the cycle continues.

There are two periods of double support, each accounting for 10% of the cycle, when both feet are on the ground. These are the initiation and termination of the stance phase. The two principal phases can be further subdivided as follows.

The stance phase can be divided into:

- Heel-strike;
- Foot flat;
- Mid-stance;
- Toe-off.

The swing phase can be divided into:

- Acceleration;
- Mid-swing;
- Deceleration.

It has already been noted that normal gait is energy-efficient. In fact, the typical energy expenditure in gait is less than twice that expended while sitting or standing (10.5 kilojoules (kJ) compared to 6.3 kJ/min).

It is important to understand the relationships between the various joints (Figure 22.2). A stable centre of gravity is energy-efficient, and a stable hip and knee are essential for this. The hip only flexes to about 30° in the early stance phase, extending to 6° at terminal stance. The knee functions as a shock absorber, flexing in early stance and then extending through the rest of the stance phase. The ankle plays a crucial role in meeting the ground during loading, acting as a rocker upon which the normal cycle depends. It has been estimated that approximately 85% of the power for normal walking comes from the plantar flexors of the ankle.

A strong abductor mechanism is essential for normal gait, and actively tilts the pelvis to allow the opposite limb to swing through, so clearing the ground. In addition, hip abduction and knee flexion assist in this manoeuvre. Peak flexion of the knee, for example, occurs in the early swing phase.

There are measurable differences between adult and childhood gait. Toddlers tend to have a wide-based gait in which the arms are held out to aid balance further. The body proportions of children are different to those of adults. Their knees and ankles are proportionally closer to the ground, and one consequence of this is that

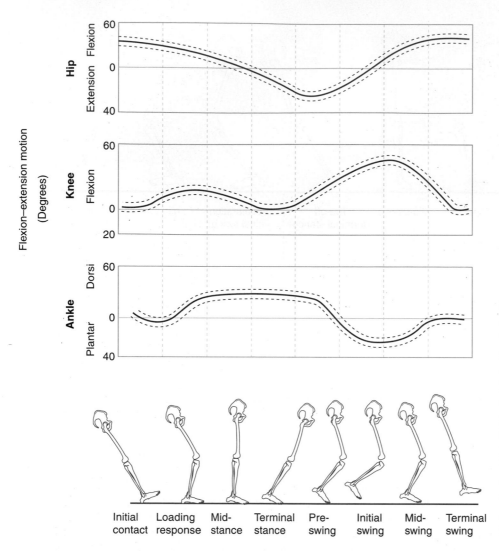

Figure 22.2 The position of the hip, knee and ankle with the stance phase divided into five segments and the swing phase divided into three segments. The curves represent the normal patterns of motion for the hip, knee and ankle. The limb below the curves illustrates the position of the pelvis, thigh and shank as they would be observed during each of these segments of the gait cycle.

adults have greater ground clearance during the swing phase than do children. Children tend to take short abrupt steps, and they trip and fall easily.

The prerequisites of normal gait include stability of the lower limb in the stance phase, clearance of the ground by the foot in the swing phase, proper pre-positioning of the foot in the terminal swing, adequate step length and maximization of energy conservation.

THE TRENDELENBURG TEST

The Trendelenburg test enables gait disturbance to be assessed by physical examination. Originally described by Friedrich Trendelenburg in 1897, it was a test he found useful for determining hip abductor muscle function, with specific reference to congenital dislocation of the hip and progressive muscular atrophy. Ultimately, the manoeuvre is a test of hip stability, in which the stance phase of gait is reproduced, particularly when looking at the effect of disturbance to the abductor lever

arm. The latter consists of the motor (abductor muscles) and the lever (the femoral neck and trochanter) acting through a fulcrum (the hip joint). Injury or disease at any of these points can lead to a positive test (Figures 22.3 and 22.4).

Performing the test The patient is exposed so that the iliac crest is visible, with the examiner usually standing behind him or her. The patient is first asked to lift the affected limb from the ground (flexing the hip to 30° only). They are then asked to lift the pelvis further on the non-stance side. The intact abductors on the unaffected side should easily allow tilting of the pelvis above an imaginary line drawn parallel to the ground. The patient is then asked to repeat the manoeuvre, this time lifting the unaffected side off the ground. The weakened abductor mechanism is unable to stabilize or tilt the pelvis, and the pelvis drops below the imaginary parallel line. The so-called *sound side sags in a positive test*.

Special points Care should be taken to prevent the lateral shift of body weight to the affected side beyond the new mechanical axis that characterizes the 'lurch' of the

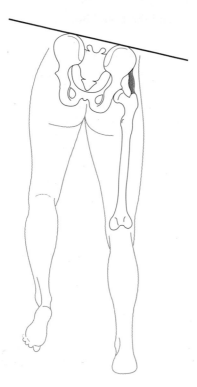

Figure 22.3 A negative Trendelenburg test. The abductor lever arm is functioning normally, and the pelvis tilts on the opposite side during single leg stance.

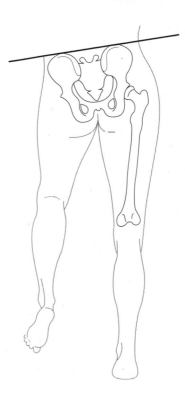

Figure 22.4 A positive Trendelenburg test. The abductor lever arm is not functioning and the pelvis falls on the opposite side during single leg stance.

Trendelenburg gait (Figure 22.5). Similarly, the patient should not be allowed to be supported by a walking aid or table through the non-stance side, or a false-negative test may result. A period of 30 s should be allowed to elapse before the test is considered negative, as a 'delayed abnormal' response may occur.

ABNORMAL GAIT

Gait is normally highly efficient, and there is a relatively large reserve of joint movement and muscle strength. This may mean that gross structural abnormalities are not apparent to the casual observer. The reserve of muscle power is very great, and only considerable loss of it will affect gait. Gravity may also help to conceal significant weakness. Similarly, the joints of the lower limb form a linked movement in which afflictions of one joint may be well hidden. For example, increased movement at the sub-talar and talo-navicular joint may make the effect of an ankle arthrodesis difficult to detect. A similar relationship exists between the hip and the lumbo-sacral junction. However, an arthrodesis of the knee is not well compensated for as it is a relatively independent joint, and little adaptive change can conceal it.

There are four main ways in which musculoskeletal disease may affect gait:

1. pain;
2. loss of control of the joint;
3. abnormality of the joint itself;
4. injury or disease causing bending or shortening of bones.

Abnormal gait will increase energy expenditure, sometimes remarkably. Estimates of increased energy expenditure have included walking with a below-knee brace (10% increase), walking with a 15° fixed flexion contracture of the knee (25%), fast walking (60%), walking after a below-knee amputation (60%) and walking after an above-knee amputation (100%) or with crutches (300%).

A PROBLEM-BASED GAIT ASSESSMENT

1. Antalgic (Lt: against pain) gait This is the most common gait disturbance, and elements of an antalgic gait will be seen in any unilateral painful condition. This is characteristically a pain-relieving gait in which weight-bearing on the affected limb is minimized. It is therefore characterized by a short stance phase on the affected side. The normal rhythm of gait is lost and the affected side is 'favoured', the step length is reduced, and the limb will swing slowly and be loaded carefully.

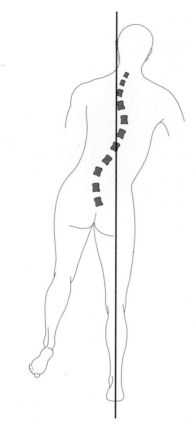

Figure 22.5 In a Trendelenburg gait, the upper body might swing excessively past the centre of gravity to provide a mechanical advantage to the abductor lever arm.

2. Loss of muscle power of the hip Loss of muscle power around the hip may lead to inability to stabilize this joint (see the above section on the Trendelenburg test). Characteristically this gait (a Trendelenburg gait) is a waddling or swinging one in which the shoulders cross the centre of gravity during the stance phase ('lurching'). This lurch partly compensates for weakness, conferring a mechanical advantage by shifting the centre of gravity past its usual point, thus aiding pelvic tilt. The shoulder is not seen to rise with pelvic tilt, but rather it falls on the unaffected side or lurches across during the stance phase. The use of a stick or aid for the contralateral limb will often mask this gait.

3. Loss of muscle power of the knee Quadriceps weakness will often lead to difficulty in stabilizing the knee in extension, especially if it is linked with weakness of hip extensors when associated with poliomyelitis. The patient may back-knee or hyper-extend, sometimes using their hand to assist this manoeuvre.

4. Loss of muscle power of the ankle Often a common peroneal nerve palsy will affect gait in this way. The absence of active dorsiflexion leads the patient to over-flex the hip to clear the foot during swing. This leads to a high-stepping or 'drop-foot' gait. In addition, the foot is supinated and the lateral border contacts the ground first.

5. Abnormality of the joint itself Mechanical derangement of the hip itself will lead to a situation in which the fulcrum will not be stabilized. The typical example of this occurs in developmental dysplasia of the hip (DDH) in which complete dislocation has occurred. A stable hip centre does not exist, and the hip often forms a false joint both superiorly and laterally. The mechanical lever arm is foreshortened and the abductor muscles act inefficiently and over a much shorter distance. These patients often have a marked Trendelenburg gait which may be bilateral. In addition, they have significant fixed flexion deformities of the hip and, to enable upright stance, they will have marked increased lumbar lordosis.

With ankylosis or arthrodesis of the hip joint, gait disturbance may be relatively hidden, especially if it is unilateral. A degree of compensation can occur by allowing flexion and extension to take place at the junction between the pelvis and the lumbar spine. Such adaptation cannot occur at the knee, where an ankylosed joint is very obvious, but may occur at the ankle or smaller joints of the mid-foot.

6. Injury or disease causing shortening or bending of bones Shortening is a not uncommon cause of limp, and its causes are many. Infantile poliomyelitis is now rare in the developed world, but on a world-wide basis it must be regarded as a common cause. Developmental dysplasia of the hip with dislocation may account for a significant unilateral shortening (of around 5 cm). Smaller degrees of shortening may arise from growth-plate arrest after injury, rare congenital conditions, or from malunion of a long-bone fracture. Not uncommonly, smaller degrees of inequality are seen after joint replacement arthroplasty (usually of the hip).

The short leg gait is usually (although not always) painless, and is characterized by a gait in which the shoulder on the affected side drops during stance.

7. Central causes of a limp There are many neurological causes of limp or gait disturbance. Hemiparesis after stroke may cause a unilateral weakness in which both upper and lower limbs are affected. The affected lower limb may drag and not clear during the swing phase. The affected upper limb is usually held flexed and adducted close by the side. It does not swing freely with the contralateral limb, resulting in a clumsy dysrhythmic gait.

Cerebellar conditions may lead to a broad-based unsteady ataxic gait in which balance is seriously affected. For example, there may be a persistent deviation to one side. Conditions of the posterior columns, including tabes dorsalis, may lead to a slapping, high-stepping gait which lacks proprioceptive feedback (spinal ataxia).

A wide range of gait disturbance is seen in cerebral

palsy. In mild hemiplegia the difference may be subtle, appearing similar to hemiplegic gait after stroke. Running may reveal the less obvious disability. With more severe involvement the arm will be flexed, adducted and internally rotated at the shoulder. The forearm is pronated, the wrist flexed, the thumb adducted and the fingers flexed.

Abnormalities in the legs vary. In mild cases, toe walking may be difficult to spot, but in severe cases severe bilateral 'scissor gait' may occur, in which the hips are held adducted and internally rotated, and the knees may cross over or be held against each other. Frequently there is a 'crouched' posture with flexion deformities at the knees throughout all phases of walking. This gait has a high energy requirement, and walking is often abandoned in late adolescence.

Conversion reactions are very rarely responsible for limp or gait abnormality. The gait is usually bizarre and unlike anything experienced before. It is possible to judge that the changes are inconsistent and not in keeping with physical signs. A careful history will reveal that some secondary gain is to be obtained, such as school avoidance or occupation-related compensation.

LIMP AND GAIT DISTURBANCE IN CHILDHOOD

Limp in childhood is both a common presentation and a diagnostic challenge. Often the parents are concerned about the manner in which a child walks, or the fact that they walk with a limp.

IN-TOEING AND OUT-TOEING

Once children begin to stand, many will show an out-toed stance. This is often observed at a peak age of 12 months, and there is excellent longitudinal evidence that most cases will tend to disappear by the age of 18 months. The theory that this stance is derived from a frog-leg sleep posture is generally accepted.

In-toeing of gait is slightly more common, affecting about 1 in 10 young children. About 40% will recover completely and, of the rest, few require treatment. There are three major causes:

1. *metatarsus varus* (in the newborn);
2. *internal tibial torsion* (in the toddler);
3. *internal femoral torsion or inset hips* (in the primary school-aged child).

These are usually caused by a mixture of genetic and postural factors. The relationship between internal tibial torsion or excessive femoral anteversion of the hip and the knee is uncertain. In non-neuromuscular disease

most cases will improve spontaneously to some extent. In neuromuscular disease osteotomy is usually required, and spontaneous improvement is the exception.

FLAT FEET

The medial longitudinal arch develops with age. At the time when a child is beginning to walk, at about 18 months, the foot appears flat. In the majority of individuals the arch will continue to form 'normally', but about 15% of Australians will remain flat-footed throughout life. There is no evidence that pain-free flexible flat foot should be treated, or that orthotic insoles will affect the natural history of this condition. Occasionally the child with painless flat foot will have a tight Achilles tendon, forcing a plano-valgus deformity. In those with a painful or rigid flat foot there may be another cause – which will require treatment – including tarsal coalition (originally known as peroneal spastic flat foot) or an underlying neuromuscular disorder.

KNOCK KNEES – GENU VALGUM

Many children between the ages of 2 and 7 years have knock-knee deformity. Longitudinal population-based studies have shown that the majority will grow out of this condition without the need for bracing or surgery. Certainly some cases will persist into adulthood, although in the absence of a significant cause most will be mild (but beware the unilateral case).

CAUSES OF LIMP IN CHILDHOOD

Although postural disturbance is common and relatively benign, there are many other possible causes of limp in childhood (see Table 22.1).

GAIT ANALYSIS AND GAIT LABORATORIES

The scientific study of gait may prove helpful in the management of disorders of gait. Gait analysis is an evaluation of a subject's walking pattern by systematic measurement and description. At its simplest, this may involve an experienced examiner observing a person walking the length of a long corridor, and at its most sophisticated assessment is made within a gait laboratory, where measurements can be taken by means of video analysis, force-plate measurement, electromyographic data and other sophisticated methods.

It is possible to measure the spatial movement of the body independently of the forces which cause that movement. Such measurement is known as *kinematics*.

Table 22.1 Causes of childhood limp (adapted from Rang)

	Region	Causes
1. Anatomical causes	Spine	Spondylolisthesis, spinal osteomyelitis, spinal dysraphism
	Hip	CDH, synovitis, Perthes' disease, slipped capital femoral epiphysis
	Knee	Osteochondritis, tumour
	Leg	Toddler's fracture, stress fracture, pathological fracture, bone cyst, short leg
	Foot	Kohler's disease, tarsal coalition
2. General causes	Muscle disease	e.g. Duchenne muscular dystrophy
	Disease of bone	Leukaemia, rickets, renal failure
	Infection	Osteomyelitis, Brodie's abscess
	Joint disease	Rheumatoid arthritis, septic arthritis
	Others	Polio, clubfoot, cerebral palsy
	Hysteria	Rare

Measurement of the forces that produce movement is known as *kinetics* (the study of the relationship between force and motion). Kinetics involves the measurement of ground-reaction forces, joint moments and joint power.

The motion of the skeletal system is the result of a balance between external and internal forces. The external forces on the skeletal system include gravity, inertia, and foot–ground reaction forces during walking. Internal forces are generated by muscular contraction, passive soft-tissue stretching, and bony contact at the articulations of joints. At any instant during gait, the external forces and moments must be balanced by internal forces or moments (Newton's third law). Remember that muscles always work as a motor unit to a lever arm acting on a joint. This action is referred to as an *internal joint moment*, and is a product of force and distance. It is possible to calculate the net moment acting across a joint, and thus to plot its relationship to the gait cycle for all joint levels in all planes of movement, so providing a framework for understanding the process of normal walking.

Gait analysis has a proven role in pre-operative planning for the surgical management of cerebral palsy in particular. In addition, it plays an important part in research on the effect on ambulation of surgery to and disease of the lower limb. Research applications have included studying the effects of amputation, the efficacy of prosthetic limbs and orthotic devices, arthroplasty, ligament repair, and arthrodesis in the lower limb. Gait analysis has also been used to monitor the progress of neuromuscular disease and as a diagnostic tool. The cost of setting up a gait laboratory and the complex nature of the analysis have meant that this facility is usually only available in highly specialized centres.

FURTHER READING

Andriacchi TP. 1996: Biomechanics and gait. In Kasser JR (ed.), *Orthopaedic knowledge update 5*. Rosemont, IL: The American Academy of Orthopaedic Surgeons, 29–40.

Gage JR, De Luca PA, Renshaw TS. 1995: Instructional Course Lecture of the American Academy of Orthopaedic Surgeons. Gait analysis: principles and applications. Emphasis on its use in cerebral palsy. *Journal of Bone and Joint Surgery* 77, 1607–23.

Hardcastle P, Nade S. 1985: The significance of the Trendelenburg test. *Journal of Bone and Joint Surgery* 67, 741–6.

Rang M. 1993: Toeing in and toeing out: gait disorders. In Wegner DR, Rang M (eds), *The art and practice of children's orthopaedics*. New York: Raven Press, 50–76.

Williams PF. (ed.) 1982: *Orthopaedic management in childhood*. Oxford: Blackwell Science.

Sore mouth and oral mugcosal disorders

Sheila E. Fisher

Introduction

The mouth can often serve as a guide for the careful and astute clinician. The conditions which affect the oral mucosa are often linked to systemic disorders, and the mouth has the advantage of being easily accessible for clinical examination.

In this chapter, the common and important disorders which may present as oral conditions, as well as those in which the oral mucosa may give clues to systemic disease, will be considered.

These fall into the following main categories:

- sore mouth;
- ulcers and vesicles;
- white and red patches;
- oral cancer.

SORE MOUTH

Complaints of sore mouth are common. As a symptom, it is most often a side-effect of drug therapy, but may also be linked to haematological abnormalities or present as an idiopathic condition.

BURNING MOUTH SYNDROME/ HAEMATOLOGICAL CONDITIONS

To distinguish between these two conditions clinically can be difficult, as both tend to affect middle-aged or elderly patients, and women more than men. A list of conditions which may present as a sore or burning mouth is shown in Table 23.1.1.

Usually when the mouth is examined no obvious pathology can be seen. Classical associations, such as a beefy red tongue in vitamin B deficiency, are described, but usually the practical course is to test for the conditions listed and to consign those patients without

demonstrable abnormalities to the idiopathic group. Sometimes the sore mouth clarifies the whole picture. For example, this complaint linked to vague neurological symptoms in the lower limbs raises a strong suspicion of subacute degeneration of the cord. Rare but important conditions, such as Plummer-Vinson syndrome, alternatively known as Patterson-Kelly-Brown syndrome, in which iron-deficiency anaemia is linked to oesophageal webbing and the development of post-cricoid carcinoma, should not be forgotten.

XEROSTOMIA

Complaints of dry mouth are not uncommon, and again may often be linked to drug therapy or may be idiopathic. Where the patient also complains of dry eyes, the diagnosis of Sjögren's syndrome should be considered. This diagnosis can often (but not invariably) be confirmed by biopsy of a labial minor salivary gland. Treatment is aimed at control of symptoms, but patients with Sjögren's syndrome should be kept under review, as

Table 23.1.1 Possible aetiological factors involved in burning mouth

Haematological
  Vitamin B complex deficiency
  Iron or ferritin deficiency
  Folic acid deficiency

Systemic
  Diabetes

Iatrogenic
  Drugs

Local
  Candidiasis
  Poorly fitting dentures
  Xerostomia (possible idiopathic or Sjögren's syndrome)
  Parafunctional habits

Psychological
  Cancer phobia
  Depression
  Anxiety

approximately 6% of them will develop B-cell lymphoma in a major salivary gland.

ULCERS AND VESICLES

People seek treatment primarily because of pain. Where pain may be a late feature, which is particularly true in the case of malignant ulcers, delays in presentation have serious consequences. A simple rule is that all patients with mouth ulcers which do not show signs of healing after 2 weeks of observation should have a specialist opinion. The main differential diagnoses are trauma, recurrent oral (aphthous) ulceration and vesicular disorders.

RECURRENT ORAL (APHTHOUS) ULCERATION

This is probably the commonest of all mucosal disorders, affecting 15–20% of the population, especially the young. The peak age at onset is 10–19 years. Most cases are of minor aphthous ulceration, in which the ulcers are shallow, less than 5 mm in diameter, and heal in 10–14 days without scarring. Most of the remainder are major aphthous ulcers, which are larger, usually 1–3 cm in diameter, deeper, often with rolled edges, last up to 4–6 weeks and heal with scarring. A definitive diagnosis between a major aphthous ulcer and carcinoma often requires a biopsy. The least common group are herpeti-

form ulcers, where up to 100 tiny ulcers may appear simultaneously.

Important clinical associations

1. Behcet's disease consists of oral ulceration together with two of the following: recurrent genital ulcers, skin and eye lesions, arthritis and cardiovascular disease.

2. Recurrent oral ulceration has been linked to Crohn's disease, ulcerative colitis and gluten-sensitive enteropathy. In each of these disorders, a higher than expected number of patients suffer from aphthous-like ulcers.

Pathophysiology Despite much research, no definitive cause has been established. The appearance of ulcers may be linked to haematological deficiencies, stress (typically examinations), local trauma, hormonal variation (especially the luteal phase of the menstrual cycle), allergy to foods, cessation of smoking, familial and variations in immune response.

Treatment Control of symptoms is the main aim of treatment. Some reduction in the severity and duration of ulceration can be achieved by the use of topical steroids in the 'prodromal' phase, when the patient is usually aware of a prickling sensation at the site of the developing ulcer. Pain is due to secondary infection, which can be controlled by the use of analgesic and antiseptic mouthwashes or, in severe cases, tetracycline capsules dissolved and used as a mouthwash. Recently, various immunomodulators have been tried, and thalidomide has been shown to control severe ulceration. However, the ulcers recur on stopping treatment, and none of these agents has gained an accepted place in the management of recurrent oral ulceration. Very occasionally, admission of the patient for adequate analgesia and intravenous hydration may be required.

VESICULOBULLOUS DISORDERS

The important distinction to be made lies between the potentially fatal autoimmune disease, pemphigus, and the other main vesiculobullous condition, pemphigoid. The critical distinction is made on the basis of histological examination of a bulla. In pemphigus the bullae are intra-epithelial, and immunofluorescence demonstrates epithelial-bound auto-antibody. Recent studies have shown that the antigen is a protein, belonging to the cadherin family, which is a component of the desmosome.

In pemphigoid, the bulla is subepithelial and linear binding of IgG can be demonstrated in the basement membrane zone.

The other form of oral bullous disorder with which

the clinician should be familiar is angina bullosa haemorrhagica. In this curious condition, blood-filled bullae develop spontaneously, usually in the palate. No cause has ever been identified, although it is thought probable that they are related to trauma and that they may arise after intubation. They are harmless and the patient can be reassured of this.

WHITE AND RED PATCHES

The important distinction to be made here is between patches which are benign and those which are premalignant or malignant. In this chapter they will be divided into idiopathic, infective, autoimmune and premalignant categories.

IDIOPATHIC

Geographic tongue/migratory glossitis

This condition is common, and is characterized by irregular depapillated areas on the dorsal aspect and lateral margins of the tongue. The patient may complain of discomfort, especially on eating hot or spicy food. The pattern of depapillation alters, often over a period of days.

It is advisable to carry out a full blood count and to exclude dietary deficiency by testing for vitamin B_{12}, folate, ferritin and zinc. Where these tests are normal, the patient can be reassured that the condition is harmless.

INFECTIVE

Oral candidiasis

Candidal species are found as part of the normal oral commensal flora in about 40% of patients. Any kind of underlying illness or debilitating condition can be associated with proliferation of *Candida* in the oral cavity. Because of this, oral candidiasis is common in all types of surgical patient. In its acute form, it causes soreness, and because of this may interfere with the re-establishment of oral nutrition in surgical patients.

Acute pseudomembranous candidiasis (thrush) is most common in very young, very old or very debilitated patients. It is characterized by creamy-white patches which can easily be wiped off, leaving a sore and bleeding area. Treatment may be topical or systemic. Traditional remedies such as nystatin have been superseded by modern agents, especially the imidazoles. Acute pseudomembranous candidiasis is a frequent complication of radiotherapy to head and neck lesions.

Chronic erythematous (atrophic) candidiasis is the form most frequently seen in adults, and it affects approximately 25% of the denture-wearing population. Continuous coverage of the palatal mucosa is a recognized factor. To eradicate the condition it is necessary to persuade the patient to leave the dentures out at night, and to treat both patient and denture.

Candidal hyperplasia usually affects the corners of the mouth, although it can be widespread, particularly in patients who are immunocompromised. It appears as a speckled white patch, and is important because it is this type of candidiasis which is associated with dysplasia and malignant transformation. Treatment may involve prolonged (up to 3 months) antifungal therapy. Persistent lesions, especially if they are localized, can be treated using a carbon dioxide laser.

AUTOIMMUNE

Oral lichen planus

Oral lichen planus affects approximately 1% of the population in the UK, with a slightly higher incidence in females than in males. It is a mucocutaneous disorder, with approximately one-third of patients having both oral and skin lesions. Other mucosal surfaces, notably the vulva, can be involved.

The clinical appearance is variable, ranging from white striae in the buccal mucosa to florid atrophic glossitis (see Plate 23.1.1 in the colour plate section). Whether or not lichen planus is premalignant is a contentious issue. The author believes that it is in cases where the condition is erosive in nature and when the tongue is affected. The case shown in Plate 23.1.1 has developed squamous-cell carcinoma.

Pathophysiology The disorder is generally considered to be of autoimmune origin. The classical histological picture is of a clearly defined band of T-cells in the submucosal area (see Plate 23.1.2 in the colour plate section).

Treatment The mainstay of treatment is steroid therapy, usually topically administered, although systemic therapy may be required for severe exacerbations. Good oral hygiene is important for control of symptoms.

PREMALIGNANT

Leukoplakia/erythroplakia

The presence of either leukoplakia (white patch) or erythroplakia (red velvety patch) places patients at higher risk of developing oral cancer. The rate of malignant change is variable, but on average is around 6% for leukoplakia. Erythroplakia should be considered malignant until proven otherwise.

Pathophysiology The aetiology is likely to be multifactorial. Tobacco is the most important agent, whether smoked or chewed. Viruses may also be important. In hairy leukoplakia, the type seen in HIV-positive and other immunosuppressed patients, an association with the Epstein-Barr virus has been demonstrated. High-risk subtypes of human papilloma virus may also play a part in the development of some leukoplakias. In addition p 53 mutations have been shown, especially in cases where patients are heavy smokers or drinkers.

Pathological grading In common with other dysplastic conditions, the degree of epithelial disturbance can be graded (see Plate 23.1.3 in the colour plate section). In mild dysplasia few cellular abnormalities are seen, and the normal structure of the epithelium is largely preserved. In carcinoma *in situ*, organization of the epithelium is disrupted and many cellular abnormalities are apparent, but the basement membrane is not breached. Lesions falling between these two extremes may be graded as moderately or severely dysplastic.

Treatment Where a cause can be identified (usually smoking), the patient is encouraged to stop. This may be enough to induce regression of the lesion. Clinical appearance is not a reliable guide to malignant transformation. Where there are wide areas of change, regular surveillance is necessary. For smaller, isolated areas and for all erythroplakias, excision is advised. Carbon dioxide laser treatment is useful, as it can achieve ablation of the lesion with minimal scarring.

ORAL CANCER

Each year approximately 2000 new cases of oral cancer are diagnosed in the UK. Of these, approximately 50% will survive for 5 years. In some parts of the world, especially the Indian subcontinent, the incidence is much higher. Although oral cancer is most common in middle-aged and elderly patients, and is linked to smoking and heavy drinking, there is clear evidence of an increasing incidence in young patients without demonstrable risk factors.

Despite the accessibility of the mouth for examination, cancers of the oral cavity usually present late. They can often mimic benign disease (see Plate 23.1.4 in the colour plate section), and pain is not a feature until comparatively late. Neural transmission pathways are such that the presenting feature may be intractable otalgia. Approximately one-third of UK cancers arise in areas of documented premalignant change.

Pathophysiology p53 mutations have been conclusively implicated in the development of oral cancer, especially in smokers. Viruses, such as high-risk subtypes of the human papillomavirus, may also be involved, but further research is needed to confirm this relationship.

Staging This is done according to the TNM classification (see Table 23.1.2).

Table 23.1.2 Staging of oral cancer

T stage

T1	Tumour 2 cm or less in greatest diameter
T2	Tumour more than 2 cm but less than 4 cm in greatest diameter
T3	Tumour more than 4 cm in greatest diameter
T4	Tumour invades adjacent structures, e.g. bone
TX	Tumour cannot be assesed

N stage

N0	No regional lymph node metastasis
N1	Metastasis in a single ipsilateral node, 3 cm or less in diameter
N2	Metastasis in a single ipsilateral node, more than 3 cm but less than 6 cm in diameter, in multiple ipsilateral nodes, or in bilateral or contralateral nodes, none more than 6 cm in diameter
N3	Metastasis in a lymph node more than 6 cm in diameter
NX	Lymph nodes cannot be assessed

M stage

M0	No distant metastasis
M1	Distant metastasis
MX	Metastasis cannot be assessed

Treatment T1 and some T2 lesions can be cured by either surgery or radiotherapy. Larger lesions, those invading bone and those with nodal metastases are treated surgically, with adjuvant radiotherapy in cases where nodal involvement or the presence of close surgical margins are seen histologically.

Survival The 5-year survival rate ranges from 80% for T1N0 lesions to less than 40% for T4N0 lesions. The presence of nodal metastases reduces survival by a further 50%, and the presence of extracapsular spread of tumour is a further adverse sign. The degree of differentiation, the pattern of invasion and the speed of tumour growth can all be linked to prognosis.

Although survival rates have not changed greatly in recent years, advances in surgery, especially microvascular soft-tissue and bone transfer, have led to a much better level of function and a much decreased level of deformity in these patients.

ACKNOWLEDGEMENTS

The author wishes to thank Dr NR Griffin, Consultant Histopathologist, for the histopathological slides illustrated in this chapter.

FURTHER READING

Langdon JD, Henk JM. (eds) 1995: *Malignant tumours of the mouth, jaws and salivary glands.* London: Edward Arnold.

Lewis MAO, Lamey PJ. 1993: *Clinical oral medicine.* Oxford: Butterworth Heinemann.

Infections

Sheila E. Fisher

Introduction

Infections affecting the teeth, jaws and other parts of the oral cavity are common. Consideration of local and general factors is important to secure best management. The general factors are those which are relevant to all surgical fields (Table 23.2.1) and which not only render the patient more susceptible to the infective process, but allow it to develop to a more serious degree than in healthy patients. In this chapter the local processes will be considered, but attention will also be drawn to general aspects where these are of particular or specific relevance.

Table 23.2.1 Local and general factors implicated in oral infections

Local factors	General factors
Sources of infection	Factors which predispose the patient to infection
Teeth and their surrounding structures	Immunosuppression (diabetes, tumours with or without chemotherapy, transplants, HIV)
Bone – cysts, trauma, radiation	Medical therapy (steroids)
Soft tissues	Debilitation (serious systemic disturbance, malnutrition)
Salivary glands, including calculi	Factors which put the patient at risk from the infection
Waldeyer's ring – tonsils, adenoids	As above
Paranasal air sinuses	Valvular or other congenital heart defect
Predisposing factors	Surgical prosthetic materials
Poor oral hygiene	
Radiotherapy	

ACUTE ODONTOGENIC INFECTIONS

Most acute infections are odontogenic, i.e. related to the teeth or surrounding structures. They range from pulpitis (inflammation of the pulp of the tooth) and periodontitis (inflammation of the supporting tissues of the tooth) to severe and life-threatening infections of the deep tissue spaces. The surgical anatomy of severe bacterial infection is summarized in Figure 23.2.1.

Pathophysiology Acute pyogenic infections such as dento-alveolar abscesses, pericoronitis (inflammation around the crown of a tooth, most commonly the third molar or 'wisdom tooth') and actinomycosis are usually endogenous, being caused by organisms that constitute part of the normal flora of the oral cavity. Dental caries

(a)

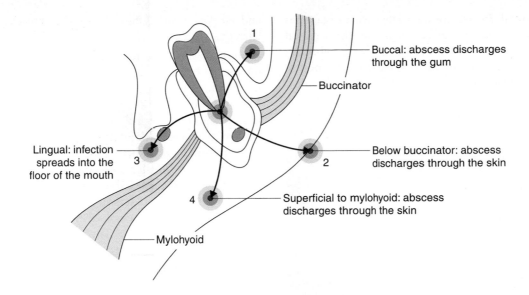

1

Buccal: abscess discharges
through the gum

Buccinator

Lingual: infection
spreads into the
floor of the mouth

3

2

Below buccinator: abscess
discharges through the skin

4

Superficial to mylohyoid: abscess
discharges through the skin

Mylohyoid

(b)

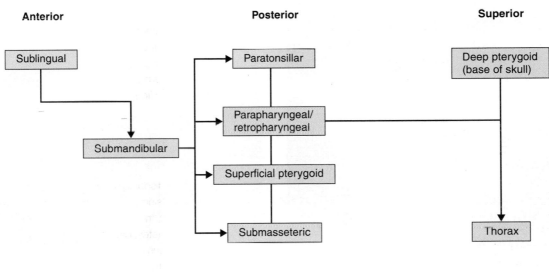

Anterior

Posterior

Superior

Sublingual

Paratonsillar

Deep pterygoid
(base of skull)

Parapharyngeal/
retropharyngeal

Submandibular

Superficial pterygoid

Submasseteric

Thorax

Inferior

(c)

Clinical relevance

Airway control: Trismus
                  Soft-tissue swelling and oedema – floor of mouth
                                                – pharyngeal wall
                  Displacement of key structures – trachea

Relation to major structures – pus closely related to – airway
                                                     – major vessels

Rare but important complications – cavernous sinus thrombosis

Figure 23.2.1 Surgical anatomy of oral infection: (a) routes by which infection spreads; (b) spread of infection into the deep
tissue spaces of the head and neck; (c) clinical relevance.

and periodontal disease are associated with organisms that are present on the surface of the tooth in dental plaque. In studies of healthy subjects, at least 30 bacterial genera have been commonly isolated from the mouth. Of these, *Streptococcus mutans* appears to be the most important in the development of dental caries. The species involved in periodontal disease are less well established, but *Actinobacillus actinomycetemcomitans*

and *Porphyromonas gingivalis* are the subject of much current study.

Clinical relevance For the practising surgeon, the direct relevance of these processes lies in the progression from pulpitis to dento-alveolar abscess, with diagnostic and treatment considerations. When an abscess discharges intra-orally, there is little confusion about its source. However, an abscess pointing externally must be distinguished from skin conditions such as sebaceous cyst and also from more sinister pathology (Figures 23.2.2 and 23.2.3). If a tooth-related abscess or sinus is treated without attention to the underlying cause, the infection will invariably recur, with the risk of morbidity such as multiple scars and facial nerve damage from multiple ineffective interventions. In the early stages most dento-alveolar infections will respond well to oral penicillin V or intravenous benzyl penicillin, with the addition of metronidazole if early resolution does not occur. Once an abscess has formed, drainage is mandatory, but it can be hazardous, as outlined in Figure 23.2.1. Involvement of these tissue spaces may lead to extreme degrees of trismus and the risk of direct rupture of the abscess into the laryngopharnyx on attempted intubation. Anaesthesia for these patients requires a senior

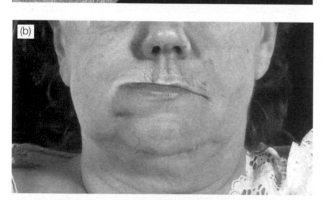

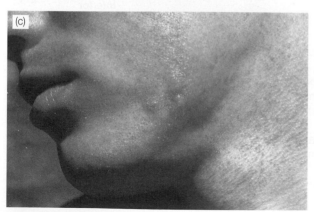

Figure 23.2.2 Differential diagnosis of extra-oral swellings: a difficult area. (a) Dental abscess. (b) Fungating squamous-cell carcinoma. (c) Cervicofacial actinomycosis.

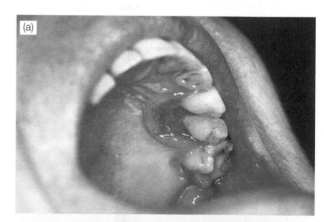

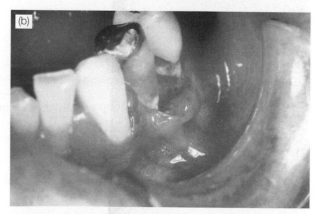

Figure 23.2.3 Differential diagnosis of intra-oral swellings: benign and malignant pathology. (a) Pyogenic ulcer. (b) Squamous-cell carcinoma.

anaesthetist and maxillofacial surgeon. Facilities for the provision of an emergency tracheostomy with placement of a cuffed tube to protect the lungs from direct aspiration of purulent material are mandatory.

Ludwig's angina is a rare cellulitis which involves all of the tissue spaces on both sides of the mouth. The patient is extremely unwell, with a massive brawny swelling which raises the tongue up towards the palate and back towards the pharynx (Figure 23.2.4). Management is controversial, with some advocating high-dose antibiotics and steroids, and others advocating surgical decompression in addition. Pus is seldom found. However, in the author's experience the patient starts to recover rapidly once the tissue spaces have been carefully and fully opened and through and through drains inserted from the neck to the floor of the mouth. Even with optimal management the mortality rate is about 4%.

CHRONIC ODONTOGENIC INFECTION

The most common type is chronic periodontitis, which leads to the progressive loss of tooth support. Loose teeth are a hazard at intubation, and it is sensible to check for loose teeth when clerking pre-operative patients.

Cervicofacial actinomycosis (Figure 23.2.2) presents as a symptomless localized swelling, usually in the submandibular region. It is not uncommon to elicit a history of surgery within the mouth or tooth extraction during the few weeks preceding presentation. Drainage may produce characteristic 'sulphur granules', and after confirmation of the diagnosis the patient is treated with long-term penicillin or ampicillin.

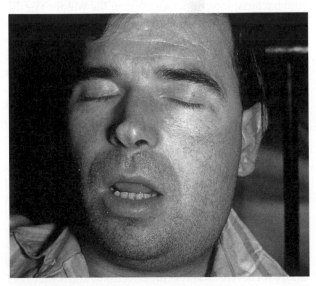

Figure 23.2.4 Ludwig's angina.

NON-ODONTOGENIC INFECTIONS

Occasionally a similar clinical picture to the above can occur due to atypical mycobacterial infection of the submandibular nodes. This can occur in children and adults, and should be suspected when the clinical picture does not fit the more common infective processes.

Suppurative lymphadenitis is an unusual condition which affects young children and can be difficult to manage. It follows an apparent viral infection of the upper respiratory tract, and the affected nodes require surgical drainage. The pathogen involved is *Staphylococcus aureus*, and antibiotic treatment (flucloxacillin or other antibiotics as advised after culture and sensitivity tests on pus obtained at operation) must be given in high doses and for an adequate period, otherwise other cervical nodes will become involved.

INFECTIONS INVOLVING BONE

Infection is usually secondary to pathology within bone. Common precipitating causes include retained tooth roots and cysts. Infection can complicate the fixation of facial fractures with titanium miniplates, but this is uncommon (less than 4% in most published series). In patients where the bone is otherwise normal, management is according to standard surgical principles, namely elimination of the cause and antibiotic therapy for systemic symptoms. The bacteriological spectrum is as discussed above.

Following radiotherapy, osteoradionecrosis can represent a considerable surgical challenge. Bone vascularity is severely impaired because of endarteritis obliterans, and the bone becomes susceptible to low-grade spreading infection after mucosal breach or tooth removal. For this reason, most maxillofacial surgeons will electively remove teeth in an area that is planned to receive radiotherapy. Often a specific organism cannot be identified. Treatment consists of maintenance of oral hygiene, antibiotics (tetracycline, penicillin or metronidazole) and hyperbaric oxygen therapy. Where sequestration occurs, the necrotic bone should be removed, and this will not infrequently require replacement with a composite microvascular free flap to provide well-vascularized bone and covering soft tissue. The principal differential diagnosis is from recurrent bony tumour, and biopsy is required to confirm the absence of neoplasia.

Chronic osteomyelitis may occur in the facial skeleton, especially in the mandible, but is rare and will not be discussed in this chapter.

SOFT-TISSUE INFECTIONS

Unlike the odontogenic infections, those that directly affect the oral mucosa are usually viral or fungal. As they present as a sore mouth, they are discussed in Chapter 23.1.

SALIVARY GLAND INFECTIONS

These may involve the gland directly or be due to a precipitating factor, the most common of which is the presence of a calculus.

CALCULI

About 80% of calculi are found in the submandibular duct and 20% in the parotid duct. The reasons why salivary calculi form are unclear. The fact that the submandibular gland produces a mucous secretion, as well as the length and course of its duct have been cited as reasons why this gland is particularly susceptible to calculus formation. Blockage of the duct results in swelling associated with eating, and stasis results in episodes of acute infection. Episodes of infection usually respond to antibiotic therapy (penicillin and/or metronidazole). In suitable cases the stone may be allowed to pass spontaneously and can sometimes be 'milked' along the duct. If this is inappropriate, where accessible the stone is removed by an intra-oral approach. Otherwise, for stones in the proximal part of the submandibular duct or in the gland, the gland itself is excised. Parotid stones are sometimes amenable to removal by a limited approach, the main requirement being to protect the facial nerve, and the most suitable operation may thus be a superficial parotidectomy. Short-wave lithotripsy has been attempted with some success, allowing the fragments to pass.

BACTERIAL INFECTION

This can occur in the young or the old as recurrent acute suppurative parotitis. Young patients usually outgrow the condition, and in the elderly it is important to look for systemic precipitating factors, especially dehydration. The organisms associated with the condition are *Staphylococcus aureus*, *Streptococcus pneumoniae* and β-haemolytic streptococci. Antibiotic therapy and massage of the gland after meals constitute the accepted therapy. In cases where a gland is non-functional because of sialectasis, it may be necessary to remove it because of the frequency of infective episodes.

Chronic sialadenitis presents as recurrent, tender enlargement of the affected gland associated with sialectasis, stones and strictures. Conservative therapy is as described above, but surgery will involve excision of the affected gland. For the parotid gland, a subtotal parotidectomy, in which as much secretory tissue is removed as possible whilst preserving the facial nerve, is performed. This operation can be technically challenging, and should only be considered in severe and intractable cases.

VIRAL INFECTIONS

The most common of these is mumps, which is usually a disease of the young. It is important for the surgeon to be aware that mumps can initially present as a unilateral swelling.

Human immunodeficiency virus (HIV) infection can present as bilateral parotid gland enlargement, and this usually coincides with the stage of persistent generalized lymphadenopathy in the AIDS-related complex. The pathological features are lymphocytic infiltration and benign lympho-epithelial cyst formation. This presentation is common in HIV-infected children.

WALDEYER'S RING

Anatomy Waldeyer's ring consists of lymphoid tissue which encircles the junction of the nasopharynx and hypopharynx. It produces B-cell lymphocytes, and is subdivided into the adenoid, palatine or faucial tonsil and lingual tonsil.

Pathophysiology Because of its physiological function, the tonsil and adenoidal tissue are often the site of viral and bacterial infection, especially in the young. The difficulty lies in determining the cause and whether antibiotic therapy is indicated. Common viral conditions include infectious mononucleosis, and streptococci and *Haemophilus influenzae* are the bacteria most likely to be implicated. A throat swab is useful as an aid to diagnosis. Hyperplasia of adenoidal tissue can obstruct the inner end of the Eustachian tube, leading to otitis media. Tonsillectomy is now limited to cases of gross hypertrophy and intractable symptoms.

Paratonsillar abscess or quinsy is a unilateral abscess in the supratonsillar fossa which displaces the tonsil medially, inferiorly and anteriorly. It may track through the superior constrictor muscle to the parapharyngeal space. In cases where an abscess has formed, it must be drained. For extensive infections involving the parapharyngeal space, the risks are the same as those outlined above for severe odontogenic infections, and senior ENT and anaesthetic staff must be involved.

PARANASAL AIR SINUSES

Streptococcus pneumoniae and *Haemophilus influenzae* are the most common pathogens, but *Staphylococcus aureus* is implicated in complex cases. Treatment consists of control of the infective process by appropriate antibiotics, and encouragement of drainage by inhalants. In cases of complex sinusitis, it is essential to check the patient's visual status. If there is no visual compromise, parenteral antibiotics may be used for a short time, but if there is no response after 24 h, surgical drainage should be performed. Functional endoscopic surgery has much improved the assessment and treatment of sinusitis.

GENERAL CONDITIONS

INFECTIVE ENDOCARDITIS

Despite advances in management, this condition continues to have a mortality rate of the order of 30%, and all patients suffer a degree of morbidity. Patients at risk are those with heart-valve pathology or prosthetic heart valves, and also those with coarctation of the aorta and shunts for haemodialysis.

The pathophysiology is of both progressive cardiac damage and damage to other organs due to septic emboli. The pathogenesis is unknown, and the condition has been reported to affect normal valves. It is not usually possible to relate an episode of infective endocarditis to a specific surgical procedure.

Although dental causes are often quoted, only 5–10% of cases are preceded by dental treatment, and the likelihood of infective endocarditis developing as a result of a single tooth extraction has been estimated to be 1 in 3000. Other surgical manipulations, especially urinary catheterization, are well-documented risk factors.

Streptococcus viridans is isolated in approximately 40% of cases, although a large number of organisms have been implicated.

CLINICAL RELEVANCE

Patients listed for heart-valve replacement and other cardiac sugery which may place them at risk should have an oral assessment, and eradication of sources of oral sepsis should be carried out prior to surgery. Post-surgery patients require an excellent level of oral care and prompt attention to any septic foci with appropriate antibiotic cover as listed in the British National Formulary.

OTHER PROSTHESES

The position with regard to antibiotic prophylaxis and the presence of hip and other joint prostheses has been the subject of considerable study and debate. A consensus view has not been expressed, and there is little firm evidence of protection by the use of prophylactic antibiotics during dental treatment or surgery to the mouth.

FURTHER READING

De Stefano F, Anda RF, Kahn HS *et al.* 1993: Dental disease and risk of coronary disease and mortality. *British Medical Journal* **306**, 688–91.

Walsh TLP. 1998: Periodontitis for medical practitioners. *British Medical Journal* **316**, 993–6.

Working Party of the British Society for Antimicrobial Chemotherapy. 1992: Antibiotic prophylaxis of infective endocarditis. *Lancet* **339**, 1292–3.

Part 2

Clinical Practice

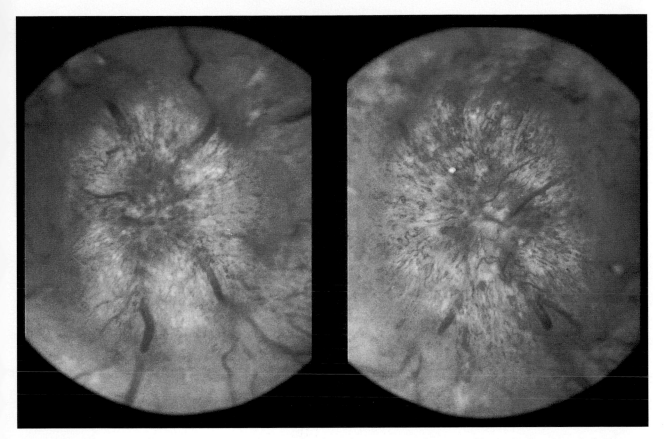

Plate 1.2.1 Bilateral papilloedema associated with long-standing raised intracranial pressure. The optic discs have indistinct margins, dilated capillaries on the surface and tortuosity of the retinal veins, which are buried in the thickened retinal nerve-fibre layer in places.

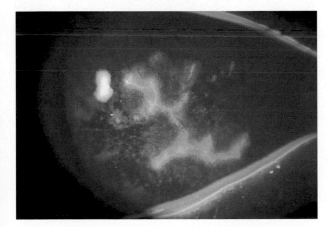

Plate 1.3.1 Dendritic ulcer stained with fluorescein 2 per cent eyedrops and illuminated with cobalt blue light.

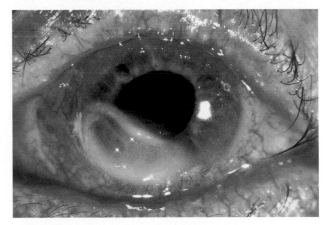

Plate 1.3.2 Bacterial corneal ulcer due to *Pseudomonas aeruginosa* in an eye predisposed to infection due to previous corneal surgery. There is extensive opaque stromal suppuration. A central desmatocele (forward bulging of cornea which has thinned to the level of Descemet's membrane) is also present.

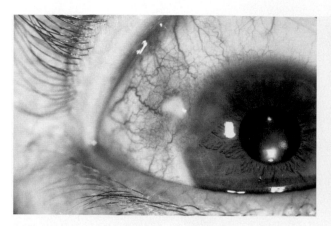

Plate 1.3.3 Anterior scleritis presenting in a patient with rheumatoid arthritis. Localized scleral injection is associated with a scleral nodule.

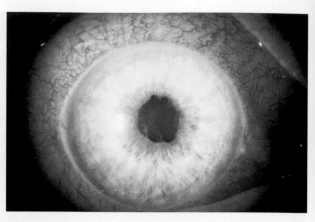

Plate 1.3.4 Acute anterior uveitis occurring in a patient with ankylosing spondylitis. There is intense ciliary injection and a small irregular pupil.

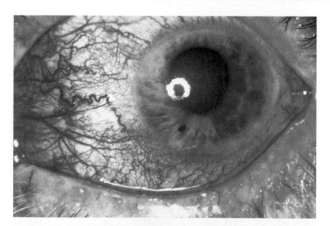

Plate 1.3.5 Acute angle-closure glaucoma. Marked ciliary injection, corneal haze and a mid-dilated pupil are observed.

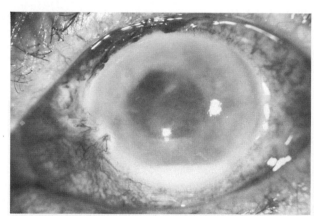

Plate 1.3.6 *Staphylococcus epidermidis* endophthalmitis presenting 1 day after routine cataract extraction with intra-ocular lens implantation. The fresh wound is visible just below the upper lid. There is conjunctival hyperaemia and chemosis, corneal clouding and a hypopyon.

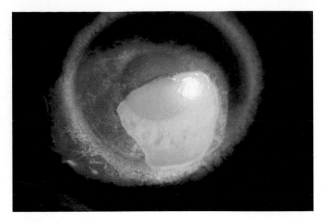

Plate 1.3.7 Corneal abrasion stained with fluorescein 2 per cent eyedrops and viewed using a cobalt blue light.

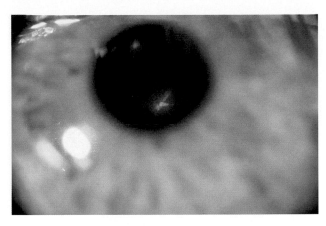

Plate 1.3.8 Wood splinter embedded in the cornea.

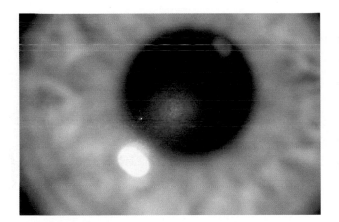

Plate 1.3.9 Residual rust stain following removal of a metallic corneal foreign body.

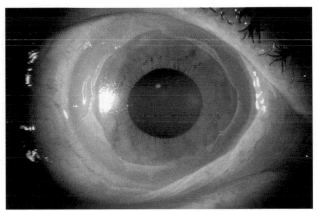

Plate 1.3.10 Alkali burn. There is a large corneal epithelial defect with chemosis. Minimal redness is an ominous sign, signifying significant ischaemia of the anterior segment.

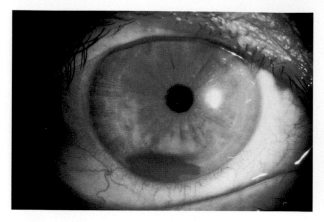

Plate 1.3.11 Hyphaema. Blood in the anterior chamber collects inferiorly.

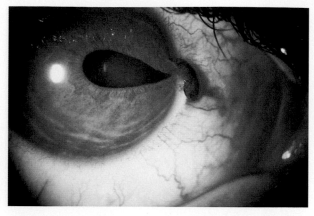

Plate 1.3.12 Penetrating eye injury. The pupil has a tear-drop shape, and the iris tissue is protruding through a corneal puncture.

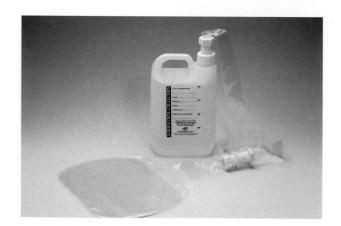

Plate 2.3.1 'Megostomy' device.

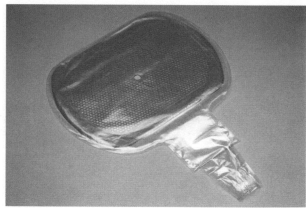

Plate 2.3.2 Eakin bag.

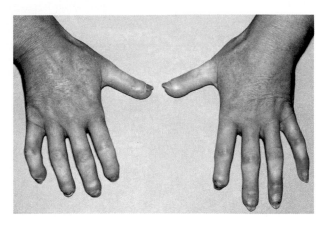

Plate 11.1 Scleroderma of hands.

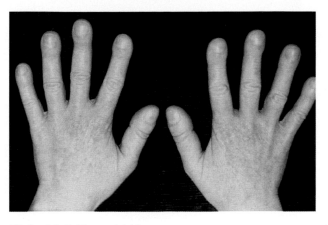

Plate 11.2 Finger clubbing.

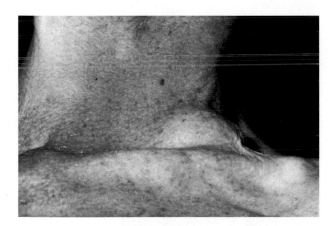

Plate 11.3 Virchow's node.

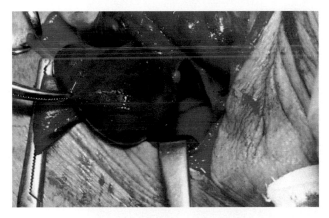

Plate 11.4 Thyroid nodule.

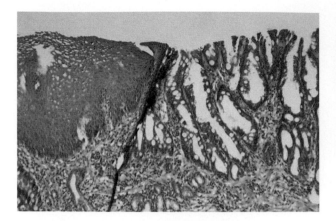

Plate 11.5 Barrett's oesophagus.

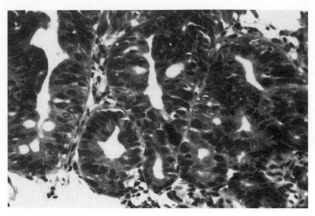

Plate 11.6 Severe dysplasia in a Barrett's oesophagus.

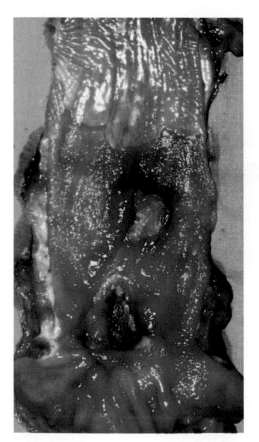

Plate 11.7 Barrett's oesophagus with two carcinomas; the lower at the oesophagogastric junction and the upper at the junction between squamous and columnar epithelium.

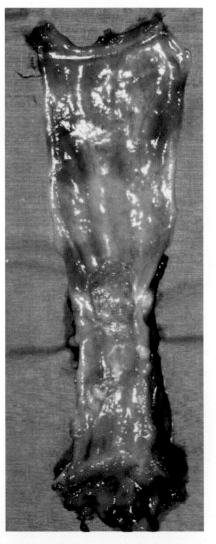

Plate 11.8 Obstructing carcinoma well above the oesophagogastric junction.

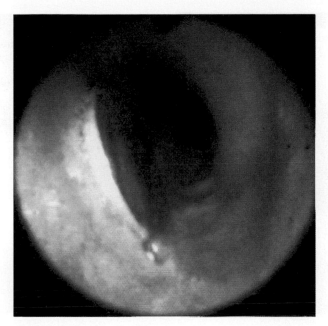

Plate 11.9 Coin in oesophagus.

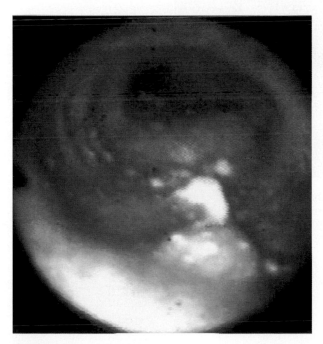

Plate 11.10 Candidiasis.

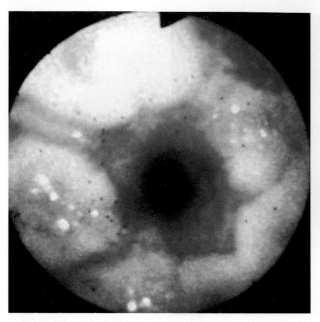

Plate 11.11 Endoscopic view of a peptic stricture near the lower end of the oesophagus.

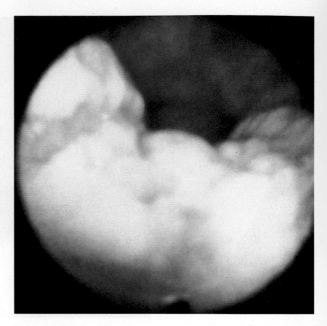

Plate 11.12 Endoscopic view of cacinoma of the oesophagus.

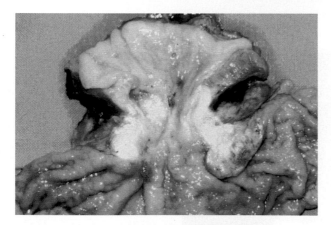

Plate 11.13 A stenosing carcinoma at the cardia.

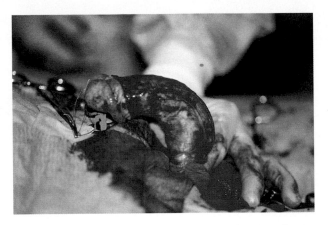

Plate 18.1 Artificial erection demonstrating dorsal penile deformity of Peyronie's disease.

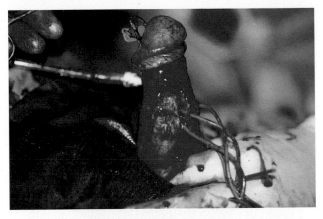

Plate 18.2 Repeat artificial erection after excision of ellipse of tunica albuginea.

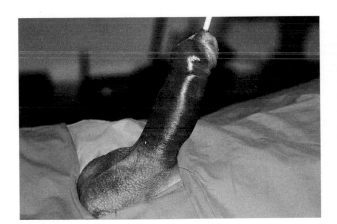

Plate 18.3 Priapism following self-injection of papaverine – aspiration and instillation of phenylephrine were unsuccessful, and the patient needed a penile prosthesis.

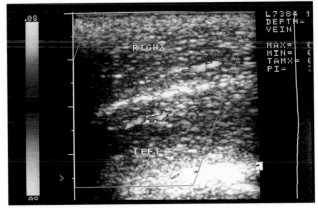

Plate 18.4 Colour Doppler ultrasound defining both cavernosal arteries separated by the mid-line septum.

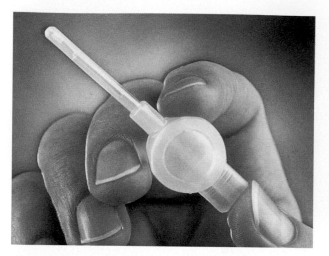

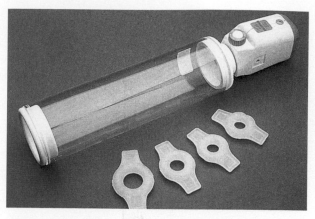

Plate 18.5 The Medicated Intra-urethral System of Erection (MUSE), in which prostaglandin E₁ is administered intra-urethrally.

Plate 18.6 A vacuum device with different-sized compression rings.

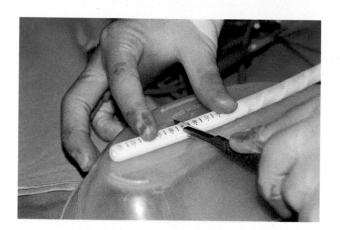

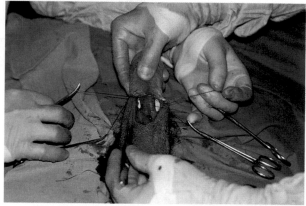

Plate 18.7 A malleable prosthesis being cut to size.

Plate 18.8 A malleable prosthesis inserted into each corpus cavernosus through a penoscrotal incision.

(a)

(b)

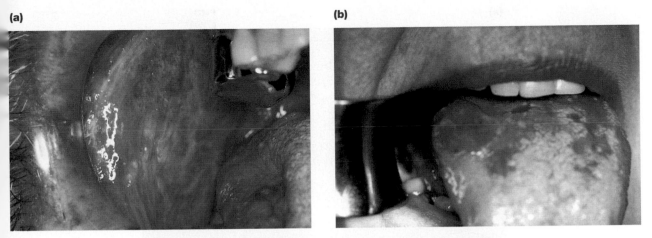

Plate 23.1.1 Oral lichen planus. (a) Typical striae of non-erosive lichen planus. (b) Squamous-cell carcinoma in a case of atrophic erosive lichen planus.

(a)

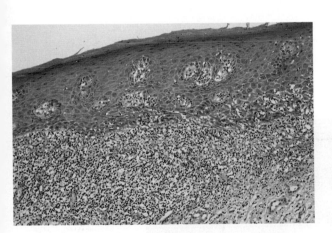

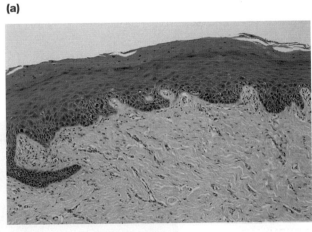

Plate 23.1.2 Typical histological appearance in oral lichen planus.

(b)

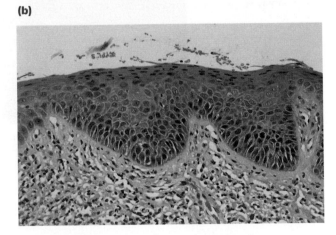

Plate 23.1.3 Grading of dysplasia. (a) Mild dysplasia. (b) Severe dysplasia.

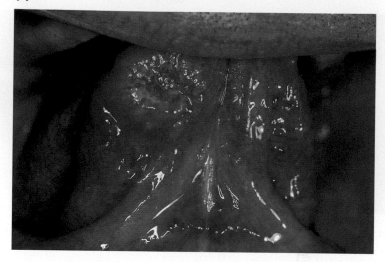

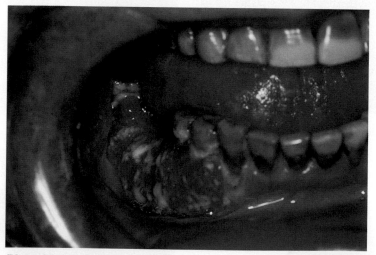

Plate 23.1.4 Oral cancer. (a) Exophytic oral cancer. (b) Cancer of the alveolus.

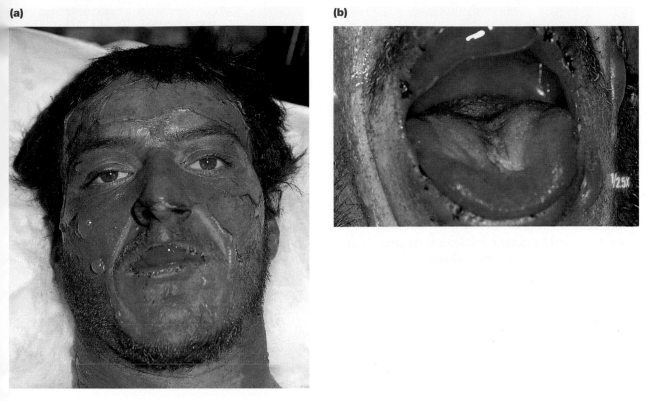

Plate 25.1 (a) Facial burns. (b) Soot on tongue and erythema of oropharynx. Facial burns and redness/blisters with soot in the oropharynx are very strong indicators of airway injury and smoke inhalation.

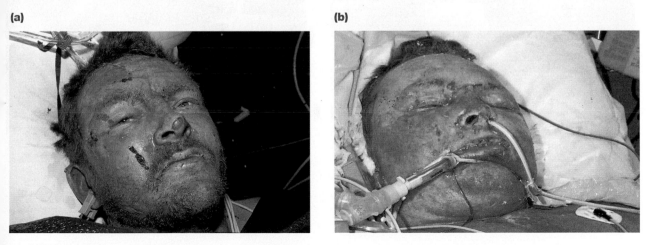

Plate 25.2 (a) and (b) Oedema formation can be immense in large burns as has occurred with this young man with 68 per cent TBSA flame burns – *intubate early*.

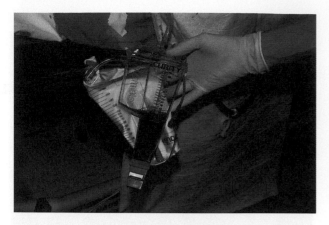

Plate 25.3 Haemoglobin and myoglobin are present in the urine. Urine output should be doubled until the urine is cleared. A mannitol infusion may be required.

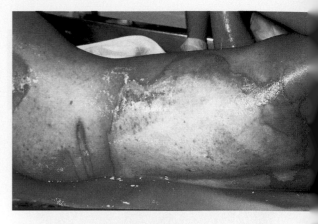

Plate 25.4 Superficial dermal burns are pale pink, moist and sensate. They can be seen around the periphery of the burn on this patient's back and on his buttocks. These sections heal quickly. Deep dermal burns are white, moist and retain some sensation. Surgery is usually indicated.

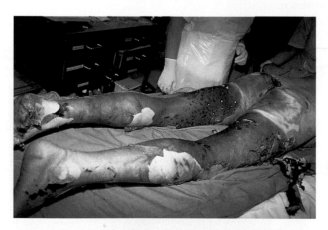

Plate 25.5 Full thickness burns are thick, leathery and white or tan in appearance.

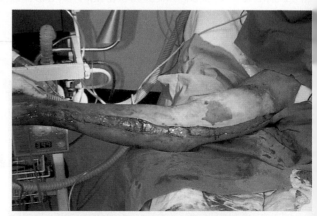

Plate 25.6 Mid-medial escharotomy of the arm. Note the way the incision has sprung apart.

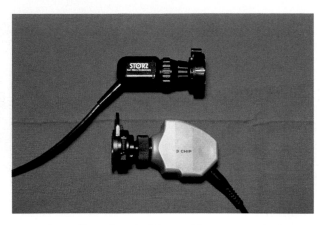

Plate 31.1 Examples of miniature video cameras designed for endoscopic surgery. The smaller camera (above) is a single-chip camera, and the larger camera (below) is a 3-chip camera.

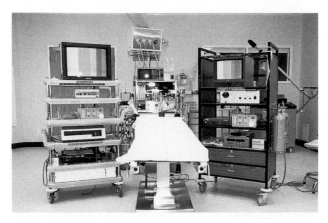

Plate 31.2 Instrument trolleys for endoscopic surgery. Both trolleys contain a video monitor, camera control box, intense light source, laparoscopic insufflator and video recorder.

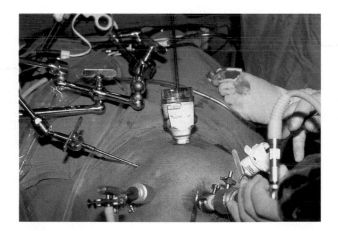

Plate 31.3 Cannulas placed for laparoscoic surgery. In this photograph a laparoscopic anterior spinal fusion is in progress. Two 11-mm ports, one 5-mm and one 15-mm port have been sited in the abdominal wall. In addition, an 'Iron Intern' is holding a retraction device used to lift the sigmoid colon away from the operative field.

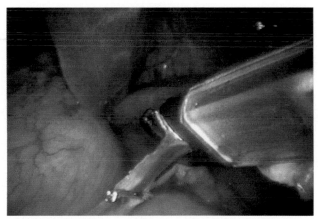

Plate 31.4 Laparoscopic view during laparoscopic Nissen fundoplication. The stomach is pulled towards the midline to place the short gastric vessels on stretch. The liver is seen above the stomach, and the spleen is present in the background. A laparoscopic haemoclip has already been placed across a short gastric vessel, and a second clip is being placed before dividing the vessel.

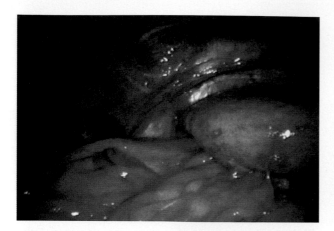

Plate 31.5 Laparoscopic view of the spleen at the commencement of laparoscopic splenectomy. The patient is positioned laterally to enable the stomach, liver, bowel and omentum to fall away from the spleen, faciliatating the surgical approach.

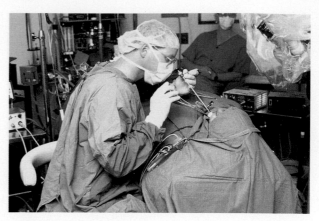

Plate 31.6 Otorhinolaryngologist performing functional endoscopic sinus surgery.

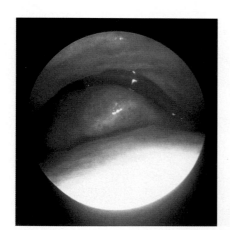

Plate 31.7 Endoscopic view of middle turbinate.

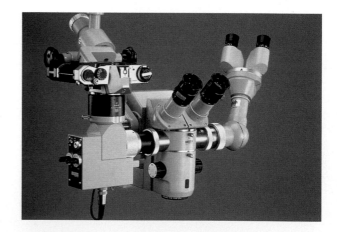

Plate 35.4.1 Operating microscope fitted with a beam-splitter that permits attchment of a 35-mm camera and a co-observation tube.

Continuing education

Jenepher Ann Martin

I am master of my fate, I am captain of my soul.
W. E. Henley

Introduction

There is now world-wide recognition that all medical graduates will need to participate in a programme of continuing education to keep up with changing medical knowledge. Public concern about the ongoing competence of medical practitioners has led to Government interest in re-certification processes. The current trend is to formalize this process. Many medical accrediting and licensing bodies now require practitioners to submit documentation of ongoing educational activities. In some cases re-certification or continued accreditation to practice is dependent on the accrual of educational points over a set period of time. This approach may lead to a narrow view of continuing medical education (CME), such that the objective becomes the achievement of maximum points rather than true educational value. The real value of CME is realized when a broad view is taken and specialist trainees are equipped with the skills to pursue meaningful lifelong learning.

WHAT IS CONTINUING EDUCATION?

Medical education must be considered as a continuum. In surgery, this continuum encompasses medical school, internship, basic training, advanced training and consultant surgical practice. The needs of surgical trainees should be relatively easy to identify and fulfil. However, the individual educational needs of practising surgeons are varied, and trainees must develop the skills to undertake effective CME after Fellowship.

The maintenance of knowledge and skills is a professional responsibility. Every surgeon needs to learn new information as it becomes relevant, discard obsolete practices and evaluate the ever expanding literature. At one end of the spectrum of CME are compulsory, structured programmes or interventions which are implemented across a particular specialist or interest group. The effectiveness of this type of formal CME programme or intervention, targeted as it is at large groups of specialists without regard for educational need, is doubtful. Targeted interventions where individual practitioners have not been made aware of their own deficiencies have not been shown to result in long-term practice behaviour change or changed patient outcomes. At the other end of the CME spectrum are the informal 'keeping up to date' activities in which most medical practitioners engage as a matter of course. This *ad-hoc* educational activity has the disadvantage of not being specifically designed to meet individual needs. Activities may be undertaken simply out of interest or to fulfil requirements for re-certification, rather than to address a specific learning need.

The 1997 Royal Australasian College of Surgeons (RACS) re-certification manual states that the goal of the re-certification programme is to enable 'Fellows to demonstrate that they are engaged in a range of activities which assist them to improve their knowledge and skills and so provide their patients with quality health care'. The three arms of the programme are continuing education, audit and credentialled practices at an approved hospital. CME is defined as 'educational activities... which serve to increase, maintain and develop the knowledge, skills and attitudes needed to provide safe, effective surgical care'. Four categories of CME activity are required for each re-certification period. These are hospital and committee meetings, scientific meetings, self-education activities and other activities. Of the total required number of hours, 47% is accounted for by the first two categories. Although the activities included in each of the four categories are very varied, and the manual states that Fellows may choose activities to suit their own needs, it would be easy to fulfil the requirements by undertaking activities not specifically aimed at addressing learning needs. Apart from information obtainable from audit, which may be of limited value if appropriate data are not collected, there is no requirement for Fellows to measure the outcome of their continuing education activities. This fails to close the educational loop of identification of a learning need, learning activity, and assessment and reappraisal of needs, leading to a new learning programme (Figure 24.1.1).

Continuing medical education should involve much more than just 'keeping up to date' (see Appendix A). All Australian surgeons must fulfil the requirements for re-certification of their respective Colleges, but a comprehensive CME programme will encompass an individualized, needs-based and continuous learning experience. This will result in the maintenance and development of existing knowledge and skills, as well as the acquisition of new skills.

A much broader but highly structured model for continuing education in surgery would involve each individual identifying his or her own learning needs, identifying methods to address these, and determining learning outcome by assessment. This model is elaborated below with strategies to achieve an effective individual CME programme for each trainee and surgeon (see Appendix B).

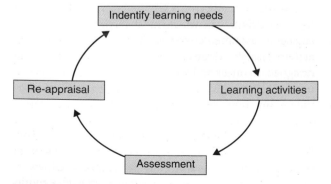

Figure 24.1.1 The educational loop. A programme which conforms to this will ensure maximum effect of continuing education.

EFFECTIVE CONTINUING EDUCATION

The principles of adult learning theory should guide the development of continuing education programmes. A deficiency of many medical school curricula in the past has been the emphasis on passive learning, which has resulted in many medical graduates having poorly developed active learning skills. Newer curricula are designed to foster active learning so that graduates have the skills to undertake effective CME. Adults learn most effectively when they are given responsibility for their own learning. Learning then becomes student centred and active, in contradistinction to being teacher centred and passive. Adult learners need to be involved in planning their learning, to be able to identify the relevance of learning to their current or future activities, and to have well-developed information-seeking skills and early opportunities to apply new knowledge and skills in practice. If these conditions are met, effective self-directed learning should occur. Trainees embarking on a career in surgery will require these active learning skills to allow them to become independent learners.

To be effective, CME must be relevant and the learner must be motivated. If individual learning needs are identified and addressed, the educational programme becomes relevant to the learner. New knowledge can be applied immediately to the current working situation, providing a powerful motivation to succeed. The final requirement for effective CME is feedback. Some measure of success in achieving the learning goals must be provided. This may range from a formal test or examination to audit and review of changed practice.

SKILLS FOR CONTINUING EDUCATION

Effective CME requires specific skills, and all surgical trainees should acquire these prior to completing Fellowship training. The immediate goals during basic and advanced training are the acquisition of the knowledge and skills and development of the professional attitudes needed to pass the required assessments. The adult learning skills essential for effective CME can be developed in the context of basic and advanced surgical training. These skills are the self-directed learning skills of identification of learning needs, accessing and appraising information, familiarity with various learning methods and assessment of progress.

Identification of learning needs/objectives

Surgical trainees may perceive their learning objectives to be clearly articulated by the syllabuses of basic and advanced training. At the post-Fellowship stage, however, specific individual objectives need to be developed.

Learning objectives should be fairly detailed statements of what is to be achieved as a result of the learning exercise, and they must be achievable in the allocated time. There is no point in setting impossible tasks. Techniques that are useful for developing both long- and short-term learning goals are career planning, critical incident analysis and audit.

Career planning Most surgeons will have some longer-term career aspirations in terms of a special interest or type of practice by the time they complete the Fellowship. A 12-month, 2-year and 5-year career development pathway can then be developed, outlining goals to be achieved along the way. This should be reviewed each year and some flexibility maintained, particularly if interests and opportunities change. The assistance of a long-term mentor in developing a career pathway may be invaluable. The specific goals of the current 12-month career plan can then be used to develop learning objectives for the short term. The 2- or 5-year goals may indicate the need for some long-term educational strategy, such as undertaking a period of research or a higher degree.

Critical incidents/reflection Critical incident analysis has been used in business to improve practice, and is now being introduced into the health system at an organizational level. A critical incident is an omission or poor practice which results in a less than ideal outcome. In surgical practice an omission which led to significant morbidity or to mortality would be a critical incident. Analysis of poor outcomes to identify omissions or poor practice can indicate learning needs. At a personal level, critical incident identification will depend on a reflective approach to practice. Poor outcomes can be easily noted on cards or in a diary and the management of the case then reviewed. This may be done with all involved or at a unit level, but it can also be conducted alone or with a mentor colleague. This case-management review is a constructive exercise for identifying errors or omissions that can be remedied for future practice. It is not an exercise in apportioning blame. The learning needs identified in this way can then form the basis of a planned educational programme.

Audit The process of audit is a requirement of re-certification by the RACS, and is central to surgical quality assurance. Audit is also a powerful way of identifying group and individual educational needs. Audit commonly takes the form of a unit- or specialty group-based review of practice incorporating outcomes analysis. The outcomes assessed in the audit need to be reviewed by peers and compared with standards for the particular procedure or area of practice under audit. The results of the audit can then inform individual or group practice. If audit reveals deficiencies such as unacceptably high mortality or complication rates, then clearly practice must change. This may translate into the need for a group or individual educational programme.

A personal audit may take the form of a total practice audit or a selected audit for a particular procedure. Individual outcomes are compared with local and/or international standards and discussed with peers in a non-threatening environment. Higher than expected rates of poor outcome may indicate a need for personal practice change and education. However, when small numbers of cases are reviewed, the results may be unduly influenced by very small numbers of adverse outcomes, and this needs to be taken into consideration.

Accurate data collection is essential for meaningful audit. Information should be easily retrievable and stored in a database that enables multiple outcomes to be analysed. Computer-based systems are ideal. Personal logbook statistics are the responsibility of every surgeon, the minimum requirement of the logbook being to allow retrieval of detailed information from larger databases.

Information access and appraisal

All trainees should become familiar with a number of learning resources that are easily accessible. The most efficient use of these will depend on the development of clear learning objectives. Learning resources commonly used include textbooks, journals, information databases and expert colleagues, and each has advantages and drawbacks. Surgeons must cultivate efficient information-search strategies using diverse sources. Critical appraisal of information is essential, with the aim of achieving evidence-based practice.

Learning methods

Targeted reading This is probably the most familiar and widely used method for surgeons and trainees. The goal of targeted reading is to address a specifically defined knowledge deficit. The scope of reading will be determined by the deficit, but very large tasks should be broken down into smaller components. An efficient targeted reading strategy will access up-to-date, accurate, relevant and balanced information. The information-search strategy must have defined boundaries in order to limit the information accessed, and the temptation to access great detail outside the specified area of learning must be avoided. Targeted reading is best achieved using a work-to-task strategy. The reading for one topic is completed before commencing the next one, and all readings for the topic should be identified at the beginning, thus clearly defining the task. Large reading loads should be broken down into manageable segments, and time allocated to the latter. A written commentary in the form of an annotated bibliography will reinforce learning, particularly in large reading programmes.

Task-based learning The service commitments of most trainees and the practice commitments of surgeons make the allocation of time for study a challenge. Task-based learning (TBL), in which tasks encountered in practice form the focus for learning, can overcome this. TBL is an effective method of learning with a sound educational basis, and it constitutes efficient on-the-job learning and is relevant. TBL does not simply involve mastering the task, but is a much more in-depth approach to learning. Principles and concepts underlying the task are learned, as well as skills that can then be transferred to other tasks. For example, a trainee learning an inguinal hernia operation would take the opportunity to study hernia in depth. Themes to be covered might include clinical skills, anatomy, normal structure/function, pathophysiology, etc.

It is easier to develop TBL for surgical trainees than for practising surgeons. Most rotations have tasks that are commonly encountered, and around which themes of learning can be developed. A training guide could be provided with suggested resources. Practising surgeons may find TBL useful when learning new procedures, developing a new area of interest or resuming practice after a break.

Courses Many courses are available to surgeons who wish to learn new skills. Courses have the advantage of providing access to experts, potential 'hands-on' experience and the opportunity to practise new skills in a non-threatening and safe environment (see Appendix C). Attendance at a course should be planned to fulfil a current learning need. Information should first be sought from course organizers about the objectives of the course, methods of instruction, the instructors and the materials provided. Maximum benefit will be obtained if new knowledge and skills can be applied in practice soon after the course.

Learning contracts Contract learning is increasingly being used in postgraduate settings, and has been introduced to postgraduate medical education in the UK. A learning contract is an explicit statement of the knowledge and skills to be learned, the time-frame for learning, the resources to be used, the evidence to be produced that learning has occurred, and the assessment of this evidence. The negotiation of the contract depends on a trusting trainee/supervisor-mentor relationship. The role of the supervisor is to provide guidance and to facilitate learning. The responsibility for the learning contract is shared by both the learner and the supervisor. The supervisor's responsibilities are to provide assistance and guidance in identifying learning objectives and a realistic time-frame, to indicate likely resources, to assess the outcomes of learning and to provide feedback. The learner's responsibilities are to identify relevant learning objectives and a realistic time-

frame, to access the necessary resources, to provide evidence that learning has occurred, and to use feedback to guide further learning.

Formative assessment during the course of the contract is essential, and can result in a renegotiation of the contract. Despite this flexibility, which is one of the advantages of contract learning, some summative assessment should occur to ensure that specified end-points and standards are achieved.

Assessment

Assessment must be incorporated into any learning programme, and it can take many forms, ranging from self-assessment to formal examinations.

Self-assessment Self-assessment is not easy for medical practitioners. Multiple studies have documented major discrepancies between medical students' and doctors' self-assessment ratings and ratings by others. A number of strategies may be useful to increase the accuracy of trainees' and surgeons' self-assessment, including personal audit, reflection, critical incident analysis and learning diaries.

Mentor/supervisor assessment Surgical trainees are formally assessed every 6 months by their immediate supervisor(s). The performance feedback received from this assessment may not be particularly useful educationally. Practising surgeons have even less opportunity for performance feedback.

The only way in which a trainee or surgeon can know whether or not he or she has achieved specific learning objectives is by seeking feedback on performance. Medical practitioners are not very good at seeking feedback or performance appraisal, nor are they good at delivering it. Good feedback is honest, constructive and non-threatening. Discussion is very specific, emphasizing positive features and outlining strategies to overcome deficiencies. It is essential that feedback is timely, with an opportunity for remediation or improvement in performance if necessary. There is no point in delivering or receiving feedback at the end of a rotation.

When seeking feedback it is essential that the learner specifies a detailed analysis of his or her performance, including strengths and weaknesses. Ideally, a dedicated meeting is arranged. The person giving feedback must have appropriate knowledge of the student's performance. If the student has discussed specific learning objectives with the supervisor prior to the meeting (as in a learning contract), this can form the starting point for discussion. Alternatively, the in-training evaluation form can be used as the framework for discussion.

Good feedback closes the educational loop. Students can assess their achievements and use information obtained from feedback to set new learning objectives.

External assessment Formal testing of knowledge and skills can be undertaken in the CME setting. Often this is in the context of a course such as Early Management of Severe Trauma (Advanced Trauma Life Support), but self-administered examinations are another option. Maximum benefit will only be obtained if an opportunity for question-and-answer review exists (see Appendices D and E).

DESIGNING AN INDIVIDUAL EDUCATION PROGRAMME

Given that relevant information is learned best, it is imperative that surgical trainees take advantage of their current work situation when designing a learning programme. By following the steps shown in Box 24.1.1, a 3- or 6-month programme can be developed. It is important not to be over-ambitious. Achievable goals are best!

The education of a surgeon does not stop with admission to Fellowship or consultant appointment. It is a lifelong process. The continuing education outline described above can be applied by practising surgeons who identify a learning need. Examples include learning a new procedure, developing a special interest, undertaking research or a sabbatical, and returning to practice after a significant break.

BOX 24.1.1 STEPS TO AN EFFECTIVE INDIVIDUAL CONTINUING EDUCATION PROGRAMME

Indentify learning objectives/needs
  Career planning
  Critical incident analysis
  Reflection
  Audit
  Performance appraisal/feedback

Determine suitable learning methods
  Targeted reading
  Courses
  Task-based learning
  Contract learning

Access information
  Textbooks
  Journals
  Databases
  Expert colleagues

Access learning
  Self-assessment activity
  Performance appraisal/feedback
  Formal tests

Surgical trainees who develop the skills outlined above and actively plan their educational programme will develop learning habits that serve them for the whole of their career.

FURTHER READING

Grant J, Stanton F. 1998: *The effectiveness of continuing professional development*. London: Joint Centre for Education in Medicine.

Harden RM, Laidlaw JM, Ker JS, Mitchell HE. 1996: *Task-based learning: an educational strategy for undergraduate, postgraduate and continuing medical education*. AMEE Education Guide Number 7. Dundee: Association for Medical Education of Europe.

Knowles M. 1986: *Using learning contracts*. San Francisco, CA: Jossey-Bass.

Knowles M. 1990: *The adult learner. A neglected species*, 4th edn. Houston, TX: Gulf Publishing Company.

Royal Australasian College of Surgeons. 1997: *Continuing medical education and recertification program information manual and diary*. Melbourne: Capitol Press.

Sackett D, Richardson W, Rosenberg W, Haynes R. 1996: *Evidence-based medicine. How to practice and teach evidence-based medicine*. Edinburgh: Churchill Livingstone.

APPENDIX A

In the UK the surgical Royal Colleges expect their consultant Fellows to attend at least 50 h of recognized CME each year. For the Royal College of Surgeons of England this should include 25 h of internal CME (at one's place of work) and 25 h of external CME. Internal CME can include postgraduate meetings, journal clubs, audit meetings and personal reading time. External CME includes attending meetings, conferences or courses that have been approved for the purpose by the College, or visits to other centres to learn new techniques. At the end of each year, consultant Fellows must send a record of their CME activity for the year to the College. The CME tutor at the College maintains these records, and writes back to inform any individual who has not attended an adequate amount of recognized CME activities during the year. At present in the UK, as in Australia, there is no system for measuring the educational outcome of surgeons' CME. The introduction of clinical governance in the UK (defined as a framework to enable continual improvement in the quality of health care, and involving personal responsibility for managers as well as clinicians to ensure delivery of quality health care) may provide a stimulus to develop the necessary educational audit tools to determine the relative value of differing types of CME activity.

APPENDIX B

Continuing education should address the broader professional developmental needs of the surgeon, as well as those required to develop clinical skills and knowledge. These broader needs might, for example, include teaching skills or management training. Continuing professional development in such areas can benefit both the surgeon and the employing authority by preparing surgeons adequately to take on educational or service management roles. This can enable surgeons who wish to change the focus of their work at different stages of their careers. For example, an older surgeon might wish to reduce his or her emergency on-call commitment, but instead take on a greater role in managing service development.

Continuing professional development, encompassing CME, is a joint responsibility of surgeons and their employers. Patients and the public have a right to know whether specialists are properly trained and accredited. It is a prime responsibility of any profession to ensure self-regulation to satisfactory standards of practice.

APPENDIX C

Distance learning courses, such as the STEP course of the Royal College of Surgeons of England, can be valuable training aids. In continuing education there are also examples of interactive distance learning, such as that offered by the Royal College of Pathologists (in which histopathologists are sent multiple-choice tests to complete, and then receive confidential feedback on their marks).

APPENDIX D

The reflective practitioner may see areas for improvement in quality. However, peer review with colleagues, not necessarily working in the same institution, may provide a better objective view of the quality of performance. Peer group discussion, as well as formal comparative audits such as that offered by the Royal College of Surgeons of England, can be valuable. Another educational support system which works for many surgeons is that of mentorship, where a less experienced surgeon seeks advice on either clinical matters or personal professional developmental plans from a more experienced colleague.

APPENDIX E

In some other specialities, such as general medical practice in the UK, doctors have found it valuable to keep a personal portfolio of their CME activity and to use this to plan their future CME, either by personal reflection or jointly with a colleague using a 'buddy' system.

Outcome measurement

Mark Emberton

Introduction

The aims of this chapter are as follows:

1. to discuss what is meant by operative success;

2. to recognize that operating on someone can result in a wide range of outcomes or end results;

3. to recognize that different types of surgical outcomes are important to different parties;

4. to highlight the problems associated with using outcome alone as an index of quality;

5. to explore the relationships between measures relating to structure, process and outcome;

6. to introduce the idea of patient-defined outcomes such as health-related quality of life.

Patient:	*I'm still not sure about this operation which you're all telling me I need. Will you clarify a few things for me?*
Surgeon:	I'll try.
Patient:	*What kind of complications should I expect?*
Surgeon:	About 8 in 10 patients don't have any complications.
Patient:	*What are the chances that I'll get back to living the kind of life I was used to a year ago?*
Surgeon:	Well that's a little more difficult, and depends very much on what you were doing a year ago.
Patient:	*Will the 'op' affect my sex life in any way?*
Surgeon:	It might, but this hasn't been studied particularly well.
Patient:	*How will I feel in myself afterwards?*
Surgeon:	You might feel a little weak and perhaps a little tired for about a month.
Patient:	*Is there any risk of incontinence?*
Surgeon:	No, I'm not aware of anybody reporting

this as a problem – but I'll tell you what I'll look it up.

Patient:	*When will I be able to get back to earning a living?*
Surgeon:	Most patients can get back to work after about 2 months, but people vary quite a lot.
Patient:	*Oh, one last thing – will it make me live longer?*

These are not unreasonable questions. They address potential consequences or outcomes that might result from an impending operation, and they include a variety of end-points (economic, sexual, survival, risk and in addition general well-being).

Some of the questions could be answered quite well, while others could not. Most readers will accept, perhaps with a slight shudder of guilt, that we often do not have the necessary answers to these very real questions, and at times we gloss over them or (if we are totally honest) manage to fabricate our responses (admittedly with the very best of intentions). Such a position is becoming increasingly untenable as we enter the new millennium. Surgeons, like all professionals, have to respond to the changes in society that have characterized much of the second half of this century. Developments such as consumerism, patient sovereignty, informed consent, the trend away from the implicit and towards the explicit, the increase in accountability, the erosion of professional opinion (beliefs) by demonstrable achievement (evidence-based medicine) could be listed endlessly.

As if this were not enough, the nature of most of the surgery that we undertake has been slowly changing. At the beginning of this century a patient usually chose to have an operation because not having it meant that he was almost certain to die. Today most of the operations that we perform do not aim to make patients live longer. Instead, they have as their principal aim an improvement in the quality of the patient's remaining life. Hip replacement reduces pain and improves mobility and productivity (however we choose to define it). Cataract surgery improves visual acuity and takes an individual from dependence to independence. Coronary artery revascularization can get rid of debilitating angina and improve exercise tolerance. Prostatectomy improves urinary symptoms and results in better sleep, less reliance on public toilets and fewer laundry bills. To this undeniable and highly valued 'up-side' to effective operations that are appropriately administered there is an inevitable 'down-side'. Hip prostheses can fail, heart surgery is associated with small risk of dying, and prostatectomy affects men's fertility and sexual function.

Measuring these outcomes or the end results of operations is becoming an increasingly important part of evaluating the surgery that we undertake. Patients increasingly choose to play an active part in the decision of whether or not to have an operation. Their ability to make this decision depends on having an accurate estimate of the outcome of the surgical intervention (both good and bad) they are contemplating. Like most things in medicine, there is nothing new about all of this. Healers during the Hippocratic period would accept a cure as having occurred when the four bodily humours were restored to a harmonious balance. Symptoms (an individual's idiosyncratic response to humoral disruption) were regarded as markers of this imbalance. When the symptoms got better the healer assumed that humoral harmony had been restored.

The case-books of John Hunter FRS (often described as the father of modern surgery) illustrate how keen he was to measure and record the outcome of his operations. The outcome of two cases of lithotomy performed in the 1720s were recorded as follows. The outcome of the first case pleased him: '10th (postoperative day) better, and continued so till he went out'. The result of the second case was not so good: 'She went to the country and stayed 2 months; I then saw her at the hospital: she was better, but on walking, the water dropped from her'.

Although these descriptions do enable the observer, a few centuries later, to classify the outcome as either good or poor, with time more objectivity was sought. By the middle of this century this was achieved by using tests or physiological measurements to define the outcome of interventions. This 'objectivity' was made possible by exploiting the burgeoning technology that was becoming increasingly available. A reduction in forced expiratory volume (FEV_1) was preferred to a patient's report of dyspnoea. Tinsley Harrison's critique of this 'modern' medical practice in 1944 gives us some idea how much physicians relied on technology. He describes a typical consultation as follows:

'a five-minute history, followed by a five-day barrage of tests in the hope that the diagnostic rabbit may suddenly emerge from the laboratory hat'.

However, since then we have all become increasingly sceptical about relying on technology alone. Resolution of a lesion seen on X-ray does not always mean that a patient is cured. Left ventricular ejection fraction does not always correspond to a person's exercise tolerance. Urinary flow rates and urodynamics correlate poorly with urinary symptoms. These last few observations have all been made fairly recently, and they result from health professionals taking another look at patients' own descriptions of the course of their disease. Some have called this the 'outcomes movement'.

THE MODERN OUTCOMES MOVEMENT

The modern outcomes movement has been described as the third revolution in medical care this century. Relman has argued that it arose because the first two revolutions failed. The 'era of expansion' and burgeoning cost of medicine in the USA came under close scrutiny when analysts began to realize that there was little evidence to demonstrate the benefit of a service to the community that was costing 11% of the gross national product by the early 1980s. The 'era of expansion' was followed by the 'era of cost containment'. It was not long before it was realized that cost control alone would not provide the answers to either escalating health care costs on the one hand, or issues of effectiveness and appropriateness on the other. Expensive technologies were being commissioned and implemented with little in the way of prior assessment.

The debate was not a new one. It was started by a surgeon from Boston, Ernest A. Codman, in a now often quoted lecture to The Philadelphia County Medical Society just before the First World War:

'We must formulate some method of hospital report showing as nearly as possible what are the results of treatment obtained at different institutions. This report must be made out and published by each hospital in a uniform manner, so that comparison will be possible. With such a report as a starting point, those interested can begin to ask questions as to management and efficiency. In a similar way, all the important by-products depend in the end on demonstration that the patient can be helped.'

At the time, Codman was ridiculed for trying to bring industrial standards of quality control into medicine. Now he is regarded as a visionary by those who acknowledge the problems described above.

The US Health Care Financing Administration (HCFA), probably unaware of Codman's writing, and not knowing how to proceed, organized a conference. Representatives from government, private insurers, major corporations, community agencies and the medical profession were invited to address the escalating problem of health-care financing. In his report of the conference, Relman was surprised that a consensus was possible between these traditionally disparate groups. It was founded on two broad areas – first, that more knowledge was needed about the performance differences between practitioners and between institutions, and, secondly, that more knowledge was needed about the relative safety, effectiveness and costs of physicians' actions. The policy statements that resulted from the meeting were summarized in an important editorial by Ellwood, which recommended a process of 'outcomes management' which linked medical management decisions to systematic information about outcomes. In choosing the title for this editorial, 'A technology of patient experience', the author alluded to an increasingly strongly held belief that patients' views would have to play an increasingly important role.

In his editorial, Ellwood referred to the work of Jack Wennberg. For years, Wennberg had tried to explain why rates of operation varied by factors of five- to eight-fold between institutions, and why these differences persisted despite controlling for different levels of provision and case mix. He showed that the greatest variations were in areas where there was considerable professional uncertainty about when to intervene. Hysterectomy, coronary artery bypass grafting and prostatectomy were classic examples. With such wide variation in professional opinion (opinions that were usually very strongly held), would it ever be possible to identify a correct or appropriate rate of operation? One way around this problem would be to share this uncertainty with patients who were being considered for an operation, and to allow them to make the final decision. Given the professional uncertainty, a patient's

preference for treatment could reasonably be given greater weighting than the preference of the physician. Work on men undergoing prostatectomy has shown that patients are well placed to make these choices. If patients' views are considered to be useful in helping to decide whether or not to undergo a certain treatment, it would also seem reasonable to solicit their views on the outcome of that procedure. The patients' own views of the outcome of the procedure could then be viewed as a measure of its success.

Although the renewed interest in measuring outcome was initiated in the USA, it was soon embraced by opinion leaders in Europe and elsewhere. Most of them agreed that biomedical researchers had to broaden their definition of medical and surgical outcome. One important review on the management of sub-fertility acknowledged that the most obvious outcome might not be the most important one. They concluded their report:

'The management of infertility should be evaluated according to the degree to which it has been successful in reducing stress, distress or social handicap [and not just] ... on reproductive outcomes.'

Effective Health Care Bulletin, University of York, 1992

In this example the researchers thought that psychological/sociological factors were the pertinent endpoints to measure, e.g. 'perceived health status' rather than conception rates or maternity rates. This preoccupation with measuring the impact of our interventions on a person's general well-being has led to something akin to an industry whose aims are to create valid, reliable and responsive instruments that can measure the effects of interventions on individuals. These instruments seek to measure and record changes in people's health status by using symptom scores and health-related quality of life measures which are either designed specifically for one disease process or operation (disease specific), or for any of them (generic).

A description of these measures is beyond the scope of this article, but the reader is referred to the recommended Further Reading at the end of the chapter. It is truly amazing how quickly such measures have become incorporated into mainstream surgical thinking. In the late 1980s, surgeons who were interested in issues of quality of life were difficult to find. Today, at the very end of the century, try submitting a research protocol comparing two treatment strategies without including some measure of the effect of those treatments on the patients' quality of life, and you will almost certainly be asked to revise it.

INPUTS VS. OUTPUTS: STRUCTURE, PROCESS AND OUTCOME (BOX 24.2.1)

Most of us would agree that the only true measure of whether a treatment has worked is an assessment of the effect of that treatment on an individual or a population. Do we then have to record the outcome of all our operations all of the time? Do we have to ask every single patient about the immediate results of their surgery and its impact on their lives? After all, these things are difficult to measure and would require a battery of questionnaires if we were to do the job properly. Could there be any easier way of predicting the outcome of our interventions?

Like most developments in medicine, a period of reappraisal follows the introduction of novel ideas. The precise role of outcome in assessing or auditing the quality of medical care has yet to be defined. It has been argued that it may be more feasible and equally valid to focus attention on other variables which are more easily measured. Could attention to structural components (characteristics of physicians and hospitals, e.g. specialists/non-specialists, teaching/non-teaching) help to predict outcomes and obviate the need to measure them? Might attention to data about process – components of the encounter between a heath-care professional and the patient (e.g. tests ordered, operation performed, details of post-operative care) – help to predict outcome? These questions need to be addressed because outcome measures have inherent weaknesses that are being increasingly recognized.

PROBLEMS WITH MEASURING OUTCOME (BOX 24.2.2)

The first and probably most important problem is that of attribution. Is the outcome being measured a specific consequence of the type of operation performed and the skill with which it was undertaken? Clearly this is not so. Many factors other than these might affect a patient's outcome. To make the situation even more complicated, the more general the outcome (i.e. the more divorced it is from the disease process), the more difficult it will be to attribute any effect. For example, consider a patient who had a mixed outcome following a total hip replacement. Her hip pain might be better but her mobility was not as good as it should be for someone of her age. Closer questioning revealed that her mobility was now not limited by any restriction in hip movement, but by

---

BOX 24.2.1 STRUCTURE, PROCESS AND OUTCOME (these terms have been borrowed from industrial quality-control programmes, and have been applied to health care)

Structure

The idea of structure relates to the framework in which an operation is carried out. Structural components are often determined by resources.

What kind of hospital is it? How is it accredited? What grade is the operating surgeon? What type of training is given to the surgeons, nurses and technicians?

Process

Process refers to patterns of practice that can be modified within one institution (the implication being that structural elements are less amenable to change).

What are the criteria for operating? What type of information is given to patients? How is the waiting-list managed? What type of hernia repair is performed? How are antibiotics used? What types of anaesthetics are administered?

Outcome

The term outcome refers to the demonstrable consequences of an operation.

Usually these are seen or defined from the physician's perspective, e.g. radiological union or non-union of a fracture, blood loss, biochemical remission (PSA) following radical prostatectomy.

Outcomes of direct consequence to patients are considered to be increasingly important. Randomized studies are usually powered to a primary end-point that is of direct consequence to patients. This might be symptom reduction, improvement of quality of life, or survival.

Some outcomes can be of importance to society as a whole, or to those who pay for health care. Economic outcomes such as cost-effectiveness, cost-benefit and cost-utility are of consequence to society but not directly to individuals. The outcome of mass screening programmes is often seen from this perspective.

BOX 24.2.2 PROBLEMS ENCOUNTERED WHEN USING OUTCOME ALONE

1. Attributing an outcome to a specific action is difficult
2. Case mix is always a problem
3. Statistics are difficult to apply to rare outcomes
4. Outcomes tell us how well something works, not why it works
5. Measuring outcome at different times will give different results
6. Details of structure and process impact directly on patients

her shortness of breath on exertion. This was subsequently improved by attention to her diuretic medication. The lack of mobility was not due to poor surgery, but to other pre-existing factors.

The above example also serves to illustrate the second problem, which concerns case mix. No matter how good the diagnostic facilities, surgical expertise and post-operative care, the most important predictors of surgical outcome are not under the direct control of the surgeon. Patient factors such as age, social class, fitness and disease severity are much more powerful determinants of outcome than whether, for example, a cholecystectomy is performed using a laparoscope instead of a mini-incision.

Third, some outcomes are so rare that they provide little power for statistical analysis. Death within 30 days after prostatectomy is a rare event (0.5–1.2%), and this makes comparison – even within series of moderate size – somewhat difficult. With such a low incidence, four-, five- or sixfold differences between providers may just be due to chance alone, unless vast numbers of patient episodes are compared.

Fourth, outcomes as a single measure are limited in the extent to which they can inform clinical decisions – analysis of outcomes tells us how well it worked, not why it worked. For instance, suppose surgeon A has a postoperative wound infection rate three times that of his colleague, surgeon B. This difference was found following a prospective audit on a large number of patients, and was therefore considered to be a real difference. Somehow the local newspaper got hold of this information and ran a story about differences in surgical competence – much to the astonishment of the hospital Chief Executive. The newspaper editor was quite happy to report the difference and allude to a scandal. The Chief Executive, on the other hand, wanted to find out why there was a difference. Both surgeons' practices required close scrutiny (something close to detective work) in order to try to explain the difference. Was surgeon B omitting to do things he should have been doing based on traditional standards of evidence? After all, had not all surgeons recently agreed on a set of guidelines to which they were all committed? Perhaps there was poor attention to asepsis, or perhaps surgeon B was not using antibiotic prophylaxis appropriately. This did not prove to be the case.

On close examination, surgeon B's technique and adherence to the previously agreed guidelines were found to be beyond question. However, the Chief Executive's investigations did reveal other differences between the two surgeons. Surgeon B was operating on a greater proportion of emergencies and contaminated cases than his colleague, surgeon A. Perhaps there was indeed an explanation for the difference in infection rates. Surgeon A's much lower infection rate may be entirely appropriate, given the lower comorbidity and disease severity of her patients. Indeed, once these case-mix factors were controlled for, the differences magically disappeared.

Fifth, it is sometimes difficult to agree when an outcome should be measured. The interval between an intervention and the time when the effect of that intervention is measured appears to be important. In one study looking at total hip replacement, it was found that the longer the interval, the greater the perceived gain reported by patients. Just when outcome should be measured after an operation is clearly important. For instance, should mortality figures be obtained prior to discharge, at 30 days, at 90 days, or by actuarial means?

Sixth, the details of structure and process of health care matter a great deal to patients. In other words, patients like to know, at the time of service delivery, that services are being delivered in a way that maximizes their chances of an ultimately favourable outcome. The environment in which they are treated and the way in which they are treated (the delivery of care) are usually rated by patients as being most important. These issues are also significant to parties interested in monitoring or auditing the quality of medical care. The problem lies in the relationship between structure, process and outcome. Critics of outcome measures believe that most differences in outcome between patients receiving the same treatments are due to factors that are not under the control of the health-care provider. Several factors may confound the association between the exposure of a patient to a health-care institution and the ultimate outcome. These might include hospital admission practices, case-mix differences, patient comorbidity, case severity, and many factors which are either unknown, unmeasurable or missing. For outcomes to be useful, one of their attributes should be that differences in outcome will result if the processes of care (which are under the control of health professionals) are altered. For instance, if a genuine difference in mortality is found between two units, in order to improve the results of the unit with the higher mortality rate it would be necessary to identify what processes (that have been shown to influence mortality in experimental settings) were different.

On the other hand, if we decided not to use outcome as a determinant of the quality of surgical care, then we must be able to demonstrate that differences in the variable that we do choose to measure inevitably lead to differences in outcome. Outcomes are considered important by many because they believe that process data does not necessarily predict desired outcomes. If this is the case, considerable time, effort and money might be spent on ensuring that a particular process is carried out (e.g. heparin DVT prophylaxis) with little certainty that an improvement in health (a reduction in fatal pulmonary embolism) had resulted.

On the other hand, concentrating on the outcomes rather than the processes of care allows effects from process variables that are thought to exist, but are difficult to measure, to be assessed. For example, several processes of care have been shown to be important determinants of myocardial death following coronary artery bypass surgery. However, concentrating on these processes may result in other factors being overlooked (e.g. the surgeon's skill in the operating room – which is notoriously difficult to measure). By concentrating on mortality rates as an outcome measure, and adjusting for factors that are known to influence those rates, unknown factors which influence mortality may be incorporated. By using surgeon-specific adjusted mortality data as an outcome measure, O'Connor and his colleagues managed to reduce mortality rates. The outcome measure was used to stimulate discussion between providers, in the hope that practices conferring decreased mortality rates would be disseminated to other surgeons.

Problems in using mortality as an outcome measure, this time after myocardial infarction, have been highlighted by Mant and Hicks, who reviewed aspects of hospital care (process) that have been shown through meta-analysis or randomized controlled trials to have an impact on survival after myocardial infarction, namely beta-blockade, aspirin administration, thrombolysis, and angiotensin-converting-enzyme inhibitors. They estimated the impact that optimal use of these interventions would have on mortality in a typical district general hospital. Sample size calculations were used to determine how many years of data would be needed to detect significant differences between hospitals. They then compared this with the amount of data that would be needed to detect significant differences if process data were being used. They concluded that process measures (when based on the results of randomized controlled trials) were able to detect relevant differences between hospitals that would not be identified using hospital-specific mortal-

ity, which was thought by the authors to be an insensitive indicator of the quality of care. Such an approach is only useful when there is good evidence that a discrete process of medical *care* leads to better outcomes. A typical example is thrombolytic therapy after myocardial infarction in patients for whom this treatment is not contraindicated.

SUMMARY

Measuring and recording the outcome of surgical care, whether it is of direct or indirect consequence to the patient, is still the only way to be certain that a patient has benefited from surgery. However, a large number of outcomes might be considered important following any particular procedure. Outcomes can often be difficult to measure. Moreover, they may not always be sensitive indicators of the quality of care, and if real differences are detected between providers, it is usually difficult to know why these differences have occurred. There is still much work to be done before outcomes can be used as a routine index of the quality of surgical care.

FURTHER READING

Bowling A. 1991: *Measuring health: a review of quality of life measurement scales.* Milton Keynes: Open University Press.

Bowling A. 1995: *Measuring disease: a review of disease-specific quality of life measurement scales.* Buckingham: Open University Press.

Delamothe A (ed.). 1994: *Outcomes into clinical practice.* London: BMJ Publishing Group.

Chapter 24.3

Audit

Jean Simpson

Introduction

Clinical audit is defined as 'the systematic, critical analysis of the quality of medical care, including the procedures used for diagnosis and treatment, the use of resources, and the resulting outcome and quality of life for the patient'. It is a clinically led initiative with the primary objectives of improving:

- quality of care for patients;
- outcomes of care for patients;
- professional development and education for clinicians.

In the UK, medical audit was introduced into the NHS as part of the reforms proposed in the Government's White Paper, *Working for Patients*, which took effect from 1991. Audit for nurses and professions allied to medicine (PAMs) developed separately, but now most audit is clinical audit based on an assessment of care given by the whole multiprofessional health-care team.

Further developmental goals for audit were identified in 1996, and the important role of clinical audit in improving the clinical effectiveness of services was stressed. Audit should aim for the following objectives:

- a clear patient focus;
- greater multiprofessional working;
- patient care managed across primary, secondary and continuing care;
- closer links with education;
- better integration of effectiveness information.

The new White Paper issued at the end of 1997, *The New NHS; Modern, Dependable*, identifies a central role for clinical audit as part of the quality improvement processes that fall within the umbrella of 'clinical governance'. Chief executives and trust boards will be held accountable for the quality of services that they provide, and will be expected to have robust systems for clinical audit, adverse incident reporting, clinical risk management and evidence-based practice.

BACKGROUND

The roots of modern audit lie in the regular morbidity and mortality meetings held in many hospitals in the UK and the USA in the 1950s and 1960s. The value of these meetings as a means of learning was recognized, and they formed the basis of broader audit activities. Following the reorganization of the health service in 1991, every hospital in England was responsible for ensuring the development of medical audit in which all doctors participated. Whereas previously audit was practised predominantly by enthusiasts, the requirement for audit is now written into the job descriptions of all new medical staff. Participation in audit meetings is a mandatory requirement for the educational approval of surgical training posts by the Royal College of Surgeons of England, and consultants recognized as trainers must actively participate. By 1995, a survey by the National Audit Office confirmed that more than 80% of doctors were involved in audit, and that clinical audit was generally accepted as having become embedded in the NHS as part of routine clinical practice. However, the effectiveness of this activity in securing worthwhile and lasting improvements in the quality of care for patients is still very variable.

There have been several studies examining the reasons why audit programmes have been successful in some trusts and not in others. Key factors include close links with other quality activities, a respected audit lead supported by an effective committee, good monitoring and reporting mechanisms, and a high level of audit activity leading to change.

After the NHS reorganization, dedicated funding was available for the first time for audit. This was allocated directly to hospital, community, mental health trusts and primary care groups via regional health authorities. Following the transfer of funding responsibility in 1995, health authorities were required to agree plans for audit addressing local service and clinical priorities with trust managers and audit groups. As part of the audit contract with hospitals, health authorities can request audit of specific clinical areas. These topics are frequently chosen in areas where there is evidence of what good quality care should entail. An effective clinical audit programme can provide the necessary reassurance to patients, clinicians and managers that an agreed quality of service is being given within the available resources.

Many deficiencies revealed by audit relate to the organization of care and, although audit must remain clinically led, greater involvement of managers is vital if it is to achieve the necessary changes in practice. Separate funding for audit has often led to it being viewed as a peripheral activity – solely the province of clinicians, and with few links to the business of the hospital.

CLINICAL EFFECTIVENESS

There is a growing need to base clinical practice on the knowledge obtained from rigorous research into the effectiveness of health-care interventions. Clinically effective interventions maintain and improve health and secure the greatest possible health gain from the available resources. Clinical audit has a crucial role to play in this, namely:

- assessing current practice;
- identifying and bringing about the necessary changes in practice;
- monitoring to check that the expected outcomes have been achieved.

Clinical staff should aim to review care against agreed clinical standards, evidence-based clinical guidelines and systematic reviews of research. Clinicians are increas-

ingly being asked by managers and purchasers to develop evidence-based guidelines for the delivery of care, and to audit care against locally developed or nationally commended guidelines. All hospital libraries should have easy access to information both in printed form (e.g. Effective Health Care bulletins) and in the form of electronic media (e.g. the Cochrane Library) with trained staff to help in its use.

IMPACT OF AUDIT

In the early 1990s, at the start of the formal audit programme, there were many doctors who argued that they already practised audit – that ward rounds, clinical presentations, research and morbidity and mortality meetings fulfilled this function. However, there are differences between all of these and audit. Audit must be seen as a systematic approach to the review of clinical care to highlight opportunities for improvement and to provide a mechanism for bringing about such improvement. As such, it endeavours to get away from the 'single interesting case' and to look for patterns of care which should ideally be evaluated against research-based evidence or accepted best practice. Audit should initiate investigation into those areas of clinical care that are considered to be:

- high risk;
- high cost;
- very common;
- issues of local interest.

The rare and clinically interesting case should be left for the clinical conference.

Some staff still feel that the time spent on audit could be better devoted to other activities, such as treating more patients. Audit was introduced without any prior evaluation, and although there have been several subsequent evaluations, as yet the results have failed to demonstrate clear value for money. Although the overall impact of audit may be difficult to quantify, there have been clear demonstrations of its effect in individual trusts on, for instance, reducing inappropriate test requests, cost-effective use of blood supplies, and lower infection rates. Most would agree that it is beneficial for clinical staff to review practice regularly, either as a professional group or as part of the team, against agreed standards of best practice, and that this can lead to improved standards of care for the patient. Furthermore, clinical audit can improve patient care not only through direct changes in clinical practice, but also through indirect effects such as professional education and team development.

THE IMPLEMENTATION OF CHANGE

If audit is to be effective, it must lead to change. Audit may be viewed as a cycle, the first component of which is the observation of existing practice to establish what is actually happening. Standards of practice are then set to define what ought to happen, and a comparison is made between observed practice and the standard. Finally, change is implemented. Clinical practice is observed again to see whether what has been planned has been achieved. A decision can then be made as to whether practice needs to change further, or whether the standards were unrealistic or unachievable. This process has become known as the 'audit cycle' and the achievement of change as 'closing the audit loop' (Figure 24.3.1).

The implementation of change is the most difficult part of the audit cycle. A systematic review of 160 interventions directed at changing clinical behaviour or health outcomes showed that effects were small to moderate. Effective strategies included outreach visits, opinion leaders, patient-mediated interventions and physician reminders. Variable results were found for audit with feedback. The provision of information on clinical activity, without any evaluation, has been judged to have almost no effect on clinical practice, but it is effective if targeted at clinicians who had agreed to review their practice.

The most commonly used approach to initiate change involves the publication of guidelines. This has been shown both to change practice and to affect outcomes. Guidelines are more likely to be effective if they have local involvement and take into account local circumstances, and if they are supported by active educational interventions and use patient-specific reminders (e.g. in the medical notes or as computer prompts). Guidelines need to be reviewed regularly to establish 'ownership' and to incorporate the latest research findings. National guidelines have been produced, many of them in collaboration with the medical Royal Colleges. These can prove valuable in establishing the main evidence-based principles of care, thereby short-cutting some of the development process while still allowing ownership by integration with local service arrangements.

EDUCATION AND TRAINING

It is now considered vital that doctors in training are taught the basic principles of audit. Equally, conclusions drawn from the audit process should be viewed as an important feeder into education and training. Self-evaluation and peer review (common activities in audit) are important components of postgraduate education. There can be little doubt that the critical review of current practice and comparisons against predefined standards encourage the acquisition and updating of knowledge. The audit process also enables the identification of key features of clinical practice which should help to make teaching more explicit.

Through audit it is possible to identify particular areas where knowledge could be improved or is deficient, suggesting the need for research. It must be remembered that audit itself will not lead to new clinical knowledge. Research aims to identify 'the right thing to do', while audit assesses whether 'the right thing has been done' and whether further improvement is required. In order to realize fully the educational potential of audit, it is essential that the lessons arising from previous audit meetings are reviewed, and the conclusions acted upon.

SUPPORT FOR AUDIT

Audit staff Most hospitals now have an audit officer and/or audit co-ordinator. Audit staff should be able to provide support in helping to plan audit studies, literature searches, retrieval of data from medical notes against clinically determined criteria, and preparation of audit reports.

Audit committees The majority of hospitals have a clinical audit committee that reports to their unit management.

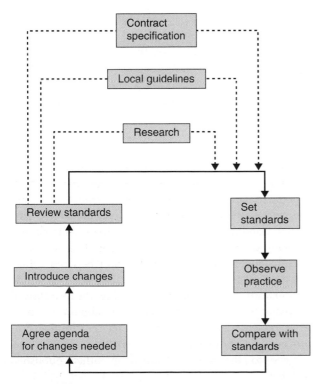

Figure 24.3.1 Clinical audit cycle.

Membership should be multidisciplinary and include directorate managers and audit staff. The chairman needs to be well motivated and prepared to devote time to the task on a regular basis. The committee should co-ordinate and foster clinical audit for everyone involved in patient care, ensure that changes (where indicated by the outcome of audit) are implemented, ensure that all clinical staff are trained in audit, and prepare an annual report and forward programme. Some audit committees have extended their role to integrate audit actively with clinical effectiveness, clinical risk management or complaints monitoring.

National Centre for Clinical Audit (NCCA) This was established in 1995, and absorbed into the National Institute for Clinical Excellence (NICE) in June 1999.

AUDIT TECHNIQUES

Donabedian has identified three main elements in the delivery of health care, namely structure, process and outcome.

Structure This includes the quantity and type of resources available, and is generally easy to measure. It is not a good indicator of the quality of care, but should be taken into account in the assessment of process and outcome.

Process This refers to what is done to the patient. It includes consideration of the way in which an operation was performed, what medications were prescribed, the adequacy of notes, and compliance with consensus policies. There is an underlying assumption that the activities under review have been previously shown to produce an optimal medical outcome. An increasingly important part of this process is to inform patients of probable risks and outcomes, and to involve those who wish it in making treatment choices. The process of care is the area that is most open to change by the clinician.

Outcome This is the result of clinical intervention, and it may represent the success or failure of process. For example, outcome could be measured by studies of surgical fatality rates, the incidence of complications, or patient satisfaction. It can be considered to be the most relevant indicator of patient care, but it is the most difficult to define and quantify. Mortality and length of stay in hospital are very easily measured outcome indicators, but variations in these outcomes are rarely related directly to the quality of the service being delivered. It may be more important to consider whether patients perceive that their problems have been solved and that their quality of life has improved and, where

appropriate, to take into account the duration of their survival.

The following audit techniques are commonly used when reviewing clinical practice.

Basic clinical audit This involves an analysis of throughput, and a broad analysis of case type, complications and morbidity and mortality. This could be undertaken by each clinical firm at regular intervals (e.g. every 3 months). This enables the team to identify any notable deviations from an accepted 'norm' and then to investigate the reasons for such observations.

Incident review This involves the discussion of strategies to be adopted in the context of certain clinical scenarios. An incident may be taken to be anything from a patient suffering from a leaking aortic aneurysm to the use of a department for an investigation (e.g. emergency intravenous urography). It is expected that such discussions will lead to clear policies for future use, and may result in the production of local guidelines.

Clinical record review A member of another firm of the same or similar specialty is invited to review a random selection of case-notes. Where possible, criteria should be established for this review purpose. Clinical record audit has the advantage of simplicity and requires relatively little additional time or other resources. However, there is a potential disadvantage in that discussion might concentrate too much on the quality of record-keeping and not enough on patient care – these two are distinct facets of the clinical process.

Criterion audit This is an approach that can be viewed as a more advanced and structured form of incident audit. A retrospective analysis of clinical records is made and judged against a number of carefully chosen criteria capturing the key elements in management of a particular topic. Ideally, information should be available in the medical record for documentation by an audit assistant. All cases that fail to meet any of the criteria are brought forward for further clinical review. The criteria may relate to administrative elements (e.g. waiting time), investigations ordered, treatments given, outcome, follow-up strategies, etc. Criteria for adequate management of a particular condition can be easily derived from clinical guidelines. Criterion audit is applicable to a variety of circumstances and allows comparison between different hospitals. The criteria can be used for the setting of standards, with targets identifying the proportion of patients in whom the criterion should be met. After review, new targets can be set to stimulate improvement (e.g. to reduce infection rates in colorectal surgery to the levels obtained in other published studies).

Adverse occurrence screening A clinical firm decides on a short-list of events that should be avoided (e.g. wound infections, unplanned readmissions, delay or error in diagnosis). Details of occurrences are recorded, and complex or serious occurrences are reviewed by clinicians. A database is compiled which can then be interrogated to identify trends, perform comparative analyses, etc. Cases can be selected by considering either all admissions or a sample of them. This technique is also valuable in clinical risk management.

Comparative audit In any one hospital the number of departments undertaking similar work is often very small. Even between two firms of general surgeons the case mix may be sufficiently different to make comparisons difficult. Comparative audit implies the collection of data and its comparison across units, health authorities or regions. In 1991, the Royal College of Surgeons set up a comparative audit service in which all surgeons are requested to supply information under a confidential number for comparison with their peers at regular meetings. Data presentation techniques allow information to be widely disseminated and discussed, while maintaining an individual clinician's confidentiality. In Scotland, a computerized audit system, maintained by general surgeons in the Lothian region over 15 years and recording clinical data which is regularly reviewed in a peer-group setting, has provided clear evidence that regional audit can significantly influence and improve surgical practice.

National studies These were first used over a decade ago to address the question of perinatal mortality in obstetric units. The report of the first confidential enquiry into peri-operative deaths (CEPOD) considered the factors involved in the deaths of patients who died within 30 days of surgery in three regional health authorities. This exposed the need for doctors in the training grades to be given adequate support and supervision. It was clear that disaster frequently occurred when surgeons attempted procedures for which they possessed insufficient skill or training. The enquiry has since developed into a national annual review (NCEPOD) to which data is submitted on a voluntary confidential basis by surgeons and anaesthetists. The findings can identify remedial actions and indicate appropriate topics for local audit. Issues of particular concern have been dealt with in separate reports (e.g. *Who Operates When?* – a review of out-of-hours surgery issued in 1997).

Outcome audit Outcome will depend on the whole of the process of health care delivery during a patient's episode in hospital and, as such, is a measure of the spectrum of the skills of the medical and nursing staff, the hospital administration and, indeed, every person or department with whom the patient comes into contact. Information used in audit about patients must protect the confidentiality both of individual patients and of the professionals involved.

CONFIDENTIALITY

With regard to patient confidentiality, it is important that all those involved do not talk about what was discussed in an audit meeting outside that meeting. Unless an explicit and convincing case can be made for inclusion of identifying details of a patient in verbal or written presentations, these should be excluded.

The confidentiality of the professionals involved also requires protection. This is likely to be difficult in some types of audit (e.g. where one consultant reviews the clinical records of another consultant's patient). Nevertheless, this type of audit can be successful, provided that the necessary atmosphere of trust and collaboration is fostered. It is always necessary to obtain permission from all consultants involved before starting an audit exercise.

It is important to consider what should happen if audit reveals problems of deficiencies in a given individual's clinical practice. Such a situation is likely to occur infrequently, if at all, but this makes it all the more important to anticipate such an eventuality and to make explicit provision for it. The Joint Consultants Committee has recommended that clinicians develop a local protocol for action, and in 1996 they identified a suggested course of action.

FURTHER READING

Aitken RJ, Nixon SJ, Ruckley CV. 1997: Lothian surgical audit: a 15-year experience of improvement in surgical practice through regional computerised audit. *Lancet* 350, 800–4.

Campling EA, Devlin HB, Hoile RW, Ingram GS, Lunn JN. 1997: *Who operates when? A report of the national confidential enquiry into perioperative deaths.* London: National Confidential Enquiry into perioperative deaths.

Department of Health. 1996a: *Clinical audit in the NHS.* Leeds: National Health Service Executive.

Department of Health. 1996b: *Clinical guidelines.* Leeds: National Health Service Executive.

Donabedian A. 1966: Evaluating the quality of medical care. *Millbank Memorial Federation of Quality* **3**, 166–203.

Emberton M, Rivett RC, Ellis BW. 1991: Comparative audit: a new method of delivering audit. *Bulletin of the Annals of the Royal College of Surgeons* **73**, 117–20.

Royal College of Surgeons of England. 1994: *Guidelines for clinicians on medical records and notes.* London: Royal College of Surgeons of England.

Royal College of Surgeons of England. 1995: *Clinical audit in surgical practice.* London: Royal College of Surgeons of England.

Trent Regional Health Authority. 1993: *Guidelines on confidentiality and medical audit.* Sheffield: Trent Regional Health Authority.

Rehabilitation and the surgical patient

Paul Finucane and Maria Crotty

Introduction

Rehabilitation is a process which aims to minimize the disability (loss of function) and handicap (social consequences) of impairment (the defect in an organ). As a practical example, a woman with a fractured neck of femur (an impairment) may have mobility problems and be restricted in undertaking daily activities (i.e. be disabled) even after surgical fixation. This is likely to interfere with her role in society (i.e. cause handicap). A rehabilitation programme will aim to restore mobility and functional competence, thereby reducing or eliminating the patient's handicap.

THE SCALE OF THE PROBLEM

Approximately 500 million people (10% of the world's population) have a disability, of whom 80% live in developing countries and one-third are children. In the UK, Australia and other developed countries, the prevalence of disability increases exponentially with age, so childhood disability is relatively uncommon. Among adults in developed countries:

- one-third have an impairment;
- of impaired adults, one-third are disabled; and
- of disabled adults, one-third are handicapped.

Impairment is due to sensory problems (especially visual and hearing loss) in 16% of adults, mental illness and retardation in 10% and congenital or acquired physical disease in 8%. However, physical diseases account for more handicap (1.8%) than do mental disorders (1.2%) or sensory problems (0.5%).

THE RELEVANCE OF REHABILITATION TO SURGERY

Rehabilitation is most relevant to surgery when a person has residual disability and handicap following a surgical procedure. As most surgical morbidity resolves quickly and spontaneously, referral for specialized rehabilitation is only appropriate when:

- post-operative disability and handicap is substantial; and
- spontaneous resolution is unlikely; or
- the time to spontaneous recovery is likely to be prolonged.

Surgery can be an integral part of rehabilitation and relieve disability and handicap, as occurs, for example, when hand deformities in chronic rheumatoid arthritis are surgically corrected.

SOME IMPORTANT REHABILITATION PRINCIPLES

A number of principles underpin the clinical practice of rehabilitation for surgical patients. These include the need for:

- pre-operative assessment in elective surgery. The pre-operative physical, mental and functional status will greatly influence the post-operative rehabilitation programme. Many operative and post-operative problems can be anticipated and prevented, cardiorespiratory fitness can be maximized and preventive strategies can be introduced, e.g. strengthening the quadriceps muscles prior to knee replacement;

- early post-operative mobilization. Deconditioning and the complications of immobility (e.g. chest infections, thrombo-embolic disease, pressure ulcers) are reduced if time in bed is minimized;

- a multidisciplinary team approach. The skills of a variety of health professionals (e.g. doctors, nurses, allied health staff, social workers) are required;

- a rehabilitation programme which is customized to the individual.

THE REHABILITATION PROCESS

As the abilities, needs and goals of each individual in rehabilitation are unique, the programme designed to address them must be targeted at the individual. However, all rehabilitation programmes tend to proceed in recognized stages, as summarized in Box 24.4.1.

Assessing the patient

The factors which should be considered are outlined in Table 24.4.1. Much depends on the pre-operative status, and in this regard two main categories of patients are recognized, namely the young and previously fit and the

---

BOX 24.4.1 THE ESSENTIAL STEPS IN A REHABILITATION PROGRAMME

- Assessing the patient
- Setting rehabilitation goals
- Providing therapy
- Use of aids and appliances (including prostheses and orthoses)
- Monitoring progress
- Education and secondary prevention
- Psychosocial support
- Discharge planning and follow-up

---

old and previously frail, although many people do not fit either stereotype. Among other factors, these groups tend to have different social supports and different expectations of rehabilitation.

Setting rehabilitation goals

At an early stage it is essential to ensure that the key individuals (i.e. the patient, rehabilitation team members and 'significant others') are working towards common goals. Formal team meetings help to define such goals, which need to be both realistic and sufficiently flexible to allow modification in the light of progress. It is sometimes useful to set interim as well as long-term goals, and to set a flexible time-frame within which they might be achieved.

Providing therapy

Well-resourced rehabilitation teams have access to a variety of therapists (e.g. physiotherapists, occupational therapists, speech pathologists, clinical psychologists, dietitians, social workers) in addition to nursing and medical staff. A description of what each has to offer is beyond the scope of this chapter. The level of input from each is highly dependent on the individual's needs, and these may change over time. For example, physiotherapy may be particularly important in the early stages following lower limb amputation, while social work and occupational therapy input may be crucial prior to hospital discharge.

Table 24.4.1 Assessment of rehabilitation needs

The principal impairment
Nature (e.g. acquired brain injury, limb amputation)
Severity

Other impairments
Patient's general medical status

Patient's premorbid physical status
Cardiorespiratory fitness
Mobility

Mental factors
Cognition
Mood (e.g. depression)

Patient's premorbid social status
Family supports (e.g. spouse, other family)
Community supports (friends and neighbours)
Employment
Financial supports (income)

Use of aids and appliances

These range from aids and appliances that are cheap and simple (e.g. a raised toilet seat to relieve disability following hip surgery) to the complex and expensive (e.g. a prosthetic limb). Aids and appliances should be used judiciously, as inappropriate use promotes dependence and can reinforce a disability. Advice from allied health staff reduces this risk. An occupational therapist home visit to assess a patient in their usual environment prior to hospital discharge will often clarify the need for home modifications (e.g. shower facilities, ramps and railings).

Monitoring progress

Rehabilitation teams hold regular (at least weekly) formal meetings to inform each other of the patient's progress, to ensure that the rehabilitation goals are being met, to identify the factors inhibiting progress, and collectively to plan further care, including discharge and follow-up.

Education and secondary prevention

The relationship between impairment, disability and handicap is often complex. Disability can be a cause as well as a consequence of impairment. For example, in an amputee patient with peripheral vascular disease, the added physical stress placed on the remaining limb can exacerbate ischaemia. A focus of rehabilitation is to educate the patient so as to minimize the risk factors for further impairment, disability and handicap. Psychological morbidity (e.g. anxiety, depression, loss of confidence) is a particular concern, and may require an approach varying from simple reassurance to sophisticated psychotherapy.

Discharge planning and follow-up

This step is essential for ensuring that the gains made in rehabilitation are maintained and further enhanced. Some individuals who do well in a structured hospital environment falter on return to the community, especially if their social supports are tenuous. The demands of caring for a disabled person can also produce stress in carers unless their needs are anticipated and addressed. In many cases, the rehabilitation process needs to continue following hospital discharge, although usually at a less intensive pace than in hospital. Good discharge planning also improves hospital efficiency. It has been estimated that 30% of all hospital discharges are delayed for non-medical reasons.

REHABILITATION FOLLOWING LIMB AMPUTATION

The incidence of amputation increases with age, and the average age of amputees is rising with the ageing of the general population. In Western societies, about 80% of individuals undergoing lower limb amputation are aged over 60 years; most have peripheral vascular disease and many have significant comorbidity, particularly other vascular problems. A smaller and younger group have amputation following trauma, and about 5% have malignancy. Elderly amputees are a high-risk group; 50% of patients die within 3 years and, of the survivors, 25% of non-diabetics and over 50% of diabetics will require a second amputation within 5 years. Their functional outcome depends on the level of amputation (Table 24.4.2), their premorbid health (particularly cardiovascular status) and their level of motivation. With appropriate rehabilitation and social support, the majority of elderly amputees can return home. Rehabilitation programmes consist of pre-operative conditioning, post-operative care, prosthetic training and community reintegration.

Pre-operative conditioning aims to:

- maintain mobility and activity of the other limbs. The presence of joint contractures or arthritic change will preclude prosthetic fitting;
- improve general conditioning and maximize cardiac and pulmonary reserve;
- provide psychological support and education.

Post-operative care aims to:

- desensitize the stump (e.g. with massage or transcutaneous electric nerve stimulation – TENS);
- stabilize residual limb volume, decrease oedema and promote healing (e.g. with rigid or soft dressings – shrinkers and elastic bandaging);
- increase muscle strength, maintain joint mobility and avoid contractures;
- maximize independent living skills;
- facilitate transfers from bed to chair;
- facilitate wheelchair mobility. The base of the wheelchair is displaced posteriorly to accommodate the posteriorly displaced centre of gravity.

Prosthetic training focuses on:

- balance re-education;
- the ability to transfer (e.g. bed to chair, chair to toilet, etc.);
- general conditioning and fitness;
- stump care, including bandaging of the stump;

Table 24.4.2 Probable outcomes for amputee patients

Level of amputation	Probable outcome
Unilateral transradial or transhumeral	Independent with ADLs; able to drive; able to work with some restrictions
Bilateral upper limb	Will require assistance with donning prostheses, but then independent with ADLs, able to drive and work despite many restrictions
Trans-tibial	Energy requirements 24–40% higher than normal. Requires no gait aids; stands and walks continuously for over 2 h; climbs stairs step over step; works with some restrictions
Transfemoral	Energy requirements 60–100% above normal. Otherwise as for trans-tibial amputation
Bilateral transfemoral	Energy requirements 100% above normal. Can stand or walk for up to 1 h continuously; can climb stairs one at a time; can return to restricted work; needs an amputee wheelchair

- fitting an interim/temporary prosthesis. Fitting a definitive prosthesis is deferred until stump oedema has resolved;
- gait training;
- hopping with the use of an aid (crutches or frame), a skill that is useful when the prosthesis is being repaired or when the patient gets up at night;
- walking on slopes or rough ground.

Lower limb amputations

In non-traumatic situations the level of amputation is a clinical decision, usually based on vascular status. If possible the knee should be preserved, as this greatly reduces the energy subsequently required for walking. Walking is generally attainable in unilateral trans-tibial (below-knee) amputees who walked before surgery, and in selected bilateral trans-tibial amputees. In transfemoral (above-knee) amputees, walking can generally be achieved in those aged under 80 years and in fit older people. A below-knee amputee expends less energy walking with a prosthesis than with crutches. Bilateral transfemoral prosthetic use requires energy expenditure of which individuals over 40 years of age are often incapable. However, training is trialled if the patient is motivated.

Upper limb amputations

The main surgical consideration is the preservation of maximal possible length – the longer the residual limb, the greater the control of prosthetic components that can be achieved. Amputation at shoulder level rarely results in functional prosthetic use, although a shoulder cap is often prescribed to restore shoulder contour. The range of pronation and supination decreases rapidly as the length of the residual limb decreases, and when 60% or

more of the forearm is lost, no supination/pronation is possible.

Rehabilitation programmes for upper limb amputees teach one-handed functional techniques and transfer of dominance when the dominant limb has been amputated, and promote a rapid return to bimanual activities with a prosthesis. Research indicates that only 37% of upper-limb amputees use their prostheses for 8 h per day. A 30-day 'golden period' has been described; upper limb protheses fitted within 1 month of amputation are more likely to be used than those fitted several months later.

Pain after amputation

A variety of pains occur after amputation, and these need to be correctly identified.

Phantom limb sensations occur in about 70% of amputees, and these usually become more proximal (i.e. telescope) when patients start walking, and they eventually disappear. Conventional management involves massage, vibration, percussion and TENS.

Stump pain is felt in the residual limb, and may be due to ischaemia, infection, neuroma (up to 25% of cases in upper-limb amputations) or a poorly fitting prosthesis.

Phantom pain is a burning knife-like pain felt in the missing limb, which tends to begin post-operatively and to subside during subsequent months. Its pathophysiology is unclear. Pain that persists beyond 6 months is difficult to treat. Physical treatments such as desensitizing massage and TENS should be taught. Walking on a temporary prosthesis often reduces pain, and psychological interventions (e.g. relaxation therapy, biofeedback) sometimes help. Pharmacological treatment favours agents used for neurogenic pain, such as a membrane stabilizer (e.g. carbamazepine) and/or a tricyclic antidepressant. The incidence of phantom pain is related to the duration and severity of pre-operative limb pain, and can be reduced by aggressive pre-operative pain control with epidural blocks.

REHABILITATION FOLLOWING SPINAL CORD INJURY (SCI)

The typical SCI patient is a young male injured in a motor-vehicle accident. However, SCI is increasingly common in elderly people who fall. To achieve maximal independence compatible with the level of injury, patients require intensive and prolonged in-patient rehabilitation in a specialized unit. On average, paraplegic patients require over 3 months of intensive in-patient rehabilitation, while tetraplegic patients require about twice this.

Rehabilitation programmes emphasize patient education and focus on the following:

- neurogenic bladder and bowel management;
- spasticity management;
- skin care and prevention of ulceration;
- prescription of appropriate equipment (e.g. wheelchairs, cushion, shower chairs, feeding aids);
- sexuality and fertility;
- psychological adaptation.

Spinal cord injuries are classified according to the level of motor and sensory loss and mobility and self-care outcomes are often predictable (see Table 24.4.3), although individual variation can be considerable. As an approximate rule, it is possible for individuals with injuries at C7 or below to live alone without help largely because retained triceps function facilitates transfers and mobility. 'Trick' movements and adaptations are often possible and can increase independence. Tendon transfer surgery to provide pinch and grasp or to improve elbow function offers further opportunities to increase function and independence.

Common problems encountered in SCI rehabilitation include the following.

- *DVTs*, which develop in 10–64% of cases, are more common with complete injuries and tetraplegia. Their incidence decreases after 8 weeks, so prophylaxis with warfarin or low-molecular-weight heparin is given for 8 weeks post injury in most units.
- *Orthostatic hypotension* is more likely with high injuries and is managed by gradually increasing tilt on a tilt table, together with elastic binders and stockings, and possibly adding ephedrine sulphate or fludrocortisone.
- *Autonomic dysreflexia syndrome* of massive reflex sympathetic discharge in patients with a lesion above

the splanchnic outflow (T5–6) typically presents with headache, sweating, hypertension and bradycardia. Removal of noxious stimuli (e.g. blocked catheter, faecal impaction) usually relieves the problem. Otherwise the head of the bed should be elevated and glyceryl trinitrate spray given and, if necessary, repeated after 5 min, followed by nifedipine 10 mg orally.

- *Heterotopic ossification* (the formation of bone in soft tissues) usually begins 1–3 months after injury, usually below the level of the injury and in large proximal joints (especially the hip, knee and shoulder). Physiotherapy helps to maintain a range of movements and NSAIDs relieve pain. Progress should be monitored using serial bone scans, and when the problem is 'mature' (i.e. alkaline phosphatase is normal and the bone scan is cold) the problem can be treated surgically.

REHABILITATION FOLLOWING TRAUMATIC BRAIN INJURY (TBI)

Early prognostic indicators include the severity and duration of coma and the duration of post-traumatic amnesia (PTA). The prognosis is best in patients under 40 years of age, those with intact brainstem function and those receiving early specialized care.

About two-thirds of survivors of severe TBI have significant residual physical, emotional and cognitive problems. The core elements of TBI rehabilitation include:

- maximization of natural recovery processes;
- teaching compensatory techniques;
- provision of appropriate adaptive equipment (e.g. wheelchairs, orthotics) and adaptive environmental modifications (e.g. transport, home modifications);
- education of patients and their families.

Common problems encountered in TBI rehabilitation include the following.

- *Post-traumatic amnesia*, a subtype of delirium unique to TBI survivors, is usually the first issue to be dealt with in rehabilitation. It involves behavioural excesses including aggression, disinhibition, emotional lability and akathisia. Management involves strategies which reduce the level of stimulation, minimize the risk of self-injury and educate families.
- *Spasticity* after severe head injury may result in painful spasms and functional impairments such as gait disturbances. Treatments include positional and handling techniques, stretching, casting with orthoses, drugs such as dantrolene and baclofen, motor point injections or nerve blocks, intrathecal

Table 24.4.3 Probable outcomes for tetraplegic (complete) patients

Functional spinal cord level	Key muscles	Muscle function	Feeding	Bladder and bowel care	Weight shifts	Chair transfers	Locomotion	Driving
C4 and above	Sternomastoid, trapezius	Neck control	Possible	Dependent	Dependent unless using powered equipment	Dependent	Dependent unless using powered equipment	Unable to drive
C5	Deltoid, biceps	Partial shoulder control, elbow flexion, supination	Independent with equipment	Dependent	Dependent unless using powered equipment	Assisted	Independent with manual wheelchair with lugs or plastic rims on level surfaces for short distances	Unable to drive
C6	Extensor carpi radialis longus and brevis Pronator teres	Wrist extension and pronation	Independent	Independent with bowel, assistance with bladder	Independent	Independent with transfer board	Independent with manual chair and plastic rims on level surfaces	Specially adapted van
C7	Triceps Latissimus dorsi	Shoulder depression, elbow extension	Independent	Independent	Independent	Independent	Independent with manual chair except kerbs	Car with hand controls or adapted van
C8	Flexor digitorum profundus	Some hand function Finger flexors	Independent	Independent	Independent	Independent	Independent	Car with hand controls

pumps and surgical inverventions such as tenotomy and tendon transfers.

- *Cognitive rehabilitation* aims to establish new strategies to compensate for cognitive problems, and is directed at deficits in attention, concentration, initiation, judgement, communication, learning and memory. 'Internal' strategies involve self-talk to enhance skills (e.g. repetition, association, categorization, imaging) and 'external' strategies (e.g. lists, alarm watches) and task analysis, in which the task is broken down into simple, logically sequenced steps.

- *Post-traumatic epilepsy* develops in about 5% of hospitalized patients with closed head injury, and this risk increases to 35–50% with open head injury. Prophylaxis is generally not used in patients with closed head injury who have not had seizures after the first 2 weeks.

REHABILITATION OF THE ELDERLY SURGICAL PATIENT

The number of elderly people undergoing surgery is increasing because:

- their number in Western societies is rapidly increasing;

- they have high prevalence rates for problems which are surgically treatable;

- better anaesthetic and surgical techniques have lowered the risk–benefit ratio of surgery;

- elderly people have increasing health expectations and are more willing to consider undergoing surgery.

From a rehabilitation perspective, elderly surgical patients differ from the young in the following ways.

- Several disease processes are likely to be active simultaneously. Thus the elderly patient with a fractured neck of femur following a fall may have coexisting Parkinson's disease, postural hypotension, cerebrovascular disease and dementia.

- Cardiorespiratory and other physiological reserves become attenuated with ageing, such that the patient can decompensate when stressed by illness and/or surgery.

- Elderly patients become more readily deconditioned by the rigours of surgery and by post-operative immobility.

Because the likelihood of spontaneous recovery is lower, it can be argued that rehabilitation has more to offer elderly surgical patients than those who are younger. It is also cost-effective, as successful rehabilitation will reduce the length of hospital stay and, by help-ing elderly individuals to regain their former functional status, will often obviate the need for long-term institutional care. It follows that early access to rehabilitation is particularly important for elderly surgical patients. Surgical services who deal predominantly with elderly patients (e.g. orthopaedics, vascular surgery, urology) should have close functional links with physicians in geriatric or rehabilitation medicine, and models of shared care are increasingly being developed.

Falls are of particular importance, as it is estimated that 90% of fractures in elderly people result from falls. While physiotherapy alone has not been shown to reduce the incidence of falls, a package of interventions which include balance and strength training programmes, treatment of postural hypotension and review of medications and environmental hazards does reduce the number of falls in elderly people.

Common problems encountered in rehabilitation of the elderly surgical patient include the following:

- *post-operative delirium* – while this can be the first overt presentation of confusion, delirium is more often an acute exacerbation of underlying chronic confusion (dementia). Precipitating factors other than the surgical procedure should be sought (e.g. infection, drug treatment, electrolyte imbalance, stroke, myocardial infarction). Use of psychotropic drugs (e.g. benzodiazepines, major tranquillizers) should be avoided, as these tend to exacerbate and prolong the delirium;

- *post-operative pain* – although pain is no more prevalent than in the young, older people are more susceptible to the side-effects of analgesics. Constipation frequently results from opiate use, particularly when mobility is reduced. NSAIDs are more likely to cause acute gastrointestinal problems, and some analgesics (e.g. dextropropoxyphene) cause confusion. While post-operative pain must be adequately controlled, such problems should be anticipated and minimized. For example, aperients should generally be prescribed with opiate drugs;

- *constipation and/or urinary retention* – these are often atypical in their presentation and therefore liable to be overlooked. A high index of suspicion is needed, and abdominal and rectal examinations together with abdominal X-ray and/or ultrasound examination may be required to confirm the diagnosis;

- *undernutrition* – this commonly compromises recovery in elderly surgical patients, whose nutritional requirements increase as their ability to eat is reduced. In this context, even people who appear obese can be undernourished. For the elderly surgical patient, the importance of routine nutritional assessment and dietetic advice is increasingly recognized.

FURTHER READING

Braddom RL. 1996: *Physical medicine and rehabilitation*. Philadelphia, PA: W.B. Saunders.

Chadwick SJD, Wolfe JHN. 1992: Rehabilitation of the amputee. *British Medical Journal* **304**, 373–6.

Cope DN. 1995: Effectiveness of TBI rehabilitation: a review. *Brain Injury* **9**, 649–70.

DeLisa JA, Gane BM. 1993: *Rehabilitation medicine: principles and practice*, 2nd ed. Philadelphia, PA: J.B. Lippincott.

Jennett B, Teasdale G. 1981: *Management of head injuries*. Philadelphia, PA: F.A. Davis.

Leonard JA. 1994: The elderly amputee. In Felsenthal G, Garrison SJ, Streinberg FU (eds), *Rehabilitation of the aging and elderly patient*. Baltimore, MD: Williams & Wilkins, 397–406.

Nickel VL, Botte MJ. 1992: *Orthopaedic rehabilitation*, 2nd ed. New York: Churchill Livingstone.

Sandel ME, Mysiw WJ. 1996: Agitated brain injured patient. Part 1. Definitions, differential diagnosis and assessment. *Archives of Physical Medicine and Rehabilitation* **77**, 617–23.

Chapter 24.5

Statistical analysis, statistical inference and surgical clinical trials

John C. Hall and John Ludbrook

Introduction

Trainee and trained surgeons should have an understanding of statistical analysis, if only in order to be able to evaluate the published clinical trials that have an important influence on the practice of surgery. In this chapter we give a broad overview of the field, with emphasis on some of the difficulties that surgeons and surgical trainees encounter in understanding the statistical content of published papers, or in evaluating the results of audits, surveys and clinical trials.

EXPERIMENTAL DESIGN AND STATISTICAL INFERENCE

EXPERIMENTAL DESIGN

Proper statistical analysis of the results follows logically and automatically from the design of an experiment or set of observations. The most important consideration in design is to eliminate all sources of systematic bias. This can only be done prospectively. It involves either *random sampling* of the experimental units (humans, animals, tissues or cells) from defined populations, or non-random sampling followed by *randomization* to treatments (using the term 'treatments' in the broad sense of medical, surgical or pharmacological therapies, or other sets of conditions). It is quite rare to be able to perform random sampling of populations in biomedical research. Randomization of non-random samples is the much commoner approach (as, for instance, in clinical trials). Retrospective studies of patients can never involve genuine randomization or random sampling, and are invariably attended by a greater or lesser degree of systematic bias.

SCALES OF MEASUREMENT

There are three recognized scales of measurement:

1. *interval* – this is used, for example, in measurements of continuous variables such as age, weight, pressure or plasma concentration;

2. *ordinal* – this involves assigning a rank between 1 and n to each experimental unit in a sample or group of size n;

3. *nominal* – the experimental units are placed in two or more mutually exclusive categories, e.g. alive or dead, infection or no infection. Sometimes the categories may be ordered, e.g. excellent, good, fair, poor.

It is a general rule that if an interval scale of measurement can be employed, the subsequent process of statistical analysis is more powerful than if an ordinal scale is used, and that ordinal scale measurements result in more powerful statistical analyses than those made on nominal scales.

STATISTICS AND STATISTICAL ANALYSIS

A *statistic*, or *summary statistic*, is a numerical characteristic of a sample, such as the arithmetic mean. A *parameter* is a numerical characteristic of a population. However, the distinction is somewhat blurred because sample statistics are also used as best estimates of parameters of populations from which the samples were randomly drawn. Thus the sample mean is the best estimate of the population mean, and the corresponding standard error or confidence interval indicates the range within which the 'true' population mean is predicted to lie.

The term *statistical analysis* is usually used to refer to the process of making comparisons between populations, by subjecting samples from those populations to statistical tests. The outcome of such comparisons is a *statistical inference*.

MODELS OF STATISTICAL INFERENCE

It is important to appreciate that there can be no valid statistical inference unless there has been random sampling of defined populations (*population model*), or division of non-random samples into randomized groups (*randomization model*). The latter is the norm in biomedical research, and statistical inferences under this model apply only to the specific experiment or trial that has been conducted.

HYPOTHESIS-TESTING VS. ESTIMATION

A statistical inference depends on the outcome of testing a statistical hypothesis. Statistical hypotheses are *null hypotheses*. Statisticians postulate that there is no difference, whereas investigators postulate (even if only privately) that there *is* a difference. The outcome of testing a statistical null hypothesis is given as a P (probability) value. Under the population model of inference, the value of P indicates the probability of obtaining the same or a more extreme outcome if a large (infinite) number of random samples was to be taken from the same populations. More simply, although not quite so accurately, it indicates the probability that the null hypothesis is true.

P has a somewhat different meaning under the randomization model of inference. There is no reference to populations, and P merely indicates the probability that the observed differences between randomized groups could have occurred by chance in the experiment that was performed. It makes no reference to other hypothetical experiments that might be performed (the basis for the population model).

However, a P-value is not in itself an inference. Some critical value of P must be selected that distinguishes rejection from acceptance of the null hypothesis. It is customary to specify this as $P = 0.05$. That is, if $P \leqslant 0.05$ the null hypothesis is rejected. If $P > 0.05$ the null hypothesis is accepted. $P \leqslant 0.05$ is often described as indicating a *significant difference*. However, it is far better to present the actual P-value and to let the reader judge whether it is significant. $P < 0.05$ may mean that $P = 0.04999$, or that $P = 0.00001$.

There is another approach to statistical inference. It is usually described as *estimation*, in contrast to *hypothesis-testing*. This approach can only be used under the population model of inference. It involves the construction of *confidence intervals* (also known as *confidence limits*), commonly referred to as CIs, for population parameters such as the mean, or the difference between means. The usual convention is to use 95% confidence intervals. These indicate the range of values within which the corresponding parameters of the randomly sampled populations are estimated to lie.

Some medical editors insist that the outcome of statistical testing (e.g. for a difference between two means) must be presented in the form of the observed difference plus the CI. However, this is not a view shared by all medical editors, nor by all statisticians. For instance, there has been no serious attempt to discover whether clinicians or investigators find it easier to interpret P-values or CIs. Nevertheless, it is generally agreed that the P-value for a difference must be accompanied by an indication of the size of the observed difference and an estimate of the range of that size in the population (e.g. mean difference $\pm$ standard error). This information can be presented either in tabular form or graphically.

STATISTICAL VS. BIOLOGICAL INFERENCES

It is important to make this distinction. The statistical inference that there is a difference (e.g. in duration of survival following two different cancer treatments) only partly takes into account the magnitude of that difference. For instance, $P = 0.01$ invites the inference that there is a 'significant' difference. However, a difference in mean survival of 2 years would have important clinical implications, whereas a difference of 2 days would have none. This is one of the reasons for advocating the use of CIs, or for supplementing P-values with statements of means $\pm$ standard errors (see above).

ERRORS IN STATISTICAL INFERENCE

These are of two main types. The *Type 1* error rate is the probability of falsely rejecting the null hypothesis, and corresponds to the P-value attached to the null hypothesis. Thus the Type 1 error rate can be regarded as the probability of making a false-positive inference. There are several ways in which the Type 1 error rate can be inflated beyond that stipulated by the investigator (usually $P = 0.05$, or 5%). In practice, the commonest source of excessive Type 1 error is the use of the results of a single experiment to test multiple hypotheses. There are several techniques for controlling this *experiment-wise*, or *family-wise*, Type 1 error rate. The most conservative – and it is sometimes over-conservative – is to use the one-step Bonferroni adjustment in which the P-values are multiplied by the number of hypotheses tested. Thus if 10 hypotheses are tested, then in the worst case the resultant P-values are inflated 10-fold. That is, $P = 0.05$ should in reality be $P' = 0.5$. A better technique is the Holm step-down Bonferroni procedure, which provides as effective control over the Type 1 error rate as the one-step procedure, but is more powerful.

The other important error in statistical inference is *Type 2*. The Type 2 error rate is the probability of falsely accepting the null hypothesis, and thus making a false-negative inference. The commonest source of this type of error is the use of experimental groups that are too small. Estimation of the minimal group size that will result in an acceptable risk of Type 2 error should always be part of designing an experiment or clinical trial. There is no hard and fast convention that dictates an acceptable risk, although $P = 0.20$ (20% risk) is commonly used. *Power* (to reject a null hypothesis) is defined as $(1 - P)$ for Type 2 error.

Opinions vary as to whether excessive Type 1 or Type 2 error is the more reprehensible. This involves a non-statistical judgement. Our argument is based on the Hippocratic principle of *non nocere* – that is, in the setting of clinical research, it is more important to guard against excessive Type 1 error. A false-positive inference may result in the introduction of a new therapy into clinical practice that is in reality no better (or even worse) than current therapy.

CLINICAL TRIALS

Clinical trials evaluate the effects of an intervention in a predetermined manner. There are essentially only two types of clinical studies, namely *explanatory* (mechanistic) and *pragmatic* (empirical) studies. Explanatory studies look at underlying processes, whereas pragmatic studies provide management recommendations that are relevant to clinical practice.

PROSPECTIVE, RANDOMIZED, COMPARATIVE CLINICAL TRIALS

These are generally regarded as the benchmark for evaluating treatments and providing sound recommen-

dations about patient management. Patients are recruited into the trial in a non-random but clearly defined manner, and are then randomly allocated to two or more treatment groups. One group will be exposed to the intervention under study while the other group or groups may be exposed to a placebo treatment or to other conventional forms of medical or surgical treatment. Because of the randomization process, all of the observed differences in outcome between the groups will be attributed to the intervention. Statistical inferences based on the outcome will be made under the randomization model of inference.

When designing and executing prospective, randomized, comparative clinical trials (including trials of surgical therapy), the overriding goal of design is to minimize bias. Some of the more important considerations in achieving that goal are calculation in advance of minimal group sizes, the use of a secure method for randomizing patients to those groups, maximum blinding of all those involved in a trial to the treatments received by individual patients (thus single-blind, double-blind or even triple-blind trials), choice of an appropriate endpoint to the trial, and rigorous statistical analysis of the outcome of the trial. No clinical trial, however modest in size, should be undertaken without prior consultation with an experienced statistician.

OTHER DESIGNS FOR PROSPECTIVE CLINICAL TRIALS

Readers should be aware that there are other ways of designing prospective clinical trials. These include *sequential trials* (legislated testing for statistical significance at set intervals throughout the study) and *crossover studies* (in which each of the patients receives each of the treatments in random sequence). *Case–control studies* are neither prospective nor randomized, for they involve comparing a contemporary group of patients with historical controls, which leads to a high risk of biased conclusions.

ETHICAL ISSUES IN CLINICAL TRIALS

It is essential that every clinical trial, however small, be approved in advance by a properly constituted institutional ethics committee. This protects the interests of the patients participating in the trial, protects the health-care personnel involved, and is a prerequisite for publication of the results in a reputable journal. This places a heavy responsibility on ethics committees. To allow a trial to proceed, they must not only ensure patients' safety, but they must also assure themselves that the question asked is worthwhile and original in terms of improving clinical practice. In addition, they have to decide whether the design of the trial, including its planned size, is appropriate for answering the clinical question.

INTERPRETING THE OUTCOME OF CLINICAL TRIALS

In the simplest cases, evaluation of the outcome takes place at a predetermined, unique time after completion of treatment. Relatively simple statistical techniques are used to evaluate the outcome, the specific techniques employed depending on the scale of measurement used. However, analysing the results of clinical trials is not always as simple as analysing the results of laboratory experiments, on several counts.

Intention to treat Particulary when one arm of a trial is a surgical operation and the other is a more conservative form of therapy, a special problem may occur. For instance, patients assigned to conservative treatment may, part of the way through their course of treatment, develop a complication that requires more or less urgent surgical intervention. It is in response to such cases that most trialists code such patients according to intention to treat. That is, even though the patients undergo surgery, in the analysis of the results of the trial they are counted according to their original assignment to the conservative arm of the trial.

Follow-up It may not be possible to trace some patients at the time or times when the end-point is to be determined. How does one cope with this situation? One approach is merely to delete such patients from the trial as if they had never entered it. This may be satisfactory if (a) the rate of loss to follow-up is very low (e.g. < 2%) and (b) the rate of loss to follow-up of each arm of the trial is equal. A more rigorous approach, but one that goes further towards reducing bias, is to declare patients who are lost to follow-up as 'failures' of the treatment to which they were assigned. In survival analysis (see below), special techniques are used to allow for loss to follow-up.

Withdrawal For a variety of reasons, patients may withdraw or be withdrawn from the trial. These include a patient's refusal to continue or an attending doctor's decision to withdraw the patient on grounds of side-effects. What is to be done with these patients? If the results of the trial are to be analysed at the end of a fixed period of time, the safest approach is to count withdrawal as a failure of the treatment to which the patient was assigned. In survival analysis (see below), special techniques are used to allow for withdrawal.

STATISTICAL ANALYSIS OF RESULTS WHEN THERE ARE TWO ARMS TO THE TRIAL

It is paradoxical that the simpler the design of an experiment or clinical trial, and the more explicit the main hypothesis, the greater the risk of false-positive statistical inference (Type 1 error).

Outcome expressed on an interval scale Usually the results are analysed by *Student's t-test*, most commonly for independent groups, but for related groups in crossover trials. There are two sources of difficulty with this approach. The *t*-test for detecting a difference between population means (and the corresponding technique of constructing confidence intervals) assumes that there has been random sampling of two normally distributed populations with equal variance (scatter). The normality assumption is not of great importance, but the equality of variance is. If there is a suspicion of inequality of population variances, then a modified form of the *t*-test (e.g. the *Welch–Satterthwaite procedure*) or *data transformation* (usually logarithmic) should be used. However, when randomization rather than random sampling has been employed, and when the group sizes are small or unequal, the *t*-test is notoriously inaccurate. Instead, a *permutation (randomization)* test for the difference between means should be employed, in which no assumptions are made about normality or equality of variance.

Outcome expressed on an ordinal scale The standard tests are the non-parametric *Wilcoxon–Mann–Whitney procedure* for two independent groups, and the *Wilcoxon matched-pairs, signed rank-sum procedure* for two related groups. Investigators sometimes use these rank-order tests to analyse data expressed on an interval scale when it is suspected that there are breaches of the assumptions for classical tests. This approach is wrong, and general permutation tests are more informative.

Outcome expressed on a nominal scale. Traditionally, the results are analysed by a test that uses the chi-squared distribution (*Pearson's χ^2 test*) as an approximation to the double-binomial distribution. This test is notoriously inaccurate when entries in some cells of the 2×2 table are small. The appropriate test is then *Fisher's exact test*. If the two groups are related (before/after), the *McNemar test* in an approximate or exact form can be used.

STATISTICAL ANALYSIS WHEN THERE ARE MORE THAN TWO ARMS TO THE TRIAL

Outcome expressed on an interval scale The classical test under assumptions of random sampling, population normality and equality of variance is *analysis of variance (ANOVA)*. This is cast in a one-way form when the groups are independent, and in a two- or multi-way form when the groups are related. Global ANOVA detects any inequality among population means, so there must be some assurance that population variances are equal. Following ANOVA, it is possible to make specific pairwise comparisons between treatment groups, but a correction for multiple comparisons must be made. If the observations have been made serially (e.g. over time) rather than independently, then a modified form of ANOVA, namely repeated-measures analysis of variance, should be used.

Outcome expressed on an ordinal scale If there are more than two independent groups, the non-parametric *Kruskal–Wallis test* can be used. If the various groups are related, the *Friedman test* is appropriate. Both of these tests are part of the family of rank-order procedures.

Outcome expressed on a nominal scale The results can usually be tabulated as an $r \times c$ table of frequencies, in which case *Pearson's χ^2 test* or, better still, the exact *Fisher–Freeman–Halton test*, can be used to detect any inequality among the cells of the table. There is a special test for cases in which one of the nominal categories is an ordered one, e.g. grades of severity (*Cochran–Armitage test*). There are also special tests for cases in which the tabulated data take the form of stratified 2×2 or $2 \times c$ tables.

REGRESSION AND CORRELATION

We mention here only cases in which measurements have been made on an interval scale. This comes into play when two or more variables are studied at the same time to determine whether they are interrelated. Regression analysis is a very powerful technique for resolving this issue. Unfortunately, it is also open to a variety of serious abuses.

Linear regression analysis: comparison of methods of measurement As a preliminary to a trial, one method of measurement (one that is new or non-invasive) may be compared with another well-established, benchmark or 'gold-standard' method. It is common, and unequivocally wrong, to use the Pearson correlation coefficient as a test of equivalence of the two methods. Rather, the *Altman–Bland method of differences, or least-products regression analysis*, should be used.

Multiple linear regression analysis This is a powerful technique for identifying categorical variables (e.g. age or stage of disease) that are important predictors of outcome when this is expressed on an interval scale.

Logistic regression This is almost a mirror image of multiple linear regression. It identifies continuous variables (e.g. age or a plasma concentration) or categorical variables (e.g. gender) that are important predictors of outcome when this is expressed on a binomial scale.

SURVIVAL ANALYSIS

In many clinical trials a binomial categorical variable is selected as the primary end-point. Common examples are dead/alive, or recurrence/recurrence-free. Entry into such trials occurs over a prolonged period of time, so that at any particular moment in the course of the trial some patients will have died, some will be lost or will have withdrawn, and the remainder will have been under review for different periods of time. The simple comparison of mortality rates at any specified time is an inadequate expression of how the patients have responded. It is much better to compare the survival experience of the two or more groups of patients over the total period of review (survival analysis). The techniques used for survival analysis contain two steps. The first of these is the estimation of survival experience for each group of patients in the form of a graph or table. Plotting of survival curves by the *product–limit (Kaplan–Meier) technique*, in which there is a step in the survival curve each time a death occurs, has replaced the classical *life-table*, which tabulates survival at fixed intervals of time. Secondly, comparison of the survival experiences is used to test whether there is a 'significant' difference between the two or more groups. Several statistical techniques are available for carrying out this step. The most popular is the *log-rank (Mantel–Haenszel)* technique. Others that are encountered from time to time include the *Wilcoxon–Gehan, Breslow–Gehan* or *Tarone–Ware procedures*, and *Cox's proportional hazards regression analysis*. All of these are readily executed by computer programs. They all require three pieces of information about each patient:

1. the treatment to which the patient was assigned;

2. the duration of 'survival' of the patient from his or her entry to the trial, in the smallest possible unit of time (hours, days, weeks or months);

3. whether the patient's survival can be described as 'uncensored' or 'censored'. *Uncensored* observations are those in which the patient is known to have reached the end-point (e.g. death or recurrence). An observation is *censored* if the patient's future behaviour is unknown – that is, if he or she has been lost to follow-up, has withdrawn from the trial, or had not reached the end-point at the last time of attendance.

All of the techniques mentioned above for comparing survival experience depend on the test statistic being distributed according to the chi-squared distribution. This assumption may sometimes be grossly breached, so empirical techniques that are based on permutation or bootstrapping have recently been developed.

META-ANALYSIS

This is a relatively new but increasingly popular statistical technique for evaluating in a relatively objective manner the overall outcome of several clinical trials that address the same question and which have been conducted in the past. Ideally, meta-analysis takes into account unpublished as well as published trials. The technique is undeniably useful in deciding whether large-scale clinical trials should be conducted or not. However, it is arguable whether meta-analysis of several small clinical trials provides a sounder guide to clinical practice than a single well-designed and well-conducted large-scale clinical trial.

EVIDENCE-BASED MEDICINE

This has been defined by Sackett and colleagues as 'the conscientious, explicit and judicious use of current best evidence in making decisions about the care of individual patients'. It is important to appreciate that, for the good surgeon, neither individual expertise nor external evidence is enough. What is required is a thoughtful evaluation of published research so that useful information is rapidly incorporated into clinical practice. This is not easy, because there is a dearth of new information that is both reliable and useful. On the other hand, it is important not to persist with established practices when they are futile. This dilemma is now being approached in a more formal manner. Greater emphasis is being placed on determining the validity of the results of clinical research. Some groups are creating catalogues of publications on specific topics, and attempts are being made to construct clinical guidelines. However, as the above definition implies, evidence-based medicine is not about having clinical practice rigorously governed by protocols.

EVALUATING PUBLISHED REPORTS

It is desirable to sift out reliable and relevant information from the deluge of publications that are available for study. An essential component in this process is the critical appraisal of written information. The results of a clinical trial can be evaluated only after the methods used in the study have been subjected to scrutiny. Regrettably, many clinical trials fail to fulfil important criteria for study design and analysis. Before discussing approaches to the evaluation of published research, we shall review the limitations of clinical trials.

LIMITATIONS OF CLINICAL TRIALS

One of the fundamental problems associated with clinical trials is that they often ignore information that relates to aspects of everyday clinical practice. This is because entities such as 'quality of life' are difficult to measure, and are therefore scientifically 'soft'. Currently, there is a concerted effort to establish standards for such information (clinimetrics). Clinical trials are also limited in their ability to test for safety, because they may evaluate relatively small numbers of patients and they tend to exclude patients who are susceptible to complications (selection bias).

Only a limited number of clinical situations can be evaluated by clinical trials. If prophylaxis is being investigated, it is necessary to study very large numbers of patients in order to detect a clinically (or statistically) significant treatment effect. It may be unwise to embark on a clinical trial when the treatment for the condition under study is still evolving, as by the time the study is completed that form of intervention may have been superseded. In addition, there are many situations in which ethical issues reduce the likelihood of performing a successful clinical trial.

EVALUATING PUBLISHED CLINICAL TRIALS

New advice needs to be treated with caution. A number of operations that were introduced with optimism were eventually rejected after the performance of prospective clinical trials. Examples include nephropexy for 'floating-kidney', colectomy for epilepsy, gastric freezing for peptic ulcer disease, internal mammary artery ligation for angina pectoris, carotid body extirpation for asthma, extracranial–intracranial arterial bypass to reduce the risk of ischaemic stroke, and prefrontal lobotomy for schizophrenia. Now there are second thoughts about laparoscopic surgery – is it really a surgical revolution, or is it just an expensive luxury?

The first step when evaluating a clinical trial is to decide whether the study has any relevance to your particular area of interest. A value judgement must then be made about the need for such a study. A number of published studies have compared the efficacy of antimicrobial agents with similar spectra of activity, but the clinical reality is that a choice of which antimicrobial agent to use must be influenced by the incidence and nature of its side-effects, its cost, and the risk that resistant micro-organisms will emerge. In addition to this, a number of studies are directed towards facts that are already well established. It is surely unethical to engage in yet another study to determine whether antimicrobial agents are more effective than a placebo in preventing wound infection after contaminated abdominal surgery.

There are two useful guides to the validity of a clinical trial. The first is that the trial has been supported by a reputable grant-giving body, or has been conducted under the auspices of a reputable society or institution. Trials that are likely to be invalid are of small size and conducted by doctors who have no documented previous experience or affiliation with a reputable institution. The second guide is that the outcome of the trial has been published in a high-quality, international journal whose policy is to submit manuscripts to criticial peer review.

Once such issues have been considered, a number of specific factors concerning the mechanics of the trial must be considered.

1. *Aims.* Is there a clear statement of the aims of the study? These should not be ambiguous, nor should they be expressed too generally to allow a specific study design to be formulated.

2. *Eligibility criteria.* How were the patients selected for study? Are the characteristics of the patients similar to those found in your clinical practice? What percentage of the patients who were eligible for study did in fact enter the study? How many patients were excluded from the analysis, and why? Answers to these questions will clarify the relevance of the study and indicate the appropriateness of extrapolating the findings to everyday clinical practice.

3. *Baseline equivalence.* There must be firm evidence that all the groups were similar before the start of the study. Known risk factors should be equally distributed between them.

4. *Group size.* There should be a statement that the minimal group size was determined before the start of the study. The criteria and methods used to estimate this should be documented. If this has not been performed, a declaration of 'no significant difference' must be interpreted as indicating that an incomplete evaluation has been performed. Negative results should be accompanied by a declaration of the probability of Type 2 error or, inversely, calculation of the power of the study to reject the null hypothesis.

5. *Randomization.* Was there adequate random allocation of patients to treatment groups? Are there explicit statements about the technique of randomization?

6. *Control group.* Was there a control group, so that it is possible to make valid interpretations of the results obtained in the active treatment group? If a placebo was used, is it appropriate? If a placebo has not been used, has the control group been subjected to a therapy that is acceptable as the optimum form of current clinical practice?

7. *The intervention.* Has this been clearly defined, so that the methods can be reproduced by others? Are criteria for stopping or modifying treatment stated? Has compliance been measured?

8. *Assessment of outcome.* Is there a clear definition of study end-points, so that it is unnecessary for discretionary judgements to be made by the assessor? Has the assessment been performed by someone who does not know to which groups the patients belong?

9. *Patient blindness.* Did the patients know to which treatment group they belonged? If so, is it possible that this could have influenced the outcome of the study?

10. *Treatment complications.* The presence or absence of side-effects must be clearly documented. Unless this information is provided, it is difficult for a reader to estimate the clinical utility of the intervention.

11. *Loss to follow-up.* Information about the number of patients who were lost to follow-up, and the reasons for this, must be included in the publication. If a substantial proportion of the patients failed to complete the study, the analysis of the remaining patients may be over-optimistic. Analysis should be performed on an 'intention-to-treat' basis, and include all patients who were randomized, regardless of the incompleteness of their therapy.

12. *Data analysis.* The statistical methods that have been used should be clearly stated. Variables that are important for the validity and interpretation of the study should be presented using graphical methods (e.g. scatter plots, histograms or survival curves), or by using summary statistics. The level of statistical significance (usually $P \leq 0.05$) must be declared in advance, and the assumptions that underlie the methods of analysis must be fulfilled (e.g. normally distributed data with equal variance for parametric tests). Look for skewness of the data and inequalities of variance, which would disqualify conventional t-tests or ANOVA. There should be an explicit statement that two-sided tests were used – it is usually ethically unjustifiable to use one-tailed tests. If multiple tests of statistical significance have been performed, the P-values must be adjusted by a multiple comparison procedure. Actual P-values should be declared, together with the observed values of the test statistic, the number of observations on which it is based, statements of effect size, and either standard errors or confidence intervals. If correlation coefficients are used, the observations must be

derived from independent populations (no biological or mathematical coupling). If regression equations are used, then the confidence intervals or standard errors of the regression coefficients must be stated.

13. *Study conclusions.* Were the differences detected of clinical as well as statistical significance? Are the conclusions drawn by the authors within the limits of the data?

14. *Ethics.* Is the study ethically sound? A good indication of this is whether you would be happy to include a close family member in such a study. Remember that a study which is methodologically unsound is also unethical. Is there a statement that the study was approved by an institutional ethics committee? Multicentre studies pose special problems, especially if the analysis is performed by a group that has a vested interest in the outcome of the study.

FURTHER READING

Aickin M, Gensler H. 1996: Adjusting for multiple testing when reporting research results: the Bonferroni vs Holm methods. *American Journal of Public Health* 86, 726–8.

Armitage P, Berry G. 1994: *Statistical methods in medical research*, 3rd edn. Oxford: Blackwell Science.

Bailor JC. 1997: The promise and problems of meta-analysis. *New England Journal of Medicine* 337, 559–61.

Begg C, Cho M, Eastwood S *et al.* 1996: Improving the quality of reporting of randomized controlled trials: the CONSORT statement. *Journal of the American Medical Association* 276, 637–9.

Friedman LM, Furberg CD, DeMets DL. 1995: *Fundamentals of clinical trials*, 3rd edn. Boston, MA: John Wright.

Hall JC, Mills B, Nguyen H, Hall JL. 1996: Methodologic standards in surgical trials. *Surgery* 119, 466–72.

Motulsky H. 1995: *Intuitive biostatistics*. Oxford: Oxford University Press.

Sackett DL, Rosenberg WMC, Gray JAM, Haynes RB, Richardson WS. 1996: Evidence-based medicine: what it is and what it isn't. *British Medical Journal* 312: 71–2.

Siegel S, Castellan NJ. 1988: *Nonparametric statistics for the behavioral sciences*, 2nd edn. New York: McGraw-Hill.

Walter SD. 1995: Methods of reporting statistical results from medical research studies. *American Journal of Epidemiology* 141, 896–906.

Chapter 25

Trauma

Ian Civil, Michael Rodgers, Michael Hulme-Moir, James Hamill, Michael Muller and Peter Freeman

Introduction

Trauma is one of the most common causes of death and disability throughout the world. Among the younger population it outranks all other causes in industrialized nations, and is the third most common cause after cardiovascular disease and cancer in the older population. Unlike most other areas of clinical practice, trauma patients often have to be treated on the basis of the signs that are evident, without a definitive diagnosis being made. This chapter outlines the common causes of injury, the early treatment strategies, and some guidelines for the management of specific problems.

OVERVIEW AND ORGANIZATION OF TRAUMA SERVICES

Although active promotion of injury prevention strategies will reduce the incidence of accidental and self-inflicted injuries, a significant number of patients suffering the effects of some form of externally applied force will continue to present for medical care. The appropriate environment in which this care should be provided is a *trauma system* (Figure 25.1).

A trauma system embraces the whole spectrum of injury, from trivial to catastrophic, and functions from the moment of injury until the full potential from re-habilitation has been achieved. The trauma system is the framework in which institutions and individuals provide care within a broad geographical area.

The trauma system consists of all those elements which interact with the injured person throughout the continuum of care. Thus it includes:

- prehospital care;

- hospital care (emergency department, intensive care and definitive surgical and medical care);

- rehabilitation.

Within a trauma care system there is stratification of care. Broadly speaking, more complex and advanced services are required to care for patients with major or more complex injuries. The capability of any given location of care can be classified according to its resources. Throughout the world there is a range of systems to classify trauma care locations. Some are descriptive (e.g. major urban trauma service), and some are numerical (e.g. Level 1 trauma centre). Patients are also categorized according to their injuries, with a range of triage criteria being used to determine whether a patient has a 'major' or less severe injury. The premise underpinning this categorization and that of the facilities is the importance of getting the right patient to the right hospital.

It is also implicit in a trauma system that the injured patient will be transported to hospital 'at the right time'. Trauma is one of a small group of acute conditions that can be described as 'time-critical'. This means that there is a time imperative in the assessment of the patient, with swift institution of resuscitation and management of life-threatening conditions.

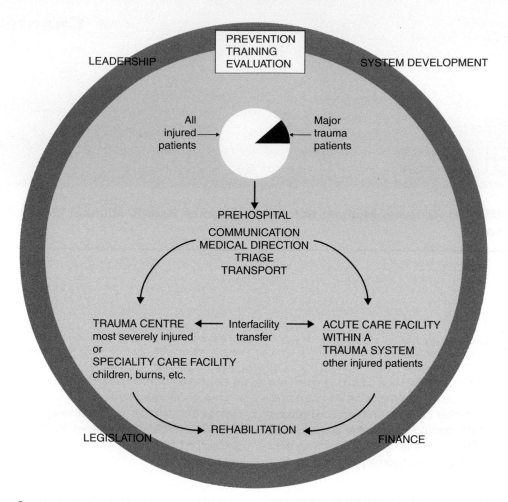

Figure 25.1 Components of an inclusive trauma care system.

PREHOSPITAL CARE

Prehospital care is a fundamental component of the system of care, and it is the process by which an injured patient enters and first interacts with the trauma system.

While most prehospital care will be provided by ambulance personnel, the participation of medical practitioners in this process is both desirable and necessary.

An effective and efficient prehospital care service ensures that patients are treated promptly and appropriately. Essential elements of such a service include the following:

- ready access by the public via the use of a well-known single emergency telephone number. Calling a single number, such as 111, should immediately put the caller on line to an experienced prehospital care provider who can interpret the request for assistance, and who is familiar with the vehicles and personnel available to respond;

- prompt dispatch and arrival of appropriately trained and staffed prehospital care resources, including ambulances with two crew members;

- ready and immediate communication between the providers of prehospital emergency care and the hospital to which the patient is being transported;

- clinical outcome and peer review of the process of prehospital care.

TRIAGE

Once a basic assessment of a patient's injuries has been made, it is possible to undertake a triage process. Depending on the triage assessment, the patient may need to be transported by the most rapid means available to the most specialized hospital, or may be safely taken by the most readily available vehicle to the nearest hospital. Broadly speaking, there are three forms of triage, based on mechanism of injury, physiology or nature of injuries.

Mechanism of injury criteria

The mechanism of injury should always be taken into account when considering the potential for serious injury. Patients may be identified because the mechanism of the injury that they sustained means they have a high probability of harbouring occult severe injury. In particular the following mechanisms, which imply high energy transfer, should trigger very careful evaluation of the patient:

- vehicle crash at over 60 km/h;
- major deformation of the vehicle;
- fatal injury in the same vehicle;
- ejection from the vehicle;
- unrestrained child in a motor vehicle crash;
- cyclist or pedestrian hit by a vehicle travelling at over 30 km/h;
- a fall from a height of over 5 m;
- any mechanism causing injuries to multiple body regions.

Physiological criteria

Physiological triage is based on the present state of vital signs of the patient. It thus categorizes patients according to the immediate threat to life. This is usually appropriate in the field, as it is simply performed and requires no investigative process.

Prehospital care providers can assess vital signs and level of consciousness, including the following:

- respiratory distress – less than 10 or more than 30 breaths/min and/or cyanosis;
- systolic blood pressure less than 90 mmHg or pulse greater than 130 beats/min;
- difficulty in arousal, or falling level of consciousness.

If any of the above criteria are met, the patient should be regarded as having potentially major trauma with immediate threat to life, and should be taken directly to a facility identified as having the capability for stabilizing or definitively managing severe trauma.

In children the same general principles apply. However, physiological criteria must be considered in the context of both the age and the physical size of the child. The Paediatric Trauma Score (PTS) is one triage tool which uses both physiological and anatomical criteria to identify severe injury. A PTS of < 8 identifies the subset of paediatric trauma victims with severe injury, including those with the highest potential for preventable morbidity and mortality.

Anatomical criteria

Specific injuries or injury complexes signify that major forces have been involved and that there is potential threat to life. These are not usually apparent in the field, and this form of triage has particular relevance when the patient is being assessed at the first hospital.

Some specific injuries are apparent in the field, and patients with these injuries should be transferred to the most advanced hospital. Examples include the following:

- penetrating injury to head, neck, chest, abdomen, perineum or back;
- head injury with coma, a dilated pupil, open head injury or severe facial injury;
- chest injury with flail segment or subcutaneous emphysema;
- abdominal injury with distension and/or rigidity;
- spinal injury with weakness and/or sensory loss;
- limb injury involving vascular injury with ischaemia of the limb, amputation, crush injury of the limb or trunk, or bilateral fractures of the femur;
- burns, partial or full thickness, more than 20% in adults or 10% in children.

If any of these anatomical factors are recognized, the patient should be transferred to a facility with the capability for dealing not only with these problems but also with the likely associated injuries.

HOSPITAL CARE

In-hospital management of the injured patient requires integration of all aspects of the delivery of care. This includes ready availability of relevant specialists and a smooth transition between the emergency department, operating room, ICU and other sites at which care is delivered. Procedures must exist for the co-ordination of the various surgical and non-surgical specialists, not only in the initial assessment and early definitive care phases, but also in the intensive-care units and surgical wards. Such co-ordination has the potential to improve outcomes, facilitate early rehabilitation, minimize the length of stay in hospital and optimize the use of other hospital resources.

A critical element in matching health-care resources to severity of injury is the ability to categorize hospitals and other location-based providers of injury care according to their capabilities. This process has been undertaken in many countries and has resulted in a description of 'levels of care'. One of the principles underlying such categorization is that any given facility should receive enough trauma patients to be able to maintain the skills, experience and expertise of both the staff and the system.

TRAUMA CENTRES

Hospitals categorized according to their ability to provide trauma care are known in some areas of the world as 'trauma centres'. This term applies not only to the most advanced level of care, but also to every facility that has organized its services to deal with injured patients within its capability.

TRAUMA TEAMS

Integral to the ability to provide care for the trauma patient is an organized response when the patient arrives in hospital. This response is often called a 'trauma team' and, depending on the type of trauma centre, it may involve just a few people or many (Figure 25.2). The smallest trauma team consists of a doctor with knowledge of resuscitation techniques, a nurse, and an orderly, clerk or other form of assistant. In more advanced centres the trauma team may consist of the following types of personnel:

- medical – surgeon, anaesthetist, emergency physician;
- nursing – up to three nurses;
- radiographer;
- laboratory technician;
- orderly – porter.

All members of the team should be aware of when they are on call, and should be available immediately. Advanced warning of the impending arrival of a major trauma case should be a prearranged system with the ambulance service. One member of the team should be designated the team leader. His or her responsibility is to ensure the smooth running of resuscitation by delegating appropriately with regard to the tasks to be performed.

THE TRAUMA SERVICE

While all of the elements of hospital care already mentioned deliver care to injured patients, none of them necessarily integrates the care of the patient between services and between locations of care. All injured patients, especially those with multiple or severe injuries, have requirements which span numerous physical locations and many personnel. Optimal care is provided when all of these resources are matched with the patient's needs. This task can be complex, and requires both experience and knowledge of injury care and the available resources. The key person is usually known as a trauma co-ordinator.

A trauma service must have medical leadership, and the director of a trauma service may be a surgeon or another specialist with expertise in the management of injured patients. In order to ensure that patients are managed according to Advance Trauma Life Support (ATLS®) guidelines, a quality assurance process must be in place. In general this is achieved by regular educational meetings between trauma care providers, with discussion of broad trauma care areas or specific cases. Most trauma services strongly encourage participating doctors to have undertaken an ATLS® course.

DATA SYSTEMS

For a trauma service and trauma system to work effectively, information must be collected about the number of injured patients managed, the nature of their injuries, the process of care and the outcome. These data are essential for resource allocation, for developing and evaluating trauma services and for clinical audit.

A number of data collection models are possible, ranging from a national minimum data set on injury to detailed epidemiological register-based data sets (e.g. the American College of Surgeons Major Trauma Outcome Study, MTOS). A range of commercially available software programs is available which incorporate relevant data fields together with a computerized injury severity calculation facility. Certain clinical indicators which flag potential preventable morbidity or mortality (e.g. delays to surgery for intracavitary haemorrhage) may be highlighted by registry programmes.

SUMMARY

Optimal trauma care requires prompt accurate assessment and provision of a level of care that is matched to the patient's needs. A trauma system provides this

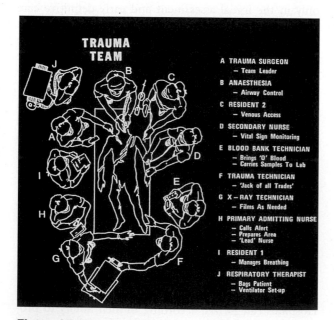

Figure 25.2 Typical trauma team in a US Level 1 trauma centre.

response. States and regions have trauma committees who are responsible for ensuring adequate integration of the various components of the trauma system. Although a trauma system consists of a range of clinical care providers, their excellence alone is not sufficient to ensure adequate overall management. Unless their efforts are co-ordinated, the ultimate result may be inadequate care. The trauma service co-ordinates the overall delivery of care.

EPIDEMIOLOGY AND MECHANISM OF INJURY OF THE TRAUMATIZED PATIENT

Trauma is a common phenomenon. In a typical New Zealand metropolitan hospital, 15% of admissions are trauma related. Much of this is not major trauma, with only 16% of patients having an Injury Severity Score (ISS) of ≥ 16. None the less, it accounts for a very significant consumption of resources.

Trauma is also a significant cause of mortality. Causes of death in New Zealand are summarized in Table 25.1. As can be seen, trauma is a significant cause of death overall, and particularly in the younger age group.

Trauma is the third most common cause of death in all age groups, and it is the leading cause of death in the age group under 45 years. Approximately 60% of the deaths in this age group are trauma related, and males are over-represented, with about 72% of the trauma-related deaths occurring in men.

Motor vehicle accidents account for 45% of trauma-related deaths in New Zealand. The trend is for a decrease in road fatalities overall. Changing social perceptions about drinking and driving, and intense campaigns to increase public awareness of alcohol-related accidents have contributed to this. Again, young males predominate, constituting 67% of the total. The type of vehicle may also be implicated – motorcycles are associated with a higher fatality rate per crash. Various car manufacturers offer assurance that their vehicles are safer. Interestingly, the large four-wheel drive vehicles, although safer in the perceptions of many, are associated with high rates of accident but not of fatality in many areas of New Zealand.

Who sustains significant trauma in Australasia? Young aggressive males are most at risk of suffering traumatic injuries in our society. A combination of natural recklessness, an attraction to high-risk activity and a tendency to combine such activities with recreational drugs all contribute to this phenomenon. The male: female ratio of patients suffering significant trauma (ISS of ≥ 16) is 3:1 in a trauma registry maintained at a typical metropolitan hospital in New Zealand.

In recent years there has been a trend for women to become better represented in the trauma statistics. It is speculated that this may be a result of women indulging in more high-risk activities, including sports.

Mechanisms of injury

There are various ways of classifying trauma, but the most common starting point is penetrating vs. blunt

Table 25.1 Age-standardized death rates in New Zealand per 100 000 population

Year	IHD M	IHD F	Cancer M	Cancer F	CVD M	CVD F	Unintentional trauma* M	Unintentional trauma* F	Suicide M	Suicide F	RTC M	RTC F
1987	219	103	171	128	52	50	54	16	32	7	35	15
1988	204	95	173	125	51	45	48	19	21	5	32	10
1989	195	89	171	129	50	45	49	17	21	–	–	–
1990	181	87	170	129	46	44	50	20	20	5	31	12
1991	173	84	168	129	46	43	45	18	21	5	26	11
1992	181	82	173	118	47	42	–	–	23	5	26	11
1993	167	81	178	127	45	44	–	–	19	5	25	10
1994	157	75	167	121	44	39	–	–	24	5	25	12
1995	158	72	168	127	42	38	–	–	23	6	23	11
1996	150	69	162	125	40	36	–	–	22	6	17	15

Source: Mortality and Demographic Data 1990–1999 New Zealand Information Service.

*Unintentional trauma includes RTC in those years it is specified.

CVD, cerebrovascular disease; IHD, ischaemic heart disease; RTC, road traffic crash.

trauma. In Australasia, blunt trauma (e.g. car crash, fall, blunt weapon) is the most common form. Conversely, in North America and South Africa the high numbers of guns available account for a steady stream of devastating penetrating trauma. In these regions the injured patients bear many similarities to those injured in military conflicts. Other forms of trauma include thermal injury and blast injury.

This classification can then be subdivided into more specific subgroups depending on the exact mechanism. In Australia and New Zealand the mechanism of injury is heavily weighted in favour of blunt trauma and motor vehicles. The frequency of motor vehicle-related fatality has decreased somewhat in the last decade, but has remained fairly constant in recent years. The correlation with alcohol is well known, with one-third of car crashes being associated with alcohol.

Falls are a common cause of admission for trauma. The elderly are particularly at risk and suffer a high mortality rate, with those over the age of 75 years having a 12-fold higher risk of death from a fall compared to younger patients.

Homicide is a relatively uncommon cause of traumatic death, with rates of 0.3 per 100 000 in New Zealand. This is in marked contrast to the USA, where rates from 8–9 per 100 000 are the standard each year. In the USA there is also marked racial variation, with murder being the 14th most common cause of death among whites, but the fifth most common cause among blacks.

Suicide is a cause of death that may often go under-reported, with some car crashes, falls and house fires being attributed to accident. While women have a higher rate of parasuicidal behaviour, men have higher rates of successfully completing suicide. New Zealand has the unfortunate distinction of having one of the highest youth suicide rates in the world.

PATTERNS OF INJURY

When a patient with trauma first presents, certain factors relating to the nature of the injury may raise clinical suspicion and direct certain paths of investigation. These factors include the following:

- factors in the history;
- the mechanism of injury;
- the speed involved;
- the direction of energy transfer;
- associated injuries.

It is important to obtain as clear a story as possible about the circumstances of the injury. Several clues in the history should alert one to both the type of injury to expect and the probable severity of it. As discussed in the section on triage, a number of clues may suggest a more serious injury when at first glance the situation appears minor. These include the history of a death at the scene, ejection of the patient from a moving vehicle, major damage to the vehicle, including damage to the steering wheel in the case of the driver and a smashed windscreen in a patient with facial injuries, prolonged extraction

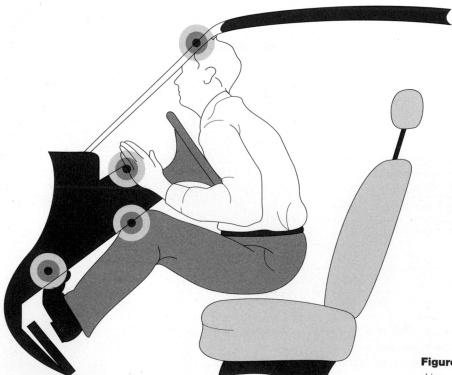

Figure 25.3 Frontal impact, unrestrained driver.

time, and the use of intoxicants. These clues are particularly important in the case of a young adult who may compensate physiologically but have serious underlying injury. It must also be borne in mind that the elderly, although exposed to less major trauma than the young, are much more likely to die from it. A number of studies have shown that the rate of fatality for trauma in those over the age of 70 years is fourfold higher than that of their younger counterparts with the same ISS. The young tend to bend and the elderly to break. However, young people, particularly children, may suffer a surprising amount of underlying visceral damage while maintaining their bony integrity.

The mechanism of injury may be penetrating, blunt, blast or thermal. With penetrating injury, the direction of the penetrating object must be ascertained and, in particular, which body cavity has been entered. It is also vital to establish the trajectory of a bullet and its final location as determined on X-ray. The calibre, velocity and type of ammunition used in gunshot wounds may give clues to the expected severity of injury.

Blunt injury, particularly in a road traffic crash (RTC), can result in four different types of injury. First, direct impact applies a crushing or compressing force to the body, and this is the major transference of energy. Secondly, the victim may sustain injury from striking body parts against the interior of the vehicle (face to windscreen, seatbelt injury, etc.). Thirdly, mobile internal organs may strike their hard bony containers (classically this is the brain against the cranium in a contra-coup injury, but it may also occur with the heart and other mobile internal organs). Finally, deceleration forces may cause tearing of organs as a relatively mobile part of an organ moves on a relatively immobile one. This classically occurs at descending thoracic aorta, but also at the duodenal-jejunal junction, renal pedicle, ligamentum teres, C7–T1 junction (accounting for 25% of C-spine injury in road traffic crashes) and at a microscopic level with diffuse axonal brain injury.

Specific activities are associated with particular injuries. The neck injury in the rugby scrum, the head injury from a 'spear' tackle, the wrist injury from the outstretched fall, and the Achilles tendon rupture from sudden jumping, as in netball, are well-known sporting injuries. The pedestrian struck by a car is known to be at risk from a triad of injuries involving the lower leg, head and wrists as they are struck, hit the bonnet of the car and then fall to the ground, respectively. Head injury occurs in one-third of bicycle-related injuries and is directly related to 85% of the fatalities. Some of the common road traffic crash injury patterns are listed in Table 25.2.

The speed of the injury is the key determinant of the energy imparted to the casualty's body. This may be reflected in the velocity of the bullet, the height of the fall

Table 25.2 Correlations between the mechanism of trauma and certain injury patterns

Mechanism	Injuries
Unrestrained driver, frontal impact	Head injury (windshield)
	Maxillofacial fractures
	Cervical spine fracture
	Thoracic injury (steering column)
	Liver, spleen, duodenum and small-bowel injury
	Pelvic fracture
	Posterior dislocation of the hip
	Tibia, fibula and femoral fractures
Rear impact	Head injury
	Cervical spine fracture
Direct blow to abdomen ('handlebar injury')	Duodenal rupture
	Pancreatic transection
Direct blow to flank or back	Renal injury
Straddle	Anterior urethral injury
Pedestrian vs. car	Tibia and fibula fracture (bumper)
	Thoracic injury (car bonnet)
	Head injury (as patient hits the ground)
Fall on to feet	Calcaneal fracture
	Femoral neck fracture
	Anterior vertebral compression fracture
	Avulsion of abdominal viscera
Fall on to torso	Head injury
	Cervical spine fracture
	Pulmonary contusion
	Thoracic aortic rupture
	Pelvic fracture

or the speed of the moving car. Kinetic energy is directly related to the mass involved, but is related to the square of the velocity, and this is why speed is the key factor. This is responsible for such statistics as the risk of death in a road traffic crash doubling with an increase in speed from 50 to 70 km/h.

The direction of energy transfer is best thought of as a wave of force spreading out from the point of impact and dissipating as it spreads out. In the case of a bullet, this wave is perpetuated along the entire tract of the bullet. As a result of this dissipation of force, those structures closest to the point of impact receive the highest energy and are the most damaged. Hence information about the location of the patient in the vehicle and the point of impact on the car is extremely important. The use of a seatbelt is also a clue as to likely injury, and has now been conclusively shown to decrease the risk of death overall by 75%.

In a road traffic crash, four main patterns of injury can be described in relation to the direction of impact. Direct frontal impact carries the highest mortality rate, probably as head-to-head collision results in the highest combined speeds and the highest energy transference. The pattern of injury (Figure 25.3) may involve fracture/dislocation of the ankle, knee dislocation or posterior dislocation of the hip. Head impact on the windscreen and chest impact on the steering wheel complete the picture. The degree of injury will be related to the total energy transfer. Rear impact is relatively safe in relation to overall injury severity, but is particularly likely to result in soft-tissue and ligamentous cervical spine injury. Lateral impacts cause injury of varying severity depending on whether the impact is to the left or the right, and whether or not the occupant is immediately adjacent to the striking force. A typical right-sided impact into the driver's side may well cause a head injury, flail chest, liver laceration, fractured pelvis and ipsilateral femur fracture to an occupant on the right hand-side of the vehicle.

SEVERITY OF TRAUMA AND TRAUMA SCORING

The severity of trauma is clearly as relevant as the raw number of patients presenting. This is a key determinant of resource consumption. It is also highly relevant to the level of trauma care required in a particular area, and to the type of specialist equipment and staff allocated to a particular centre. Figure 25.4 illustrates some of the estimated costs for a given severity of injury (based on the Abbreviated Injury Severity Score).

In the 1980s there was much debate about the need for specialist trauma centres and whether such expensive 'state of the art' care was cost-effective, or indeed simply whether it was better than standard care. Much autopsy data was accumulated showing 'preventable' deaths at non-specialist centres. Of course there was debate about the comparisons that were made. This was one factor in the development of scoring systems for assessing trauma severity. Such systems are necessary both for comparing different centres and for determining the effectiveness of new interventions and strategies. Scoring systems may be useful primarily for research, or may be used for triaging. They may be based on physiological parameters (e.g. APACHE II and the Revised Trauma Score), or they may be based on the anatomical description of injuries (e.g. ISS).

Injury Severity Score

The most widely used scoring system is the Injury Severity Score (ISS). This is an anatomical scale based on scores being given to each of the injuries which are shown to be present in an individual patient. Injuries are graded on a scale from 1 to 6, where 1 = trivial injury and 6 = unsurvivable. The ISS is then composed of the sum of the squares of the three highest individual scores for injuries to six body regions (the head and neck, face, thorax, abdomen and pelvis, extremities, and external). The maximum possible score is 75, and an individual score of 6 is automatically credited with an ISS of 75.

For example, a multiple trauma might be scored as follows:

Minor liver laceration	2
Haemothorax	3
Grade IIIc compound tibia	3
Fractured jaw	2

$$ISS = 2^2 + 3^2 + 3^2 = 22.$$

Using such a scoring system, it is possible to check its validity in predicting outcome, e.g. mortality. Figure 25.5 shows the mortality rates for particular scores in US data.

Figure 25.6 shows the range of ISS based on the Auckland Hospital data accumulated over a 3-year period and including over 5000 patients.

Revised Trauma Score

Another function of scoring systems is the rapid and consistent communication of information concerning a patient's status. A simple example is the Ambulance

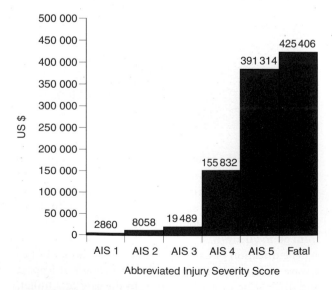

Figure 25.4 Costs per injury in the USA in 1989.

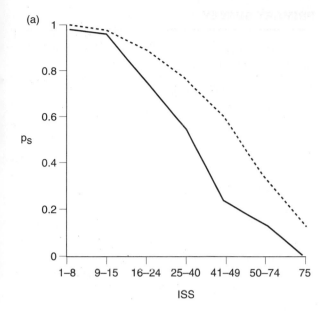

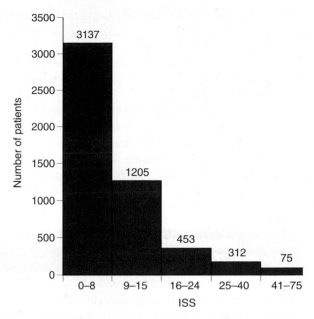

Figure 25.6 ISS breakdown based on data from over 5000 patients over a 3-year period.

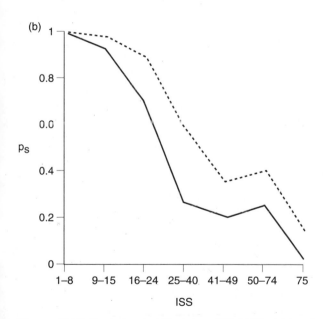

Figure 25.5 Survival probability (p_s) vs. ISS. (a) Blunt-injured patients. (b) Penetrating-injured patients. ——, younger than 55 years; ----- 55 years or over. Feliciano DV, Moore EE, Mattox KL (eds). 1996: *Trauma* 3rd edn. Stanford, CT: Appleton & Lange, p. 56.

Service's assignment of a status number when they radio the hospital, with status 1 indicating cardiopulmonary resuscitation (CPR) in progress, status 2 indicating instability, status 3 indicating the potential to become unstable and status 4 being stable (usually minor injury).

A commonly used field triage system for medical staff is the Revised Trauma Score. This uses three key para-

meters, namely the Glasgow Coma Scale (GCS), respiratory rate and systolic blood pressure. It has been shown to be reasonably accurate in predicting severity and outcome for serious head injury and trauma in general, and it can be used as a research tool. Table 25.3 shows how the score is calculated.

APACHE II (Acute Physiology And Chronic Health Evaluation)

This system is based on 12 physiological parameters (temperature, mean blood pressure, heart rate,

Table 25.3 Revised Trauma Score (triage)

Parameter	Variables	Score
Respiratory rate	10–29	4
(breaths/min)	> 29	3
	6–9	2
	1–5	1
	0	0
Systolic blood pressure	> 90	4
(mmHg)	75–90	3
	50–75	2
	< 50	1
	0	0
GCS	13–15	4
	9–12	3
	6–8	2
	4–5	1
	3	0

respiratory rate, alveolar–arterial (A–a) gradient, arterial pH, serum Na^+ and K^+, creatinine concentration, haematocrit, white cell count and GCS). It is used as a research tool, primarily in the intensive-care setting, to predict outcome and to stratify patients for assessment of therapeutic manoeuvres.

Generally speaking APACHE II is not considered to be particularly useful in the trauma setting, perhaps because it is too blunt an instrument and does not really give injury-specific information. However, it is used to compare trauma patients with other intensive-care patients.

INITIAL MANAGEMENT OF THE ACUTELY TRAUMATIZED PATIENT

This section on the early management of trauma deals with the initial assessment and management of trauma victims within the 'golden hour'. While this chapter deals mainly with in-hospital practice, the basic principles apply anywhere that early management of trauma is performed. Some of the causes of death that occur in the first few minutes after an accident are not treatable. However, this is not the case with the majority of conditions that require diagnosis and treatment in the 'golden hour'. Many of these conditions are easily treated, often with spectacular results. A systematic sequential approach to the initial assessment will help to minimize the misdiagnosis of potentially fatal but treatable conditions. It follows that the aims of the initial assessment and management of trauma victims are as follows:

- to diagnose life-threatening conditions;
- to stabilize and/or treat these conditions;
- to initiate a secondary survey, laboratory and radiological investigations and/or specialist referral.

The initial rapid part of the assessment and management of trauma is known as the primary survey. Once the primary survey is complete, the next phase is the secondary survey, during which the patient is examined from head to toe. Appropriate investigations and referrals are then initiated. If at any stage the patient becomes unstable, attention must immediately be directed back to the basics of the primary survey.

In order to help create a logical approach to the primary survey, one needs to remember that people will die sooner of some conditions than of others. For example, respiratory obstruction is a terminal event within a few minutes, while this is seldom true for haemorrhage. This enables one to create a sequence of priorities that require attention during the primary survey. The approach to be outlined in this text is as follows.

PRIMARY SURVEY

The points to cover in the primary survey are usefully summed up by ABCDE.

- A for airway management with cervical spine control.
- B for breathing.
- C for circulation and control of haemorrhage.
- D for disability.
- E for exposure and temperature control.

If during the primary survey the patient appears to deteriorate, then it may be necessary to return to the beginning of the assessment to make sure nothing has been missed or has changed. Each of these topics will be considered in more detail, examining the life-threatening conditions that may be encountered and how to assess and manage them.

Airway

Assessment of the airway starts when the patient arrives in the Emergency Department. A person who can talk freely is unlikely to have significant airway obstruction, but this situation may change rapidly. Major facial injury, swelling, subcutaneous emphysema, burns, depressed level of consciousness and stridor are all indications for rapidly securing an airway. It is a mistake to attribute confusion or agitation to alcohol or drugs before establishing that the patient is not hypoxic.

Management of potential or existing airway compromise starts with simple manoeuvres, and progresses to more complex procedures, ending with intubation or surgical airway. In all cases one needs to protect the cervical spine with in-line traction or a stiff cervical collar. It is imperative to avoid hyperextension, hyperflexion and rotation of the neck until the cervical spine is cleared. All patients should be given high-flow oxygen at the rate of at least 10 L/min. As a first step, the patient's mouth needs to be cleared of debris/secretions and the tongue pulled forward. A chin lift or jaw thrust will open the upper airway and facilitate respiration. If further support is needed, an oropharangeal or nasopharangeal airway can be inserted. Care needs to taken when inserting a nasopharangeal airway, as significant damage can be inflicted if too much force is used.

In certain circumstances a definitive airway is essential. This may be either an endotracheal tube or a surgical airway. Briefly, the indications can be divided into two broad groups, namely those patients who cannot be ventilated without a definitive airway and those who are at risk of obstructing or aspirating due to their injuries. The first group includes patients with apnoea, and severe head, neck and facial injuries. Cases that are at risk of obstructing include facial burns, depressed levels of consciousness and patients who are vomiting. Trauma intubation is not an easy undertaking, and should preferably not be attempted by inexperienced personnel.

Occasionally intubation is not possible, and in this situation a surgical airway is required. Almost without exception the appropriate technique is the cricothyroidotomy. After fixing the trachea between the fingers and thumb of the left hand, the notch between the thyroid and cricoid cartilages is palpated with the right forefinger. A stab incision is then made through all layers into the trachea. By rotating the blade through 90° the incision is enlarged enough to slip a curved haemostat into the opening. This is used to dilate the opening to allow insertion of a small cuffed endotracheal tube (size 5 to 6) or a small tracheostomy tube. This technique is not recommended in children under the age of 12 years. An alternative to cricothyroidotomy is jet insufflation of the airway. This technique utilizes a percutaneous cannula of a large calibre inserted into the upper airway. High-flow oxygen is provided by way of plastic tubing (15 L/min), and insufflation is provided for 1 s alternating with 4 s without. Oxygenation can be maintained for a maximum of 30–40 min.

Breathing

Assessment of the patient's respiratory status is the next step, after their airway is secure. After establishing that the trachea is central, the chest must be examined. Particular attention should be paid to respiratory rate, chest movement and obvious chest injuries. Subcutaneous emphysema is usually a marker of significant underlying injury. Rib fractures can be palpated or occasionally seen when a flail segment is present. Percussion and auscultation help to assess the presence or absence of equal air entry. Cyanosis of the lips or fingertips is an ominous sign and reflects hypoxaemia at a cellular level for whatever reason. Pulse oximetry is a very useful adjunct to clinical assessment, although it has its limitations.

A number of injuries can interfere with a patient's ability to breathe. In the context of trauma, tension and simple pneumothorax must be looked for and treated appropriately. The cardinal signs of a tension pneumothorax include distended neck veins, tracheal deviation to the normal side, hyper-resonance, decreased breath sounds, tachypnoea and hypotension. Fractured ribs with or without internal injury are very painful and will prevent adequate chest movement. Compound and sucking chest wounds require an occlusive dressing while the underlying pneumo/haemothorax is treated. A large haemothorax may interfere with a patient's breathing as well as being a cause of hypovolaemia. This problem might be suggested by hypovolaemia combined with decreased breath sounds and dullness to percussion. Towards the end of the primary survey it is routine to obtain a trauma series of X-rays. This will include a supine chest film which will pick up potentially life-threatening problems that may have been missed clinically.

The management of breathing difficulties during the primary survey will be focused on the specific cause. As mentioned above, all patients should first have a secure airway and be receiving high-flow oxygen. If a tension pneumothorax is suspected, the first step is the immediate insertion of a 16-G cannula into the chest via the second intercostal space in the midclavicular line. The hissing of air under tension confirms the diagnosis and can be followed by the insertion of an intercostal drain. As mentioned above, open wounds require dressings with or without intercostal drains. Occasionally the injuries sustained by an individual to their chest are such that they require intubation and mechanical ventilation. This would be the case for major chest wall damage, including large flail segments.

Circulation

Assessment of the circulatory status of a trauma victim should focus on the question of whether or not they are in shock. Shock is the inadequate tissue oxygenation and organ perfusion that results from a defect in circulation. It manifests as a whole host of non-specific signs, and can be multifactorial in origin. It is worth considering the basics of circulatory physiology, as this will help to clarify shock management.

Cardiac output is determined by heart rate and stroke volume. Stroke volume in turn is determined by preload, afterload and the contractility of the myocardium. Broadly speaking, the venous return to the heart is the preload. This is determined by venous capacitance, intravascular volume and the pressure differential between the right atrium and the venous compartment. Starling's law relates the length of the myocardial fibres to their contractility. Myocardial fibre length is determined by the volume of venous return at the end of diastole. The peripheral resistance to forward flow equates to the afterload. Adults have approximately 70 mL/kg (ideal body weight) of blood in circulation, which corresponds to 5 L of blood in a 70-kg man.

The physiological responses to haemorrhage are compensatory mechanisms which attempt to maintain circulation. Heart rate increases to maintain cardiac output. Selective vasoconstriction leads to preferential perfusion of vital organs such as the brain, kidneys and heart. This occurs at the expense of blood flow to the viscera, peripheries and musculature. Associated with the increase in peripheral resistance is an increase in the diastolic pressure, leading to a reduced pulse pressure (i.e. the difference between systolic and diastolic pressures). A whole host of vasoactive hormones, including the catecholamines, bradykinin, histamine and other cytokines, are released into the circulation.

At a cellular level the metabolism switches from aerobic to anaerobic metabolism. This generates lactic acid as a by-product, with a resulting metabolic acidosis. In time the homeostatic mechanisms that maintain cell membrane integrity fail. With the loss of membrane integrity, the electrical gradients in turn fail, and sodium and water enter the cell, causing swelling and eventual cell death. The combination of this process and release of vasoactive hormones leads to leaky capillaries. Toxic metabolites from anaerobic metabolism also exacerbate this problem, the net result of which is tissue oedema.

Shock is manifested in a number of ways and can be caused by several different mechanisms. Depending on the degree of shock, different symptoms and signs will be more or less evident. It follows that in the trauma situation one needs to have a low threshold to diagnose and treat shock. The commonest cause of shock in trauma victims is haemorrhage, but the other causes must be considered and treated. These include cardiogenic shock, shock due to a tension pneumothorax, septic shock and neurogenic shock. Cardiogenic shock can arise from myocardial contusion, ischaemia, embolus (fat or air) and tamponade. Beck's triad of muffled heart sounds, hypotension and engorged neck veins is a useful indication of cardiac tamponade. Some or all of the signs may be absent, and if tamponade is suspected then it is better to perform pericardiocentesis 'on spec'. Acute cardiac enzymes seldom alter the acute management of a trauma patient. However, ECGs are a useful adjunct to the clinical examination during a primary survey.

Neurogenic shock is characterized by hypotension without tachycardia and cool peripheries. It is caused by loss of sympathetic tone following transection of the spinal cord. As with all forms of non-haemorrhagic shock, it can coexist with true hypovolaemia due to bleeding. Septic shock is caused by established sepsis, often due to Gram-negative organisms. It is not seen that often in the context of acute trauma. Delayed presentation of trauma victims, especially those with penetrating injuries to the abdomen, is one situation in which it may be encountered. Tension pneumothorax has already been covered in the preceding section.

The early signs of shock are cutaneous vasoconstriction and tachycardia. Pulse rates over 100/min in an adult are abnormal and must not be attributed to pain until shock has been excluded or treated. Tachypnoea is another early sign of shock and is not necessarily due to respiratory distress. As the degree of shock progresses the patient becomes more anxious, confused, then lethargic and finally unrousable. A drop in systolic blood pressure is an ominous sign suggesting significant blood loss. Up to 30% of the total blood volume can be lost without any drop in systolic pressure. Before this occurs the patient's pulse pressure will drop as their diastolic pressure rises in response to peripheral vasoconstriction. All trauma victims require assessment of their urine output. Urethral catherization should only be performed after adequate assessment of the patient's urethra. Volumes of less than 0.5 mL/kg/h of urine suggest hypovolaemia.

Occasionally patients are seen who do not respond to shock in a normal way. People on beta-blockers will not develop the normal tachycardia seen in the early stages of shock. This may also occur in an otherwise normal older patient. Also found in older people are pacemakers which may prevent a normal response to haemorrhage. Athletes tend to have lower resting pulse rates and blood pressures. They can also compensate for larger volumes of blood loss, and may not manifest any signs until they are critically hypovolaemic. Pregnancy causes profound circulatory changes, the most notable being the increased maternal blood volume. Hypothermic patients will not respond to fluid resuscitation as a normal person would. They are also predisposed to developing coagulopathies. Finally, haemoglobin and haematocrit are not reliable indicators of blood loss in the early post-trauma period.

The management of shock in the context of the primary survey consists of volume replacement and control of external haemorrhage. Actively bleeding wounds require a quick inspection and then the use of pressure to control ongoing blood loss. Splinting of long-bone fractures reduces both bleeding and pain. After ensuring that the patient's airway and breathing are secure, vascular access is obtained with at least two large IV cannulae. At a minimum, 16-G cannulae should be used. Good access can usually be obtained in the antecubital fossa or forearm. If this fails, then large-calibre central lines need to be inserted into the jugular, femoral and/or subclavian veins. An alternative to central line placement is the use of venous cut-down techniques. In this situation, the long saphenous vein is exposed 2 cm above and anterior to the medial malleolus. It is then tied off distally and a large-calibre cannula is inserted into the vein for fluid infusion. At the same time that vascular access is obtained, it is important to take blood for chemistry, haematology and cross-matching. Pregnancy tests and toxicology analysis can also be performed on the same sample.

Several ancillary procedures form part of the initial management of shock. ECGs and pulse oximetry are fairly standard in most resuscitation rooms. Nasogastric or orogastric tubes should be passed in all trauma patients unless there is a compelling reason not to do so. Untreated gastric dilatation can alter the way in which a patient responds to otherwise appropriate treatment. Catheterization of the bladder is also essential in order to monitor urine output in response to treatment. Care must be taken in cases where urethral injury is suspected. Central venous monitoring can be a helpful adjunct to clinical assessment.

Fluid resuscitation forms the backbone of shock management. In the first instance a warm isotonic solution such as normal saline or Ringer's lactate is used. A bolus dose of 1–2 L is given rapidly and the patient's haemodynamic status is then reassessed. For every 1 mL of blood lost, approximately 3 mL of fluid replacement will be required. However, it can be difficult to assess true blood loss accurately, and ongoing monitoring of the response to fluid is more helpful. Persistent tachycardia, hypotension, cool peripheries or low urine output suggest inadequate treatment. This may be due to ongoing bleeding or another cause of the patient's shocked state.

The bottom line in shock management is that the underlying cause for the shock must be fixed. Patients who respond to the initial resuscitation rapidly and then remain stable are likely to have lost less than 20% of their blood volume. If they have no further losses, they will only require maintenance fluid replacement. Others will respond transiently, suggesting that their initial volume replacement was inadequate or that they have ongoing losses. Blood should be made available and used if they remain unstable. A small group of patients will show no response to the initial resuscitation. These people have usually sustained losses of more than 40% of their circulating volume and urgently require blood. It is highly likely that they have ongoing losses, and urgent surgical intervention is required to stop this. As mentioned above, it is imperative not to forget that another cause for their shock is possible.

Disability

Assessment of the patient's neurological status is an essential component of the primary survey. Once their airway, breathing and circulation are under control, their level of consciousness and pupils need to be examined. The gold standard is the Glasgow Coma Scale (GCS), which scores the patient with respect to three variables, namely vocal ability, pupillary function and motor function (Table 25.4). In the case of the GCS assessment it is important to use the best score obtained initially. As with any clinical examination, ongoing assessment is essential to detect improvement and deterioration. A score of ≤ 8 is regarded as a definition of coma or severe head injury. Scores of 9 to 13 are classified as moderate head injuries, and scores of 14 and 15 as minor head injuries.

Changes in the level of consciousness in a trauma patient may be due to direct head injury or to alterations in their cardiac or respiratory systems. Abnormalities should lead to immediate assessment of the patient's

Table 25.4 Glasgow Coma Scale (GCS)

Assessment area	Score
Eye opening	
Eyes open spontaneously	4
Eyes open to voice	3
Eyes open to pain	2
Eyes do not open	1
Vocalization	
Oriented	5
Confused conversation	4
Inappropriate words	3
Incomprehensible sounds	2
No sounds	1
Movement	
Obeys commands	6
Localizes pain	5
Withdrawal to pain (normal flexor response)	4
Abnormal flexion to pain (decorticate response)	3
Extensor response to pain (decerebrate response)	2
No movement	1

oxygenation. If this appears to be adequate, then the status of their circulation should be checked. Once these two areas are stable, then alcohol, drugs and blood glucose can be investigated. In cases where alterations of consciousness have occurred and head injury is suspected, CT scans and/or neurosurgical referral may be indicated. Two important factors that help to prevent ongoing brain injury are adequate oxygenation and maintenance of adequate blood pressures.

Exposure and temperature control

Complete exposure of trauma patients is mandatory, and this is the bridge to the secondary survey. The patient's clothing is removed in such a way as to avoid further injury. This means protecting the cervical spine and any injured limbs, and is usually accomplished by cutting clothing off. In the process of fully exposing the patient they must not be allowed to become hypothermic. Not only do patients often arrive hypothermic, but many of our therapeutic measures can exacerbate their low body temperatures. Massive transfusion of cool solutions and exposure of the patient for protracted examination will certainly drop their temperature further. Warmed solutions or blood-warming devices can help in this situation. Warm blankets, prompt removal of wet clothing and a warm ambient temperature are other simple effective measures that must be taken. Measurement of core body temperature via rectal or oesophageal probes is the most accurate technique.

Hypothermia needs to be reversed because of its

detrimental effects on many normal physiological functions. The coagulation cascade and platelet aggregation are adversely affected by hypothermia. Shocked patients will not respond as well to appropriate therapeutic measures if they are hypothermic. Peripheral vasodilatation associated with excess alcohol consumption can lead to profound hypothermia in trauma patients. CNS function will also be adversely affected.

SECONDARY SURVEY

At the end of the primary survey the patient will either be in need of an urgent life-saving intervention or stable enough for a secondary survey. This is an exhaustive top-to-toe examination of the patient looking for all injuries. It must include re-evaluation of all the vital signs and a return to the ABCs if the patient deteriorates. An adequate history, including medications, allergies, past medical history, last food and the events of the accident itself, must be taken. Hidden areas such as the back and the perineum must be examined. An old dictum suggests that tubes and fingers need to be inserted into every orifice. This is the time when extra investigations such as diagnostic peritoneal lavage, X-rays and CT scans are performed. Detailed legible documentation is essential, and will be very helpful in any future medico-legal investigations.

In order to avoid missing anything, it is worth running through a set list of areas to be examined during the secondary survey. The following is based on that suggested by the ATLS® manual.

Head and skull

This must include the scalp, skull, eyes and maxillofacial structures. Cranial nerves need to be formally examined in some situations. Mid-face fractures mandate orogastric as opposed to nasogastric intubation.

Cervical spine and neck

Protect the cervical spine until fractures have been excluded by a combination of clinical and radiological examination. Tenderness and crepitus should be looked for as well as swelling, bruising and/or lacerations. Penetrating injuries require surgical referral. Auscultation of the carotids may reveal unexpected bruits from vessel wall damage.

Chest

Much of this examination is conducted during the primary survey but needs to be repeated. Palpation of the entire chest wall is important to look for occult fractures. Chest X-rays and ECGs are carried out if not performed already. A high index of suspicion is required in order not to miss significant intra-thoracic injuries.

Abdomen

Like the chest, significant injuries can exist with very few external signs. Penetrating abdominal injury mandates laparotomy in most centres. In cases where blunt trauma is present the situation is more complex. Patients fall into two groups, namely those who are conscious and alert and can thus be assessed by repeated clinical examination, and those who for one reason or another cannot be assessed clinically. These can be divided into two further groups, namely those who are stable and can be safely CT-scanned, and those who are unstable and require an urgent laparotomy or a diagnostic peritoneal lavage (DPL). Ultrasonography is being used more frequently as a baseline investigation to look for free intraperitoneal fluid. The reasons why clinical assessment may be inadequate include depressed levels of consciousness, pelvic fractures, spinal injuries and lower rib fractures. In cases where unexplained hypotension is a problem, the abdomen must be cleared by more than just a clinical examination.

No abdominal examination is complete without a thorough inspection of the perineum. In males the genitalia need to be examined for signs of urethral injury such as meatal bleeding and scrotal bruising. This is completed by a rectal examination to look for normal tone, PR blood and a high-riding prostate. It is often easiest to perform the rectal examination while the patient is log-rolled. Females do not sustain the same degree of urethral injury but still require both rectal and vaginal examination. At some stage their pregnancy status needs to be established with a urine or serum βHCG.

Musculoskeletal examination

Soft-tissue and bony injuries are often forgotten in the rush of a trauma resuscitation. Detailed inspection, palpation, tests of function and appropriate radiology are utilized to detect these injuries. Excessive palpation and stressing of possible pelvic fractures will hurt patients unnecessarily and possibly cause bleeding. All patients must be log-rolled to allow a complete inspection and palpation of their backs.

Neurology

The GCS should be repeated as part of this examination. Head injuries are often unstable and deterioration may necessitate early CT and neurosurgical intervention. Spinal cord injuries must be recognized and, at the very least, lead to immobilization of the patient. Peripheral nerve injuries are usually associated with lacerations, but closed fractures can also lead to severe injury.

Table 25.5 Summary of principles of early trauma management

Primary survey
  Airways with cervical spine control
  Breathing
  Circulation and control of external bleeding
  Disability
  Exposure without hypothermia

Adjuncts to the primary survey
  Trauma views, chest X-ray, lateral cervical spine and
    pelvis
  Urinary catheter and gastric tube
  Blood and urine tests including cross-match and
    pregnancy test
  Other diagnostic tests, such as DPL
  Monitoring

Secondary survey
  Head and scalp
  Neck and cervical spine
  Chest
  Abdomen and perineum
  Musculoskeletal
  Neurology

Adjuncts to the secondary survey
  CT scan
  Contrast radiology
  Echocardiography
  Specialist referral

Extras

If this has not already been done, insert a gastric drainage tube and a urinary catheter. CT scans are often required at this stage. Contrast studies of the genito-urinary system may be required if urethral injury is suspected. Arteriography is helpful in cases where vascular injury is suspected, or as therapy for pelvic bleeding. Occasionally echocardiography is useful in cases of suspected cardiac injury.

SUMMARY

The early assessment of trauma lends itself to a systematic approach. This consists of a primary survey consisting of ABCDE (see above) and a secondary survey in which the patient is examined from top to toe. A team approach is the most efficient way to manage severe trauma. Team members must have clearly defined roles prior to the arrival of the trauma patient.

DEFINITIVE CARE OF TRAUMA

After the primary survey, resuscitation, history, secondary survey and appropriate investigations, one or more diagnoses will have been made. The treatment of these injuries is based on a knowledge of the relevant anatomy, physiology and the available treatment modalities. The appropriate management of some injuries can follow any of a variety of pathways depending on the patient's state, and for this reason the decision tree for managing these injuries will be presented in algorithm form. What follows is a brief outline of the pertinent features of the history, examination, anatomy, physiology and management of injuries in seven major body regions, namely the head, neck, thorax, abdomen, pelvis, spine and extremities.

HEAD

Head injury occurs as either a primary or secondary event, and primary head injury may be blunt or penetrating. The three main patterns of blunt primary head injury are direct contusion, contra-coup contusion and diffuse axonal injury (DAI). A fourth mechanism is compression (e.g. when the head is crushed under a car), but while this may cause cranial nerve palsies, it is rare for it to result in brain injury. Following the primary survey and history, a brief neurological examination is performed, the essentials of which are the Glasgow Coma Scale (GCS), pupil size and response, and motor responses of the extremities. The cranium consists of the scalp, skull and intracranial contents. The layers of the scalp are remembered by the mnemonic 'SCALP' – skin, subcutaneous tissue, aponeurosis, loose areolar tissue

---

BOX 25.1 INDICATORS OF AN INCREASED RISK OF A SIGNIFICANT INTRACRANIAL LESION IN A PATIENT WITH APPARENTLY MILD HEAD INJURY

Penetrating head injury
Moderate to severe headache
Amnesia
History of loss of consciousness
Deteriorating level of consciousness
Alcohol or drug intoxication
CSF leak, rhinorrhoea or otorrhoea
Abnormal CT scan
No CT scanner available
Skull fracture
Significant associated injuries
No reliable companion at home
Unable to return to hospital (or medical facility) promptly

and periosteum ('pericranium'). A scalp injury can result in significant blood loss, especially in children, because of its rich vascular supply. Scalping injuries occur in the loose areolar plane.

Skull fractures of the vault can be classified as linear, comminuted or depressed. Depression greater than the thickness of the skull may require surgical elevation in an attempt to avoid secondary epilepsy. Both vault and basal skull fractures can also be classified as open or closed. The term 'open' or 'compound' skull fracture specifically refers to a fracture in which the dura is torn. The fracture can be externally open (associated with a scalp laceration) or internally open (a basal skull fracture into a sinus). An open basal skull fracture may be associated with cerebrospinal fluid (CSF) leakage, and may predispose to infection of the central nervous system. However, prophylactic antibiotics for basal skull fracture patients have now been shown to be ineffective. The clinical signs of a basal skull fracture include periorbital haematoma ('racoon eyes'), post-auricular ecchymosis (Battle's sign), CSF leakage and facial nerve palsy.

The primary goal in the management of the patient with a significant head injury is to prevent secondary brain injury, which may result from systemic or local events. Adverse systemic events include hypotension and hypoxia. A single hypotensive episode in a head-injured patient significantly increases morbidity and mortality. Local factors include raised intracranial pressure (secondary to brain swelling and intracranial haematomas), ischaemia and brain shifts.

The four types of intracranial haematoma are extradural, subdural, subarachnoid and intracerebral. Extradural haematomas arise from the bleeding from meningeal arteries which run between the periosteum and the dura. Subdural haematomas arise from bleeding from the bridging veins that cross the subdural space. The midbrain (containing the corticospinal tract) and the occulomotor nerve (cranial nerve III) pass through the incisure in the tentorium. Brain swelling or an intracranial haematoma may cause herniation of the uncus of the temporal lobe through the incisure (tentorial herniation), resulting in an ipsilateral fixed dilated pupil (third nerve palsy) and contralateral arm and leg weakness (corticospinal tract compression). Compression or ischaemia of the brainstem results in a decreased level of consciousness, hypertension and bradycardia (Cushing's response), and eventually death.

Because the intracerebral contents are contained in a solid 'box' – the skull – the total volume, usually composed of brain, cerebrospinal fluid (CSF) and blood, must remain constant. This is the basis of the Monro-Kellie principle, which states that in the presence of an expanding mass (oedematous brain or intracranial haematoma), an equal volume of CSF or venous blood must be squeezed out of the 'box' to maintain the same

intracranial pressure (ICP). When this compensatory mechanism is overcome, ICP begins to rise exponentially. ICP is normally about 10 mmHg, and an ICP of 20 mmHg is definitely abnormal and should be treated. The treatment modalities for raised ICP are medical and surgical (evacuation of intracerebral mass lesions). Medical modalities include hyperventilation to a $PaCO_2$ of 30–35 mmHg to cause mild intracerebral vasoconstriction, mannitol (1 g/kg) in the case of patients with localizing signs prior to CT and theatre, hypertonic saline to reduce cerebral oedema, and sedatives to reduce the cerebral metabolic rate.

Cerebral blood flow (CBF) is related to cerebral perfusion pressure (CPP) and cerebral vascular resistance (CVR), such that CBF = CPP/CVR. CPP is related to mean arterial pressure (MAP) and intracranial pressure, such that CPP = MAP − ICP. In the presence of raised ICP, CBF is maintained by ensuring a MAP with the judicious use of fluids and vasopressors.

NECK

The patient who is exsanguinating from a major vascular injury to the neck requires emergency surgery. The portion of the neck between the cricoid cartilage and the hyoid bone (zone 2; Figure 25.7) is easily accessible surgically, and all wounds deep to the platysma in this region should be explored without further investigation (Figure 25.8). Wounds in zone 3, between the clavicles and the cricoid, may involve the great vessels at the thoracic inlet (brachiocephalic, subclavian, carotid, vertebral, etc.), and require a thoracic incision for proximal control. Vascular injuries in zone 1, between the hyoid

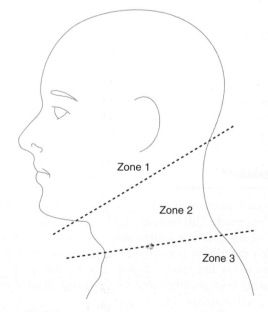

Figure 25.7 Location of the three zones of the neck.

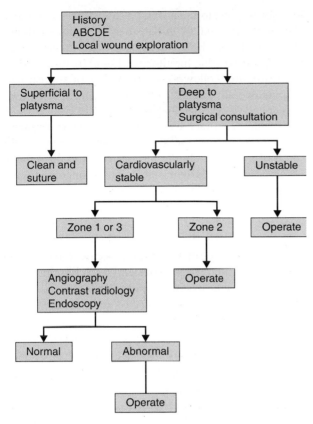

Figure 25.8 Management of penetrating injury to the neck.

Table 25.6 Correlation of chest X-ray findings with internal injuries

Radiographic finding	Association
Fractured rib 1, 2 or 3 Sternoclavicular fracture or dislocation	Airway or great vessel injury
Fractured left lower ribs 9–12	Splenic injury
Fractured right lower ribs 9–12	Liver injury
Two or more rib fractures in two or more places	Flail chest and pulmonary contusion
Scapular fracture	Brachial plexus injury Pulmonary contusion Great vessel injury
Sternal fracture	Cardiac contusion
Widened mediastinum	Aortic arch rupture
Mediastinal air	Oesophageal injury Tracheal injury
Gastrointestinal gas in chest	Ruptured diaphragm
Nasogastric tube in chest	Ruptured diaphragm or oesophageal rupture

bone and the base of the skull, can be difficult to access surgically. If the stability of the patient allows, wounds in zones 1 and 3 should be carefully investigated with angiography, contrast swallow, bronchoscopy and/or oesophagoscopy as appropriate. A surgical procedure can then be performed in a carefully planned manner.

THORAX

The thorax is commonly injured in blunt and penetrating trauma. The mechanism of injury, as ascertained from the history, can provide important clues about the presence of more serious internal injuries (Table 25.6). A chest X-ray should be obtained in all patients.

Indications for the insertion of a chest (thoracostomy) tube in trauma include the presence of a pneumothorax, significant haemothorax, any penetrating chest wound, and selected patients with suspected severe lung injury who will be undergoing positive pressure ventilation or are to be transferred to another hospital by ground or air.

Rib fractures in themselves may cause severe pain, which inhibits coughing and deep breathing. This leads to atelectasis and pneumonia. The keys to treatment are adequate analgesia and chest physiotherapy. Two or more rib fractures in two or more places result in a flail

segment of chest wall. A large flail segment may result from an unrestrained driver's chest impacting on the steering column during a head-on collision, or passenger compartment intrusion impacting on the occupant's lateral chest during a side impact ('T-bone') collision. A large flail segment interferes with respiration in three ways. The mechanical 'bellow' action of the chest wall is impaired, severe pain causes splinting of the muscles of ventilation, and the associated pulmonary contusion interferes with gas exchange. In addition to providing analgesia (often a thoracic epidural is the best option) and physiotherapy, intubation and ventilation are sometimes required to provide adequate ventilation.

A simple pneumothorax may interfere with ventilation by increasing the intrathoracic pressure (normal intrathoracic pressure is −2 to −6 mmHg) and by allowing lung to collapse. A ventilation–perfusion (V/Q) mismatch occurs, causing a physiological right-to-left shunt and systemic hypoxia. A tension pneumothorax develops if a lung leak with a one-way valve effect forces air into the pleural space. A simple pneumothorax may be converted into a tension pneumothorax, especially during positive pressure ventilation or air transport. Both the ipsilateral and contralateral lungs are compressed, the mediastinum is displaced to the contralateral side, the venous return to the heart via the superior and inferior vena cava is reduced, and cardiac output falls. The clinical signs are a pentad, namely respiratory distress, shock, distended neck veins, trachea deviated to the contralateral side, and ipsilateral hyper-resonance and absent breath sounds. Treatment is by emergency needle thoracocentesis using an over-the-needle catheter, followed by insertion of a chest tube.

Open pneumothorax is a life-threatening condition. If the opening in the chest wall is more than two-thirds the diameter of the trachea, air preferentially passes through the chest wall. Ventilation is then impaired, resulting in hypoxia and hypercarbia. Treatment is by the application of an occlusive dressing taped on three sides to provide a flutter-valve effect, chest-tube insertion at a site away from the wound, and surgical repair of the defect.

Tracheobronchial tree injury is usually fatal at the scene, and patients who make it to the hospital have a high mortality from associated injuries. The diagnosis is suggested by haemoptysis, subcutaneous emphysema and a persistent large air leak from the chest tube. Confirmation is by bronchoscopy, and treatment is by surgical repair.

Pulmonary contusion is a common and potentially lethal injury. In adults it is usually associated with rib fractures, but in children the compliant chest wall may transmit large forces to the lungs, resulting in severe pulmonary contusion without rib fracture. Respiratory failure may develop insidiously. Management consists of careful monitoring, ventilatory support as required, the avoidance of fluid overload and the treatment of associated medical conditions.

Myocardial contusion should be suspected in the blunt trauma patient with a sternal fracture. It may cause hypotension, electrocardiographic changes (unexplained sinus tachycardia, atrial fibrillation, premature ventricular contractions, bundle-branch block and ST changes) and wall motion abnormalities on echocardiography. These must be distinguished from ischaemic changes. The patient should undergo continuous cardiac monitoring for 24 h because of the risk of arrhythmias.

Cardiac tamponade is usually the result of penetrating trauma involving the heart, coronary vessels or roots of the great vessels. However, it can also follow blunt trauma. Clinically the diagnosis is suggested by Beck's triad, namely hypotension, raised jugular venous pressure and muffled heart sounds. Pulsus paradoxus, the normal rise in systolic blood pressure on expiration, is abnormally raised to higher than 10 mmHg. A rise in venous pressure with inspiration (Kussmaul's sign) is a true paradoxical sign associated with cardiac tamponade. The condition may present with pulseless electrical activity (PEA). In practice, in the trauma scenario these signs may be either absent or difficult to elicit. Transthoracic echocardiography or focused abdominal ultrasonography may help to confirm the diagnosis. However, a high index of suspicion in the patient who does not respond to the normal resuscitative measures is all that is required to initiate needle thoracocentesis, which may be both diagnostic and therapeutic. Electrocardiographic monitoring should be used during the procedure. Following confirmation of the cardiac tamponade, all patients require surgery to expose, inspect and, if necessary, repair the heart.

Internal mammary artery, intercostal artery or penetrating lung injuries may cause a significant haemothorax. A thoracotomy should be considered in the patient who is cardiovascularly unstable, has an ongoing transfusion requirement, drains 1500 mL of blood initially from the chest tube, or continues to drain over 200 mL of blood per hour for 2–4 h.

Traumatic aortic rupture is a relatively common cause of death at the scene of a road traffic accident or fall from a great height. In those patients who reach hospital alive, the rupture is almost invariably contained within a sac of adventitia or pleura. If unsuspected and untreated, 80% of the remaining patients die each day. The diagnosis is made on a high index of suspicion based on the mechanism of injury, suggestive findings on chest X-ray and the findings of an arch aortogram. Treatment is by surgical repair.

BOX 25.2 SIGNS OF AORTIC DISRUPTION ON CHEST X-RAY

Widened mediastinum > 8 cm
Depressed left main bronchus
Obliteration of aortic knob
Deviation of oesophagus (NGT) or trachea (ETT) to right
Left apical haematoma
Double contour to the aorta
Fractured ribs 1 or 2
Multiple left rib fractures
Fractured scapula or sternum

ABDOMEN

The abdomen consists of the peritoneal cavity, retroperitoneum and pelvis. The peritoneal cavity is further subdivided into upper (thoracic) and lower (abdominal) regions. The upper abdomen extends from the level of the dome of the diaphragm, which reaches the fourth intercostal space in full expiration, to the costal margin. It contains the diaphragm, liver, gall-bladder, spleen, stomach, part of the duodenum (most of it being retroperitoneal) and transverse colon. The abdominal cavity contains the small bowel and sigmoid colon. The retroperitoneum contains the aorta, inferior vena cava, kidneys, ureters, duodenum, pancreas, and ascending and descending colon. The pelvis contains the pelvic and sacral plexuses, iliac vessels, rectum, bladder and female

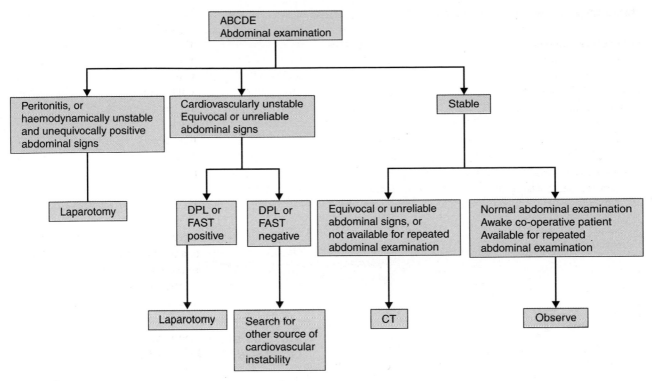

Figure 25.9 Abdominal evaluation in the blunt trauma patient. DPL, diagnostic peritoneal lavage; FAST, focused abdominal sonogram for trauma.

internal genitalia. In order to evaluate the abdomen completely, the thorax, abdomen (inspection, palpation, percussion and auscultation), pelvis (perineum, genital, vaginal and rectal examination) and back must be examined (Figure 25.9).

The management of stab wounds to the abdomen or thorax below the level of the nipples (fourth intercostal space) is outlined in Figure 25.10.

Laparoscopy is not sensitive for the diagnosis of bowel or retroperitoneal injuries. For this reason, the role of laparoscopy is limited to diagnosing peritoneal penetration, which in turn mandates laparotomy. The danger of pneumoperitoneum in the presence of an undiagnosed diaphragmatic laceration is the development of a tension pneumothorax, or rarely a tension pneumopericardium. For this reason a chest tube must be in place in all penetrating chest injuries.

Gunshot wounds to the abdomen are treated by laparotomy. This includes wounds to the flank, back and buttock, which may result in retroperitoneal colorectal injuries that may be fatal if not detected and treated early.

PELVIS

Pelvic fractures are generally the result of blunt trauma. The history of the mechanism of injury may indicate the

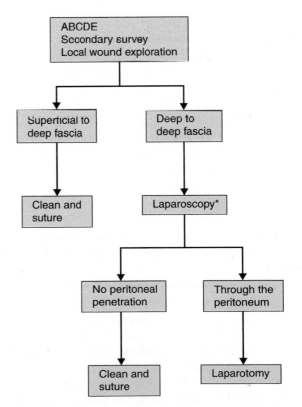

Figure 25.10 Management of penetrating lower chest or abdominal stab wounds. *Chest tube *in situ* for all chest injuries.

Table 25.7 Classification of major pelvic fractures and associated injuries

Fracture pattern	Mechanism	Associated injuries
AP compression		
Open book	Crush	Pelvic vascular injury
	Road traffic crash,	Multi-organ injuries
	especially motorcycle or pedestrian	
Straddle		Anterior urethral injury
Lateral compression		
Anterior and posterior	Crush	
Miscellaneous	Road traffic crash	Multi-organ injuries
	Fall from a height	
Vertical shear	Road traffic accident,	Multi-organ injuries
	especially motorcycle or high-speed car	
	Fall from a height	

likely fracture pattern and possible associated injuries (Table 25.7). During the examination, each anterior superior iliac spine is gently grasped and rotated medially to detect mechanical pelvic instability. This manoeuvre is performed only once because it can dislodge clot and lead to further bleeding into the pelvic haematoma. The external genitalia, perineum and buttocks are examined. It is essential to perform rectal and vaginal examinations to detect rectal or vaginal laceration. The management of the multitrauma patient who has been shown to have a pelvic fracture on the routine pelvic X-ray (one of the three standard 'trauma views') is outlined in Figure 25.11.

Early review by an orthopaedic surgeon is essential, especially in AP compression and vertical shear injuries in which early pelvic reduction and stabilization can help to tamponade the pelvic haematoma and significantly reduce transfusion requirements. Exsanguinating haemorrhage may result from pelvic vascular injury, especially in AP compression fractures. Angiography with embolization of bleeding arteries is an extremely useful treatment modality in the treatment of these patients.

SPINE

A knowledge of the mechanism of trauma is extremely useful in detecting the multitrauma patient with a spinal injury, especially if unconscious. Any patient involved in a high-energy collision should be immobilized on the suspicion of a spinal injury. The presence of a head injury or any injury above the clavicles raises the suspicion of a cervical spinal injury. The presence of arthritic changes in the spine (especially rheumatoid arthritis or ankylosing spondylitis) increases the likelihood of cord damage.

BOX 25.3 GUIDELINES FOR READING THE LATERAL CERVICAL SPINE X-RAY

Adequacy*
Vertical lines
  Soft-tissue line
  Retropharyngeal space ≤ 6 mm
  Retrotracheal space ≤ 22 mm in adults, ≤ 14 mm in children
  Anterior vertebral body line
  Anterior spinal canal line
  Posterior spinal canal line
  Tips of the spinous processes

Odontoid peg
Alignment
Atlanto-odontoid gap ≤ 2.5 mm in adults, ≤ 4 mm in children
Each vertebra
Body
Disk
Pedicle
Facets
Lamina
Spinous process

*An adequate lateral cervical spine X-ray will have imaged C1–T1.

The objectives of the physical examination during the secondary survey are to detect the presence of a fracture, the presence of any neurological defect, its sensory and motor level, and whether it is a complete or incomplete cord injury. The spine is inspected and palpated during the log-roll, noting tender areas, skin markings,

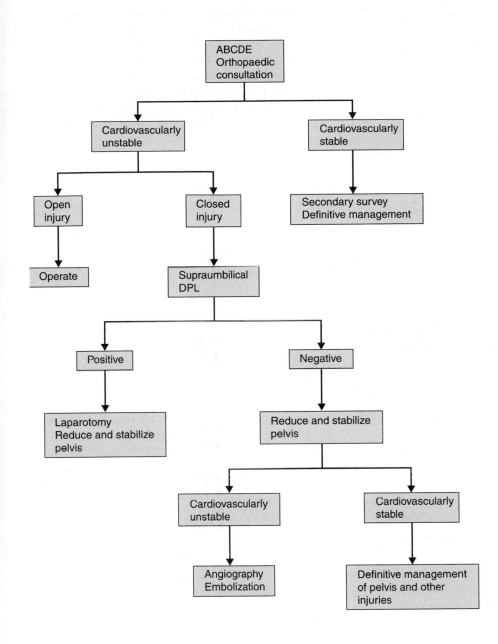

Figure 25.11
Management of the trauma patient with a fractured pelvis. DPL, diagnostic peritoneal lavage.

swellings and deformities. Sensory testing begins at the head and progresses downwards. Arm and leg movements to command, or in response to pain in the uncooperative patient, are noted. Perineal sensation must be examined because sacral sparing may be the only indication of an incomplete injury. Rectal examination for tonic and voluntary anal sphincter tone is performed. Priapism is an uncommon but important sign, indicating spinal shock. The lateral cervical spine X-ray is one of the three standard 'trauma views'.

If there is clinical suspicion of a thoracic or lumbar spine fracture, a 'shoot-through' lateral thoracolumbar spine X-ray can be taken in the resuscitation room at the same time as the other three views. The management of

the trauma patient's cervical spine is outlined in Figure 25.12.

The aims of treatment in the spine-injured patient are primarily to avoid further cord damage. Together with the ABCs of resuscitation, the spine is immobilized using a semi-rigid collar, spinal board and straps, to avoid causing mechanical damage to the cord. Fluid resuscitation is instituted, as with any trauma patient, in order to maintain organ perfusion. The patient with a neurological defect should be considered for treatment with methylprednisolone, which may improve neurological outcome by preventing secondary injury. Treatment should be instituted within 8 h, and in consultation with an orthopaedic or spinal surgeon.

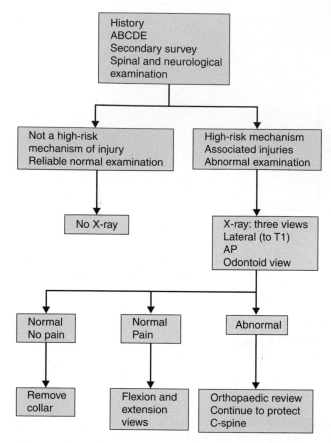

Figure 25.12 Management of the cervical spine in trauma.

EXTREMITIES

Fractures of the extremities are present in over 50% of all patients admitted for trauma, and in 35% of all severely injured patients (those with an injury severity score of > 15). Certain injury patterns should be borne in mind:

- frontal-impact road traffic crash and fractured ankle, knee injury, femoral fracture and posterior hip dislocation;

- pedestrian vs. car and fractured tibia, fibula, and upper extremity fractures;

- fall from a height and calcaneal fracture, femoral neck and anterior vertebral compression fracture.

A history inconsistent with the injury may indicate a pathological fracture or non-accidental injury. The time of injury and degree of contamination are particularly important for determining the management of open fractures.

During the primary survey, management of the circulation may include the control of external bleeding from extremity injuries, using direct pressure or occasionally the judicious use of a pneumatic tourniquet. The use of a tourniquet will mandate urgent transfer to the operating room for definitive treatment of the vascular injury.

During the secondary survey, extremity injuries are assessed using the standard examination technique of 'look, feel, move' and neurovascular assessment. Open wounds are inspected but not probed, and a sterile dressing is applied. Fractures are aligned and immobilized using either a plaster of Paris cast or a commercially available splint. Dislocated joints may be relocated by an experienced medical attendant, or immobilized until surgical relocation is performed.

Peripheral vascular injuries may be the result of blunt or penetrating trauma. Since muscle necrosis occurs after 6 h of warm ischaemia, prompt diagnosis is paramount. 'Hard' signs of vascular injury include the following:

- pulsatile bleeding;

- expanding haematoma;

- palpable thrill;

- audible bruit;

- evidence of regional ischaemia (pain, pallor, poikilothermia, paraesthesia, paralysis, pulselessness).

Positive 'hard' signs of vascular injury are an indication for urgent surgical exploration with either pre-operative or on-table angiography. 'Soft' signs include the following:

- history of haemorrhage;

- injury in proximity to a major artery (e.g. dislocated knee);

- diminished but palpable peripheral pulses;

- peripheral nerve deficits.

These indicate a need for further evaluation using ankle-brachial index measurements, duplex ultrasonography or angiography.

Compartment syndrome is the ischaemia caused within a body compartment by either increased pressure from within (e.g. following revascularization or after a crush injury) or by constriction from without (e.g. by tight bandages or casts). The long-term result of compartment syndrome is Volkmann's ischaemic contracture. The cardinal signs are severe pain exacerbated by passive stretch of the muscle group involved, paraesthesias, loss of sensation, and a tense swelling. Loss of a peripheral pulse is a late sign. Compartment pressures over 35–45 mmHg are sufficient to reduce capillary blood flow and cause compartment syndrome. Treatment involves the immediate release of any constricting dressings or casts, and fasciotomy (incision of the fascia that envelops the involved compartment).

SUMMARY

The management of injuries in seven body regions has been presented. Emphasis should be placed on rapid diagnosis based on the history and examination, the efficient use of appropriate investigations, early consultation with specialty services, and development of a treatment plan that will minimize morbidity and the risk of mortality for the patient.

BURNS

Modern burn care involves prompt attention to respiratory support, fluid resuscitation, wound care and excision, nutritional supplementation, adequate pain management, intensive physical therapy and proactive scar management, and emotional and psychological support in specialized units where a team of interested professionals can deliver all of these diverse aspects of care in a co-ordinated manner. Patients treated in burn centres are more likely to survive, and their treatment is cost-efficient. The Australian and New Zealand Burn Association (ANZBA) guidelines for referral to a Burns Centre are listed in Box 25.4.

The management of a severely burned patient is complex, but can be simplified by following a sequence of priorities in exactly the same way as for any other injured patient.

INHALATION INJURY

Airway obstruction and systemic intoxication are the most immediate life-threatening conditions found in burn patients. Victims who are 'overcome by smoke' at

---

BOX 25.4 ANZBA GUIDELINES FOR REFERRAL TO A BURNS CENTRE

- Burns greater than 10% of total body surface area (TBSA)
- Burns of special areas – face, hands, feet, genitalia, perineum and major joints
- Full-thickness burns greater than 5% of TBSA
- Electrical burns
- Chemical burns
- Burns with an associated inhalation injury
- Circumferential burns of the limbs or chest
- Burns at the extremes of age – children and the elderly
- Burn injury in patients with pre-existing medical disorders which could complicate management, prolong recovery or affect mortality
- Any burn patient with associated trauma

---

the scene of a fire have usually succumbed to carbon monoxide poisoning or asphyxiation. Carbon monoxide has a 240-fold higher affinity for haemoglobin than oxygen, leading to hypoxia. Carboxyhaemoglobin levels greater than 10–15% are abnormal, with neurological dysfunction developing at levels greater than 15–20%. Loss of consciousness is usual at levels in the range 40–60%, and death or brain injury is common with > 60% levels of carboxyhaemoglobin. Cyanide poisoning can also occur. Treatment of systemic intoxication is by delivery of 100% oxygen, which in patients whose carboxyhaemoglobin levels are > 20% is best achieved by intubation and mechanical ventilation. The classic 'cherry-red' colour of the skin in cases of carbon monoxide poisoning is in fact uncommon. Therefore this condition needs to be excluded by measuring carboxyhaemoglobin levels in any patient who has been in a confined space with smoke/flames present.

Supralaryngeal injury is due to inhalation of hot gases which do not pass the vocal cords. The upper airway is actually burned. A history of being burned in a confined space, such as a structural fire or a burning car, burns of the head and neck, burned nasal hairs and lips, soot in the mouth, redness or blistering of the posterior pharynx, stridor, hoarse or weak voice and brassy cough are all indicators of the possibility of an airway injury (see Plates 25.1 and 25.2 in the colour plate section).

As airway obstruction only ever gets worse due to oedema, early endotracheal intubation is wise. If any doubt exists about the continued patency of the airway, and certainly prior to transfer, intubate.

Infra-laryngeal inhalation injury is associated with an increase in mortality by up to 20% among the severely burned. The products of combustion dissolve in the lower airways to form acids and aldehydes which, together with soot, lead to tracheobronchitis. Bronchoscopy will often establish the presence and severity of inhalation injury. Ventilation–perfusion radioisotope scanning is indicated for patients in whom clinical suspicion remains following negative bronchoscopy. Tracheobronchitis leads to cast formation from aggregation of sloughed mucosa and inflammatory exudates. This in turn leads to atelectasis, pneumonia and air trapping. This is especially prevalent in small airways such as the terminal bronchioles. Neutrophil and pulmonary macrophage actuation leads to increased pulmonary endothelial permeability and susceptibility to the development of pulmonary oedema. Treatment includes warmed, humidified supplemental oxygen, vigorous chest physiotherapy, incentive spirometry, early aggressive antimicrobial treatment of pulmonary sepsis when it develops at about day 5 to 7, and ventilatory support as needed for respiratory failure. Oxygen saturation monitoring with pulse oximetry, regular blood gas analysis, daily chest X-ray and frequent sputum microbiology is indicated. Nebulized heparin (5000 units in 3 mL of saline) every 4 h loosens secretions and decreases cast formation, with a subsequent improvement in pulmonary function. The presence of an inhalation injury indicates the need for an additional 50% volume of resuscitation fluid.

BURN SHOCK

Circulatory collapse is the next life-threatening condition following burn injury, and it develops within hours without fluid resuscitation. The burn wound initially causes microvascular changes in its immediate vicinity, and then more generally as a result of elaboration of inflammatory mediators. These microvascular changes include increased negativity of interstitial hydrostatic pressure due to denaturation of collagen, and a decrease in the osmotic reflection coefficient, which leads to increased permeability to plasma proteins. Histamine causes an increase in pore size in post-capillary venules. This alteration in capillary endothelial integrity leads to a phenomenon usually known as permeability oedema. This process becomes widespread as a result of elaboration of vasoactive substances from the burn wound when the burn size is larger than 25% of total body surface area (TBSA). Naturally, increasing burn size increases the severity of the response. In addition to histamine, arachidonic acid metabolites – thromboxane A2 and leukotriene, platelet-activating factor, substance P and oxygen radicals – superoxide anion O_2^-, hydrogen peroxide (H_2O_2) and the hydroxyl ion OH^-, all play a role. Oedema formation peaks between 8–12 h post burn in smaller burns and 12–24 h in large burns, and then diminishes as capillary integrity is restored.

Increased systemic and pulmonary vascular resistance that follows the release of huge amounts of catecholamines together with angiotensin II, antidiuretic hormone and neuropeptide Y can lead to right heart overload and left–right ventricular desynchronization. Myocardial depression, probably due to oxygen-radical-mediated myocyte dysfunction, is seen in some patients with very large burns in whom fluid resuscitation is delayed. It is known that in burns involving > 30% TBSA, there is a systemic decrease in cellular transmembrane potential due to a decrease in sodium ATPase activity and a consequent increase in intracellular sodium levels. This effect is partially reversed by adequate fluid resuscitation.

Clinical and experimental studies have addressed the type of fluid and volume required to resuscitate a burn patient successfully. These studies have established that during the early post-burn period the type of fluid used (crystalloid or colloid) did not affect changes in plasma volume. However, after 24 h post-burn, colloid fluid

infusion was more effective in increasing plasma volume. This coincides with the restoration of capillary integrity. Furthermore, colloid fluid resuscitation has been shown to have no extra effect on cardiac output compared to crystalloid resuscitation during the first 12 h post-burn.

Post-burn permeability oedema becomes generalized when the burn size is greater than 25% of TBSA, and is due to increased interstitial osmotic pressure and increased capillary endothelial permeability to macromolecules of up to 250 000 daltons. This allows free egress of all components of the vascular space except red cells. This in part explains the phenomenon of fluid resuscitation having no effect on haemoconcentration. Certainly a haemoglobin concentration of 180 g/L is commonplace and should be expected. Extracellular sodium loss into the burned tissues leads to extracellular sodium depletion and explains the necessity for 'salty' fluid resuscitation.

FLUID RESUSCITATION

The optimal volume of fluid resuscitation is the least amount of fluid necessary to maintain adequate organ perfusion that will also limit unnecessary oedema formation.

This can be achieved by close attention to response and very regular alteration of infusion rates. In fact, reassessment and adjustment of fluid volume should occur every 30 min during resuscitation of a patient with a large burn. Many fluid resuscitation regimens have been published. The factors that they all have in common are that they are only a starting point, and the volume of fluid infused is then titrated to give the response required. This response is a urinary output of 0.5 mL/kg/h for adults and 1.0 mL/kg/h for children. The Australian and New Zealand Burn Association recommendations for fluid resuscitation as taught in the Emergency Management of Severe Burns (EMSB©) course are as follows.

For adults (> 30 kg), give Hartmann's solution, 3–4 mL/kg/% TBSA burned, over the first 24 h – half of this volume to be given over the first 8 h. This calculation is made from the time when the burn occurred. If fluid resuscitation has been delayed, then the first quantum is divided between the remaining time. The volume of fluid delivered is then adjusted to maintain a urine output of 30–50 mL/h. Additional fluid will be required for patients in whom resuscitation has been delayed, where pre-existing dehydration is likely (e.g. firefighters, or cases of heavy alcohol consumption), when a coexisting inhalation injury is present, when haemochromogens are present in the urine, and in children. Inhalation injury has been shown to necessitate a 50% increase in the volume of fluid resuscitation. Therefore, 6 mL/kg/%

TBSA burned of Hartmann's solution over 24 h will be required for the largest burns with inhalation injury. A urine output of 60–100 mL/h should be achieved in these patients.

Discoloured, dirty, 'port-wine stained' urine indicates the presence of haemoglobin and myoglobin (see Plate 25.3 in the colour plate section). Haemoglobin and myoglobin are produced by destruction of red cells and muscle cells by heat, and are most commonly encountered following high-voltage electrical injury, but are also seen with deep thermal burns, delayed fluid resuscitation and limb necrosis when escharotomy has been inadequate or not performed. Unconjugated free haemoglobin/myoglobin passes through the glomeruli and leads to cast formation and tubular occlusion. The renal tubular epithelium is also damaged by oxygen radicals released by haem from haemoglobin degradation. Acute tubular necrosis and renal failure is the end result. Treatment includes increased urine flow to 100 mL/h. An osmotic diuretic such as mannitol can be given to initiate urine flow. The addition of 12.5 g mannitol to each 1-L flask of resuscitation fluid is recommended. Once the urine has cleared, urine output can be decreased to 30–50 mL/h as the pigment will not recur. If a diuretic is used, then other forms of monitoring such as central venous and pulmonary artery wedge pressure will be required, as urine output will be an unreliable guide to adequacy of resuscitation.

Children require additional fluid resuscitation, as they have a larger surface area to body weight ratio and less physiological reserve. This additional volume just happens to coincide with their maintenance fluid requirements. Children also require carbohydrate, as their hepatic glycogen stores are limited. Therefore, in addition to 4 mL/kg/% TBSA burned as Hartmann's solution, maintenance fluid in the form of half normal saline (0.45%) with 5% dextrose (or similar) is given: 100 mL/kg for the first 10 kg, 50 mL/kg for the next 10 kg and 25 mL/kg thereafter. A urine flow of 1.0 mL/kg/h is appropriate for children. Hyponatraemia is common in children and should be monitored. If the sodium concentration falls below 130 mEq/L, the maintenance fluids should be changed to a more concentrated salt solution. The urine output remains the best guide to adequacy of organ perfusion and fluid resuscitation. The pulse rate is always elevated due to pain, fear and catecholamine release. The blood pressure should be measured by an intra-arterial line in burns of > 40% TBSA. It is usually low due to the obligated decrease in intravascular volume, as explained earlier. Burn shock fluid resuscitation is a form of minimal volume fluid resuscitation with slow restoration of intravascular volume. Patients with burns of < 40% TBSA without inhalation injury can be adequately resuscitated with Hartmann's solution alone. In other patients, and especially in children, the elderly

and the malnourished, colloid fluids need to be introduced in order to restore a colloid osmotic pressure and plasma volume after permeability oedema has ceased. Therefore 4% albumin solution, 0.5 mL/kg/% TBSA burned is given in the second 24 h in addition to glucose-containing maintenance fluids titrated to maintain adequate urinary output. In practice, a gradual decrease in the amount of fluid administered each hour in the second 24-h period can be achieved by decrements of 25% of the hourly rate each 3 h while observing whether urinary flow remains adequate. In patients with very large burns of > 50% TBSA, evidence exists to support the use of mildly hypertonic (180 mEq/L) salt solution until acidaemia is corrected. The addition of 50 mEq of sodium bicarbonate to each 1-L bag of Hartmann's solution is followed by adjustment of the volume infused to give a urine output of 30–50 mL/h. Hartmann's solution is always appropriate in emergency and retrieval settings.

BURN SIZE

Determination of body weight and burn size is obviously vital to appropriate fluid resuscitation. Burn size can be quickly estimated by using the Rule of Nines (Figure 25.13a and b).

In an adult, the front and back of the torso, from the tops of the shoulders to the gluteal or groin crease, is 18% each. Each arm, including the hand, is 9%. The lower limbs are 18% each, with the genitalia accounting for 1%. The head is 9% in an adult. Children have disproportionately larger heads and smaller lower limbs, with a 1-year-old infant having a head that accounts for 18% TBSA and each lower limb representing 14%. With each year of life, 1% is taken from the head and distributed to both lower limbs. Therefore a 4-year-old child will have 15% TBSA in its head and 15.5% in each lower limb. Scattered burns can be estimated by using the area of the palmar surface of the patient's outstretched hand.

BOX 25.5 ANZBA-EMSB FLUID RESUSCITATION RECOMMENDATIONS

Adults   3–4 mL/kg/% TBSA burned over 24 h, half in first 8 h
Urine output 30–50 mL/h

Children 3–4 mL/kg/% TBSA burned
(< 30 kg) plus maintenance
          0.45% saline with 5% dextrose
          100 mL/kg for first 10 kg body weight
          50 mL/kg for second 10 kg
          25 mL/kg thereafter
Urine output 1.0 mL/kg/h

This area is slightly less than 1% TBSA. Estimation of burn area is more accurate when a body chart is used. An alternative method is that described by Lund and Browder (Figure 25.13c). Photography is also an essential element in burn wound assessment.

DIAGNOSIS OF BURN DEPTH

Accurate diagnosis of the depth of burn injury allows appropriate calculation of fluid formulae and has great prognostic significance. The Australian and New Zealand Burn Association uses a descriptor based on the anatomy of the skin (see Plate 25.4 in the colour plate section).

Epidermal burns are the equivalent of sunburn with pain, redness and sometimes tiny, vesicular epidermal blisters. This area is not included in calculations of fluid resuscitation, and will heal in 3–5 days without residual scar formation. Dermal burns are further subdivided into superficial and deep dermal burns (Figure 25.14). Superficial dermal burns are blistered, with the blisters

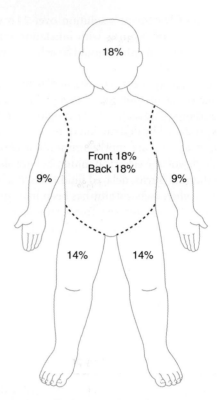

Figure 25.13b Body proportions of a 1-year-old infant according to the 'Rule of Nines'.

often remaining intact. The rapidity with which the blisters form and burst gives a further clue to depth. Superficial dermal burns are moist, red, painful and sensate, and blanch on digital pressure. As the burn becomes deeper, the surface assumes a white appearance (see Plate 25.5 in the colour plate section) until, with deep dermal burns, the surface is homogeneously white, moist and feels thickened, but remains sensate to the sterile gloved hand (leave the hypodermic needle in the drawer).

Superficial dermal burns should heal in 10–14 days, while deep dermal burns may take 4–6 weeks to heal. Hypertrophic scar formation becomes common if burns take longer than 14 days to heal, and are the norm if healing is delayed beyond 21 days. Accurate early diagnosis of burn depth will allow excision and skin grafting of these deeper burns within 7 days of injury, and thereby minimize scar formation. Full-thickness burns look leathery, have a dry surface and are insensate, feel thick and immalleable, and are white, charred or tanned (chemical injury). Difficulties arise with dark-skinned individuals where the feel of the wound becomes important, as well as removing residual pigmented epidermis to reveal the wound surface, which can then be assessed in a similar manner to that for fair-skinned people. Full-thickness burns in young children can often appear red due to coagulated blood in the subdermal plexus seen through their thin skin. The colour is therefore fixed and

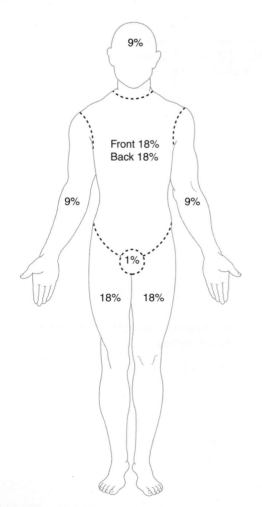

Figure 25.13a Adult body surface area according to the 'Rule of Nines'.

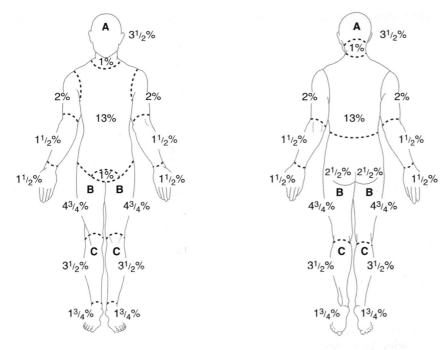

Figure 25.13c
Estimation of burn size using the Lund and Browder method.

Body proportions in children

Age (years)	0–1	2–4	5–9	10–14	15
A – front of head	$9^1/_2$%	$8^1/_2$%	$6^1/_2$%	$5^1/_2$%	$4^1/_2$%
B – front of one thigh	$2^3/_4$%	$3^1/_4$%	4%	$4^1/_4$%	$4^1/_2$%
C – front of one leg	$2^1/_2$%	$2^1/_2$%	$2^3/_4$%	3%	$3^1/_4$%

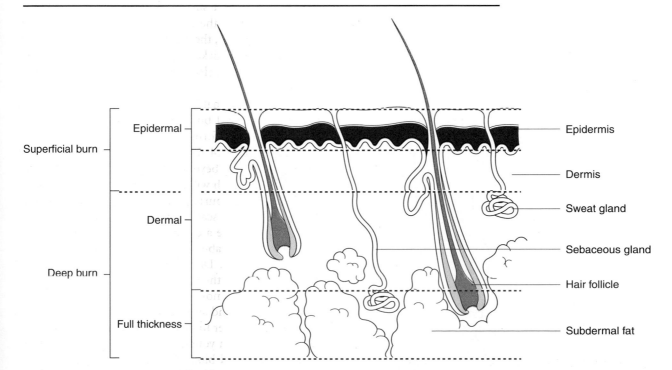

Figure 25.14 Schematic cross-section of skin.

does not blanch. Full-thickness burns require excision and skin grafting.

ESCHAROTOMY

An escharotomy is an incision placed in the burned, dead layer of skin. It does not and should not routinely include the underlying fascia. Escharotomies are required when circumferential burns are present around a limb or the thorax and oedema formation becomes so marked that the pressure inside the unyielding, tight eschar rises above perfusion pressure in the limbs or causes restriction to ventilation. Elevation of the limbs, active exercises and limitation of excessive fluid administration can ameliorate this situation. Escharotomy is indicated when distal pulses begin to decrease. A conscious patient will complain of a cold, painful extremity, and cyanosis, pallor, prolonged capillary blanch test and coolness can be observed. Deep muscle pain, tenderness and pain on passive stretching of the muscle group combined with paraesthesia/anaesthesia are all late signs. These occur about 2–6 h post-burn. Escharotomy is an emergency bedside procedure that can be performed without a general anaesthetic because the eschar is insensate. Intravenous narcotic and sedation combined with selective infiltration of spared skin or sensate partial-thickness burn result in the procedure being very well tolerated. The lines of incision are the mid-axial planes of the limbs (Figure 25.15a).

In the upper limb the forearm needs to be returned to the anatomical position with the palm facing upwards (supinated) for correct placement. The incision is made starting from normal skin, or the upper extent of the limb proximally, and continued down across the mid-medial and mid-lateral aspects of the joints down to the base of the digits. The incision is carried through the full depth of skin until subcutaneous fat appears (see Plate 25.6 in the colour plate section). The eschar will spring open and the pulse should be restored. The incisions are covered by an alginate dressing and the limb loosely dressed and elevated. Occasionally the incision needs to be taken into the underlying subcutaneous fat, which will lead to venous haemorrhage that needs to be controlled by ligation/diathermy. Finger escharotomies are seldom necessary, and should be left to a burn surgeon. Fasciotomies are performed for high-voltage electrical injury, and should be carried out in an operating theatre under anaesthesia with cross-matched blood available. Chest escharotomy is placed lateral to the nipple vertically on each side. These incisions are then joined by two horizontal incisions – below the sternal notch and at the level of the costal margin, thereby lifting a plate (Figure 25.15b). In children especially, the vertical incisions are extended down over the abdomen where eschar can restrict abdominal breathing.

WOUND CARE – FIRST AID

Wound management involves cooling the burn wound for 20 min with tap water (8–15°C). Ice must not be used and wet dressings lead to hypothermia if left in place. The wound is cleaned with water or saline to remove dirt or other forms of contamination (e.g. material used to extinguish flames). The burns can then be covered with

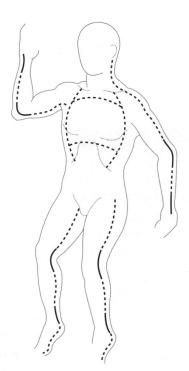

Figure 25.15a Anatomical landmarks for escharotomy.

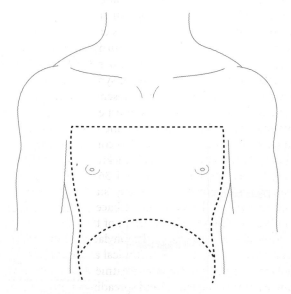

Figure 25.15b Chest escharotomy sites.

a clean dry sheet or plastic clingfilm until transfer to the burn unit is effected. Patients with small superficial dermal burns who are to be treated as out-patients require an absorptive, non-adherent dressing that excludes air. Blisters in this patient group can be left intact unless movement is restricted. If burn depth is uncertain or the burn size is more than trivial, Silvazine™ (silver sulfadiazine with chlorhexidine) cream is indicated for the first few days. When exudate is settling and wound infection is not apparent, a plastic film dressing is well tolerated.

Burns are tetanus-prone wounds and patients should be treated according to their immunization status. In-patient wound care involves daily or twice daily wound cleaning by shower with a chlorhexidine sponge, or bathing immersed in a weak chlorhexidine solution. Wounds are cleaned and Silvazine cream applied to a depth of 4–6 mm. Non-stick absorbent material such as Melolin™ is then loosely bandaged. Silver nitrate 0.5% solution is a good alternative antimicrobial agent. Progression of burn depth over the first 3–5 days post-burn is a well-known phenomenon, and is explained by the target theory of burn injury.

If concentric globes are considered in three dimensions, the central zone is the area of coagulative necrosis where the tissue is dead. The outer zone is an area of mild inflammatory response characterized by erythema. The intermediate zone is known as the zone of stosis, where the microcirculation becomes progressively impaired, leading to further cell death. The zone of stosis is adversely affected by inadequate or excessive fluid resuscitation, dessication, infection and pressure. Optimal patient and wound care can reverse these changes in the zone of stosis, with prevention of further necrosis. Agents such as non-steroidal anti-inflammatory drugs (NSAIDs) that affect platelet adherence and vaso-constriction caused by thromboxane A2 and prostaglandin F2 have had partial success in reversing this effect. Burn wound infection is common and can be life-threatening in patients with burns of > 20% TBSA, although deaths in children from overwhelming Gram-positive infection, or toxic shock syndrome, in smaller burns are not unknown. The presence of necrotic and partially devitalized tissue in a moist environment, when combined with the cellular immune depression seen in patients with large burns, leads to conditions that allow microbial proliferation. Partial-thickness burns are more likely to become infected around 36 h post-burn with Gram-positive organisms (usually staphylococcal) that were resident in the sweat and sebaceous glands. These glands become blocked as a result of the burn, and bacterial proliferation is rapid. Prophylactic antibiotics do not ameliorate this situation. Topical antimicrobials and vigilance are the mainstays of treatment. An increase in pain of a throbbing nature and spreading erythema combined with fever are the hallmarks. Rest, elevation and

intravenous antistaphylococcal antibiotics are indicated. Deep burns become infected around days 5–7, often with a combination of organisms such as *Pseudomonas* or *Klebsiella* and staphylococci. The general signs of burn wound infection are gastroparesis with intolerance of nasogastric feeds, mental obtundation, hyper- or hypothermia (body temperature > 39.5°C or < 36.5°C), thrombocythaemia, hyperglycaemia and leucocytosis (white cell count $> 16 \times 10^9$/L). Local signs of burn wound infection include conversion of dermal to full-thickness burns, development of black or brown spots, and peri-eschar cellulitis.

Punch biopsies should be taken for quantitative culture and antibiotic therapy commenced. Wound excision should follow shortly thereafter.

PAIN MANAGEMENT

Burns hurt! Pain relief should be provided early and liberally, and should have sufficient scope to control background, breakthrough and procedural pain. Anxiolytics and hypnotics are essential, as is attention to bowel care. Professor T. Crammond, Director of the Chronic Pain

---

BOX 25.6 PAIN MANAGEMENT FOR ACUTE BURN INJURY

Morphine intravenous injection (IV) 0.1 mg/kg bolus given slowly and repeated until pain is controlled. (Remember, IV morphine takes 15–20 minutes to take effect.)

If the oral route is available:

- oxycodone (orally) 0.5–1 mg/kg per day divided into 4–6 hourly doses.

When pain is controlled, IV morphine infusion, preferably patient-controlled if a limb is not burned, with a background infusion each hour slightly less than the final bolus dose that was required and additional bolus doses of 1–2.5 mg/h as needed. An anti-emetic should routinely be added and laxatives commenced immediately.

As tolerance develops quickly with the intravenous route, change to a subcutaneous infusion via a 'Grasby' pump.

Add paracetamol, 1 g four times a day, and change to an oral form of morphine as soon as possible:

- MS Contin or Kapanol (N-G tube compatible).

Dressing changes:
- subcutaneous/oral morphine and midazolam premedication
- 'Entonox' – patient-administered and premixed nitrous oxide/oxygen
- have an anaesthetist deliver a low-dose ketamine infusion i.e. 20 µg/kg per min.

Service, Royal Brisbane Hospital has provided guidelines (see Box 25.6), which have proved effective over a number of years.

The use of intravenous lignocaine and oral mexilitene is effective in about 80% of patients to control the 'burning' pain of partial-thickness burns and donor-site wounds. As one of the earliest clinical signs of sepsis is confusion, this aetiology should be actively sought as a cause while temporarily interrupting the pain management regimen.

NUTRITIONAL SUPPORT

Nutritional support should be commenced as soon as is practicable in the form of enteral feeding. This helps to control stress ulceration in the stomach and duodenum, keeps the intestinal mucosa proliferating, and so controls bacterial translocation and provides support for the hyper-metabolic response to injury. Energy provision is best estimated by use of a metabolic computer, but is usually around twice the basal requirement.

EXTREMITY CARE

Physiotherapy with both active and passive activity should commence from the time of admission, and is particularly important to maintain mobility of the fingers. This is aided by the use of proprietary glove dressings or by bandaging the fingers individually. The position of comfort of a joint is the position of contracture. Appropriate positioning and splinting from the time of admission is vital to prevent contracture. In short, shoulders are abducted, elbows straight, wrist extended, fingers (ready to accept a beer glass) straight at the interphalangeal joints and flexed at the metacarpophalangeal joints, hips extended, knees extended and ankles at least plantigrade. Thermoplastic splints should be requested from an occupational therapist to maintain the positions described.

OPERATIVE MANAGEMENT

Burn wound excision and grafting can be a major physiological insult. Hypothermia, blood loss and prolonged anaesthesia all combine to stress the patient. These factors can be ameliorated by ensuring that sufficient blood and products are available, and by warming the operating theatre sufficiently to maintain normothermia. A core temperature monitor is essential, and devices such as a Bair Hugger™ make life more tolerable for the staff. On average, a unit of blood should be cross-matched for each 1% of burn wound to be excised. For a large burn

excision, 10 units of blood, 10 units of fresh frozen plasma and 10 units of platelets form a good starting point. The mainstay of surgical excision is tangential removal of eschar with sequential slices performed until a viable, and therefore bleeding, wound bed is obtained.

Preservation of at least some of the dermal elements at the bases of the rete pegs enhances long-term functional and cosmetic results (Figure 25.16). Bleeding is controlled by application of 1:20 000 adrenalin solution and calcium-enriched alginate dressing. Donor skin is harvested with a mechanical dermatome usually set at 0.001 inches. Donor sites are dressed with an alginate. If the burn size is small, the donor skin or autograft is applied as a sheet graft and held in place by sutures, staples, adhesive dressings or biological glue. If possible, a pressure dressing is then applied. In any case, the graft needs to be inspected regularly and any seromas or haematomas expressed.

When the burns are more extensive and donor sites are limited, meshing of the autograft becomes necessary. Mesh dermatomes are available in ratios of 1:1 to 1:9. Expansion ratios of 4:1 or greater require overgrafting with either allograft or a skin substitute such as Biobrane™ or Dermagraft TC™. These techniques become necessary when operating on very large burns. In these cases, fascial excision is often indicated, as grafts frequently fail on the relatively avascular subcutaneous fat. These operations are performed in the first few days post-burn, before sepsis develops and the patient becomes too unstable for surgery. Early operation also halves the blood loss. A recently available skin substitute called Integra™ has a definite role in the operative man-

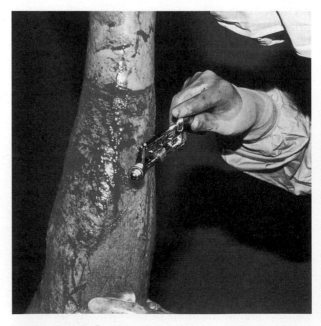

Figure 25.16 Operative excision of burn tissue to achieve a viable, bleeding wound bed.

agement of large burns. It is bovine dermal collagen bonded with shark chondroitin sulphate as a neodermis that becomes vascularized. It has a layer of silicone press-sealed as a neo-epidermis, which is removed about 3 weeks after application, when vascular ingrowth is fully established. An epithelial graft in the form of cultured epithelial autograft or ultra-thin, widely meshed skin graft is then applied.

BURN SCARS

Wound contraction is a normal part of wound healing that produces cosmetic and functional deformity after burn injury. A wound continues to contract until it is opposed by an equal force. The degree of contraction is proportional to the amount of fibrosis, and the latter is the result of inflammation and granulation tissue. Therefore delayed wound healing in deep burns that have been allowed to heal spontaneously, wounds covered with insufficient skin (e.g. when wide-meshed skin grafts are necessary), or failure of engraftment all lead to ongoing inflammation, granulation tissue formation and collagen deposition in whorls. This whorl-like pattern is characteristic of hypertrophic scars, which are by convention defined as scars confined to the original boundaries of the wound. These whorls progress to nodules as the scar matures. The maturation process transforms the wound from a vascular, itchy, raised, angry, red turgid scar to a flat, soft, pliable and pale residuum with collagen arranged in parallel. This process can take years. Custom-made pressure garments are the mainstay of burn scar management, and are indicated for all grafted burns and also for those dermal burns that have taken longer than 14 days to heal. Topical application of silicone sheets is added for unresponsive areas, together with intralesional injection of triamcinolone. Burn scar release is indicated for contractures that do not respond to stretching regimens. If the scar is broad, then skin grafting is indicated, while z-plasty release is reserved for bands of scar.

ELECTRICAL INJURY

Electrical burns are classified into high- and low-voltage injuries, with the division occurring at 1000 volts. Below this level, charring occurs at the cutaneous contact point and current flow is decreased because of increased resistance. Above 1000 volts, both current and injury continue. The smaller the cross-sectional area through which the current flows, the greater the injury. Bone/periosteum is the least electrically resistant tissue, leading to the greatest current flow. As deep tissues cool more slowly, the worst injuries are therefore found in the middle of the limbs. High-voltage electrical injury is characterized by damage to the limbs rather than the trunk, muscle injury with liberation of myoglobin, and rapid increases in compartment pressures, swiftly leading to ischaemic necrosis of the contents of the affected compartment. As so much tissue damage cannot be seen, fluid resuscitation needs to be guided by response, rather than estimated from the visible burn, as this may represent only a fraction of the problem. Haemochromogens in the urine, with the risk of acute renal failure, should be expected and actively sought and treated. Cardiac arrhythmias are commonplace. An abnormal electrocardiogram or history of loss of consciousness indicates the need for cardiac monitoring. Fasciotomies are usually required following high-voltage electrical injury. An injured hand that is held in flexion should have a carpal tunnel decompression as well as forearm fasciotomies. If the leg has been injured, all four compartments will require decompression. The muscles closest to bone should be assessed for viability, and non-viable tissue should be excised. This should be repeated daily until all non-viable tissue has been removed. Amputation is a common sequela. Another scenario is a 'flash-over' of current across the skin, which burns the skin and ignites the clothing.

Neurological dysfunction with personality changes and memory and speech loss can be disabling consequences of high-voltage electrical injury to the head. Spinal cord lesions should be sought. Immediate lesions are usually in the form of transverse defects, and most of them usually recover. Long tract signs can appear late due to arteritis of nutrient vessels to the cord. Late lesions are often permanent. Another problem of late onset, 6–48 months post-injury, is that of cataract formation. Ophthalmological assessment should be arranged during follow-up for all patients who have received a high-voltage injury to the head and neck region.

CHEMICAL INJURY

Most chemical injuries are actually thermal burns caused by the liberation of heat from strong acids and alkalis. Some substances, such as hydrofluoric acid, have cytotoxic effects in their own right. In general, neutralizing solutions should not be used, as the chemical reaction involves the liberation of even more heat. The solution here is dilution. Copious irrigation with any available fluid should commence immediately and continue until the pH of the effluent has returned to normal. Strong alkalis, such as sodium hydroxide and lime, lead to saponification of fat, desiccation of cells and dissolution of proteins. This allows the hydroxyl (OH^-) ions to penetrate more deeply, causing further tissue injury. Copious irrigation may need to continue for several hours, especially if the eye is involved.

Hydrofluoric acid is used in the petroleum industry, and for etching glass, as well as for cleaning metal. The hydrogen ions cause corrosion of tissue, while the fluoride ions bind to bivalent cations such as calcium and magnesium. Local cell death and generalized hypocalcaemia follow. The problem is very serious, and death frequently follows a major burn. Major hydrofluoric acid burns are defined as exposure to > 1% TBSA with > 50% HF or > 5% TBSA with any concentration of HF. Excruciating pain is a major feature, while the first sign of hypocalcaemia is ventricular fibrillation. Cardiac monitoring and intravenous calcium infusion should commence early. Serum calcium levels are required every 30 min, and prolongation of the Q-T interval on ECG should be sought. Treatment commences with copious irrigation followed by topical application of calcium gluconate as a solution or mixed with water-soluble gel. Dimethyl sulphoxide (DMSO) can be added to enhance calcium penetration.

SUMMARY

Modern burn care has resulted in marked improvements in survival following burn injury, such that most children and young adults can be rehabilitated to lead a fruitful and productive life, no matter how large the burn. Inhalation injury, increasing age and burn size remain the principal determinants of mortality.

Good functional and cosmetic outcomes are best achieved in specialized burn centres that can address the varied physiological, surgical and emotionally complex problems that a patient with a burn injury poses.

SOFT TISSUE, HAND, LIMB, FACE AND EYE

Kinetic forces applied to human tissue result in varying degrees of cellular injury. An understanding of the effects of injury must be based on an awareness of the mechanism of injury and a knowledge of the relevant anatomy.

GENERAL PRINCIPLES

Skin injuries are some of the most common presentations of trauma to the Emergency Department. In the context of major trauma, wounds may be a distraction from more serious life-threatening injuries. Wounds may be associated with underlying pathology, such as long-bone fractures, penetrating visceral injuries or neurovascular damage. Simple wounds should initially be dressed with a moist sterile dressing until such time as attention is indicated. Once major injuries have been dealt with in a systematic manner (ATLS®), attention

may then be paid to the superficial soft-tissue injuries. It is important to note that these injuries may leave scars and disfigurements and therefore, after full recovery from major internal injuries, a facial scar may be all that remains to remind the individual of their trauma. Incorrectly managed soft-tissue injuries therefore carry a significant psychological and medico-legal burden.

SKIN

The first point of contact will be skin or mucous membrane, and the body surface may show evidence of injury. Terms such as contusion, bruising, incised wounds and lacerations are all used to describe different appearances of cutaneous injury. Wounds may be caused by direct trauma (e.g. as with incised wounds or lacerations). Damage may result from shearing forces resulting in tearing of tissue planes. Compressive forces cause rupture or disruption of viscus and solid organs. Blast injuries cause devastating tissue damage due to the sudden explosive release of kinetic forces on the fragile human structure. Missiles that tumble as they pass through tissues cause more extensive local disruption than high-velocity bullets that pass through structures. However, the high-velocity missiles produce temporary cavitation which sucks debris into the wound. Shock waves result from the transference of energy, causing extensive cellular injury that extends beyond the permanent cavity of the missile track.

Descriptive terms need to be used precisely in order to provide an accurate record of the injury sustained. Correct use of terminology is a vital skill in the context of trauma (Table 25.8), where the effects of injury are variable. The terms 'laceration' and 'incised wound' in particular are often used incorrectly.

SURGICAL MANAGEMENT OF SOFT-TISSUE INJURIES

Before any traumatic wound is sutured, the extent of the wound must be fully assessed.

This information is obtained by:

- taking a clear history, including 'mechanism of injury';
- examining the patient;
- inspecting the wound;
- exploring the wound.

This process allows the astute clinician to gain a fair expectation of the kind of wound and associated injuries that are likely to be found during exploration. 'A good surgeon anticipates problems rather than stumbling on them'. A brief medical history needs to be taken in the

Table 25.8 Correct use of terminology in the context of trauma

Terminology	Description	Mechanism of injury
Laceration	Tearing of skin	Blunt implement
Incised wound	Division of skin	Sharp implement
Contusion	Capillary haemorrhage	Local pressure
Defect	Loss of skin	Gouging
Deformity	Misplaced structures	Traction/rotation
Swelling	Oedema of tissues	All mechanisms
Haematoma	Subcutaneous clot	Shearing forces and direct pressure effects

context of the injury, including ascertaining the status of tetanus prophylaxis. Drug allergies should be sought and pre-morbid conditions (e.g. diabetes) discussed. Any medications taken should be noted. Conscious patients need to be advised of the treatment planned and verbal consent obtained. Patients who require a general anaesthetic for wound care or other surgical procedures need to give their full informed consent.

Children may be frightened and their parents will be anxious and concerned. Some wounds in children may require repair under general anaesthesia in order not to traumatize the family further. All patients and next of kin should be kept informed of the treatment plan and likely duration of care.

SUTURING

Suturing is a skill required by all clinicians who deal with trauma.

Traumatic wounds differ from surgical wounds in the following respects.

- They are not planned.
- They are usually contaminated.
- They are often irregular and complex.
- The depth of penetration is unknown.

Local anaesthetic is appropriate for the management of the majority of soft-tissue wounds in adults (Table 25.9).

It is pointless to cause further local damage by injecting local anaesthetic through intact skin unless the wound is grossly contaminated. Local anaesthetic is injected as soon as the needle is introduced into the wound for early comfort, and then infiltrated as the needle is advanced along the wound margins (Figure 25.17). Intravascular bolus injection will be avoided if the needle is kept moving during infiltration.

Time should be allowed for the anaesthetic to take effect. This is particularly important in the case of nerve blocks. Loss of sensation should be elicited before commencement of the procedure. Occasionally in anxious patients a small intravenous dose of a benzodiazepine may be titrated for sedation.

The following basic surgical principles must be applied to soft-tissue injury.

- Remove all foreign material from the wound.
- Remove all obviously devitalized tissue.
- Treat tissues with respect and care.
- Cause no further harm to the tissues.
- Close wounds by primary intent if possible.
- Leave wounds open if closing the tissue planes is likely to compromise circulation.
- Use suture material judiciously.
- Apply a suitable sterile dressing.
- Consider the tetanus status of the patient.
- Routine use of prophylactic antibiotics is not indicated.

EXPLORATION

The traumatic wound should be gently explored to remove contaminated material (e.g. glass or gravel) and

Table 25.9 Local anaesthetics

Type of local anaesthetic	Duration of action
Lignocaine 1%	Short (30 min)
Prilocaine 0.5%	Short
Bupivacaine 0.25%	Long (30–120 min)
Lignocaine and adrenalin (for a blood-free field)	Extended to 90 min
Contraindicated around blood vessels (i.e. digital vessels)	
Maximum dose for lignocaine is 200 mg for a 70-kg adult (20 mL 1%)	

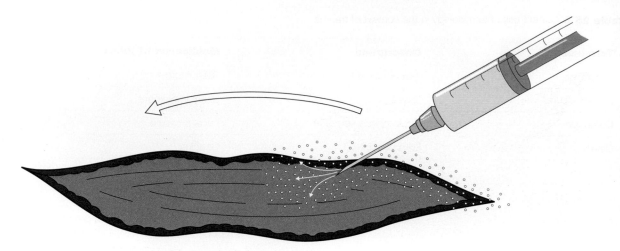

Figure 25.17 Technique of local anaesthetic wound infiltration.

irrigated. Prior radiology may be indicated if glass contamination is suspected. Local anatomy should be inspected, bearing in mind the expected findings from the history and mechanism of injury.

A specialist opinion may be sought at this stage if the operator feels uncertain about their own personal capabilities or is suspicious of deep structural injury.

SUTURING

Closure of traumatic wounds requires the same skills as those utilized in the surgical field. The difference is that ingenuity may be required to approximate an irregular unplanned wound.

Simple sutures are indicated in the majority of cases. Occasionally a vertical mattress is helpful when wound margins tend to fold under. Subcutaneous sutures are rarely indicated unless they are needed to close a defect or muscle fascia. No suture should be inserted that does not positively contribute to the wound closure.

CORNER SUTURES

Traumatic wounds often have irregular margins, and the corner suture is extremely useful in incised wounds. This preserves the circulation to the tip of a flap by placing the suture through the subcutaneous tissues (Figure 25.18).

Sutures should be secured so that the wound margins are gently approximated. Blanching of the skin edges indicates overtightening of sutures. Adhesive skin tapes may be applied to help to close difficult wounds. Sutures should be avoided if at all possible in wounds with compromised blood supply, such as pre-tibial lacerations.

DRESSINGS

Sterile dressings should be applied to all wounds. When granulation tissue is expected, a tulle dressing may be appropriate, otherwise a non-adherent layer with some suitable padding (gauze) is applied and a firm pressure bandage held in place with tape. Hand injuries usually require rest in a high sling until the swelling has subsided.

SPECIFIC SOFT-TISSUE INJURIES

Hand

One of the commonest areas for trauma is the hand, and good soft-tissue care is essential if a return to useful function is to be achieved. It is important to know the basic anatomy and function of the hand in order to assess and treat hand injuries correctly and appropriately.

Functional anatomy

There is no part of the body for which a knowledge of anatomy is more important than the hand. There is little subcutaneous fat in the hand, and therefore vital structures are easily damaged during trauma. The skin, particularly in the palm and fingertips, is densely innervated for tactile sensation. This also renders hand and finger injuries particularly painful.

The thumb is highly mobile and opposes against all four fingers. The resting position of the uninjured hand is such that the thumb approximates to the radial border of the index finger, and the remaining fingers lie in gently increasing flexion. On full flexion the fingertips point towards the scaphoid carpal bone. The functional plane of the thumb lies at 90° to the remaining fingers.

Three major sensory nerves supply the hand (Figure 25.19).

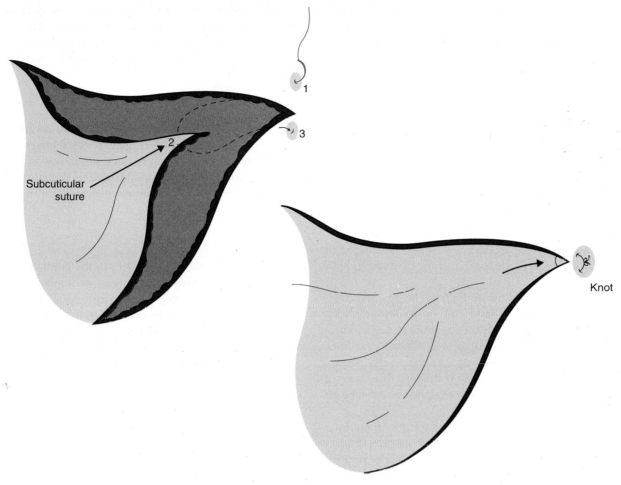

Figure 25.18 Technique for placing a corner suture.

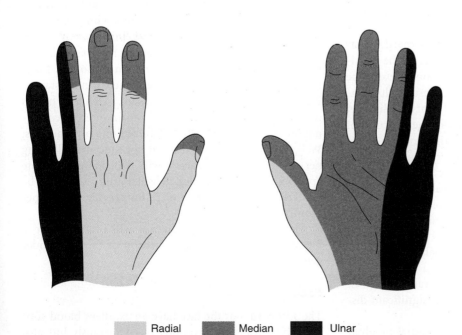

Radial   Median   Ulnar

Figure 25.19 Cutaneous nerve supply to the hand.

The *ulnar nerve* has a motor branch which supplies the following:

- hypothenar muscles;
- medial two lumbricals;
- adductor pollicis muscles;
- interosseous muscles.

The *median nerve* enters the hand through the carpal tunnel and supplies motor fibres to the following:

- thenar muscles;
- abductor pollicis brevis;
- flexor pollicis brevis;
- opponens pollicis;
- first and second lumbricals.

The *radial nerve* is purely sensory in the hand.

These nerves may be damaged by wounds around the wrist, in the palm of the hand or along the margins of the fingers.

The extensor tendons in the hand lie subcutaneously on the dorsum of the hand and are readily divided by transverse incised wounds such as those caused by knives or glass. These tendons have extensive lateral attachment and therefore tend not to retract far from the point of division. The exception to this is the long thumb extensor, which passes around Lister's tubercle and can be difficult to locate when divided.

Extensor tendon tears around the proximal interphalangeal joints are notorious for causing buttonholing of the head of the proximal phalanx. The resulting Boutonnière's deformity can be difficult to repair later if these injuries are missed.

Flexor tendons lie deep within the palmar compartment. They are complex and operate within a synovial sheath through a mechanism of pulleys. When divided these tendons retract, and specialist expertise is required for repair and rehabilitation.

The profundus tendon passes through the decussation of the superficialis tendon at the level of the proximal phalanx. The superficialis tendon flexes the proximal interphalangeal joint and the profundus tendon flexes both of the interphalangeal joints. A clinician skilled in examination is able to test for the function of these two tendons separately. To test the function of the profundus tendon the proximal interphalangeal joint needs to be immobilized. To test the function of the superficialis tendon the distal interphalangeal joints of the other fingers are immobilized to isolate the function of the profundus tendon from the superficialis tendon at the level of the proximal interphalangeal joint.

Ligaments around the metacarpo-phalangeal joint of the thumb are vulnerable in abduction (e.g. skiing) injuries, and rupture of the ulnar collateral ligament of the thumb (gamekeeper's thumb) causes significant disability if not treated early.

Blood supply to the hand is via the radial or ulnar arteries which join in an anastomosis of the deep and superficial palmar arches. This anastomosis allows the blood supply to be maintained despite loss of one of the arteries. Arteries in the hand may bleed from both divided ends.

Limb

The upper and lower limbs are both vulnerable to trauma, which often involves fracture of the long bones.

However, soft-tissue injury can result in skin wounds, nerve or tendon injury or muscle damage. Compartment syndromes result from swelling, causing compromise of nerve and artery function.

Arteries

Lives are lost when major arteries in the groin or axilla bleed without immediate attention. All limb haemorrhage can be arrested with firm local pressure. Tourniquets should not be utilized, as they often cause more harm than good, and they may merely prevent venous return, resulting in even greater blood loss. Major arterial disruption will require urgent surgical repair. Arteriography may be required to establish the full extent of arterial injury, particularly in the context of complicated long-bone fractures.

Nerves

Distal anaesthesia or functional loss will draw attention to nerve injury. A knowledge of local anatomy in the vicinity of the wound or fracture will indicate the nerves likely to be involved. Early correction of gross deformity is essential to prevent neurovascular complications. Crush injury of the soft tissues may result in neuropraxia. Neurotmesis may be associated with penetrating wounds and comminuted fractures. Initially, both result in motor or sensory loss. Neuropraxia resolves with conservative treatment, allowing a return to normal function within several weeks so long as there is no sustained increase in compartment pressure. Divided nerves require surgical exploration and repair, often in combination with orthopaedic stabilization of fractures. Wallerian degeneration of distal fibres occurs following nerve division, so recovery will depend on accurate approximation of bundles. Regenerating axons can be expected to grow at a rate of 1 mm per day (1 inch per month).

The repair of limb structures will often require a bloodless field using exsanguination of the area under general anaesthesia.

Face

The soft tissues of the face have an excellent blood supply. This means that wounds bleed furiously but also heal well. Major facial injuries often involve damage to the underlying bony structures. Meticulous repair of facial lacerations and attention to surgical principles are necessary if unnecessary facial scarring and deformity are to be avoided. Contours need to be maintained and landmarks re-established. Wounds around the lips need to be carefully approximated in order to avoid steps in the vermilion border. Underlying facial muscles may need to be sutured to maintain facial expression and movement. Haemorrhage around the nose and mouth may compromise the airway, and requires urgent establishment of a definite airway if this is threatened.

Scalp lacerations may cause significant blood loss and require urgent suturing to achieve haemostasis.

Facial wounds should be thoroughly cleaned to remove all traces of foreign material which may otherwise result in wound tattooing. Fine sutures (6.0) are carefully placed to approximate wounds, and these are removed early (after 5 days) to reduce scarring.

Eye

Penetrating eye injuries should be expected in any patient with visual loss following trauma. Some wounds may be obvious because of loss of the aqueous humour. High-speed metal fragments may puncture the globe with little sign of the point of entry. These cases are identified by recognizing the mechanism of injury (high-speed metal fragments) and X-rays of the orbit to identify intra-ocular foreign bodies.

Examination of the eye includes examination of visual acuity, eye movements, pupil reaction and fundoscopy. Blood in the anterior chamber (hyphema) usually indicates significant intra-ocular disruption. About 7% of patients with hyphema go on to develop glaucoma. Laceration of the eyelid may involve the tarsal plate and require expert repair. The lacrimal puncta on the inferior and superior medial margin of the eyelid drain tears via the lacrimal canaliculus into the lacrimal sac. The nasolacrimal duct is 2 cm long, slopes downwards from the lacrimal sac and drains into the anterior part of the inferior nasal meatus. Damage to this structure must be considered in wounds that affect the inferomedial border of the eye.

FURTHER READING

American College of Surgeons Committee on Trauma. 1997: *Advanced Trauma Life Support® Program for Doctors.* Chicago, IL: American College of Surgeons.

Baker SP, O'Neill B, Karpf RS (eds). 1984: *The injury fact book.* Lexington, MA: Lexington Books.

Feliciano DV, Moore EE, Mattox KL (eds). 1996: *Trauma*, 3rd edn. Stanford, CT: Appleton & Lange.

National Road Trauma Advisory Council. 1993: *Report of the Working Party on Trauma Systems.* Canberra: Australian Government Publishing Service.

Royal Australasian College of Surgeons. 1997: *Policy on trauma (injury)*, 3rd edn. Melbourne: Royal Australasian College of Surgeons.

US Department of Health and Human Services. 1992: *Model trauma care system plan.* Rockville, MD: Bureau of Health Resources Development.

Oncology

John Slavin and John P. Neoptolemos

Introduction

World-wide at least 7.5 million new cases of cancer are reported each year (Table 26.1.1). In developed countries the lifetime risk of cancer is 1:3, and the lifetime mortality risk from cancer is 1:4. In the UK there are just over 270 000 new cases of cancer and over 160 000 deaths from cancer each year (Table 26.1.2).

The incidence of cancer is rising throughout the world due to environmental factors and an increasingly older population. The most significant factors contributing to the increase in cancer are the spread of westernized lifestyles (especially smoking) and viral infections. Interestingly, gastric cancer is on the decline, in contrast to most other cancers.

The vast majority of cancers involve solid organs, poten-tially amenable to resection, and are therefore classed as surgical cancers. In developed countries the death rate from cancer has become static despite a continuing rise in incidence. The objectives of surgery are to cure by complete resection (when possible), to debulk the tumour volume (for palliation or as a prelude to adjuvant treatment – palliative or curative), to stage the cancer and to provide tissue for diagnosis and/or staging.

Improvements in outcome have arisen because of better surgical care (reduced post-operative mortality, increased resection rates and improved 'surgical' cure rates), pre-symptomatic diagnosis through screening (for cervical and breast cancers) and improvements in radiotherapy and chemotherapy (most notably for testicular tumours).

NATURE AND CAUSES OF CANCER

WHAT IS CANCER?

A neoplastic tumour is an uncontrolled growth of tissue without useful function. A benign tumour grows by expansion without invasion of the adjacent extracellular matrix. A malignant tumour or cancer grows by invasion into the extracellular matrix; most solid cancers also invade the basement membrane of the endothelium and metastasize. Carcinomas are cancers of epithelium, adenocarcinomas are cancers of mucus-secreting epithe-lium, sarcomas arise from mesothelial elements, and germ-cell tumours are referred to according to the tissue of origin.

The basic unit of organization and control in the human body is the cell. The four-dimensional organiza-tion of cells to form functioning organs and, at a higher level, a healthy individual is dependent on the ability of each cell to control its structure and function, and to communicate with adjacent cells. Genes make proteins which govern the structure and function of a cell. Cancer is a disease of genes which determine processes funda-mental to cell proliferation. For comparison, cystic fibro-sis is an inherited disorder of cell-membrane chloride channels due to a mutation in the *CFTR* gene which codes for the chloride-channel protein. Although this

Table 26.1.1 The 10 commonest cancers world-wide*

Cancer	New cases per year
Lung	896 000
Stomach	755 000
Breast	720 000
Colorectum	678 000
Cervix uteri	437 000
Oral	412 000
Lymphoma	316 000
Liver	315 000
Oesophagus	304 000
Prostate	291 000
Total	7 620 000

*Estimated for 1985 (adapted from Cancer Research Campaign Factsheet 22.1, 1995).

protein serves a vital function in numerous organs sufficient to lead to death by the second or third decade of life in most affected individuals, it does not alter cell proliferation or cause cancer.

GENES AND CONTROL OF THE CELL CYCLE

Each healthy individual has the same number of genes as every other individual, located within every nucleated cell. Altogether there are approximately 100 000 genes constituting the human genome; within 5 years or so all of these genes will be sequenced and mapped by the Human Genome Project. Genes are composed of DNA organized in a double helix, and are usually found within the cell nucleus. Nuclear DNA are extremely long and tangled molecules, only being grouped into chromosomes during cell division. DNA with sequences which code for gene expression represents only 10% of all nuclear DNA. In each cell, genes exist in pairs, one of each pair being of paternal origin and one of maternal origin. Depending on the cell type, 6–10% of the genes within the nucleus will be expressed, and thus 6000–10 000 genes will define a particular cell type. However, given the appropriate stimuli, any of the remaining genes can be expressed. DNA is highly stable – a prerequisite for constituting the genetic code.

Each gene produces one type of protein molecule. Proteins can contribute to the architectural intra- and extracellular framework or possess functional activity (growth factors, cell-surface receptors, transmembrane channel proteins, immunoglobulins, chaperone molecules, enzymes and enzyme cofactors). Enzymes will catalyse reactions that alter proteins or enable the synthesis of other types of molecule, namely carbohydrates and lipids.

Transcription of a gene to messenger RNA (mRNA) requires the enzyme RNA polymerase II to engage at the promoter site (Figure 26.1.1). Each gene has a specific promoter, usually upstream of the start site. Specific protein cofactors known as transcription factors will form a unique complex with RNA polymerase II prior to engagement of the promoter site, leading to DNA strand separation and transcription. Because mRNA contains powerful information (the programme for synthesizing proteins) it has a short half-life and is highly labile, enabling tight control of gene expression by the nucleus.

Response elements (RE) are often associated with genes, usually lie upstream of the promoter, and constitute additional protein-DNA binding sites that enhance promoter activity. Hormone-responsive genes will contain hormone response elements (HREs), resulting in greatly increased transcription activity once they are activated by appropriate ligands such as hormone–hormone receptor complexes. Any one hormone is responsible for modulating the expression of numerous genes.

As well as controlling cellular function and intercellular communication, genes will regulate the cell cycle (Figure 26.1.2). Replication of cells is essential to replace cells which have been shed (e.g. from crypt villi into the gut lumen), destroyed by external forces (due to trauma or disease) or which have become dysfunctional due to irreparable nuclear damage (due to senescence or carcinogenesis). In the latter case a genetically programmed sequence is activated, leading to apoptosis or cell suicide. This physiological process results in an implosion of cellular organelles, in contrast to the cellular swelling and necrosis associated with pathological processes. The neatly compact apoptosed body is phagocytosed by neighbouring cells and, if present, macrophages. In contrast, necrosis excites an inflammatory response. A prerequisite for carcinogenesis is an excess of cellular proliferation over cell death.

Prior to cell division, all genetic DNA must be replicated, and this process begins at the highly regulated cell-cycle checkpoint known as the restriction point (or START) (Figure 26.1.2). Completion of the cell cycle requires progression through several checkpoints controlled by cyclin-dependent protein kinases (CDKs), which are part of the cell-division cycle (CDC) gene family. CDKs form complexes consisting of a catalytic (kinase) unit and a regulating (cyclin) unit (Figure 26.1.3). Activity of CDKs also requires that they are both phosphorylated on a threonine residue and dephosphorylated on a serine residue, offering a means of regulation

Table 26.1.2 Incidence and mortality of cancer in the UK*

Cancer	New cases per year	Rank	Deaths per year	Rank
Lung	43793	1	37128	1
Skin (non-melanoma)	36284	2	489	25
Colorectum	30932	3	18089	2
Breast	30075†	4	14534‡	3
CIN-cervix	21987	5	–	–
Prostate	13974	6	9635	4
Bladder	12901	7	5309	8
Stomach	12815	8	8542	5
Pancreas	7048	9	6505	7
Non-Hodgkin's lymphoma	6981	10	4317	10
Oesophagus	5908	10	6579	6
Ovary	5832	12	4393	9
Leukaemia	5832	12	3889	11
Cervix	4943	13	1561	16
Melanoma	4438	14	1521	17
Kidney	4330	15	2910	13
Uterus	4179	16	834	19
Brain	3573	17	2965	12
Multiple myeloma	3096	18	2384	14
Larynx	2376	19	951	18
Liver	1597	20	2030	15
Gall bladder	1447	21	748	21
Hodgkin's disease	1430	22	328	26
Testis	1418	23	90	32
Pharynx	1241	24	826	20
Connective tissue	1230	25	727	22
Mouth	1053	26	541	23
Thyroid	928	27	321	27
Pleura	854	28	517	24
Tongue	761	29	–	–
Bone	588	30	230	29
Eye	467	31	103	31
Small intestine	430	32	232	28
Penis	420	33	129	30
Lip	342	34	–	–

*Incidence of all neoplasms = 305726; incidence of all malignant neoplasms = 271833. Incidence data for United Kingdom of Great Britain and Northern Ireland for 1988, population = 57065400 (adapted from Cancer Research Campaign (CRC) Factsheets 1.2 and 1.3, 1994). All deaths from cancer = 160676. Mortality data for United Kingdom of Great Britain and Northern Ireland for 1994, population = 58394600 (adapted from CRC Factsheets 3.2 and 3.3, 1995). CIN = cervical intra-epithelial neoplasia.

† Includes 205 cases in men.

‡ Includes 91 deaths in men.

by cyclin-dependent kinase-inhibiting proteins (CDKIs) such as p21, p15, p27 and p16. The transcription factor E2F is crucial for the expression of several genes required for cell-cycle activation, but is otherwise sequestered by being bound to hypophosphorylated retinoblastoma protein (pRb). The Cdk4/Cyclin D or Cdk2/Cyclin E complexes can phosphorylate pRb releasing E2F. The Cdk/Cyclin complexes can be activated by intracellular signals generated by extracellular growth factors acting on cell-membrane receptors, or they may be activated

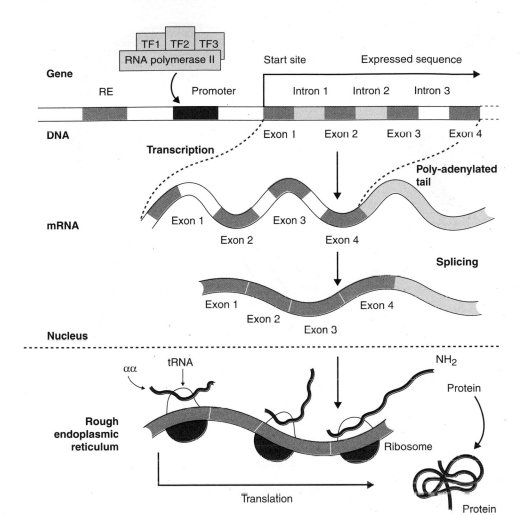

Figure 26.1.1

Transcription and translation.

permanently by mutant signal transducers such as K-Ras.

In the same way that the switch mechanism at START is controlled by positive and negative regulatory proteins, programmed cell death is controlled by pro-apoptotic (Bax, Bak and p53) and anti-apoptotic (Bcl) proteins.

The α-helix double strand of DNA is separated every time a sequence is transcribed (for gene expression) or replicated (for cell division). This can cause supercoiling of the DNA molecule, and this problem may also arise during exchange of genetic material between chromosomes (recombination) during meiosis (germ-cell proliferation). Topoisomerases are enzymes which correct undue DNA coiling. DNA topoisomerase I can break only one strand of the DNA duplex, and is involved in the correction of supercoiling during transcription. DNA polymerases II (α and β isoforms) can cleave both strands of the DNA duplex, knot and unknot circular DNA, and are essential for chromosomal segregation.

The formation of chromosomes during meiosis potentially leaves the DNA duplex at each end 'open'. This could lead to abnormal hybridization or enzyme activity. Telomerase is an enzyme which synthesizes a DNA sequence, enabling it to form a stable hairpin.

The genetic code consists of triplets of nucleotides (each of which is known as a codon), each coding for an amino acid. The sequence of codons thus determines the amino-acid sequence of a protein molecule. During replication the duplex DNA strands are separated, followed by synthesis of nucleotide sequences which are an exact mirror image of the template strands. A single nucleotide error within one codon of a transcribed gene can give rise to one of several functional mutations. A stop codon will produce a shortened (truncated) protein. A shift in nucleotide triplet recognition (frameshift mutation) will result in a completely different amino-acid sequence, a full-length protein being produced, but with a different amino acid corresponding to the altered codon (point mutation). If a mutation occurs during meiosis, this may be passed on to an offspring and then to subsequent generations (germ-cell mutation).

A series of DNA repair genes are responsible for checking the fidelity of replication and replacing incorrectly matched nucleotides.

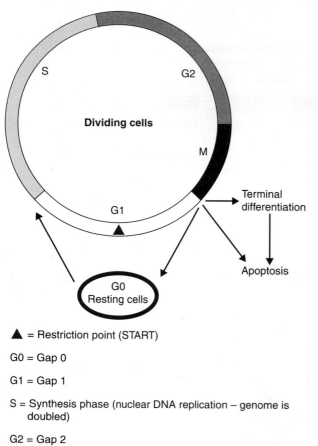

Figure 26.1.2 The cell cycle.

▲ = Restriction point (START)

G0 = Gap 0

G1 = Gap 1

S = Synthesis phase (nuclear DNA replication – genome is doubled)

G2 = Gap 2

M = Mitosis

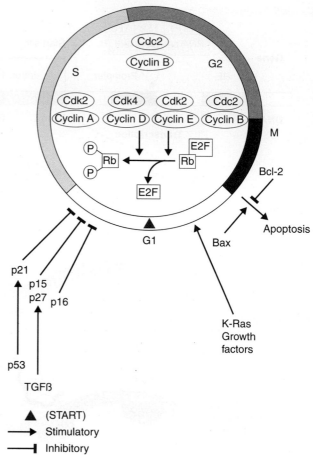

Figure 26.1.3 Control of the cell cycle.

Mutations may arise spontaneously or because of chemical carcinogens, or ionizing or UV radiation. The more often a cell divides, the greater the opportunity for mutations to occur and for these mutations to be transferred to daughter cells. A crucial role is played by p53 in guarding the integrity of the genome. If during G1 of the cell cycle excess mutations are recognized, increased p53 expression will inhibit progression to the S-phase to enable elimination of mutations. If there is an accumulation of mutations which cannot be repaired, p53 will induce apoptosis.

In cancer, the p53 check system may be overridden either by mutations in p53 *per se*, or by one or more mutations which stress the system sufficiently to overwhelm the security capacity of p53. Eventually clones of daughter cells with advantageous survival, invading and metastasizing properties become self-selected.

MOLECULAR BIOLOGY OF CANCER

In 1971, Knudson proposed the 'two-hit' hypothesis that cancer arises when two genetic mutations occur. In 1973, Cummings clarified the hypothesis by proposing that the two hits had to be against respective homologous genes, so that the mutations affected each of the maternal and paternal gene pair. In familial cancers one inherited gene mutation was already present (in all cells), the second mutation being acquired in the somatic cell, leading to malignant transformation and establishment of the cancer-cell clone. In sporadic cancers both mutations were acquired in the same somatic cell. Thus in familial disease the cancers arise in much younger individuals and are multifocal (and, in the case of symmetrical organs, bilateral). In the commoner sporadic forms, the cancers occur much later in life and are usually single. A first hit will predispose to a second hit; the exact mechanisms are not completely defined, an important one being homologous recombination during mitosis. The affected gene is often identical in equivalent familial and sporadic cancers. Knudson developed the hypothesis on the basis of retinoblastoma. In the inherited form of the latter, the tumours arise in young children and affect both eyes. In sporadic retinoblastoma only adults are affected, and only in one eye.

The gene which is mutated in retinoblastoma is *RB1*. Mutation of both genes results in absent/dysfunctional protein (pRb) with the consequence that the E2F

Table 26.1.3 Examples of tumour suppressor genes (TSGs) in inherited and sporadic cancers

TSG	Function of gene	Inherited cancer syndrome	Sporadic cancer(s) commonly affected
TP53	Cell-cycle/ apoptosis control	Li-Fraumeni	Pancreas, colorectum, lung, skin, breast, head and neck, oesophagus, prostate, bladder
RB1	Cell-cycle control	Retinoblastoma	Retinoblastoma, sarcoma, prostate, bladder, lung
APC	Cytoskeleton/ cell-cell interaction	Familial adenomatous polyposis (FAP)	Colorectum
p16 (CDKN2)	Cell-cycle control	Familial atypical multiple mole and melanoma (FAMMM)	Pancreas, head and neck, malignant melanoma
DCC	Adhesion molecule	–	Colorectum
MCC	Unknown	–	Colorectum
MSH LMH1, PMS	Mismatch/ DNA repair	Hereditary non-polyposis colon cancer (HNPCC)	–
BRCA1/2	Unknown	Breast/breast-ovarian	–
NF1/2	Cell signalling	Neurofibromatosis	–
VHL	Unknown	Von Hippel-Lindau	–
MEN1/2	Unknown	Multiple endocrine neoplasia 1/2	–
WT1	Transcription repressor	Wilm's tumour	–
SMAD4/DPC4	Cell-cycle control	Juvenile polyposis	Pancreas

transcription factor is always present at high levels, sufficient to stimulate continuous cell-cycling, irrespective of the protective activity of p53. Increased patient survival and preservation of sight in inherited retinoblastoma are now possible using laser surgery/chemotherapy, often avoiding ocular enucleation altogether. Unfortunately, since mutation of *RB1* is present in every cell in the body, cancers will arise in other organs. There is a high incidence of osteosarcoma in inherited retinoblastoma, but not in the sporadic form in which the *RB1* mutations are present only in the tumour.

RB1 is one of a class of genes known as tumour suppressor genes (Table 26.1.3). Their functional loss results in cancer, and their reintroduction results in reversion of the cell clone from a cancer to a non-malignant cell clone and/or complete destruction of the cell clone. All cancers are characterized by mutational inactivation of at least one tumour suppressor gene.

In sporadic cancer, increased cellular activity often precedes tumour suppressor gene loss. Increased intra-cellular downstream signalling may arise from mutational activation of oncogenes. Growth factors are proteins which bind to a transmembrane receptor, usually situated at the cell surface. Ligand-receptor binding results in transduction of the signal to the cytosolic domain of the receptor. The activated receptor sends the signal to a second intracellular messenger which it activates, commonly by phosphorylation. Most strongly implicated in neoplasia are the tyrosine kinase receptors (TKRs) which phosphorylate intracellular signalling molecules on tyrosine residues. This activated molecule may now participate in amplification reactions, generating additional signalling molecules such as those in the K-Ras system. Further downstream, signals involve a sequential series of kinase reactions. In the nucleus, transcription factors (c-fos, c-jun, c-myc, S6 kinase, etc.) are activated, resulting in increased expression of genes that control proliferation. Genes representing such signalling pathways may be mutated, resulting in increased un-regulated expression. If this increased expression can contribute to the development of neoplasia, the gene is termed an oncogene. The normal (or wild-type) gene is known as a proto-oncogene. An oncogene *per se* will not cause cancer – mutation of at least two oncogenes seems to be necessary.

The *K-RAS* oncogene is frequently activated by a point mutation (at codons 12, 13 and 61) in many surgical cancers, including those of the pancreas (100%), colorectum (40%) and lung (30%), frequently being the earliest observed genetic mutation. *TP53* is unusual in that it can also undergo mutational activation to function in a dominant manner. Thus it can function as an oncogene as well as a tumour suppressor gene. Erb-b2 is a receptor of the epidermal growth factor receptor (EGFR) group of TKRs. In breast cancer, over-expression of Erb-b2 (up to 60%), an important prognostic variable, is partly due to transcriptional activation and partly due to gene amplification (expression of multiple copies of the *ERB-B2* gene within each nucleus). Amplification of the transcription factor v-, n- and c-myc variants occurs in 5, 10 and 15% of cases, respectively, in lung cancer.

However, in most cases of human cancer, there is over-expression of growth factors and their respective receptors due to transcriptional activation, rather than to mutational activation or gene amplification.

SPREAD OF CANCER

Tumour cells need to acquire a considerable number of genetic characteristics to enable invasion and metastasis to occur. The high cellular proliferation rate and reduced level of apoptosis appear to be sufficient to permit clonal selection of cells with these characteristics.

The process of metastasizing has a symmetrical dynamic, namely loss of cell–cell adhesion, breakdown of the extracellular matrix (ECM), angiogenesis, motility, breakdown of the basement membrane, diapedesis into the vessel lumen, detachment and spread to a distant site, reattachment to the endothelial surface, diapedesis into the ECM and establishment of a new cancer focus, requiring stroma–tumour cell co-operation, and angiogenesis.

Important cell-adhesion molecules and receptors are the cadherins (Ca^{2+} dependent), the integrins (VLA1–6, LFA-1 and CR3), proteoglycans, notably CD44s (s = standard variant), the immunoglobulin superfamily (ICAM, VCAM and MAdCAM) and the lectin–cell adhesion molecule (LEC-CAM) family. Breakdown of the ECM involves a proteolytic cascade initiated by cysteine (cathepsin B) and serine (tissue- and urinary-plasminogen activator) proteases. The matrix-metalloproteinases (MMPs) break down specialized ECM molecules and are physiologically antagonized by specific tissue inhibitors (TIMPs). Vascular endothelial growth factor (VEGF) is a powerful angiogenic factor, and scatter factor or hepatocyte growth factor (HGF) is a potent motility factor. In cancer there is impaired function of cell-adhesion molecules (by gene loss or mutation) and over-expression of MMPs, VEGF and HGF.

Patients with cancer frequently produce showers of hundreds or thousands of cancer cells into the circulation, but very few of these are successful in establishing a metastasis. Interestingly, some tumours have a predilection for certain metastatic sites. Common routes of spread include local invasion, and lymphatic, perineural, haematogenous and transcoelomic routes.

IMMUNOLOGY OF CANCER

Destruction of cancer cells by the immune system requires recognition of cancer-related antigens.

Cancer-related antigens can induce:

1. production of antibodies (Abs) from B-cells;

2. cellular cytotoxicity by cytotoxic T-cells (TCs), macrophages and natural killer (NK) cells; and

3. Ab-dependent cellular cytotoxicity (ADCC).

The structures of Abs and T-cell receptors (TCRs) show many similarities. The genes encoding the heavy and (κ and λ) light chains of immunoglobulins (Igs) contain V, D and J gene segments which undergo recombination to produce a vast number of variable domains. Similarly, the genes encoding the α and β chains of TCRs (γ and δ chains in the small population of thymus-derived T-cells) also have V, D and J gene segments which undergo recombination. The huge diversity of Igs and TCRs is such that any natural antigen will be recognized by (at least) several different Ig- and TCR-expressing clones. Appropriate antigen recognition will result in a large clonal expansion, provided that an adequate co-stimulus is given at the same time by specific co-stimulating molecules or cytokines.

The clonal expansion of Ab-forming cells (AFCs) requires two processes (Figure 26.1.4), namely binding of *native* antigen by B-cell Ig-receptor, and stimulatory signals from T-helper (T_H) cells generated by the presentation of *processed* antigen to virgin T-cells by professional antigen-presenting cells (APCs). The latter include mononuclear phagocytes, dendritic cells and B- and T-cells in lymphoid tissues.

T-cells can usually recognize antigens only when they are presented in association with major histocompatibility complex (MHC) class I or II molecules (MHC-restricted T-cells). *Endogeneously produced antigens* and those associated with *viruses* are processed from the native antigen (protein) by cleavage in proteasomes to small peptides, and are presented at the cell surface

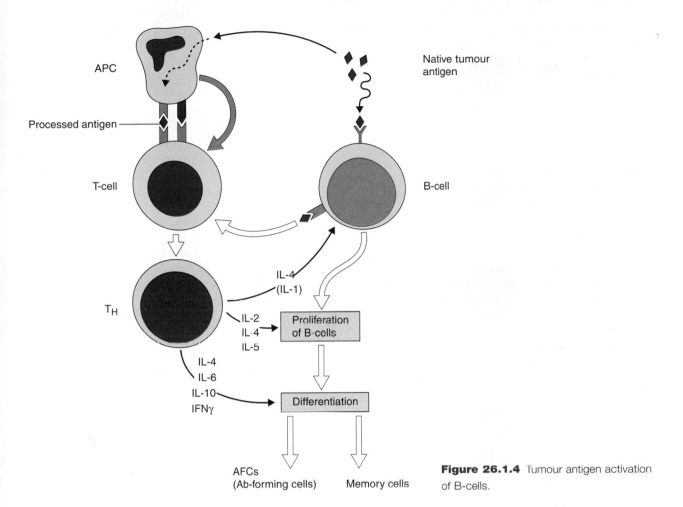

Figure 26.1.4 Tumour antigen activation of B-cells.

complexed with MHC class I α1–3 chains and β2-microglobulin (β2m). *Exogenously produced antigens* are endocytosed, cleaved into peptides in MIIC vesicles and presented at the cell surface complexed with MHC class II α1–2 and β1–2 chains. CD8[+] T-cells recognize only Class I complexed antigen, whilst CD4[+] T-cells recognize only Class II complexed antigens.

Most CD8[+] T-cells are TC lymphocytes, whilst CD4[+] T-cells are T_H lymphocytes. Suppressor (TS) lymphocytes, which modulate T_H and B-cell activity, are also CD8[+]. T-cells will infiltrate tumours, becoming activated by cell–cell interactions (TILs). Circulating cytokines may also have a stimulatory effect on T-cells, producing cytokine (lymphokine)-activated killer cells (LAKs), but to a lesser degree.

Tumours produce a very poor antibody response. Antigen presentation by tumour cells with appropriate expression of co-stimulatory molecules (notably B7) will promote TC activity. An even more powerful response may be evoked if T_H cells are activated by interaction with APCs (Figure 26.1.5).

Tumours evade the immune system by multiple mechanisms:

1. lack of co-stimulatory molecule expression during tumour-cell antigen presentation, resulting in anergy;

2. lack of MHC class I alleles (more than 50% of tumours) preventing antigen presentation. The genes include those involved in the proteasome complex (LMP2/7), intracellular antigen transport by the ABC superfamily (TAP1/2), and surface α-chain and/or β2m complex expression;

3. lack of cell–cell adhesion molecules (LFA-1/3, ICAM-2);

4. expression of anti-adhesive molecules, such as mucins or variant forms of CD44(v);

5. secretion of immunosuppressive cytokines (TGFβ).

Immune surveillance At one time immune surveillance was believed to play a crucial role in preventing cancer. Now it is recognized that the immune system usually only becomes active when a cancer is already well established. There is one exception to this – the immune system plays a pivotal role in preventing viral infection and hence in controlling cancers caused by viruses.

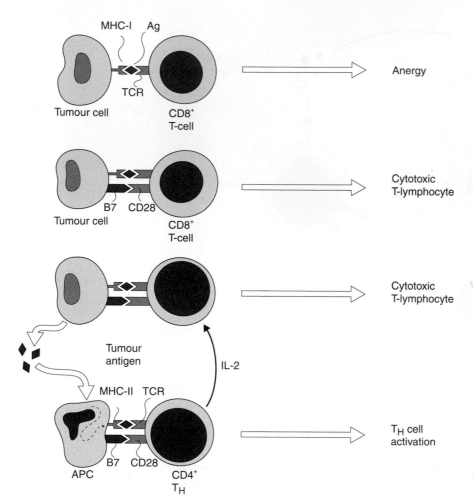

Figure 26.1.5 Tumour antigen presentation by T-cells.

CAUSES OF CANCER

Cancer is a disease of genes, and it may be inherited or acquired.

Inherited cancer A specific DNA mutation of a tumour suppressor gene (TSG) is inherited in all cells through the parental germ-cell line. A second hit knocks out the function of the second homologous gene in a somatic cell, initiating a sequence of genetic mutations, culminating in the formation of a cancer cell. The TSG mutation is then passed on to siblings through the germ-cell line.

Chemical carcinogens These probably account for the majority of sporadic cancers. The tobacco-associated nitrosamines cause lung cancer, and the aromatic amines (α- and β-napthylamine and benzidrine) cause various cancers in workers in chemical and manufacturing plants. Aflatoxin, produced by the mould *Aspergillus flavens*, is a cofactor in liver cancer caused by viral infection. The exact mechanisms of action are not understood, but the *K-RAS* oncogene and the *TP53* tumour suppressor gene are often affected by mutations. Differences between individuals in the expression of

isoforms of detoxification enzymes such as glutathione-S-transferase account for some of the variance in susceptibility to exposure.

Ultraviolet (UV) radiation UV radiation consists of three regions of wavelength, namely UV-A (320–400 nm), UV-B (280–320 nm) and UV-C (200–280 nm). The ozone layer absorbs all of UV-C and some of UV-B, the remainder reaching the earth's surface. DNA is damaged by UV light, which causes pyrimidine dimers to be inserted into the DNA, and repair normally takes place by sequential endonuclease, DNA polymerase and DNA ligase activity. Within $1\,\mathrm{cm}^2$ of human skin exposed to UV radiation there may be several clones of cells with p53 mutations, all of which are eliminated normally. Skin cancers and malignant melanomas arise from an inability to repair mutations in key genes or to eliminate the clones.

Ionizing radiation Electromagnetic waves (γ-particles) generated by radiation penetrate deeply into tissues, causing direct damage to DNA bases and DNA strands and, by radiolysis of water, generating reactive O_2 species which subsequently damage DNA. Although the great majority of cells die, or the DNA defects are repaired,

Table 26.1.4 Viruses that cause cancer in humans

Virus	Cancer	Viral gene implicated	Mode of action	Cofactors
Epstein-Barr virus (EBV)	Nasopharyngeal carcinoma	*LMP-1*	Intracellular signalling	Genetic Dietary
Herpes virus group (172-kb DNA)	Endemic Burkitt's lymphoma (B-cell)	*EBNA-1*	Expansion of B-cell clone with translocation (t[8:14])	Malaria
	Hodgkin's disease (40%) (?Rare lymphoid cell)	*?LMP-1*	Intracellular signalling	?
	Myosarcoma	?	?	?
	Post-transplant lymphomatous proliferative disease (PTLPD) (B-cell)	*EBNA-2*; *3a,b,c*; *LP*; *LMP-1*	Transcriptional activation D-cyclins	Immune suppression
Kaposi's sarcoma herpes virus (KSHV; HHV8)	Kaposi's sarcoma	Numerous genes implicated	?Inhibition of apoptosis D-cyclins, signal transduction	Human immuno-deficiency virus (HIV)
	Body-cavity-based lymphoma	?		?
	Multicentric Castlemen's disease	Several genes		?
Human papilloma viruses (HPV) Types 16–18, 33, 69 (8-kb DNA)	Cervical cancer Cervical intra-epithelial neoplasia (CIN)	*E6, E7*	E6 → p53 E7 → pRb	Smoking
Human T-cell leukaemia virus type I (HTLV-1) C-type retrovirus (RNA)	Adult T-cell leukaemia lymphoma (ATLL) (CD4⁺ T-lymphocytes)	*TAX*	Transcriptional activation, IL-2, IL-2-R p53, p16, D-cyclins	?
Hepatitis B virus (HBV)	Liver	X-protein	?Transcriptional transactivation	Aflatoxins
Hepatitis C virus (HCV)	Liver	None	Uncontrolled replication	?
HEPADNA family (small DNA, replicate using reverse transcription of RNA)				

some may survive and become clonally selected as cancer cells.

Cellular instability Ageing of a stem-cell line (as in many common cancers) or chronic inflammation (as in Marjolin's ulcer) will result in cellular instability, causing increased proliferation and decreased apoptosis. Increasingly the acquisition of more mutations which go uncorrected leads to malignant transformation. Telomerase is involved, as its activity is steadily impaired with increasing age.

Viruses Once thought not to be implicated in cancers in humans, viruses are now known to cause several cancers which account for at least 20% of the world-wide incidence of cancer (Table 26.1.4).

Many of the mechanisms and causes of cancer are not understood clearly. *Helicobacter pylori* is strongly associated with gastric cancer to the extent that it is regarded as a Class I carcinogen by the World Health Organization (WHO), but the detailed mechanism of cancer pathogenesis is not yet known.

SURGICAL TREATMENT OF CANCER

SURGERY: RESECTION FOR CURE

Malignant tumours vary greatly in their behaviour. At one end of the spectrum are those of low-grade malignant potential with a restricted ability to metastasize. In such cases, complete surgical removal usually results in cure. At the other extreme are tumours that metastasize early, often before they are clinically detectable. However, most tumours lie somewhere between these two extremes and, in the absence of overt metastatic disease, surgery offers the best hope of cure.

At the turn of the century, Halsted proposed that tumours metastasize in a systematic manner and that the regional draining lymph nodes are involved before the tumour becomes widely disseminated. Based on this theory, and in an attempt to improve survival, he popularized the concept of radical mastectomy. This involved removal of the breast together with all of the regional draining nodes and the pectoral muscles. The surgical community embraced his ideas and operation. However, many patients underwent radical resection only to develop recurrent disease at a local or distant site. One approach was to adopt even more extensive surgery, involving partial excision of the chest, including the ribs. Another approach was to develop the hypothesis that micrometastases were present in a significant proportion of patients at the time of diagnosis, in which case aggressive local resection as advocated by Halsted was unlikely to improve survival.

In 1985 the results of a US multicentre randomized controlled trial (RCT) sponsored by the National Surgical Adjuvant Breast and Bowel Project (NSABP) (B-06) in 2163 patients comparing lumpectomy, lumpectomy and radiotherapy to the breast, and mastectomy for early carcinoma of the breast were reported. All patients underwent axillary lymph-node dissection. There was no difference in survival rates between the three groups. Although the rate of local recurrence was higher in patients treated with lumpectomy alone, local control could be achieved by delayed radiotherapy.

Resection of a primary tumour with its draining nodal groups is widely practised in a range of malignancies – quite rightly so since a certain proportion of patients with involved nodes go on to become long-term survivors. Identification of lymph-node involvement provides important prognostic information and can be used to select patients who are suitable for adjuvant therapy. The extent of surgical resection and its associated morbidity is the point at issue. Beyond the immediate local lymph nodes, there is no strong evidence that extensive resection with wide lymphadenectomy improves survival (in cancers of the oesophagus, stomach, liver, pancreas, colon, rectum and breast). However, there are apparently better results associated with radical resection of gastric, oesophageal, pancreatic and rectal cancers from some centres in Japan compared to results from Europe, and a number of randomized controlled trials are examining this issue.

Complete resection of the primary tumour is essential for cure. The radical margins should be macroscopically and microscopically clear of tumour and, if possible, adjacent involved organs should be taken *en bloc*. In principle, a margin of 2–3 cm is the minimum distance between the resected edge and the cancer required to effect local cure. In the stomach, oesophagus and lower rectum it is important to ensure that margins are clear microscopically at the time of resection, because of submucosal infiltration.

Tumour mobilization may seed tumour cells into the circulation and promote metastasis. To avoid this, early vascular exclusion of the tumour and dissection with a no-touch technique as far as is possible is advocated. It has also been suggested that dissemination of tumour cells in an aerosol form can occur at the time of laparoscopic surgery, and may lead to recurrence, particularly at port sites. Biopsy of a potentially resectable cancer should be avoided if the needle tract transgresses tissue planes or cavities (such as liver or pancreas) unless the needle tract is to be excised (e.g. in cancer of the breast).

Pre-operative staging Radical resection of a tumour is inappropriate in the presence of metastatic disease. In order to reduce the numbers of patients undergoing unnecessary surgery, various staging protocols have been introduced. These utilize techniques such as computerized axial tomography (CT), magnetic resonance imaging (MRI), laparoscopy, and endoscopic and laparoscopic ultrasound (EUS, LUS). Pre-operative staging may identify patients who will benefit from other more appropriate palliative procedures. In advanced local disease without metastases, pre-operative radiotherapy or chemotherapy (neoadjuvant therapy) may convert a locally advanced tumour into one that is resectable (e.g. in breast, oesophageal and rectal cancers). Local recurrence may on occasion be amenable to further potentially curative resection (e.g. in breast, stomach, colon, pancreatic, liver and rectal cancers).

Follow-up Although follow-up at regular intervals can be justified to some extent for detection of local recurrence, there is no strong evidence in favour of aggressive follow-up of patients following curative resection of a malignant tumour in terms of cost-benefit/survival. This issue is well illustrated by colorectal carcinoma, in which there is a 1–5% rate of metachronous tumours, and up to 70% of cases develop liver metastases. It is still unclear how often colonoscopy should be performed postoperatively, and the percentage of lives saved is not known. Only about 5% of liver metastases are isolated to a single lobe and amenable to 'curative' resection. There is no evidence that aggressive follow-up with US, CT, MRI or tumour markers improves the overall detection rate of favourable liver metastases, let alone demonstrates an overall improvement in longer-term survival.

Follow-up is important for monitoring results, providing supportive care to patients (quality of life) and investigating symptoms which may be related to the original cancer (including/excluding recurrence).

Causes of failure The reasons why patients with an apparently localized cancer are not cured by surgery are as follows:

1. micro-metastases are widely disseminated already;

2. the resection margins of the tumour are not clear or adequate (< 2–3 cm);

3. the tumour has been breached and cells disseminated by biopsy or cutting into the tumour and/or excessive handling of the tumour during surgery;

4. failure to include locally draining lymphatics, lymph nodes, neural and fascial tissue in an *en-bloc* resection with the main tumour. Inevitably this means cutting across these structures, which may contain malignant cells, leading to spillage and dissemination;

5. development of a similar cancer *de novo* (i.e. second primary).

Tumour cells which have invaded locally or metastasized may remain dormant for many years after the primary has been removed. For example, patients with breast cancer may present 20 years after the initial surgery. Neo-angiogenesis around a colony of metastatic cells is a key mechanism for increased growth and reactivation of disseminated disease (upregulatation of VEGF is involved).

SURGERY FOR CURE: METASTASES AND LOCAL RECURRENCE

In certain situations, resection of localized metastatic disease may be justified. For example, patients with liver metastases from colorectal carcinoma limited to one or other lobe, without other evidence of disease, may benefit from resectional surgery. The 5-year survival rate in this group is about 20%. These patients self-select into two groups, namely those that have fairly rapid recurrence (and it is likely that in these individuals occult metastases were present at the time of the original procedure), and those that become long-term survivors. Only around 5% of all patients with colorectal liver metastases are eligible for resection. A similar proportion of patients with solitary lung metastasis are eligible for resection, with a similar prospect of long-term cure.

Local recurrence is rarely an isolated event but, if so, resection can lead to cure or improvement in symptoms (e.g. in rectal cancer and breast cancer). In metastatic disease or locally advanced recurrence, *chemotherapy* may improve survival and quality of life, even in the absence of symptoms. The improvement in median survival achieved by chemotherapy is of the order of 6–12 months for colorectal cancer and 2–3 years for breast cancer.

SURGERY FOR PALLIATION AND TUMOUR DEBULKING

From Table 26.1.2 it can be observed that a high proportion of patients with surgical cancers (most of whom have resection) still die of the cancer. Although the intention is to cure by resection, often this must be regarded as a palliative measure. At one end of the spectrum, most non-melanoma skin cancers can be cured by surgery alone. At the other end of the spectrum, virtually no patients with pancreatic ductal adenocarcinoma are ever cured by surgery.

The concept of 'debulking cancer' is crude, but nevertheless appears valid on empirical grounds. Thus testicular malignancies now have a very high cure rate, but only if resection is followed by appropriate chemotherapy (and/or radiotherapy). On the other hand, chemotherapy (and/or radiotherapy) will not be effective without resection ('debulking'). The value of 'debulking' only applies if the primary cancer and any metastatic disease can be removed completely macroscopically. Thus removal of a pancreatic cancer is of no value if there are peritoneal metastases, liver metastases or lung metastases, as symptoms are not improved (quality of life) and survival time is not increased (it may well be decreased by post-operative deaths).

Palliative resection is justified only if there is a significant improvement in symptoms and/or survival. Thus resection of a rectal cancer is often justified to improve symptoms (e.g. rectal bleeding, incontinence, diarrhoea and pain) even in the presence of advanced local disease and/or metastases. Bypass of luminal obstruction improves symptoms for gastric outlet malignancy, small-bowel disease, large-bowel cancer and bile-duct obstruction. An internal intestinal bypass or a colostomy may be required.

Non-surgical methods of relieving obstruction may be more desirable than surgery in many cases, as they avoid the morbidity and mortality associated with the latter. Important examples include the following:

1. endoscopic or percutaneous stenting of biliary obstruction;

2. endoscopic stent insertion in oesophageal, duodenal or distal colon obstruction;

3. laser treatment of oesophageal or colon cancers;

4. photodynamic therapy, which is a more selective form of laser treatment in which cancer cells take up a photosensitive dye (administered intravenously). The dye absorbs the energy of the laser source of a particular wavelength, leading to death of those cells. The normal cells which have not absorbed the dye are therefore protected.

RADIOTHERAPY OF CANCER

PRINCIPLES OF RADIOTHERAPY

Decay of radioactive isotopes produces radioactive particles, e.g. β-particles (electrons) or γ-particles (electromagnetic radiation). β-particles have poor penetration and are rarely used for therapy. The use of natural sources of radiation is now mostly limited to intra-cavity irradiation (brachytherapy) and the treatment of thyroid disease. Linear accelerators allow the production of high-energy X-rays (which are synonymous with γ-particles). These can be focused and combined with targeting modalities such as CT for accurate delivery of radiation. High-energy beams have high tissue penetration and reduce the cutaneous erythema seen after treatment.

Excess energy destroys the complex molecular structure of cells, and the type of damage depends on the nature of the energy and its intensity. For example, thermal energy coagulates proteins and destroys other large macromolecules, as a consequence of which a tissue is immediately and irrevocably damaged. The damage inflicted by short-wave electromagnetic radiation (X-rays) is initially much less apparent. This is because at the doses of radiation conventionally used, damage is primarily to DNA, with relative sparing of other molecules, and cell division is required to reveal the consequences.

Damage to normal surrounding tissue limits the dose of radiation that can be safely delivered to a tumour. Rapidly dividing cells are more sensitive, so normal tissues that are particularly affected include the gastrointestinal tract and the bone marrow. However, cells that are dividing slowly may exhibit the effects of radiation damage at a later date. One particular long-term problem is vascular damage, with narrowing and occlusion of small vessels. This can cause ischaemia, fibrosis and even necrosis. Such changes can be particularly debilitating if they involve the gastrointestinal tract.

Radiotherapy impairs healing. A number of different mechanisms may be involved. Following high-dose radiotherapy there is systemic immunosuppression, decreased migration of monocytes and reduced wound cytokine levels. Radiation damages tissue fibroblasts, resulting in collagen-deficient weak scars. The vascular changes described above lead to chronic tissue ischaemia, and this in turn causes deficient repair. This last mechanism is probably the most important in clinical practice. Thus if surgery is performed soon after a course of radiotherapy, healing will be relatively preserved. However, if there has been a long delay, chronic ischaemia may lead to impaired healing and wound failure.

There is a critical balance between a tumour and the surrounding tissue and their relative rates of cell division and DNA repair. Normal cells divide more slowly and often have more efficient DNA repair mechanisms. If the interval between doses is correctly chosen to allow DNA repair in the normal cells but not in the malignant ones, then destruction of tumour with preservation of normal surrounding cells can be optimized. This is one of the reasons why radiotherapy is given in fractionated doses that are spread over a number of weeks. Parts of a large tumour are often hypoxic, and cells in these areas will be dividing less rapidly and will therefore be relatively radio-resistant. Breaking up a course of radiotherapy into a number of doses may allow revascularization and increased tumour kill in these areas. The effects of radiotherapy will be enhanced by treating hypoxia or administering radiosensitizing agents such as 5-fluorouracil (5FU).

Radiotherapy is quantified by the gray (Gy), which is defined as one joule per kilogram (1 Gy = 100 rads).

MOLECULAR TARGETS OF RADIOTHERAPY

Damage is caused by collisions with electrons, causing their excitation or displacement. Damage to DNA arises by direct ionization of DNA itself, or as a consequence of radiolysis of water. The latter results in the formation of highly reactive species (hydroxyl radical OH^-, hydrated electron e_{aq}^- and hydrogen peroxide, H_2O_2). Phosphodiester bonds are cleaved and sugars and bases damaged in DNA. A dose of 1 Gy will produce thousands of damaged DNA bases, 1000 single-strand breaks, 150 DNA-protein cross-links and 40 double-strand breaks. Repair of DNA is effected by DNA repair enzymes (redoxyendonuclease, AP endonuclease, DNA polymerase β and DNA ligase). Ionizing radiation will inhibit DNA synthesis – p53 is activated, inducing G1 arrest and Cdc2/Cyclin B is inhibited, producing G2/M arrest. In addition, DNA repair genes, the growth arrest protein Gadd-45 and cytokines are induced. The result will be either complete repair, induction of apoptosis, or necrosis and induction of the inflammatory response, depending on the dose administered and the susceptibility of the particular cell to the ionizing radiation. Radiosensitizing agents presumably act by further inhibiting the induced repair mechanisms.

CLINICAL APPLICATIONS OF RADIOTHERAPY

Complete cure is possible in certain tumour types by radiotherapy alone (Table 26.1.5). Primary treatment in anal cancer (with chemotherapy) can lead to complete cure, avoiding the need for an abdomino-perineal excision. The disadvantages of radiotherapy are the lack of excised tissue for histological purposes and the lack of accurate staging data. Increasingly, the tendency is to combine radiotherapy, chemotherapy and surgery in an attempt to optimize the treatment of individual cancers.

Adjuvant radiotherapy is often given to reduce local recurrence following surgery. Neoadjuvant therapy given before resection may allow the downstaging of an otherwise irresectable primary tumour. Alternatively, radiotherapy may be delivered after resection. One advantage of delaying therapy is that more accurate staging data will be available from histopathology. Concerns previously expressed about impaired healing have been dispelled. Reduced local recurrence rates following adjuvant radiotherapy have been shown in controlled clinical trials of early breast cancer treated by lumpectomy and radiotherapy compared to lumpectomy alone (NSABP), and in advanced (Dukes C) cancer of the rectum (MRC). However, a reduction in local recurrence rates by adjuvant therapy does not equate to a reduction in long-term mortality because of coexisting distant metastases.

Table 26.1.5 Role of radiotherapy in cancer treatment

Primary treatment (potentially curative)
Squamous-cell carcinomas
  head and neck cancer
  oesophageal cancer
  anal cancer
  squamous-cell skin cancer
  cervical cancer
Basal-cell carcinoma (skin)
Bladder cancer
Lymphomas

Adjuvant treatment (increased survival)
Breast cancer
Rectal cancer
Astrocytoma
Endometrial cancer

Palliation (improved symptoms)
Bony metastases
Pain from infiltrating lesions
Spinal cord compression

Radiation can be used to palliate advanced disease (e.g. pain from bony metastases or acute spinal cord compression). In this situation, radiotherapy can be given as a short course or even as a single dose, since the overriding aim is to palliate rather than to eradicate a tumour.

CHEMOTHERAPY OF CANCER

BASIC CONCEPTS

Skipper's laws Since all tumour cells are dividing, growth will be exponential, resulting in a straight line on a semi-log plot. A cytotoxic drug will follow first-order kinetics and kill the same proportion of cells each time. From these values it is possible to determine how many doses are needed to eradicate a particular tumour with a particular drug. These laws were determined in the 1970s using various numbers of L1210 mouse leukaemia cells injected into mice followed by observation of growth with and without injected drugs. In human cancer these laws do not strictly apply.

Gompertzian growth Cancers that develop *in vivo* follow a sigmoid curve when the number of cells is plotted against time. Factors which contribute to this type of growth curve include the fact that not all tumour cells are dividing, and the fact that in solid tumours growth may outstrip angiogenesis, leading to areas of hypoxia or necrosis in which cells are dividing poorly.

Goldie-Coldman hypothesis This hypothesis proposes that drug-resistant clones of cells will develop spontaneously and/or in response to chemotherapy. Macroscopic detection of tumours requires the presence of $> 10^9$ tumour cells, and resistant clones occur after every 10^5 cell divisions. Thus resistant clones are present at the time of clinical diagnosis. The larger the tumour, the more resistant clones it contains.

MECHANISMS OF ACTION

Neoplastic cells divide more rapidly than normal cells. Chemotherapy involves the use of drugs which interfere with cell division and take advantage of this difference to selectively kill the cancer cells (Table 26.1.6). The action of a particular drug may be improved by giving another agent which modulates its action: 5-fluorouracil (5FU) is converted into the active form (5-fluoro-2'-deoxyuridylate monophosphate, FdUMP) to bind covalently with thymidylate synthetase, inhibiting pyrimidine synthesis and blocking cell division. Folinic acid, which is a substrate for this reaction, potentiates inhibition of thymidylate synthetase and hence cell division.

Since cytotoxic drugs produce their effects by inhibiting cell division, at therapeutic doses their principal side-effects are on normal cells which have a naturally high cell proliferation rate. Thus the haematopoietic system (mainly consisting of white cells and platelets) and cells lining the gastrointestinal tract (leading to mucositis and diarrhoea) are mostly affected.

CLINICAL APPLICATIONS OF CHEMOTHERAPY

Modern chemotherapy regimens can now cure a high proportion of certain types of malignancy (Table 26.1.7). For some of the commoner malignancies cure is not possible with chemotherapy, but high ($> 50\%$) response rates can be achieved with prolongation of life. Chemotherapy may have a dual role for these cancers, first as adjuvant treatment following resection, and secondly as palliative treatment in the presence of recurrence or metastases. Patients with advanced colorectal cancer may have improved quality of life and survival (approximately 6–12 months) if chemotherapy is administered even in the absence of symptoms. In advanced breast cancer, an extra 2–3 years of life may be observed with chemotherapy. In many cancers the response rates are poor ($< 30\%$), with no influence on survival. The clinical role of chemotherapy in this setting is marginal.

WHO response criteria In assessing the response rate to any non-resectional form of treatment (radiotherapy, chemotherapy, biological therapy, gene therapy, etc.) the World Health Organization (WHO) criteria should be used (see Table 26.1.8).

COMBINED CHEMOTHERAPY AND RADIOTHERAPY

Chemotherapy may be given at the time of radiotherapy in order to increase the sensitivity of the tissues to ionizing radiation. The most widely used drug is 5FU, given with external beam radiotherapy. This form of treatment has been shown to reduce local recurrence rates following resection of rectal cancer given either before surgery (neoadjuvant treatment) or after excision (adjuvant treatment).

In addition, chemotherapy courses may be given subsequent to surgery and radiotherapy, an important example being node-positive women with breast cancer (CMF – see Table 26.1.6). Adjuvant treatment for cancer may not translate across all stages and sites. Thus 5FU and folinic acid improve survival in Dukes C colon cancer, but this has not been demonstrated for Dukes B colon cancer or for Dukes B or C rectal cancer. Trials are ongoing to establish any potential value of this treatment.

Randomized controlled trials As for any condition, treatment regimens (of chemotherapy and/or radiotherapy) for cancer which have not been shown to have a benefit as demonstrated by at least two randomized controlled trials should not be used routinely, in general terms. Since the benefit of any adjuvant treatment over resection alone is only of the order of 10%, very large numbers of patients (a minimum of 400–500) are required to show a benefit in randomized controlled trials. If two adjuvant modalities are used, such as radiotherapy and then chemotherapy, over 1000 patients are usually required in randomized controlled trials. The numbers required for statistical significance rise dramatically as the perceived benefit decreases.

ENDOCRINE THERAPY

This form of treatment relies on selectivity by targeting the HREs on DNA or cell-surface receptors of tumours derived from cells which are especially hormone sensitive.

BREAST CANCER

Tamoxifen is an anti-oestrogen that produces responses in 60% of oestrogen receptor-'positive' breast cancers. The tamoxifen–oestrogen receptor complex will not bind to nuclear DNA HRE elements, and thus

Table 26.1.6 Classification and mechanisms of action of chemotherapy drugs

Class of drug	Name of drug	Tumour targets	Mechanism of any action
Antimetabolites (DNA synthesis)	5-Fluorouracil	Gastrointestinal cancers	Inhibits pyrimidine synthesis
	Cytosine arabinoside	AML	Inhibits pyrimidine synthesis
	6-Mercaptopurine	Leukaemias	Inhibits purine synthesis
	Methotrexate	Breast (CMF)	Inhibits dihydrofolate reductase
		Gastric (FAM)	
Camptotecans	Irinotecan	Under evaluation	Inhibits DNA topoisomerase I
	Topetecan		
Chloroethyl nitrosureas	BCNU	Brain tumours	Inter-strand DNA cross-linking
DNA cross-linking agents	Cisplatin	Germ cell, ovary, SCLC, lymphoma	DNA cross-linking
	Mitomycin C	Gastrointestinal cancers, breast, NSCLC	DNA cross-linking
Epipodophyllotoxins	Etoposide	SCLC, lymphomas	Inhibits DNA topoisomerase II
Glycopeptides	Bleomycin	Germ-cell tumours, pleural cavity (effusions)	Free radicals causing DNA strand breaks
Intercalating agents	Adriamycin	Breast, lung, sarcomas	Inhibits DNA topoisomerase II and generates free radicals
	Mitoxantrone		
Oxazaphosphorins	Cyclophosphamide	Breast, lymphomas, leukaemias, soft-tissue sarcomas	Inter- and intra-strand DNA cross-linking
	Ifosfamide		
Simple alkylating agents	Streptozotocin	Endocrine	Base alkylation
Taxanes	Paclitaxel	Breast, ovary	Dysfunctional microtubule assembly
Vinca alkaloids	Vincristine	Wilm's, Ewing's, rhabdomyosarcoma, ALL, lymphomas, myeloma	Inhibits microtubule assembly (binds to tubule molecules, preventing polymerization)

CMF = cyclophosphamide, mitomycin C, 5-fluorouracil; FAM = 5-fluorouracil, adriamycin, methotrexate; BCNU = *bis*-chloroethyl nitrosurea; AML = acute myeloid leukaemia; SCLC = small-cell lung cancer; NSCLC = non-small-cell lung cancer; ALL = acute lymphatic leukaemia.

Table 26.1.7 Spectrum of responses to chemotherapy

Potentially curable
Testicular germ-cell tumours
Choriocarcinoma
Childhood cancers
Leukaemias
Lymphomas

High response rates, prolonged survival
Breast cancer
Bladder cancer
Colorectal cancer
Ovarian cancer
Small-cell lung cancer

Poor response rates, survival little changed
Pancreatic cancer
Malignant melanoma
Hypernephroma
Non-small-cell lung cancer

transcription of a wide range of oestrogen-dependent genes is reduced. Tamoxifen also acts via other mechanisms, as about 20% of oestrogen receptor-'negative' breast cancers also respond.

Tamoxifen may be used in four situations:

1. for prevention of breast cancer. A trial in the USA has shown a reduction in overall and breast-cancer-related deaths in high-risk individuals. There is an increased risk of endometrial cancer, but this seems to be outweighed by the reduction in breast-cancer deaths. The results of a long-term UK trial are awaited;

2. as adjuvant treatment. Widely used in post-menopausal cancer, there is now strong evidence that it should also be used in pre-menopausal women. The proportion of lives saved is of the order of 6–10% at 10 years. Although the proportional benefit is small, thousands of lives are saved because

breast cancer is a common condition. The drug has minimal side-effects, it is easy to administer (oral tablets) and is relatively cheap;

3. in advanced disease, endocrine therapy is applicable if there are mild to moderate symptoms, a previous response to endocrine treatment, a long disease-free interval and an oestrogen receptor-'positive' tumour. In the absence of these criteria, systemic chemotherapy is recommended;

4. if given to elderly patients who are unsuitable for surgery and/or chemotherapy, tamoxifen will result in tumour regression (and occasionally complete disappearance), improving the quality of life.

Failure of first-line endocrine therapy after an initial response indicates a likely response to second- and third-line drugs which have been designed to interfere with and/or inhibit the metabolism of oestrogen and other steroids (medroxyprogesterone, megestrol acetate, aminoglutethimide, hydrocortisone, nandrolone decanoate and LHRH analogues).

Ovarian ablation by surgery or radiotherapy is equally effective, and this approach may be particularly attractive in less affluent countries.

PROSTATE CANCER

These cancers are usually androgen dependent. The management of prostate cancer is complicated by the fact that it is extremely common in older men (60–80%) but runs a fairly indolent course in the majority of cases. Unfortunately, at the present time it is not possible to predict which cancers are aggressive and which are relatively benign. Thus a common approach is to use anti-androgens in symptomatic patients.

About 80% of prostate cancers are responsive to endocrine therapy, but the extent and duration of the response are unpredictable. However, all tumours eventually progress to an androgen-independent state. There

Table 26.1.8 World Health Organization (WHO) classification of responses to (non-resectional) cancer therapy (this can only be applied to tumours with at least two measurable dimensions)

Response	Definition
Complete response (CR)	No residual disease
Partial response (PR)	A reduction in tumour volume of >50% using the two greatest dimensions
Stable disease (SD)	A reduction in tumour volume of <50% or an increase of <25% using the two greatest dimensions
Progressive disease (PD)	An increase in tumour volume of >25% using the two greatest dimensions

is no obvious relationship between androgen-receptor 'positivity' and response using similar receptor detection techniques to those used for the oestrogen receptor. This may be related to clonal selection of androgen receptors with mutations in the hormone-binding domain. These receptors therefore give rise to transcriptional activation of androgen-dependent genes following receptor binding not only of androgen but also of the anti-androgen, oestrogen and progesterone.

Commonly used drugs include stilboestrol and LHRH analogues. Bilateral orchidectomy is an alternative.

GASTROINTESTINAL ENDOCRINE TUMOURS

Distinct syndromes may be produced by a variety of gastrointestinal endocrine tumours. Many of them possess one or more of the five somatostatin receptors (SMSR1–5). In the presence of symptoms and functioning SMSRs, the function and/or growth of the tumour may be blocked by the administration of appropriate somatostatin (SMS) analogues. The half-life of physiological SMS is too short to be of pharmacological value.

Like all cells, non-endocrine cells of the gastrointestinal tract also possess hormone receptors. Attempts at hormonal manipulation of these tumours have not proved successful, because hormonal sensitivity is slight (e.g. tamoxifen given for pancreatic cancer) and/or because the hormone has been targeted against tumours which lack the designated receptors (e.g. octreotide, an SMS analogue, directed against pancreatic cancer).

THYROID CANCER

Follicular papillary and anaplastic cancer arises from the thyroid follicular cells. In physiological states, follicular cells are under growth control by the action of TSH. Following TSH receptor (TSHR) binding at the cell surface, the signal is transduced via adenyl-cyclase to activate secondary messengers (cyclic AMP and protein kinase A), leading to increased nuclear transcription, cell activity, growth and division. Following complete resection of thyroid cancer, the lifetime administration of thyroxine (T_4) is important. T_4 renders the patient euthyroid and suppresses the production of TSH from the pituitary gland (acting on TRH at the level of the hypothalamus), removing the major growth factor for any residual thyroid cancer cells.

IMMUNOTHERAPY

PASSIVE IMMUNOTHERAPY

This involves the use of specific allogenic antibodies directed against tumour antigens, which are used to destroy cancer cells (Table 26.1.9). This therapy depends on the existence of tumour-associated antigens, i.e. antigens that are expressed selectively on tumour cells, or tumour-specific antigens. Many tumour-associated antigens are expressed at low levels in adult life, and are more commonly seen during early development. Tumour-specific antigens have been more difficult to identify, but there is some recent evidence for their existence. The main problem with passive immunotherapy is the immune response to allogenic anti-tumour monoclonal antibodies. Thus recent developments have focused on the development of human instead of mouse monoclonal antibodies, and the use of fragments instead of the whole immunoglobulin molecule.

ACTIVE IMMUNOTHERAPY

This involves stimulation of those components of the immune system that are most likely to be responsible for

Table 26.1.9 Immunotherapy of cancer

Class of action		Description	Tumour target
Active			
	Non-specific	BCG	Bladder
		Levamisole*	Colon
	Specific	Preventative vaccines of tumour cells (K-Ras)	Pancreas
		Purified antigens (*H. pylori*)	Gastric
Passive			
	Non-specific	LAK cells	Renal
		Cytokines (IL-2, INF-α)	
	Specific	Antibodies	Colon

*With 5FU.

anti-tumour activity. Various strategies have been employed. Vaccination with non-specific promoters of immunity (e.g. BCG) has been shown to have some anti-tumour activity. Vaccination with disabled tumour cells or antigens can stimulate or promote a specific anti-tumour response. Stimulation of the immune response with cytokines (IL-2, INF-α) has been used to augment an innate anti-tumour response. Most clinical experience to date has been with IL-2, which has been shown to be of some benefit in the treatment of renal-cell carcinoma and melanoma.

ADOPTIVE IMMUNOTHERAPY

This involves the transfer of macrophages or immunocompetent cells from one individual to another. Normally such cells have little in the way of anti-tumour activity, but if they are stimulated in culture with IL-2, LAK cells with anti-tumour activity are produced. Stimulation of and replacement with autologous lymphocyte fractions is also possible. LAK cells have been shown to have anti-tumour activity in a similar range of tumours to that seen with IL-2 therapy.

GENE THERAPY AND NOVEL BIOLOGICAL DRUGS

GENE THERAPY

Of many different approaches (Table 26.1.10), gene-directed enzyme prodrug therapy (GDEPT) and the replacement of TSGs have progressed to early clinical studies. GDEPT involves delivery of an alien gene (usually cloned from a bacteria or virus) into the tumour cells. A harmless prodrug is then given which is converted by the transduced gene product to a powerful cytotoxic agent. Thus cytosine deaminase (CD) converts 5-fluorocytosine to 5FU. Concentration increases of the order of 500-fold can be achieved by gene therapy (GDEPT), compared to the conventional administration of 5FU. Prodrugs for TK include ganciclovir, and for β-nitroreductase the prodrug CB1954.

Bystander effect Many more cancer cells are killed than are transduced by the gene. In the case of GDEPT, only some of the bystander effect can be accounted for by 'leakage' of activated drug. For reasons that are not yet fully understood, the death of cancer cells by gene therapy results in a powerful anticancer immune response.

Targeting vectors The principal limitation of gene therapy at present is targeting vectors. The best way to introduce genes into mammalian cells is by the use of disabled viruses. Unfortunately, adenoviruses stimulate a large immune response, so that repeated delivery may not be possible. Retroviruses are only able to carry smaller gene constructs, and are more difficult to culture for large titres. *Tumour-specific targeting* is not possible at present, and the development of modified viruses or 'synthetic' viruses is ongoing. *Tumour-specific expression* is possible by linking the promoter of a tumour-specific gene (such as *CEA* or *AFP*) in the gene construct.

NOVEL BIOLOGICAL DRUGS

Conventional cytotoxic therapy relies on disabling the more rapidly dividing cancer cells. Novel biological approaches interfere with the behaviour of cancer cells. Anti-angiogenesis drugs (e.g. TI470, angiostatin, endostatin) inhibit the development of new blood vessels induced by tumour cells, thus impairing viability. General inhibitors of MMPs (marimastat) prevent the breakdown of the ECM, thereby impairing invasion, and they also demonstrate moderate anti-angiogenetic activity. The principal clinical benefits of these new classes of

Table 26.1.10 Gene therapy approaches

Gene therapy approach	Genes used or targeted
Gene-directed enzyme prodrug therapy (GDEPT)	Cytosine deaminase (*CD*) Thymidine kinase (*TK*) β-Nitroreductase (*β-NTR*)
Replacement of tumour suppressor genes	*TP53, p16, APC*
Co-stimulatory genes	*B7.1*
Lymphokine genes	*IL-2*
Antisense (to mRNA)	*K-RAS, TP53, BCL-2*
Ribozymes (to mRNA)	*K-RAS*

compound may be cytostatic and antimetastatic, rather than cytotoxic. Because they have different actions from each other and from conventional cytotoxic drugs, there is considerable scope for multiple drug therapy.

PALLIATIVE CARE

Many patients with cancer die from this disease, and thus palliation forms a major part of cancer care. Multidisciplinary teams which span the hospital and the community, and include specialists in palliative care, nurses who specialize in caring for those dying from cancer, and general practitioners, can provide support in a seamless fashion. Wherever practicable, and if it is the wish of the patient, they should be allowed to die at home or in a hospice. The treatment of pain (Table 26.1.11) and other specific symptoms (Table 26.1.12) similarly requires a multidisciplinary approach.

Respecting the autonomy and dignity of the dying patients and their relatives requires honesty about the diagnosis and prognosis, as well as considerable kindness and tactfulness, with kindness being the overriding factor. Life should be allowed to take its natural course with optimum palliation. Frequent mouthwashes are preferred to IV fluids for untreatable internal obstruction. Ureteric stents are often best avoided, despite uraemia. On the other hand, chest infections are usually worth treating because of the symptom improvement that can be achieved. Total parenteral nutrition will do little to relieve the cachexia of cancer and gives rise to other complications and anxieties.

SCREENING FOR CANCER

The aim of screening is to identify asymptomatic patients who either do not have cancer but will develop it, or who have developed an early form of cancer, before dissemination. In the first type of screening no patient should die from cancer, but in the second type only a reduction in the death rate can be achieved. By definition, screening cannot be applied to individuals with symptoms.

Table 26.1.11 Pain relief in advanced malignancy

Method of pain relief	Comment
Analgesic drugs	
NSAIDs	Gastrointestinal complications
Opioids	Give laxatives and anti-emetics for opioid-resistant pain
Co-analgesics (amitriptyline, etc.)	
Injection neurolysis	
Intrapleural blockade	Mesothelioma
Coeliac plexus block	Stomach, oesophageal and pancreatic cancers
Nervous system stimulation	
Transcutaneous electrical nerve stimulation (TENS)	β nerve-fibre stimulation inhibits A and C nerve-fibre transmission (gate
Dorsal column stimulation	theory of pain)
Ultrasound, infrared, ice, acupuncture	
Radiotherapy	
Surgery	
CNS destruction	
Cordotomy	
Thalamic nuclei	
Pituitary	Breast, prostate and thyroid cancers
Orthopaedic	Stabilizing pathological fractures, spinal cord decompression

Table 26.1.12 Symptom management in terminal malignancy

Symptoms	Management
Anorexia	Small regular meals; dexamethasone may help; TPN, etc., of little value
Nausea and vomiting caused by:	
Drugs	Anti-emetics: metoclopramide and domperidone (also gastrokinetic); cyclizine; haloperidol; phenothiazines
Brain metastases	Dexamethasone
Squashed stomach syndrome	Activated dimethicone and metoclopramide
Metabolic	Treat cause (hypercalcaemia or uraemia)
Hiccough	Peppermint water; activated dimethicone; chlorpromazine
Constipation	Senna; magnesium hydroxide; co-danthrocate; lactulose; glycerine suppositories; enemas
Diarrhoea	
General	Loperamide; codeine phosphate
Pancreas cancer	Pancreatic enzyme supplements
Caused by constipation, subacute obstruction, drugs, infection, radiotherapy	Treat cause if possible
Untreatable intestinal obstruction	Diamorphine; hyoscine; haloperidol; cyclizine; ± NGT; ± IV or SC fluids; mouthwashes
Ascites	Spironolactone and frusemide; peritoneovenous shunt
Symptoms due to advanced pelvic cancer	Colostomy; urinary catheter; ± ureteric stents
Bronchial obstruction	Radiotherapy; endobronchial treatment (lasers, stents, etc.)
Untreatable breathlessness	Benzodiazepines; morphine
Untreatable cough	Morphine
Lymphoedema	Compression bandaging; support garment
Pruritus	Relieve biliary obstruction – give androgens if not possible; chlorpheniramine; promethazine; acrivastine; loratadine
Hypercalcaemia	
Caused by increased osteolytic activity or parathyroid-hormone-related protein (pTHrp) produced by the tumour	Frusemide; dexamethasone; phosphate tablets; pamidronate

PREDICTIVE DIAGNOSIS

This method of screening involves DNA testing of individuals from families with a known or possible familial cancer syndrome (Table 26.1.3). Tests are now widely available for these cancer syndromes. Identification of an 'at-risk' family is crucial before DNA testing. Although there are specific tests for different types of mutation if there is reasonable certainty about a family being at risk, it is impractical for DNA laboratories to undertake extensive analyses in dubious families. Some of the cancer syndromes have a distinct phenotype. In familial adenomatous polyposis (FAP), for example, there are more than 100 polyps (usually more than 1000 polyps) in the colon, with symptoms developing in the first or second decade of life. Once the type of mutation in the adenomatous polyposis coli (*APC*) gene has been identified in the presenting individual from the family (i.e. the index case), other family members can be tested much more easily for the same mutation. A disease such as FAP has about 100% penetrance, meaning that the disease will invariably develop in offspring if a mutation is present. In FAP, the rate of development of colon cancer and death if untreated is also 100%. Thus predictive diagnosis will prompt secondary screening and a prophylactic total proctocolectomy at the appropriate age to prevent the development of colon cancer.

Other cancer syndromes are associated with a 'non-classical' TSG, such as the DNA repair genes in HNPCC (non-FAP familial colon cancer) or the *BRCA1/2* genes in breast and breast/ovarian cancer families. In this instance, the familial phenotype may easily be confused with the sporadic (non-inherited) phenotype. For example, the incidence of breast cancer in women is approximately 1:12. By chance alone, two or more women in one family may have the cancer, but not due to inherited breast cancer gene mutations. Once a potential index case has been identified, the joint involvement of a clinical geneticist is vital in order to determine whether the individual(s) of a family meet the clinical genetic criteria to justify DNA screening. There are special ethical issues relating to DNA testing. For example, it may not be possible to obtain life insurance if the individual is known to have a cancer-carrying gene mutation. Prenatal diagnosis is (potentially) possible for any of the cancer syndromes, and hence the option of early termination in selected cases.

SECONDARY SCREENING

This refers to screening for cancer in a group of patients who will definitely develop the disease or who are at very high risk. For example, a young teenager with FAP may elect for annual sigmoidoscopy (to look for polyps) in order to delay total proctocolectomy until completion of a university or apprenticeship course.

Certain conditions are associated with a very high risk of cancer. For example, hereditary pancreatitis (caused by a mutation of the cationic trypsinogen gene) has a 40–70% likelihood of leading to pancreatic cancer. Secondary screening in patients with mutations might involve regular radiology or repeated pancreatic juice sampling for DNA analysis of pancreatic cancer-carrying genes (*K-RAS*, *p53*, *p16* and *SMAD4*) at the presymptomatic stage as an alternative to total pancreatectomy.

Other examples in which secondary screening for cancer may be developed in the future include Barrett's oesophagus and gastric dysplasia once appropriate molecular tests have been defined.

PRIMARY SCREENING

This refers to the screening of all or more usually part of the population for a common condition. The best established programmes are for cervical cancer and breast cancer. In the UK, all sexually active women are screened for cervical cancer by cervical scrape cytology. Each year there are 22 000 positive cases of cervical neoplasia *in situ* with no deaths. Of 5000 cases diagnosed because of symptoms with invasive cancers, there are over 1500 deaths (see Table 26.1.2). Since the introduction of breast screening by mammography for women aged 55–64 years in 1988 in the UK, there has been a reduction in the age-standardized mortality of approximately 10%, a similar figure to that observed in other countries with similar programmes.

Primary screening is only feasible for cancers which are common, carry a high mortality and can be diagnosed accurately by simple testing (e.g. cervical and breast cancer). On the other hand, less common cancers for which there is no simple test are not diagnosed accurately. For example, the prevalence of pancreatic cancer in individuals aged over 40 years is approximately 20 per 100 000. The best screening tests currently available (ultrasound, computerized tomography, or tumour markers) have a sensitivity and specificity of 85% each. For every 17 (85/100 × 20) true positives (out of 100 000 individuals screened) there would be 15% false-positives, i.e. 15 000 individuals without the disease (but wrongly detected). Only if a test is 100% sensitive and more than 99.98% specific would the true-positives equal the false-positives. Screening would be feasible for cancer in general if a shared set of characteristics could be defined – appropriate cost-effective tests would be developed (since the prevalence would be very high). For example, non-white-cell plasma testing for DNA shed by tumour cells (mutations of TSGs or oncogenes) may be a real option in the near future.

Colorectal cancer screening may be introduced more widely and be based on a combination of faecal occult blood testing and colonoscopy or once-only flexible sigmoidoscopy. Although these approaches may reduce the rate of death from colorectal cancer to a similar extent to that from breast cancer, there are many more 'false-positives', which may render this approach to screening non-cost-effective and therefore impractical.

FURTHER READING

Lemoine N, Neoptolemos J, Cooke T. 1994: *Cancer: a molecular approach*. Oxford: Blackwell Scientific Publications.

Roitt I, Brostoft J, Mole D. 1998: *Immunology*, 5th edn. London: Mosby.

Strachan T, Read AP. 1996: *Human molecular genetics*. New York: BIOS Scientific Publishers.

Taylor I, Cooke TG, Guillou P. 1996: *Essential general surgical oncology*. London: Churchill Livingstone.

Chapter 26.2

Palliative care and communication

Robert George

Introduction

There is rather more to being a good surgeon than simple technique. Remember that regardless of our chosen speciality, we are also doctors. The way we treat patients as people is every bit as important to the role of healer as the way we treat a pathology. This chapter deals with two aspects of care that are essential to being a good surgeon, namely how to care for and communicate with dying patients. I would like to start by making three points.

First, it is essential to recognize that often treatments are bound to fail, for no other reason than that the patient's illness will kill them. We can influence the time and mode of that death, but we cannot stave it off for eternity. Sadly, a substantial percentage of patients who clinicians see during their career are seeking help for diseases that will ultimately kill them. At best, then, our treatment of these patients is palliative, i.e. it is not performed with cure as a realistic expectation, yet the procedures such patients undergo at our hands are usually necessary and justified.

Second, medicine is changing and practice is rightly becoming a partnership in which the doctor–patient relationship is evolving from the paternalistic view that doctor knows best to one in which there is genuine honesty between clinician and patient. For us to reach the ideal, where uncertainties surrounding all diagnoses and the limitations of treatments are routinely discussed, is still unacceptably rare. As the next generation of clinicians, it is your responsibility to move this important matter forward.

Third, patients will respond far better when they are aware of the uncertainties surrounding their illness and can become truly involved in their care and the decisions that are being made around them. It is also the ethical way to practise – patients have a moral and legal right to know the truth and to base their consent and refusal to treatment on full, accurate and comprehensible information.

Palliation and communication are closely associated. Indeed, many referrals to our specialist service are for assistance not with pain or symptom control, but to unravel some complexities of communication between patients, families and professionals when these have reached an impasse.

This chapter focuses on these 'soft issues', which are often at the centre of hard decisions, but seldom find their way into medical let alone surgical texts. The bibliography at the end of the chapter expands on the issues that we touch on here. After a short explanation of palliative care and the basics of communications, I shall draw the two together, ending with a case study to examine:

- how to find common communication ground;
- truth-telling;
- making therapeutic choices;
- withdrawing and withholding treatment;
- the last few days of life.

WHAT IS PALLIATIVE CARE?

Palliative and terminal care are often confused with each other. Historically, palliative care has been seen as necessary pain and symptom control at the very end of life when 'proper measures' are futile and there is nothing more to be done. Palliative care *actually starts* at the time of the first decision that a treatment is not curative. In short, some clinicians are practising palliative care all of the time, and many of them are palliating most of the time. Hardly any are practising it none of the time. This is the reason why the definitions descriminate between three levels of palliative care, as described below.

The palliative care approach

This is the minimum standard of care and skill that is to be expected of all clinicians. A palliative approach is the attitude and quality of practice that manages incurably ill patients sensitively and effectively throughout their illness, not just during their remaining months. It ensures that pain and symptoms are managed as a priority and that patients do not suffer unnecessarily. It places an expectation on all to understand the principles and application of full palliative care and to ensure that those needing it have access to specialist palliative care if necessary.

Palliative interventions

This is the area of specialist practice where technical skills and treatments may have a place. Surgery is an important element of this and has varying roles according to the problem in hand. Examples would include debulking procedures, bypasses, reconstruction, etc.

Surgery is often seen as representing hope, because operations are equated with cure in the public mind. What is essential is that these interventions must always be performed in open and complete knowledge of the reality of the overall clinical situation. Overly optimistic short-term interventions can undo months of benefit achieved by a careful counselling strategy.

Specialist palliative care

This is the interdisciplinary speciality that extends beyond symptoms to practical, social, psychological and spiritual care of the patient and their family through the dying process and into bereavement. Specialist palliative care is one of the core services of all cancer centres. All clinicians should have access to advice and help through either the acute centres or the local hospice facility.

So much for the conventional definitions used. However, palliation is better understood by taking a look at its aims, character and elements in more detail.

A BROAD DEFINITION

The aims of palliation are as follows:

- to relieve suffering in whatever form it takes;
- to optimize quality of life;
- to use time for maximum benefit;
- to help people to find meaning in completing and concluding their lives;
- finally, whilst we affirm life and have no place for the capitulation of euthanasia, palliative care sees death as a natural end.

This is the broad definition of palliative care that sees therapeutics as a tool to achieve these ends. Hence there should be no tensions between curative and palliative measures, interventions or omissions. Whatever is necessary to achieve a realistic outcome is a legitimate palliative measure. Aggressive and invasive measures are perfectly justified in cases where:

- strategies are centred on the needs and wishes of the patient and family;
- there is a clear and good reason;
- there is a clear goal in view; and
- the clinical situation is reviewed once the objective is met.

We shall return to these points in the case study.

Characteristics

These are, of course, all interconnected.

Taking a pragmatic approach and prioritizing need
Fundamentally, palliative care is needs based. It is therefore independent of both diagnosis and prognosis, as there is no logical reason why palliation and symptom control should be confined to the dying. Much of what we are saying in this chapter is applicable to anyone with symptoms or complex psychological and social needs.

Focusing on outcome
Palliative care is problem-solving. It looks well beyond the immediate need to focus care on meaningful outcomes. In other words, we only see value in an action if it is going to make a genuine difference to a patient's quality of life and the time that they have left.

Looking beyond pathology
The trendy word at the moment is 'holistic'. Holism refers to an integration and cohesion in the individual. Health also derives from '*holos*', which translates literally as 'everything in its right order'. For example, problems with symptom control, and especially pain, may be due to psychological distress. If the latter is not resolved, then no form of medication will relieve the situation ade-

quately. One of the commonest reasons why patients need excessive sedation as they die is that insufficient time has been given to these areas. It is important to ensure that the appropriate assessments are made early in the case.

Seeing your patients in context

Patients and families form a complex 'universe' of relationships that can have profound and fundamental effects on clinical care. Individuals cannot be separated from their social setting, although it is easy to forget this when we are based in hospitals. However, any decisions must take these wider considerations into account.

Teamwork: using your colleagues

With all of these complexities it is clear that no single person can manage a case comprehensively. By this I mean that the broader aspects of care, counselling, practical and social care, etc., are all important to improving independence and quality of life. They may in fact be more important than the clinical problem in hand. Do not fall into the trap of thinking that because you are good at your job, you are therefore good at everybody else's. You are not, and teamwork is essential.

Elements

Symptom control by whatever means

I am not going to list symptoms or their management. They appear elsewhere in the book, and can also be found in the further reading section. However, there is one comment worth making on symptoms in general.

A symptom is a complex integral of a stimulus, its context and its interpretation by the patient (Figure 26.2.1). The pathological stimulus need only be trivial. This is because the symptom only becomes problematic when it exceeds a threshold that cannot be ignored. It is the level of this threshold in relation to the intensity of the stimulus that is influenced by non-physical factors such as emotional and family conflicts, fear or guilt ('spiritual' matters), and so on. This is the domain of specialist practice, but all good clinicians need to be able to recognize when a symptom is complicated by an unexpectedly low symptom threshold and to make a referral. This ability will develop with experience, but is probably an issue when:

- the patient cannot specify the problem clearly;
- the problem fluctuates without obvious physical reasons;
- nursing staff report that the symptoms worsen when doctors or certain individuals (family, friends, etc.) are around;
- there is evidence of tensions or difficulty elsewhere in the patient's life.

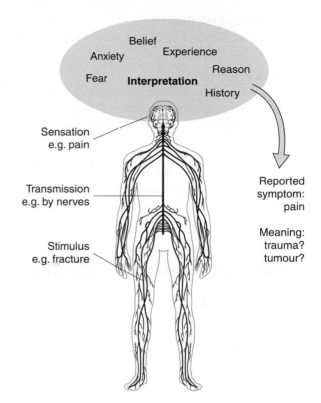

Figure 26.2.1 The factors that make up a reported symptom. In this example, a patient presents with leg pain due to a fracture. They will respond differently if they are young and have had a road accident, rather than if the fracture is preceded by a history of malignancy.

Finally, 'not knowing' is a potent reducer of symptom thresholds, especially pain, nausea, vomiting and breathlessness. One simple way of influencing thresholds is therefore to provide information. Ignorance or inaccurate knowledge leads to anxiety and fantasies about diagnosis or the likely course of events. These fears may develop a life of their own and become increasingly irrational. Although psychological and spiritual care is really the domain of specialist care, it is possible to observe real results in terms of improved symptoms with effective communication and clear information exchange. Here, then, we see one clear overlap between simple communication and palliation that puts a responsibility on the non-specialist.

Summary of goals

It is useful to think of three headings when managing patients palliatively.

Completion of tasks

Whatever 'jobs' are outstanding in a person's life are the ones that matter. Regardless of how strange they may be, prioritize your therapeutic options with these in mind.

Reconciliation of relationships

Saying one's goodbyes, sorry's and thank-you's is essential.

Resolution of beliefs

We all have our own view of the material world, our death and what may come after that. This goes beyond conventional religion as people seek some meaning for themselves.

We shall return to palliation and express these three areas diagrammatically in the third section. Before that, we need first to look at the broad principles of communication.

WHAT IS COMMUNICATION?

SOME BASELINES

Doing to others as you would have them do to you

There is no difference between communicating with patients and communicating with anyone else. Consider what you expect when a friend or colleague speaks to you.

- You expect that they are saying what they mean and that you are hearing what is meant.

- You expect them to tell the truth as far as they are able to know it, and to use language that you can understand.

- You do not expect to be manipulated or conned into a course of action that is foolish or not in your own interest, nor do you expect to be patronized or humiliated.

- You expect and appreciate respect for who you are.

- You expect the conversation to be a dialogue in which you have an opportunity to contribute to the conversation and influence it in some way.

- You expect to be heard.

The doctor–patient relationship

The doctor–patient relationship should be no different. It lies at the heart of clinical practice and must therefore be taken extremely seriously. It is a contract that is confidential, based on trust, and exclusively for the benefit and best interests of the patient.

It should be a partnership to help the patient to make free, real and informed decisions about their care. Ingredients for this come from the patient who brings a problem, its context and their needs. The doctor in turn provides information from diagnosis or investigation, and advice based on his or her expertise. Out of the partnership should come understanding of the facts and the truth of a situation (these are not necessarily synonymous) and some options for a way forward, both in terms of a plan and how to execute it. The patient is then in a position to make an informed decision (Figure 26.2.2).

The days of consultants being perceived and acting as demigods are over. Patients are no longer passive or submissive to the idea that 'what the doctor says is best'. Of course, a patient may choose to have the doctor take a decision on their behalf, but that is an entirely different matter. A paternalistic view of our role towards our patients has in fact always been unethical, but our patients now know it to be so.

SOME THEORY

To be perfectly blunt, communications theory does not say a great deal more than what common sense tells us is

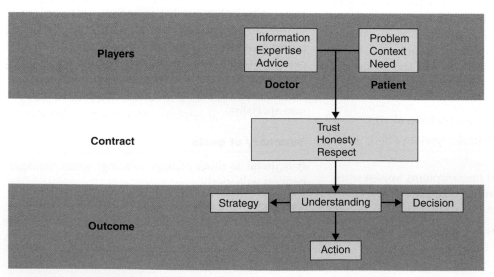

Figure 26.2.2 The doctor–patient relationship expressed diagrammatically. Essentially the doctor's role is to assist with strategy. The patient takes the decision on the doctor's recommendations and an action ensues.

good and effective dialogue, namely that what is understood is what is meant. Between the two is what is said and what is heard. The skill is to ensure that the four correspond. Below are annotations of the classical elements relevant to our discussion.

The purpose and objective of communication

To develop the doctor–patient relationship

This has two components. The first is to develop trust. Without trust there is no certainty that one is being told the truth, and one may feel unable to disclose important information. Consequently decisions may be neither real nor informed.

The second aspect is to express mutual respect. Doctors only have status in so far as their patients and society give it to them. Do not forget this. Patients are often made very angry by the discovery that they may be dying, and are apt to place blame anywhere they can. This is an aspect of denial known as transference. Clinicians are in the frame for taking the blame, so if we treat our patients badly, there is a case for saying that we deserve everything we get!

To promote informed choice

Patients have the right to consent to or refuse treatment, and these decisions are valid only if they are informed and freely made. It is our obligation to ensure that all of the relevant information is available and understandable to our patients.

To act in a patient's best interest

To know what is a patient's best interest requires at least some level of relationship, particularly in the grey areas of opinion.

The process of communication

This is the 'guts' of communication and is where it succeeds or fails. Try always to have a nurse present to follow up on discussion in support or interpretation. There are three basic ingredients.

Context

This includes considerations such as the level of relationship that you have with the patient, whether you are able only to give a few minutes in out-patients and should therefore arrange more appropriate surroundings and time, whether the patient is post-op, and so on.

People involved

Does the patient want their family to be involved in discussions? If so, then this should be arranged.

Anticipated effects

Is the patient likely to react badly to the information that is given?

The variables in communication

The importance of these is fundamental. Remember that anyone in distress will hear only a fraction of what is said. Remember also that, when stressed, the person concerned is likely to fall back on their own way of communicating. In the case of doctors, this is usually with complex and technical language which is entirely foreign to the patient.

Language, culture, values, etc.

People from different cultures are 'wired' differently, and it is possible to cause terrible offence unintentionally. Violating some dimension of personhood in communication can set you back enormously. Take great care to obtain as much information as possible from other clinical colleagues if matters of culture are at stake. Nursing staff are the most consistent source of wisdom here.

Level of understanding and mental capacity

Take care not to patronize the patient, but always check the degree to which they understand you. You will probably need to repeat conversations several times and in several ways. Be patient, as your relationship with the patient will benefit from this approach and any difficult times ahead will be eased.

Stage of illness

This aspect is relatively straightforward and, in essence, is a reflection of the margins of uncertainty about prognostication. However, avoid being drawn about exact time-scales. It is far better to break the future into blocks of time that are appropriate to the situation in hand. For example, a patient facing a prognosis of 3–6 months is best given 1-month blocks in which he or she can think of being relatively stable or facing deterioration. This will be expanded on more in the case study, but first we need to draw the concepts of palliative care and communication together.

DRAWING THE CONCEPTS OF COMMUNICATION AND PALLIATION TOGETHER

We ended the last section by saying that we are motivated to help patients to complete tasks, resolve relationships and find peace.

MORE ON PERSPECTIVE: THE MEANING–MECHANISM GAP

One of the stumbling blocks to an effective relationship with patients is that we have fundamentally different perspectives. The doctor's surgical training and scientific method are rightly preoccupied with the mechanisms that underlie a clinical problem. Their motives are being cultivated to unravel its elements by assessment and investigation, and then to achieve a balanced and correct analysis of therapeutic options. Conversely, a patient is usually asking what a problem means. Will their work be affected? Can they afford to be ill? What will happen to the family? If the clinical problem is curable, these two views do not conflict. However, if uncertainty or in particular chronicity develop, we need to break free from our cycle of mechanism to be of greater help in the patient's cycle of meaning. The three outcomes are illustrated in Figure 26.2.3; namely, the patient is cured, they resolve their conflict or they begin to suffer.

Clinicians are susceptible to entering into a denial cycle with patients by colluding with vain hopes of cure and increasingly extreme treatments whilst failing to speak about the source of distress (helplessness and progressive deterioration, etc.). Because no one wants to be the bringer of bad news, we either collude with vain hopes or present the available options in inappropriately optimistic ways. We may even lie, and overtly deny that someone is dying, saying 'of course you will get better' when this is clearly nonsense. We have all done this with the best intentions, but it is never helpful in the long term. The longer an individual has a chance to accommodate or address bad news, the greater the chance they have of being successful. Thus the sooner they know the facts the better.

In these circumstances hope cannot be placed in treatment, but must emerge from other sources of meaning, such as important tasks completed, relationships healed and beliefs about the future resolved. By giving the patient control in these areas, quality can be gained and positive things can come out of the dying process. These points are summarized in Figure 26.2.4 (the three cycles that lead to miscommunication) and Figure 26.2.5 (the clinical balance for managing uncertainty). Cost and benefit links these two diagrams.

FINDING COMMON GROUND

The central fact is that, much as we would like it to be otherwise, many of the conversations that we have with our patients, although they perhaps involve presenting therapeutic options, are in reality moving towards the possibility of deterioration or incurability. The only meaningful way forward is to seek means of presenting the truth in an accessible and audible way. The easiest approach here is to present the problems as being shared and the best solutions as those that serve the needs of the patient and their family.

Telling the truth and partnership

If we are honest, none of us like relationships that involve lying. It demeans us and leaves us uncertain. Relationships are only real when their currency (what we say to one another) is reliable. If this is so for one set of

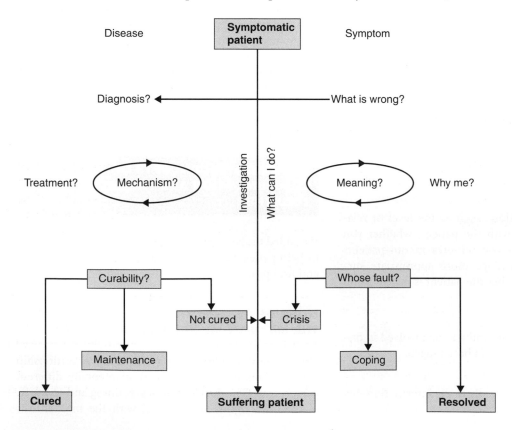

Figure 26.2.3 The problem of perspective.

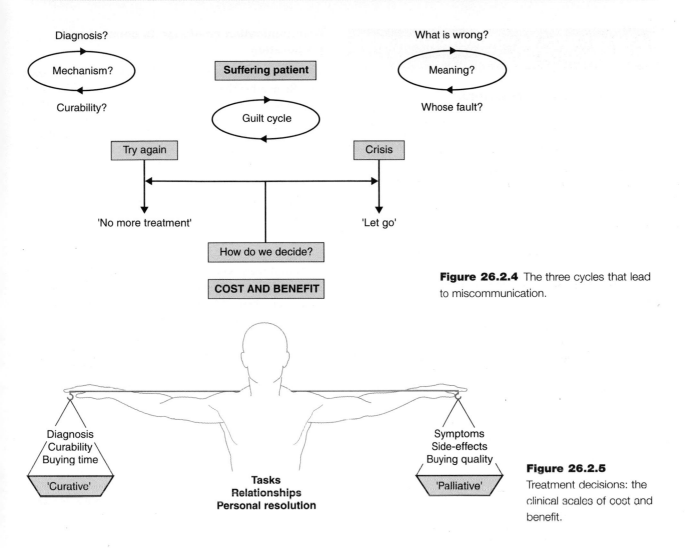

Figure 26.2.4 The three cycles that lead to miscommunication.

Figure 26.2.5
Treatment decisions: the clinical scales of cost and benefit.

relationships, why should it not be so for others? What makes a doctor–patient relationship less unsatisfactory if there is lying and collusion in it? There needs to be sensitivity to process and an understanding of the impact of both the truth and the way in which it will be delivered. This is the matter of communicating uncertainty.

Communicating uncertainty

Although banal, it is a truism to say that none of us knows whether we are going to take another breath. Arrhythmias, subarachnoid haemorrhages, etc., are no respecters of profession or status. Bearing that in mind, it is self-evident that we can say, as fellow humans, to any patient that we are unable with certainty to predict the future. Everything is a matter of probability. It is approaching certainty that being young and healthy trainees, you as readers of this text (subarachnoids, etc., notwithstanding) will survive to the end of the chapter. Equally, it is approaching certainty that your patients

with hepatic metastases from colonic cancer will die (despite the latest chemotherapy). However, these certainties may be dissembled into elements that are in themselves far less certain. Uncertainty can be used positively as well as negatively. Here we can use uncertainty to help a patient to move towards a real understanding of their future in a way that liberates them to make use of their time, rather than to create a prison of false hope or a paralysing fear that death is just around the next corner. For example, although the patient may die in the medium or short term, we can be fairly sure of being able to buy some time, even though its quality may be less certain. However, we can also do our very best to ensure that the time that remains is as free of symptoms as possible, and that it is available to the patient, not wasted by us on some frivolous investigations or futile treatment.

We shall now examine a case in order to try to give form to the preceding discussion and examine this way of communicating.

A CASE STUDY OF COMMUNICATION WITH THE DYING

DECISION POINT 1: THE OPENER

> A young man in his late thirties presents with weight loss, lower abdominal discomfort and some blood in his stool. You perform a sigmoidoscopy and biopsy his malignancy.
>
> He wants to know what you have found and what it means.

Communication challenge 1: giving the diagnosis

This finding is highly likely to be malignant, so you might as well say so, because by doing so you have signalled that you are a truth-teller. In my opinion, the wisest approach is to gauge your patient's fears first. I usually ask what they think is happening and whether they have a worst fear. I have even opened such conversations with the question: 'Do you think that you are dying?' Interestingly, one patient concerned said how helpful the question was, as it made her step back and really wonder what was going on. You can then follow up with openers like 'I hope I am wrong, but this is probably going to be a type of cancer,' or 'Of course I can't be sure until we have looked under the microscope, but this looks like an active cancer.'

The patient is then clearly in a position to take or leave the comment. They may say nothing, they may quiz you or they may become upset. However, they know that you are not afraid to tell it how it is. Furthermore, if the news is good, then it is easy to back off, and if it is bad, then you have already prepared the ground.

Eye contact is important. As a tip, if you find looking into someone's eyes is a problem, then focus on the bridge of their nose. They cannot tell the difference, and it resolves the dilemma of where to look.

Phase 1

Assuming that the biopsy is a poorly differentiated adenocarcinoma, the decision is to perform staging and surgery. You set this in train and plan to review matters pre-operatively.

DECISION POINT 2: PRE-OP

> We know from staging that there is a questionable area in the liver, but aggressive management is warranted. However, the patient's consent is needed.

Communication challenge 2: consent and preparation

Your patient has the right to full disclosure, and quizzes you. Remember that because you have been straight with him so far, the currency is established. Anything you say he will believe anyway, but the important thing is that you have already established that it is truth in which you are dealing. You are now in a position to discuss uncertainties and probabilities. Keep it simple, give ballpark probabilities, set aside plenty of time (this will require an absolute minimum of 15 min) and sit down beside the patient. Consider an approach similar to the following.

'There are probably four scenarios we have to prepare for.

1. At best there will be a cancer that is confined to the inner lining of the bowel, but we shall only be sure of that when we have had the tissue examined under the microscope.

2. There may be spread through the bowel wall.

3. There may be spread into the surrounding tissues.

4. This is the worst scenario (always give advance warning of bad news). The area in the liver or other areas in the abdomen may be involved. This is bad news because it means that, in effect, the cancer cannot be cured. However, it does not mean that nothing more can be done.'

Phase 2: hope for the best and prepare for the worst

You may then go on to discuss surgical options, adjuvant chemotherapy, radiotherapy, etc.

DECISION POINT 3: POST-OP

> Successful local resection.
>
> Dukes C with palpable liver metastasis and some peritoneal seeding.
>
> Trials of chemotherapy represent one option. Plan to refer the patient to oncology.

Communication challenge 3: breaking bad news

Take time again (you will need at least half an hour, probably on two or three occasions), ensure privacy and, depending on the opinion of the nursing staff and your relationship with the patient, you may wish to set up a meeting with their family. However, you cannot do the latter until you have spoken to the patient. (Families, even spouses, have no legal rights to prevent disclosure of information without the permission of the patient – it is simply wrong to try things out on the family first.)

Again, give warning and frame the news as a shared problem. As I have said, it may take several sessions, with or without the patient's family. The following approach could be used. 'Well, this is the conversation I was hoping we wouldn't have. You will recall our last conversation, I am afraid we are facing the worst . . .'

1. Ask how much the patient wants to know.

2. Give a clear account of your findings. Diagrams are often helpful here.

3. Make sure that a nurse is present.

4. Arrange a follow-up meeting explicitly for you to answer the patient's and/or their family's questions.

Phase 3: refer on to oncology

This man is going to die from his disease regardless, and the only variable is when. We have some ideas of median survival periods, etc., but this patient needs options for refusing treatment, looking at a clear palliative approach, and a chance to use his time in his own way. You will be standing aside from the case at this stage. To make a proper handover, it is important to obtain an assessment by specialist palliative care services or a liaison nurse at the very least.

DECISION POINT 4

The patient has refused support from specialist palliative care services, believing that he could manage things with maximum 'chemo' and diet.

Objectively, however, 'chemo' has not been going well and there is clearly active disease.

The patient has requested another referral to you because he has local recurrence and intermittent obstruction. This episode has not resolved conservatively. He is now uncomfortable, vomiting and dry. In his view things have been going fine and his weight loss and anorexia are due to the chemotherapy and latterly 'this local problem'.

Communication challenge 4: an operation and some bottom lines

This patient is now almost certainly in his last months. One commodity that all dying patients lack is time. Because time cannot always be bought with treatment, and never with certainty, the benefit of any treatment must be set against its potential cost. Put simply, there is no point in spending 3 weeks in hospital having a treatment that will only promise a month or two of extra life. The patient is guaranteed to 'waste' 3 weeks in hospital, but we cannot guarantee that those 3 weeks will be recouped later. This time might well have been better spent enjoying being at home with friends or family, a final trip, and so on. The same may be said of unnecessary out-patient visits, monitoring, etc., all of which cost precious energy and time.

As a reminder, palliative care is a tool for achieving ends. Whatever is necessary to achieve a realistic outcome is a legitimate palliative measure, provided that:

● it is seen as such;

● the indication is a need or wish of the patient and/or their family;

● there is a clear goal in view; and

● the clinical situation is reviewed once the objective has been met.

The question is what is realistic.

Evaluating realism/testing benefit

In the case of this patient, we need immediate benefit and minimum time in hospital. In all probablity a defunctioning procedure will be the solution. The patient needs a quick turnaround and decisive help, but he also needs to face the truth. You, as his initial contact, may be the best person to do this because of the level of trust and truth-telling that you established in the initial consultations.

It is often wise to conduct a joint consultation with a specialist in palliative care in order to give a clear message to the patient that other help is necessary. The responsibility then falls to them to look at the tasks, relationships and personal resolution necessary (Figure 26.2.4). However, the patient *must* know that continued denial of the state of affairs is futile and self-defeating. It is probably the last time that you will be involved directly in the care of this patient, so you can be very helpful to those taking the case on by being very clear with the patient about the real issues. For example, you might consider the following approach.

'I am pleased to say that we can help this time with some limited surgery. However, I have to say that this is not a long-term solution. It really is time for you to begin looking at the future and the reality that you will die from this disease sooner or later. We need now to involve the experts to help you and the family to manage at this very difficult time.'

You will see here that the first statement is positive, but that the truth is also being stated clearly and unequivocally.

You are unlikely to be involved again, but I have included what follows to show what is likely to happen from a specialist perspective.

DECISION POINT 5

> The patient is admitted with multiple obstructions via the casualty department.
>   He does not want acute treatment, but wishes to die.

Communication challenge 5

Life of itself has value, but it is the experience of it that matters most, and by and large our physical health is there to allow that experience.

We are now at the end of the road. Is there anything useful left therapeutically? Probably not in terms of prolonging life, but we can make a difference to the quality of the patient's life. He is miserable, dehydrated, vomiting and in pain.

Much work has probably already been done with the family. Hopefully there is relatively little or nothing left in terms of major projects. It may appear that there is nothing more that can be done. However, from our perspective this is not the case.

First, we need to know exactly what our patient means by saying that he wants to die. Does this mean no more treatment or no more pretending? Does it mean that he wants only symptom control or that he literally wants nothing? (It may surprise you to know that some people *do* want nothing.) We shall be able to unravel this issue quite quickly.

Interestingly, at this stage in a person's life one can talk quite normally about dying. I would want to know directly and explicitly what was being meant. It is astonishing to experience the depth and calm of communication at this time, even with patients who up until now have been hostile to the idea of looking at the reality of dying. I would probably end up saying the following.

'If we leave things as they are, you are likely to die in the next few days. We should certainly be able to control your symptoms. If you wish, we may be able to buy you a bit more time – days or even weeks – but this will need some different treatments. Are you game for this?' Examples of such conversations can be found in some of the books listed in the Further reading section at the end of this chapter.

From a physical point of view, patients with complete obstruction can be managed medically for many weeks in relative comfort and still find themselves able to move around and function at home. Obstruction is not an indication to stay in hospital

1. The patient has probably been on steroids to manage the obstructive episodes. This should continue, as mood, appetite and general well-being are significantly enhanced by even a small dose of dexamethasone (2–6 mg in the morning).

2. Obstruction can be managed very effectively using medication to produce a pharmacological ileus. The conventional regime is an opiate such as diamorphine for analgesia, an anticholinergic (hyoscine butyl-bromide or glycopyrrolate) and an anti-emetic. These can all be given subcutaneously by a continuous infusion cocktail.

3. Large-volume vomits can be reduced by octreotide, 200–600 mg per 24 h administered by subcutaneous infusion. We may have to opt for a venting gastrostomy if this does not work, when we would come back to you.

4. Hydration can be managed effectively with about 1 L of liquid a day by mouth in the form of anything the patient fancies drinking.

WITHDRAWING AND WITHHOLDING TREATMENT

The time has come to be very explicit about what is left to do or say. The patient's family may need to be gathered, religious rites may be appropriate, and so on. Most of all, clinical activity is kept as much in the background as possible. It is purely there to make the time that is left as comfortable, peaceful and useful as possible.

GENERAL POINTERS

Every aspect of care must be examined for its benefit and burden, so that nothing remains which is burdensome. Withdrawing treatment in these situations is usually not a problem, and if communication is good, then the question of withholding any invasive support is usually not an issue. However, if there is some dissent within the family, or the patient is still wedded to the idea that he will get better, then matters may be different, and decisions may need to be made.

One advantage of evidence-based medicine is that we are expected to operate within clear parameters. In addition, one cannot be forced to treat a patient against one's clinical judgement. That said, it is often very difficult to refuse, and if there is no clear clinical indication, continuing treatment while a patient or their family adjust to events may be reasonable. What is not reasonable is to continue or initiate treatment as a substitute for communication.

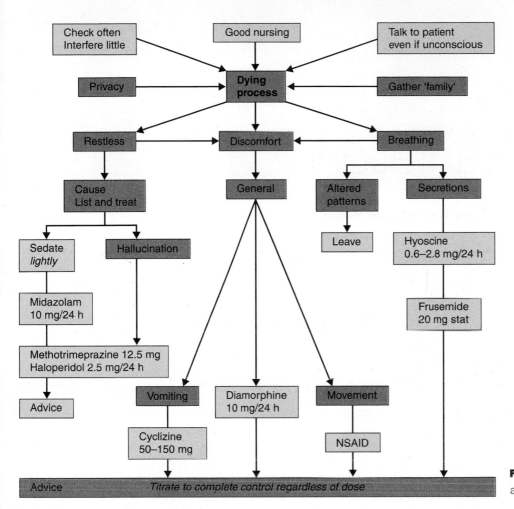

Figure 26.2.6 An algorithm for terminal care.

MANAGING THE LAST FEW DAYS OF LIFE

Memories of the last few days will endure for the patient's family, and may redeem or destroy what has gone before. Complete symptom control is the goal. An algorithm that summarizes the basics of our approach is shown in Figure 26.2.6.

CONCLUSIONS

We have reviewed the basic principles of both communication and palliation, and seen a simple application in the management of a common general surgical problem. The purpose has been to demonstrate that the two areas are central to the art of our profession. If we cannot relate to and gain the confidence of our patients, and be sure that at the time of their greatest need – their final illness – we are going to be effective, then our profession has sunk to the level of arid technicalities. There is nothing then to distinguish us from a commercial utility.

FURTHER READING

Cassell E. 1991: *The nature of suffering and the goals of medicine.* Oxford: Oxford University Press.

Doyle D, Hanks G, MacDonald N (eds). 1998: *The Oxford textbook of palliative medicine*, 2nd edn. Oxford: Oxford University Press.

George R, Houghton P, Robinson V. 2000: *Healthy dying.* London: Jessica Kingsley Publishers.

Murray Parkes C, Laungani P, Young B. 1997: *Death and bereavement across cultures.* London: Routledge.

Twycross R. 1997: *Symptom management in advanced cancer*, 2nd edn. Oxford: Radcliffe Medical Press.

Twycross R, Wilcox A, Thorp S. 1998: *PCF1, Palliative Care Formulary.* Oxford: Radcliffe Medical Press.

Chapter 27

Transplantation

Anthony K. House, Anthony Kierath and Roger Bell

Introduction

Transplantation has become a universally accepted modality of treatment for disease that has resulted in failure of tissues, cells and organs throughout the body. It is a relatively new science, founded in Greek mythology, but based on scientific principles to obtain a standard of care that is surpassed by few other discplines. The solutions to problems that have allowed transplantation to proceed include the development of vascular suturing in the early 1900s, and recognition of the biological difference between species and individuals, highlighted by John Hunter (in the 1760s), Baronio (in 1804) and later by Williamson (in 1926). It is the genetic difference between the donor and the recipient that is responsible for graft failure. Murphy (in 1926), Gibson, Medawar and Billingham (in 1940–54) further emphasized the nature of this biological difference, and the fact that the capacity for graft rejection resided in the lymphocytes. The difference between individuals was recognized by Murray and Merrill (in 1954), with a successful kidney transplantation between identical twins.

This successful transplant shifted the emphasis in transplantation away from the technical problems of the transplant operation to the recognition that the biological difference between individuals was expressed as organ rejection that had to be controlled with adequate immunosuppression before transplantation between non-identical individuals could occur. Many contributors, including Sir Roy Calne, Tom Starzl, the Boston Transplant Group and others, have been responsible for developing a plethora of immunosuppressive agents. The early drugs, azathioprine and prednisolone, superseded total body irradiation and other aggressive treatments that resulted in kidney graft survivals, but severely compromised the patient's ability to avoid septic complications. The more recently developed and successful agents include cyclosporin, tacrolimus (FK506), mycophenolate mofetil and antilymphocyte antibodies. The advent of cyclosporin and tacrolimus has enhanced kidney graft survival to 5-year rates of 80% compared to 65% in the azathioprine/corticosteroid era.

Two other developments occurred concurrently with the development of rejection-controlling immunosuppression. These involved the recognition that:

- the viability and quality of the graft were paramount to successful organ transplantation. In this regard, ischaemia, both cold and warm, and the preservation of the organ, had a profound effect on subsequent graft function and survival;
- recipient and graft outcome is influenced by the recipient's primary disease and the timing of transplantation during the progression of that disease.

These scientific developments have necessitated concurrent changes to the law relating to the diagnosis of brain death, the management of donors and recipients, and defining the ethical considerations relevant to these issues.

Present problems mirror the historical evolution of transplantation.

- Which cells, tissues or organs can and should be transplanted?
- Who should receive a transplant, and what is the definition of the pathologies that initiate end-stage organ failure and that preclude patient transplant listing?
- At what time in the progression to end-stage organ failure should the transplant occur?

- Who are the donors, how should they be managed, and how should the donated cells, tissues or organs be processed and re-implanted?
- Are the laws pertaining to these activities adequate and focused without being restrictive?
- What are the ethical considerations, and how should they be addressed?

Organ and tissue transplantation is now an enormous international clinical commitment, with 8598 kidneys, 3882 livers and 2360 hearts transplanted in 1995 in the USA. The other nations of Europe, the Americas, Australasia and South Africa have an equivalent for population requirement. The equatorial and Southeast Asian countries are similarly committed. Numbers will increase particularly as nations such as Japan have adopted a policy of brain death for certifying death. All forms of transplantation are a multidisciplinary process which requires that all of those involved act as supporting team members. Failure of any member of the team will compromise the patient outcome.

DONORS AND DONOR PROCUREMENT

The aim of organ donation or procurement should be to provide an organ of perfect function to the recipient. Organs for transplantation are derived from two major donor sources, namely live (either related or unrelated) or cadaveric heart beating (i.e. brain dead). Of these, organ donation from heart-beating brain-dead patients remains the most common source of grafts for all forms of transplantation. The concept of brainstem death is essential to this process. Potential donors include any patient who is deeply unconscious as a result of severe irreversible brain injury. The commonest causes of irremediable brain damage include cerebrovascular accidents and severe head injury.

In the potential brain-dead organ donor, irremediable brain damage is confirmed directly and by appropriate imaging (e.g. computerized tomography (CT) scans). The presence of confounding factors which may affect the levels of consciousness is excluded. Such confounding factors include the presence of sedative medication, metabolic or endocrine derangement (e.g. hypothyroidism) or hypothermia.

Once the above factors have been attended to, then clinical testing to confirm the absence of brainstem function is carried out. This testing is performed by two medical practitioners who are proficient in the process (usually intensive-care specialists or neurologists). The testing is performed by each practitioner independently (i.e. on two separate occasions).

The criteria for absence of brainstem function are as follows:

- no motor response to painful stimuli within the cranial nerve distribution (i.e. the face);
- fixed and dilated pupils not responding to light;
- absent corneal reflexes;
- no oculo-cephalic reflex (doll's eye);
- absent vestibulo-ocular reflex;
- no gag or cough reflex;
- no respiratory movements if mechanical ventilation is ceased for long enough to ensure that arterial pCO_2 rises above the threshold for stimulation of ventilation;
- as further evidence of brain death or clinical testing is not possible (e.g. due to severe facial injury), the absence of cerebral blood flow may be confirmed by four-vessel cerebral angiography or nuclear scintigraphy.

Once the diagnosis of brain death has been made, the process of organ procurement should begin as soon as possible, to spare the relatives from further emotional trauma. The doctors involved in determining brainstem death of a donor should not be involved in organ retrieval or the subsequent transplantation.

ORGAN DONATION

Over the past 5 years there has been a fall in the number of donors due in part to a reduction in the number of deaths from road traffic accidents and from intracranial haemorrhage. There is considerable variation in donor rates between different countries. Organ donation rates in Australia of approximately 10 per million population (pmp) compare unfavourably with those in many Western countries, such as Spain (28 pmp). The high rate of organ donation in Spain is linked to the establishment of a single organ donor agency with regional donor co-ordinators, the majority of whom are doctors who co-ordinate and organize daily visits to all hospitals and intensive-care units, identifying appropriate donors.

Organ donation has been encouraged by schemes such as 'donor cards' which indicate that the carrier is willing to act as a donor in the event of untimely death. However, in Australia this can be overruled by the next of kin. It would seem that the most important aspect of this difficult area is to improve the ways in which families are asked about organ donation and, although time-consuming and emotionally demanding, the need for professionally trained co-ordinators to approach the relatives of brain-dead patients cannot be overstated.

TRANSPLANT CO-ORDINATORS

At present, the most successful organ procurement and donation model is in Spain. This model consists of an independent agency staffed by a director and medically and non-medically qualified transplant co-ordinators. The medical co-ordinators are drawn from many disciplines and are usually working part-time in their discipline as well as acting as co-ordinators. All of them are well trained in interpersonal skills to discuss organ donation empathetically with the next of kin, which results in organs being donated on a high number of occasions.

The responsibility of the co-ordinators is to identify the potential donor, obtain consent for the donation, and organize within a defined and restricted time-frame the complex processes of organ retrieval and implantation. The groups to be co-ordinated include the donor caring, retrieval, operating-room and implantation teams, and the recipients for each of the organs. This may necessitate shipment of organs to other centres nationally or internationally.

MEDICAL MANAGEMENT OF THE DONOR

Correct medical management of the donor is vital in order to obtain optimal use of all donor organs. This involves the early recognition and treatment of haemodynamic instability and the maintenance of an adequate systemic perfusion pressure to ensure the best possible function of the graft on transplantation.

The most common haemodynamic abnormality seen in brain-dead patients is hypotension due to destruction of the brainstem vasomotor centres. Maintaining a minimum systolic pressure of 90–100 mmHg is necessary to ensure adequate perfusion of all vital organs. This involves correction of hypovolaemia using central venous pressure monitoring in association with catecholamine infusions. Dopamine is the preferred vasopressor because of its potential to maintain renal and mesenteric blood flow. High-dose inotropic support will have a detrimental effect on the perfusion of various viscera, and should be avoided.

Destruction of the hypothalamic–pituitary axis results in diabetes insipidus. None the less, it is important to maintain a urine output of at least 100 mL/h, especially in the hour preceding retrieval. This has been shown to have an important effect in determining renal allograft function following transplantation. If the urine output is inadequate after volume expansion, mannitol or frusemide should be administered to establish a diuresis.

Maintenance fluids should contain dextrose to ensure preservation of adequate stores of intrahepatic glucose, especially if the donor has not received any nutrition during the preceding 24 h.

Ventilation should be maintained to ensure arterial saturation of 95–100% with positive pressure ventilation to maintain lung expansion. Maintenance of the core body temperature above 33°C is necessary to ensure an accurate diagnosis of brainstem death, and it also reduces the risk of cardiovascular instability. This can be achieved through the use of radiant warmers and thermal mattresses. This care is extended into the operating theatre during the donor surgical procedure, and is governed by all of the principles associated with other major surgical operations.

ASSESSMENT OF POTENTIAL DONORS

There are a number of conditions which exclude a donor from further consideration. These include severe untreated systemic sepsis, HIV positivity, active viral hepatitis B or C, malignancy (excluding primary brain tumours), systemic disease, hypertension, diabetes, disseminated intravascular disease, any patient who is at risk of rare viral diseases such as Creutzfeldt-Jakob disease, and recipients of human pituitary growth hormone.

The tests required in the evaluation of the donor include the following:

- ABO and rhesus blood match;
- haemoglobin, platelets and white cell count;
- urea, creatinine and electrolytes;
- liver function tests;
- chest X-ray;
- ECG
- blood and sputum cultures;
- viral studies.

There are also organ-specific requirements, which are described below.

Lung

The requirements of lung donation are difficult to meet, and consequently only 25% of cadaver donors satisfy the criteria. Pneumonia is common with brain death, and in addition many fatal events, drowning, severe asthma, older donors and smoking preclude lung donation. Intubation is associated with an increased risk of nosocomial infection and is suggested by a high polymorphonuclear count with bacteria and oedematous mucosa on bronchoscopy. Other lung function features of PaO_2 and body size will contribute to exclude a potential lung donor. These features all contribute to the immediate and long-term outcome of the recipient.

Heart

The general criteria for organ donation apply, but the age of acceptance is under 55 years. There should be no evidence of coronary artery disease, ventricular function should be normal without excessive inotropic support, and the body weight of the donor and recipient should be comparable. Ischaemic time, older donor age, small donor (particularly female to large male), greater inotropic support, diabetes mellitus and diffuse donor heart wall motion all contribute to a poorer outcome in the recipient.

Kidney

Pre-existing renal disease, acute tubular necrosis (ATN), impaired glomerular function and severe vascular disease may exclude kidney donation or require further delineation by biopsy when kidneys with 20–30% glomerulosclerosis, glomerular thrombi, severe ATN, interstitial infiltrates or fibrosis are exclusions from transplantation. Older or very young donors, poor human leucocyte antigen (HLA) complex, DR (a class II antigen) matching and cold ischaemic time of > 18 h are all adverse donor factors for graft survival. A history of cardiac arrest and systemic hypotension does not necessarily contraindicate organ donation. Over the years there has been a gradual rise in the maximum age for organ donations, with more and more units tending to use more elderly donors (e.g. over the age of 70 years).

Liver

A history of chronic disease affecting the liver is a contraindication to donation. Alcohol abuse and potential liver disease are difficult to assess from the liver function tests alone, unless they are very deranged. The most common abnormality of the liver at the time of retrieval is the presence of fatty change or steatosis which can be observed on inspection. This mandates liver biopsy, and if on frozen section examination more than 30–40% of the parenchyma has been replaced by fatty change, then that liver should not be used for transplantation. Fatty change and prolonged cold ischaemic time of > 12 h, donor hypotension and the use of inotropes are all associated with poorer graft survival.

ORGAN PRESERVATION

Effective organ preservation facilitates the transplantation process. Indeed, without it the possibility of cadaveric organ transplantation would be extremely limited and distant procurement would not take place. In other words, effective organ preservation substantially increases the potential pool without which the problems associated with a shortage of donor organs would be even further compounded.

Optimal organ preservation requires the preservation of the viability of the parenchymal cells such as the hepatocyte in the liver and the renal tubular cells of the kidney, but even more importantly the non-parenchymal elements, particularly the microvasculature. Its effect on antigenicity should at the very least be that the organ does not become more immunogenic.

Whilst immediate function is desirable for organs such as the kidney and pancreas, it is essential for the heart, lungs and liver.

What are the benefits to be gained by effective organ preservation?

Effective organ preservation restores order to the process of transplantation. Extending the time of tolerable ischaemia allows for careful selection of the recipient, which is important in circumstances where a large number of recipients might require an organ (e.g. in renal transplantation). In addition, it provides ample time for preparation of the recipient for surgery, such as preoperative dialysis.

Currently the preservation times for heart and lungs are of the order of 6 h, whereas for pancreas and liver the preservation interval can be extended to 18 h. For renal allografts preservation times of up to 48 h have been reported, but longer preservation times have been associated with compromised graft function and reduced graft survival.

HYPOTHERMIA AND ISCHAEMIA

All modalities of organ preservation utilize hypothermia as the most important element in the preservation process. In order to understand how preservation works, it is useful to review briefly the effects of ischaemia and hypothermia.

Under normal aerobic conditions the milieu of the cell is maintained through function of the ATP-dependent sodium/potassium pump. This pump effectively extrudes sodium from the cell and at the same time prevents egress of potassium. Within the cell the potassium cations are balanced by large intracellular protein anions which are incapable of crossing the cell membrane.

In ischaemia, high-energy phosphates cannot be supplied to drive the sodium/potassium pump. High-energy phosphates are rapidly depleted from the cell, which then switches to anaerobic glycolysis. Paralysis of the sodium/potassium pump results in a loss of potassium from the cell in association with an influx of sodium. Chloride ions follow sodium from the extracellular fluid, but as the large intracellular protein anions are incapable of escaping from the cell, water moves into the cell to restore osmotic equilibrium. Consequently the cell swells and cellular and organellar membranes become disrupted. As the cells revert to anaerobic respiration there is an accumulation of lactic acid.

Other changes also occur during the ischaemic interval, setting the scene for further damage by oxygen free radicals on reperfusion. During the ischaemic interval the enzyme xanthine dehydrogenase is converted to xanthine oxidase, which later catalyses the production of free radicals. In addition, the breakdown of nucleotides provides ample substrate in the form of hypoxanthine. With the introduction of oxygen to ischaemic tissue on reperfusion there is a burst of free radicals which causes injury to the organ. This injury produced by free radicals and seen only on reperfusion with the reintroduction of oxygen is therefore often referred to as a *reperfusion injury*.

Hypothermia also paralyses the functioning of the sodium/potassium pump and therefore produces a similar effect to ischaemia, but the process is slowed considerably. Oxygen consumption and the metabolic functions of the cell fall exponentially with a decrease in temperature. For every 10°C fall in temperature, oxygen consumption is halved such that, for a fall from 37°C (normothermia) to 0°C, oxygen consumption falls by a factor of 12. In the context of organ preservation this means that if an organ is capable of withstanding 1 h of normothermic ischaemia, then it should be able to survive 12 h of hypothermic ischaemia.

METHODS OF ORGAN PRESERVATION

All methods of organ preservation utilize hypothermia, but the method used almost exclusively in clinical practice is that of cold storage. Interestingly, longer periods of organ perfusion can be achieved in the experimental laboratory using machine preservation whereby the organ is maintained under hypothermic conditions, with continuous perfusion supporting some metabolism, albeit reduced. However, this technique is cumbersome and fraught with problems, and is therefore unsuited to distant procurement. However, there are still some centres that utilize this process for the rejuvenation of organs that have been damaged by prolonged preservation.

Static preservation or cold storage is simple, relatively cheap and ideally suited for distant procurement. Organs are flushed with a cold solution *in situ* during the procurement procedure in order to minimize the effects of warm ischaemia. This initial cooling process is supplemented by the application of ice packs to the organ. Once the organ has been removed from the donor it is reflushed and stored in a preservation solution in which the organ is transported.

These solutions include the University of Wisconsin (UW), Ross, Marshall and Collin solutions, and, for the heart, St Thomas or Stanford Cardioplegic solutions, and the flushing solution for the lungs should contain prostaglandin. These solutions have different components but share a number of common properties. UW solution, originally developed for pancreas preservation, is now regarded as the best preservation solution for liver, pancreas and kidney retrieval, while Collin's solution is still used for heart and lung preservation.

In order to understand the concepts embraced in preservation research, it is useful to look at UW solution and examine how it functions as a preservation solution. In simple terms, the various components of UW solution counteract the solute and water shifts which occur when the cell is rendered hypoxic. Thus the relatively high concentrations of potassium and low concentrations of sodium help to offset the natural tendency for diffusion of these ions across the cell membrane along a concentration gradient following paralysis of the cell-membrane pump. The prevention of cell swelling is accomplished by the presence of effective impermeants as key components in storage solutions. This forms the rationale for the selection of the large saccharides raffinose and lactobionate as impermeants in UW solution.

In order to prevent the development of intracellular acidosis, the inclusion of buffers such as phosphate is considered to be important. Moreover, as the cell is rapidly depleted of high-energy phosphates during hypoxia, the inclusion of adenosine and phosphate provides substrate to help to offset this loss. The potential for damage on reperfusion by oxygen free radicals is offset by the presence of glutathione, a free-radical scavenger, and allopurinol, a xanthine oxidase inhibitor, which blocks the enzyme responsible for the production of the supra-oxide radical.

A large pentastarch fraction which provides oncotic support was originally included in the solution so that it could be used for both static storage and machine perfusion. It is in fact an unnecessary component of the solution when used for static storage alone, but nevertheless it has been retained. Indeed, a number of the components selected for theoretical reasons alone may not in fact be necessary for optimal function of the preservation solution.

CARE OF THE DONOR

The care of the donor in theatre follows the same basic physiological principles as for other major surgical procedures. This involves optimal oxygenation and maintenance of cardiac output, regular measurement of arterial blood gases and haemoglobin, replacement of blood loss with blood or colloid to maintain a haematocrit of approximately 30%, and maintenance of urine output in excess of 60 mL/h. Blood pressure should be maintained with adequate fluid replacement and appropriate inotropic support.

SURGICAL TECHNIQUE OF CADAVER ORGAN RETRIEVAL

The surgical procedure of organ retrieval from brain-dead donors requires techniques that aim to minimize warm ischaemic damage to the organ(s) being retrieved. Nowadays the operation is performed as a multi-organ procurement in which one or more surgical teams may be involved. This requires close co-ordination between teams (in most situations an abdominal and cardiac retrieval team).

The operation commences with a median sternotomy and midline laparotomy. All viscera in the abdomen and chest are inspected for suitability for organ procurement. In the abdomen the distal aorta and portal system are prepared for cannulation. In the chest the proximal aorta and pulmonary artery are cannulated for cardioplegic and pneumoplegic solutions, respectively. When all is prepared, the organs are cooled *in situ* with a cold flush which both cools the organs and washes out the blood within the organ, the effluent draining to waste. The cooling process is supplemented by the application of ice packs and slush to the external surface of the organs.

The abdominal and thoracic viscera are removed, with care taken to preserve the vascular structures supplying the organs. Each organ is reflushed with preservation solution and then placed in a bag immersed in preservation solution and stored in an ice chest ready for transportation.

OTHER ORGAN DONORS

The shortage of cadaver donor organs is the most significant limiting factor for organ transplantation. It has been postulated that animal or living organs may be used in transplantation.

With regard to xenotransplantation, there are still a number of problems to be conquered before animals as a source of organs become a reality. These difficulties relate to:

- scientific conquest of the hyperacute rejection associated with cross-species transplants;
- defining and understanding the impact of potential cross-species transfer of infections, particularly viruses;
- defining the pathophysiological impact of an animal organ functioning in the human recipient;
- development of specific breeding programmes and environments for donor animals;
- modification of transplant laws to enable the use of animal organs;
- development of appropriate ethical codes of practice for xenotransplantation.

LIVING ORGAN DONATION

The shortage of cadaver organs has led to a demand for increased use of living and, where possible, cut-down donated organs. Despite the theoretical and practical advantages of living related organ donation, reservations remain about the effects of subjecting a healthy donor to surgery for the benefit of a relative with end-stage organ failure. There are risks associated with living related kidney donation, but these are small. Complications such as peri-operative bleeding, wound infection, prolonged paralytic ileus and pulmonary embolus have been described. The long-term problems might include emotional and psychological trauma, but progressive deterioration in renal function after kidney donation does not appear to occur.

Living related liver donation usually involves resection of the left lateral segment, but may utilize the right lobe. Again there is potential for complications, including bile leakage, bleeding, small-bowel obstruction, wound infection and incisional hernia, which have been reported from over 1000 living donations.

However, the current rise in the number of liver transplants being performed is placing increased demands on a scarce resource, especially for paediatric patients. Split liver transplantation, whereby the donor organ can be divided and offered to two recipients, is helping to offset some of these problems, but children who face a potentially long wait for liver transplantation should be offered living related liver transplantation if their families are considered suitable. Living donor organ procurement provides the best opportunity to supply the perfect organ to the recipient.

Living related lung donors are suitable for lung transplantation when the donor is larger than the recipient. The lower lobes are utilized for this purpose.

Living related pancreatic donation has taken place, using the tail of the pancreas. However, there has been a high incidence of subsequent diabetes and pancreatitis in the donor.

ETHICS IN TRANSPLANTATION

GENERAL CONSIDERATIONS

The basis for the ethical management of recipients and donors centres around the principles of *informed consent*, the conveyance of valid, relevant information, and the prosecution of the wishes of individuals within the moderating interests of society. This is embodied in the concept of 'do no harm, aid or benefit others, provide greatest good for the greatest number, distribute benefits and burdens in an equal and fair manner, and respect the individual'. These principles are only enacted if the data relating to transplantation is accurate and timely and the programme and its staff have appropriate credentials.

Cadaver organ donation requires that:

- death has occurred and that this is diagnosed with certainty;
- donated organs will benefit and not harm a recipient;
- the wishes of the donor are sought from or, if known, conveyed to the next of kin;
- informed discussion is entered into with the next of kin, with an empathetic and sensitive understanding of their grieving process, conveying the wishes of the donor, the benefits of organ donation, and preserving ethnic, religious and burial rights;
- there is an equitable allocation and distribution of transplantable organs;
- there will be no financial or pecuniary gains.

Living donors require that:

- organ donation is appropriately discussed, leading to informed consent;
- recipients will benefit and the donor will not suffer harm and will emotionally benefit from the process;
- they are motivated by altruism;
- there has been no financial or emotional coercion;
- the donor has been evaluated by a third party independent of the transplant team;
- there is provision to opt out with dignity, and strict privacy is retained.

The *recipient* requires that:

- informed consent should be based on an understanding of the underlying disease process and best medical treatment with transplantation as an alternative;
- they appreciate the projected intermediate and long-term outcomes, and the process of surgery and aftercare, together with the possibility of re-operation;
- they must fully understand the organ donation process, the allocation of organs and the waiting periods;
- there is a requirement for compliance with treatment;
- there is a possibility of recurrent disease where applicable;
- they can anticipate returning to normal health, work and family life.

Patients who do not qualify for transplantation have to be informed of the process and the reasons for their non-eligibility.

Transplantable organs should be distributed to those with the highest medical priority, determined by guidelines established by the collective transplantation units, but preserving the principles of fairness and equality to all, including minority groups. This requires that patients are carefully evaluated to determine those who are best able to utilize a valuable and limited resource.

The *community* has the ethical dilemma of allocating financial resources to groups who might superficially appear to expend resources on small numbers of recipients, at the expense of a wider community disbursement. New evaluation tools that equate expenditure to outcome and quality of life will aid these difficult and ethically directed financial deliberations.

TRANSPLANTED ORGANS AND TISSUES

Who should receive a transplant and when?

Any individual whose bone marrow, cornea, heart valves, bones, skin and solid organs – heart, lungs, liver, kidney, small bowel and pancreas – have failed so that life is threatened, or the quality of life is severely impaired, is entitled to be considered for transplantation as a modality of therapy. If the underlying condition of the patient is such that remedial treatment by transplantation will not alter or influence the outcome for the patient, transplantation should not be recommended. For example, transplantation for primary liver tumours as a single entity is now seldom advocated, as the long-term patient and graft survival is considerably less than for many other diseases causing end-stage liver failure. This is despite the knowledge that the outcome for hepatoma treated by transplantation is often better than that for resection or other modalities of treatment. Priority is determined by transplant outcomes in allocating a valuable and limited resource.

Thus for each organ or tissue the indication for transplantation is end-stage disease wherein, without transplantation, the patient will shortly succumb. This is modified in the case of kidney, pancreatic and small-bowel failure, where life can be maintained with dialysis, treatment with insulin, or intravenous hyperalimentation.

THE RECIPIENT

Next to blood transfusion, the most common cell transplant is that of bone marrow.

BONE MARROW

The indications for this transplant are for a number of haematological disorders, including lymphoma, aplastic anaemia, acute and chronic leukaemia and other malignancies. The best results occur when there is a close HLA match between the donor and the recipient, and when the disease process has been brought into remission. Adverse outcomes are associated with the transplanted bone marrow establishing a severe graft vs. host response, the original disease process recurring, and the development of lymphoproliferative disease.

Graft vs. host disease occurs when the donor-derived T- and B-lymphocytes are stimulated by the recipient antigens to proliferate actively to repopulate the host (recipient) lymphoid tissue. This results in immunologically based donor anti-recipient immune antibodies and responses. It may be controlled by immunosuppression.

Lymphoproliferative disease occurs when immunosuppression augments lymphoid proliferation as a neoplastic-like change which is often initiated by a virus (e.g. the Epstein-Barr virus).

CORNEA

This is the most commonly transplanted tissue and has restored vision to thousands of recipients. The ischaemic time for this tissue is not as critical as it is for organ donation. The outcome for corneal transplantation is very good, with a 10-year graft survival rate of 62%. The major causes of graft loss are rejection (30%), endothelial cell failure (20%), infection (14%) and glaucoma (8%).

HEART VALVE

Heart valve transplants have similar ischaemic requirements to those of the cornea, and make a significant contribution to cardiac surgery.

SKIN

Skin is highly antigenic and accordingly is readily rejected, but on occasion is required for severely burned patients. It may be used as split skin or as cell-cultured strips or cells. The latter technique has greatly increased the availability of autologous skin, even from the most severely burned individual.

BONE

Bone transplants are used to augment bone formation with fracture union, and in addition they permit extensive long-bone resection. The defect is bridged with a bone graft, so avoiding the need for amputation.

SMALL BOWEL

Small-bowel transplantation is limited to a few select units, and is undertaken when there has been extensive small-bowel injury, loss due to volvulus, or inflammatory bowel disease requiring the patient to be maintained with parenteral nutrition. The specific and significant complications of small-bowel transplantation are sepsis, and graft vs. host disease, in assocation with the amount of lymphoid tissue transplanted with the graft. The other complicating response is that of lymphoproliferative disease precipitated by the high level of immunosuppression required in these patients.

PRINCIPLES OF SUITABILITY

The whole organs kidney, pancreas, liver, heart and lungs are transplanted on the basis of the general criteria of end-stage organ failure, and that there will be optimal patient survival, quality of life and allocation of scarce donor organs.

The criteria include the following.

1. The recipient must not have an excluding disease entity:
   - malignancy or uncontrolled infection, as both are likely to be exacerbated by immunosuppression;
   - severe cardiopulmonary disease that will threaten survival at operation or be exacerbated by immunosuppressive medication. Ischaemic heart disease requires evaluation;
   - multisystem organ failure, particularly renal impairment, which deteriorates with immunosuppression (unless for renal transplantation);
   - bone-marrow failure;

- cirrhosis of the liver (unless considered for liver transplantation);

- HIV seropositivity;

- viral infections of hepatitis B or C (HBV, HBC) (modified for liver transplantation), Epstein-Barr or cytomegaloblast virus, which are all relative contraindications. HBV-negative patients require immunization;

- type 1 diabetes – this can be a relative contraindication;

- nutritional states: obesity is a contraindication, and neurasthenic individuals may not have the reserve to withstand the procedures;

- medication regimes (e.g. anticonvulsant) that conflict with cyclosporin and tacrolimus;

- peripheral vascular disease, particularly if associated with cerebrovascular disease;

- gastrointestinal disease, such as diverticular and peptic ulcer disease, which requires prior treatment;

- hepatobiliary disease, such as cholecystitis or cholelithiasis, may require pretransplant treatment.

2. The recipient must have stable social support and not have any psychiatric illness that may be associated with non-compliance. They must not have current alcohol, tobacco or drug abuse.

3. The recipient must be within set age limits, but is usually younger than 65 years.

Ideally, organ transplant recipients are normal individuals except for their single failed organ. Their failed organ pathology determines transplantation outcomes and contributes to the decision process in listing patients for transplantation and organ allocation.

ORGAN-RELATED SUITABILITY

Kidney

The general criteria for suitability for transplantation apply, although the urgency for operation is modified because life can be maintained on a kidney machine, but transplantation promotes a better quality of life and a substantial saving in health-care costs. Organ pathologies are recognized and relate to transplantation outcome measured by graft and patient survival. Primary and secondary hyper-parathyroidism associated with renal failure may require treatment prior to transplantation.

Renal-specific factors causing end-stage renal failure that have to be considered include the following:

- disease processes that result in damage to the glomerular basement membrane;

- urological disease – kidney parenchymal infection, stones, intractable hypertension and large polycystic kidneys may necessitate pretransplant nephrectomy. Bladder voiding function requires evaluation and may need treatment;

- systemic disease – diabetes mellitus type 1 with diabetic nephropathy requires critical evaluation and consideration for combined kidney–pancreas transplantation.

The best renal transplant outcomes are achieved in ABO-compatible, negative lymphocytotoxicity cross-matched grafts with close HLA DR-matched donor and recipient pairs. Hence HLA-identical related living donors or six antigen-matched cadaver donors are sought.

Liver

Any patient with end-stage liver disease is considered for transplantation, given the general suitability for transplantation criteria and the relative contraindications for transplantation, which include the following:

- the presence of haemochromatosis, for which there is a poor prognosis in transplantation;

- replicating HBV has a very poor graft outcome, but treatment may control this to allow transplantation; HCV patients are not excluded;

- hepatobiliary malignancy and acute liver failure are both associated with poorer outcomes, and hepatobiliary malignancy seldom qualifies in the face of organ shortages.

The factors associated with end-stage liver failure leading to transplantation include the following:

- recurrent spontaneous bacterial peritonitis;

- progressive hyperbilirubinaemia;

- uncontrolled encephalopathy;

- poor synthetic function expressed as decreased albumin and fibrinogen or elevated prothrombin time;

- portal hypertension causing intractable ascites, hypersplenism and/or bleeding varices;

- inability to function or maintain normal activity (fatigue);

- paediatric metabolic disease associated with chronic liver disease.

The above represent two basic groups, namely those associated with a prognosis of less than 50% survival at 1 year (particularly the first four factors above) or severe impairment of the quality of life (the last three factors above). In each group there is an overlap and difficulty in predicting when quality-of-life considerations will become a life-threatening indication. Hepatorenal syndrome, recurrent spontaneous bacterial peritonitis, serum albumin levels of < 25 g/L, prothrombin time prolonged by more than 5 s and serum bilirubin levels of > 85 μmol/L all suggest severe disease and the need for imminent transplantation.

Unfortunately there are few reliable predictive models which can be used to determine the precise time at which transplantation should take place. The more reliable indications are seen in the cholestatic forms of liver disease, primary biliary cirrhosis and primary sclerosing cholangitis. The outcome for liver transplantation is such that transplantation can now be considered for genetic metabolic disorders manifesting outside the liver (e.g. familial hypercholesterolaemia and hereditary oxalosis).

Heart

The indications for transplantation are cardiac disease causing a threat to life or severe impairment to the quality of life that cannot be corrected by alternative surgery or medical therapy such as:

- revascularization for significant reversible ischaemia;
- valve replacement for critical aortic valve disease;
- valve replacement for repair of severe mitral regurgitation.

This group includes patients with severe functional limitation from heart failure, refractory angina, life-threatening arrhythmia or cardiomyopathy.

The general suitability criteria for transplantation apply, but additional features contraindicating transplantation include pulmonary disease associated with high vascular resistance and FEV_1 < 1 L or < 50% of predicted value, excessive body weight > 150% of ideal body weight, and impaired renal function (serum creatinine > 250 μmol/L).

Lung

The indications for lung or heart–lung transplantation relate to pulmonary parenchymal or vascular disease causing a projected life expectancy of < 2 years. The patient is unable to perform daily living activities of eating, dressing and washing, each of these causing dyspnoea, fatigue, palpitations or chest pain.

The specific relative contraindications for lung transplantation include excessive weight in the recipient, previous cardiopulmonary surgery resulting in pleurodesis, mechanical ventilation, impaired left heart function (unless considered for heart–lung transplantation), symptomatic osteoporosis, severe chest wall deformity, sputum with resistant bacteria and *Aspergillus*.

The disease-specific indications for suitability include the following:

- idiopathic pulmonary fibrosis where FVC is < 65% of the predicted value or the patient is a steroid non-responder;
- cystic fibrosis where FVC is < 40% of the predicted value, FEV_1 is < 30% of the predicted value and in room air the PaO_2 at rest is < 60 mmHg;
- symptomatic primary pulmonary hypertension;
- emphysema after using a bronchodilator FEV_1 is < 25% of the predicted value.

In each of these conditions the 2-year survival rate for transplanted vs. non-transplanted patients is similar, and hence optimal medical care should have been delivered, and careful evaluation made in terms of transplant waiting time, and quality-of-life factors considered in the decision for transplant listing.

Pancreas

These patients are insulin-dependent diabetics, usually between the ages of 20 and 40 years, either with end-stage renal failure or with poorly controlled insulin-dependent diabetes. There should be minimal evidence of secondary diabetic complications. Indeed, advanced changes of blindness, major amputation, neuropathy or heart disease are regarded as a contraindication to pancreatic transplantation, but the initial presence of these complications can be modified by a transplant.

COMPLICATIONS OF WHOLE ORGAN TRANSPLANTATION

Surveys of all whole organ transplant patients and graft survival curves suggest that the greatest loss of organs occurs in the 12-month interval immediately after the procedure. Beyond this time graft function and survival become stable, with a slower and more predictable rate of attrition. The complications resulting in early graft loss are cited below.

Primary non-function of the graft

In the kidney this can manifest as total anuria or relatively poor urine output with a slow decline in serum creatinine and the patient controlled by dialysis. This state may persist for 2 or more weeks, usually as acute tubular necrosis, and must be distinguished from the other causes of poor urine production and persisting elevation of serum creatinine levels, namely:

- vascular complications of the renal artery or vein;
- early severe rejection;
- external compression of the kidney;

- hypovolaemia;

- urinary obstruction or leakage;

- intravesical bleeding with clot formation and catheter obstruction.

In *pancreatic* graft failure the serum glucose level does not fall, and if there has been bladder drainage of the graft the urinary amylase activity is low. The other causes that need to be excluded are similar to those for the kidney, but the following are particularly important:

- vascular problems;

- early severe rejection;

- hypovolaemia or external graft compression with poor graft perfusion.

In the other organs, namely *heart, lungs and liver*, primary non-function is uncommon, but when it occurs is a devastating event that results in death unless a graft becomes available for regrafting within 24–48 h. Less than optimal early graft function, due to a number of contributing factors, may occur in up to 20% of grafts.

Primary non-function may be related to donor factors, poor graft perfusion secondary to hypovolaemia or the use of inotropes, graft factors, preservation injury, prolonged ischaemic time (either warm or cold) or, in the recipient, poor graft perfusion secondary to hypovolaemia often associated with excessive bleeding, with a prolonged patient recovery and poor graft revascularization secondary to problems at the anastomosis site.

Technical problems

Technical problems are seldom directly responsible for graft failure or compromised function. However, a less than optimal technical outcome may occur in up to 10% of graft implantations. This varies depending on the complexity of the transplanted organ, and relates to the vascular (arterial or venous) or drainage system anastomoses.

Kidney Primary graft loss due to vascular or ureteric mechanical problems occurs infrequently in the short term, but accounts for the loss of 1–2% of organs in the long term.

Bleeding with resulting haematoma still accounts for 1–2% of returns to the operating room, depending on the amount of anticoagulant used in association with surgery. In the long term, renal artery stenosis may give rise to hypertension in 2% of cases and ureteric obstruction from ischaemia (either primarily or secondarily to chronic rejection) will occur in an equally small number of patients.

Pancreas Vascular occlusion, particularly venous thrombosis (6%) is more common due to the slow venous blood flow. Consequently patients are often treated with anticoagulation with a commensurate increase in bleeding and haematoma formation. Leakage from the exocrine drainage of the graft to either bowel or bladder occurs in up to 6–10% of cases. The latter may be associated with metabolic acidosis, urethritis or cystitis, and necessitates conversion to an enteric anastomosis in 10–20% of patients. Pancreatitis occurs in up to 3–4% of grafted organs.

Liver Stenosis and/or thrombosis may occur in any of the vascular anastomoses, but the more severe sequelae result from hepatic artery stenosis or occlusion (in approximately 5% of adults and 30% of children). Occlusion is often associated with graft necrosis, recurrent sepsis or major biliary complications followed by the need for regrafting. Lower levels of arterial occlusion are complicated by ischaemia of the bile duct with leaks or strictures. Portal vein thrombosis occurs in up to 2% of grafts.

The incidence of bleeding resulting in re-operation is in the range 3–15%. Biliary problems, leaks, strictures and obstruction occur in up to 20% of patients and are secondary to hepatic artery stenosis, bile duct ischaemia from excessive dissection, rejection or, in late disease, recurrent primary pathology (e.g. primary biliary cirrhosis), stone formation, cholangitis or as a complication of removing the T-tube drain.

Heart The vascular problems include pseudoaneurysm formation with rupture of the cannulation or anastomosis site, valvular regurgitation, pulmonary artery torsion and haemorrhage. Rhythm disturbance of both atrial or ventricular asystole and right or left ventricular dysfunction also occurs. Bleeding may cause cardiac tamponade.

Lung Anastomotic problems occur in 2–3% of early and 7–15% of late complications. These mainly relate to the bronchial anastomosis. The bronchial arteries are too small to identify and anastomose, and in this regard are analogous to the blood supply of the bile duct. Thus the problems of the bronchus are thought to be ischaemic in nature and include dehiscence, leaks and stricture formation. Venous strictures may cause pulmonary vein occlusion with pulmonary oedema or thrombosis and death. Pulmonary artery stricture is associated with pulmonary artery hypertension.

Rejection

The experimental work initiated by Sir Peter Medawar established that graft rejection is donor specific and occurs as a cell-mediated response on first exposure of the recipient to donor antigen. On a second or subsequent graft, the process is accelerated due to an antibody-mediated interaction between the donor and the recipient. These responses are now better understood and involve varied lymphocyte populations, antigen-processing cells, cytokines, adhesion molecules and major histocompatibility antigens. Clinically, rejection results in graft dysfunction, which has to be distinguished from other causes of organ function deterioration.

Hyperacute rejection

On account of donor and recipient matching for lymphocytotoxicity antibodies, hyperacute rejection is seldom seen in organ transplantation. It is an antibody response in which endothelial cells become disrupted, platelets marginate along the vessel wall, complement is activated and thrombosis occurs with consequent acute swelling, cyanosis and death of the organ.

Acute rejection

This is the more common rejection response in all organ transplants and frequently manifests between days 5 and 14 after organ implantation. Histologically it is recognized by infiltration of the organ with lymphocytes. The location of the infiltrate is specific to the implanted organ. Later rejection episodes may be precipitated by septic episodes (viral or bacterial) such as CMV infection.

Chronic rejection

Chronic rejection is expressed as a vascular response which tends to be organ specific. In each instance, the characteristic feature is of ischaemic changes secondary to sclerosis of the microcirculation. In the heart this is seen as accelerated arteriosclerosis, in the kidney ischaemic change is seen in the glomerulus, and in the liver the change is featured by vanishing bile ducts. The process is probably mediated by antibody-induced cytokine activity causing smooth muscle intimal hyperplasia.

Organ-specific changes of rejection

In the *kidney* this is most frequently a cellular response affecting the glomerulus, but it may also have a vascular component and accounts for the majority of organs lost in the first year. It is minimized in well HLA/DR-matched donor recipient pairs and a negative lymphocytotoxic antibody cross-match. Acute rejection occurs in 20–60% of renal transplant recipients, and is readily reversed with steroid treatment in 70% of these cases.

In the *pancreas* acute rejection is difficult to diagnose because, by the time hyperglycaemia has occured, much of the islet cell mass has been destroyed. Hence the indices for rejection are those of the associated kidney transplant if this has occurred concurrently (most have) and the decline in urinary pancreatic enzymes (amylase). Confirmation is by percutaneous needle biopsy. Rejection of this graft often requires more vigorous treatment to bring it under control than is experienced in other organ transplants. ABO and HLA/DR matching with a negative lymphocytotoxic cross-match are important in managing acute rejection.

In the *liver*, acute rejection does occur but appears to be less severe than in the other organ transplants. Nevertheless it accounts for more early graft losses than does primary non-function. Grafts are matched for ABO compatibility but not for HLA/DR or negative lymphocytotoxity matching. In urgent circumstances, ABO compatibility is ignored, but with a significantly greater graft loss. Chronic rejection is less common for the liver (< 10% of patients) than for the kidney or heart, and leads to bile duct obliteration which is difficult to distinguish from recurrent primary disease.

In the *heart*, acute rejection episodes occur at a high rate (54%), or 1.3 episodes for cardiac transplant recipients at 12 months. These episodes are difficult to diagnose from functional studies, and require diagnostic endomyocardial biopsy. Rejection is most frequently seen in younger recipients receiving a female donor organ. Other matching combinations have been sought and designed to guide anti-rejection strategies. Chronic rejection is associated with allograft arteriopathy (accelerated coronary artery disease) in 30–50% of patients at 5 years, and is a leading cause of death.

In the *lung*, acute rejection occurs as early as 4 days post-transplant, and is difficult to distinguish from lung infiltrates of donor or recipient origin; it depends on transbronchial biopsy for confirmation. Steroid treatment may influence the bronchial anastomosis and its complications, but chronic rejection is associated with morbidity and mortality in 15–30% of patients.

Anti-rejection therapy

Immunosuppressive therapy has made organ transplantation possible, but suppression of the host response to all antigens, including those of viruses, fungi, bacteria, parasites, foreign tissues and malignancies has a cost in terms of septic and malignancy complications. The broad grouping of currently used medications is as follows.

Glucocorticoids

These are an important immunosuppressive adjunct. Because of the multiplicity of side-effects with prolonged administration, glucocorticoids are given in large doses initially and then on a reducing regimen to a low maintenance dose of 10–15 mg/day. The predominant immunosuppressive effect is prevention of the release of interleukins 1 and 6. Larger doses are given at the time of transplantation and for bouts of acute rejection.

Azathioprine

This drug is a common analogue of mercaptopurine, and because of its ability to inhibit nucleic acid synthesis it has been the backbone of therapeutic immunosuppression, and remains very much a part of the current pharmacological armamentarium. Currently it is used in doses of up to 2 mg/kg/day in combination with cyclosporin to allow lower cyclosporin doses and toxicity.

There is no serum assay for azathioprine. However, a falling platelet count necessitates a reduction in the dosage.

Cyclosporin

This fungal extract has a potent immunosuppressive effect. Since its introduction in the early 1980s, a major improvement in graft survival has been achieved by better immunosuppression. Significant side-effects include nephrotoxicity, neurotoxicity, hepatotoxicity and endocrine abnormalities which necessitate combination immunotherapy with glucocorticoids and azathioprine. The mechanism of action involves disrupting transcription of mRNA for interleukin-2 and other cytokines influencing the immunological response. T-cell proliferation is inhibited as a result. The immunosuppressive effect of cyclosporin is enhanced by glucocorticoids. Serum assays exist for this drug. The blood level must be titrated against renal function and the dose reduced in the face of a rising creatinine concentration.

Tacrolimus (FK506)

Tacrolimus is a fungal peptide, similar to cyclosporin, although it is much more potent, with a mode of action and side-effects paralleling those of cyclosporin. Diabetes tends to be a greater problem than with cyclosporin. Serum assays are more difficult to perform and not as widely available as those for cyclosporin, but they are used to regulate the dosage.

Mycophenolate mofetil

The mode of action of this drug is similar to that of azathioprine, and in some cases it is used to replace azathioprine when it has less platelet suppression. Its main advantages are its simplicity and dosage (2 or 3 g/day). Compared to azathioprine it has an increased 'anti-rejection' effect, with few side-effects. There are no widely used serum assays in clinical practice.

Serolimus (rapamycin)

This is another fungal extract that is currently being tested in clinical trials. In combination with cyclosporin it appears to have a beneficial effect. The action of this drug is to inhibit the T-cell response to cytokines and inhibit the smooth muscle proliferation that is seen in chronic rejection.

Anti-lymphocyte antibodies

Human lymphocytes/thymocytes injected into target animals (horses, rabbits, mice and goats) produce anti-human lymphocyte serum. The separation and subsequent injection of the globulin fraction (anti-thymocyte or anti-lymphocyte globulin) enhances graft survival. The efficacy is unpredictable and depends in particular on the source of the globulin. Mouse monoclonal antibodies against particular T-cell lymphocyte subsets are a refined source of this therapy. OKT3 is an antibody in common use. The mechanism of action is targeted at CD3 molecules in the T-cell antigen-receptor complex. The expansion of this form of therapy against other molecules in the receptor complex has further potential for immunotherapy.

The antibodies can be antigenic and can cause anti-mouse antibody formation that will limit the duration of treatment effectiveness.

Treatment of acute bouts of rejection

Once a patient's post-operative condition has stabilized, maintenance therapy with two or three drugs is continued indefinitely. In most cases this is a combination of cyclosporin and azathioprine with or without glucocorticoids. Acute rejection episodes require additional therapy, usually in the form of methylprednisolone, 1–3 g IV for 2–3 days or, if the patient is unresponsive to this regimen, the institution of tacrolimus or an OKT3 infusion.

Infection

Infection as a cause of graft loss acts in the acute early period, most commonly as bacteria entering through drains, catheters, T-tubes, wounds and the airways. These infections become more severe in the presence of leaks, haematoma, obstruction to hollow organs or in cases where there is ischaemic damage to the mucosa. The particularly susceptible areas include the biliary tree in the liver, the bronchi in the lung, and the region in and around the pancreas with a pancreatic transplant (most serious when complicated by pancreatitis). Prophylactic antibiotics are given to help to control these early infections.

Later infections and those associated with increased immunosuppression are viral (cytomegalovirus (CMV) Epstein-Barr and herpes virus), fungi (candida, aspergillosis), cryptococcus and *Pneumocystis carinii*. Of these, CMV is most common, and particularly severe in lung transplantation. Matching CMV is needed, with CMV positive donor to positive recipient or negative donor to positive or negative recipient, but preferably not positive donor to negative recipient. Aciclovir or ganciclovir may reduce the severity of this infection and prevent herpes infection. Trimethoprim prophylaxis will substantially reduce pneumocystis infection.

Impaired renal function, hypertension and progressive vascular disease

These are common to all transplant recipients and relate to the undesirable side-effects of immunosuppressive agents, particularly cyclosporin, tacrolimus and steroids. The associated dyslipidaemia of some immunosuppressives contribute to these changes, and in the heart may be a feature of chronic rejection.

Malignancy in transplantation

Skin cancers and lymphoproliferative disease have part of their genesis in immunosuppression. Most units report long-term patient and graft loss to early-onset cardiovascular and neoplastic disease of 3–5 times that found in an equivalent non-transplant population.

The drugs implicated in this process include cyclosporin, tacrolimus and azathioprine. The mechanism of action is unknown. Epstein-Barr virus is implicated, but the magnitude of its effect is difficult to determine. In some cases there has been a linear relationship between immunosuppression and lymphoma, with the lymphoma responding to a lowering of the immunosuppressive regimen. The risk of lymphoproliferative disease is of the order of 5%. The risk of other neoplasms, including carcinomas, is also elevated. Rarely, malignancies of donor origin have been transmitted to the recipient by the allograft.

Retransplantation and surgery in the previous operative field

Retransplantation is possible for graft failure in each area of organ transplantation, but is associated with high initial graft loss and mortality rates due to complications and often more difficult rejection. Similarly, with transplantation in any body cavity, the site of previous surgery is accompanied by increased technical difficulty, greater bleeding and often a more complicated post-transplant recovery secondary to bleeding and sepsis.

Recurrence of underlying disease

Some conditions, particularly arteriosclerosis, are accelerated in transplant recipients, and in others diabetes is induced by immunosuppression. Whenever transplantation has been performed for neoplasia there has been a high recurrence rate in the recipient, and in some cases also in the graft.

In *kidney* transplantation, diseases that have resulted in damage to the glomerular basement membrane, focal and segmental glomeruloscleroses, IgA nephropathy, mesengial proliferative glomerulonephropathy types I and II and membranous glomerulonephropathy can have an increased risk of recurrence. This risk may be in the range of 10–80% of patients, particularly those who require regrafting.

In *pancreatic* transplantation, damage to the islet cells as a consequence of the original disease results in recurrent diabetes.

In *liver* transplantation, the diseases that are most likely to recur include hepatitis B (90%; this may be reduced with prior and continuing treatment with the antiviral agent lamivudine), hepatitis C (52%; however, the need for retransplantation is low), autoimmune hepatitis (20%), sclerosing cholangitis (12%), primary biliary cirrhosis (7%) and alcoholic disease (7%). Recidivism for alcoholics is more likely in those with a short period of total abstinence from alcohol before transplantation. Most units require a period of at least 1 year.

In *lung* transplantation the diseases that recur include sarcoidosis, lymphangioleiomyomatosis and giant-cell interstitial pneumonitis. These are an infrequent indication for transplantation.

In *heart* transplantation the principal recurrent disease is arteriosclerosis, which may be either part of chronic rejection or a progression of the atheromatous change that is seen following all transplantation.

OUTCOME FOR TRANSPLANT PATIENTS

The survival outcome for transplant patients is organ dependent. In the kidney, a failed graft is treated by the patient returning to dialysis, and hence graft and patient survival are different. Patient survival is always better than graft survival, by approximately 10% in the short term (5 years). In the other organ transplants there is no equivalent to a dialysis machine, and hence graft and patient survival are very similar. However, for all organs, patient and graft survival is dependent on a number of factors.

The era of transplantation

Liver patients who were transplanted in the 1970s and 1980s had a 20–30% probability of graft and patient survival at 5 years, but many of those who survived are still alive and pursuing normal work and social activities. In 1998, up to 90% of transplant recipients could be expected to be alive in 12 months, with little change in their survival over the next 5 years. These survival changes are reflected in the United Network for Organ Sharing (UNOS) published data (Table 27.1).

The present outcomes compare very favourably with the outcome for other disease modalities treated by surgery (e.g. colorectal cancer with an overall survival rate of 50%, peripheral vascular disease (50%), and gastric carcinoma with a survival rate of under 15% at 5 years).

The following factors influence patient and graft survival:

- *donor factors* – living vs. cadaver (see Table 27.1 for kidney), donor age and organ ischaemic time. Extremes of age adversely influence recipient outcomes, as does a prolonged ischaemic time;

Table 27.1 Comparisons of 1-year graft survival in relation to the year of transplantation*

Graft	Year 1989	Year 1994
Cadaver kidney	76	84
Living kidney	89	93
Liver	64	76
Pancreas	63	79
Heart	81	84
Lung	42	74
Heart–lung	51	71

*Data from United Network for Organ Sharing (UNOS), 1996.

- *recipient matching* – all mismatches of the ABO system adversely affect all organ transplants. Close HLA/DR matching benefits kidney graft outcomes, and may confer similar benefits on heart transplants. However, the ischaemic time constraints prevent sophisticated matching for hearts;
- *CMV infection* appears to affect graft survival adversely in all transplants;
- *very ill patients* (e.g. those on ventilation) have a poorer prognosis;
- *graft loss* is greatest in the first 12 months due to a number of factors, including rejection and primary diseases (Table 27.2). Subsequently the attrition rate is 2–5% per year, due mainly to chronic rejection or recurrent diseases;

Table 27.2 Graft survival in relation to primary disease causing organ failure*

Organ	Pathology (pre-transplant)	Survival rate (%) at 1 year
Kidney	Polycystic disease	68
	Diabetic nephrosis	52
Liver	Cholestatic liver disease	85
	Fulminant liver disease	70
Lung	Emphysema	78
	Primary pulmonary hypertension	65

*Data from United Network for Organ Sharing (UNOS), 1996.

- *retransplantation* is associated with an adverse outcome;
- *new immunosuppressive medications* which inhibit acute and chronic rejection will probably influence chronic rejection and benefit survival.

Survival and quality of life post-transplantation

There are a limited number of comprehensive studies defining quality of life, but in general terms the transplanted patient returns to normal social and work practices, rather than facing death in 6–18 months without surgery. Normal children have been born to patients of both sexes without loss of the graft in women, and without evidence of a teratogenic effect in the infant from the immunosuppresive treatment of the parent. Paediatric patients have grown and developed normally.

Summary synopsis of patient management

1. Factors that require vigilance:
   - patients who might be suitable for transplantation need to be identified early in the progression of their disease;
   - patients with substantial comorbidity who would not ultimately benefit from organ transplantation are excluded.
2. Positive influences on outcome:
   - the best available donor organ, live related donation;
   - close donor/recipient match;
   - minimal graft ischaemic time (both cold and warm ischaemia);
   - a technically precise procedure associated with minimal blood loss;
   - tailoring immunosuppression to minimize the side-effects associated with over-immunosuppression.
3. Factors requiring early recognition and treatment:
   - deteriorating graft function due to rejection;
   - over-immunosuppression, particularly in association with deteriorating renal function, bone-marrow suppression and sepsis;
   - lymphoproliferative disease, neoplasia, hyperlipidaemia, diabetes or rising blood pressure all suggest that immunosuppression should be changed to lower doses or alternative medication;
   - chronic rejection defined by biopsy is more difficult to manage, but altered immunosuppression may help.

4. The depressed immune system in the transplant patient demands constant assessment for:

- neoplasia, particularly of the skin and lymphoid tissues, but all tumours have a higher prevalence that is time and immunosuppression related;

- the risk of infection (bacterial or viral infections are more common, but organisms such as *Mycobacterium, Listeria, Nocardia, Candida, Aspergillus* and *Pneumocystis* must be considered).

Chapter 28

Blood transfusion: blood products and alternatives

Laurie Catley, John V. Lloyd and Ken Davis

Introduction

Blood transfusion therapy utilizes an expensive resource, and in most countries the blood is donated by volunteer donors. There is usually a fine balance between the numbers of donors available and the amount of product required. In addition, transfusion of blood products is not without risk, including transfusion reactions and the transmission of infection. For these reasons it is important that surgeons prescribe the infusion of blood products with a proper knowledge of the benefits and risks involved. In many cases there is still not a direct charge to the hospital for the supply of blood products. In this situation it is important to make a special effort to maintain an awareness of their cost to the community.

BLOOD PRODUCTS

Modern transfusion therapy is based on the need for specific components. In many countries, whole blood is now rarely if ever given. Instead, it is fractionated into red cells, platelets and plasma. Some plasma is used as fresh frozen plasma, and the remainder is processed by fractionation to produce components such as albumin, gammaglobulin, and factor VIII and factor IX concentrates.

PATIENT CONSENT

Before transfusion of blood products, the reason for the transfusion must be discussed with the patient, and their consent obtained. This information, including the indication, should be documented in the case file. Whenever possible, the patient should be well informed of the risks, benefits and possible alternatives to blood transfusion.

RED CELLS

Red cells are the most commonly transfused blood product. This relates in part to the fact that stored red cells are relatively stable for some weeks, and that their lifespan in the circulation (120 days) is much longer than that of platelets (8–10 days) or neutrophils (8–12 h). In addition, it is usually possible to transfuse red cells regularly and indefinitely without inducing severe problems of incompatibility due to the development of alloantibodies. This contrasts with platelet transfusions where, because of the diversity of the HLA antibody system, alloantibodies can severely compromise their effectiveness.

The red cells are prepared by centrifugation of the donor unit, followed by removal of plasma or platelet-rich plasma. A buffer solution is then added to decrease viscosity and improve shelf-life. To preserve their viability, and to inhibit the growth of microbial organisms, they must be stored under strict conditions at 4–6°C in controlled refrigerators, and must on no account be stored in ward refrigerators.

For all donor units the ABO and Rh blood groups are determined. This is also performed on the blood of the recipient to ensure that the units to be transfused are compatible with the ABO and Rh group of the recipient. In addition, it is essential to ascertain whether the recipient's plasma contains any antibodies that could potentially agglutinate or lyse the donor red cells.

In most centres, requests for the majority of patients are dealt with by a 'type and screen' procedure. This means that the patient's blood is typed for ABO and Rh groups, and the plasma is screened for antibodies which may cause incompatibility with the donor red cells. If the antibody screen is negative, cross-matched compatible blood can be available within 10–15 min. For urgent specimens, group-specific, unmatched blood can be made available within 5–10 min. In emergency situations, O-negative blood can be issued immediately.

When the antibody screen is positive, further tests are required, and blood that has been shown to be fully compatible by cross-match is supplied.

Indications for red cell transfusion (see also Box 28.1)

Prior to surgery, the decision to transfuse a specific patient should take into consideration the following factors:

- the duration of anaemia;
- intravascular volume depletion, such as occurs in blood loss;
- the extent of any operation planned;
- the probability of massive blood loss;
- the presence of coexisting conditions such as impaired pulmonary function, inadequate cardiac output, myocardial ischaemia, or cerebrovascular or peripheral circulatory disease.

In many patients who are found to be anaemic during recovery from surgery, red cell transfusion is not indicated. Clinical grounds for deciding that post-operative anaemia is making a significant contribution to delayed recovery would include the presence of cardiovascular or respiratory compromise, or the threat of continued bleeding. This should be balanced against the potentially adverse effects of homologous blood.

Protocols for transfusion indicators provide a guide for decision-making. However, practices vary widely between centres, and lack standardization in both Europe and the USA.

The decision to transfuse red cells should be individualized as much as possible. Risks and benefits need to be considered, and the overall benefit to each individual patient should exceed the potential risks. This requires judgment based on a knowledge of the detrimental effects of anaemia, and the risks vs. the benefits of red cell transfusion.

In general, 2 to 4 units of red cells are required to increase the haemoglobin concentration by a clinically significant amount. The haemoglobin level should rise by about 1 g/dL for each unit of red cells transfused.

BOX 28.1 GUIDELINES FOR TRANSFUSION (DEVELOPED AT THE ROYAL ADELAIDE HOSPITAL)

Red cells

1. *Haemoglobin value < 7.0 g/dL*
2. *Peri-operative haemoglobin value < 8.0 g/dL*
3. *Haemoglobin value 7.0–10.0 g/dL if any of the following are present:*
   - **3.1.** Ongoing bleeding
   - **3.2.** Dyspnoea, lethargy or weakness, poor effort tolerance, angina, syncope
   - **3.3.** Cardiac ischaemia or cardiac failure due to anaemia
4. Rapid blood loss leading to hypovolaemia and shock

Platelets

1. *Prophylactic transfusion before surgery or other invasive procedure that could result in significant bleeding*
   - **1.1.** Platelet count $< 50 \times 10^9$/L
   - **1.2.** Platelet count $> 50 \times 10^9$/L, but evidence of platelet dysfunction
2. *Therapeutic transfusion for uncontrolled haemorrhage*
   - **2.1.** Platelet count $< 100 \times 10^9$/L and/or evidence of platelet dysfunction
3. *Prophylactic transfusion in marrow failure (leukaemia and other malignancies causing a regenerative megakaryocytopenia) when no procedures are planned*
   - **3.1.** Platelet count $< 10 \times 10^9$/L, or $< 20 \times 10^9$/L if the patient is febrile (except in patients in palliative phase, where platelet transfusion is given only for clinically significant bleeding)
4. *ITP*
   - **4.1.** Only if visceral or mucosal bleeding is present

Fresh frozen plasma

1. *Massive transfusion (> one blood volume per 24 h)* 4–5 units of fresh frozen plasma (FPP) for each 10 units of red cells. Increased amounts are indicated if the INR

BOX 28.1 *(Continued)*

(prothrombin time) > 1.5 or APTT (activated partial thromboplastin time) > 40 s*

2. *Prophylactic transfusion before surgery or other invasive procedure that could result in significant bleeding*
   2.1. Urgent correction of prolonged INR or APTT* in warfarin overdose or vitamin K deficiency
   2.2. Correction of prolonged INR or APTT* in liver disease
   2.3. Correction of inherited coagulation factor deficiencies in cases where specific coagulation factor concentrates are not available

3. *Therapeutic transfusion for uncontrolled haemorrhage in*
   3.1. Warfarin overdose
   3.2. Liver disease
   3.3. Vitamin K deficiency
   3.4. Inherited coagulation factor deficiencies in cases where specific coagulation factor concentrates are not available

4. *Plasma exchange in thrombotic thrombocytopenic purpura (TTP)*
   In TTP platelet transfusions are contraindicated as they aggravate intravascular thrombosis. Plasmapheresis with FFP replacement is the appropriate therapy for patients with thrombotic thrombocytopenic purpura

Cryoprecipitate
1. *Diffuse microvascular bleeding and fibrinogen < 1.0 g/L in*
   1.1. DIC
   1.2. Massive transfusion
   1.3. Hereditary hypofibrinogenaemia

---

*Values for APTT vary between laboratories.

Detrimental effects of post-operative anaemia

When assessing a patient with anaemia, it should be remembered that physiological mechanisms serve to compensate for anaemia and improve oxygen delivery to tissues by:

- increased cardiac output by increased stroke volume and tachycardia;
- decreased blood viscosity;
- right shift in the oxygen dissociation curve increasing oxygen extraction by cells;
- regional microcirculatory vasodilatation.

Cellular oxygen utilization is only impaired when delivery is reduced to a critical level and physiological compensatory mechanisms are maximized. Patients in shock may therefore achieve adequate tissue oxygenation by inotrope and haemodynamic volume resuscitation alone. In this setting, red cell transfusions given for haemoglobin values of approximately 80 g/L have been shown not to improve the shock state, regardless of the aetiology of the shock.

The consequences of forgoing blood transfusions can be assessed by examining the experiences of surgery performed on Jehovah's Witnesses. These patients observe the strict religious practice of refusing all blood products, including autologous transfusions. Apart from this, they have similar characteristics to the general population.

Operations traditionally associated with high transfusion requirements have been performed on Jehovah's Witnesses. These operations include coronary artery bypass grafts, adult and paediatric cardiovascular operations, and total hip replacements, and there has been an estimated 0.5–1.5% increase in mortality by forgoing red cell transfusion.

Strokes, myocardial infarction, acute renal failure, post-operative infection, delayed wound healing, length of stay and other maladies were not increased in Jehovah's Witness patients compared to other patients. Hypotensive anaesthetic techniques resulted in significantly less blood loss and a shorter operative time for these patients. Using normovolaemic haemodilution techniques, paediatric heart bypass with intra-operative haematocrits of 15% was tolerated without ill effects.

It can be concluded that operations which traditionally result in anaemia and require a blood transfusion can be well tolerated without transfusions. It is therefore likely that in general patients are transfused more often than is necessary. This results in an increased risk of transfusion-related complications. There is also a significant cost to the community in terms of the logistics of blood collection, storage and administration. Widespread agreement about the indications for transfusions and standardization of transfusion practices are needed to address this issue.

Transfusion of red cells

Transfusion should commence within 30 min of the pack leaving the transfusion department. Intravenous medications should never be put in blood packs or the infusion line when blood is running. An acceptable way of administering an intravenous drug while a transfusion is in progress is to temporarily cease the transfusion, flush with 0.9% saline, inject the drug, repeat the flush and then continue the transfusion.

PLATELETS

Platelet packs are prepared from whole-blood donations after low-speed centrifugation, or by higher-speed centrifugation followed by harvesting of the buffy coat. For an adult patient a dose is usually 5 or 6 donor units. Alternatively, apheresis can be used to collect enough platelets from a single donor. Platelets are stored at room temperature. At this temperature they are metabolically active, and gas exchange is necessary. To facilitate this, the plastic of the storage bag is permeable to O_2, and they are continually agitated on a rocking device. Under these conditions their shelf-life is 5 days.

The HLA class I antigen is the main antigenic determinant of the platelet. This antigen is extremely heterogeneous in the general population. This is in contrast to red cells, where the antigenic determinants are the ABO and Rh groups, which are relatively homogeneous. Because of the heterogeneity of the HLA antigen, it is generally not possible to provide patients with HLA-matched platelets. In special circumstances, however, they may be obtainable from an HLA-compatible donor, often a family member.

Therefore, in routine transfusion practice, platelets are chosen without regard to their antigenic determinants. Platelets do weakly express red cell antigens, and better recovery is obtained if the units are ABO blood group compatible. In addition, there may be intact red cells contaminating the platelet preparation. Therefore RhD immunoglobulin should be administered to RhD-negative females who are at or below childbearing age and who are receiving platelets from RhD-positive donors.

Platelet refractoriness

Patients who have received a number of platelet or blood transfusions may become refractory to platelet transfusions due to the development of antiplatelet antibodies. This is usually a result of the development of antibodies against HLA antigens. The platelet count fails to rise in response to transfusion of platelets, or the survival time of transfused platelets may be very short. In this situation, platelet transfusion may be ineffective. It may be possible to provide compatible platelets from HLA-antigen-compatible family members.

Platelet refractoriness due to antibodies should be distinguished from non-immune causes of increased platelet consumption, such as disseminated intravascular coagulation, sepsis and trauma (see Table 29.3.3 in Chapter 29.3).

Indications and dosage

A therapeutic dose is 3×10^{11} platelets. This should raise the platelet count by approximately 60×10^9/L. The half-life of normal platelets is about 3–4 days. Therefore repeat doses of platelets are usually required.

In surgery, platelets may be given pre-operatively, particularly in cases where the platelet count is less than

50×10^9 L. In these situations, a haematologist should be involved in management. In addition, platelets may be appropriate in the management of intra- or post-operative bleeding where there is thrombocytopenia, or where platelet dysfunction is suspected. A more detailed list of indications is given in Box 28.1.

FRESH FROZEN PLASMA (FFP)

Plasma is separated from whole blood by centrifugation and then stored in the frozen state within 6 h of blood collection. Fresh frozen plasma contains the labile as well as stable components of the coagulation, fibrinolytic and complement systems. It is mainly used to supply the coagulation factors. There is no justification for the use of fresh frozen plasma as a volume expander or nutritional source. Indications for the use of fresh frozen plasma are outlined in Box 28.1.

CRYOPRECIPITATE

Cryoprecipitate is prepared by centrifugation of fresh frozen plasma that has been allowed to thaw at 0–4°C. In the past it was used as a source of factor VIII and von Willebrand factor in the treatment of haemophilia A and von Willebrand's disease. In developed countries it has now been replaced for the treatment of these conditions by factor VIII concentrate. It is occasionally used as a source of fibrinogen.

COMPONENTS OF PLASMA

Factor VIII concentrate

Factor VIII concentrates are available either derived from plasma, or produced by recombinant technology. In the past the plasma-derived products have transmitted viruses such as HIV and hepatitis C to large numbers of patients. The plasma-derived products are of either intermediate or high-grade purity. The potential for virus transmission by these products has been greatly reduced by a number of processes, including treatment by heat and solvent detergent during manufacture. Recombinant products are more expensive than those derived from plasma. They provide a higher degree of safety with regard to virus transmission, but those currently available contain albumin derived from human plasma.

Factor VIII concentrates are used mainly for the treatment and prevention of haemorrhage in patients with haemophilia A. Many plasma-derived factor VIII concentrates also contain von Willebrand factor, but the multimeric structure of this von Willebrand factor may be suboptimal. Therefore, although they may be used in von Willebrand disorder, care should be taken to choose a brand of concentrate that is thought to be suitable for this indication. Elective surgery in patients with haemophilia and von Willebrand's disease should be carried out in close consultation with a haematologist, and in a hospital with ready access to a nearby, preferably onsite, specialized haemostasis laboratory.

Factor IX concentrate

Purified factor IX concentrates are now available in most developed countries for the treatment and prevention of haemorrhage in haemophilia B. At the present time, these products are almost all plasma derived, but recombinant factor IX is available on a small but increasing scale. Where they are available in sufficient quantity, the purified factor IX concentrates replace prothrombin complex concentrates, which are more primitive products also containing factors II and X. In high doses the prothrombin complex concentrates predispose to thrombosis. However, prothrombin complex concentrates still have a place in treatment, e.g. in the emergency management of severe haemorrhage in some cases of warfarin overdose or vitamin K deficiency, and are used in patients with haemophilia A who have developed inhibitors to the factor VIII in factor VIII concentrates. As with factor VIII concentrates, the plasma-derived factor IX concentrates are treated to reduce greatly the likelihood of virus transmission.

Albumin

Albumin is infused to increase intravascular volume in patients who are hypovolaemic. In many countries synthetic alternatives, such as hydroxyethyl starch or dextran polymers, are preferred because of their lower cost and wider availability.

Immunoglobulin

Preparations of gammaglobulin for intravenous infusion have become available in increasing quantities. Initially these were primarily used to treat patients with hypogammaglobulinaemia. However, the product is of benefit in a variety of autoimmune conditions, and the number of disorders in which it has been shown to be effective continues to expand, putting increasing pressure on a limited resource.

COMPLICATIONS OF BLOOD TRANSFUSION

The risks of blood transfusion are mainly immune, infective and metabolic in nature (Box 28.2).

BOX 28.2 TIME COURSE OF COMPLICATIONS

During transfusion

Bacterial infection, acute haemolytic transfusion reaction, non-haemolytic non-infective febrile reaction, fluid overload, metabolic derangements, dilutional coagulopathy, urticaria, anaphylaxis, phlebitis, air embolism, transfusion-related acute lung injury.

Within days

Delayed haemolytic transfusion reaction, passive alloimmune thrombocytopenia, post-transfusion purpura.

Within weeks

Viral hepatitis, HIV, CMV, graft vs. host disease, HLA and rhesus alloimmunization.

Within years

HIV, chronic hepatitis B and C, as yet unknown blood-borne infections, iron overload.

INFECTION

Donor eligibility

The transmission of viral and bacterial disease by blood transfusion has been significantly reduced over the years by following rigorous protocols. Donors are required to declare high-risk activity for the transmission of blood-borne viruses, including use of intravenous drugs and high-risk sexual activity. Donors who respond in the affirmative are excluded. Each donor is tested for syphilis and blood-borne viruses (including HIV, CMV and hepatitis B and C).

The risk of viral transmission still exists due to the window period, i.e. the time between a blood donor contracting a virus and developing a positive serological test. The window period has been reduced to approximately 16 days for HIV by testing for p24 viral antigen. The emergence of a new as yet undiscovered virus always remains a threat. The risk of viral transmission is increased with repeated transfusions and use of pooled products, because there is exposure to a greater number of donors.

To eliminate further the possibility of viral contamination, products derived by fractionation of plasma, such as albumin and factor VIII concentrate, are subjected to heat treatment, solvent detergent treatment and often nanofiltration.

Bacterial contamination

Handling of blood products should always be by means of a sterilized closed collection system. Meticulous hygiene, cleaning and antisepsis are paramount at all stages of blood collection and storage. Storage at 4–6°C does not completely eliminate the risk of bacterial infection, especially with cryophilic organisms such as *Pseudomonas*, *Serratia* and *Yersinia*. These may flourish at 4°C, and if transfused may result in endotoxic shock syndrome and septicaemia.

Virus transmission

HIV Allowing for donations made during the window period and laboratory error in testing for HIV seropositivity in the donor unit, it has been estimated that the risk of HIV transmission in the USA is 1 in 493 000 donations of screened blood. In Australia the risk is 1 in 1.27 million, and in France it is 1 in 571 000.

Hepatitis Hepatitis viruses A, B, C, D and E have been identified. Hepatitis A and E viruses are transmitted enterically and induce acute hepatitis, but only rarely cause chronic hepatitis. Hepatitis B virus (HBV) and hepatitis C virus (HCV), by contrast, are primarily blood-borne, cause acute as well as chronic hepatitis, and can lead to cirrhosis and hepatocellular carcinoma. Hepatitis D, or delta virus, is exceptional in that it is dependent on HBV and can modify the disease associated with that virus.

Hepatitis B The transmission rate has been dramatically reduced with surface antigen testing, and is approximately 1 in 200 000.

Hepatitis non-A non-B The transmission rate has been dramatically reduced since testing for hepatitis C antibody was introduced in 1990. The transmission rate of hepatitis C is now approximately 4.27 per million donations.

Hepatitis G (HGV) The recently identified HGV virus is a flavivirus like hepatitis C. It is common among volunteer blood donors, and can be transmitted by transfusion. No causal relationship between HGV and hepatitis has been established.

Cytomegalovirus (CMV) An estimated 3–12% of blood donations can potentially transmit CMV. In almost all cases infection is asymptomatic, but CMV may cause life-threatening disease in allogeneic transplant recipients and children with severe combined immune deficiency. These patients need CMV-negative products if they are CMV-negative.

Prion disease Creutzfeldt-Jakob disease, bovine spongiform encephalopathy, kuru and scrapie are transmitted by ingestion of or injection with infected neural tissue. They have not been shown to be transmitted by blood transfusion. However, donor declaration excludes anyone who has received pituitary hormone extract and all donors with a past or family history of such a debilitating neurological disease.

Summary

Blood products currently appear to be very safe from viral transmission. However, the possibility of a new infectious agent appearing cannot be excluded. Although blood products may never be completely safe, the aim is to maximize their safety. Transfusion services must be prompt in recognizing potential risks, and introduce relevant screening procedures as soon as these are available. World medical and health literature should be continually under review, and new information acted upon without delay.

Only use blood transfusions for potentially debilitating or life-threatening diseases and conditions.

HAEMOLYTIC REACTION – IMMUNE SEROLOGICAL INCOMPATIBILITY (ABO INCOMPATIBILITY)

Immediate transfusion reaction

A common error leading to the potential for transfusion of ABO-incompatible red cells is the taking of blood from the wrong patient. To avoid this, it is very important to check the information on both the specimen container and the sample with the information on the patient identification wrist band. The information on the sample and on the request form must include the surname, given name, hospital record number and/or date of birth. Similarly, an error involving incorrect patient identification may be made when blood is administered. Careful checking against the patient wrist band is again mandatory.

A haemolytic transfusion reaction may result in intravascular haemolysis due to complement activation. Symptoms include shock, chills, fever, dyspnoea, haemoglobinaemia, haemoglobinuria, hyperbilirubinaemia and renal failure (Table 28.1). Disseminated intravascular coagulation may occur, and the first sign of a transfusion reaction may be excessive blood loss during an operation.

A transfusion reaction is a medical emergency. Rapid action is required, with expert advice from the transfusion service. The blood infusion must be stopped immediately, and the identity of the blood and patient checked.

The transfused unit should be sent back to the transfusion laboratory for repeat typing and bacteriological culture. The patient's pre- and post-transfusion specimens must be checked for blood group, antibody screen and direct Coomb's test.

The patient plasma and urine must be examined for free haemoglobin indicating intravascular haemolysis. Disseminated intravascular coagulation may occur, and is a poor prognostic sign.

Acute haemolytic transfusion reaction must be distinguished from:

Table 28.1 Diagnosis and treatment of transfusion reactions (developed at the Royal Adelaide Hospital)

Type	Signs and symptoms	Treatment	Prevention
Febrile	Pyrexia Rigors/chills Anxiety Restlessness	Discontinue. Investigate as for haemolytic reaction. *Mild fever without other symptoms may be treated by slowing infusion. An antihistamine may be helpful*	Consider use of leucocyte-poor filtered blood if a recurrent problem
Circulatory	Distension of neck veins Pulmonary oedema Dyspnoea Headache Heaviness in the limbs Pyrexia and rigors may be a manifestation	Discontinue. Institute treatment for fluid overload, e.g. diuretic	Give all fluids slowly to patients with normal blood volume and compromised cardiac status. Use concentrated red cells. If anticipated, give diuretic
Allergic	Urticaria Facial oedema	*Slow rate of infusion.* Consider antihistamine. Watch for laryngeal oedema	When anticipated, use prophylactic antihistamines
Anaphylaxis	Dyspnoea, sometimes cyanosis and peripheral collapse	Discontinue immediately. Institute treatment for anaphylaxis (e.g. adrenalin, steroids)	Transfuse with washed blood products
Haemolytic	Pyrexia Rigors/chills Lumbar pain Hypotension Pain along vein Jaundice Haemoglobinuria Oliguria – later uraemia	Discontinue transfusion. Get expert advice immediately. Do not give IV fluids.* Save all urine. Save all used bottles, packs and blood samples. Collect fresh blood samples	Careful blood grouping and cross-matching. Careful technique in storing and labelling blood. Care in identifying the patient
Infected	Hyperpyrexia Pain in limbs and chest Headache Pallor Burning along injected vein Low blood pressure Rapid pulse Profound collapse and shock	Discontinue infusion. *Acute medical emergency – get advice immediately* Save all urine. Save used bottles, packs, and all blood samples, with labels. Give anti-shock treatment	Careful technique in collecting blood. Storage at correct temperature. Do not remove from refrigerator until immediately before transfusion

* Expert advice should be sought for subsequent management. Adequate renal perfusion must be maintained, but if oliguria develops there is a high risk of pulmonary oedema. Haemodialysis may be indicated.

- transfusion of infected blood;
- transfusion of lysed red blood cells (thermal damage or mechanical damage during infusion);
- other causes of haemolysis occurring coincidentally (e.g. *Clostridium perfringens* septicaemia).

Delayed transfusion reaction

This reaction is an anamnestic immune response that occurs several days after the transfusion in patients who have been previously exposed to a red cell antigen (e.g. during pregnancy or a previous transfusion). Upon re-exposure, these antibodies are reactivated and may cause a delayed haemolytic reaction. Clinically, there is continued anaemia despite transfusion therapy, with haemoglobinuria with or without hyperbilirubinaemia.

NON-HAEMOLYTIC, NON-INFECTIVE FEBRILE TRANSFUSION REACTIONS

These are due to:

- donor cytokines;
- sensitization of the recipient to contaminating donor white cells; or
- an aetiology unrelated to the transfusion but occurring coincidentally.

Donor white-cell contamination

Febrile non-haemolytic reactions to donor white cells occur in 1% of all transfusions. They are the result of sensitization to Class I HLA A and B antigens on donor white cells, and to a lesser extent platelets. Fever and chills occur, often towards the end of infusion. Multiparous females and patients undergoing multiple transfusion are most at risk. In sensitized individuals, centrifuged and filtered products reduce the rate of febrile reactions from 25% to 3%.

Cytokines

Cytokines are produced *in vitro* during storage and *in vivo* by transfused or recipient leucocytes. There is increasing evidence that production of cytokines during storage can be prevented by processes that deplete the leucocytes in donated blood prior to production and storage of red cells or platelets.

ALLERGIC REACTIONS

Urticaria during transfusion of whole blood or plasma is relatively common, and probably represents an allergic reaction to one or more plasma proteins. Rarely there may be an anaphylactic type of reaction, and in some cases an antibody against IgA has been identified.

MASSIVE TRANSFUSION

Massive transfusion may be regarded as replacement of more than one blood volume in 24 h. Although in earlier times there was marked depletion of factors V and VIII in stored blood, with modern methods of blood collection and blood storage the levels of these are reasonable, as are the levels in fresh frozen plasma. Initially, during massive transfusion one pack of fresh frozen plasma

should be transfused for every 2 units of red cells. More fresh frozen plasma should be given if there is a significant prolongation of the prothrombin time or APTT. If hypofibrinogenaemia develops, cryoprecipitate can be used as a source of fibrinogen (see Table 28.1).

Platelets from blood stored for more than about 24 h do not circulate after blood transfusion. Therefore, after the transfusion of 10 to 20 units of blood, thrombocytopenia is common. After the transfusion of about 15 units of red cells, platelet transfusions should be given as required to maintain the platelet count above about 100 000.

METABOLIC COMPLICATIONS

Citrate intoxication and hypocalcaemia

This may occur if blood is infused at a very rapid rate. Patients with liver impairment are more at risk due to decreased metabolism of citrate. The resulting hypocalcaemia may cause perioral paraesthesia, tetany and ECG changes. Treatment is by slowing the infusion. If symptomatic, 10 mL of 10% calcium gluconate administered intravenously is a rapid antidote.

Hypothermia

Massive transfusion of refrigerated products can cause hypothermia. Warming all intravenous fluids by passing them through a blood-warming device helps to prevent unwanted heat loss. It is important to monitor the patient's body temperature and maintain normothermia at 37°C. Hypothermia impairs immune function and decreases subcutaneous oxygen tension. This may promote surgical wound infection and dehiscence, with the added risk of increased blood loss.

CIRCULATORY OVERLOAD

This is particularly a problem in patients with cardiovascular compromise. In such patients infusion rates should be slower, and diuretics should be used judiciously.

IRON OVERLOAD

Each unit of red cells contains approximately 250 mg of iron. There is no significant biological mechanism for iron excretion apart from minimal loss through senescence of gut epithelium. Therefore, in the absence of blood loss, the transfusion of 40 units of red cells leads to the accumulation of 10 g of iron, which deposits in organs, causing tissue damage. Therefore multiple transfusions may lead to cardiomyopathy, cirrhosis and endocrinopathy.

Patients who are transfusion dependent should be considered for regular iron chelation therapy. This is administered in the form of desferrioxamine as a slow subcutaneous infusion overnight, usually for 4 to 6 nights per week.

ACUTE LUNG INJURY

This uncommon and life-threatening complication is characterized by respiratory insufficiency with pulmonary infiltrates occurring within 1–6 h of blood transfusion. The clinical features are indistinguishable from adult respiratory distress syndrome. It is caused by leucoagglutinins that can be present in donor plasma with high levels of leucocyte-associated antibody.

TRANSFUSION-RELATED GRAFT VS. HOST DISEASE (GVHD)

GVHD occurs when donor T-lymphocytes engraft in an immunodeficient recipient, causing an immune reaction against the recipient. Donor T-lymphocytes infiltrate the liver, skin and bowel, resulting in jaundice, rash and diarrhoea. This most commonly occurs following allogeneic marrow transplantation.

It may also occur in normal individuals after blood transfusion when the donor and recipient are of similar HLA composition. For example, when a father donor is homozygous for a haplotype for which the recipient son is heterozygous, the recipient does not recognize the donor as non-self, and allows engraftment. Directed blood donations between close relatives are therefore at risk of causing transfusion-related GVHD.

For random blood donations in homogeneous populations (e.g. as in Japan and Israel), the incidence is approximately 1 in 600 per year. Otherwise, the incidence among immunocompetent recipients is rare. Immunosuppressed patients are at increased risk of transfusion-related GVHD.

In contrast to marrow transplantation-related GVHD, transfusion-related GVHD responds poorly to therapy. The mortality rate has been reported to be up to 100%.

In situations where there is a risk of transfusion-related graft vs. host disease, this can be prevented by irradiation of blood products prior to transfusion.

MINIMIZING HOMOLOGOUS BLOOD TRANSFUSIONS

Many transfusions are initiated in the intra- or post-operative period. It is important to minimize the use of homologous blood transfusion in order to reduce the likelihood of complications and to conserve resources.

REDUCING INDICATIONS FOR ALLOGENEIC BLOOD

Adoption of strict transfusion criteria

Predetermined criteria leading to more optimal therapy should be adopted as a guide to decision-making when contemplating blood transfusion (see Box 28.1). Combined with education of medical staff, this will probably reduce the number of unnecessary transfusions given.

On-site testing

Modern devices allow haemoglobin to be monitored in theatre. Haemoglobin measurements during surgery, together with assessment of haemodynamic status and ongoing bleeding, can provide more precise information to guide ongoing transfusion requirements.

Autologous blood donation

This procedure should in general be reserved for those procedures in which it is likely that the extent of blood loss will be sufficient to render blood transfusion desirable.

Usually the patient is required to attend weekly for the collection of 1 unit of blood, and is given concomitant oral iron during this time. Therefore, depending on the number of units required, collection of blood must commence 1 to 4 weeks prior to surgery. Prior to embarking on the programme, the patient must have been determined to be medically fit to undergo the procedure.

Although autologous is safer than homologous blood transfusion, the provision of autologous blood does not avoid all the risks of blood transfusion, and there are still some potential complications.

Vasovagal reactions during blood donation are not uncommon. Although these reactions are well tolerated by healthy donors, they may endanger certain patients, particularly those with cardiovascular compromise.

Errors of identification leading to administration of an incorrect unit can still occur.

Autologous blood is more expensive than the provision of homologous blood. It requires that a system is set up for proper collection, labelling, transport and storage. Nevertheless, particularly in places where an autologous blood collection service is properly set up, it is wise to inform the patient of its availability along with a discussion of the risks and benefits compared to homologous blood.

Erythropoietin

The use of recombinant erythropoietin (r-HuEPO) to stimulate red cell production by the bone marrow can reduce the need for homologous transfusion. If administered to patients enrolled in autologous transfusion programmes it can increase the amount of blood available. It may also be given before surgery to increase the pre-operative haematocrit.

R-HuEPO treatment prior to orthopaedic and cardiac surgery has been shown to significantly reduce exposure to homologous blood without the use of autologous blood donation. R-HuEPO has also been shown to be effective in combination with acute normovolaemic haemodilution in reducing patient exposure to homologous blood.

R-HuEPO was approved for use in non-cardiac, non-vascular surgery in 1996 in the USA and Canada. Approval for use with autologous blood donation was passed in Canada in 1996, and in the European Union in 1994. Cost remains the major drawback.

REDUCING BLOOD LOSS

Peri-operative haemodilution

This technique involves exchanging blood for a volume expander immediately prior to surgery. Any blood subsequently lost will be of a lower haematocrit, resulting in red cell conservation.

For example, it is estimated that if a 100-kg man has 3 units of blood replaced, the haematocrit will drop from 44% to 32%. A loss of 2600 mL of blood during the operation will result in a loss of 732 mL of red cells, compared to a loss of 947 mL without the haemodilution. The net saving of 215 mL is equivalent to only 1 unit of blood. [Paragraph taken from 'Erythropoietin therapy' by Goodnough *et al.* in the *New England Journal of Medicine*, March 27, 1997 **336**(13). Copyright © 1997 by the Massachuetts Medical Society.]

Intra-operative blood salvage

With the use of modern blood salvage devices that produce washed red cells, intra-operative blood salvage is safe and effective. Although current technology is costly in terms of equipment, disposable supplies, and personnel, it reduces the need for homologous blood.

Correction of coagulation dysfunction

To prevent excessive bleeding during and after surgery, coagulation factor deficiencies, platelet dysfunction or thrombocytopenia may require the use of allogeneic blood products such as fresh frozen plasma or donor platelet concentrates. In such cases advice should be obtained from a haematologist. Pharmacological agents such as desmopressin, aprotinin, tranexamic acid and aminocaproic acid may be of value.

CONCLUSIONS

It is important that surgeons have an understanding of the basic principles of transfusion therapy. Correct prescribing and administration of blood products depends on a knowledge of both the indications and the side-effects. Documentation and the obtaining of patient consent are important parts of the process. In clinical situations where further advice is required, consultation with a haematologist or a specialist in transfusion medicine is encouraged.

FURTHER READING

American Society of Anesthesiologists, Inc. 1996: Practice guidelines for blood component therapy. *Anesthesiology* **84**, 732–47.

Anderson K, Weinstein H. 1990: Transfusion-associated graft versus host disease. *New England Journal of Medicine* **323**, 315–21.

Dietrich KA, Conrad SA, Herbert CA, *et al.* 1990: Cardiovascular and metabolic response to red blood cell transfusion in critically ill volume-resuscitated nonsurgical patients. *Critical Care Medicine* **18**: 940–4.

Goodnough L, Monk T, Andriole G. 1997: Erythropoietin therapy. *New England Journal of Medicine* **336**, 933–8.

Goodnough LT, Brecher ME, Kanter MH, AuBuchon JP. 1999: Transfusion medicine (first of 2 parts). *New England Journal of Medicine* **340**, 438–47.

Hondow JA, Russell WJ, Duncan BM, Lloyd JV. 1982: The stability of coagulation factors in stored blood. *Australia and New Zealand Journal of Surgery* **52**, 265–9.

Levinsky L, Srinivasan V, Choh JH *et al.* 1981: Intracardiac surgery in children of Jehovah's Witnesses. *Johns Hopkins Medical Journal* **148**, 196–8.

Mannucci PM. 1998: Hemostatic drugs (review article). *New England Journal of Medicine* **339**, 245–53.

Metz J, McGrath KM, Copperchini ML, *et al.* 1995: Appropriateness of transfusions of red cells, platelets and fresh frozen plasma. An audit in a tertiary care teaching hospital. *Medical Journal of Australia* **162**, 572–7.

Mollison P, Engelfreit C, Contreras M. 1997: *Blood transfusion in clinical medicine.* Oxford: Blackwell Science.

Mongan P. 1995: Optimizing erythrocyte conservation and transfusion practices in cardiac surgery. *Current Opinion in Anaesthesiology* **8**, 41–8.

Nelson CL, Bowen WS. 1986: Total hip arthroplasty in Jehovah's Witnesses without blood transfusion. *Journal of Bone and Joint Surgery* **68**, 350–3.

Sanguis Study Group. 1994: Use of blood products for elective surgery in 43 European hospitals. *Transfusion Medicine* **4**, 251–68.

Schreiber GB, Busch MP, Kleinman SH, Korelitz JJ. 1996: The risk of transfusion-transmitted viral infections. *New England Journal of Medicine* **334**, 1685–90.

Whyte G, Savoia H. 1997: The risk of transmitting HCV, HBV or HIV by blood transfusion in Victoria. *Medical Journal of Australia* **166**, 584–6.

Radiological organ imaging

Alison R. Gillams

Introduction

A good understanding of radiology will improve the clinical practice of any aspiring surgeon. The technology has become increasingly varied and sophisticated and continues to evolve and develop all the time. Different tests offer many different types of information with a variable degree of accuracy. The surgeon needs to understand the information being offered to him. He needs to ask what information do I need to manage this patient? What technology will provide that information and how accurate is the result in any given clinical situation?

This chapter deals with the major imaging modalities used in organ imaging. The basic principles are described and the findings in typical, common surgical pathologies are outlined; some advice as to the relative role of each modality is offered.

PLAIN X-RAY

The plain film has almost no role in solid organ imaging and has been supplanted by cross-sectional imaging techniques. Occasionally plain films will show organomegaly, but they do not provide any information about internal architecture. Plain films are still indicated for the detection of renal and ureteric calculi, the first-line assessment of large- and small-bowel gas patterns, particularly in suspected bowel obstruction, and the detection of free air. Plain films may show abnormal air collections, e.g. in abscesses or the biliary tree, and calcifications in liver, spleen, adrenal glands or pancreas.

TRANSABDOMINAL ULTRASOUND

BASIC PRINCIPLES

The ultrasound (US) transducer consists of a piezoelectric crystal which vibrates in response to a change in voltage, emitting acoustic energy of a particular frequency. After a short delay the transducer collects the returning acoustic signal for analysis. Signal analysis is performed along multiple individual lines, and these constitute the US image. In tissue, acoustic energy may be absorbed, reflected or transmitted, but only the reflected signal is detected and contributes to the image. Acoustic impedance is a fundamental property of tissue, and is derived from the product of density and the velocity of sound in the tissue. Acoustic energy is reflected where there is a change or mismatch in acoustic impedance. This is most marked at air or bone interfaces, where the resulting total reflection of sound produces a large echo or bright signal on the image, with complete loss of signal beyond that point. Other tissues attenuate the US beam by varying degrees. The signal processing of the returning beam imposes a standard compensation for attenuation. This is to compensate for loss of signal from more distant structures. Therefore, those tissues that transmit less will demonstrate acoustic shadowing, and those that transmit more will produce distal acoustic enhancement. Fluid-filled structures transmit sound, producing distal acoustic enhancement, and are clearly delineated by US, so fluid-filled structures such as blood vessels and ducts provide the major anatomical landmarks.

CLINICAL UTILITY

Ultrasound is often the first line of organ-imaging investigation. It is widely available, quick, cheap and non-invasive, and has no absolute contraindications and no side-effects. The patient experiences only mild skin pressure, so US has a high level of patient acceptability. The main technical failures are in obese patients where an inadequate return signal from deep structures results in poor image quality. The other major technical problem is bowel gas. Sound is reflected by gas, so structures deep to a gas-filled bowel loop are not seen. The most common difficulty arises in visualizing the pancreas. This may be exaggerated in the presence of ileus or bowel obstruction, or in distressed patients who have swallowed a lot of air. Similarly, lesions high in the liver under the dome of the diaphragm can be obscured by air in the costophrenic recess. It is preferable to study patients after a 4-h fast in order to minimize the effects of bowel gas.

As previously mentioned, US readily detects fluid, and as little as 10 mL of free intra-peritoneal fluid can be seen. US will detect the majority of fluid collections, but occasionally gas obscures a collection which is subsequently detected by computed tomography (CT). Within a complex inflammatory mass, US remains one of the best methods by which to determine the presence and size of any fluid component. Only magnetic resonance imaging (MRI) offers better differentiation of the solid and cystic components of, for example, a pancreatic phlegmon (see Figure 29.1.5). This can be important in identifying the reason for failure of percutaneous drainage. This same feature allows US to distinguish readily between cystic and solid lesions.

Bilary tract, liver and pancreas

US is the investigation of choice in the diagnosis of gallstones, which do not generally calcify and are iso-attenuating to bile in 23% of cases and therefore not detected by CT. On US, gallstones are seen as echogenic foci with distal acoustic shadowing. The gall bladder volume, wall thickness (normal thickness is < 3 mm) and function can all be evaluated. In acute cholecystitis, the gall bladder wall appears thickened and sometimes layered due to oedema (Figure 29.1.1). An echo-poor rim of pericholecystic fluid may be present. The causative stone is often seen impacted in the cystic duct or Hartmann's pouch, and a sonographic Murphy's sign is usually present. US sensitivity for acute cholecystitis is 90%. In chronic

cholecystitis the gall bladder appears shrunken, thick-walled (mean thickness is 5 mm), is often non-functioning and contains stones. Sometimes a small gall bladder packed with stones can be difficult to find, particularly in obese patients. US will reliably detect focal or generalized bile-duct dilatation and show the level of biliary obstruction. The common hepatic duct is usually measured in the sagittal plane at the liver hilum, anterior to the portal vein (normal diameter is < 6 mm). The cause of obstruction is seen in 80% of patients. Following biliary stenting, bilio-enteric anastomosis or sphincterotomy, brightly echogenic air may be seen outlining the biliary tree. However, the presence of aerobilia does not exclude partial or functional biliary obstruction.

In liver imaging, US can define the size (normal longitudinal diameter is < 15.5 cm), shape and contour of the liver, focal atrophy or hypertrophy, and the echogenicity relative to adjacent kidney, and will detect the majority of focal lesions. Simple liver cysts are not an uncommon, incidental finding. If they are homogeneous and well defined, with no solid component, these are most often benign and of no significance. Most liver metastases are hypoechoic or of mixed echogenicity (75% of cases). Echogenic lesions (25%) are seen in colorectal, neuroendocrine and treated breast metastases and some hepatocellular carcinomas. Calcification occurs in 2–3% of metastases, most commonly in mucinous carcinomas of the gastrointestinal tract. The most common benign liver tumour is the haemangioma, which occurs in 4% of the population. These are usually well defined, hyperechoic lesions which remain stable over time. About 10% of them are multiple. CT or MRI is required to differentiate haemangiomas from metastases. The echogenicity of the liver is diffusely increased in fatty infiltration, chronic hepatitis or cirrhosis, and may be decreased in acute hepatitis. The echo texture becomes coarse in chronic diffuse parenchymal liver disease. The presence, direction and quantity of portal and hepatic venous flow can be assessed using Doppler. In the presence of portal hypertension, US may detect varices at the liver or splenic hilum, and along the lesser curve of the stomach and in the intra-abdominal oesophagus.

The majority of the pancreas is seen in up to 95% of patients, but visualization of the whole of the pancreas is rare. Normal pancreatic echogenicity is homogeneous and slightly higher than that of liver. Echogenicity increases with age due to fatty infiltration. The pancreatic duct is usually seen (normal diameter is < 4 mm), tapering from head to tail, and again the duct diameter increases with age. US will show duct dilatation, focal calcifications, focal fluid collections or pseudocyst formation. In acute pancreatitis the gland may appear swollen and of reduced echogenicity either in part or throughout. Focal fluid collections, phlegmon and

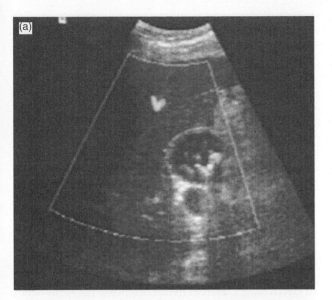

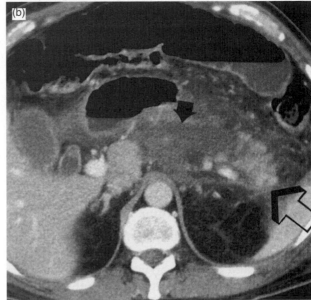

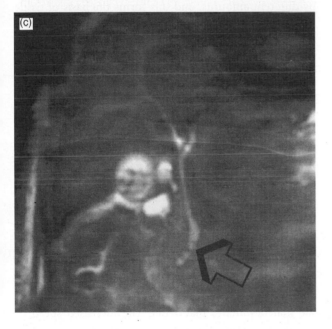

Figure 29.1.1 A 52-year-old man presenting with acute abdominal pain secondary to acute pancreatitis. (a) Transabdominal ultrasound image showing multiple stones in a thick-walled gall bladder. The wall of the gall bladder demonstrates a layered appearance with a central hypoechoic layer consistent with oedema. This appearance is typical of acute inflammation. (b) Axial contrast-enhanced CT scan demonstrating inflammatory phlegmon in the body of the pancreas (solid arrow). Normal enhancing pancreatic parenchyma is seen in the tail (open arrow). Note the normal right adrenal gland. (c) MRCP shows multiple common bile-duct stones in a non-dilated system (arrow), the cause of the acute pancreatitis. Note the multiple gallstones in the gall bladder.

abscesses may be seen as may pseudocyst formation. In approximately 33% of patients with mild, acute pancreatitis, the pancreas appears normal on US. In chronic pancreatitis calculi, duct dilatation and increased parenchymal echogenicity can all be seen on US. Tiny flecks of calcification will only be appreciated on unenhanced CT. Subtle changes in the pancreatic duct require a pancreatogram. Carcinoma of the head of the pancreas causes obstructive jaundice in 80% of cases, producing the double duct sign (i.e. a dilated pancreatic and common bile duct). By tracing the ducts to the point of obstruction, it is often possible to identify the obstructing lesion. Pancreatic adenocarcinoma is seen as an irregular, hypoechoic mass lesion. US may show evidence of vascular encasement or invasion, local adenopathy, ascites or hepatic metastases. More accurate

staging is provided by CT or MRI. Benign neuroendocrine tumours of the pancreas are infrequently shown by transabdominal US, partly because of their small size (< 10 mm) at presentation and partly because they are isoechoic with normal pancreatic parenchyma.

Reticulo-endothelial system

US will accurately detect splenomegaly, defined on US as a longitudinal diameter of > 15 cm. The normal spleen is homogeneous, with slightly higher echogenicity than adjacent kidney. US will show focal lymphoma deposits or metastases as rounded poorly echogenic lesions. Diffuse lymphomatous involvement does not alter splenic echogenicity and only causes splenomegaly in 50% of cases, i.e. 50% of patients with splenic lymphoma will have a normal US. Splenic calcifications are occasionally seen and are usually due to old granulomas. Infarction, if focal, is seen as a peripheral wedge of low echogenicity. US can rapidly assess the presence of trauma to the spleen, and will detect subclinical, subcapsular haematoma in 10–20% of cases. Serial US can be used to monitor conservative management. US is less reliable than CT in the detection of enlarged intra-abdominal lymph nodes (short axis diameter > 1 cm), but mildly enlarged nodes may be detected at the liver hilum and in the retroperitoneum, and gross adenopathy is readily seen.

Renal and adrenal systems

The normal kidney measures 11–14 cm in bipolar diameter, and has a smooth contour and a characteristic echo pattern derived from the brightly echogenic fat in the renal hilum. Failure to detect a kidney in the renal bed, despite an adequate study, is most commonly due to ectopia, but may be due to congenital absence or end-stage renal disease. US is very effective in detecting pelvicalyceal system dilatation, and even mild degrees are shown. In patients with distal renal obstruction, it may be possible to trace the dilated ureter down to the level of the obstruction and define the cause. More often only the dilated proximal ureter is seen, and it is necessary to resort to IVU or CT in order to define the level and cause of obstruction more clearly. The kidney appears normal in most cases of acute pyelonephritis; occasionally, mild renal enlargement with a slight reduction in echogenicity is seen. Progression to focal nephritis results in the development of an ill-defined, poorly echogenic mass. Simple renal cysts are a common incidental finding and of no clinical significance unless they are extremely large. Polycystic kidney disease causes bilateral renal enlargement and a characteristic appearance of multiple small cysts. Renal calculi appear as brightly echogenic foci with distal acoustic enhancement. Calculi that are > 1 cm in diameter are easily detected, but tiny flecks of calcification may not be seen. US will demonstrate renal tumours as solid, mixed, echogenic masses, and at the same time the renal vein and inferior vena cava can be assessed for tumour extension. Chronic renal disease has a similar appearance regardless of aetiology, with small, brightly echogenic kidneys which can be difficult to distinguish from adjacent fat.

The normal adrenal glands can be seen on US if they are meticulously sought, and the right gland is easier to see than the left one. Benign adenomas are usually less than 15 mm in diameter, and are better detected by CT or MRI. Larger adrenal masses can be seen with US. There is overlap in the US appearances of benign and malignant lesions, and CT or (better still MRI) offers improved specificity.

COMPUTED TOMOGRAPHY (CT)

BASIC PRINCIPLES

The CT scanner uses multiple, finely collimated X-ray beams to produce a series of attenuation profiles through the patient, from which cross-sectional images are computed. The scanner consists of a moving X-ray table and a CT gantry which rotates around the patient. Within the gantry is the X-ray generator and multiple X-ray detectors which record the attenuation value of the X-ray beams as they emerge from the patient. The attenuation value will depend on the energy of the X-ray beam and on the tissues that the X-ray beam has encountered *en route*. The three tissue properties that affect X-ray attenuation are density, atomic number and the number of electrons/g. Different tissues attenuate the X-ray beam by different amounts, and this forms the basis of tissue contrast. Fat, air, haemorrhage and calcification have specific attenuation values or CT numbers. CT numbers are measured in Hounsfield units (HU) and are expressed relative to water. Unlike US or MRI signal measurements, attenuation values are absolute and highly reproducible between patients.

Older CT scanners produced sequential two-dimensional cross-sections through the body. The most recent technology, namely spiral CT, produces a volume of contiguous data with image acquisition times of less than 1 s per revolution. Volume data acquisition is important, as this improves multiplanar and three-dimensional reconstruction, increases lesion detection by allowing image reconstruction at different intervals (thus reducing partial volume effects), and pre-empts the possibility of misregistration. Partial volume is the term applied to a lesion that occupies only a small part of an imaging voxel and is effectively hidden by the tissue that dominates that voxel. The increased speed of acquisition allows the whole abdomen to be scanned within a single breath-hold, permits image acquisition to be timed to the optimal phase of contrast enhancement, and reduces examination time.

CLINICAL UTILITY

CT provides more reproducible image quality and more complete anatomical coverage than US. Whereas for US, image quality is degraded by larger patients, CT image quality is only degraded for the very large patient. In fact, a modicum of intraperitoneal fat is useful in CT, as the fat outlines the surfaces of the different organs. Some difficulties in interpretation arise in the very cachectic, because of the absence of intraperitoneal fat. Bowel gas does not interfere with CT images, so CT is ideal for examining the pancreas and retroperitoneum. Oral contrast, traditionally in the form of dilute barium, but currently using water, can be of value in distending the bowel (e.g. the duodenum) when studying the pancreas. Unenhanced CT is required for the identification of calcification, acute haemorrhage or the measurement of liver attenuation values (e.g. in haemachromatosis). Most other CT studies are performed after the administration of a bolus of IV iodinated contrast. Image acquisition can be timed to different phases of the contrast cycle (e.g. arterial, venous or the equilibrium/parenchymal phase). Optimization of the timing of contrast administration will improve detection of certain lesions, and will aid lesion characterization (Figure 29.1.2).

Biliary tract, liver and pancreas

Biliary tract

Normal intrahepatic bile ducts are seen as small lucencies measuring 1–3 mm in diameter, running adjacent to portal venous radicles. The normal common hepatic duct measures 3–6 mm and has a thin, smooth wall best seen after IV contrast. The normal common bile duct measures < 8 mm diameter and has a wall thickness of < 1.5 mm. CT is very sensitive to bile duct dilatation, and will show the level and almost always the cause of biliary obstruction. Although CT is less reliable than US in the detection of gallstones, it is more likely to show common bile-duct stones. Calcified stones are readily detected, but account for only 20%, and the more common soft-tissue density stone is seen as a faint density surrounded by a rim of bile. The most frequently occurring bile-duct malignancy, namely cholangiocarcinoma, usually arises in the proximal extrahepatic ducts, but can be entirely intrahepatic or confined to the distal common bile duct. Three morphological patterns are recognized, namely a central, infiltrating type; a peripheral, dominant mass; or a rare polypoid, intramural tumour. The mass lesions are usually seen as low attenuation on portal venous phase images, but may show abnormal enhancement on delayed images, 15–20 min after administration of IV contrast. The infiltrating lesion poses diagnostic difficulties on all imaging modalities, with no identifiable tumour mass, the only detectable abnormality being eccentric bile-duct wall thickening.

Focal liver lesions

CT will detect more than 90% of focal lesions in the liver, and will detect more liver metastases than US. Lesions as small as 5–6 mm in diameter are seen. CT not only detects more and smaller lesions but also, by studying the vascularity of the lesion, can offer some specificity. The most reliable sign for the diagnosis of haemangioma is the presence of nodular, discontinuous, peripheral contrast enhancement, which is equal in intensity to adja-

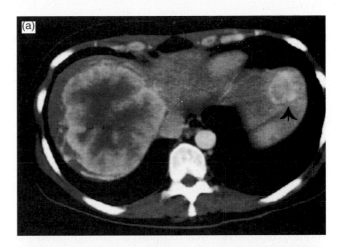

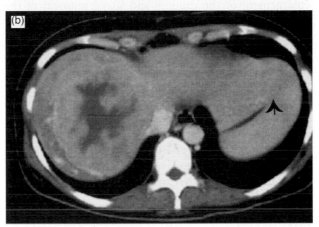

Figure 29.1.2 Axial contrast-enhanced CT in a patient with multiple hypervascular hepatic metastases. The smaller lesion in the left lobe has central necrosis (arrows). (a) During the arterial phase. (b) During the portal venous phase. Note the difference in appearance with bright peripheral enhancement in the tumour in the arterial phase but loss of contrast between the normal liver parenchyma and the tumour on the later scan, such that the smaller lesion in the left lobe is more difficult to visualize (arrow).

cent vessels. Hypervascular lesions (e.g. hepatocellular carcinoma or neuroendocrine metastases) will show marked enhancement during arterial phase imaging (Figure 29.1.2). By timing image acquisition to this phase of enhancement, more lesions can be detected. The portal venous phase is optimal for the detection of hypovascular metastases (e.g. colorectal secondaries). Delayed images may be required for the diagnosis of haemangioma, which become partially or completely isodense (to adjacent liver parenchyma) in 93% of cases, and demonstrate characteristic incremental, centripetal enhancement in 72% of cases. Abscesses, unlike simple cysts, have a thick enhancing wall. The presence of gas is the most useful diagnostic sign, but is only present in 20% of cases. Where doubt remains, aspiration is required. *Echinococcus granulosus* produces well-defined, uni- or multi-loculated cysts, sometimes with septae, calcification (rim or septal) and daughter cysts. The daughter cysts have a lower attenuation value than the mother cyst, and this is a specific diagnostic sign.

Diffuse liver disease

Diffuse fatty infiltration of the liver produces a reduction in attenuation value, whereas raised attenuation values occur in haemachromatosis, Wilson's disease or haemosiderosis. The attenuation value may be mildly elevated in cirrhosis, but is usually normal. Although the liver may appear entirely normal in some patients with cirrhosis, there are often changes in contour, size and homogeneity. A well-recognized configuration is enlargement of the caudate and lateral segment of the left lobe, with shrinkage of the right lobe. Associated findings include ascites, portal hypertension, varices, hepatocellular carcinoma or regenerating nodules. Regenerating nodules are usually isointense to normal liver and detected by contour abnormality, but occasionally they are hyperattenuating and can simulate a mass lesion. It may then be difficult to differentiate regenerating nodules from hepatocellular carcinoma. Portal venous patency can be established on CT (Figure 29.1.3). Varices are seen as round, serpiginous, enhancing structures in the porta hepatis, perigastric, oesophageal, periumbilical and splenic regions.

Liver trauma

CT is precise in depicting disruption of hepatic architecture and haemorrhage following acute trauma. Lacerations appear as linear or branching, poorly demarcated, low-attenuation lesions that are either isolated or in continuity with haematoma. Haematomas can be either focal, intraparenchymal or subcapsular, lenticular. The attenuation value depends on the age of the haematoma – initially there is high attenuation secondary to clotted blood, with surrounding low attenuation due to liquid blood, oedema and contused liver. With time the central clot lyses and the attenuation value falls.

Acute pancreatitis (Figure 29.1.1)

Diffuse or focal swelling of the gland is one of the most common manifestations. Other common CT signs are blurring of the pancreatic margins and thickening of Gerota's fascia. Focal thickening of the gastric wall occurs in 70% of cases. Peripancreatic fluid or pancreatic fluid collections are well delineated on CT. These are often complex and multiloculated, and may track as far as the thigh or extend up into the chest. Pancreatic phlegmon is seen in more than 50% of severe attacks, and has an overall incidence of 18%. A phlegmon is seen as a boggy, oedematous, soft-tissue mass composed of inflammation, exudate and retroperitoneal fat. In mild cases of

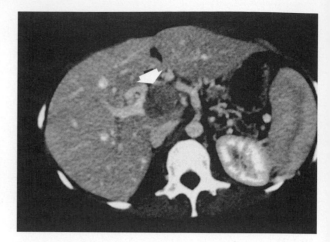

Figure 29.1.3 Axial contrast-enhanced CT showing tumour expanding and occluding the portal vein (arrow).

acute pancreatitis the CT can be normal. The specific role for CT is in defining the complications of acute pancreatitis, haemorrhage, venous thrombosis, pseudoaneurysm, abscess or pseudocyst formation. Haemorrhage is seen in 5% of cases, and appears as a focal collection of high attenuation (> 60 HU). Venous thrombosis is seen as non-enhancement of the vein or, if partial, as filling defects within the vessel. Pseudoaneurysms are seen as densely enhancing structures. Pseudocysts form in 10% of cases when pancreatic or peripancreatic fluid collections become loculated and fixed by a dense fibrous capsule. The presence of gas suggests fistulation to bowel, abscess formation or prior intervention. If gas is not present, abscesses are indistinguishable from non-infected phlegmon or pseudocysts. In suspected infection, image-guided fine-needle aspiration and microbiological analysis are recommended. CT also has a role in predicting prognosis, where early CT findings, at 72 h, correlate with the severity of the attack and the development of complications.

Chronic pancreatitis

Non-enhanced CT will detect tiny flecks of pancreatic calcification that are not apparent on any other imaging modality. Normal pancreatic ducts are seen in 70% of cases (diameter < 4 mm). CT detects 100% of dilated ducts, and often shows the relationship of calculi to the pancreatic duct. Atrophy of the parenchyma is a common sequela of chronic inflammation, and is readily detected by CT.

Neoplasms

Changes in the size and contour of the gland are the most frequent features of pancreatic cancer. However, the high incidence of normal variation in pancreatic size and shape can generate diagnostic confusion. Differential contrast enhancement patterns can be helpful.

Ductal adenocarcinoma is hypovascular relative to normal pancreatic parenchyma, 25–30 s after the injection, but rapidly becomes iso-attenuating, and therefore early scans are essential. CT is more accurate than US in staging pancreatic cancer, but consistently underestimates the extent of tumour spread. In cases where CT shows evidence of inoperability it is more than 95% accurate. Where CT suggests an operable lesion, 65% of cases prove to be operable at surgery. Obliteration of peripancreatic fat planes is most commonly due to direct tumour invasion, but the fat planes can appear normal in the presence of microscopic invasion. Involved vessels can be displaced, narrowed, irregular or occluded, but even loss of the fat plane between tumour and vessel indicates vascular invasion. Regional lymph node metastases occur in 38–65% of cases, and hepatic metastases in 17–55% of cases. Neuroendocrine tumours will demonstrate a characteristic dense, homogeneous, hypervascular pattern. As patients with secreting neuroendocrine lesions present when the tumours are very small, CT may fail to demonstrate the lesion. In these cases the most sensitive method for detection is invasive US (either endoscopic or intra-operative).

Reticulo-endothelial system

CT is highly sensitive and specific (> 95%) in diagnosing splenic injury. Unenhanced CT is required to detect hyperdense haematoma. The use of IV contrast increases the detection of splenic injury, as normal spleen enhances and subcapsular and intrasplenic haematomas do not. Even when parenchymal laceration is not seen, the presence of perisplenic clot, a heterogeneous collection (CT value > 60 HU), indicates splenic trauma. Cysts, abscesses, metastases and infarcts have similar appearances to those described in the liver. Lymphomatous involvement of the spleen is usually diffuse, and the majority of cases demonstrate homogeneous splenic parenchyma. CT offers similar information to US in the detection of enlarged lymph nodes, but more reliably detects even mildly enlarged nodes in the retroperitoneum, small-bowel mesentery, or adjacent to the lesser curve of the stomach. None of the cross-sectional imaging studies offer information about internal nodal architecture. The criteria used for detection of neoplastic involvement of lymph nodes are based on the increasing statistical likelihood of involvement with increasing size. Normal-sized nodes containing tumour may be seen on CT, but cannot be differentiated from normal nodes. Similarly, inflammatory nodal enlargement generally looks the same as metastatic enlargement.

Kidney

Focal lesions

CT is useful in the detection, characterization and staging of renal masses. Simple renal cysts occur in over 50% of patients above the age of 50 years. A typical benign cyst is round or oval, with no measurable wall thickness, and is of uniform low attenuation with no enhancement after contrast (Figure 29.1.4). Atypical cysts (e.g. haemorrhagic, infected or calcified cysts) can cause diagnostic confusion and fine-needle aspiration may be required to confirm their benign nature. These cysts are readily differentiated from the renal appearances of polycystic kidney disease, in which the kidneys are enlarged and contain multiple small cysts that distort the collecting system. Renal-cell carcinomas appear as solid masses, often irregular or ill-defined, that disrupt the normal renal contour. For staging, CT will show the relationship of the tumour to Gerota's fascia, invasion of adjacent structures including venous invasion, either renal vein or cava, and detection of local adenopathy. Local adenopathy occurs in 9–20% and caval extension in 4–10% of cases. The accuracy of diagnosis of venous invasion is good (78–93%). At the same time, the contralateral kidney can be evaluated. Renal pelvic tumours (transitional cell or squamous cell) are detected as filling defects on late scans when the renal pelvis contains IV contrast.

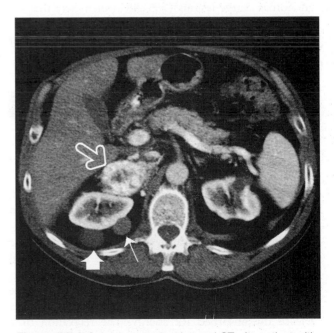

Figure 29.1.4 Axial contrast-enhanced CT of a patient with phaeochromocytoma seen as a large, hypervascular enhancing mass in the right adrenal gland (open arrow). In addition, there are multiple renal cysts, and the more lateral cyst (white arrow) on the right kidney has all the features of a typical benign cyst. The more medial cyst (long arrow) is of high attenuation, probably due to haemorrhage within the cyst.

Angiomyolipoma is a benign tumour with a specific CT diagnosis. It contains varying amounts of smooth muscle, blood vessels and fat. The detection of low-attenuation fat is pathognomonic for angiomyolipoma.

Infection

CT is not indicated in uncomplicated acute pyelonephritis, but if performed will demonstrate patchy, linear, radially oriented, low-density material in the renal parenchyma on contrast-enhanced scans. In more severe cases, CT may show a solid mass secondary to focal bacterial nephritis or even frank abscess formation.

Trauma

CT is very sensitive in detecting the degree and extent of renal trauma. Subcapsular haematoma, perinephric haematoma, renal contusion, laceration, fracture or shattered kidney are all readily demonstrated.

ADRENAL SYSTEM

CT will show the normal adrenal gland, the body and the medial and lateral limbs. It will also detect adrenal masses (Figure 29.1.4) and can attempt to differentiate benign from malignant lesions. Usually small lesions (< 2 cm in diameter) that are well defined, homogeneous, low-attenuation lesions or have a rim represent adenomas. Large lesions (> 5 cm in diameter) that are irregular and of mixed attenuation are usually malignant. These criteria are not absolute, and MRI will offer better specificity.

MAGNETIC RESONANCE IMAGING (MRI)

BASIC PRINCIPLES

MRI images are derived from the returning radiofrequency (RF) signal released from previously excited, relaxing hydrogen nuclei (protons). In order to obtain an MRI image, the patient is placed within a uniform magnetic field which will cause protons to align with the main magnetic field. The protons are then displaced from their aligned position by an RF pulse of a particular frequency. When the RF pulse is switched off, the protons relax back to their original alignment and release the absorbed RF energy. The relaxation time depends on both the molecule and the matrix environment of the proton. Two relaxation constants commonly referred to are T1 and T2, usually measured in milliseconds. T1 refers to the time it takes for the protons to return to their original aligned position, while T2 refers to the length of time for which the returning protons maintain coherence with each other. These relaxation times vary for different tissues, and this forms the basis

of MRI tissue contrast. The MRI scanner can be programmed to produce images which emphasize different features of tissue, e.g. a T2-weighted image emphasizes differences in tissue T2. Other sequences look specifically at flowing blood or stationary fluid, or conversely suppress signal from fat or from fluid. By using techniques such as these, MRI offers a tissue specificity that is not realized by other imaging technologies.

CLINICAL UTILITY

The first MRI scanners were very slow, with protracted image acquisition times, and consequently body imaging was severely impaired by motion artefact. Improvements in the last 2 to 3 years in both hardware (stronger gradients and reduced gradient rise times) and software (with the development of new sequences) have resulted in breath-hold imaging. This has revolutionized the role that MRI can now play in the abdomen. The liver or the pancreas can be imaged in 2–3 breath-holds. MRI, like US, is multiplanar in a way that CT has yet to rival. MRI provides much greater soft-tissue contrast than either CT or US, and today the spatial resolution is nearly as good as that of CT. The drawback of MRI is the need for a reasonably co-operative patient who can cope without claustrophobia in an enclosed environment. There are some absolute contraindications. Some electronic and metallic implants do not operate within the magnetic field or are interfered with by the changing RF pulses and localizer gradients (e.g. cochlear implants, some artificial heart valves and most types of pacemaker). Lack of MRI availability compared to both CT and US results in MRI being used for complex or problem cases, or to solve specific problems that other imaging tests cannot address.

Liver and biliary tract

The MRI sequences that show signal from stationary fluid while suppressing signal from parenchyma can be used to define the ductal anatomy of the biliary system or pancreas, without the injection of any contrast media. These sequences provide images non-invasively with very similar information to that obtained at ERCP. Duct dilatation, strictures and calculi are demonstrated (Figure 29.1.1). MRCP can be combined with MRI images of the liver and pancreatic parenchyma, and provide in one examination the type of information that previously required CT and ERCP. MRCP has 100% sensitivity for obstruction, > 93% sensitivity for the detection of calculi and > 95% sensitivity for establishing the cause of obstruction, but will not show subtle duct changes (e.g. minimal-change pancreatitis or early primary sclerosing cholangitis). MRCP could replace diag-

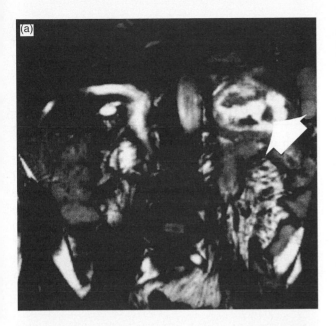

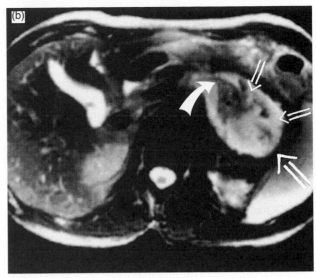

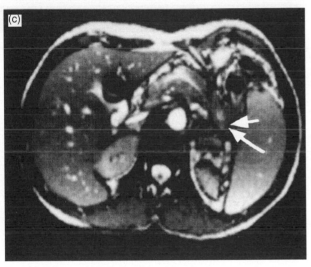

Figure 29.1.5 (a) Coronal T2-weighted image showing a mixed-signal-intensity pancreatic fluid collection (arrow). High signal intensity on this sequence represents fluid or flowing blood. Note the normal right portal vein, aorta and fluid in the duodenum. (b) Axial T2-weighted image showing the pancreatic fluid collection in the tail of the pancreas (arrows). The dominant component of the phlegmon is fluid. A percutaneous drain has been inserted, giving a curved low signal (curved arrow). (c) Axial T2-weighted image several weeks later, showing successful resolution of the collection (arrow).

nostic ERCP for most applications if sufficient MRI capability was available. ERCP will increasingly be used as a therapeutic procedure.

Historically, CT was better than MRI for liver imaging, but the introduction of liver-specific contrast agents (e.g. super-paramagnetic iron oxide particles (SPIO), which are taken up by normal Kupffer cells) has resulted in MRI having superior sensitivity and specificity. It is proposed that SPIO-enhanced MRI is reserved for those patients in whom the size, number and distribution of the metastases are critical for patient management. Fat suppression sequences can be used to differentiate focal fat deposition from other focal lesions. MRI is very sensitive to iron deposition in the liver, either in cirrhosis or in haemachromatosis.

Pancreas

MRI tissue specificity allows differentiation of the solid and cystic components of a pancreatic phlegmon (Figure 29.1.5). CT will show which areas of the phlegmon enhance with contrast, but this does not distinguish fluid and non-viable, necrotic but solid pancreatic tissue. Therefore MRI offers an advantage over CT, and can be used to direct drainage procedures. Currently MRI is competitive with CT in the staging of pancreatic cancers.

Reticulo-endothelial system

MRI is very similar to CT for the assessment of the spleen and regional lymphadenopathy, and does not offer any specific advantages over CT in these areas. Like CT, MRI currently uses size criteria in the assessment of lymphadenopathy. A search for an MRI lymphographic agent has been in progress for some time, but has not yet proved successful.

Renal and adrenal systems

CT is more accurate than MRI in the staging of renal tumours, with the exception of identification of venous invasion, where sagittal and coronal images of the vena cava are advantageous. MRI pyelography can be performed using a similar technique to MRCP. The images produced are similar to a slightly crude IVP. MRI pyelography is most commonly performed in pregnancy to avoid the use of ionizing radiation.

MRI can improve the specificity of imaging assessment of the adrenal gland. Benign adenomas, which are the most common cause of an adrenal mass even in patients with a primary malignancy, have specific signal characteristics on MRI, due to the presence of intracellular fat. Similarly, the majority of phaeochromocytomas demonstrate a very high signal intensity on T2-weighted images.

POSITRON EMISSION TOMOGRAPHY (PET)

BASIC PRINCIPLES

PET is a non-invasive technique for the *in-vivo* examination of metabolism and blood flow. A positron matter–antimatter annihilation reaction with an electron produces 'annihilation photons' which are emitted in exactly opposite directions with an energy of 511 keV each. These photons are detected by coincidence circuitry using simultaneous arrival at detectors on opposite sides of the patient. PET uses cyclotron-produced agents, most commonly F18 fluorodeoxyglucose (FDG) for scanning glucose metabolism and N-13 ammonia for perfusion. PET can be used to detect active tumour by mapping FDG uptake and therefore glucose metabolism.

CLINICAL UTILITY

Much of the original work has been in neuroimaging, but more recently there have been a number of studies of PET in the abdomen. PET studies can differentiate focal pancreatitis from carcinoma, which can be impossible with other imaging modalities, and even a negative biopsy can be misleading due to sampling variability. Similarly, PET should be of value in differentiating scar or post-surgical change from recurrent tumour. Preliminary data suggest that PET has a potential role in detecting lymph-node metastases.

FURTHER READING

Curry TS, Dowdey JE, Murry RC. 1994: *Christensen's physics of diagnostic radiology*. Philadelphia, PA: Lea & Febiger.

Dahnert W. 1996: *Radiology review manual*. London: Williams & Wilkins.

Grainger RG, Allison DJ. 1997: *Diagnostic radiology; an Anglo-American textbook of imaging*. London: Churchill Livingstone.

Sutton D. 1998: *A textbook of radiology and imaging*. London: Churchill Livingstone.

Biochemical investigations

David W. Thomas

Introduction

Analysis of the constituents of blood and other body fluids, an activity variously described as clinical chemistry, clinical biochemistry or chemical pathology, has a long history in the diagnosis and management of surgical diseases. Biochemical investigations can provide quantitative data that not only indicate the presence of disease, but also its extent and severity. Organ function can be assessed and the degree of disease-induced compromise measured. However, despite the seeming accuracy of the numerical values generated in the biochemistry laboratory, it is important for clinicians to be aware of the limitations of commonly performed tests. The objective of this chapter is to outline some basic principles which must be kept in mind when ordering laboratory tests and interpreting test results.

Laboratory tests are used for diagnosis and management. The clinician is interested in establishing the cause of a patient's illness and treating it. This often requires laboratory tests for the confirmation or exclusion of specific conditions, an assessment of disease complications, monitoring of treatment (which includes therapeutic response, side-effects and complications) and an indication of prognosis. Laboratory data is rarely used in isolation; it complements clinical observations and other information to provide an extensive database which the clinician can then use to make decisions on patient management. It is important that the clinician understands the reliability of the information in the specific context of the clinical situation being managed, particularly its validity and limitations.

TEST SELECTION

When ordering laboratory investigations, the clinician must first decide what specific information is required for patient management and then select the appropriate tests, rather than adopt a standardized approach. This may require tests not only for diagnostic purposes but also for assessment of vital organ function, particularly if the patient is unstable or being prepared for surgery. Having decided what information is required, the clinician is then more likely to interpret the results correctly and utilize the information appropriately when proceeding with patient management. Familiarity with the tests available from the laboratory, both during and after normal working hours,

is essential, and when tests are required which are not routinely available it is the clinician's responsibility to discuss this with laboratory staff. It is also the laboratory's responsibility to ensure that someone in authority is always available and easy to contact.

There are several books which provide helpful information on the selection and interpretation of tests for a wide range of clinical conditions (see the Further Reading section at the end of this chapter). Many laboratories provide similar information in their handbooks, but not in as much detail. It is also important to be aware of the clinical validity of the tests selected, particularly in the clinical setting for which they are being used. This will be discussed in greater detail in the Test Result Interpretation section.

PATIENT PREPARATION AND SPECIMEN COLLECTION

Some tests require that the patient should meet certain criteria prior to testing. Most commonly, fasting for specific periods is required for assessment of carbohydrate tolerance (8 h preliminary fasting) and lipid abnormalities (12–14 h preliminary fasting). Fasting itself may cause increases in urate and bilirubin values in some individuals. Dynamic tests for endocrine assessment often involve complex protocols which describe the conditions under which specimens must be collected. Failure to adhere to these requirements will invalidate the test, cause inconvenience to the patient and nursing staff, and impose unnecessary work and expense on the laboratory.

Each laboratory test requires a specimen which has been collected properly, placed in an appropriate container and delivered to the laboratory under specified conditions. Collection of blood usually involves venepuncture, which should be performed with minimal tourniquet pressure. Raising the venous pressure causes haemoconcentration (due to increased retention of water in the extravascular space), with artefactual increases in cell counts and concentrations of high-molecular-weight proteins and protein-bound substances. A variety of specimen containers is available, each with a specific purpose, to provide the laboratory with the sample it requires for testing. In particular, tests using plasma will require the addition of an appropriate anticoagulant (e.g. lithium heparin for most biochemical tests, potassium EDTA for cell counts, sodium citrate for coagulation studies). Unstable constituents may require the addition of a suitable preservative (e.g. a glycolytic inhibitor such as sodium fluoride for glucose measurements) and/or transport to the laboratory at 4°C (e.g. a capped syringe in a container of water with adequate ice for pH and blood gas studies).

Most laboratories publish a handbook which provides information on available tests, the volumes of specimens required, the types of containers to be used and any special conditions for the collection of specimens and transport to the laboratory. Where doubt exists, information should be sought from the laboratory, as inappropriately collected, preserved or transported specimens are not tested.

BIOLOGICAL VARIABILITY, PRE-ANALYTICAL ERROR AND LABORATORY ERROR

All laboratory measurements are subject to errors that compound normal biological variability. In assessing the significance of fluctuations in laboratory measurements, some understanding of biological variability, pre-analytical error and laboratory error is required. For example, how significant are fluctuations in plasma glucose observed from day to day in a patient recovering from upper abdominal surgery?

The concentrations of most substances in blood vary over time as a result of normal daily activities such as eating, drinking, exercising and sleeping. These changes are referred to as normal *biological variation*, and are often distorted as a result of illness, hospitalization, drug treatment and surgical intervention. Factors contributing to the normal biological variation of commonly measured blood constituents are listed in Table 29.2.1. Some of these cannot be controlled (e.g. the individual's gender, age, race, etc.), and must be taken into account when interpreting test results. Others can be controlled (e.g. dietary intake, physical activity, posture, etc.) and, where appropriate, modified prior to the collection of specimens for testing.

From the moment a specimen of blood or any other body fluid is removed from the body until it is analysed in the laboratory, changes occur which may influence the results. Errors resulting from such changes are referred to as *pre-analytical errors*, and in some circumstances they can be quite significant. The artefacts mentioned above introduced as a result of specimen collection and transport are examples of pre-analytical error. Incorrect handling and storage in the laboratory prior to analysis are also sources of pre-analytical error.

Any measurement process itself is subject to error, and laboratory testing is no exception. Analytical error in the laboratory can be of two types, namely inaccuracy or systematic deviation from the true value, and imprecision or random deviation. Accuracy is established by correct calibration using standards which are traceable to certified reference materials, and is regularly assessed by participation in external quality assurance programmes. Automated instrumentation and standardized testing procedures minimize imprecision, which is assessed on an ongoing basis by regular measurement of internal quality control materials at a minimum of two concentration levels (normal and abnormal). Analytical precision is indicated by the coefficient of variation (CV%) of a test. This is the standard deviation of repeat measurements on the same specimen divided by the mean value and expessed as a percentage. These quality control procedures are mandatory for laboratory accreditation.

TEST RESULT INTERPRETATION

The interpretation of tests usually involves comparing the patient's results with the reference intervals provided

Table 29.2.1 Biological variability – factors influencing composition of body fluids

Short-term biological variables (controllable, short-acting or self-limiting)

Posture	Recumbency increases plasma volume by 10%; haemodilution reduces cell counts, protein, protein-bound, and other non-diffusible constituents
Exercise/physical training	Muscle release of K^+, lactic acid, AST, LD and CK; hypoglycaemia; increased fibrinolytic activity
Circadian rhythms	Affect urea, creatinine, phosphate, urate, cholesterol, AST, ALT, LD, ALP, acid phosphatase, iron and many hormones
Food ingestion	Increased glucose, urea, phosphate, urate, iron, triglycerides, ALP (intestinal)
Caffeine	Increased glucose, cortisol and catecholamine release and 5-HIAA excretion
Smoking	Increased glucose, cortisol, growth hormone and catecholamine release, erythrocyte and leucocyte counts, and carboxyhaemoglobin
Alcohol	Increased glucose, triglycerides, GGT, cortisol and catecholamine release; hypoglycaemia when hepatic glycogen is diminished
Drug administration	Can cause *in-vivo* and/or *in-vitro* effects; intra-muscular delivery releases AST, LD and CK from muscle
	Oral contraceptives affect many constituents depending on the oestrogen and progestin combination
	Diuretics reduce sodium and potassium and increase glucose, calcium and urate
	Opiates increase amylase, ALP, GGT, AST, ALT and LD
Fever	Releases cortisol, growth hormone and glucagon with increased glycogenolysis, gluconeogenesis, protein breakdown and negative nitrogen balance resulting in hyperglycaemia, insulin resistance, raised urea/creatinine ratio and urate; increases aldosterone and ADH release resulting in retention of sodium and water; increases hepatic synthesis and plasma concentrations of acute-phase proteins; reduces T_3 and T_4
Trauma, surgical stress and shock	As for fever, together with release of catecholamines, extravasation of vascular fluid and proteins into extracellular space, reduced blood volume and glomerular filtration rate resulting in reduced plasma proteins and raised urea and creatinine; release of intracellular constituents from damaged tissues resulting in raised potassium, phosphate, AST, LD and CK
Environmental factors	Heat exposure promotes fluid loss, dehydration and haemoconcentration

Long-term biological variables (not controllable, long-acting or permanent)

Age, gender, race	Where significant these are usually allowed for in reference intervals (if any doubt, check with laboratory)
Environmental factors	*High altitude* increases urate, growth hormone, erythrocyte count and haemoglobin
Seasonal influences	Sunlight exposure in summer increases vitamin D_3 and reduces bilirubin
Menstrual cycle	Cortisol and aldosterone increase during the luteal phase with sodium retention
Obesity	Increased glucose (insulin resistance), urate, cholesterol, triglycerides, T_3 and cortisol; reduced phosphate and growth hormone
Malnutrition	Reduced urea, creatinine, cholesterol, triglyceride, total protein, albumin, complement C3, retinol-binding protein, transferrin, prealbumin, TSH, T_4, T_3 and vitamins A and E; increased cortisol

by the laboratory and identifying 'abnormal' values. Table 29.2.2 lists the reference intervals for biochemical measurements commonly performed on plasma, serum or whole blood. Some laboratories flag abnormal results as high (H) or low (L). Most laboratories report population-based reference values which have been determined from a group of individuals who were fit, healthy, eating a 'normal' diet, not suffering from any acute or chronic illness and not taking any drugs at the time of testing. To minimize biological variability (see Table 29.2.1) and pre-analytical error, individuals are requested to fast for 8 h beforehand and to rest quietly for 20 min in a seated position prior to testing. A standardized procedure is used to collect specimens. It is common practice to base

Table 29.2.2 Reference intervals* for tests commonly performed on plasma, serum or whole blood

Analyte	Reference interval	Units	Comments
Sodium	137–145	mmol/L	
Potassium	3.1–4.2	mmol/L	Plasma
	3.8–4.9	mmol/L	Serum
Chloride	101–109	mmol/L	
Bicarbonate	22–32	mmol/L	
Anion gap	10–18	mmol/L	Calculated (see text)
Glucose	3.8–5.4	mmol/L	Fasting
Urea	2.7–7.2	mmol/L	
Creatinine	0.05–0.12	mmol/L	Units may be µmol/L
Urea/creatinine ratio	35–80		Calculated
Osmolarity	265–285	mmol/L	Calculated (see text)
Calcium			
Total	2.20–2.55	mmol/L	
Ionized	1.07–1.27	mmol/L	
Magnesium	0.70–0.95	mmol/L	
Phosphate	0.80–1.45	mmol/L	Age related
Urate	0.25–0.50	mmol/L	Males
	0.15–0.40	mmol/L	Females
Liver tests			
Protein – total	60–80	g/L	
Albumin	36–48	g/L	
Globulin	22–35	g/L	Calculated
Bilirubin – total	6–24	µmol/L	
Bilirubin – conjugated	1–4	µmol/L	
γ-Glutamyl transpeptidase (γGT)	5–60	U/L	Males
	5–40	U/L	Females
Alkaline phosphatase (ALP)	30–110	U/L	Age related
Alanine aminotransferase (ALT)	12–50	U/L	Males
	8–29	U/L	Females
Aspartate aminotransferase (AST)	13–45	U/L	Males
	10–28	U/L	Females
Lactate dehydrogenase (LD)	110–230	U/L	
Miscellaneous enzymes			
Lipase	25–130	U/L	Method dependent
Amylase	20–100	U/L	Method dependent
Creatine kinase	60–270	U/L	Males
	40–180	U/L	Females
Arterial pH and blood gases			
Base excess	−2–2	mmol/L	
PaO_2	90–110	mmHg	
$PaCO_2$	35–45	mmHg	
pH	7.35–7.45		
Hydrogen ion	35–45	nmol/L	
Bicarbonate	22–31	mmol/L	Calculated
Lipid studies			
Triglycerides	0.3–2.0	mmol/L	
Total cholesterol	Desirable < 5.5	mmol/L	NHF recommendation
HDL – cholesterol	0.9–2.0	mmol/L	Males
	1.0–2.2	mmol/L	Females
LDL – cholesterol	Desirable < 3.7	mmol/L	Calculated

* Reference intervals given in this table are for adult men and (non-pregnant) women aged ⩾ 17 years.

reference intervals on the central 95% interval (bounded by the 2.5 and 97.5 percentiles) of the distribution of results observed in the reference population. Usually, separate reference intervals are provided for neonates, children, adults and pregnant women. Even within these groups, separate reference intervals may be provided for certain tests, according to the individual's age and gender (see Table 29.2.2).

It must be appreciated that the reference intervals are broad, and include intra- and inter-individual biological variation as well as pre-analytical and analytical errors. Results within the reference interval may be abnormal for a particular patient. Changes between sequential results may be significant, despite all being 'normal', particularly if they are in the same direction. However, the interpretation of small differences between sequential test results requires a knowledge of analytical precision (see above). A difference greater than $3 \times CV\% \times$ initial value/100 is considered to be significant, i.e. when the difference is not entirely due to analytical imprecision. Laboratory measurement of plasma glucose has a typical CV of 3%, and thus a value of 5.0 mmol/L has to be exceeded by 0.45 mmol/L before being significantly different just on the basis of analytical imprecision. However, the biological variability in plasma glucose values is even larger, depending on whether the patient is fasting, has recently ingested food containing carbohydrate, or is receiving dextrose intravenously. It is important to assess whether the differences in sequential test results are clinically significant, or just the result of 'normal' biological variability or analytical imprecision.

Special attention is required when test results are inconsistent with the patient's clinical condition, or with previous results obtained from the same patient. In the latter circumstance, most laboratories compare the current result with the patient's previous result prior to reporting (delta check), and initiate checking procedures to eliminate laboratory error when the difference exceeds acceptable limits. Furthermore, when results are considered to be life-threatening or indicate a serious abnormality, the laboratory contacts the clinician urgently to discuss the result and any further action that is required. Grossly abnormal results should always be confirmed on a new specimen collected from the patient. Similarly, when test results are inconsistent with the clinical situation, the clinician must contact the laboratory and discuss the issue. Usually it is necessary to repeat the test on a freshly collected specimen.

When interpreting test results, it is also important to be aware of the diagnostic capabilities of the tests used (see Table 29.2.3). As an example, a group of participants in a screening programme for colorectal cancer have been identified with neoplastic lesions (either carcinoma or adenoma). Tests A and B have been carried out to

Table 29.2.3 Test sensitivity, specificity, positive predictive value and likelihood ratio

	Number of participants with positive test result	Number of participants with negative test result	Total
Number of participants with disease	TP	FN	TP + FN
Number of participants without disease	FP	TN	FP + TN
Total	TP + FP	FN + TN	TP + FP + TN + FN

TP = true-positives (number of diseased participants correctly identified by the test)
FP = false-positives (number of non-diseased participants incorrectly identified by the test)
TN = true-negatives (number of non-diseased participants correctly identified by the test)
FN = false-negatives (number of diseased participants incorrectly identified by the test)

Sensitivity	Percentage of participants with disease who test positive	$= \dfrac{TP}{TP + FN} \times 100$
Specificity	Percentage of participants without disease who test negative	$= \dfrac{TN}{FP + TN} \times 100$
Positive predictive value	Percentage of participants with positive results who have disease	$= \dfrac{TP}{TP + FP} \times 100$
Positive likelihood ratio		$= \dfrac{Sensitivity}{1 - Specificity}$

Table 29.2.4 Hypothetical test to diagnose colorectal cancer

	Carcinoma* (positive test)	Adenoma (negative test)
Test A (%)	49	92
Test B (%)	80	68
Diagnostic validity	**Test A**	**Test B**
Sensitivity (%)	49	80
Specificity (%)	92	68
Positive predictive value (%)	61	39
Likelihood ratio (positive test)	1.8	3.4

* Prevalence of carcinoma = 20%

identify those individuals with carcinoma (results shown in Table 29.2.4). Which is the best test for detecting carcinoma? Whereas test B detects 80% of those with carcinoma, with 32% false-positives, test A detects only 49% with carcinoma, but with only 8% false-positives. In fact, the same testing procedure has been used but with different 'cut-off' values for the diagnosis of carcinoma. Test A has a high cut-off value (low sensitivity and high specificity) and Test B has a low cut-off value (high sensitivity and low specificity). Neither test is perfect. Test A could be used as a diagnostic test and Test B could be used as a screening test if the large numbers of false-negatives and false-positives, respectively, were acceptable.

It is also important to be aware of the prevalence of the condition in the population being tested. Using test A in the above example, 61% of individuals with a positive test result will actually have cancer (positive predictive value). The incidence of carcinoma in this group is 20%. Using the same tests, but in a group in which the prevalence of carcinoma is only 5%, the positive predictive values for tests A and B will be 24% and 12%, respectively, i.e. for each test there will be fewer true-positives and more false-positives.

Despite the quantitative nature of biochemical investigations, the traditional approach to the interpretation of results remains qualitative. Additional information can often be obtained by interpreting results in a quantitative

manner. For example, in a shocked patient with a low plasma bicarbonate level, calculation of the unmeasured anions and determining what substances are contributing to the increased anion gap may provide information critical to patient management. Alternatively, calculation of the osmolar gap (measured osmolality − calculated osmolarity) may indicate the presence of non-ionized substances such as ethanol, methanol, ethylene glycol, etc., and indicate the need for specific investigation.

In the current climate of economic constraint, clinical biochemists and chemical pathologists expend considerable effort in providing a basic range of laboratory tests which are reliable, provided in a timely manner and cost-effective. Additional services are often available but not provided for the initial assessment of patients. In some instances, when the laboratory is provided with the appropriate clinical information, such tests will be performed when considered appropriate by the laboratory staff. More often than not, the clinical information provided to the laboratory is sparse or non-existent. Here it is essential that the clinician is prepared to seek the advice of laboratory staff, particularly when there is uncertainty about which tests to perform, the interpretation of laboratory results or the need for additional tests.

FURTHER READING

McPherson J (ed.). 1997: *Manual of use and interpretation of pathology tests*. Sydney: Royal College of Pathologists of Australasia.

Tietz NW (ed.). 1995: *Clinical guide to laboratory tests*. Philadelphia, PA: W.B. Saunders.

Young DS. 1993: *Effects of preanalytical variables on clinical laboratory tests*. Washington, DC: American Association for Clinical Chemistry.

Young DS, Bermes EW. 1996: Specimen collection and processing: sources of biological variation. In Burtis CA, Ashwood ER (eds), *Tietz: fundamentals of clinical chemistry*. Philadelphia, PA: W.B. Saunders, 33–52.

Zweig MH, Campbell G. 1993: Receiver operating characteristic (ROC) plots: a fundamental evaluation tool in clinical medicine. *Clinical Chemistry* **39**, 561–77.

Haematological investigations

Laurie Catley and John V. Lloyd

Introduction

The most important haematological tests in surgical practice are the complete blood examination and the simple coagulation tests. Other tests of interest include bone-marrow biopsy and some more specialized coagulation tests.

COMPLETE BLOOD EXAMINATION

In the laboratory, the complete blood examination (CBE) is almost invariably performed by automated methods. Modern analysers can vary considerably, but all of them use either electrical impedance signalling or light-scatter flow cytometry.

NORMAL RANGES FOUND BY CBE

Haemoglobin, 11.5–16 g/dL (female), 13.5–18 g/dL (male)
Platelets, 150–400 × 10^9/L
Total white cell count, 4–11 × 10^9/L
Neutrophils, 2.5–7 × 10^9/L
Lymphocytes, 1–4 × 10^9/L
Monocytes, 0.2–0.8 × 10^9/L
Eosinophils, 0.04–0.44 × 10^9/L
Basophils, 0.01–0.1 × 10^9/L

In addition, further information may be obtained by inspection of the blood film for changes in morphology of the red cells, white cells and platelets.

A reticulocyte count may provide further important information. Reticulocytes are immature erythrocytes, and their numbers are increased when the marrow is able to respond to anaemia by increasing red cell production. This may occur in:

- acute or chronic blood loss;
- haemolysis;
- response to iron, vitamin B_{12} or folate therapy in patients who are deficient.

Common abnormalities revealed by the CBE are an increase or decrease in the haemoglobin, white cell count or platelet count. The causes of these are listed in Tables 29.3.1 and 29.3.2. Important abnormalities are microcytic and macrocytic anaemias. These are discussed in more detail below.

MICROCYTIC ANAEMIA

Microcytic anaemia is a commonly encountered clinical problem. The differential diagnoses are anaemia of chronic disease, iron-deficiency anaemia, sideroblastic anaemia and thalassaemia.

The initial investigation of microcytic anaemia consists of serum iron studies, which include serum ferritin, transferrin, transferrin saturation and serum iron.

Serum ferritin reflects iron stores. It is reduced in iron depletion and raised in iron overload and chronic disease.

Table 29.3.1 Causes of an increased or decreased haemoglobin concentration

Elevated concentration

Reduced plasma volume (patient dehydrated)
Check patient for thirst, diuretic use
- hypotension, tachycardia, reduced skin turgor
- measure urea, creatinine ($\uparrow$ urea:creatinine ratio)

Increased red cell mass (polycythaemia)
Measure red cell mass, serum erythropoietin, arterial
   oxygen pressure

Primary polycythaemia (myeloproliferative disorder)
   Decreased serum erythropoietin
   Splenomegaly, leucocytosis and thrombocytosis

Secondary polycythaemia
   Increased serum erythropoietin due to decreased tissue
      oxygenation or erythropoietin-producing tumou
   History of smoking, cardiac or pulmonary disease

Reduced concentration

Spurious result
Clotted specimen
Dilutional (e.g. from site of intravenous therapy)

Anaemia – increased loss
Blood loss
   Occult if silent peptic ulcer or within a body cavity
   Can be insidious in gastrointestinal malignancy
   Normochromia initially, later hypochromia if iron deficiency
      develops
   Test for faecal occult blood. Red-cell scan for site of
      bleeding. Upper and lower gastrointestinal endoscopy
      should be considered for all cases of unexplained iron
      deficiency
Haemolysis (intravascular and extravascular)
   Intravascular:
   - haemolytic transfusion reaction
   - extensive burns
   - traumatic (cardiac valve, DIC, TTP, HUS)
   - lysins – snake venom, *Clostridium perfringens* bacteraemia
   - paroxysmal nocturnal haemoglobinuria (PNH)
   Extravascular:
   - autoimmune
   - hereditary conditions (e.g. hereditary spherocytosis,
      G6PD deficiency)

Anaemia – decreased production
Anaemia of chronic disease
Chronic renal failure
Iron, vitamin B_{12} or folate deficiency
Malignancy – primary (e.g. leukaemia) or secondary
   (e.g. metastatic carcinoma)
Toxic injury, especially chemotherapy or radiotherapy
Aplastic anaemia

In patients with chronic disease who also develop iron deficiency, the ferritin may still be within the normal range, making interpretation of iron studies difficult.

Serum transferrin is the circulating iron-transport protein. It is raised in iron deficiency, and lowered in iron overload and chronic disease.

Serum transferrin saturation is raised in iron overload, and is a sensitive early marker of haemochromatosis.

Serum iron is sensitive to diurnal variations and changes with inflammation. Alone, it gives very little useful information.

THALASSAEMIA AND HAEMOGLOBINOPATHIES

The normal haemoglobin molecule is a tetramer consisting of two alpha chains and two beta chains ($\alpha_2\beta_2$).

Abnormalities of haemoglobin synthesis lead to thalassaemia or haemoglobinopathy. Haemoglobin electrophoresis is useful in the diagnosis of these disorders.

Alpha and beta thalassaemia are characterized by a deficiency of α- or β-globin chains, respectively. Heterozygous carriers of β-thalassaemia usually have a mild microcytic anaemia, with a disproportionately low MCV. Homozygous β-thalassaemia results in transfusion-dependent anaemia within the first few months of life.

In the normal individual there are four α-globin genes. Patients with α-thalassaemia have one to four genes deleted. This results in a spectrum of clinical presentations. When only one gene is affected there are no clinical consequences. However, when all four genes are affected, death occurs *in utero*.

Haemoglobinopathies are characterized by structurally

Table 29.3.2 Causes of an increased or decreased white blood cell and platelet count

	Neutrophils	**Lymphocytes**	**Monocytes**	**Eosinophils**	**Platelets**
Elevated count	Infection	Acute viral infections	Chronic bacterial infections	Allergic conditions	*Primary* Infarction
	Infarction	TB, toxoplasmosis, syphilis	Protozoan infections	(e.g. asthma, drug reactions)	Myeloproliferative disorder
	Malignancy	Chronic lymphocytic leukaemia	Chronic neutropenia	Infections (e.g. parasites)	*Secondary* Leukaemia
	Leukaemia	Acute lymphocytic leukaemia	Hodgkin's disease	Skin disorders	Inflammation
	Inflammation	Non-Hodgkin's lymphoma	Myelodysplasia	Collagen vascular disease	Post-splenectomy
	Haemorrhage	Hairy cell leukaemia	Cytokines (GM-CSF or M-CSF)	Hepatitis – cholestatic	Iron deficiency
	Haemolysis			Neoplasia (e.g. Hodgkin's disease)	
	Cytokines (G-CSF or CM-CSF)			Immunodeficiency syndromes	
	Smoking			Interstitial nephritis	
	Metabolic derangements			Post-splenectomy	
	Steroids			Following marrow suppression or viral illness	
Reduced count	*Increased loss*	*Increased loss*			*Decreased production*
	Severe bacterial sepsis	Severe marrow failure			Vitamin B_{12} or folate deficiency
	Viral infection	Immunosuppressive therapy			Malignancy – primary (e.g. leukaemia) or secondary
	Hypersplenism	Hodgkin's disease			(e.g. metastatic carcinoma)
	Autoimmune	Widespread radiotherapy			Toxic injury, especially chemotherapy
	Decreased production	Immunodeficiency syndromes (e.g. AIDS)			or radiotherapy
	Vitamin B_{12} or folate deficiency				Idiosyncratic drug reactions
	Malignancy – primary (e.g. leukaemia) or secondary				Aplastic anaemia
	(e.g. metastatic carcinoma)				Hereditary thrombocytopenia
	Toxic injury, especially chemotherapy or radiotherapy				*Increased consumption*
	Idiosyncratic drug reactions				Severe bacterial sepsis
	Aplastic anaemia				Trauma
					Disseminated intravascular coagulation
					Thrombotic thrombocytopenic purpura
					Haemolytic uraemia syndrome
					Immune
					Idiopathic thrombocytopenic purpura
					Human immunodeficiency virus
					Drugs (e.g. heparin)
					Abnormal distribution
					Hypersplenism
					Dilutional
					Massive blood transfusion

abnormal haemoglobin, resulting in a characteristic migration pattern on haemoglobin gel electrophoresis. The commonly encountered haemoglobinopathies are β-chain variants (e.g. HbC, HbS, HbE).

Sickle-cell anaemia is the most important and prevalent type of haemoglobinopathy. Homozygous sickle-cell anaemia (HbSS) or double heterozygous sickle-cell disease (e.g. HbSC, HbSβ) results in severe anaemia. Sickle cells are seen in the peripheral blood. Painful crises are common in sickle-cell anaemia.

ANAEMIA OF CHRONIC DISEASE

The anaemia of chronic disease may be either normocytic or microcytic. Typically, the serum ferritin level is normal or raised and the serum transferrin level is low normal. Examples of chronic diseases include rheumatoid arthritis, infection, renal disease and malignancies.

MACROCYTIC ANAEMIA

A macrocytic anaemia is commonly caused by deficiencies of vitamin B_{12} or folic acid, liver disease, alcohol consumption, or reticulocytosis following blood loss or haemolysis. Hypothyroidism, pregnancy, marrow failure and certain drugs may also cause a macrocytosis.

Vitamin B_{12} and folate deficiencies are diagnosed by reduced serum B_{12} and folate levels. Serum folate levels are influenced by recent intake, and body stores are most reliably reflected by fasting samples. Red-cell folic acid can also be measured, and is less influenced by recent intake.

HAEMOLYTIC ANAEMIA

Haemolysis classically causes anaemia with reticulocytosis and reduced plasma haptoglobin. There may also be elevation of lactate dehydrogenase and unconjugated bilirubin.

The Coomb's test, or direct antiglobulin test, detects antibodies on the red-cell surface. It is almost always positive in cases of autoimmune haemolysis or incompatible blood transfusion.

There are many causes of haemolysis. Further investigations should be dictated by the initial history, examination, blood film appearance and other findings.

BONE-MARROW BIOPSY

Bone marrow is sampled by aspiration, commonly from the posterior superior iliac spine. A core of bone (trephine) is also usually taken. The sternum (and/or tibia in children) can be used for aspirating marrow, but not to obtain a trephine. The procedure takes about 20 min and is performed as an out-patient procedure.

INDICATIONS FOR BONE-MARROW BIOPSY

Bone-marrow examination is indicated mainly for the diagnosis of some peripheral blood abnormalities and for the staging of haematological malignancies.

Common abnormalities for which marrow biopsy is generally recommended include the following:

1. immature myeloid or erythroid precursors in the blood (leuco-erythroblastic blood picture);

2. severe unexplained cytopenias (neutropenia, thrombocytopenia, anaemia);

3. paraprotein in the blood or urine;

4. suspected leukaemia, lymphoma or myeloma.

COMMON FINDINGS

These include the following:

1. *hyperplasia* indicating peripheral loss of haemopoietic cells (e.g. megakaryocyte hyperplasia in immune thrombocytopenic purpura, or erythroid hyperplasia in haemolysis);

2. *hypoplasia or aplasia indicating aplastic anaemia* – this may be primary, or more commonly secondary to toxic exposure (especially to chemotherapy or radiotherapy) or to an idiosyncratic drug reaction;

3. *abnormal cellular infiltrates,* which may be haematological (leukaemia, lymphoma, myeloma) or metastatic (carcinoma).

There are many other situations in which a bone-marrow examination may be indicated. Consultation with a haematologist is advisable when ordering a bone-marrow biopsy.

COAGULATION DISORDERS: BLEEDING AND THROMBOSIS

THE COAGULATION CASCADE

Traditionally the coagulation cascade has been arbitrarily divided into the intrinsic or contact pathway, and the extrinsic or tissue-factor pathway (Figure 29.3.1). Behind this artificial subdivision of the coagulation process lies a much more intricate and complicated process. For practical purposes, the contact and tissue-factor pathways provide a simple means of measuring

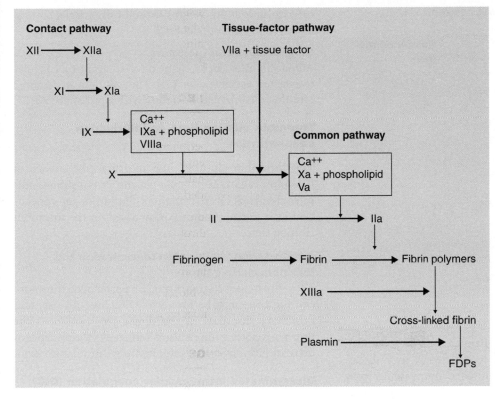

Figure 29.3.1 The coagulation cascade. FDPs, fibrin degradation products. Factors V, VIII, XI and XIII are activated by thrombin. Phospholipid is provided by the platelet external membranes. Platelets are activated to aggregate while releasing the contents of their storage granules, including fibrinogen and von Willebrand factor. They form a primary haemostatic plug, which is then strengthened by fibrin strands formed by the coagulation process.

coagulation activity when diagnosing bleeding disorders and monitoring therapy for haemorrhagic and thrombotic disorders.

INVESTIGATION OF A BLEEDING DISORDER

History

A stepwise approach to bleeding disorders should begin with a thorough history covering the following points:

- bleeding after previous surgery or dental extraction, previous transfusion;
- easy bruising, bleeding after trauma;
- spontaneous haemorrhage into joints or muscle, spontaneous epistaxis, unexplained haematuria;
- primary menorrhagia;
- family history.

Investigations

Screening tests that are available in all laboratories include the following:

- platelet count;
- INR, APTT, fibrinogen, FDP and thrombin clotting time.

Special tests that are available only in reference laboratories include the following:

- coagulation factor assays;
- von Willebrand factor;
- platelet function tests.

Caution is required because normal screening tests do not rule out a bleeding disorder. In addition, an abnormal test result should be interpreted in the context of the patient's clinical history and circumstances.

Bleeding times are measured in some specialized centres for assessment of selected patients with hereditary bleeding disorders. There is substantial operator and laboratory variability in assessment of the bleeding time.

COAGULATION TESTS

The most common tests are the prothrombin time and activated partial thromboplastin time (APTT).

An abnormal clotting time (INR or APTT) may be artefactual. The test should therefore always be repeated with a carefully collected fresh specimen to check an abnormal result.

Prothrombin time

The prothrombin time is prolonged in deficiencies of coagulation factors in the tissue-factor pathway or common pathway. The results are usually expressed as the INR, which is a calculation based on the prothrombin time (Table 29.3.3).

Table 29.3.3 Oral anticoagulation therapy

Clinical indications	Recommended INR*
Venous thrombosis High-risk atrial fibrillation Rheumatic heart valve Tissue prosthetic heart valve After myocardial infarction	2.0–3.0
Mechanical prosthetic heart valve (low risk)†	2.5–3.5
Mechanical prosthetic heart valve (high risk)†	3.0–4.5

*Australian Society of Thrombosis and Haemostasis Working Party.
† Consult the patient's cardiologist.

Interpretation

The prothrombin time may be increased in oral anticoagulation therapy, vitamin K deficiency, liver disease, hypofibrinogenaemia, disseminated intravascular coagulation (DIC), massive blood transfusion or *in-vitro* artefact.

Clinical uses

The prothrombin time is most often used to monitor warfarin therapy. It is relatively insensitive to heparin.

Activated partial thromboplastin time (APTT)

The APTT is prolonged in deficiencies of coagulation factors in the contact pathway or the common pathway.

Interpretation

The APTT can be increased in liver disease, DIC, oral anticoagulants, heparin, newborn, *in-vitro* artefact, standard heparin therapy, von Willebrand's disease, antiphospholipid antibodies, and deficiency of or an inhibitor against factors VIII, IX, XI or XII.

Clinical uses

The APTT is most often used to monitor standard heparin therapy. Low-molecular-weight heparins do not generally affect the APTT. However, because they have very predictable pharmacokinetics and *in-vitro* activity, monitoring is not required.

Lupus anticoagulant

Patients with the lupus anticoagulant may also show positivity for anticardiolipin antibodies. The lupus anticoagulant and anticardiolipin antibodies often occur in individuals with no apparent underlying illness. They are common in systemic lupus erythematosus, and also occur in other autoimmune disorders, in inflammation, and may be secondary to certain drugs. Important clinical associations are venous thrombosis, arterial thrombosis and recurrent fetal loss.

Coagulation factor inhibitors

Autoantibodies can rarely be directed against a coagulation factor, usually factor VIII. They result in an acquired bleeding disorder in association with a prolonged APTT.

Thrombin clotting time and fibrinogen concentration

The thrombin clotting time measures the ability of thrombin to clot the patient's plasma. Prolongation indicates abnormal fibrin formation. The fibrinogen concentration is measured by an assay based on the thrombin clotting time.

Interpretation of fibrinogen concentration and thrombin clotting time

A low fibrinogen concentration or a prolonged thrombin clotting time may be found in DIC, liver disease, and hereditary disorders of the fibrinogen molecule. The thrombin clotting time is also prolonged by the presence of heparin. Fibrinogen levels are often raised in inflammation.

Disseminated intravascular coagulation (DIC)

In disseminated intravascular coagulation there is overactivity of the coagulation cascade with enhancement of fibrinolysis. Widespread intravascular thrombosis occurs. There is depletion of clotting factors and platelets, resulting in a bleeding disorder. The diagnosis of DIC involves a combination of clinical suspicion and confirmatory laboratory results. Characteristically there is elevation of fibrin degradation products (FDP), prolongation of the INR, APTT and thrombin time, and reduced fibrinogen levels and platelet counts.

D-dimer In many laboratories the FDP level is estimated by the D-dimer test. The D-dimer is produced during fibrinolysis by degradation of cross-linked fibrin polymer. The D-dimer level reflects both coagulation and fibrinolytic activity. It is highly sensitive but non-specific for DIC.

Interpretation of D-dimer The D-dimer is increased in DIC, but is also raised in acute venous thromboembolism, acute myocardial infarction, severe pneumonia, after major surgery, or in association with any cause of inflammation. Very high levels (above about 3.2 mg/L in the author's laboratory) are unlikely to be due to conditions other than DIC.

Platelet function tests

Platelet function can be assessed by platelet aggregation studies and the template bleeding time. The role of these tests is mainly in the diagnosis of those hereditary bleeding disorders in which there is a defect of platelet function. Performance of the tests should be accompanied by careful assessment by a haematologist of the patient's personal and family history of bleeding.

Tests for heparin-induced thrombocytopenia (HIT)

This syndrome is caused by antibodies to heparin–platelet factor 4 complexes. The patient develops thrombocytopenia (usually $< 100 \times 10^9/L$) while on heparin. The syndrome may be complicated by extensive and life-threatening venous or arterial thrombosis. Tests are available to detect the heparin-associated antibodies.

TESTS FOR A THROMBOTIC TENDENCY

For patients with venous thrombo-embolism it is important to consider tests for predisposing conditions. It is possible to identify a predisposing condition in about 50% of cases.

The lupus anticoagulant is an acquired condition and was discussed earlier in the section on APTT. A common hereditary condition is the heterozygous state for activated protein C resistance, also known as the factor V Leiden gene mutation. It is present in about 3–5% of the normal Caucasian population, and has been found in about 30–40% of cases of hereditary thrombophilia. Other important hereditary conditions predisposing to thrombosis are deficiencies of antithrombin III, protein C or protein S. It is becoming increasingly important to screen for these disorders. A careful family history is important, but is negative in many cases.

Inherited thrombotic syndromes should be tested for in the following circumstances:

- patients who present with spontaneous thrombosis;
- young patients;
- unusually severe or extensive thrombosis;
- unusual site;
- family history of thrombosis.

Advice to the affected patient depends on a careful evaluation of the personal and family history of venous thrombo-embolism. In many cases it is sufficient to counsel the patient about situations that are associated with a high risk of venous thrombo-embolism, and to recommend appropriate prophylaxis where indicated (e.g. for major surgery). In some cases the test results may contribute to a decision to embark on long-term anticoagulation.

CONCLUSION

A basic understanding of haematology testing is important in surgical practice. Many patients have an abnormality in the CBE on presentation. These abnormalities may be important for diagnosis, and may require correction prior to surgery. Abnormalities of haemostasis must be identified and treated before surgery. In addition, venous thrombosis is a frequent and often life-threatening complication in the post-operative period, and it is important to identify patients who are at risk.

FURTHER READING

Brandt J, Barna L, Triplett D. 1995: Laboratory identification of lupus anticoagulants: results of the Second International Workshop for Identification of Lupus Anticoagulants. *Thrombosis and Haemostasis* 74, 1597–603.

Chui D, Waye J. 1998: Hydrops fetalis caused by α-thalassemia: an emerging health care problem. *Blood* 91, 2213–22.

Dacic J, Lewis S. 1995: *Practical haematology*, 8th edn. Edinburgh: Churchill Livingstone.

Griffiths E, Dzik W. 1997: Assays for heparin-induced thrombocytopenia. *Transfusion Medicine* 7, 1–11.

Goodeve A. 1998: Laboratory methods for the genetic diagnosis of bleeding disorders. *Clinical and Laboratory Haematology* 20, 3–19.

Isselbacher KJ, Braunwald E, Wilson JD, Martin JB, Fauci AS, Kaspar DL (eds). 1998: *Harrison's principles of internal medicine*, 14th edn. New York: McGraw-Hill.

Hillarp A, Dahlback B, Zoller B. 1995: Activated protein C resistance: from phenotype to genotype and clinical practice. *Blood Reviews* 9, 201–12.

Hoffbrand A, Pettit J. 1993: *Essential haematology*, 3rd edn. Oxford: Blackwell Scientific Publications.

Mazza J. 1995: *Manual of clinical haematology*, 2nd edn. Boston, MA: Little, Brown & Co.

Rosendaal FR. 1997: Risk factors for venous thrombosis: prevalence, risk and interaction. *Semin Hematol* 34, 171–87.

Sadler JE, Matsushita T, Dong Z, *et al.* 1995: Molecular mechanism and classification of von Willebrand disease. *Thrombosis and Haemostasis* 74, 161–6.

Simioni P, Prandoni P, Lensing AWA, *et al.* 1997: The risk of recurrent venous thromboembolism in patients with an $Arg^{506} \rightarrow$ Gln mutation in the gene for factor V (factor V Leiden). *New England Journal of Medicine* 336, 399–403.

Warkentin T, Chong B, Greinacher A. 1998: Heparin-induced thrombocytopenia: towards consensus. *Thrombosis and Haemostasis* 79, 1–7.

Microbiological investigations

John M.B. Smith

Introduction

While the laboratory services available to surgeons vary tremendously from one hospital to another, a few basic points concerning the type of specimen required and the time and interpretation of subsequent laboratory-generated information deserve comment.

SPECIMENS

Although the classical 'swab' sent to the laboratory in an appropriate transport medium is the easiest specimen to obtain, it should be possible with most infections encountered in surgery to send pus or other fluid/secretions, or even tissue, to the laboratory. These are vastly superior to the 'swab'. In cases where anaerobes are likely to be involved, care should be taken to exclude air from the specimen. Simply plugging the end of a syringe, in which an aspirate has been obtained, with a rubber stopper or cork is adequate in this respect.

In most situations, expectorated sputum is sufficient for investigations involving possible pulmonary infections. More aggressive and invasive techniques (e.g. bronchial brushing and lavage, trans-tracheal aspirates) are only warranted in a few situations (e.g. possible pneumocystis pneumonia) – and even then not as the initial line of investigation.

Where lesions are absent and/or bacteraemia is suspected, blood cultures are mandatory. Although blood-culture techniques differ widely between laboratories, the basic principles remain constant. The important points are summarized below.

1. Blood may contain fewer than one microbe/mL. It is therefore important to obtain as much blood as is practicable, usually a minimum of 10 mL from an adult. Some laboratories recommend a minimum of 20–30 mL, especially where non-automated culture systems are employed.

2. Blood should be obtained from a new 'clean' venepuncture site. Intravenous catheters readily become colonized by bacteria and are unsuitable sites for obtaining blood.

3. Blood is obtained aseptically in a syringe and immediately placed in a 'set' of warmed blood-culture bottles at the bedside. This set contains two bottles – one aerobic and one anaerobic. Up to 10 mL (maximum) of the blood is placed in each bottle, giving a dilution of medium to blood of around 5:1. This stops the blood clotting, and also helps to dilute out any antimicrobial substances present in the blood. It is important not to overfill bottles associated with automated machines, as this may result in false-positive readings. If in doubt, consult the medical microbiologist.

4. As bacteria may be only transiently present in the blood, 3 sets (i.e. 6 bottles) of cultures taken over a 24-h period or at fever spikes are recommended.

Increasing this number has been shown to have little effect on the final result. In cases where patients are seriously ill and the clinician is anxious to commence antibiotic therapy, the 24-h period can be dispensed with or shortened to a few minutes. In such cases, one or two sets are probably sufficient.

5. Although blood should ideally be taken before any antibiotic therapy has been commenced, it can still be obtained and processed after this has been instituted. In such cases, the laboratory must be informed (preferably before the blood is taken), so that appropriate measures can be implemented to neutralize any residual antibiotic remaining in the blood.

6. Where fungi are suspected of being the causal microbe, special techniques and/or increased incubation periods may be required. The laboratory should be notified of this possibility.

Specimens for virological and chlamydial studies must include cells scraped from the lesion (as the causative microbes are intracellular). Special transport media are also required (check with the local laboratory).

All specimens should be transferred to the laboratory as soon as possible. This is especially important for urine samples, where a delay of 2 h or more can seriously affect the subsequent laboratory findings.

Serological tests for the detection of circulating antibody or antigen are available for many microbial infections. These are of most use in cases where the causative microbe is non-culturable or presents other problems with regard to its growth and isolation in the laboratory, and where the pathological significance of an isolate is in some doubt. This applies to many viral infections and to a few other infectious diseases (e.g. invasive candidosis, rheumatic heart disease). Of the antibody tests that are currently available, enzyme-linked immunosorbent assays (ELISAs) lend themselves well to automation and large-scale surveys. These sensitive tests are available for detecting antibody levels in a variety of infectious diseases, including human immunodeficiency virus (HIV) infection. While it is usual to demonstrate a significant (i.e. fourfold) rise in antibody titre between sera obtained in the acute and convalescent phase of the illness, infections where the causal microbe is not part of the normal flora can often be confirmed with a 'one-off' specimen. ELISAs are able to distinguish antibody to the different immunoglobulin classes (e.g. IgM, IgG). The results are expressed as a titre, which is the reciprocal of the last positive dilution. Thus a titre of 256 implies that the last positive serum dilution was 1 in 256.

Unfortunately, antibody tests are seldom 100% sensitive or specific – a feature that is usually related to the crude nature of the antigen employed. Where false positivity may create concern (e.g. in HIV infection), confirmatory tests which detect antibody against purified microbial antigens can be considered. The immunoblotting tests currently used to detect antibody against unique HIV antigens (e.g. gp120, p41) are a classical example of such a test.

In the early phase of infection, or in patients who fail to mount a significant antibody response following infection, or where such a response is delayed (e.g. in immunocompromised patients), detection of circulating microbial antigens may aid the diagnosis (e.g. chronically infected hepatitis B patients, and surgical patients with possible invasive candidosis). Assays ranging from crude latex agglutination using antibody-coated (sensitized) latex beads to more sensitive ELISAs, in which plates are coated with antibody rather than antigen as in the antibody tests, are available.

In addition, specific microbial antigens can be detected in tissues or similar specimens using fluorescent-antibody techniques. Such techniques have been enhanced by the availability of monoclonal antibodies against clinically relevant microbial antigens. As the number and usefulness of serological tests is continually changing, surgeons should consult with their medical microbiologist to clarify the local situation. It is not unusual for laboratories to receive totally inappropriate serological requests (and specimens) (e.g. a 'one-off' serum sample with the accompanying form simply stating 'viral antibodies').

INITIAL LABORATORY INVESTIGATIONS

With most specimens, direct microscopy or similar procedures will often provide the clinician with some idea of the likely causal organism. This is especially true for sputum, urine, aspirates including cerebrospinal fluid, and pus, where a Gram stain is an extremely quick (< 5 min) and accurate way of obtaining some knowledge of the pathological process involved. As well as providing presumptive identification of any microbes present (as judged by shape, size and Gram-stain reaction), the presence or absence of inflammatory cells (e.g. polymorphonuclear leucocytes) and other host material can be extremely informative to the clinician. The value of the direct Gram stain cannot be overemphasized.

Other useful staining and/or direct microscopic techniques include the Ziehl-Neelsen acid-fast and auramine O stains (for mycobacteria), potassium hydroxide and/or calcofluor white wet preparations for fungi, electron microscopy for viruses (e.g. rotaviruses, herpes viruses) and fluorescent-antibody techniques (FAT). The availability of specific monoclonal antibodies against important antigens of a number of microbes (e.g. herpes simplex viruses, chlamydiae) has allowed their rapid visualization in appropriate specimens.

In cases where bacteria are not visible in specimens, an indication of their presence may be obtainable by the detection of antigenic material or by the demonstration of microbial metabolic by-products (e.g. increased lactate levels) in the specimen. The demonstration of capsular antigens from bacteria such as *Streptococcus pneumoniae* in clinical material can now be achieved by a variety of serological techniques (e.g. latex agglutination). Apart from the polymicrobial appearance on Gram staining, an indication that pus from an abscess contains anaerobes can be obtained by the demonstration of characteristic fatty acids in the specimen using gas–liquid chromatography (in addition to its foul smell).

Molecular techniques are now widely employed for detecting unique microbial DNA or RNA sequences in pathological specimens. These have proved extremely useful with infections where the causal microbes are present in low numbers and/or difficult to culture (e.g. viral infections of the central nervous system). The polymerase chain reaction (PCR) amplification of specific nucleotide sequences is perhaps the most widely used of the molecular techniques. This permits the detection (by amplification) of small amounts of unique DNA in specimens. Detection of specific gene sequences (e.g. by gene probes, nucleic acid probes) has also been employed in the identification of microbes, and in the detection of antibiotic resistance in bacteria such as methicillin-resistant *Staphylococcus aureus*, where interpretation of the usual laboratory techniques may be troublesome. Gene probes usually lack an amplification step, but are readily applicable to cultures of the isolated pathogen or to some pathogens *in situ*. Although expensive, nucleic acid probe and amplification technology is now widely employed in many laboratories.

In addition, DNA fingerprinting of isolates using a variety of techniques (e.g. pulsed-field gel electrophoresis of endonuclease-cleaved DNA) has greatly facilitated epidemiological studies and our ability to identify strains or biotypes at a molecular level. Another increasingly widely used typing procedure is ribotyping, which involves analysis of restriction fragments with probes that detect rRNA sequences. Molecular biological techniques are now an integral part of the modern day microbiological laboratory, but perhaps beyond the scope of smaller units.

CULTURE AND OTHER INVESTIGATIONS

Provided that adequate information is conveyed on the requisition form accompanying specimens, the laboratory will carry out the appropriate culture and other investigations (e.g. antibiotic sensitivities). In most laboratories, sensitivity testing is only performed on isolates which the laboratory staff consider to be potentially significant – hence the need for adequate information on requisition forms. Any 'unusual' sensitivities must be specifically requested. With the Vitek automated system, the Gram-positive susceptibility card (GPS-IX) includes the following antibiotics: ciprofloxacin, clindamycin, erythromycin, fusidic acid, gentamicin, nitrofurantoin, oxacillin, penicillin G, rifampicin, tetracycline, vancomycin and a β-lactamase detector.

Catheter-related sepsis is a potentially life-threatening infection caused by microbial colonization of an indwelling intravenous catheter. A variety of laboratory techniques are available for the microbiological investigation of this problem. In the past these quantitative tests required removal of the catheter, and were designed to distinguish significant disease-associated colonization from insignificant low-level contamination. Recent studies have shown that by using an endoluminal brush technique, it is possible to detect infected central venous catheters *in situ*. The brush, which has nylon bristles wound tightly around the distal end of a stainless steel wire, is passed down the catheter to the inner end, withdrawn and then cultured. Such a procedure has the potential to reduce removal of non-colonized catheters that are wrongly suspected of being the source of an infection.

Antimicrobial sensitivity testing

Determining the antibiotic sensitivity of an isolate is important in situations where the incidence of potentially resistant strains is high or increasing, where potentially life-threatening illnesses are involved, and where it is important to know accurately the susceptibility (in mg/L of antibiotic) of an isolate to particular antibiotics. Although the laboratory conditions employed with sensitivity testing are far removed from those which occur in the body, there does appear to be a reasonable correlation between the results generated and subsequent clinical outcome. A variety of techniques are available for sensitivity testing, such as disc diffusion, liquid and agar dilution tests, and the E test (Figure 29.4.1), details of which need not be repeated here. Dilution and E tests are quantitative and allow determination of minimum inhibitory concentrations (MICs), and in some cases can be extended to establish minimum bactericidal concentrations (MBCs).

In the laboratory reports that are given to clinicians, sensitivity results for isolates considered by laboratory staff to be potentially significant are simply listed as susceptible, intermediate or resistant to the drug in question. Only in exceptional circumstances will actual MIC figures expressed in mg/L be quoted. The term 'susceptible' implies that the infection should respond to normal doses/regimens of that particular antibiotic. The term 'intermediate' (or 'moderately susceptible') indicates that doses above those normally given are probably required for a satisfactory outcome, or that a

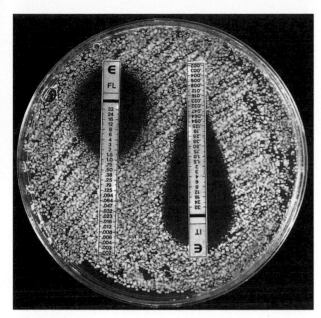

Figure 29.4.1 E-test sensitivity on a strain of *Candida albicans*. The MICs for the antifungals shown are 1.5 mg/L for fluconazole (FL) and 0.064 mg/L for itraconazole (IT).

favourable response can be expected only if infection occurs in an area of the body where natural concentration of the drug occurs (e.g. in the bladder/urine). The term 'resistant' indicates that the microbe will be unaffected by any safely achievable drug levels. In practice, many laboratories only report susceptible and resistant categories. Antibiotics that are demonstrated to be ineffective (resistant) should be withdrawn as soon as possible, and replaced by those listed as potentially effective (susceptible) in order to reduce the risks of morbidity and mortality.

In general, sensitivity testing presents few problems for laboratory staff in terms of procedure and interpretation, although detection of potential resistance in some microbes (e.g. methicillin resistance in *Staphylococcus aureus*) relies heavily on the use of appropriate techniques. Demonstration of the *mec*A gene using recently developed molecular techniques is now clearly the most appropriate way to confirm the methicillin-resistant potential of isolates.

In addition to the tests mentioned above, rapid tests are available for detecting β-lactamase activity in bacteria (e.g. the chromogenic cephalosporin assay). The clinical use of these assays is to provide a rapid indication of β-lactamase activity, which may not always be apparent with more conventional sensitivity tests.

Serum assays on patients during antibiotic therapy

In seriously ill patients who are not responding to an expected adequate antibiotic-dosing regimen, it is often necessary to monitor blood levels to show that the therapy being used is achieving a suitably 'high' antibiotic blood level. With bacterial endocarditis (one of the few diseases thoroughly studied), a satisfactory clinical response is known to be associated with serum antibiotic levels at least 8 times the MBC at all times. There is currently some debate about the need for and/or usefulness of serum assays, especially in patients who are responding well to therapy. Tests known as serum bactericidal assays (SBAs) are usually performed on blood specimens obtained immediately before the next antibiotic dose (i.e. when levels will be at their lowest).

All patients who are receiving aminoglycosides *must* have blood levels determined at regular intervals. The methodology and interpretation of results varies depending on the dosing regimen being used. With 24-h dosing schedules, patients receive between 5 and 7 mg/kg of gentamicin (or tobramycin or netilmicin) as a single 30-min infusion every 24 h. Peak serum levels are in the range 15–25 mg/L and clearly well above minimum therapeutic levels (5 mg/L), and do not need to be measured. However, in order to minimize potential nephro- and ototoxicity, it is important to maintain the 24-h trough levels below 0.5 mg/L. As this level is difficult to measure, blood levels are measured at some convenient time during the 24-h cycle, and by the use of a computer or other methodologies the level that is likely to be present after 24 h is calculated. An indication of the recommended 'safe' levels at various times during the 24-h period is shown in Table 29.4.1. If trough levels are observed to be exceeding the safety level, increasing the time interval between doses, rather than lowering the next dose, is recommended. Regular monitoring, especially in cases where renal function is poor or deteriorating, is mandatory. Although clearly less toxic than multiple daily dosing schedules, unacceptably high levels of drug accumulation and related toxicity can occur with once-daily routines. Amikacin dose and trough levels vary to those for the three aminoglycosides mentioned above (e.g. 15 mg/kg once daily with safe levels at 18 h post-infusion being < 2 mg/L; see also Table 29.4.1).

TIMING AND INTERPRETATION OF LABORATORY REPORTS

Like other branches of medicine, microbiology has advanced and changed dramatically in the last decade – and continues to do so. It is therefore imperative that clinicians be in constant communication with the laboratory and its staff. Failure in this respect will undoubtedly result in errors in patient management, especially with regard to antibiotic therapy.

Direct microscopy/Gram-stain results can be avail-

Table 29.4.1 Suggested 'safe' aminoglycoside serum levels with once-daily dosing schedules

Time post-injection (h)	Serum level (mg/L)*
6	4–7
8	3–5
10	2–3
12	1–2
14	0.5–1

*Figures shown apply to gentamicin, tobramycin and netilmicin; double these levels for amikacin (see Bailey TC, Little JR, Littenburg B, Reichley RM, Dunagan WC. 1997: A meta-analysis of extended interval dosing versus multiple daily dosing of aminoglycosides. *Clinical Infectious Diseases* **24**, 786–95).

able within minutes of the specimen reaching the laboratory – these can easily be collected and examined by junior medical staff. Preliminary culture results should be available after overnight incubation, and confirmation of the identification may take a further 24 h or longer. It generally takes a minimum of 48 h for anaerobe culture results to become available.

Antibiotic sensitivities on potentially significant isolates should be available within 24 to 48 h depending on the sophistication of the laboratory. While isolates may be tested against a range of eight or more potentially useful antimicrobials (see above), most laboratories restrict their reporting to just a few of these, although information regarding the others will be available on request. Important implications may be drawn from reports. For example, methicillin (oxacillin) resistance in *Staphylococcus aureus* implies that the microbe is resistant to all β-lactams, including imipenem and co-amoxiclav. Listing a Gram-negative bacillus as ampicillin (amoxycillin) susceptible suggests that it will also be susceptible to co-amoxiclav. Not all laboratories examine Gram-negative coliforms for potential extended-spectrum β-lactamase (ESBL) activity, even though about 2% of routine isolates are likely to be positive. Clinicians should bear this in mind in the case of patients who are responding poorly to apparently appropriate cephalosporin therapy. High-level gentamicin resistance in enterococci means that the synergistic properties of combined penicillin and aminoglycoside therapy are lost. In addition, enterococci resistant to amoxycillin are unlikely to respond to co-amoxiclav, as resistance is usually mediated by alterations to the penicillin-binding protein target site, rather than β-lactamase production. One additional word of caution – many laboratories test only one example of a group of antibiotics against the isolated pathogen (e.g. cefotaxime as the third-generation cephalosporin). While susceptibility or resistance to this example invariably implies a similar result to others in the group (e.g. ceftriaxone), this may not always be the case. Surgeons should check with their own laboratories to clarify individual reporting idiosyncrasies.

Where automated blood-culture machines are used, bacterial growth may be confirmed within 6–8 h. Non-automated systems require overnight or longer incubation. At this stage a Gram stain on positive bottles will give a clue as to the nature of the bacterium, although culture and sensitivity results require a further 12–24 h. After this initial 24-h period, blood-culture results are notified only if they are positive, with the final report being available at around 5–10 days, depending on the system employed. As a general rule, most cases of bacteraemia reveal positive blood cultures within 24 h; specimens from possible cases of infective endocarditis may take longer to reveal microbial growth.

When a report is received, the clinician must review the laboratory findings in the light of the patient's clinical condition and ongoing therapy, and decide whether or not antimicrobial therapy should be initiated or changed.

FURTHER READING

Emori TG, Gaynes RP. 1993: An overview of nosocomial infections, including the role of the microbiology laboratory. *Clinical Microbiology Reviews* **6**, 428–42.

Kite P, Dobbins BM, Wilcox MH, *et al.* 1997: Evaluation of a novel endoluminal brush method for *in situ* diagnosis of catheter-related sepsis. *Journal of Clinical Pathology* **50**, 278–82.

Koneman EM, Allen SD, Janda WM, Schreckenberger PC, Winn WC. 1997: *Color atlas and textbook of diagnostic microbiology*, 5th edn. Philadelphia, PA: Lippincott-Raven.

LaRocco MT, Bugert SJ. 1997: Infection in the bone marrow transplant recipient and role of the microbiology laboratory in clinical transplantation. *Clinical Microbiology Reviews* **10**, 277–97.

Reimer LG, Wilson ML, Weinstein MP. 1997: Update on detection of bacteremia and fungemia. *Clinical Microbiology Reviews* **10**, 444–65.

Chapter 29.5

Surgical pathology and cytology

John Blennerhassett

Introduction

The professional interaction between the surgeon and the pathologist is based on ensuring that pathological examination and interpretation provide maximum benefit for the patient. The methods used to examine a particular pathology specimen thus depend on what clinical problem requires resolution.

The surgeon must therefore attempt to address the following question. 'What clinical information about this patient, what specimen and what detail about that specimen should I supply so that the pathologist can give me the pathological interpretation that I need for the best management of this patient, and will this require special laboratory techniques and therefore special handling of the tissue?' Often these requirements are simply met by use of an 'inter-expert shorthand' between colleagues who have long worked together and where, together with demographic data, the terse information 'R hemicolectomy . . . SBO asc. col., unsucc. colonosc., presumed Ca.' when skilfully interpreted means 'Right hemicolectomy in a . . . patient with subacute (colonic) obstruction in whom attempted colonoscopic visualization of the lesion was unsuccessful; I presume it to be carcinoma. If so, I want a thorough assessment for tumour type and grade, extent of local spread (including lymph and blood vascular channels) and lymph-node involvement, a synoptic report and a staging (Dukes/Aster-Coller/TNM). If not carcinoma, I need to know the nature of the disease process, its extent and complications, an interpretation and, if possible, reference to a comprehensive summary of the nature and natural history of the disease.' On the other hand, with a complex and/or obscure clinical problem, more extensive clinical information (often including pre- and/or post-operative

interdepartmental consultation) will pave the way for the most useful interpretation possible by the pathologist, including the use of special techniques. In some instances, pre-operative consultation is essential (e.g. for immunoflow cytometry, cytomolecular and/or ultrastructural studies).

In turn, the surgeon should be confident that the pathologist will address the questions 'What information and interpretation can I supply in order to allow optimal management in this clinical situation? What techniques are appropriate (out of all those that are available) in assembling my report?' It is reasonable for the surgeon to expect the use of appropriate pathology techniques to supply maximum useful information (e.g. specimen radiology for certain breast biopsies) and to remonstrate if failure to apply such techniques compromises the examination. However, it is often the case that much more is possible than is appropriate. Expensive and time-consuming examinations (e.g. special studies for possible micrometastases in lymph nodes draining a cancer) which give data that are not known to influence either therapy or prognosis are properly regarded as research activities and treated as such.

Therefore the pathologist should view the request for an opinion as a clinical consultation from a surgical colleague, as do other clinical colleagues, including being supplied with appropriate demographic and clinical data. While it is the duty of the pathologist to seek and consider relevant clinical details in formulating an opinion, the surgeon cannot escape some responsibility if an erroneous opinion is given because important clinical information, known to the clinical team, was not supplied to the pathologist. Finally, there is no place for the following clinical attitude towards the pathology consultant: 'We wanted your unbiased opinion, so we withheld the clinical information.' Litigation money has changed hands and professional collegiality has been forfeited because of such an approach to consultation.

THE ROLE OF TISSUE SAMPLING IN SURGICAL PRACTICE

Anatomical pathology subserves several roles in surgical practice. Excluding consideration of the roles of planned (as distinct from day-to-day) clinical research and autopsy in clinical audit, the study of structural and functional morphology subserves any combination of three major purposes, namely pathological diagnosis (pathology, pathogenesis and aetiology), assessment of the likely adequacy of the surgical therapy, and staging of the extent of disease process (commonly, but not exclusively, cancer).

ESTABLISHING A PATHOLOGICAL DIAGNOSIS

Exfoliative cytology

The commonest sites that are suitable for exfoliative, touch preparation or brush sampling cytology are genital, respiratory, body cavity (including subarachnoid) and oesophago-gastro-duodenal. Other sites are sampled relatively infrequently except in special units. The information sought is generally twofold, namely diagnosis of malignancy or infection. Techniques for cell collection and fixation are standard and simple, and they are also critical for optimal study and must be understood by those obtaining the specimen and followed with care. Standard stains are usually used solely for morphological evaluation. Special techniques (e.g. for viral identification) require prior consultation and planning.

Fine-needle aspiration (FNA) biopsy

Breast, lung, liver, thyroid, lymph node and other sites are popular for sampling by this technique, which provides well-preserved cells with potentially minimal artefact when appropriate preparation techniques are used. With the added advantage of precise localization by standard radiographs, computerized tomography, ultrasound and other imaging techniques, it appears that few sites in the body are beyond the scope of fine-needle aspiration sampling. This technique also lends itself to more extensive special testing than does most exfoliative cytology.

There is little doubt that 'the better the preparation, the better the interpretation' and, in general, slide preparation is best left to the cytopathology technologist and the pathologist who perform the technique frequently and adeptly, and who bear the ultimate responsibility for the quality of the preparations and their interpretation. It is probably less important who performs the actual biopsy. In personally carrying out the needle placement and sampling, the clinician knows precisely what tissue needs to be sampled, the pathologist will gain added knowledge of the macroscopic and textural features of the sampled tissue, and the radiologist can best guide localization of the sampling device within deep structures such as lung or retroperitoneum, as does the surgeon manipulating the endoscope. More important than who obtains the material is the critical matter of rapidity and deftness of fixation of the tissue once it has been removed. The surgeon who takes personal responsibility for this aspect must be meticulous in learning and using an appropriate technique. However, it is seldom optimally performed as a 'one-person procedure'.

There are a few essential considerations for specific sites.

Breast It is essential for the surgeon and pathologist to establish local ground rules. There can be few pathologists who are not influenced in their precise diagnostic terminology by the anticipated reaction of the surgeon. A totally objective cytological 'cancer/non-cancer' diagnostic spread might be as follows: (i) benign; (ii) suspicious for malignancy (various levels perhaps); (iii) malignant. Most pathologists show a count biased from (iii) towards (ii) if a diagnosis of (iii) will automatically lead to immediate definitive therapy such as mastectomy or wide local resection with axillary clearance. Less inhibition in the use of (iii) is more likely in situations where biopsy confirmation (e.g. core biopsy) is usually sought by the surgeon following a 'malignant' FNA call.

Lymph node It is unusual to undertake FNA biopsy of a lymph node in a situation where either malignant lymphoma or infection can confidently be excluded. The pathologist should keep samples in special media for microbial culture, immunocytological and cytomolecular genetic studies. Storage is not expensive, but failure to anticipate the need for storage may prove to be so. Material that is not required can be discarded.

Thyroid A papillary carcinoma diagnosis can usually be made or strongly suspected, as can medullary carcinoma. A distinction between follicular neoplasia and colloid nodule is usually possible, but a distinction between follicular adenoma and carcinoma is usually impossible unless the carcinoma is poorly differentiated. Therefore the non-committal term 'thyroid neoplasia' (beware interpreting this to mean malignancy) is used, and excision is the usual choice, providing both definitive diagnosis and therapy.

General It is not always possible to provide for all eventualities, but it is useful to put aside slides for possible special (e.g. immunoperoxidase) studies which may be indicated after examination of the standard stains (e.g. in the diagnosis of melanoma or neuroendocrine carcinoma). If the lesion is accessible, repeat sampling is always possible in difficult cases or for special studies.

Incision/punch/core/sample biopsy

These are commonly used to sample large or disseminated disease for diagnosis, e.g. breast masses/mammographically defined lesions, and masses/other lesions sampled by endoscopy of gastrointestinal, respiratory and urinary tracts, cervix and endometrium, peritoneal, pleural and pericardial tissues, as well as other organs and tissues accessible under imaging guidance.

The term 'sample' biopsy is used to include sampling of disseminated or extensive disease. In surgical (as opposed to dermatological) practice, common instances are lymph-node biopsy for possible lymphoma/metastatic malignancy/infective/inflammatory processes, or other tissues (usually for suspected metastatic malignant disease). Lymph-node sampling should be of one or more whole abnormal node(s), with the pathologist partitioning the freshly excised node (as for FNA). For disseminated or metastatic malignancy of unknown origin, prior consultation with the pathologist will ensure that appropriately prepared material is available for special studies (e.g. immunomorphology, including steroid receptor status, cytomolecular genetic or ultrastructural studies, etc.), should these be required.

ESTABLISHING BOTH DIAGNOSIS AND ADEQUACY OF THERAPY

This is usually accomplished by excision biopsy or regional resection.

Definitive one-stage procedure

Examples include gastrointestinal polypectomy, skin-biopsy excision, gastrointestinal regional excision (suspected, unconfirmed cancer or other, e.g. inflammatory disease) and other excisions for disease previously diagnosed by one of the methods described above (e.g. breast, bronchus, genito-urinary, musculoskeletal). Special studies to differentiate between neoplasms may be particularly useful here, including empirical histo-

chemistry such as periodic acid–Schiff and Giemsa stains, immunohistochemistry for typing of neoplasms and for identification of invasive vs. *in-situ* malignancy, etc. Despite enthusiastic published information on the subject of ultrastructural studies in surgical pathology, particularly tumour pathology, with the use of critical evaluation of cytology and architecture together with the widespread use of immunomorphology, it is rare that electron microscopy is pivotal in influencing therapy (with the exception of certain renal, dermatological and myopathic diseases). It is helpfully confirmatory in Langerhans' histiocytosis and allegedly in the differential diagnosis between pleural spread of adenocarcinoma and mesothelioma (although in reality it rarely has an effective influence on the latter in medico-legal let alone clinical decision-making).

Intra-operative consultation

The key knowledge required by the surgeon, as noted above, is pathological diagnosis together with adequacy of therapy. Either or both may require intra-operative consultation, usually with a rapid (frozen) section. The commonest and most useful consultations in our experience (mutually agreed by surgeons and pathologists) are as follows:

1. establishment of a diagnosis where pre-operative attempts were unsuccessful, but definitive therapy has been embarked upon (e.g. possible carcinoma of the head of the pancreas). These cases become more unusual as imaging techniques and interventions are refined;

2. establishment of a definitive diagnosis during craniospinal neurosurgical procedures in order to establish the need for and/or desirability of complete excision (e.g. neurilemmoma, meningioma, low-grade glioma, haemangioblastoma) vs. the need for adequate biopsy alone in order to guide future non-surgical therapy (e.g. high-grade glioma, lymphoma, metastatic malignancy);

3. mini-staging procedure to guide the decision to proceed with or abandon further surgery (e.g. intra-operative liver biopsy in bowel cancer operation or lymph-node biopsy in bronchial cancer operation);

4. tissue margin status in many cancer operations (e.g. facial skin cancer).

CANCER STAGING

This important aspect of the examination of specimens from definitive (putatively curative) cancer operations is regarded as critical in providing prognostic data and in guiding many types of adjuvant therapy. For most carcinomas and related cancers (e.g. melanoma), the microscopy description (if it is the policy of the laboratory to provide this) will provide the information from which staging and survival data may be calculated. For most extended cancer operations (primary excision and regional node excision) a synoptic summary is usual, as well as a staging shorthand. Some of these, such as Dukes staging for colorectal cancer (originally described in relation to abdomino-perineal resection for rectal carcinoma and excluding consideration of extranodal metastases), are classics from surgical pathology history. All of these are based on a **T**umour, **N**ode and **M**etastases classification. An internationally agreed system of staging is available, published both by the Union Internationale Contre le Cancer and as the *Manual for Staging of Cancer*. For details of the staging systems for breast, bladder, prostate, colorectal, lung and ovarian cancers and for lymphomas, see the Further Reading section at the end of this chapter. Reports can also include survival data (e.g. for melanoma) or other referenced derived data. This varies between laboratories, but is available and may be useful for some malignancies.

SPECIAL STUDIES

Standard staining of frozen or paraffin-embedded tissue in most laboratories is with haematoxylin and eosin (HE) or some variant thereof (Papanicolaou with or without HE, with or without Giemsa for cytological preparations).

EMPIRICAL HISTOCHEMISTRY

This includes tried and (generally) true stains, the basis for only some of which is known. The following examples illustrate some tissue components which may be demonstrated:

- neutral fat/triglyceride – frozen section/oil red O stain;
- complex lipids – various;
- glycogen – periodic acid–Schiff (PAS);
- glycoprotein/mucin – PAS with diastase digestion (PASD) – complexed carbohydrate;
- elastin – Verhoff stain
- collagen – van Giesen stain } usually combined;
- cytoplasmic components – many and various;
- iron (haemosiderin) – Perl's ferric ferrocyanide stain;
- amyloid – Congo red stain and others;

- parasites – Giemsa, Gram, PASD, methenamine silver and others.

ENZYME HISTOCHEMISTRY

This technique is in common use only for leukaemia/lymphoma classification (terminal deoxytransferase, TdT) and for muscle biopsies.

IMMUNOMORPHOLOGY

This depends on the binding of a specific (usually monoclonal) antibody to a particular antigen being sought in the tissue, with demonstration of that reaction by an indicator system.

Immunofluorescence

This is used for demonstration of plasma proteins (immunoglobulin, complement, fibrinogen, etc.).

Immunoenzyme (immunoperoxidase; other enzyme-activated markers)

This development has been a great boon with regard to the recognition and classification of neoplasms (especially lymphomas, endocrine and 'para-endocrine' neoplasms) and recognition of viral and bacterial pathogens in tissues.

The principle may be applied to frozen sections, but its popularity and ready application have been markedly enhanced by its application to paraffin-embedded tissues and its increasing reliability. It is also the basis for (immuno)fluorescence-activated cell sorting (FACS). Commonly investigated/demonstrated tissue components include the following:

- membrane antigens – surface Ig, cluster designation (CD) markers;
- cytoplasmic components – Ig, hormones, other;
- cytoplasmic filaments – keratins, vimentin, neurofilaments, etc.;
- nuclear components – receptors for oestrogen, progesterone, etc.;
- infective agents – viral, bacterial;
- other – many and varied, including amyloid components, collagens, etc.

FLOW CYTOMETRY AND FLUORESCENCE-ACTIVATED CELL SORTING (FACS)

This includes the following:

1. DNA ploidy – never a pivotal diagnostic procedure;

2. cluster designation (CD) cell surface markers surface/cytoplasmic Ig (lymphoma);

3. cytoplasmic components.

CYTOMOLECULAR GENETIC STUDIES

These include the following:

1. cell culture chromosome studies, banding;

2. polymerase chain reaction (PCR) – gene rearrangements in neoplasms, including chromosomal translocations, point mutation associations.

ULTRASTRUCTURE

Ultrastructural studies have been important in the investigation of diagnostic problems in internal medicine and paediatrics, especially diagnosis of glomerular disease, skeletal myopathies, neuropathies, bullous skin diseases, ciliary abnormalities in sino-pulmonary disease, metabolic storage diseases, and rapid diagnosis of certain viral diseases.

In surgical practice the usefulness of electron microscopy is somewhat limited, but categories of disease of surgical interest where ultrastructural studies may be useful include the following:

1. malignancies of childhood/adolescence which include neuroblastoma, primitive neuroectodermal tumour (PNET) and Ewing's sarcoma, rhabdomyosarcoma and lymphoma are documented as capable of being solved by electron microscopic examination. Similarly, there is a range of adult poorly differentiated malignancies for which particular ultrastructural features may aid diagnosis. These include various sarcomas (e.g. the presence of myofilaments, Weibel-Palade bodies and others), carcinomas (junctional complexes) and melanoma (melanosomes);

2. diagnosis of Langerhans' cell histiocytosis (the more biologically aggressive variants) is generally considered to require demonstration of specific intracytoplasmic Birbeck granules. Some other purportedly specific cytoplasmic inclusions occur in other rare neoplasms (e.g. alveolar soft-tissue sarcoma);

3. diagnosis of mesothelioma by type of microvilli;

4. rapid diagnosis of some viral diseases (e.g. brain, skin, etc.).

In summary, it can confidently be stated that most morphological diagnoses are made on the basis of a thorough knowledge of the clinical circumstances,

macroscopic appearance (perhaps aided by the account of operation findings, or by radiological or ultrasound imaging) and standard tissue stains (e.g. HE, Papanicolaou, Giemsa), aided by the more reliable empirical histochemical stains.

Immunomorphological identification of infectious agents and types of neoplasms, including FACS, with cytomolecular genetic analysis in certain cases (e.g. lymphoma/leukaemia, neuroblastoma/PNET/Ewing's tumour) usually enhances the investigation of the more exotic diagnostic problems, with electron microscopy primarily playing a confirmatory rather than a pivotal diagnostic role.

In cases where a need for special studies is anticipated by the surgeon, pre-operative discussion with the pathologist should be the rule, not in order to prescribe particular special studies *per se*, but with the aim of reaching a consensus on an appropriate plan for tissue investigation.

CLINICOPATHOLOGICAL REVIEW

As well as departmental quality assurance programmes, interdepartmental reviews – either as a combined inter-service (surgery/pathology/radiology) or a more 'in-house' (surgical team/pathology team) working meeting – are essential. All cases should be presented, some perhaps briefly and others in detail and, if necessary, followed by further assessment ('in-house' or external) until an acceptable outcome is reached.

EXTERNAL REVIEW OF PATHOLOGICAL DIAGNOSIS

In most cases such a review will be initiated by the pathologist, who will usually seek the opinion of an acknowledged authority in that field of pathology whom the pathologist knows and/or trusts. Such a request and reply must become part of the permanent record of both patient and pathology department. Should such a review not be spontaneously suggested by the pathologist, it is perfectly appropriate for the surgeon to request an outside consultation, albeit in a tactful manner. Usually the pathologist will concur and perhaps agree to initiate the referral approach. However, if the pathologist considers that the diagnosis is perfectly straightforward, he or she may not wish to initiate referral. In such cases the pathologist should make appropriate study material available to the surgeon, together with a copy of the pathology report, whereupon the surgeon should initiate the referral consultation.

ADEQUACY OF DIAGNOSTIC REPORTING

With each examination, the goal of the pathologist must be to supply a report that is accurate, timely and provides clinically appropriate information which is applicable to patient care. Diagnoses of common conditions should be given in standard accepted nomenclature, and diagnoses of unusual conditions should be supplemented by an explanation and, where appropriate, references to useful publications on the subject.

FURTHER READING

Rosai J (ed.). 1995: *Ackerman's surgical pathology*, 7th edn. London: Mosby.

Silverberg GS, DeLellis RA, Frable WJ (eds). 1997: *Surgical pathology and cytology*. Edinburgh: Churchill Livingstone.

Normal and disordered oesophageal motility

Geoffrey S. Hebbard

Introduction

The major function of the oesophagus is to transport food from the pharynx to the stomach. This is accomplished by a stereotyped motor pattern involving co-ordinated contraction and relaxation of the muscle of the oesophageal wall and lower oesophageal sphincter, associated with relaxation of the muscle of the proximal stomach. The oesophageal musculature consists of an inner circular and an outer longitudinal layer. Above the level of the aortic arch these layers are composed of striated muscle, and below the aortic arch they consist of smooth muscle. Both the striated and smooth muscle segments of the oesophagus are innervated by the vagus nerve, which receives input from the swallowing centre in the brainstem. The swallowing centre is responsible for the central co-ordination of swallowing, which also requires control of oral and pharyngeal muscles. Transit of a bolus along the oesophagus involves a complex series of motor events (Figures 30.1.1 and 30.1.2). The well-known peristaltic contraction wave is preceded by a wave of inhibition of oesophageal motor activity, and is co-ordinated in time with a relaxation of the lower oesophageal sphincter to 0–5 mmHg above intragastric pressure. The oesophageal contraction wave has both a circular muscle component, which reduces radial diameter, and a longitudinal muscle component, which is responsible for oesophageal shortening during swallowing. Relaxation of the oesophagus is mediated by nitric oxide-dependent mechanisms. It has only recently been recognized that co-ordination of contraction of the striated and smooth segments of the oesophagus is an important predictor of bolus transit. Other causes of delayed transit of the oesophageal contents into the stomach include peristaltic failure due to simultaneous or low-amplitude contractions, or failure of the lower oesophageal sphincter to relax. Reflux of gastric contents into the oesophagus is associated with failure of the lower oesophageal sphincter.

BOX 30.1.1 SYMPTOMS OF OESOPHAGEAL DISEASE

Symptoms of oesephageal disease include:

- dysphagia
- odynophagia
- heartburn
- regurgitation
- chest discomfort

and occasionally

- nocturnal cough
- asthma
- dental problems

Obstructive lesions must be excluded before motility disorder is diagnosed.

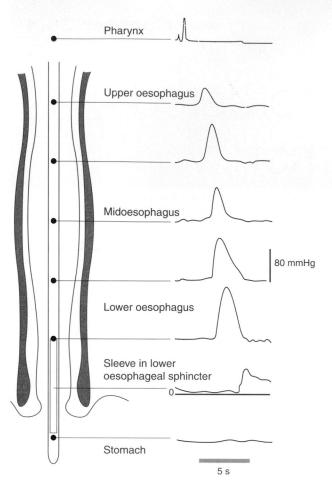

Figure 30.1.1 Pressures recorded from the oesophagus during transit of a 5-mL bolus of water. Note the complete relaxation of the lower oesophageal sphincter and the presence of a peristaltic pressure wave in the oesophageal body.

INVESTIGATION OF OESOPHAGEAL MOTILITY DISORDERS

The motor function of the oesophagus may be assessed by measuring intra-oesophageal pressure (oesophageal manometry), oesophageal wall deformation (barium swallow), oesophageal transit (barium swallow, radionuclide scans) or the reflux of gastric contents into the oesophagus (usually by measuring the oesophageal pH profile). Although oesophageal contractions are often observed at endoscopy, and suggestive abnormalities may be seen in conditions such as achalasia, the role of endoscopy in the diagnosis of oesophageal motor disorders lies primarily in excluding structural disorders which might be responsible for symptoms.

OESOPHAGEAL MANOMETRY

Oesophageal manometry involves measuring pressure at discrete points along the oesophagus using either a

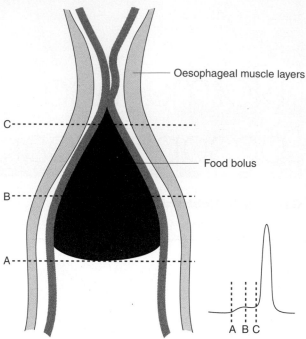

Figure 30.1.2 Components of the normal oesophageal pressure wave. Flow occurs during the low-pressure 'shelf' preceding the main pressure wave which is seen after the lumen is occluded by the advancing contraction.

water-perfused catheter and external transducers, or intraluminal transducers. The lower oesophageal sphincter (LOS) moves with swallowing, and either a perfused sleeve or closely spaced (e.g. 1 cm apart) pressure-measurement ports are required to assess accurately lower oesophageal sphincter pressure and relaxation during swallowing. During stationary oesophageal manometry, a catheter is passed into the oesophagus transnasally and positioned with the sleeve astride the LOS. After a period of accommodation, during which the basal LOS pressure (LOSP) is assessed, a series of wet swallows (5 mL of water) is performed, and the pressures generated during transit of the water down the oesophagus are recorded (Figure 30.1.1). In general, dry swallows (without water) do not add further information, but wet swallows may be repeated in different postures (e.g. sitting, right lateral), particularly if a recording artefact is suspected.

Oesophageal manometry provides information about the strength and sequencing of the pressure wave along the oesophageal body, and the degree of relaxation of the LOS. Manometry does not measure the transit of oesophageal contents, which must be inferred from the pressure patterns observed. In general, pressure waves that are peristaltic with amplitudes of 15 mmHg in the proximal oesophagus and 30 mmHg in the distal oesophagus are likely to be associated with successful transit of a liquid bolus. Oesophageal peristalsis may fail to induce transit of a bolus either because the oesophageal contractions are weak (resulting in low-amplitude pressure waves) or unco-ordinated (e.g. simultaneous, occasionally retrograde), or because the LOS fails to relax sufficiently for the bolus to pass through.

In addition to liquids, patients may be given bread to swallow during an oesophageal manometric study, particularly if this is known to cause dysphagia. However, the normal pressure patterns during solid ingestion have been poorly characterized, and this data may be difficult to interpret. On occasion, combined studies with simultaneous manometry and transit measurements (e.g. barium swallow or radionuclide transit studies) may be valuable in defining the clinical importance of specific patterns of oesophageal motility.

In general, ambulatory motility studies are combined with pH monitoring and are used in the investigation of complaints such as cough, chest pain and asthma. The major advantages of ambulatory studies over stationary studies are that the duration of recording is longer, and recordings are made in the patient's usual environment. Because of these factors it is more likely that symptoms will occur, and these can then be correlated with pressure events or oesophageal acidification.

BARIUM SWALLOW

The barium swallow provides information about the transit of a liquid (or sometimes solid) bolus and the deformation of the oesophageal wall caused by contraction of the oesophageal muscle. Relaxation of the LOS is inferred from the degree of opening of the LOS, the ease with which barium passes through (the height of the barium column supported in the upright position and the rate of clearance of the distal oesophagus) and the degree of any oesophageal dilatation. Structural lesions such as strictures, webs and tumours may be seen. Barium swallow is of most value in the assessment of dysphagia, and yields information that is often complementary to that provided by manometry. The clinical significance of gastro-oesophageal reflux induced by positioning and abdominal pressure during the barium study is questionable.

AMBULATORY pH MONITORING

Measurement of intra-oesophageal pH is used to assess the duration of acid contact with the oesophageal mucosa, a major determinant of the severity of reflux oesophagitis. A pH-sensitive electrode is passed into the oesophagus and secured in position with the recording point 5 cm above the upper border of the LOS. Positioning is most accurately determined by prior manometry, but may also be assessed by measuring the

increase in pH that occurs on withdrawal of the probe into the oesophagus from the stomach, or the distance to the Z-line at endoscopy (with a correction to allow for the extra distance from the nares when compared to the incisors). Once the probe is positioned, it is connected to a small portable recording device and the patient then undertakes their normal daily activities. If symptoms occur they are recorded in a diary or by pressing a button on the recording device. The patient returns to the laboratory the next day, and the data is downloaded from the recording device on to a computer. The latter calculates and displays the overall profile of acid exposure and the relationships between symptoms and intra-oesophageal pH.

Total oesophageal acid exposure is determined by the frequency of reflux and the duration of each episode. The duration of reflux episodes is affected by the integrity of oesophageal clearance mechanisms (primary and secondary peristalsis) and the presence of alkaline or neutral secretions (from the oesophageal glands and saliva) which buffer and wash away the acid. A pH of < 4.0 is usually taken as the level of significant acidification, as this is the pH below which pepsin becomes active and damage to the mucosa occurs. An acid exposure of $> 4\%$ over a 24-h period is usually considered to be abnormal, but the pattern of acid exposure and the correlation of symptoms with episodes of oesophageal acidification are equally important in interpreting the results of an ambulatory pH study. The 'physiological' pattern of acid exposure is that it almost all occurs in the upright position, most commonly in the postprandial period, with episodes of acidification being relatively short (ranging from seconds to minutes) (Figure 30.1.3). Abnormal patterns include increased numbers of reflux episodes, prolonged episodes of reflux (which indicate poor clearance), and nocturnal reflux (which is also often prolonged). The association of episodes of oesophageal acidification with symptoms provides an indication as to whether these symptoms are related to oesophageal acidification. It is important to note that symptoms may be due to oesophageal acidification even if total oesophageal acid exposure is within the 'normal' range. Reflux parameters may be combined in order to produce a reflux 'score'. These are used to a much greater degree in research studies than in routine clinical practice.

OESOPHAGEAL TRANSIT STUDIES

Oesophageal transit can be quantified using radiolabelled solid or liquid food. This type of measurement may be of value when the origin of symptoms or the significance of oesophageal motor abnormalities is unclear, and it provides a convenient quantification of

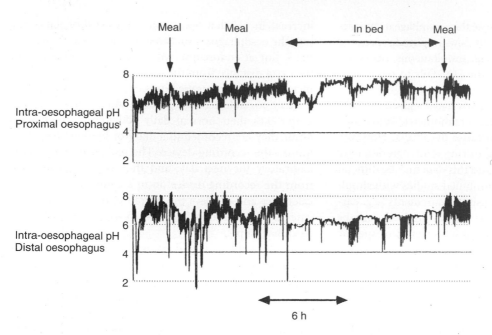

Figure 30.1.3 A 24-h ambulatory intra-oesophageal pH recording in a normal subject. Recordings are made from two sites, 5 and 15 cm above the lower oesophageal sphincter. Note the short duration and predominantly postprandial distribution of the reflux events (when pH < 4). Episodes of acidification involve only the distal oesophagus.

transit that can be used to assess the effects of surgical intervention.

OESOPHAGEAL MOTILITY DISORDERS

GASTRO-OESOPHAGEAL REFLUX DISEASE

Pathophysiology

Gastro-oesophageal reflux disease results from excessive exposure of the oesophageal mucosa to gastric acid and pepsin, and is usually due to dysfunction of the LOS. In the majority of patients the LOS dysfunction involves transient relaxation of the LOS (TLOSR) with passive reflux of the gastric contents into the oesophagus. This is particularly true in patients with mild reflux disease. However, even in patients with severe disease, TLOSR still accounts for two-thirds of episodes of gastro-oesophageal reflux. The importance of mechanical factors, such as hiatus hernia, low basal LOSP, loss of the intra-abdominal segment of the oesophagus or gastro-oesophageal angle, increase with increasing severity of oesophagitis. Transient relaxation of the LOS is a physiological event which is necessary for the venting of gas from the stomach (belching), and some degree of gastro-oesophageal reflux and oesophageal acidification is physiological (see above). The physiological stimulus for TLOSR is probably distension of the stomach in the region of the cardia. In patients with reflux disease, TLOSR occurs at inappropriate times, and this results in excessive reflux of gastric contents into the oesophagus. The pathophysiological mechanisms responsible for the inappropriate relaxation have not been defined. The contents of the refluxate which cause oesophageal dam-

age include acid, pepsin and bile (which is more injurious at acidic pH). Other factors that promote oesophagitis include poor oesophageal clearance due to dysmotility (e.g. scleroderma of the oesophagus or non-specific oesophageal motor disorders) and lack of neutralization of the acid refluxate due to reduced saliva production (e.g. Sjögren's syndrome).

Diagnosis

Patients with reflux disease typically present with heartburn, particularly after the consumption of spicy or fatty foods, and sometimes with regurgitation of gastric contents into the mouth, particularly when lying down or bending over. Dysphagia may be due to oesophagitis, but may also suggest the presence of an oesophageal stricture (usually due to fibrosis secondary to chronic inflammation). Other symptoms may include nocturnal cough, voice problems and dental changes which indicate reflux proximal to the upper oesophageal sphincter. Asthma may be aggravated by gastro-oesophageal reflux either due to aspiration of gastric contents, or to reflexes whereby oesophageal reflux promotes release of pro-inflammatory mediators into the airways. Severe reflux oesophagitis may be associated with Barrett's oesophagus, in which metaplasia of the squamous lining of the lower oesophagus is seen, and which is associated with an increased risk of adenocarcinoma.

Diagnosis of reflux disease is often made on the basis of history, and this is usually confirmed by a symptomatic response to acid-suppressive medications. Endoscopy is not necessary in young patients (< 40 years) with mild symptoms and no 'alarm symptoms' such as dysphagia or weight loss. When indicated, endoscopy may reveal anything from normal findings (endoscopy-negative reflux oesophagitis, in which microscopic changes may be present) to erythema, linear erosions, ulceration and/or stricturing of the lower oesophagus or Barrett's oesophagus. If endoscopy does not reveal any evidence of oesophagitis (or any other upper gastrointestinal lesions which might explain the symptoms), a trial of H_2-receptor antagonists is still indicated, as a significant proportion of patients with reflux disease have normal findings at endoscopy. Ambulatory pH monitoring (Figure 30.1.4) is a more sensitive test than endoscopy for the detection of gastro-oesophageal reflux disease, and allows correlation of episodes of oesophageal acidification with symptoms. Ambulatory pH monitoring is indicated in cases where symptoms are atypical or a specific symptom–reflux association is being sought (e.g. cough), in patients who do not respond to treatment, or in cases where quantitation of the degree of reflux is required (e.g. in research studies or prior to fundoplication).

Management

Medical treatment
The majority of patients with reflux disease are managed medically. Lifestyle changes include weight loss, avoidance of precipitating foods and drinks, cessation of smoking and elevation of the head of the bed. These measures may be supplemented by simple antacids (Mylanta, Gaviscon), but are usually ineffective in providing relief from significant symptoms, and many patients will not tolerate the limitations that these changes impose on their lifestyle.

H_2-receptor antagonists provide relief from mild to moderate symptoms, and the dose may be titrated up or down in order to achieve acceptable control of symptoms. Some patients may elect to take these medications in advance (e.g. before going out to a restaurant); this is acceptable in a situation where symptom control is the major aim of treatment.

Ulcerative reflux oesophagitis requires treatment with potent acid-suppressive medications, often proton-pump inhibitors, the dose of which may need to be titrated in order to achieve optimal control of symptoms. In patients with severe ulceration or stricturing disease, repeat endoscopy may be undertaken in order to check healing and to ensure that acid suppression is adequate even though symptoms are controlled. In patients who fail to respond to potent acid suppression, the diagnosis may be incorrect, acid suppression may be inadequate (a higher dose being required – but also think of Zollinger-Ellison syndrome!), or symptoms may be due to continuing reflux of non-acidic gastric contents, leading to symptoms such as chest discomfort, regurgitation and aspiration. The addition of a prokinetic agent may be helpful in some such patients, and pH monitoring whilst on therapy is useful for determining whether optimal acid suppression has been achieved. Further therapy in patients with continuing reflux of non-acidic gastric contents often involves surgery.

Surgical treatment
Surgical therapy for gastro-oesophageal reflux disease involves fundoplication, and is applicable to only a small proportion of patients. Indications for surgery include failure of medical therapy, non-compliance with medication for social or financial reasons, or continuing symptoms due to reflux of non-acidic gastric contents. Cost and the lack of knowledge of the long-term effects

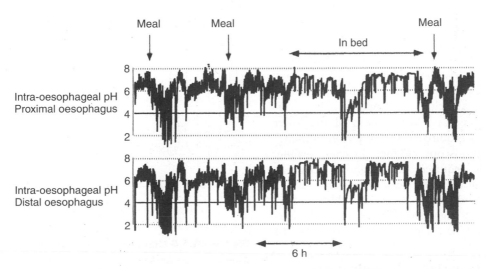

Figure 30.1.4 A 24-h ambulatory intra-oesophageal pH recording in a subject with gastro-oesophageal reflux disease. Recordings are made from two sites, 5 and 15 cm above the lower oesophageal sphincter. The intra-oesophageal pH is < 4 for 9.6% of the recording time in the distal recording electrode (normal < 4%), and a significant proportion of events also involve the proximal oesophagus. The subject reported symptoms in association with episodes of oesophageal acidification.

of proton-pump inhibitors have been proposed as reasons for favouring surgery over medical therapy in a larger proportion of patients, but these arguments are only speculative at present. Fundoplication may be achieved by either a transthoracic or a transabdominal approach (open or laparoscopic), and a variety of procedures have been developed. The major effects of fundoplication are the creation of a high-pressure zone in the lower oesophagus which reduces reflux (TLOSRs are also reduced by an unknown mechanism), repair of the diaphragmatic hiatus, and anchoring of the lower oesophagus within the abdomen. Fundoplication has a reported success rate of 90% in controlling heartburn, but recurrence of symptoms in subsequent years may be significant. Post-operative dysphagia, gas bloat, increased flatulence and early satiety generally improve with time, but may be severe and disabling.

ACHALASIA

Pathophysiology

Achalasia is a condition of unknown aetiology in which the inhibitory innervation (nitric oxide) of the LOS fails and peristalsis is absent. These changes lead to delayed passage of food through the oesophagus, with potential for aspiration, malnutrition and an increased risk of malignancy of the oesophagus.

Diagnosis

Patients with achalasia present with dysphagia for both liquids and solids. This is often associated with regurgitation (especially at night), cough and weight loss. Heartburn may be seen (possibly due to fermentation in the oesophagus), and the condition can be mistaken for reflux disease (with disastrous consequences if fundoplication is performed).

Endoscopy, with a J-turn in the fundus and also often biopsy of the cardia, is essential to exclude malignant lesions of the gastro-oesophageal junction. At endoscopy the oesophagus may be dilated and contain food and liquid. The LOS is usually closed and may be tight to traverse with the endoscope. A CT scan of the lower oesophagus may be required if the suspicion of malignancy is high but endoscopy and biopsy are unrevealing.

Manometry is required to diagnose achalasia, although the classical 'bird's beak' appearance of the lower oesophagus and lack of gastric air bubble on barium swallow are very suggestive. The manometric characteristics of achalasia (Figure 30.1.5) include the following:

1. a raised LOS pressure (often 40 mmHg or more);

2. failure or incomplete ($>$10 mmHg pressure compared to intragastric pressure) relaxation of the LOS; and

3. absence of oesophageal peristalsis, although oscillating pressure waves may be seen due to weak contractions of the wall which do not occlude the lumen.

Variants of this classical picture include patients with partial LOS relaxation, repetitive high-amplitude oesophageal contractions or partially preserved peristalsis. These may be patterns of developing achalasia and, if observed, these patients may develop a 'classical' manometric picture of achalasia over a period of months or years.

Management

Medical treatment

Medical management of achalasia with drugs that reduce LOS pressure, such as calcium-channel antagonists or GTN, is generally ineffective. More recently, trials of

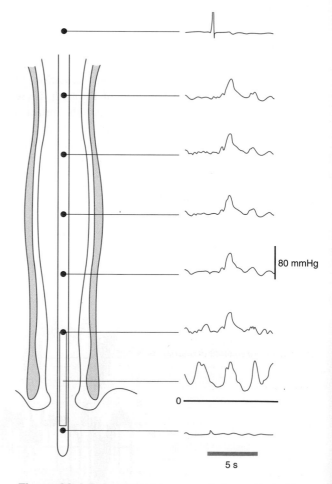

Figure 30.1.5 Oesophageal manometry in a patient with achalasia. Note the lack of relaxation of the lower oesophageal sphincter, which has a high basal pressure. Oesophageal peristalsis is absent, and simultaneous pressure waves in the oesophageal body represent ineffective, non-lumen-occluding contractions.

endoscopic injection of botulinum toxin have shown a response in 60–80% of patients, which generally lasts for several months. Injections can be repeated, but tachyphylaxis may develop. In general, botulinum toxin injection is only suitable for high-risk patients in whom short-term palliation of symptoms is sought.

Dilatation

Oesophageal dilatation is the 'traditional' definitive therapy for achalasia. Dilatation is usually performed at endoscopy, often under fluoroscopic control. The aim of oesophageal dilatation is complete or partial disruption of the LOS using balloons 30–40 mm in diameter inflated to 1–2 atm for 30–60 s. The procedure may need to be repeated in order to obtain an adequate clinical result. The major complication of oesophageal balloon dilatation is perforation of the oesophagus, which occurs in approximately 5% of patients in large series. A gastrografin swallow is often performed following dilatation in order to detect small perforations. Larger perforations may be apparent immediately following endoscopy with chest pain, pneumomediastinum, left pleural effusion and rapid deterioration. Whilst small perforations may be managed conservatively, emergency operative repair is usually required. Other complications of oesophageal dilatation include reflux oesophagitis, which occurs in 5–10% of patients.

Surgical treatment

Surgical management of achalasia involves myotomy of the LOS, which may be extended up the body of the oesophagus in the case of vigorous achalasia. In general, surgery is more effective than balloon dilatation in relieving dysphagia, but it has a higher incidence of post-operative reflux, and is thus often combined with an anti-reflux procedure. The widespread use of laparoscopic techniques has made surgery an increasingly attractive option compared to balloon dilatation, particularly as the procedure is more controlled, and any perforation can be dealt with at the time of the procedure.

DIFFUSE OESOPHAGEAL SPASM

Diagnosis

Diffuse oesophageal spasm may present as an asymptomatic abnormality found at manometry, or it may be associated with chest pain or dysphagia. The relationship between diffuse oesophageal spasm and gastro-oesophageal reflux disease – specifically whether reflux may induce the motor changes seen in diffuse oesophageal spasm – has not been definitively answered.

The diagnosis of diffuse oesophageal spasm is made at manometry, which shows the simultaneous onset of pressure waves along the oesophagus (Figure 30.1.6) in > 20% of wet swallows (with some swallows showing

normal peristalsis). Pressure waves may be prolonged and multipeaked in addition to being simultaneous. Lower oesophageal sphincter relaxation is within the normal range. Barium swallow shows simultaneous and unco-ordinated contraction of the oesophagus, and in the elderly is often termed 'presbyoesophagus'.

Management

In patients who present with dysphagia, following exclusion of a stricture, dilatation may be helpful, although the effect is usually short-lived, and a placebo effect cannot be excluded. Chest pain due to diffuse oesophageal spasm usually responds poorly to treatment. GTN may be tried, and reflux disease should be excluded by either pH studies or a trial of antisecretory agents. Occasionally, in carefully selected patients who have diffuse oesophageal spasm demonstrated as the cause of their symptoms on ambulatory motility studies, a long

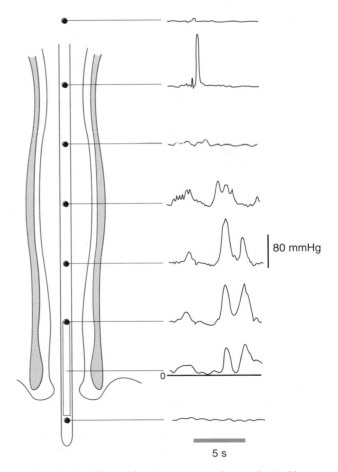

Figure 30.1.6 Oesophageal manometry in a patient with oesophageal spasm. Note the simultaneous onset of pressure waves in the distal oesophagus and multipeaked pressure waves. Relaxation of the lower oesophageal sphincter is complete.

myotomy of the oesophagus may help, but this also has the potential for significant morbidity.

NUTCRACKER OESOPHAGUS

Nutcracker oesophagus is the term given to the pattern of hypertensive peristalsis (mean pressure wave amplitude > 180 mmHg) with normal LOS pressure and relaxation. It may be a cause of chest pain, but is of uncertain clinical significance.

HYPERTENSIVE LOWER OESOPHAGEAL SPHINCTER

This is another condition of poorly defined clinical importance, in which the LOS has a high resting pressure, but relaxation is complete and oesophageal peristalsis is intact (cf. achalasia).

NON-SPECIFIC OESOPHAGEAL MOTOR DISORDER

The most common abnormality observed at routine manometry is a non-specific pattern of focal and generalized failure of peristalsis, often in the distal oesophagus. In normal subjects a relatively low-amplitude pressure wave may be seen in the region of the oesophagus where the smooth and striated muscle meet. Failure of conduction of the pressure wave across this junction, or an excessively wide region of low-amplitude pressure waves, may also be associated with failure of bolus transport. Patients often present with dysphagia, and may also have simultaneous pressure waves (oesophageal spasm) on manometry. Prokinetic agents may be tried, and are of benefit in some patients.

SCLERODERMA

Scleroderma and related conditions characteristically cause failure of peristalsis in the smooth muscle (distal oesophagus), with a low LOS pressure and commonly reflux oesophagitis. This appears to be a result of neuropathic and myopathic processes, with fibrosis of the oesophageal wall. The diagnosis may be suspected at manometry, but has usually been made on the basis of the systemic features prior to investigation of the oesophagus. Management is that of the reflux

oesophagitis (usually with proton-pump inhibitors). Because of their poor peristaltic function, these patients require a loose fundoplication if surgery is undertaken.

THE UPPER OESOPHAGEAL SPHINCTER

PHYSIOLOGY

The upper oesophageal sphincter (UES) is largely formed by the cricopharyngeus, and is a slit-like structure with a radially asymmetrical pressure profile (a higher pressure from front to back than from side to side). Techniques used to measure UES function must take into account this radial asymmetry, as well as the fact that the sphincter is mobile and pressure events in the pharynx are very rapid.

Upper oesophageal sphincter pressure changes with many factors, including state of arousal, emotion, sleep and anaesthesia, but is generally in the range 60–100 mmHg. Relaxation measured with a sleeve (relative to intra-oesophageal pressure) is usually complete. Hold-up of a bolus at the UES may be reflected by the presence of a 'ramp' in the pressure wave prior to the major upstroke (which represents mucosal contact with the catheter), and is accentuated by larger bolus sizes.

ZENKER'S DIVERTICULUM

In Zenker's diverticulum, the UES opens incompletely, resulting in increased intrabolus pressures, and a pulsion diverticulum forms at the weak area of the cricopharyngeus. Treatment is by resection of the diverticulum and myotomy of the UES. In the past this has required cervical surgery, but recently techniques have been developed for the procedure to be performed endoscopically.

FURTHER READING

Castell DO, Castell JA. 1994: *Esophageal motility testing*, 2nd edn. Norwalk, CT: Appleton & Lange.

Richter JE. 1997: *Ambulatory esophageal pH monitoring*, 2nd edn. Baltimore, MD: Williams & Wilkins.

Smout AJPM, Akkermans LMA. 1992: *Normal and disturbed motility of the gastrointestinal tract*. Stroud: Wrightson Biomedical Publishing.

Disorders of gastric motility

Geoffrey S. Hebbard

Introduction

Disordered gastric emptying is a common and clinically important problem, potentially leading to malnutrition, upper gastrointestinal symptoms, unpredictable absorption of orally administered drugs and disordered glucose homeostasis in patients with diabetes mellitus.

NORMAL GASTRIC MOTOR FUNCTION

PATTERNS OF GASTRIC MOTOR ACTIVITY

Chewed solid food must be reduced to particles of approximately 1–2 mm in diameter before entering the small intestine. This is accomplished by the movements of the stomach muscles which, in the presence of salivary and gastric secretions, break solid food into smaller particles – a process known as trituration. This food and any liquids that are ingested must then be delivered to the intestine at a rate that is optimal for absorption.

Functionally, the stomach may be divided into proximal and distal regions (Figure 30.2.1). The proximal region, which consists of the anatomical fundus and proximal corpus, receives and stores ingested food, and may modulate intragastric pressure. The distal region, which consists of corpus, antrum and pylorus, is primarily responsible for the mechanical processes of trituration and control of gastric outflow resistance.

As would be expected from its role in the storage of food and regulation of intragastric pressure, the smooth muscle of the proximal stomach contracts and relaxes slowly. Following ingestion of food, relaxation is seen (gastric accommodation), followed by a gradual return of tone during the postprandial period (Figure 30.2.1).

The motor activity of the corpus and proximal antrum is controlled by the gastric electrical slow wave, a rhythmic (3 cycles/min) depolarization of gastric smooth muscle which begins high on the greater curve, being conducted from there along the length of the stomach to the pylorus. While contractions of the distal stomach occur only in association with the gastric electrical slow wave, the electrical slow wave also occurs in the absence of gastric contractile activity, and it is therefore clear that other factors (i.e. neural and hormonal) are also involved in determining whether a contraction wave is associated with the electrical slow wave. Distal gastric contractions are of variable amplitude. The rate of propagation and vigour of the contraction wave increases towards the pylorus, and the terminal antrum contracts as a unit. While the timing and rate of pyloric contractile activity are regulated largely by the gastric slow wave, the muscle of the pylorus is specialized, and its control mechanisms appear to differ from those of the antrum.

The smooth muscle of the duodenum has a higher intrinsic rate of contraction (12 contractions/min) than that of the stomach and pylorus. Contractions of the duodenum often appear to be associated in time with those of the distal stomach, a phenomenon which has been described as 'antropyloroduodenal coordination'. Observations of the duodenum suggest that contractions may result in either clearance of the duodenum, which

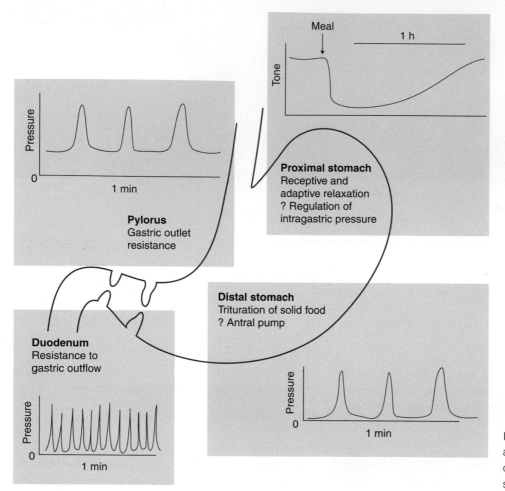

Figure 30.2.1 Anatomy and mechanical function of different regions of the stomach.

presumably facilitates gastric emptying, or segmenting or retrograde contractions, which may be associated with retardation of gastric emptying.

During fasting the stomach shows a characteristic cyclical motor activity, termed the migrating motor complex (MMC), because it subsequently progresses down the small intestine to the terminal ileum. For descriptive purposes, the MMC has been divided into phases in which the stomach is quiescent (approx 50 min, phase 1), shows irregular motor activity (approx 50 min, phase 2) and regular 3/min strong contractions (5–10 min, phase 3). During phase 3, indigestible residues are expelled from the stomach into the intestine to be carried to the colon by the small intestinal MMC. It is believed that the major functions of the MMC are to expel indigestible particles from the stomach (preventing the formation of bezoars) and to prevent bacterial overgrowth.

CONTROL OF GASTRIC EMPTYING

Gastroduodenal motor function is controlled at a number of levels by a complex neurohormonal system (Figure 30.2.2). An intrinsic nervous system, with a number of neurones similar to that of the spinal cord, is present in the wall of the gastrointestinal tract. The intrinsic nervous system of the gut communicates with the central nervous system through vagal and spinal pathways. Reflexes involving these pathways are mediated by neural circuits in the brainstem and spinal cord. Brainstem structures communicate with higher centres, including the thalamus and cortex, providing a plausible mechanism for the effects of factors such as stress and emotion on gastrointestinal motility.

The major factor controlling gastric motor function in the postprandial period is feedback from the small intestine. Observations that diversion of nutrients from the intestine results in increased rates of gastric emptying, and that infusion of nutrients into the intestine delays gastric emptying, suggest that the presence of nutrients in the intestine activates negative feedback pathways that slow gastric emptying. Other stimuli, such as distension of the intestine, and acidic or hypertonic fluids, are also capable of activating these pathways. The mechanism of sensing probably involves both neural and hormonal mechanisms. Nutrients must thus be

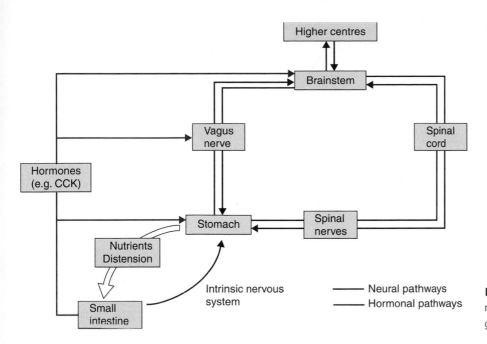

Figure 30.2.2 Control systems responsible for the regulation of gastric emptying.

digested and absorbed in order to exert negative feedback effects.

PATTERNS OF GASTRIC EMPTYING

Non-nutrient and low-nutrient liquids empty rapidly from the stomach (Figure 30.2.3), with an overall pattern that approximates to a mono-exponential curve, their rate of emptying being influenced by posture and intragastric volume. As a result of feedback from nutrient receptors in the small intestine, nutrient fluids empty at a relatively constant rate, with only minor effects of posture and intragastric volume, thus providing a steady flow of nutrients to the intestine. Emptying of ingested solids is preceded by a lag phase (Figure 30.2.3) during which some of the solids are reduced to a particle size that allows passage across the pylorus. Following the lag phase, in a similar pattern to that of a nutrient liquid, a linear phase of emptying is seen. When both liquids and solids are consumed simultaneously, liquids empty preferentially, and if a liquid is consumed after a solid, emptying of the solid slows while the liquid empties. Indigestible solids with particle sizes of *c.* 7 mm or more are emptied at the time of the next MMC. Indigestible solid particles with sizes of < 7 mm may empty with the meal; this becomes increasingly likely as the particle size decreases.

MEASUREMENT OF GASTRIC EMPTYING

Some of the earliest studies of the physiology of gastric emptying were performed in the late nineteenth century soon after the discovery of X-rays. Fluoroscopy was used to examine the emptying of barium-impregnated foods from the stomach of cats, with images being traced from a screen. Other early methods of measurement of gastric emptying involved the passage of nasogastric tubes and either aspiration of the entire gastric contents or sampling of the gastric contents after the introduction of a marker. More recently, scintigraphic gastric emptying studies using solids and/or liquids labelled with radioactive technetium or indium have come to be regarded as the 'gold standard' for the measurement of gastric emptying in clinical practice. All of the important components of a physiological meal (solids, liquids and even extracellular fat) can be labelled, and the emptying of each component can be measured separately. The stomach can be divided into proximal and distal regions, and the emptying profiles of each region can be examined for each meal component. A number of other non-invasive methods for measuring gastric emptying have been developed. These include ultrasound measurement of gastric volume, MRI, epigastric impedance, the absorption profile of drugs that are rapidly absorbed from the proximal intestine (e.g. paracetamol), and the octanoic acid breath test. In general, these tests do not have the accuracy, versatility and wide availability of radionuclide scanning, but they may be valuable in certain situations. Meals used in the measurement of gastric emptying have not been standardized, and each laboratory has developed its own normal values based on the meal and methods used. The major parameters of gastric emptying include the half-emptying time and the lag phase (usually applicable only to solids), but for research studies considerably more information may be obtained, depending on the method of data acquisition.

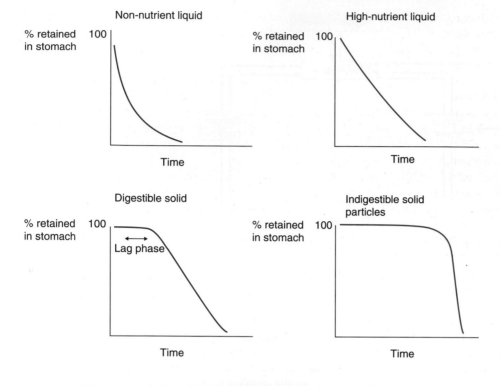

Figure 30.2.3 Schematic representation of gastric emptying of non-nutrient liquids (e.g. water), high-nutrient liquids (e.g. 25% dextrose), digestible solids (e.g. hamburger) and indigestible solid particles greater than 5 mm in diameter (e.g. some pharmaceutical preparations).

DISORDERED GASTRIC EMPTYING

Once obstructing lesions have been excluded, disordered gastric emptying may be a result of disordered motility, abnormalities of the control systems regulating gastric emptying or previous surgery (Table 30.2.1). Most disorders of gastric emptying involve delayed emptying, but in some circumstances problems may arise as a result of abnormally rapid gastric emptying. Although it is not clear to what degree this is valid, in an analogous manner to the somatic neuromuscular system, diseases affecting gastroduodenal motility have been divided into neuropathic and myopathic processes. Myopathic processes would be expected to weaken the antral contractions and reduce proximal gastric tone. Neuropathic processes affecting the enteric nervous system might be expected to influence either the force of gastric contractions (by altering the release of neurotransmitters) or the co-ordination or patterns of contraction in the gastropyloroduodenal region. The clinical significance of disorders of the conduction of the slow wave within the gastric wall, which probably involves the interstitial cells of Cajal, is unknown, but neuropathic processes would not be expected to alter the timing of contractions within the stomach. The possibility that disordered gastric electrical rhythm (i.e. abnormal pacemaker function) may contribute to disordered gastric emptying is suggested by the observation that abnormal gastric rhythm is common in some groups of patients with gastroparesis.

The pathogenesis of disorders that cause delayed gastric emptying may be classified into acute, often reversible causes and chronic, usually irreversible causes.

ACUTELY DELAYED GASTRIC EMPTYING

Gastric emptying may be affected during a generalized ileus due to surgery, severe infection or metabolic derangement (e.g. hypokalaemia). In these situations,

Table 30.2.1 Conditions associated with delayed gastric emptying

Acute conditions
Post-surgical ileus
Sepsis
Metabolic disturbance
    Hypokalaemia
    Diabetic ketoacidosis
Viral infection (may become chronic)

Chronic conditions
Diabetes mellitus
Non-ulcer dyspepsia
Gastro-oesophageal reflux disease
Chronic idiopathic intestinal pseudo-obstruction
Scleroderma
Polymyositis
Muscular dystrophy

restoration of normal gastric function usually follows the correction of the underlying problem.

Viral infections may cause gastroparesis, which appears to be reversible (although sometimes over a period of several months). The pathogenesis of these conditions has not been well defined.

Ingestion of drugs such as levodopa may be associated with delayed gastric emptying. In addition to delaying the emptying of the other gastric contents, these drugs may influence their own absorption by affecting emptying of the remaining drug from the stomach. These effects are generally reversible when the drug is stopped.

CHRONICALLY DELAYED GASTRIC EMPTYING

The incidence of disordered gastric emptying in clinical populations of both insulin-dependent and non-insulin-dependent diabetic patients appears to be of the order of 50%. Disordered oesophageal, small intestinal, gall-bladder and colonic motility are also frequently seen in patients with diabetes mellitus, indicating that any region of the gastrointestinal tract may be involved. The most common abnormality of gastric emptying observed in patients with diabetes is delayed gastric emptying, with a small subset of patients (with early type-2 diabetes) demonstrating rapid emptying. The conventional explanation for the abnormalities of gastric emptying observed in diabetes has been the presence of autonomic neuropathy. However, hyperglycaemia is also likely to be a clinically important factor, as blood glucose concentrations of *c.* 15 mmol/L slow gastric emptying in both normal individuals and diabetic patients.

A significant proportion (approx 50%) of patients with non-ulcer dyspepsia have delayed gastric emptying. Manometric studies of patients with non-ulcer dyspepsia have revealed a variety of abnormalities. However, the mechanical significance of these findings for delayed gastric emptying has not been defined.

Gastric emptying is delayed in approximately 40% of patients with gastro-oesophageal reflux disease. Proximal gastric tone is normal in the fasting state, but returns more slowly in the postprandial period than in normal subjects.

Delayed gastric emptying is a common finding in patients with scleroderma and its variants, occurring in 50–60% of patients in most series. Patients with more severe disease, especially those with systemic disease, show the most marked abnormalities. The pathogenesis of delayed gastric emptying in patients with scleroderma has not been defined, but both neuropathic and myopathic processes are probably involved.

In addition to the effects of these diseases on skeletal muscle, polymyositis and muscular dystrophies are associated with abnormalities of upper gastrointestinal motility and disordered gastric emptying. Patients with muscular dystrophy may be at risk of developing acute gastric dilatation.

Disordered gastric motor function forms an important part of the clinical syndrome of chronic idiopathic intestinal pseudo-obstruction. A variety of patterns of motor activity are seen, probably reflecting the fact that this is not a homogeneous group of patients, but rather it includes subgroups with myopathic and neuropathic diseases.

Disordered gastrointestinal motility, including delayed gastric emptying, may be seen as a paraneoplastic manifestation in patients with lung, breast and pancreatic cancer. Pathological examination of the gastrointestinal tract often reveals degeneration of the myenteric plexus with a lymphocytic infiltrate, and autoantibodies to neural structures may be present.

Delayed gastric emptying has been demonstrated in anorexia nervosa, although it is unclear whether this is a cause or a consequence of the condition. Acute dilatation of the stomach has also been reported. Possible factors contributing to delayed gastric emptying include poor nutritional status and electrolyte disturbances. Gastric emptying improves with nutritional intake and precedes weight gain. The motor abnormalities underlying these observations have not been examined.

EFFECTS OF GASTRIC SURGERY ON GASTRIC EMPTYING

Gastric surgery, especially surgery for peptic ulceration, often involves vagotomy and gastric resection or a pyloric drainage procedure. As these procedures clearly have considerable potential to interfere with the function of structures that are important in the control of gastric emptying, it is a testament to the plasticity of gastric function that more patients do not suffer debilitating post-surgical symptoms. The effects of surgery must be seen in the light of the overall control of gastric emptying, and the fact that this is probably mediated by a number of mechanisms, each of which can to some degree take over the function of others, should these be disabled. This degree of redundancy is what would be expected from a highly conserved system. In general, gastrectomy with vagotomy can be expected to result in rapid emptying of the liquid phase of a meal and delayed emptying of solids. However, the precise effects of surgical procedures are somewhat variable and appear to depend on individual factors and the operation involved. The relative contributions of vagotomy and partial gastrectomy or the drainage procedure have not been determined. In patients with post-surgical symptoms, conditions such as intra-abdominal collections, afferent loop syndrome and bile reflux gastritis should be excluded, as these may respond to revision of the surgical procedure.

MANAGEMENT OF PATIENTS WITH DISORDERED GASTRIC EMPTYING

The major clinical consequences of disordered gastric emptying include malnutrition and upper gastrointestinal symptoms. In addition, drug absorption, particularly of delayed-release preparations, may be affected, and erratic delivery of drugs and food may affect glycaemic control in patients with diabetes mellitus.

The initial management of a patient with suspected disordered gastric emptying is to optimize the nutritional status and treat any acute reversible causes (e.g. electrolyte imbalance or intra-abdominal pathology). If small intestine function is relatively normal, a feeding jejunostomy may be used to bypass the stomach and improve nutritional status.

Prokinetic agents (e.g. cisapride, metoclopramide and domperidone) act by a variety of mechanisms involving muscarinic, 5HT and dopaminergic receptors to increase the strength of gastric contractions and affect antroduodenal co-ordination. However, they are often disappointing clinically in patients with severe gastroparesis. Erythromycin acts as a motilin agonist and is a very effective prokinetic agent, increasing the rate of emptying in some patients with diabetic gastroparesis to rates that are faster than control values. This observation has fuelled the search for other motilin agonists (motilides) without the antibiotic and nauseating effects of erythromycin, some of which will be available clinically in the near future.

In several recent trials gastric pacing has been shown to improve symptoms in patients with delayed gastric emptying and, using certain stimulus parameters, the rate of gastric emptying may also be improved. The clinical role of gastric pacing has not been determined, and this technique is not currently available outside clinical trials.

Patients with chronically delayed gastric emptying which is refractory to drug therapy may be fed by a tube placed into the small intestine either surgically (via a percutaneous endoscopic gastrostomy) or via the nose. If the small intestine is also affected (e.g. in chronic intestinal pseudo-obstruction), total parenteral nutrition may be necessary. Occasionally, total gastrectomy may be helpful, particularly in patients with post-surgical gastroparesis.

FURTHER READING

Horowitz M, Fraser RJ. 1995: Gastroparesis: diagnosis and management. *Scandinavian Journal of Gastroenterology* **213** (Suppl.), 7–16.

Horowitz M, Dent J, Fraser R, Sun W, Hebbard G. 1994: Role and integration of mechanisms controlling gastric emptying. *Digestive Diseases and Sciences* **39**, 7S–13S.

Kelly K. 1981: Motility of the stomach and gastroduodenal junction. In Johnson L (ed.), *Physiology of the gastrointestinal tract.* New York: Raven Press, 393–413.

Smout AJPM, Akkermans LMA. 1992: *Normal and disturbed motility of the gastrointestinal tract.* Stroud: Wrightson Biomedical Publishing.

Szurszewski JH. 1987: Electrical basis for gastrointestinal motility. In Johnson L (ed.), *Physiology of the gastrointestinal tract*, 2nd edn. New York: Raven Press, 383–422.

Motility disorders of the biliary tract

James Toouli

Introduction

Primary disorders of the motility of the gall bladder and sphincter of Oddi are uncommon. However, when identified and treated in patients who present with symptoms, it has been demonstrated that a successful long-term outcome may be expected. The clinical presentation of pancreatobiliary motility disorders occurs in one of three forms, namely gall bladder dyskinesia, sphincter of Oddi dysfunction of the bile duct sphincter, and sphincter of Oddi dysfunction of the pancreatic duct sphincter.

GALL BLADDER

AETIOLOGY AND PATHOGENESIS

Patients with gall bladder motility disorders present with symptoms suggestive of gallstones, but on investigation do not have demonstrable stones in the gall bladder. Although the pathogenesis of the motility disorder is unknown, some clues may be deduced from the aetiology of acute acalculous gall bladder disease. There are patients who develop acute gall bladder inflammation whilst on parenteral nutrition. Often these patients are being treated in an intensive-care unit environment for an unrelated major illness. Ultrasonographic studies have demonstrated reduced gall bladder contractility and the development of 'sludge' in the gall bladder. Rarely, this may lead to cystic duct obstruction and acute gangrenous cholecystitis. More frequently, acute obstruction does not occur, but these patients are subsequently at high risk for the development of gallstones.

However, the majority of patients with acalculous gall bladder disease do not develop their symptoms following a major illness or after parenteral nutrition.

Nevertheless, the underlying motility disorder may be similar, and may reflect changes which result in relative or absolute obstruction to the normal emptying of the gall bladder.

DIAGNOSIS

Abdominal pain is the most common symptom associated with a motility disorder of the gall bladder. The pain is epigastric or in the right upper quadrant. It occurs in episodes and is quite severe, often lasting for 2–3 h or until relieved by analgesics. It may radiate to the back and under the tip of the right scapula. The pain may follow a fatty meal, and it may be associated with nausea and vomiting, although these are not diagnostic features. Occasionally the pain causes the patient to wake in the early hours of the morning, and is not relieved by a change in posture or by taking antacids. Examination during an episode of pain reveals tenderness under the right costal margin, and there may be localized guarding. The temperature is usually normal, and there are no changes in the white cell count or in liver transaminases, bilirubin, alkaline phosphatase or serum amylase. These symptoms occur most commonly in women in the 35–55 years age group, but they are also recognized in younger or older patients of either sex.

A diagnosis of gall bladder disease due to gallstones is usually made following the above presentation. The most appropriate first investigation is a biliary ultrasound examination and, in these patients, the result is that of a normal gall bladder and bile duct with no evidence of stones. When other possible causes of upper abdominal pain (e.g. peptic ulcer, irritable bowel or non-ulcer dyspepsia) have been excluded, the available options include a second ultrasound study or an oral cholecystogram.

In patients in whom the suspicion of biliary tract disease remains strong, further investigation is warranted. Endoscopic retrograde cholangiopancreatography (ERCP) is sometimes useful and may be combined with endoscopy to exclude any gastric or duodenal pathology. ERCP is mandatory in any patient with associated liver transaminase, bilirubin, alkaline phosphatase or amylase change with episodes of pain. In such patients there is a high probability of identifying small stones in either the gall bladder or bile duct by careful radiological screening of the biliary tract after the controlled infusion of dilute contrast material. Rare causes of pain, such as sclerosing cholangitis, Caroli's disease or choledochal cyst, will also be identified.

At the end of the endoscopic procedure, gall bladder contraction may be produced by the intravenous injection of cholecystokinin octapeptide (CCK-OP, 40 ng/kg). gall bladder bile which flows into the bile duct and duodenum can then be aspirated through the ERCP catheter and examined for the presence of cholesterol crystals. The finding of cholesterol crystals in gall bladder bile is strongly associated with the presence of small calculi in the gall bladder, or cholesterolosis. Such patients may benefit from cholecystectomy. Bile from the gall bladder for examination for crystals can also be obtained during a separate procedure by aspirating through a duodenal tube after the administration of CCK-OP.

An objective diagnosis of gall bladder motility disorders is made by evaluating the ability of the gall bladder to empty following a standard stimulus.

The introduction of the Tc-99m-labelled iminodiacetic acid derivatives has made it possible to study the hepatobiliary system using the gamma-camera and computer analysis (Figure 30.3.1). The gall bladder ejection fraction (GBEF) can be estimated by use of the following formula:

$$\text{GBEF (\%)} = \frac{\text{Change in GB activity}}{\text{Baseline GB activity}} \times 100.$$

It has been shown that the normal gall bladder empties in excess of 50% of its volume in response to a standard meal or a 45-min intravenous infusion of CCK-OP

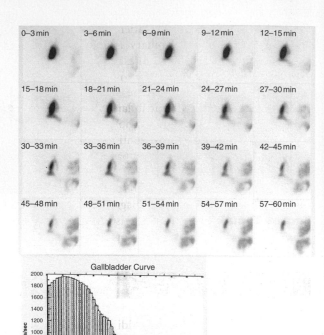

Figure 30.3.1 Gall bladder scintigraphy, illustrating a normal gall bladder ejection fraction (GBEF) in response to infusion of cholecystokinin octapeptide (CCK-OP).

(20 ng/kg/h). In a patient with biliary-type pain, if the GBEF is lower than 40% this is considered to be abnormal. One study has demonstrated a significant difference in the GBEF of patients with gallstones compared to controls. The gall bladder emptying in 14 of 20 patients with gallstones measured < 50% after ingestion of a corn oil meal. In another study, 24 patients with abnormal CCK-OP GBEF (< 40%) were identified from a group of patients presenting with biliary-type pain and no evidence of gallstones. The patients who received an infusion of cholecystokinin or a corn oil meal did not experience pain.

MANAGEMENT

The most appropriate treatment for patients with identified gall bladder motility disorder is cholecystectomy, as it permanently eliminates the organ that is producing the symptoms. However, in certain situations the disorder may be transient, and it may therefore be unnecessary to proceed to surgery.

The role of cholecystectomy was evaluated in 24 patients with abnormal CCK-OP GBEF. Patients were randomized prospectively to either cholecystectomy or follow-up. All but one of the patients who had a chole-cystectomy were cured of biliary symptoms at 3 years after the operation. Histological examination of the gall bladders removed at operation revealed features of chronic cholecystitis such as increased gall bladder wall thickness, fibrosis and chronic inflammatory cells. None of the patients had gallstones. Those patients who did not have a cholecystectomy continued to experience symptoms, and three of these patients subsequently developed gallstones.

The approach for patients with suspected gall bladder motility disorder is to make the diagnosis using CCK-OP infusion scintigraphy. If the GBEF is abnormal, it is recommended to proceed to laparoscopic cholecystectomy.

SPHINCTER OF ODDI

Over 100 years ago, Rugero Oddi proposed that the sphincter he had recently identified could malfunction, resulting in clinical symptoms. This clinical entity is known as sphincter of Oddi dysfunction.

AETIOLOGY AND PATHOGENESIS

The pathogenesis of sphincter of Oddi dysfunction is unknown. One possibility is the existence of primary disorders of motility, perhaps related to defects in the enteric nervous system. Secondary disorders also seem likely, either from direct damage or from the indirect effects on factors which control motility of the sphincter.

The sphincter of Oddi is a smooth-muscle structure approximately 1 cm in length which is situated at the junction of the bile duct, pancreatic duct and duodenum. Its function has been characterized by manometric techniques which allow direct measurement of pressure changes using a small catheter directed into either the bile duct or the pancreatic duct.

The sphincter normally produces high-pressure phasic contractions which are superimposed on a modest basal pressure. The pressure changes produce a resistance to flow whilst at the same time propelling small volumes of either bile or pancreatic juice into the duodenum. Most flow occurs in-between the phasic contractions, but the contractions also serve to keep the sphincter segment empty. An increase in flow and a decrease in resistance across the sphincter occur when there is a fall in basal pressure and a decrease in the amplitude and frequency of phasic contractions. These changes in resistance are normally produced by neural stimuli via local reflexes from the duodenum, or by circulating hormones such as cholecystokinin.

Abnormal responses to normal stimuli have been recorded. In a number of studies, cholecystokinin has been shown to produce an increase in resistance across the sphincter associated with a rise in the basal pressure and a rapid frequency of phasic contractions. This paradoxical response of the sphincter to cholecystokinin may reflect a primary motility disorder of the sphincter. Secondary damage to the sphincter may result from the passage of small stones or following inflammation in either the biliary tract or the pancreas. This may result in repair by fibrosis, which may in turn lead to a fixed stenosis reflected manometrically by a high basal pressure. However, at present, there is no direct evidence for these pathogenetic mechanisms.

DIAGNOSIS

Clinically, patients who present with sphincter of Oddi dysfunction can be divided into two broad groups. The majority of patients have symptoms which are mainly referable to the biliary tract, while a smaller group present with symptoms which are referable to the pancreas.

The majority of patients with sphincter of Oddi dysfunction are women who have had a cholecystectomy for treatment of symptomatic gallstones. The operation usually results in improvement in symptoms, but pain recurs after 2–10 years. The pain is felt in the epigastrium or right upper quadrant, often radiates into the back, and may be associated with nausea and vomiting. It generally occurs in episodes which last for up to several hours or until relieved by analgesics. These episodes may occur at intervals of weeks or months. Some patients also describe discomfort in the upper abdomen, which is more frequent and may occur every day. In addition, symptoms consistent with irritable bowel syndrome may coexist with episodic biliary-type pain. Some patients are aware that their symptoms can be precipitated or aggravated by opioid analgesics, including codeine. Indeed, the first episode of pain may have been experienced following opiate medication, usually for an unrelated procedure.

Physical examination during an acute episode of pain reveals a distressed afebrile patient who often moves on the examination couch in order to find the most comfortable position. Abdominal examination is usually non-contributory, other than revealing mild to moderate tenderness in the epigastrium or right upper quadrant. Signs of local or general peritonitis are not associated with this condition.

Blood screens reveal a normal white cell count. However, about 10–20% of patients show increases in serum concentrations of liver transaminases, particularly in blood specimens which are taken 3–4 h after the onset of pain. This is occasionally accompanied by increases in serum bilirubin and alkaline phosphatase. In a subgroup of patients, the serum amylase activity may be elevated either alone or in conjunction with changes in liver enzymes. This group of patients is often given the clinical label 'idiopathic recurrent pancreatitis'.

Initial treatment of patients presenting with the above clinical symptoms is directed at relief of pain, which is usually achieved by administration of a systemic analgesic or buscopan. Pethidine (meperidine) is thought to be the most appropriate analgesic in patients with suspected sphincter of Oddi dysfunction.

All patients who present with significant post-cholecystectomy biliary or pancreatic-type symptoms should be evaluated by endoscopic retrograde cholangiopancreatography (ERCP). The majority of patients will have a cause other than sphincter of Oddi dysfunction to explain their symptoms, particularly bile duct stones. In the performance of the ERCP, it is important to position the patient correctly in order to screen the bile and pancreatic ducts adequately. It should also be noted whether pain is produced on manipulating the sphincter of Oddi with the ERCP catheter. In addition, the rate of drainage of contrast material from the bile duct after the procedure can be evaluated. Although these signs from the bile duct have a low sensitivity and specificity for sphincter of Oddi dysfunction, they are supportive of the diagnosis in the setting of symptoms and radiological signs such as duct dilatation. A number of studies have now shown that significant bile duct dilatation does not occur following cholecystectomy, and that dilatation of the bile duct suggests a relative stenosis of the sphincter of Oddi. A corrected diameter of 12 mm is taken as the upper limit of normal for the bile duct, and duct dilatation is diagnosed if the maximum corrected diameter exceeds this value. Abnormal drainage is defined by the presence of contrast in the bile duct at 45 min after completion of the procedure.

The effect of opiates on sphincter of Oddi contractility may also be used to evaluate these patients, and serves as an additional non-specific screening test. Morphine and neostigmine are given in a dose determined by the patient's weight. Reproduction of pain as well as changes in liver enzymes and amylase are assessed.

The development of techniques to measure pressure across the sphincter of Oddi has enhanced our understanding of the normal physiology of the human sphincter of Oddi, and has also defined with accuracy and reproducibility the presence of manometric disorders of the sphincter (Figure 30.3.2). The miniaturized manometry catheters which are used for pressure measurement have three lumens and are made of either polyethylene or polytef (Teflon). The catheter is perfused with de-ionized bubble-free water at a pressure of 750 mmHg and the whole system is capable of recording accurately pressure changes of up to 300 mmHg/s.

A patient undergoing endoscopic sphincter of Oddi manometry is prepared for the procedure as for an

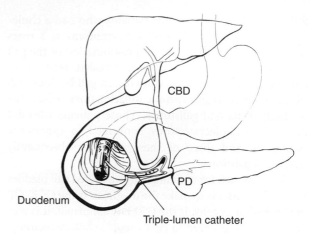

Figure 30.3.2 Endoscopic sphincter of Oddi manometry. The triple-lumen catheter is passed through the biopsy channel of a duodenoscope and inserted into either the bile duct or the pancreatic duct so that the three ports record from the sphincter. CBD, common bile duct; PD, pancreatic duct.

ERCP. Prior to and during the manometric recording, drugs which alter sphincter motility (e.g. atropine and opiate analgesics) are avoided.

When the duodenoscope is in an appropriate position in relation to the papilla, the manometry catheter is inserted through the biopsy channel. The catheter is then passed into either the bile duct or the pancreatic duct to record the duct pressure. It is then withdrawn so that all three recording ports are positioned within the sphincter segment (Figure 30.3.2). Baseline recording from the sphincter is made for approximately 3 to 5 min. The response to an intravenous bolus dose of cholecystokinin octapeptide 20 ng/kg is then assessed. Catheter position in either the pancreatic or bile duct may be assessed by injecting a small volume of contrast medium (< 1 mL) through the most distal port while briefly screening by fluoroscopy.

Endoscopic sphincter of Oddi manometry is the most objective of all available investigations for determining sphincter of Oddi motility characteristics (Table 30.3.1). Manometrically, the sphincter of Oddi is characterized by regular phasic contractions which are superimposed on a modest basal pressure (Figure 30.3.3). The majority of the contractions are orientated in an antegrade direction, but simultaneous and retrograde contractions can be recorded in control subjects.

Manometric abnormalities have been identified in patients with clinically suspected sphincter of Oddi dysfunction. Using the manometric findings, sphincter of Oddi dysfunction has been divided into two major groups, irrespective of whether the symptoms are primarily biliary or pancreatic (Table 30.3.2). This manometric division has allowed for targeting of specific therapy for patients in whom a diagnosis of sphincter of Oddi dysfunction is made. The two major groups are

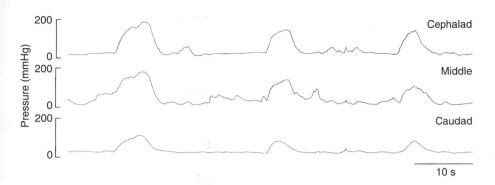

Figure 30.3.3 Manometric recording from the sphincter of Oddi. Prominent phasic contractions are superimposed on a modest basal pressure.

Table 30.3.1 Sphincter of Oddi pressures

| | Normal | | Abnormal |
	Median	Range	
Basal pressure (mmHg)	15	3–35	>40
Amplitude (mmHg)	135	95–195	>300
Frequency (number/min)	4	2–6	>7
Sequences			
Antegrade (%)	80	12–100	
Simultaneous (%)	13	0–50	
Retrograde (%)	9	0–50	>50
CCK-OP 20 ng/kg		Inhibits	Contracts

Table 30.3.2 Sphincter of Oddi dysfunction

Stenosis
   Basal pressure > 40 mmHg

Dyskinesia
   Frequency > 7/min
   Intermittent rise in basal pressure
   Retrograde contractions > 50%
   Paradoxical CCK-OP response

sphincter of Oddi stenosis and sphincter of Oddi dyskinesia.

SPHINCTER OF ODDI STENOSIS

Manometrically, these patients have an abnormally elevated sphincter of Oddi basal pressure which is defined as a basal pressure above 40 mmHg (Figure 30.3.4). Patients with manometric stenosis of the sphincter of Oddi may have a dilated bile duct at ERCP, and elevation of liver enzymes during episodes of pain. However, the correlation is not strong, so these signs cannot be used to predict those patients with sphincter stenosis.

The finding of sphincter of Oddi stenosis may involve the bile duct sphincter, pancreatic duct sphincter, or both. Stenosis in the pancreatic duct sphincter is associated with pancreatic sphincter of Oddi dysfunction, and treatment of these patients requires not only division of the bile duct portion of the sphincter of Oddi, but also division of the septum between the bile duct and the pancreatic duct.

SPHINCTER OF ODDI DYSKINESIA

This group includes a number of manometric abnormalities which have been described in patients with suspected sphincter of Oddi dysfunction. Their grouping may be inappropriate, as they may not have a common aetiology.

Rapid phasic contractions

Spontaneously occurring bursts of rapid phasic contractions may be recorded (tachyoddia). These episodes are distinct from activity fronts which relate to the migrating motor complex (MMC), as they may extend for periods of time in excess of normal MMC activity (Figure 30.3.5). Furthermore, rapid contractions may be accompanied by pain.

Intermittent episodes of elevated basal pressure

An intermittent elevation of the basal pressure may sometimes be noted in association with tachyoddia. This is unlike the stenotic recordings in that the basal pressure returns to normal, usually simultaneously, but sometimes after the inhalation of amyl nitrate.

Excessive retrograde contractions

In normal subjects, the majority of SO contractions are orientated in an antegrade direction. However, an excess of simultaneous and retrograde contractions may reflect an abnormally functioning sphincter which may impair bile flow (Figure 30.3.6). This subtle manometric finding may be of low significance, and its reproducibility is

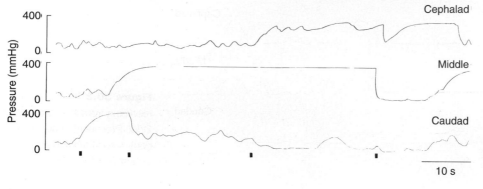

Figure 30.3.4
Manometric tracing illustrating sphincter of Oddi stenosis characterized by a high basal pressure. The black squares illustrate a stepwise withdrawal of the triple-lumen catheter across a narrow stenosis.

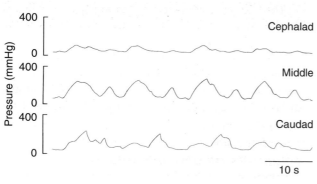

Figure 30.3.5 Manometric tracing illustrating rapid sphincter of Oddi contractions.

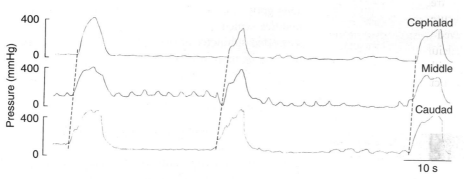

Figure 30.3.6 Manometric tracing illustrating an excess of retrograde sphincter of Oddi contraction.

poor. Taken in isolation, it should not be used to make a diagnosis of sphincter of Oddi dysfunction.

Paradoxical response to cholecystokinin

The normal response of the human sphincter of Oddi to the administration of cholecystokinin is that of inhibition of phasic contractions and a fall in basal pressure. A paradoxical response is recorded when cholecystokinin has no effect on the sphincter contractions, or produces an increase in contraction frequency and/or a rise in basal pressure (Figure 30.3.7).

MANAGEMENT AND RESULTS

The options for management of sphincter of Oddi dysfunction are either division of the sphincter or pharmacotherapy. In the past, uncertainty about the diagnosis of sphincter dysfunction has been associated with

uncertainty with regard to therapy. However, the development of sphincter manometry and the recognition of abnormal motility have led to the identification of individuals who may be cured by targeted treatment.

Prospective clinical studies in Australia, the USA and Europe have shown that patients with biliary-type symptoms and a manometric stenosis (i.e. basal pressure > 40 mmHg) are either cured or else their symptoms are significantly improved following endoscopic sphincterotomy of the biliary sphincter of Oddi. The results of treatment are sustained on long-term follow-up of these patients.

In many patients with idiopathic recurrent pancreatitis, manometry reveals sphincter stenosis. Pancreatic duct stenosis may also be found in patients who have had a biliary sphincterotomy to treat recurrent pancreatitis. Thus endoscopic sphincterotomy is often ineffective for recurrent pancreatitis, and treatment must include division of the pancreatic sphincter. This is achieved via a

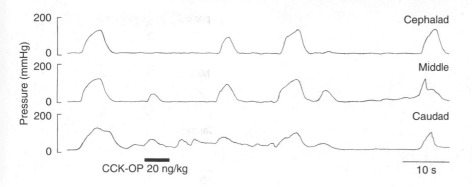

Figure 30.3.7 Manometric tracing demonstrating a paradoxical response to cholecystokinin octapeptide (CCK-OP). An increase in contraction frequency is noted instead of inhibition of contractions.

transduodenal approach at open operation, with division of the septum between the bile duct and pancreatic duct, which creates a wide opening for both ducts.

The results of this operation in producing symptomatic relief in patients with recurrent pancreatitis depend on the selection of patients. Approximately 70% of patients with an abnormally elevated basal pressure are improved by sphincteroplasty and pancreatic septoplasty.

The role of pharmacotherapy in sphincter of Oddi dysfunction is limited, as there are no drugs which are specific, long-acting and free of side-effects. Buscopan may be helpful for acute episodes of pain. However, its action is short-lived and it cannot be taken prophylactically. The calcium-channel-blocker nifedipine has also been used with some success in relieving pain, but may be associated with cardiovascular side-effects.

CONCLUSIONS

Motility disorders of the gall bladder and sphincter of Oddi are now recognized as real clinical entities. Little is known about the aetiology of these rare disorders. Diagnosis of gall bladder dysmotility is best made by calculating the gall bladder ejection fraction from cholescintigraphy with cholecystokinin octapeptide infusion. Diagnosis of sphincter of Oddi stenosis or dysfunction is best achieved by sphincter manometry. Laparoscopic cholecystectomy is recommended for patients with typical biliary symptoms and documented abnormal gall bladder emptying. Endoscopic sphincterotomy is preferred for biliary sphincter stenosis, whereas pancreatic sphincter dysfunction often requires surgical sphincteroplasty and pancreatic duct septectomy.

FURTHER READING

Bar-Meir S. 1984: Frequency of papillary dysfunction among cholecystectomized patients. *Hepatology* **4**, 328–30.

Bobba VR, Krishnamurthy GT, Kingston E, Turner FE, Brown PH, Langrell K. 1984: Gall bladder dynamics induced by a fatty meal in normal subjects and patients with gallstones: concise communication. *Journal of Nuclear Medicine* **25**, 21–4.

Geenen JE, Hogan WJ, Dodds WJ, Toouli J, Venu RP. 1989: The efficacy of endoscopic sphincterotomy in post-cholecystectomy patients with sphincter of Oddi dysfunction. *New England Journal of Medicine* **320**, 82–7.

Hunt DR, Scott AJ. 1989: Changes in bile duct diameter after cholecystectomy: a 5-year perioperative study. *Gastroenterology* **97**, 1485–8.

Nardi GL, Acosta JM. 1966: Papillitis as a cause of pancreatitis and abdominal pain: role of evocative test operative pancreatography and histologic evaluation. *Annals of Surgery* **164**, 611–21.

Rhodes M, Lennard TWJ, Farndon JR, Taylor RMR. 1988: Cholecystokinin (CCK) provocation test: long-term follow-up after cholecystectomy. *British Journal of Surgery* **75**, 951–3.

Thune A, Scicchitano J, Roberts-Thomson I, Toouli J. 1991: Reproducibility of endoscopic sphincter of Oddi manometry. *Digestive Diseases and Sciences* **36**, 1401–5.

Toouli J, Roberts-Thomson I, Dent J, Lee J. 1985: Manometric disorders in patients with suspected sphincter of Oddi dysfunction. *Gastroenterology* **88**, 1243–50.

Toouli J, Roberts-Thomson I, Dent J, Lee J. 1985: Sphincter of Oddi manometric disorders in patients with idiopathic recurrent pancreatitis. *British Journal of Surgery* **72**, 859–63.

Yap L, McKenzie J, Wycherley A, Toouli J. 1991: Gall bladder ejection fraction for acalculous gall bladder pain. *Gastroenterology* **101**, 786–93.

Chapter 30.4

Motility disorders of the colon and anorectum

David Wattchow and Nicholas Rieger

Introduction

The aims of this chapter are to describe the anatomy and physiology of the motor functions of the colon and anorectal region, and to illustrate how this knowledge contributes to the understanding of two motility disorders that present to surgeons, namely constipation and faecal incontinence.

The small intestine delivers between 1.5 and 2 L of liquid content to the colon each day (look at the output of an ileostomy!), and it is the function of the colon to propel the contents to the rectum whilst absorbing most of the fluid, thus converting the fluid to semi-solid waste.

COLON

GROSS ANATOMY AND FUNCTION

Colonic anatomy varies enormously between species depending on whether the animal is carnivorous (e.g. dogs, short and straight anatomy), herbivorous (large appendix and caecum) or omnivorous.

In the human colon the longitudinal muscle is grouped into three distinct bands termed taenia coli. These run from the caecum to the rectum, where they coalesce to form a continuous muscle coat. Because of this continuous muscle coat, diverticula are rare in the rectum, and most surgery for diverticular disease involves excision of a small portion of the upper rectum to ensure that the disease is removed. The longitudinal muscle continues in the anal canal in the intersphincteric plane, and finally fans out away from the internal anal sphincter as the corrugator ani cutis muscle. Incisions to reach the intersphincteric plane involve cutting through or around this muscle.

The colonic circular muscle is thrown into folds or haustrations. The caecum and ascending and transverse colon are relatively capacious. The descending colon is also often capacious, but the sigmoid becomes narrower, and it is preferable to remove the sigmoid colon in anterior resection so that pliable descending colon can be used for anastomosis.

A variety of *motor patterns* have been described in the colon, principally by observing the outline of the colon by instilling dilute barium and using X-ray screening. The patterns observed include peristalsis (contractions of the circular muscle that propagate anally in a slow regular fashion), retrograde peristalsis (thus barium can be moved from the rectum back to the splenic flexure) and mass movements (large, 'emptying' contractions often associated with defaecation). Latterly, similar patterns have been recorded by the use of manometry. However, manometric recordings are usually taken when the colon is empty (to enable the recording tube to be placed by colonoscopy), and they only record lumen-occluding contractions. It is possible to record relaxation of the circular muscle of the colon by the use of a barostat balloon. This is a low-compliance balloon, usually inserted into the descending colon, that can be kept at constant pressure and the volume changes recorded.

The net result of this activity is to empty the colon

from between three times a day to once every 3 days, which is the frequency of normal defaecation. *Colonic motility* can be objectified by the use of transit studies. A simple and effective technique is to ingest 20 radio-opaque markers and take an X-ray of the abdomen each day for 5 days thereafter. In most normal individuals the majority of the markers will be passed by 48 h (less than 20% should be present at 5 days). A refinement of this type of motility study is to use radioactive tracer such as indium and to scan the patient each day for 5 days (Figure 30.4.1). This approach can provide more accurate information about movements of individual regions of the colon, but for most clinical purposes the marker study is equivalent. Interestingly, in several series of 'constipated' patients only about 30% were found to be truly constipated as measured by motility studies.

These complex motor activities are a combination of spontaneous muscular activity and regulation of the muscle by the enteric nervous system, which is in turn influenced by extrinsic nerves from the spinal cord.

COLONIC MICROANATOMY AND FUNCTION

Between the taenia coli the longitudinal muscle becomes very thin. Sandwiched between the longitudinal and circular muscle layers is the myenteric plexus of nerve cell bodies and fibres (Auerbach's plexus). Then there is the submucosa, which consists of collagenous tissue (important for holding sutures in colonic anastomoses) with many blood vessels, and the submucous plexus. There are three distinct layers of the submucous plexus, with

one group of ganglia closest to the circular muscle, one closest to the muscularis mucosae, and an intermediate layer. The mucosa consists of the muscularis mucosae, the lamina propria and the epithelium (Figure 30.4.2).

The *colonic smooth muscle* demonstrates rhythmic depolarization and hyperpolarization (known as slow waves). This rhythm is generated by 'pacemaker' cells (originally described by Cajal and therefore termed interstitial cells of Cajal). The distribution of these cells varies throughout the gastrointestinal tract. In the colon they appear to be distributed around the fascicles of smooth muscle.

The importance of the *enteric nervous system* in colonic motility is illustrated by the condition of Hirschsprung's disease, in which a variable length of rectum and colon has no ganglion cells. Although there is no mechanical obstruction to the passage of faeces, this segment of bowel is aperistaltic, and the infant rapidly develops colonic obstruction.

The nerve cells of the enteric nervous system act on the smooth muscle and interstitial cells to cause contraction and relaxation of the muscle. Many *motor neurones* are found in the myenteric plexus, and in humans (and also in dogs) some motor neurones may also exist in the submucous plexus. The projection of these motor neurones is quite short, being approximately 10% of the circumference of the bowel wall, and generally less than 1 cm in an oral or anal direction. Therefore they are unlikely to be able to co-ordinate complex motor patterns such as peristalsis which occur over distances of many centimetres. This is the function of the *interneu-*

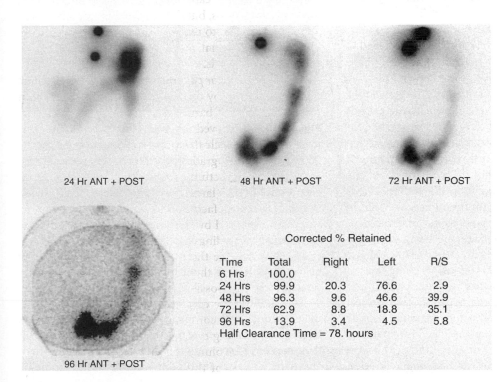

24 Hr ANT + POST   48 Hr ANT + POST   72 Hr ANT + POST

96 Hr ANT + POST

Corrected % Retained

Time	Total	Right	Left	R/S
6 Hrs	100.0			
24 Hrs	99.9	20.3	76.6	2.9
48 Hrs	96.3	9.6	46.6	39.9
72 Hrs	62.9	8.8	18.8	35.1
96 Hrs	13.9	3.4	4.5	5.8

Half Clearance Time = 78. hours

Figure 30.4.1
Radionuclide scan of colonic transit. A spot marker indicates the epigastrium. In this case tracer has moved to the splenic flexure at 24 h and outlines the left colon at 48 h. The tracer accumulates in the rectosigmoid region at 96 h. Therefore there is normal colonic transit but delayed emptying from the rectum/sigmoid.

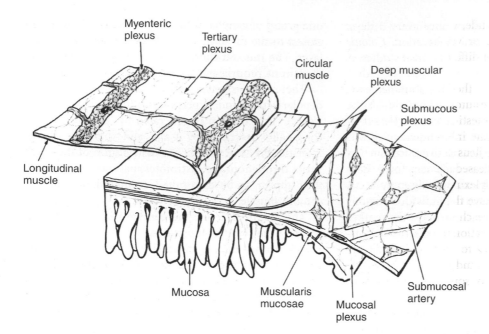

Figure 30.4.2 Microanatomy of the layers of the intestinal wall, indicating the position of the myenteric and submucous plexi.

rones, which are myenteric neurones projecting for 7 cm (or more) in an anal direction and 4 cm in an oral direction. These motor neurones and interneurones have a specific shape; their cell bodies have dendrites which are club-shaped or 'lamellar' and have a single axon (nerve cells of this shape were described by the Russian anatomist Dogiel around the turn of the century, and are termed Dogiel Type I cells).

In addition to motor neurones and interneurones, there are *intrinsic sensory neurones* in the bowel wall which transduce stretch and chemical stimuli. In small animals there is considerable evidence that nerve cells which have large, smooth cell bodies and are multiaxonal serve this function. While such cells are found in human colon, they are much fewer in number than in other species, and their function is not known.

For a long time it has been known that acetylcholine is released from motor neurones and acts on colonic smooth muscle via muscarinic receptors to cause contraction. Only recently has it been shown that relaxation is stimulated by the release of nitric oxide from enteric motor neurones. This does not account for all of the relaxation of the muscle, and it is likely that ATP is released from inhibitory motor neurones as well. In addition, a variety of peptides are found in these neurones, with tachykinins and enkephalin being present in excitatory motor neurones (Figure 30.4.3), and vasoactive intestinal peptide and neuropeptide Y being present in inhibitory motor neurones. Acetylcholine and tachykinins are found in motor neurones that project orally, and nitric oxide and vasoactive intestinal peptide are found in those that project anally. Therefore if motor neurones are fired over a short distance, the net effect is to cause contraction above the stimulus and relaxation

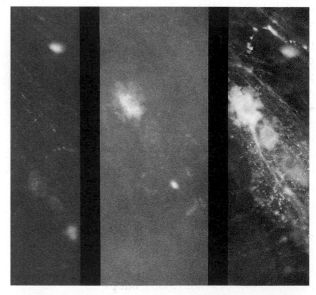

Figure 30.4.3 A photomicrograph of a circular muscle motor neurone in human colon. In the middle panel the cell body of the neurone has been identified by retrograde tracing from the circular muscle. The irregular outline of the cell can be seen (Dogiel Type I). An antiserum to substance P can be seen to identify this neurone (right panel), but an antiserum to vasoactive intestinal peptide (left panel) does not do so. This is an excitatory motor neurone to the circular muscle.

below it, thus propelling intestinal content in an anal direction.

The situation is even more complex with regard to interneuronal circuitry and chemistry. There appears to be one class of ascending interneurones characterized by their content of acetylcholine and tachykinins, but there are many classes of descending interneurones. Some of them appear to release nitric oxide, and subpopulations of these contain acetylcholine or vasoactive intestinal peptide. The functions of these different classes are not yet understood.

Extrinsic nerve fibres from the sympathetic and parasympathetic divisions of the autonomic nervous system exert their effect on the intestine by synapsing on enteric ganglia. For example, the inhibition of colonic motility observed in adynamic ileus is primarily due to the action of noradrenalin released from sympathetic nerves acting on the myenteric plexus. In addition, there are sensory nerve fibres that leave the bowel and travel with the sympathetic nerves to reach the dorsal root ganglia. These not only send information back to the central nervous system, but also appear to mediate inflammatory processes in the bowel wall (and may be involved in inflammatory bowel disease to some extent) by the release of peptides.

SLOW-TRANSIT CONSTIPATION

This disorder represents one end of the spectrum of patients who present with constipation. Typically the patient is a woman in early adulthood who has had constipation from teenage years, characterized by the passage of faeces every 2 to 3 weeks and associated distension and pain. Often the colon is of normal calibre, and motility studies reveal generalized very slow passage of content in the colon.

Just as an inability to walk may be due to any problem ranging from skeletal muscle disorder to the cortex, so the symptom of constipation may have a variety of causes. In view of the above structure and function of the bowel with regard to motility, causes may range from problems with the muscle or interstitial cells to those involving various subclasses of neurones (sensory, interneurones or motor) or their regulation by extrinsic neurones. Very little is known about patterns of motility in this disorder (e.g. whether retrograde peristalsis is more frequent or mass movements are disordered). Available measurements point to reduced power of contraction of the muscle, rather than to accentuated relaxation.

Structural abnormalities of muscle and interstitial cells have been described in some of these patients. Recently, abnormalities have also been found in excitatory motor nerve fibres (correlating closely with the known physiology), but other workers have found abnormalities in the inhibitory motor nerve fibres. There have been no studies to date on the interneurones or sensory neurones, or the *in-vitro* functions of the neurones. Until these are elucidated and effective pharmacological methods become available, surgery (subtotal colectomy with ileorectal anastomosis) will remain an effective way

of relieving constipation in these patients. However, in many patients the problem of bloating and pain is not solved, as the motility disturbance is widespread throughout the gastrointestinal tract, also affecting the small intestine or residual rectum.

RECTUM

When faeces are delivered to the rectum the circular muscle relaxes or accommodates, thus subserving a storage function. If the rectum is removed in the treatment of disease, the colon which is used in its place does not have the same ability to accommodate, so these patients often have increased frequency of defecation. This is especially true in the initial months after surgery, until some adaptation of the 'neorectum' has occurred. The creation of a colonic reservoir (J-pouch) alleviates this problem to some extent.

The circular muscle of the rectum thickens to become the internal anal sphincter (smooth muscle, involuntary). The external anal sphincter is a ring of striated muscle (voluntary) surrounding the internal anal sphincter. Between the two muscles is the intersphincteric plane. The external anal sphincter is artificially separated into three components. The subcutaneous portion lies under the skin and extends below the lower edge of the internal anal sphincter. This is apposed to the superficial portion and, at a deeper level, to the deep portion. The external anal sphincter merges with the puborectalis muscle, which is the lowermost muscle of the levator ani. The external anal sphincter is innervated by the inferior rectal nerve (a branch of the pudendal nerve), whereas the pelvic floor muscles are innervated by the perineal branch of S4. The rectal mucosa is columnar but, at the dentate line, in the mid-anal canal, changes to the stratified squamous epithelium of the skin. At the dentate line there is a zone of 'transitional' epithelium where this change takes place (Figure 30.4.4).

When gas or faeces enter the low rectum a reflex is triggered, relaxing the internal anal sphincter, which is known as the recto-anal inhibitory reflex. This is similar to relaxation induced distal to a distension in the colon. This reflex is mediated by the enteric nervous system (and is characteristically absent in Hirschsprung's disease – anal manometry can be useful in diagnosing cases where the aganglionic area is very short), and it results in relaxation of the internal anal sphincter. In a similar manner to inhibitory neurones elsewhere in the enteric nervous system, nitric oxide is the major inhibitory neurotransmitter that relaxes the internal anal sphincter. This observation has led to the development of a paste containing nitrate donors (0.2% nitroglycerine paste) that results in relaxation of the internal anal sphincter

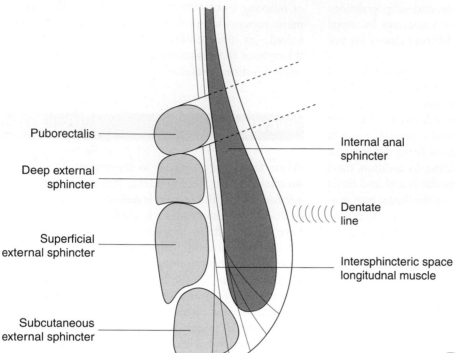

Puborectalis

Deep external sphincter

Superficial external sphincter

Subcutaneous external sphincter

Internal anal sphincter

Dentate line

Intersphincteric space longitudnal muscle

Figure 30.4.4 Anatomy of the anal canal (see description in text).

when applied to the perianal area. This has proved to be effective in relieving the spasm associated with anal fissure and accelerating healing in about 75% of these patients, thus removing the need for surgical sphincterotomy.

At rest, most (80%) of the tone of the anal canal is due to the contraction of the internal anal sphincter. When the sphincter relaxes due to the inhibitory reflex, gas or faeces enter the sensitive transitional zone and a spinally mediated reflex is triggered which results in contraction of the external anal sphincter (EAS). For defecation to occur, this muscle must be consciously relaxed in concert with straining to evacuate the rectal contents. If 3 cm or more of distal rectum is retained during a rectal resection, the sensory apparatus subserving faecal continence is reasonably well preserved, but in very low resections this may be removed and faecal incontinence may result.

The structure and function of the anorectal region can now be comprehensively assessed in an *anorectal physiology laboratory*. Digital examination of the anus gives a good impression of the resting tone (internal anal sphincter) and squeeze pressure (external anal sphincter). These pressures are accurately measured by *manometry* (Figure 30.4.5). In addition, the sensation and compliance of the rectum can be assessed by progressive balloon distension. Most often, however, disorders causing problems with compliance are evident clinically (e.g. low rectal resection, inflammation and stricturing of the rectum). The recto-anal inhibitory reflex is elicited by inflation of a balloon in the low rectum while

simultaneously recording the pressure in the anal canal. As little as 10 mL of volume in the balloon reliably triggers this reflex.

Accurate pictures of the anal muscles can now be obtained by ultrasound examination, and the presence of a defect due to surgical trauma or childbirth can be detected (Figures 30.4.6 and 30.4.7). A rotating probe is placed in the anal canal and ultrasonic waves send echoes back from the mucosa/submucosa; the internal anal sphincter is hypoechoic, whereas the external anal sphincter throws back many echoes, and the surrounding ischiorectal fat is hypoechoic.

The nerve supply to the external anal sphincter can be assessed by measuring the motor latency in the pudendal nerve. A combined stimulating and recording electrode is taped on to a gloved index finger. The region of the ischial spine (close to the pudendal nerve) is palpated while the recording electrodes are positioned at the level of the external anal sphincter. The pudendal nerve is stimulated by electrical current and the EAS can be felt to contract. The recording electrodes detect the depolarization of the muscle, and the latency between the stimulus and contraction can be determined (Figure 30.4.8). This method of study is analogous to assessing conduction delay in other nerves (e.g. median and ulnar nerves).

FAECAL INCONTINENCE

Incontinence of faeces is a very prevalent, socially disabling problem, and is estimated to affect about 2% of

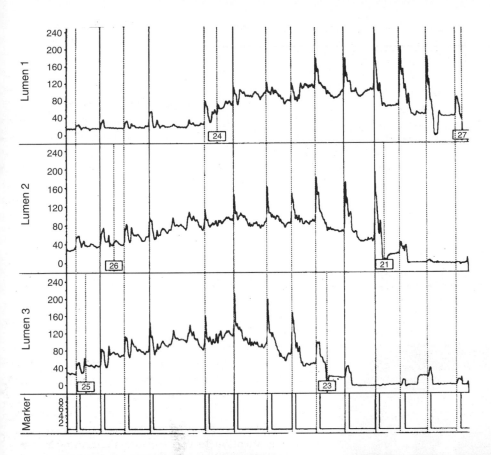

Figure 30.4.5 Manometric tracing of pressures in the anal canal obtained by multiple side-hole recordings from a perfused catheter system. As the catheter is drawn into the anal canal, the pressure is seen to rise (lumen 1 being most instructive) to about $80\,cmH_2O$. This is the resting pressure, and is largely attributable to the internal anal sphincter. The patient is then instructed to squeeze or cough, and the additional squeeze component (external anal sphincter) is recorded (in this case up to $200\,cmH_2O$).

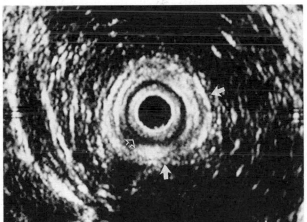

Figure 30.4.6 Ultrasound scan of the anal canal (mid-canal level). The hyperechoic zone around the probe is the mucosa/submucosa. Then there is a hypoechoic zone (dark) which is the internal anal sphincter (open arrow), and surrounding that is the hyperechoic external anal sphincter (solid arrows). The ischiorectal fat is hypoechoic.

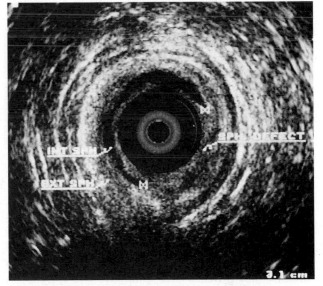

Figure 30.4.7 Ultrasound scan after internal anal sphincterotomy in the left lateral position. The internal anal sphincter edges can be seen to have retracted to 2 o'clock and 7 o'clock (as indicated by the markers). The external sphincter is intact.

the population, women being mostly affected. Problems with the colon or rectum (cancers, inflammatory bowel disease) must be looked for in the work-up of these patients. However, most cases have a reduction in anal canal pressures which can result from damage to the internal or external sphincter or their nerve supply, or a combination of the above. As the disorder mainly affects women, the events of childbirth are the main candidates

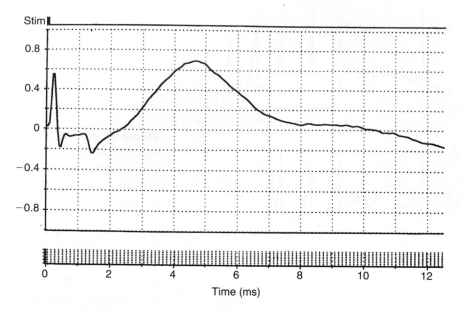

Figure 30.4.8 Pudendal nerve terminal motor latency recording. The trace is of depolarization of the external anal sphincter after stimulation of the pudendal nerve. A sharp upstroke marks the point of the stimulus, and the large, slow upstroke represents the depolarization of the external anal sphincter. The delay to the start of the muscle depolarization is the conduction delay in the pudendal nerve (in this case 2.2 ms – normal range 2.2–2.6 ms).

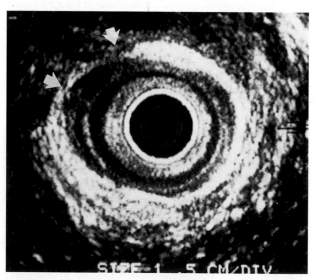

Figure 30.4.9 Anal ultrasound scan showing full-thickness defect in the external anal sphincter after childbirth (arrowed).

for damage to the sphincter. Prospective studies utilizing manometry, ultrasound and nerve conduction have shown high rates of injury (of the order of 30%) to the anal sphincter mechanism, with large tears seen in both external and internal anal sphincters and conduction delay evident in the pudendal nerves (stretched during labour) (Figure 30.4.9).

As 30% of women do not become incontinent, the clinical relevance of this pattern of damage is unclear. However, the majority of women who present later in life (it has been shown that sphincter pressures fall as a function of ageing, not just in relation to the menopause) do have demonstrable tears in the anal sphincter (most often in the anterior aspect of the external anal sphincter), and many of them also have delayed conduction in the pudendal nerves. The initial approach in these patients is to exclude any malignant or inflammatory disease of the large bowel. A cause of incontinence that is sometimes missed is rectal prolapse that has not been realized by the patient. This is an important diagnosis to make, because in about 50% of patients the incontinence will improve once the prolapse has been corrected.

Often attention to diet and the addition of a small amount of constipating medication (e.g. Imodium) are all that is required. For many patients it is the social embarrassment of the problem that is of most concern, and a small dose of constipating agent prior to a social occasion is valuable. If these measures are not successful and the problem is severe, biofeedback retraining or sphincter repair may be considered. Despite defects in the sphincter, approximately two-thirds of these patients show substantial improvement with physiotherapy utilizing biofeedback retraining of the sphincter. This is achieved by placing an electrode in the anal canal to detect depolarization of the external anal sphincter. By amplifying the signal and displaying this as an auditory and visual signal, the information is 'fed' back to the patient. As improvement is not always associated with an increase in sphincter pressure, it is likely that sensory mechanisms are also being retrained.

When surgical repair is indicated, it is usual to overlap the anterior sphincter defect (Figure 30.4.10). Prior to the development of ultrasound examination (which reveals the anterior tears), most surgery focused on plicating the external sphincter behind the anus to accentuate the anorectal angle, but there was a substantial failure rate with this procedure in the long term. If simple sphincter repair fails, other innovative procedures have been devised, such as using the gracilis muscle of the thigh to encircle the anal canal and stimulate its nerve supply to train it to have a tonic function.

Pudendal nerve conduction delay was thought to

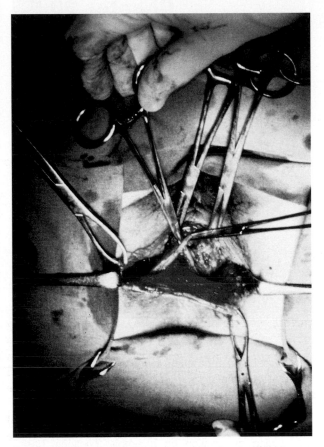

Figure 30.4.10 Photograph of an operation on a patient (who had total faecal incontinence) demonstrating the dissected-out edges of the external anal sphincter, which will be sutured in an overlapping fashion.

account for many of the failures, but the relevance of a conduction delay of the order of fractions of a millisecond has been questioned. Indeed, in many of the original studies directed towards relating conduction delay to reduced anal pressures there would have been unrecognized sphincter tears. Neverthelesss, if sphincter tears are excluded by ultrasound examination, there is still a broad correlation between conduction delay and squeeze pressures. In clinical practice, sphincter repair may still be indicated when the nerves also demonstrate conduction delay, but the functional outcome may be less successful.

CONCLUSIONS

There has recently been a large expansion in our knowledge of the nervous and muscular control of colonic and rectal functions, as well as a much more detailed appreciation of their physiology. Research in these areas is likely to provide additional insights into colorectal motor and sensory dysfunction, and therefore indicate future treatments.

Urodynamics

Villis R. Marshall

Introduction

Considerable debate and uncertainty still exist with regard to both the function and the neural mechanisms responsible for control of the lower urinary tract. However, the process of micturition undoubtedly involves two distinct processes – first, the filling of the bladder and storage of urine, and second, the appropriate and complete emptying of the bladder. In the first phase (filling and storage of urine), a number of conditions need to be met. The bladder must be able to store increasing volumes of urine at a low intravesical pressure. While this seems relatively self-evident, the functional significance of this is considerable. If the bladder is forced to store urine at high pressures, it will significantly impact on the overall renal function, as the back-pressure effect will reduce the glomerular filtration rate with a concurrent reduction in overall renal function. The other key aspect is that the bladder outlet must remain closed at rest. It also needs to remain closed or competent at times when there may be significant increases in intra-abdominal pressure. Finally, the bladder must also remain stable, i.e. not exhibit contractions other than at the time of voiding. For the bladder to enter the second phase (the expulsion of urine), there must be a co-ordinated contraction of the bladder musculature, and at the same time

there must be an appropriate lowering of the outflow resistance. All of these steps must be integrated for voiding to be normal.

As far as the function of the lower urinary tract is concerned, the International Continence Society has classified voiding dysfunction on a simple functional basis, namely failure to store or failure to empty. Failure to store may occur because of disorder of the bladder or outlet function. In the case of failure to empty, this too may be due to either bladder or outlet problems, and thus the functional classification of voiding dysfunction is disarmingly simple.

Urodynamics is the invasive system that has been developed to try to determine which of these components are faulty, and the precise nature of the fault, in individuals with voiding disorders. There has been a tendency to focus on the tubes, flows, pressures and numbers generated from these techniques, but it is important to stress that the findings of urodynamic studies cannot and should not be used in isolation. The data generated as part of the 'urodynamic assessment' need to be coupled with the detailed history and general neurological examination before a final assessment is made.

HISTORY

As part of the urodynamic assessment, a detailed history is required. Three areas are of particular importance. A history of possible neurological abnormalities

or disorders, such as a past history of back trauma, back or spinal operations, cerebrovascular accidents, multiple sclerosis or Parkinson's disease, needs to be sought. Information about previous urinary tract surgery, particularly anti-incontinence surgery, prostate surgery or pelvic surgery, needs to be obtained, and it is also necessary to enquire about the use of drugs such as anticholinergics, antidepressants, antihypertensives and, in particular, alpha-blocking drugs and psychotrophic drugs. In addition, it is important to document carefully the patient's lower urinary tract symptoms, recording frequency of micturition, volume voided each time, nature of the stream, hesitancy, feeling of incomplete emptying, urgency and incontinence. If the patient describes incontinence, then it is necessary to determine whether this is stress related or whether it is associated with urgency. It is also important to assess sexual and bowel function (particularly bowel function, as faecal incontinence associated with lower urinary tract symptoms may suggest a neurological disorder).

PHYSICAL EXAMINATION

While a full physical examination is required, special emphasis needs to be placed on the mental status, sensation, reflexes and rectal and/or pelvic examination. When assessing mental status, it is important to note orientation, intellectual performance, speech and thought content. Identification of areas of sensory loss is also important when assessing potential neurological involvement in voiding disorders. This is further enhanced by the testing of reflexes, particularly the bulbocavernosus reflex, which tests the integrity of spinal cord segments S2–S4 and is expected to be present in most normal individuals. Rectal examination also provides information about the tone of the anal sphincter, again potentially reflecting the function of the sacral nerves, and also allows the detection of rectal abnormalities capable of producing lower urinary tract symptoms.

URINE EXAMINATION

Examination of urine is vital for urodynamic assessment for two reasons. First, infection is frequently responsible for voiding dysfunction and, if overlooked, will result in abnormal urodynamic studies and possibly inappropriate interpretation being placed on those findings. The presence of infection always needs to be excluded for the simple reason that patients who require urodynamic studies will frequently have underlying pathology as well as producing urinary symptoms which will predispose them to recurrent infections. Once infection has been excluded, then the more invasive element of urodynamic studies can be undertaken.

The following tests would normally be considered part of the urodynamic armamentarium:

- uroflowmetry;
- cystometry;
- pressure-flow studies;
- video urodynamics;
- urethral pressure studies;
- sphincter electromyography.

One of the key questions, of course, concerns which patients need to have this more invasive testing.

INDICATIONS FOR URODYNAMIC STUDIES

Urodynamic testing becomes necessary when, after careful clinical assessment, the precise cause of the voiding symptoms is uncertain or the patient has undergone some form of treatment for lower urinary tract symptoms (LUTS) and there has been no symptomatic improvement. As with any investigation, it is important for the clinician ordering the test to determine what information they require to aid the diagnosis or the management of the patient's symptoms, and then only to order that test if it is believed it will be of assistance. In general, the groups for which these tests are most useful are incontinent patients, patients thought to have bladder outlet obstruction, and those for whom a neurogenic cause of their symptoms is suspected. Urodynamic investigations are also potentially useful in children who sometimes present with complex symptomatology involving both incontinence and voiding difficulties.

PATIENT PREPARATION FOR URODYNAMICS

Urodynamics, in particular the cystometry and pressure-flow studies, are invasive procedures and require careful explanation prior to the test being performed. As indicated above, invasive studies should not be performed in the presence of infection, and patients with implants such as heart valves and artificial joints should be covered with appropriate antibiotics. Although rare, autonomic dysreflexia can be a life-threatening complication of such studies. The possibility of this occurring always needs to be considered in patients who have high neurological lesions, such as cervical and upper thoracic lesions, and urodynamic studies should only be undertaken if considered absolutely necessary and in cases where appropriately experienced staff are available. Should autonomic dysreflexia occur, the bladder should immediately be emptied and appropriate antihypertensive agents given to control blood pressure.

UROFLOWMETRY

Uroflowmetry is a non-invasive test that is useful in that it measures the final result of the voiding process. In this regard, it is extremely valuable as it can be frequently repeated, if necessary, but unfortunately the flow rate is influenced by many variables, and thus a low flow rate, for example, may result from either a poorly contractile bladder or significant outflow resistance. Thus the interpretation of the significance of a particular flow rate can be difficult, which has limited the value of this test in clinical practice.

In order to measure flows, a number of devices have been developed which rely on air displacement, changes in weight or the slowing of a rotating disc by the urinary stream. The parameters that are most frequently measured by these systems are the voided volume and the maximum flow rate. Figure 30.5.1 shows a schematic of a normal flow rate. A key factor that needs to be taken into account when assessing flow rates is the voided volume. This is shown schematically in Figure 30.5.2. It is now well recognized that the maximum flow rate is dependent on the voided volume up to volumes of around 300 mL. Because of the reliance of flow rates on the voided volume, nomograms have been developed to take this into account, and one of the most commonly used sets of nomograms is that described by Siroky *et al.* in 1979. In general, however, a flow rate of > 15 mL/s is considered to be normal for a voided volume of 150 mL, although women normally have higher flow rates than men, and in young women peak flow rates of > 35 mL/s for volumes > 150 mL would be expected. Although a low flow rate is not diagnostic, it has been largely accepted, for example, that elderly men with LUTS and a flow rate of > 12 mL/s will almost invariably be obstructed, and more sophisticated urodynamic studies are not normally required. Thus in specific instances a

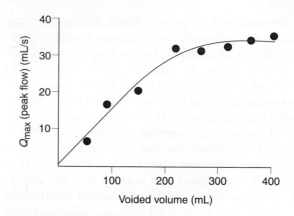

Figure 30.5.2 Influence of voided volume on flow rate.

flow rate can provide valuable contributory information in the assessment of patients with LUTS, and may preclude the need for more sophisticated tests.

CYSTOMETRY

The evaluation of bladder function is best achieved by cystometry. For an effective study, the patient must be awake, not sedated and not taking drugs that are known to influence bladder function. Bladder access is usually achieved per urethra, with most studies using two catheters, one for filling and the other for recording pressure. Gas (carbon dioxide) or liquid (water saline) is used to fill the bladder. There has been debate as to which is preferable and, while there are still proponents of gas, most systems now use a fluid medium because of its more physiological nature, and because it is much easier to demonstrate and detect incontinence. In some instances, a suprapubic catheter is used for filling and pressure recording. Although this has some practical advantages, because of its greater invasiveness it is not used routinely. Cystometry may be performed with the patient lying down, seated or standing, or in an ambulatory setting using special monitoring devices. However, for ease of calibrating the recording system, cystometry is usually performed with the patient supine, although it is recognized that this may not be the ideal method for demonstrating detrusor instability, and various provocative manoeuvres are often used in an attempt to unmask unstable contractions. Such manoeuvres may include jumping, skipping or any other activity that the patient may have described that precipitates potentially unstable contractions.

Critical to the bladder response is the filling rate. A range of filling rates have been employed, but the so-called medium fill rate of 25–100 mL/min is the rate most commonly applied. A normal cystometrogram is shown in Figure 30.5.3. When the bladder starts to fill, there is a

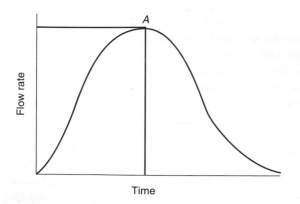

Figure 30.5.1 Urine flow rate: a normal flow curve. The area under the curve represents the voided volume. $A = Q_{max}$ or the peak flow.

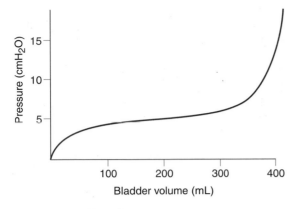

Figure 30.5.3 Normal cystometrogram.

small rise in pressure of a few centimetres of water, and the intravesical pressure rises only very slightly until the bladder-wall structure achieves maximum prolongation, and at this stage the pressure starts to rise rapidly and the patient experiences a feeling of bladder fullness. A cystometrogram provides information about the capacity of the bladder, its compliance, whether sensation is normal, and also whether involuntary contractions occur.

The maximum cystometric capacity is the volume that can be introduced before the patient is unable to defer micturition. In practice, filling usually stops before the patient reaches this point, because it is usually too uncomfortable to continue to a point where the patient is forced to void. Cystometric capacity would be expected to be greater than 350–400 mL.

BLADDER COMPLIANCE

Bladder compliance is defined as the change in bladder pressure that occurs for a given change in volume. The bladder is normally highly compliant, thus allowing filling to occur at a low pressure, and in the normal bladder the pressure rise would be expected to be no more than $10\,cmH_2O$. A poorly compliant bladder is consistent with a neurogenic abnormality. A sustained detrusor pressure in excess of $40\,cmH_2O$ is likely to be associated with significant back-pressure effects and consequent deterioration of upper tract function.

SENSATION

When assessing sensation, the patient is usually asked when they experience the first sensation of the need to void, when they feel a sensation that would normally require voiding, and when they have a strong desire to void that is uncomfortable. The latter situation would only be expected to occur when the bladder had reached its cystometric capacity. The assessment of sensation is particularly valuable, for example, in patients with

lesions leading to an acontractile bladder, as it will be possible to fill a capacity of 1000–1500 mL without any sensation of filling.

INVOLUNTARY CONTRACTIONS (UNSTABLE BLADDER)

The bladder is normally stable during filling, and for this to occur, the central nervous system connections to the bladder must be intact. An involuntary contraction is considered to be significant if the detrusor pressure rise is greater than $15\,cmH_2O$. Although the identification of an unstable bladder may be associated with significant neurological abnormalities, it is not uncommon to find bladder instability in the absence of clinically identifiable neurological lesions.

PRESSURE-FLOW STUDIES

Interpretation of flow patterns can be difficult, and cystometry examines primarily the filling and storage phase of the micturition cycle. To try to obtain a better assessment of the voiding phase of this cycle, flow rate and voiding pressure measurements have been recorded simultaneously. These combined studies have the potential, in particular, to identify obstruction. In order to achieve this as accurately as possible, it is necessary to measure the detrusor pressure. The latter is derived by subtracting the intra-abdominal pressure, measured by a rectal catheter, from the bladder pressure, measured by the intravesical catheter. Figure 30.5.4 shows the results of such a study with a low flow rate and a high voiding pressure consistent with obstruction. There are often technical difficulties associated with such studies. Patients find it difficult to void or to void to completion with catheters *in situ*, and in women in particular it may be difficult to retain the pressure-measuring catheters in the bladder during voiding.

A major problem in the interpretation of these studies has been to define what constitutes an abnormally high pressure to produce a particular flow rate. In an attempt to assist in this interpretation of pressure-flow data, Abrams and Griffiths developed a nomogram (Figure 30.5.5). Numerous subsequent attempts have been made to refine the way in which the pressure-flow data is handled. However, for practical purposes, Abrams and Griffiths' nomogram is still the one most widely used in clinical practice. As can be seen from Figure 30.5.5, it is not possible to readily separate obstructed from non-obstructed patients, and there is a large so-called 'equivocal zone'. When patients fall into this category, it is particularly important that the urodynamic findings are used in conjunction with the

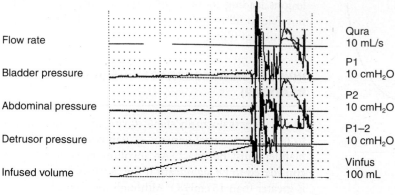

Flow rate	Qura 10 mL/s
Bladder pressure	P1 10 cmH$_2$O
Abdominal pressure	P2 10 cmH$_2$O
Detrusor pressure	P1–2 10 cmH$_2$O
Infused volume	Vinfus 100 mL

Figure 30.5.4 Normal cystometrogram, showing the minimal rise in pressure on filling in a normally compliant bladder.

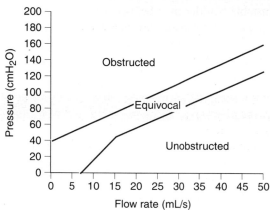

Figure 30.5.5 Nomogram developed by Abrams and Griffiths to differentiate between obstructed and non-obstructed bladders.

history and examination to determine what is the most appropriate diagnosis and hence form of management.

VIDEO URODYNAMICS

It is technically possible to visualize the lower urinary tract using either radiology or ultrasonographics at the same time as the pressure and flows are measured.

There are obvious advantages to this approach, but the cost of the equipment has precluded its widespread utilization. The other major problem is that it has been difficult to quantify and categorize the observed changes adequately. Thus while it is useful in specialized units that evaluate patients with complex lower urinary tract disorders, it has not been widely adopted in clinical practice, although it has the potential to evaluate the dynamic phase of micturition more effectively than any of the other techniques used.

URETHRAL PRESSURE STUDIES

When evaluating the function of the lower urinary tract, one of the major deficiencies is our ability to assess accu-

rately the closure function provided by the bladder neck and distal urethral mechanism. Most techniques can assess the static urethral pressure, but are unable to assess what is occurring during micturition. Thus static profilometry has been largely ignored in clinical practice, as it has not been possible, for example, to show that low-pressure profiles were associated with incontinence or, conversely, that normal-pressure profiles were associated with continence. Thus there is still a need to establish an effective method of assessing the function of the urethral closure mechanisms.

SPHINCTER EMG

This reflects another method which has been used to attempt to measure the function of the distal striated sphincter mechanism. Although valuable information has been obtained from the assessment of patients with defined neurological lesions, technical difficulties and the failure to achieve consistent clinical correlation has limited the use of this technique to research or specialized urodynamic laboratories.

CONCLUSIONS

Urodynamic studies provide valuable data concerning pressure and flow within the urinary tract. However, they constitute an invasive process which, because of its non-physiological nature, may produce artefacts which can interfere with its direct clinical application. There is evidence, for example, that even in something as non-invasive as flow rate measurement the results can vary either as a result of differences in experience in using a particular machine, or as a result of abdominal straining. The care and attention to detail practised by the staff who are performing the test is also of the utmost importance if highly reproducible data are to be obtained. Therefore, although urodynamics are a valuable adjunct in the evaluation of patients with voiding disorders, for the above reasons it is important that the significance of the findings derived from such studies are interpreted in association with the clinical data.

FURTHER READING

Abrams P, Blaivas JG, Stanton SL, Anderson JT. 1990: The standardization of terminology of lower urinary tract function recommended by the International Continence Society. *International Urogynecology Journal* **1**, 45.

Griffiths DJ. 1973: The mechanics of the urethra and of micturition *British Journal of Urology* **45**, 497–507.

Jensen KM-E, Jørgensen JB, Mogensen P. 1985: Spontaneous uroflowmetry variables in elderly males. *Urological Research* **13**, 237–9.

Jonas U, Kramer G, Höfner K. 1994: The principles and clinical application of advanced urodynamic analysis for BPH. In Kurth KH, Newling DWW (eds), *Benign prostatic hyperplasia*. New York: Wiley-Liss, 141–56.

Schäfer W. 1985: Urethral resistance? Urodynamic concepts of physiological and pathological outlet function during voiding. *Neurourology and Urodynamics* **4**, 161–201.

Siroky MB, Olsson CA, Kranc RJ. 1980: The flow rate nomogram. I. Development. *Journal of Urology* **122**, 665–8.

Siroky MB, Olsson CA, Krane RJ. 1980: The flow rate nomogram. II. Clinical correlations. *Journal of Urology* **123**, 208–10.

Webster GD, Kreder KJ. 1998: The neurourologic evaluation. In Walsh PC, Retik AB, Darracott Vaughan E Jr, Wein AJ (eds), *Campbell's urology*. Philadelphia, PA: W.B. Saunders, 927–52.

Wein AJ. 1998: Pathophysiology and categorization of voiding dysfunction. In Walsh PC, Retik AB, Darracott Vaughan E Jr, Wein AJ (eds), *Campbell's urology*. Philadelphia, PA: W.B. Saunders, 917–26.

Endoscopy

David I. Watson, John Miller, Peter C. Robinson, Suren Krishnan and Mario Penta

Introduction

Recent advances in surgical instrumentation and imaging technologies have provided surgeons from all subspecialty fields with the opportunity to perform established as well as new interventional procedures using minimal access techniques. These have the potential to reduce significantly the morbidity often associated with surgical access through conventional incisions. As a result, we have witnessed a dramatic increase in the scope and application of diagnostic and therapeutic 'endoscopic' techniques used in modern surgical practice. Significant improvements in the engineering and optics of flexible and rigid surgical endoscopes, and their application in conjunction with ever-improving miniature camera systems, now allow all members of the operating theatre team to view the operative field as a magnified video image, and to participate actively in interventional procedures.

Endoscopic interventions entail the use of these technologies to view body cavities and other inaccessible areas indirectly, without the need to resort to conventional surgical incisions. Depending on the area to be viewed, access for such techniques may require the use of small incisions, as in laparoscopy and arthroscopy, or access may be possible without the use of any incisions, as in flexible gastrointestinal endoscopy and the majority of urological and otorhinological endoscopy. In these fields, the endoscope is passed through a natural opening such as the nose, mouth, anus or urethral orifice.

An explosion in the use of endoscopic techniques has occurred since the 1980s, revolutionizing many areas of practice, with some fields of surgical endeavour (e.g. urology) now being predominantly endoscopic. Nevertheless, predictions in the early 1990s that the majority of abdominal surgery would be performed laparoscopically have not been fulfilled, as surgeons have become aware of the limitations associated with these approaches and the possibility of different complications arising due to specific aspects of laparoscopic and endoscopic approaches. Currently, almost any abdominal or thoracic procedure can be performed using an endoscopic technique. However, clinical research currently in progress will help to define which of these procedures truly represent an advance in patient care.

INSTRUMENTATION

ENDOSCOPES

An appropriately constructed endoscope is essential for endoscopic surgery, with many varieties available for different purposes. Endoscopes can be broadly classified into two types, namely rigid and flexible, with endoscopes within each broad grouping constructed in a similar way.

Rigid endoscopes

Rigid endoscopes are essential for a large range of procedures, including laparoscopy, thoracoscopy, arthroscopy and some urological applications. Although different rigid scopes generally range from 2 to 10 mm in diameter, and are now available as either reusable or disposable instruments, they are all constructed to a similar plan. This consists of a central collection of 'rod' lenses which collect light from the imaged object and transmit its image to an eyepiece (Figure 31.1). This 'rod' lens system, which was originally described by Hopkins in 1959 and adapted for clinical use by Storz in Germany, provides a magnified image of the operative field. The width of the viewing angle, and the angle of view provided, will vary with different clinical needs. Laparoscopes are available with an angle of view of 0°, 30° and 45°, whereas cystoscopes and sinoscopes have a viewing angle which ranges up to 120° relative to the endoscope shaft.

Surrounding the lens system is a sheath of fibre-optic glass fibres which transmit light from a source of intense light to illuminate the cavity into which the endoscope's tip is placed. Surrounding these fibres is an outer protective metal sheath which provides protection for the inner components, which are easily damaged by rough handling. Although most rigid endoscopes are constructed to a similar plan, an alternative system is available in which a miniature camera is sited at the end of the endoscope, with the endoscope and camera integrated into a single unit. This system eliminates any potential for image distortion due to problems at the interface between the eyepiece of the scope and the camera lens. However, its disadvantages are that the camera signal-processing unit and the endoscope must be made by the same manufacturer, it is not possible to change the endoscope angle (e.g. from a 0° to a 30° laparoscope) without changing the entire camera system as well, and angled endoscopes can only view downwards. Rotation to look around corners rotates the image viewed on the video monitor. This system is less flexible than conventional optical systems.

Flexible endoscopes

Flexible endoscopes (Figure 31.2) are conventionally used for upper gastrointestinal endoscopy, endoscopic retrograde cholangiopancreatography (ERCP), colonoscopy, cystourethroscopy, ureteroscopy, choledochoscopy and many bronchoscopic procedures. These endoscopes are constructed in one of two ways. Either a bundle of coherent fibre-optic fibres is used to transmit an image through the endoscope to an eyepiece, with the endoscopist looking directly through this, or a video endoscope is used. Video endoscopes consist of a microchip camera within the tip of the flexible scope, and the image is transmitted electronically to a processing unit and displayed on a video monitor.

Irrespective of the type of endoscope used, it must also be connected to an intense light source. This light passes down additional optical fibres within the endoscope to illuminate the field of view. Gastrointestinal endoscopes are also connected to an air pump which pumps air through the endoscope to facilitate examination by distending the gastrointestinal tract. Endoscopes used for other purposes, such as flexible choledochoscopes and cystourethroscopes, rely on the irrigation of fluid to achieve organ distension. In addition, a working channel is present in most flexible endoscopes. This

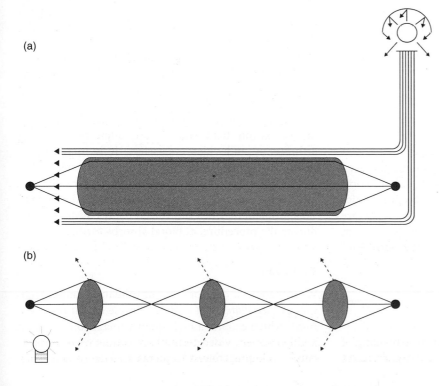

(a)

(b)

Figure 31.1 (a) Diagrammatic representation of the construction of a rigid endoscope. The endoscope incorporates an outer sheath of optical fibres, surrounding a rod lens. The rod lens transmits more light than a series of conventional lenses (b), which progressively lose light, resulting in a dimmer image. In addition, the rod lens system results in a wider angle of view.

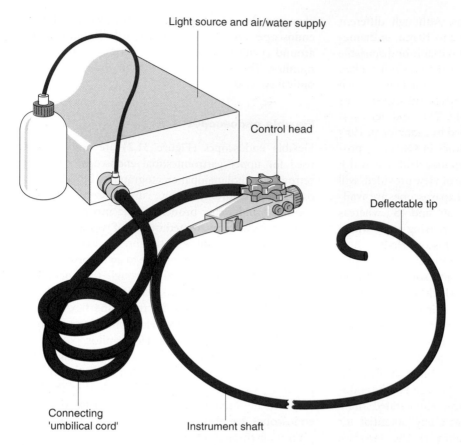

Light source and air/water supply

Control head

Deflectable tip

Connecting
'umbilical cord'

Instrument shaft

Figure 31.2 Conventional endoscope for gastrointestinal endoscopy. This type of endoscope produces an image which is viewed through its eyepiece. The endoscope consists of a control head, shaft and deflectable tip. In addition, the endoscope attaches to a light source and insufflation device.

allows various instruments, including biopsy forceps, diathermy snares and Dormier baskets, to be passed, enabling an additional therapeutic role for most flexible endoscopes.

The tip of the fibre-optic endoscope is manipulated by rotating levers which are used to achieve angulation (Figure 31.3). This enables the endoscope to be manipulated around bends in order to achieve adequate inspection of internal organs. Gastrointestinal endoscopes contain two rotating levers (up/down and left/right). Some smaller scopes (e.g. choledochoscopes and flexible cystoscopes) contain an up/down control lever only, with left/right movement achieved by rotating the flexed scope. Rotation of the shaft of a gastroscope or colonoscope is also helpful for gastrointestinal endoscopy, as it speeds the passage of the scope, and eliminates the need for an assistant to advance the scope during colonoscopy. All flexible endoscopes are end-viewing, except for side-viewing duodenoscopes used for ERCP. The latter are designed to enable good viewing of the ampulla of Vater, thereby making cannulation of this structure possible.

OTHER EQUIPMENT

Light sources

A source of intense light is essential for clear imaging of closed body cavities. The power of the light source

required for adequate imaging will depend on the diameter of the endoscope, the distance of the imaged object from the end of the endoscope, the sensitivity of the attached microchip camera system, and the integrity of the fibre-optic bundles in the light cable and the endoscope. Because smaller-diameter endoscopes, such as cystoscopes and arthroscopes, contain fewer fibre bundles for the transmission of light than larger-calibre endoscopes such as 10-mm diameter laparoscopes, a more intense light source will be more important for an adequate image to be seen through these smaller scopes. Metal halide 250-W light sources are standard for laparoscopic and thoracoscopic surgery, whereas more intense xenon light sources are often preferred for arthroscopy and video-cystoscopy. It is important to realize that broken glass fibres in the light cable and in the endoscope itself will not transmit light, resulting in less than adequate light transmission, and a dark image. This problem may be exacerbated if any bleeding occurs during the procedure, as blood absorbs further light.

Cameras

With the recent development of miniature camera technology (see Plates 31.1 and 31.2 in the colour plate section), which enables a high-quality image to be seen on a video screen, video technology is now used for most endoscopic procedures. Cameras are one of two types.

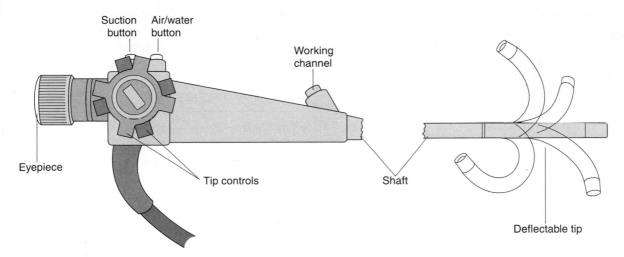

Figure 31.3 Flexible endoscopes are controlled by rotating levers which deflect the tip of the scope. Larger endoscopes have levers which bend the tip in two different directions. In addition, two buttons are used to control insufflation and aspiration functions, and to wash the lens at the instrument tip. Guide-wires and various instruments are passed though the working channel.

Single-chip cameras, which are standard for many procedures, utilize a microchip processor to produce a coloured video image. Modern versions of this system provide high-quality images, which now approach the quality provided by the more expensive triple-chip camera systems.

Triple-chip cameras achieve more accurate colour reproduction by using a prism to split the optical image into primary red, green and blue components of the spectrum. Each of these spectral components is then sensed by one of three microchip processors which are used to convert each component of the light spectrum into a separate electronic signal. The signals are recombined by a processing unit which produces a high-quality image and accurate colour rendition. Most recent variants of both types of camera are available with digital enhancement features which reprocess the electronic signal by sharpening the edges of imaged objects, thereby improving image clarity. Triple-chip cameras, being more complex than their single-chip counterparts, are usually more expensive, but are preferred by many surgeons because of their improved imaging capability. Camera choice will ultimately be determined by the nature of the surgical procedure to be performed, with many surgeons who perform complex laparoscopic and thoracoscopic procedures preferring triple-chip systems. Nevertheless, the majority of the currently available single-chip cameras provide an adequate image for most procedural work.

Insufflators

Although liquid is used as the insufflation medium for cystoscopy, choledochoscopy and arthroscopy, thoraco-scopic procedures can often be performed without the need for any insufflation, because of the rigidity of the chest wall and the ability of anaesthetists to collapse the lung temporarily, and abdominal laparoscopic surgery requires the use of a gas medium under pressure to maintain a working space for surgery. Automatic electronic insufflators are now standard. These devices are able to regulate the flow and pressure of the insufflated gas (carbon dioxide) to pre-set levels, thereby enabling the surgeon to determine a maximum flow and pressure compatible with adequate abdominal distension and patient safety. An ideal insufflator will limit the maximum intra-abdominal pressure generated by the insufflator to 15 mmHg, and will generate a high flow rate if desired (25–30 L/min). An insufflation pressure which exceeds 15 mmHg is unsafe, as it can restrict ventilation during laparoscopic surgery by splinting the diaphragm, and it can reduce venous return by compressing the inferior vena cava. High gas-flow rates assist the performance of complex procedures which can be associated with significant gas leaks due to the use of many laparoscopic ports and frequent exchanges of instruments. A high flow rate will enable the maintenance of a working space despite this problem.

PRINCIPLES OF USE

FLEXIBLE ENDOSCOPES

Flexible endoscopes are controlled by using the rotating lever(s) to deflect the tip of the endoscope. Additional manipulation is achieved by rotating the shaft of the scope, a manoeuvre which is essential for some of the narrower flexible scopes which only have one rotating lever. With practice, a combination of rotation and deflection of the tip allows good viewing of the desired area. Adequate distension of the organ lumen is also essential. Many imaging difficulties can be solved by withdrawing the scope marginally (as it may impact on the wall of the organ) and using additional insufflation.

RIGID ENDOSCOPES

When using a rigid scope, surgeons must be aware that the visualized image is magnified and peripheral vision is lost, i.e. the view is often very narrow (tunnel vision). This increases the risk of damage to organs outside the operative field of view, due to the movement of instruments outside this field (Figure 31.4). This magnification effect requires the assistant who is holding the endoscope to move it back and forth in order to accommodate different imaging requirements during the operative procedure. As the scope pivots at a fixed point where it crosses the skin and underlying fascia or muscle, movements of the scope are necessarily reversed, i.e. paradoxical. Movement of the external portion of the scope to the left manipulates its tip to the right. However, adjustment to this paradoxical movement is usually rapid. Maintaining

orientation is greatly facilitated by placing the surgeon, scope, operative field and video monitor in a relatively straight line (Figure 31.5). Variation from this results in disorientation for both the surgeon and the assistant.

IMAGING PROBLEMS

A poor-quality image, particularly when using video-assisted technology, can be caused by a range of problems. It is important to clean lens interfaces, as fogging can occur as a result of condensation, especially at the outset of surgery when the lens may be cold. If the equipment is correctly connected, and the light source is set to produce maximal light, additional difficulties can occur due to use of an old light globe which requires replacement, or due to broken or degraded optical-fibre bundles either in the fibre-optic cable connected to the light source, or within the scope.

CLINICAL INDICATIONS

Although the impetus for endoscopic surgery has been its ability to reduce morbidity associated with surgical access, for each proposed new endoscopic procedure the relative advantages should be weighed against the possibility of specific complications related to the new

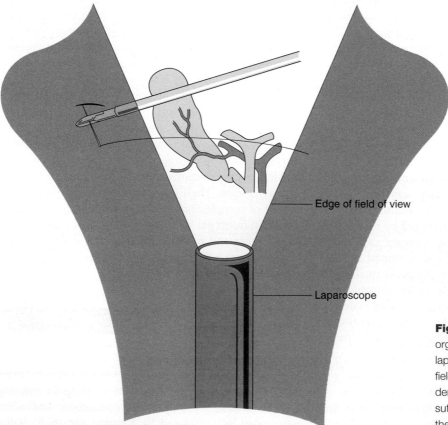

Edge of field of view

Laparoscope

Figure 31.4 Injury to intra-abdominal organs can easily occur during laparoscopic surgery due to the narrow field of view. This diagram demonstrates injury to the liver from a suture needle outside the direct view of the laparoscope.

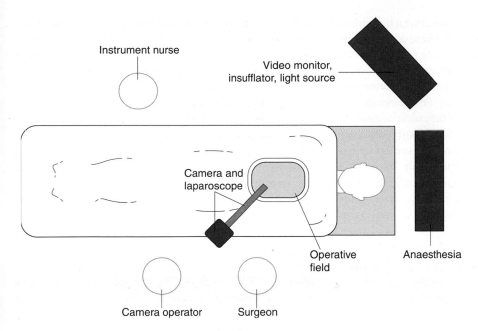

Figure 31.5 A conventional theatre set-up for laparoscopic cholecystectomy. Note that the surgeon, camera operator, laparoscope, operative field and video monitor are in a straight line, in order to facilitate the orientation of the surgical team.

technique. An endoscopic approach can be associated with specific new complications, or even mortality, which are not inherent to the conventional surgical procedure that it replaces. These possibilities are often not foreseen during the initial enthusiasm which accompanies the publicity associated with any new 'advance' in technique. Examples include the issue of port-site tumours arising following laparoscopic cancer surgery, and the potential for division of the common bile duct during laparoscopic cholecystectomy. The overall decision to choose to perform a procedure endoscopically is determined by balancing these risks against the perceived advantages of reduced morbidity and quicker recovery. Given the potential for different complications and problems, informed consent should not be forgotten, particularly as the lay public often equates endoscopy with risk-free surgery.

GASTROINTESTINAL ENDOSCOPY

Although historically rigid endoscopes were used for visualization of the proximal and distal extremities of the gastrointestinal tract, i.e. the oesophagus and rectum, the development of flexible fibre-optic endoscopes in the 1970s now enables the stomach, duodenum, colon and even the small bowel to be visualized. End-viewing flexible endoscopes are used for gastroscopy and colonoscopy. Upper gastrointestinal endoscopy is used routinely for inspection of the oesophagus, stomach and proximal duodenum, facilitating accurate diagnosis of diseases of these organs, including peptic ulceration, gastro-oesophageal reflux disease and oesophago-gastric tumours. In addition, tissue biopsies are easily obtained.

The opportunity to perform a range of interventional procedures, including dilatation of oesophageal strictures, stenting of oesophageal tumours, haemostatic injection of bleeding upper gastrointestinal lesions and placement of gastrostomy tubes, now enables flexible endoscopy to play an increasing therapeutic role.

Colonoscopy provides vision of the lumen and therapeutic access to the entire length of the colon and the terminal ileum, although manipulation of a colonoscope to the caecum in patients with a tortuous colon can be difficult, resulting in a certain percentage of examinations failing to visualize the caecum. The extent of this problem is somewhat dependent on operator experience. However, even experienced operators will sometimes be limited to an incomplete examination. Nevertheless, colonoscopy does enable a range of colonic diseases to be diagnosed accurately and, like upper gastrointestinal endoscopy, biopsy of colonic tumours and other pathology is possible. It also has an important therapeutic role for the excision of colonic polyps. This is achieved by using a diathermy snare, although the use of a 'hot-biopsy' technique for small polyps is an alternative. The latter technique involves the application of diathermy energy to colonic mucosa through the unguarded metal portion of a biopsy forceps, before the biopsy specimen is completely separated from the mucosa. A zone of diathermy necrosis around the biopsy site is achieved, and a histological diagnosis of the lesion is obtained. However, confirmation of histological margins is not possible, as the technique relies on the use of diathermy to achieve 'clearance'.

A diathermy snare is used for the excision of larger polyps, and is particularly well suited to pedunculated lesions. This technique requires the polyp to be encircled with a wire loop, which is then closed around its base.

Diathermy energy is applied to the wire, which is closed ever more tightly, cutting through the base of the polyp. Colonoscopic excision is not appropriate for large sessile polyps, which still require standard surgical resection techniques because of the increased risk of perforation of the full thickness of the colonic wall. Polypectomy carries an overall risk of perforation of the colon of approximately 0.5%. The likelihood of important pathology being missed at the time of colonoscopy is similar to that at radiological examination of the colon by barium enema, although colonoscopy is more versatile than barium enema for most clinical situations because of the opportunity to obtain a tissue diagnosis as well as its therapeutic role for colonic polyps.

ERCP requires the passage of a side-viewing flexible duodenoscope into the second part of the duodenum, visualization of the ampulla of Vater, and cannulation of this structure. Radiological contrast is then used to enable radiological imaging of the biliary and pancreatic ducts. This technique is particularly useful for the investigation of suspected bile duct obstruction. In this situation it can have an additional therapeutic role. A sphincterotomy can be performed using electrocautery, to achieve improved biliary drainage or to facilitate the passage of a Dormier basket which can be used to snare and retrieve stones from the common bile duct. In addition, rigid plastic or expandable metal stents can be placed across an area of bile duct obstruction for patients with obstruction due to malignant or benign strictures

of the common duct. Occasionally the pancreatic duct is stented to treat pain due to chronic pancreatitis, or a biliary manometry catheter is placed across the ampulla of Vater to facilitate the manometric diagnosis of biliary dyskinesia or sphincter of Oddi spasm.

A new role for flexible gastrointestinal endoscopy is small-bowel enteroscopy. This enables visual inspection of the small-bowel lumen by using a long enteroscope. The procedure requires considerable patience, as the enteroscope is passed through small-bowel lumen with the assistance of peristalsis. Deliberate, rapid manipulation of the enteroscope through the small bowel is not possible. This procedure remains under evaluation, and its role as a diagnostic tool is unclear at present.

LAPAROSCOPY

LAPAROSCOPIC ACCESS

As laparoscopy requires the placement of a cannula across the abdominal wall to provide access into the peritoneal cavity or the extraperitoneal space for a rigid laparoscope and other instruments (Figure 31.6), initial access through this barrier must be safely achieved. This can be established by using one of two methods. The open insertion of a blunt trocar and cannula system under direct vision (the Hasson technique) has become

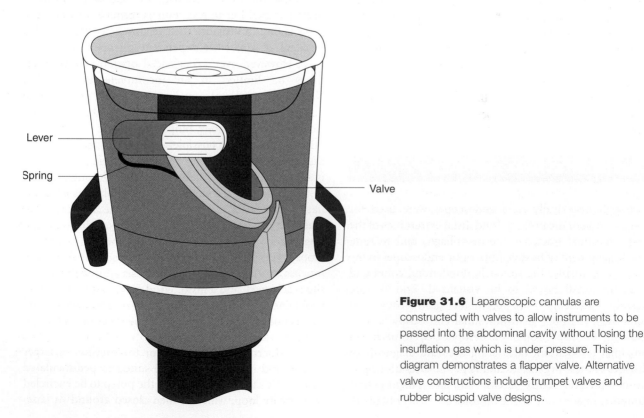

Lever

Spring

Valve

Figure 31.6 Laparoscopic cannulas are constructed with valves to allow instruments to be passed into the abdominal cavity without losing the insufflation gas which is under pressure. This diagram demonstrates a flapper valve. Alternative valve constructions include trumpet valves and rubber bicuspid valve designs.

increasingly popular with general surgeons, as it is thought to be associated with less risk of injury to the major abdominal vessels (an injury with potentially catastrophic consequences). Open insertion requires preliminary dissection of the layers of the abdominal wall under vision, usually in the periumbilical region, but at times elsewhere if umbilical access is not required. Once the peritoneum has been opened, a blunt-ended cannula is inserted and secured.

An alternative approach requires the initial use of a Veress needle. This 2-mm diameter needle consists of an outer sharp needle with a central spring-loaded blunt-ended guard. The needle is pushed through the abdominal wall, and the blunt-ended central mechanism springs out to protect underlying structures once the peritoneal cavity has been entered. It is very important to take care not to aim the needle at the major retroperitoneal vessels, to avoid serious injury. Once placed, gas is insufflated through the needle to create a pneumoperitoneum. The peritoneal cavity is usually filled by the insufflation of 2–5 L of gas, and the pressure will equilibrate at 12–15 mmHg. A sharp-pointed trocar can then be pushed through the abdominal wall. This is subsequently used for the insertion of a laparoscope.

Because this technique involves the blind passage of a sharp object on two occasions, there is likely to be a greater risk of injury to the major retroperitoneal vessels, particularly if the primary entry point is periumbilical. The use of trocars with spring-loaded safety shields for the primary trocar may reduce this risk. However, as with all areas of surgery, apparently safe instruments in unskilled hands can still cause considerable damage, and safety shields on trocars do not prevent injury if combined with poor technique. The risk of injury to the retroperitoneal vessels with the Veress needle technique is approximately 0.05–0.1%. Both the Veress and Hasson insertion techniques are associated with a low incidence of injury to intra-abdominal viscera, with the incidence reported to be in the range 0.1–0.2%.

For therapeutic laparoscopic procedures, which now represent a large part of general surgical practice, a variable number of secondary trocars must be inserted (see Plate 31.3 in the colour plate section). It is important to insert these under direct laparoscopic vision, with the trocar tip kept under observation at all times, as careless technique will again result in injury. Injury to vessels at any stage in the procedure can result in gas embolism due to introduction of the insufflant gas into the bloodstream. A sufficiently large volume of gas will impair cardiac output and lead to cardiac arrest. Fortunately, this complication is rare. It is most likely to occur if a Veress needle is introduced directly into a major vein, connected to an insufflator, and the insufflator is allowed to pump a significant volume of gas directly into the circulation.

LAPAROSCOPIC PROCEDURES

Interventional laparoscopy is feasible if surgeons are able to orient anatomy seen on a video screen. An ability to sense depth and to use both hands for the manipulation of laparoscopic instruments is essential for efficient and safe surgery. Complex manipulations can be performed, facilitating the application of laparoscopic techniques to a range of abdominal surgical procedures. For such procedures a good assistant who can manipulate the laparoscope and provide further assistance as necessary is very important.

It can now be accurately stated that the entire range of open abdominal surgery, including liver resection, aortic surgery and pancreaticoduodenectomy, can be performed laparoscopically. However, the mere fact that a procedure can be performed laparoscopically does not prove that this is better than the conventional open surgical approach. Laparoscopic cholecystectomy and laparoscopic anti-reflux surgery (see Plate 31.4 in the colour plate section) have become well established. Additional procedures such as common bile duct exploration, adrenalectomy, splenectomy, appendicectomy and nephrectomy are performed routinely in many centres, with good clinical outcomes.

Inguinal herniorrhaphy and laparoscopic colorectal surgery have been associated with more controversy, the former because the laparoscopic procedure is performed in a different way to established open techniques. This can result in unique and important new complications. In addition, unlike cholecystectomy and anti-reflux surgery, laparoscopic inguinal hernia repair has not been demonstrated within randomized trials to have significant advantages over traditional techniques. Laparoscopic surgery for colorectal cancer, on the other hand, has been associated with a worrying incidence of metastases developing in the port sites. This is of particular concern because long-term outcomes following cancer surgery are more important than short-term morbidity. Laparoscopic colectomy therefore remains under stringent evaluation, with the long-term outcomes of randomized trials awaited before its status can be confirmed.

Although procedures such as laparoscopic cholecystectomy are usually performed with the patient positioned supine, alternative patient positioning will facilitate other laparoscopic interventions. For example, exposure for laparoscopic splenectomy (see Plate 31.5 in the colour plate section), nephrectomy and adrenalectomy is improved by positioning the patient laterally. Laparoscopic upper gastrointestinal surgery is often performed with the patient positioned in the reverse Trendelenberg position. This enables the surgeon to stand between the patient's legs, and an assistant to stand on either side if necessary.

The ability of surgeons to perform laparoscopic procedures continues to improve, alongside rapid advances in surgical instrument technologies which continue to facilitate this progress. The use of stapling devices, ultrasonic dissection and coagulation devices, as well as other new technologies, will continue to open up new possibilities for interventional laparoscopy in the future.

THORACOSCOPY

As with laparoscopic surgery, thoracoscopic techniques also enable intrathoracic diagnostic and therapeutic procedures to be performed without the need for an open thoracotomy incision. Avoidance of a thoracotomy should result in a significantly more rapid recovery and a shorter convalescence following successful surgery. Positioning for thoracoscopy usually requires the patient to be in either the lateral or prone position, depending on the procedure to be performed. Although the fully prone position provides good access to the posterior mediastinum and sympathetic chains, lateral positioning is more appropriate for surgery on the lungs.

The rigidity of the thoracic cage enables most thoracoscopy to be performed using a gasless technique. This requires the anaesthetist to place a double-lumen endotracheal tube to enable deliberate collapse of the lung on the side of surgery, in order to create space for the manipulation of instruments. Alternatively, low-pressure insufflation (5 mmHg) is sometimes used, particularly in combination with the prone position. This will provide good exposure of the posterior mediastinum without the need for lung collapse, and gravity will allow the lung to fall away from the operative field. This may be important for patients with respiratory insufficiency who require a thoracoscopic procedure.

Access for thoracoscopy is conventionally obtained by using blunt dissection for the placement of thoracoscopic ports. A similar dissection technique to that used for the insertion of an intercostal drain can be safely used for initial access. Specifically modified valveless thoracoscopic trocars may be used if a gasless technique is to be performed. Alternatively, conventional laparoscopic cannulas can be used. These are essential if low-pressure insufflation is to be used. Placement of ports is more critical than for laparoscopic surgery because the trocars are restricted by the position of the spine, ribs and scapula, and the rigidity of the chest wall can further restrict instrument movement.

Established thoracoscopic procedures include sympathectomy, oesophageal myotomy and lung biopsy. Additional procedures under evaluation include thoracoscopic splanchnic nerve division for chronic abdominal pain, oesophagectomy for carcinoma, pulmonary resection for carcinoma, and lung volume-reduction surgery for emphysema. With the possible exception of oesophagectomy, initial experience with all of these procedures suggests that peri-operative morbidity is significantly reduced. The ability of thoracoscopic approaches to reduce the morbidity of oesophagectomy, however, is currently uncertain.

CYSTOSCOPY

Over 90% of urological surgery is performed using endoscopes. The earliest urological endoscope was produced in 1806, but it was not until Nitze designed an endoscope incorporating the features of the present day endoscope (lens system, distal illumination and irrigation/operating channel) in 1879 that cystoscopy became popular. The Hopkins lens system revolutionized modern rigid endoscopes in the 1960s, improving the quality, clarity and field of view for all urological endoscopes.

RIGID AND FLEXIBLE CYSTOSCOPY

Rigid cystoscopy has been used for over 120 years, and remains the most common procedure in modern urology. Fibre-optic flexible cystoscopes (similar in design to flexible bronchoscopes) have been available since the mid-1980s. These provide a safe, effective and relatively painless means of visualizing the entire lower urinary tract in male and female patients under local anaesthetic, and can be utilized for simple diagnostic and therapeutic manoeuvres such as bladder biopsy, ureteric catheterization and stent removal. Using the rigid sheath and lens system, small bladder tumours and other lesions can be removed or diathermied, and a variety of other diagnostic procedures, including retrograde visualization of the upper tracts and stent placement to relieve intrinsic or extrinsic ureteric obstruction, are made possible.

TRANSURETHRAL RESECTION

Operating telescopes with larger-calibre rigid sheaths (resectoscopes) have been utilized since the 1940s to perform endoscopic prostatectomy and bladder tumour removal via the transurethral technique. Currently the use of surgical cautery via wire loops, knives and roller balls allows safe, rapid and effective endo-urological surgery on the prostate, bladder neck and bladder proper. With the continued development of resectoscope technology, the speed of resection and safety of the surgery has improved. Camera development over the past decade has allowed this difficult surgical technique to be readily taught, whilst decreasing the risks associated with bodily fluid contact. Novel uses for the resectoscope include resection of mucosal tumours in the upper tracts of individuals with single kidneys, and endoscopic incision of urinary tract strictures (urethral, ureteric, pelvi-ureteric and calyceal).

URETEROSCOPY

Since the mid-1980s it has been possible to inspect the ureter visually with endoscopes. The small calibre of these endoscopes required the development of new operative aids, miniaturized to allow successful endoscopic treatment of ureteric calculi with basket extraction, laser-fibre stone fragmentation, ballistic ultrasonic and electrohydrolic probes designed to fit both rigid (mini-scopes) and flexible ureteroscopes. From a practical viewpoint the flexible scopes are expensive and have a short lifespan, but they enable retrograde visualization of the entire urinary tract from the urethral meatus to the renal calyces. Pressurized flow considerably improves the visualization and subsequent performance status.

NEPHROSCOPY

Associated with the development of interventional uro-radiological techniques in the 1980s was the development of endoscopes for visualization of the intrarenal collecting system via an antegrade puncture and tract dilatation. Both flexible fibre-optic and rigid versions exist. The latter is more commonly used for removal of large and small calculi, and can be combined with various forms of stone fragmentation and removing equipment.

UROLOGICAL LAPAROSCOPY

In parallel with the development of laparoscopic general and gynaecological surgery, urological laparoscopic procedures have increased in the past decade. It is now possible through both transperitoneal and retroperitoneal/extraperitoneal approaches to perform renal and adrenal surgery such as nephrectomy, pyeloplasty for pelvic ureteric junction obstruction, and adrenalectomy. Pelvic and abdominal lymphadenectomy, together with antistress incontinence procedures, have become popularized, but overall this aspect of endoscopic urology has been slow to be embraced, due to the prolonged operative times and less reliable results in the occasional operator's hands.

BRONCHOSCOPY

Fibre-optic bronchoscopy provides excellent visualization of the tracheobronchial tree, and has replaced rigid bronchoscopy for almost all diagnostic procedures. The standard fibre-optic bronchoscope is 5–6 mm in diameter, has a single instrument channel and allows angulation in one plane only. As it is manipulated within a rigid lumen, there is no requirement for an air pump to distend the operative field. The fibre-optic bronchoscope can be passed transnasally or transorally, and a good view of the nasopharynx, larynx and tracheobronchial tree down to fifth-order bronchi can be achieved. Rigid-tube bronchoscopy is still used selectively, most commonly for therapeutic procedures such as the removal of foreign bodies, laser treatment of endo-bronchial tumours, etc. However, even these therapeutic procedures can now be performed using a fibre-optic bronchoscope in most patients.

INDICATIONS

Fibre-optic bronchoscopy is used predominantly for the diagnosis of respiratory symptoms and radiological opacities. It is helpful in the evaluation of symptoms such as cough, haemoptysis, localized wheezing and stridor. Radiological abnormalities such as a lung mass, diffuse interstitial lung disease, unresolved consolidation or collapse can all be assessed bronchoscopically. Disease processes associated with the above indications include primary and metastatic carcinoma of the lung, respiratory infections, various diffuse interstitial lung diseases, asthma and bronchiectasis.

Bronchoscopy can also be used for therapeutic manoeuvres in selected patients. Bronchoscopy with washing and suction is very effective for removing excess secretions in patients with post-operative mucous retention, or in asthmatics with mucous plugging. Endotracheal tube placement can be assisted by bronchoscopy in difficult patients (e.g. patients with cervical spine or upper airway abnormalities), and the tube position can be checked after intubation. A neodymium:YAG laser can be used to photocoagulate and resect lesions obstructing major airways. This is mainly indicated in patients with primary or secondary endobronchial malignancy, but is also used for benign conditions such as bronchial webs or post-intubation tracheal stenosis.

Tracheal and bronchial stents can be inserted through either a fibre-optic or rigid bronchoscope for the treatment of benign or malignant localized airway narrowing. Another important application of fibre-optic bronchoscopy is in the assessment and management of complications associated with lung transplantation. Transbronchial lung biopsies are obtained at regular intervals to assess rejection or opportunistic infection, and the bronchial anastomosis can also be assessed for stenosis or ischaemia.

COMPLICATIONS

Excessive bleeding is the most frequent complication, and for bronchoscopy it is important to select patients who have a normal coagulation profile. Bleeding obscures the view and cannot be dealt with adequately through the small suction channel of the fibre-optic bronchoscope. There may also be worsening of respiratory failure. This occurs mainly in patients with compromised pre-operative respiratory function. Post-procedural fever is a common complication, usually short-lived, and more serious infections including pneumonia or septicaemia are rare. Pneumothorax can occur when peripheral lung biopsies are being taken.

LARYNGOSCOPY AND OTORHINOLARYNGOLOGICAL ENDOSCOPY

Modern endoscopes (both rigid and flexible) have been used in all aspects of otorhinolaryngology and head and neck surgery, as well as in facial plastic surgery. However, their most significant contribution has been to the area of sinus surgery (see Plate 31.6 in the colour plate section). The principles of sinus surgery are currently based on maximizing function, and understanding that the drainage of sinuses is not based on gravitational forces, but occurs as a result of the metachronous beat of cilia transporting a mucous blanket towards specific ostia. Rigid endoscopes allow a clear inspection of the middle meatus of the nose and its underlying anatomical structures, the uncinate process, the infundibulum, the bulla ethmoidalis and the fronto-nasal recess (see Plate 31.7 in the colour plate section). The addition of computerized tomography to image the paranasal sinuses allows an accurate determination of disease.

The use of specifically designed instruments in conjunction with endoscopes allows surgical treatment to be targeted to diseased sinuses and sinus ostia. The availability of powered instruments such as microdebriders and microdrills, which have irrigation and suction capabilities, has increased the scope of endoscopic sinus surgery. This now includes endoscopic dacryocystorhinostomy to treat obstructed nasolacrimal ducts, and endoscopic decompression of the optic nerve. These techniques have also been used in the field of operative neurosurgery to close anterior cranial fossa cerebrospinal fluid leaks, as well as to perform transphenoidal pituitary tumour surgery. The endoscope can also access regions behind the posterior wall of the maxillary sinus to facilitate surgery to the contents of the pterygopalatine fossa.

In the field of otology, rigid endoscopes have been used primarily for the purpose of inspection. Telescopes 2–3 mm in diameter with short shaft lengths can be introduced into the ear to examine the tympanic membrane. Telescopes with angled lenses can view areas of the eardrum which are retracted into the upper recesses of the middle-ear cleft. These areas are not visible to inspection by any other method. At an experimental level, some centres are using 1-mm diameter lens systems, which are introduced into the middle ear through a small incision in the eardrum, to inspect the middle ear, particularly in the search for elusive perilymphatic fistulae.

The use of endoscopes in laryngology and broncho-oesophagology has always been hampered by poor light sources. The introduction of fibre-optic light transmission in the 1960s transformed visualization of the larynx, pharynx, trachea, bronchi and oesophagus. With the development of specialized endoscopes and instruments, surgical procedures can now be performed endoscopically. In the field of laryngology, angled telescopes allow close inspection of the recess between the false and true vocal cords (known as the laryngeal ventricle), as well as close inspection of the subglottic region. More recently, contact endoscopy using a rigid endoscope has been employed with staining techniques to detect early changes in the epithelium of the vocal cords, thereby facilitating surgical treatment of early laryngeal cancer without disruption of laryngeal function. The combination of a good endoscopic light source with a laser has enabled endoscopic treatment of laryngeal tumours. Rigid and flexible bronchoscopes can also be introduced into the trachea to deal with tumours within the lumen of the trachea. These tumours can be ablated using a carbon dioxide laser with a rigid endoscope, or a Nd:YAG laser through a flexible endoscope.

In the field of oesophagoscopy it is now also feasible to treat pharyngeal pouches endoscopically. A distending Weerda diverticuloscope or the modified Dohlman's bivalved rigid oesophagoscope (Benjamin–Hollinger diverticuloscope) can be used to display the common wall between the pharyngeal pouch and oesophagus and keep it under tension. This common wall, caused by the hypertrophic cricopharyngeus, can then be divided using the carbon dioxide laser or the linear cutting and stapling devices originally designed for laparoscopic surgery.

The modern endoscope has increased the scope of surgery in the head and neck, facilitating more accurate diagnosis and improving our understanding of many disease processes. The challenge for the future lies with the development of better instruments to accompany the modern endoscope, and more accurate anatomical localization within cavities that lie close to neurological structures by using stereoscopic imaging devices.

ARTHROSCOPY

The first reported diagnostic arthroscopy of the knee was performed in 1918 by Takagi, who used a urological cystoscope, although the technique was not taken up widely at the time. Renewed interest in the mid-1970s was accompanied by scepticism about its efficiency for the diagnosis and treatment of joint disorders. However, arthroscopy has subsequently evolved to become a well-accepted and established technique. Its major advantages include accurate diagnosis of intra-articular pathology and the ability to perform precise surgical procedures, in association with rapid rehabilitation and few complications. The procedure can be performed on a day-case basis, thereby reducing hospitalization costs. However, there are some disadvantages to arthroscopic surgery. It can be a difficult technique to learn, and iatrogenic damage to articular structures in unskilled hands can be a major problem. Arthroscopic equipment is costly and easily damaged. Moreover, deep-seated joints as well as small joints may not be amenable to arthroscopic treatment of intra-articular pathology and, most importantly, major neurovascular structures can be damaged during the placement of entry portals.

INSTRUMENTATION FOR ARTHROSCOPIC SURGERY

Much of the electronic equipment for arthroscopic surgery (e.g. light sources, fibre-optic cables, miniature video cameras and video monitors) is identical to that used in other fields, while additional items of equipment are unique to this field. Arthroscopes are small-diameter rigid endoscopes. The most commonly used type is a 4-mm diameter 30° angled scope which is used routinely for intra-articular surgery of the knee and shoulder. Smaller arthroscopes (2.7 mm and 3 mm in diameter) are used for the wrist, elbow and ankle joints.

The arthroscope is used in conjunction with a sleeve of larger diameter, which is analogous to a laparoscopy trocar. This sleeve is initially inserted into the joint space using either sharp or blunt trocars. The trocar is then removed, and the arthroscope is inserted into the joint.

Fluid irrigation is required to distend the joint space. Most irrigation systems are gravity fed and involve a ball-valve for unidirectional flow. Hand pumps distal to the ball-valve are used to maintain adequate joint distension and access for intra-articular instrumentation. Various hand-held mechanical instruments are used, including right-angled blunt probes, small and large basket forceps (these can be straight, curved or up-biting), intra-articular scissors, and graspers for retrieving loose bodies from the joint. In addition, motorized cutting shavers and bone burrs of various sizes are utilized. Intra-articular cautery can also facilitate debridement of synovium and cartilage.

ARTHROSCOPIC PROCEDURES

Knee arthroscopy

The patient is positioned supine on a standard operating table. A lateral post at the mid-thigh level is used to assist distraction of the medial joint line. The lateral joint is distracted by placing the leg in a 'figure of 4' position. Alternatively, a thigh-holding device can be used to produce distraction of the joint lines. The use of a tourniquet is optional. Routine portals are made on both sides of the patellar tendon at the level of the joint line. An anterolateral portal is made first, followed by a anteromedial portal. Drainage portals are usually made in the suprapatellar region, most commonly on the lateral side.

The most common indication for knee arthroscopy is the diagnosis and treatment of suspected meniscal pathology. This may include excision or repair of the meniscus. Other indications include synovectomy, chondroplasty, lateral releases, removal of loose bodies, arthroscopic debridement of osteoarthritis, treatment of osteochondritis dissecans, drainage of septic arthritis, arthroscopically guided reduction and fixation of tibial plateau fractures, and arthroscopically assisted reconstructions of the anterior and posterior cruciate ligaments.

Shoulder arthroscopy

The patient is usually placed on a standard operating table in the lateral decubitus position. The arm is distracted using a skin traction device. Two standard skin portals are used. A posterior portal is used as the primary entry portal. This allows adequate visualization of the entire joint and also the subacromial space. An anterior portal is used mainly for instrumentation purposes. Indications include removal of loose bodies, excision of labral tears, synovectomy and biopsy, drainage of septic arthritis, debridement of biceps tendon lesions, arthroscopically assisted shoulder reconstructions and repairs of the rotator cuff.

Elbow arthroscopy

The patient is usually placed in a supine position with the arm abducted and the elbow flexed to 90°. Traction can be applied to the forearm using finger traps. Standard portals include anterolateral, anteromedial and direct lateral portals. Indications include removal of loose bodies, treatment of osteochondritis dissecans of the capitellum, division of post-traumatic adhesions, synovectomy, drainage of septic arthritis, and chondroplasty.

Wrist arthroscopy

Patient positioning is similar to that for elbow arthroscopy. Dorsal entry portals are made into the radiocarpal and intercarpal joints. The main indication for wrist arthroscopy is diagnostic evaluation of the painful wrist. Other indications include assessment of reduction of fractures of the distal radius, debridement of tears of the triangular fibrocartilage, assessment of carpal instabilities, removal of loose bodies and drainage of septic arthritis.

Ankle arthroscopy

The patient is placed in a supine position, with the optional use of an ankle-distracting device. Anterolateral and anteromedial portals are standard. Indications include treatment of osteochondritis dissecans, removal of loose bodies, debridement of osteoarthritis (which may include excision of osteophytes) and drainage of septic arthritis.

Hip arthroscopy

Indications for hip arthroscopy are not well established, and this procedure is infrequently performed.

FURTHER READING

Britton J, Barr H. 1994: Endoscopic surgery. In Morris PJ, Malt RA (eds). *Oxford textbook of surgery*. New York: Oxford University Press, 847–62.

Cotton PB, Williams CB. 1996: *Practical gastrointestinal endoscopy*, 4th edn. London: Blackwell Science.

Linder TE, Simmen D, Stool SE. 1997: Revolutionary inventions in the 20th century: the history of endoscopy. *Archives of Otolaryngology – Head and Neck Surgery* **123**, 1161–3.

Toouli J, Gossot D, Hunter JG (eds). 1996: *Endosurgery*. London: Churchill Livingstone.

Chapter 32

Vascular investigations

Irwin Faris

Introduction

Investigations are performed in vascular surgery patients to provide anatomical and haemodynamic information to support the diagnosis and to plan and monitor treatment. Technical developments continue to occur rapidly with the result that protocols for the use of investigations require frequent modification, a process which is continuing at the present time.

The introduction of *angiography* was one of the pillars which supported the development of vascular surgery. This provided anatomical but not haemodynamic assessment, which was not available outside the research laboratory. The *Doppler ultrasound* technique for measuring distal blood pressure was introduced in the early 1970s, and transformed the assessment of patients with lower limb ischaemia by providing a simple, quantitative, non-invasive and repeatable measure of the severity of the ischaemia.

This was soon followed in the mid-1970s by *duplex scanning,* which combined anatomical and haemodynamic information. This transformed vascular diagnosis and remains central to the assessment of patients. It fills the gap between clinical and laboratory data on the one hand and the medical imaging department on the other. The quality of angiography made a quantum leap forward with the introduction of *digital subtraction angiography* in the early 1980s, although the original aim of providing images of arteries following intravenous injection of contrast was only partially realized. In the late 1980s, the introduction of magnetic resonance imaging (MRI) was followed by the development of methods to examine blood vessels without the administration of contrast, namely *magnetic resonance angiography* (MRA).

DOPPLER ULTRASOUND

This approach is used in two applications:

1. as a pulse detector in the peripheral circulation;

2. to analyse the blood-flow velocity as part of a duplex scan (see below).

PHYSICAL PRINCIPLES

This method uses the principle that the frequency of sound reflected from moving structures will be changed, and that the change will be proportional to the velocity of the moving structures. This is the Doppler principle, which is expressed in the following equation:

$$F_t - F_r = \frac{2 \times F_t \times V \times \cos A}{C}$$

where F_t = frequency of transmitted sound, F_r = frequency of reflected sound, V = velocity of moving structures (in this case red blood cells), A = angle of sound incident to moving structures and C = velocity of sound in tissue (*c.* 1500 m/s).

The velocity shift and thus the potential output signal increase with increasing frequency of transmitted sound.

However, the attenuation of the sound as it passes through tissue is greater at higher frequencies, so 5–10 MHz sound is used to examine superficial vessels and 2–5 MHz to examine deeper vessels.

The simplest apparatus consists of a probe that contains two piezoelectric crystals that are continuously active (Figure 32.1). One crystal transmits sound and the other receives the reflected sound. Coupling gel is placed on the skin because the high attenuation coefficient of air substantially reduces the signals. Signals will be detected from all structures in the path of the sound. Sound reflected from stationary tissue such as the deep fascia will be unchanged in frequency and is filtered out by the apparatus. The frequency shift is generally within the audible range so that it can be amplified and played through a speaker or headphones. This is all that is needed for most applications. Alternatively, the output can be directed to a chart recorder and a permanent record of the blood-flow velocity made.

By placing the probe and coupling gel over a superficial artery, a flow signal can often be detected even though no pulse is palpable. The disadvantage of the technique is that the observer cannot be certain from which vessel or vessels the signal is arising, because there may be more than one vessel (artery or vein) in the path of the sound beam.

APPLICATIONS

The main application is the measurement of ankle blood pressure. This is part of the initial assessment of any patient who presents with lower limb pain which may be due to arterial disease.

The technique is analogous to the indirect measurement of brachial blood pressure. It involves placing a standard sphygmomanometer cuff around the lower third of the calf of the recumbent patient. The Doppler probe with coupling gel is placed over the artery to be examined, and the blood-flow signal is heard. The position and angle of the probe are adjusted until the optimum signal is obtained. The sphygmomanometer

cuff is then inflated until the signal is no longer heard. The pressure in the cuff is released slowly until the blood-flow signal is audible. The pressure in the cuff at this point is the systolic pressure in that artery. At the ankle, the dorsalis pedis, posterior tibial and sometimes the peroneal arteries are examined. The same technique is then used to measure the pressure in the brachial artery on both sides.

This technique has several limitations.

1. If the ankle arteries are calcified, as is common in diabetic patients, a falsely high reading may be obtained. In some cases it is impossible to occlude the artery even with a pressure of 300 mmHg in the cuff.

2. If there are painful ulcers around the ankle, it may not be possible to place and inflate the cuff.

3. In patients with extensive disease, there may be occlusive disease affecting both upper limbs. In such cases the brachial pressure will be falsely low.

The highest pressure measured in an ankle artery is expressed as a ratio of the higher brachial pressure. This is called the *pressure index* (PI) or *ankle brachial ratio* or *index* (ABI). Expressing the results as a ratio removes the effect of differences in systemic blood pressure either between patients or within the same patient from day to day. The usefulness of the method lies in the observation that *the level of the PI is related to the clinical severity of the disease* (Figure 32.2).

This information is used in several ways:

1. to confirm the severity of the disease;

2. to monitor the progress of the disease;

3. to determine the effectiveness of treatment.

The sensitivity of the resting ankle PI can be increased by *measuring the PI before and after exercise*. After the measurement of the resting PI, the patient then exercises. The onset of pain is noted, and on completion of exercise

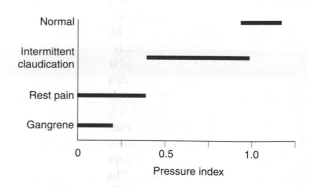

Figure 32.2 Ankle:brachial pressure index related to clinical severity of arterial disease. Note that there is a range of values for each clinical group. The lower limit of normal is 0.95, and the median value in patients with claudication is about 0.5.

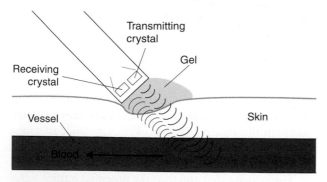

Figure 32.1 Doppler principle to detect blood flow in a vessel.

the patient lies on the couch and the ankle pressure is measured as quickly as possible. This can usually be done within 30–45 s. If the pressure has fallen, it is measured every 30–60 s until it has returned to the resting level. In patients with arterial disease, the ankle pressure falls with exercise and the level to which the pressure falls, as well as the duration of the fall, are proportional to the severity of the disease.

It is not necessary to perform this test in every case, but it is helpful in patients in whom the resting PI is higher than is consistent with the severity of the symptoms. There are two possible outcomes following exercise.

1. The PI is normal at rest and does not fall with exercise. In these patients the leg pain is not due to arterial disease.

2. The PI is normal or near normal at rest but falls steeply with exercise. This confirms the diagnosis of intermittent claudication.

Repeated measurement of the PI can be used to monitor the progress of the disease. The variability in the measurement is of the order of 0.10–0.15 units, so any change has to be greater than this if it is to be considered significant. Similarly, the success of any intervention to improve the circulation can be assessed by the change in PI produced.

DUPLEX SCANNING

The introduction of this technique has transformed vascular investigation. It combines B-mode imaging and information about blood flow using the Doppler principle. The principles of ultrasound imaging are described in Chapter 29.1. It is possible to obtain an image of the wall of a blood vessel, but images of diagnostic quality require considerable skill and patience. In some cases disease of the wall, especially calcification, may make it impossible to obtain a satisfactory image.

The duplex scanner superimposes on a real-time B-mode image information about blood-flow velocity obtained from a known site. This is in contrast to the continuous-wave Doppler described in the previous section, in which it is not possible to determine the precise site from which the signal is being obtained. The depth from which the signal is recorded is controlled by using a *pulse* of ultrasound. The ultrasound beam is of limited diameter and the time taken for the sound to return to the receiver is determined by the depth of the structure in the tissue (see formula above). Thus a crystal can be set to receive returning waves only from structures at a predetermined depth. For example, in the carotid system, samples can be obtained below, within and above a stenosis of the internal carotid artery.

In a duplex scanner the returning sound is analysed in a more sophisticated manner than with the continuous-wave instrument, which produces a single value for the velocity at any given time. In fact there is a range of velocities because different parts of the blood are moving at different velocities. These are displayed using the technique of spectral analysis, which generally employs real-time fast-Fourier transformation. In a normal artery the range of frequencies during systole is narrow because most of the red blood cells are moving at a similar velocity. There is a wider range of velocities during diastole. In a stenosed artery there are two main changes. First, the range of frequencies is wider. This is called spectral broadening, and is demonstrated by filling in of the Doppler spectrum. Secondly, the maximum frequency (or velocity) is increased as the blood flows more rapidly through the narrowed segment of artery. There is a known relationship between frequency and velocity, so either may be used. The peak systolic velocity is a commonly used criterion. The ratio of the peak velocity in the narrowed segment to the velocity in the adjacent normal artery increases with the degree of stenosis.

The utility of the method depends on the observation that the frequency spectrum changes in a predictable manner as the degree of stenosis increases. Patterns have been described for the carotid arteries (Figure 32.3), which is the commonest application, and for the iliac and femoral arteries, as well as for the renal and superior mesenteric arteries. In practice, many laboratories will be confident and competent in their examination of the carotid and superficial femoral arteries, but only a few laboratories can report authoritatively on the visceral arteries.

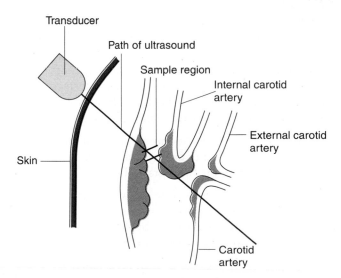

Figure 32.3 Duplex scanning of the carotid artery. The parallel lines in the lumen of the internal carotid artery represent the sample region or 'gate' from which the Doppler information is derived.

ANGIOGRAPHY

The supremacy of angiography as the 'gold standard' of vascular diagnosis has been challenged in many areas by duplex scanning (see discussion below). These changes have occurred because of the high cost of angiography and the risks of arterial puncture, which still carries a small but significant morbidity.

Access to the arterial system is most often obtained using the *Seldinger technique*. This is performed as follows.

1. Puncture the artery with a needle after infiltrating the skin with local anaesthetic.

2. Pass a guide-wire through the needle into the artery.

3. Remove the needle.

4. Pass a catheter over the guide-wire into the position in which it is desired to inject the contrast.

5. Remove the guide-wire on completion of the angiogram, and apply pressure until haemostasis is secured.

The technique has been modified in recent years to allow easier changing of catheters, guide-wires and other endovascular devices such as balloons and stents. After removal of the needle, a sheath may be inserted into the artery and left there until completion of the procedure. The sheath is a plastic tube about 10 cm long with a seal on the end which can be traversed by guide-wires, catheters, etc. A side arm allows the infusion of heparinized saline to maintain patency of the system. Thus all subsequent manoeuvres are performed via the sheath.

Any procedure involving arterial puncture carries a risk. The risk of major complications is small (about 1%), but the consequences may be catastrophic (e.g. stroke following carotid angiography), so angiography must only be ordered for good reason and the informed consent of the patient must be obtained. The major risks are *haemorrhage, arterial occlusion* and *reaction to contrast.*

1. Arterial occlusion may occur at the site of the puncture as a result of damage during the manipulation of the catheters and wires.

2. Arterial occlusion may occur anywhere that an instrument has traversed as a consequence of dissection of the arterial wall by the catheter or wire, or the injection of contrast into the wrong plane.

3. Embolism may occur as a result of dislodging atheromatous debris.

Bleeding occurs at the site of the puncture. Localized bleeding may result in the formation of a false aneurysm. This is the most common cause of arterial trauma in many major centres, and has become more common as larger devices are inserted through the femoral artery for endovascular procedures (most commonly coronary angioplasty).

Allergic reactions to contrast are less common with the use of non-iodinated contrast media (although these are substantially more expensive). Excessive doses of contrast medium may cause renal failure, and care must be taken in patients with renal impairment.

Digital subtraction angiography uses computer techniques to enhance the image by reducing the definition of the background. The principles of the technique are shown in Figure 32.4. The subtracted view (D) has been obtained by superimposing images B and C digitally. This method has allowed the use of smaller catheters and lower doses of contrast, thus improving the safety of the procedure.

The development of duplex scanning has reduced the frequency of vascular contrast studies.

1. Many patients now have carotid endarterectomy performed without cerebral angiography. The numbers vary between centres, but may exceed 50%.

2. Scanning of the superficial femoral artery may detect individuals who are suitable for angioplasty. In these cases, contrast angiography will be performed at the time of the angioplasty, and not (as formerly) at the stage of making the diagnosis.

3. In centres with special expertise, duplex scanning may be used to diagnose stenosis of the renal and superior mesenteric arteries.

4. Duplex scanning has had a major impact on the management of venous disease, and has rendered venography largely obsolete for the examination of the peripheral venous system (see below).

MAGNETIC RESONANCE ANGIOGRAPHY

(Written in collaboration with Dr N. Ferris, Radiologist, The Geelong Hospital.)

The principles of magnetic resonance imaging have been described in Chapter 29.1. In vascular surgery such imaging has been most useful in patients with aortic dissection, where the image provides an excellent demonstration of anatomy of the dissection. Magnetic resonance angiography is developing rapidly, particularly in the examination of the blood supply to the brain.

There are three major techniques for selectively imaging blood vessels with magnetic resonance techniques. Two of these, namely 'time of flight' and 'phase-contrast' magnetic resonance angiography (MRA), image the signal due to blood flow. The third and most recently devel-

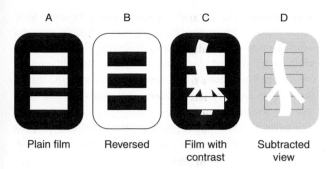

A   B   C   D

Plain film   Reversed   Film with   Subtracted
                          contrast   view

Figure 32.4 Digital subtraction angiography. A plain film (A) is reversed (B) and superimposed on the view obtained after the injection of contrast (C). In the resulting image (D) the images of structures that are the same in B and C lose their definition, and the image of the contrast is enhanced.

oped technique uses standard MR contrast agents (injected intravenously) to image the intravascular space, analogously to CT angiography or IV digital subtraction angiography.

Time of flight (TOF) MRA This has been the most widely used MRA technique. It relies on suppressing the signal from stationary tissues with a series of closely spaced radio-frequency (RF) 'saturation pulses'. Blood entering the region of interest during the acquisition has not been saturated, and is able to return a strong signal to the receiving coil after the excitatory imaging pulse. Artefacts can arise from materials of high T1 signal intensity (the sequence is inherently T1-weighted), such as extracellular methaemoglobin (found in subacute haematomas), which also appear bright in TOF images. Because of the large number of thin sections required for reasonable long-axis resolution, the technique tends to be slow (5–10 min).

Phase-contrast (PC) MRA This technique applies two additional radio-frequency pulses to the region of interest during image acquisition. These pulses vary linearly in strength along a single axis (e.g. antero-posterior). The two pulses are equal in strength but opposite in direction. Each pulse has the effect of delaying the signal ('phase delay') from tissue by an amount that is proportional to the tissue's position along the chosen 'phase-encoding' axis. For stationary tissues, the net effect of the two opposed pulses is zero. For flowing blood at any point, there is a net 'phase delay' proportional to the distance that the blood travels between the two pulses (i.e. to its velocity). The technique tends to be even slower than TOF (up to 15–20 min). It is also sensitive to signal loss from turbulent flow.

Contrast-enhanced breath-hold MRA Recent advances in MRI hardware (stronger and faster gradient systems) have made it possible to image reasonable tissue volumes at reasonable resolution in a breath-hold (15–30 s). To obtain adequate signal from blood vessels at these

speeds, MR contrast agents are required. These are chelates of paramagnetic metals (usually gadolinium) that shorten the T1 relaxation time of surrounding tissues (e.g. blood), and thus cause them to produce a brighter signal on T1-weighted images. Currently available MR contrast agents rapidly diffuse into the extracellular space, so imaging generally needs to be completed during the first (arterial) pass of contrast after injection, to avoid signal from the extracellular space (and often from veins). Note that these techniques image the intravascular space (like catheter and CT angiography), not the presence of flow (like TOF and PCMRA).

These techniques are still evolving rapidly, but usually involve a rapid intravenous bolus injection of gadolinium, followed within seconds by a breath-hold T1-weighted gradient echo sequence. Sometimes a pre-injection 'mask' image is obtained and subtracted digitally from the post-contrast image. The field of view is limited to 30–40 cm, especially if reasonable spatial resolution is required. Large volumes, as for aorto-femoral studies, require either rapid movement of the patient or table between acquisitions ('bolus-chase' techniques, similar to stepping table catheter angiography), or the use of multiple doses of gadolinium.

CLINICAL ROLE

Until now, MRA has mainly been used for non-invasive angiography of the head (two-dimensional or three-dimensional TOF techniques), for which it is well suited because there is little physiological movement outside the vessels, and little fat (T1 hyperintense) adjacent to the vessels of interest. Resolution is now only slightly inferior to that of catheter techniques. Screening for aneurysms and vertebro-basilar disease have been major indications. There may be an increasing role for 'one-stop shop' imaging consisting of MRI of the brain, intracranial MRA, and MRA of the neck. To date this has been held back by the limited accuracy of grading of stenoses by MRA, but this will improve with the use of contrast-enhanced techniques. In the USA, many groups already use MRA as the second, confirmatory test prior to surgery, although a few patients still have catheter angiography when the results of the non-invasive tests conflict. The combination of ultrasound and confirmatory MRA is reported to be more cost-effective than ultrasound plus catheter study, for similar levels of accuracy.

Elsewhere in the body, MRA has had little clinical impact. However, there is now much interest in the new contrast-enhanced techniques. Pilot studies have shown that these are quick, accurate and, despite the expense of intravenous MR contrast agents (A\$100/dose), cost-competitive with catheter techniques for diagnostic purposes. It is now widely expected that MRA will replace much of diagnostic catheter angiography over the next 10–15 years.

Development of MR contrast agents which remain in the intravascular space (e.g. gadolinium polylysine) will facilitate this advance. CT angiography may prove to be more adaptable to the abdomen than MRA (having a faster imaging time and less motion artefact), but MRA is likely to be superior in the periphery, because of its superior signal-to-noise ratio.

VENOUS SYSTEM

The surgeon may require information about the anatomy and function of the venous system in patients with venous disease, as in patients with arterial disease the surgeon obtains information about function from Doppler studies and about anatomy from angiography or ultrasound imaging. Duplex scanning is the preferred method of imaging the venous system, as described above, and provides all of the necessary information in almost every case.

Diagnosis of deep vein thrombosis Duplex scanning has been shown to have a high level of accuracy compared to venography. Veins which contain thrombus are incompressible and there is no blood flow within them. This examination is easily performed with a modern duplex scanner, especially one with a colour display. The method is not so accurate for examining thrombi in calf veins, but this condition is of less significance than thrombi in the axial veins (popliteal or above). Scanning has the major advantage that it can be repeated, daily if necessary, in patients with equivocal results, or to examine for extension of the thrombus.

Varicose veins In patients with superficial varicose veins, duplex scanning will demonstrate the presence of incompetence and localize the incompetent sites, including perforating veins in the calf. The value of the investigation is such that some authors recommend its routine use before varicose vein surgery. My view is that many patients with primary saphenofemoral incompetence do not require scanning. However, scanning should be performed if there is any doubt about the sites of incompetence, in patients with recurrent varicose veins, and in patients having operations for short saphenous varices in order to locate accurately the site of the sapheno-popliteal junction.

Assessment of venous insufficiency Duplex scanning can demonstrate both the patency of the deep venous system and the competence of the valves. These are the two major anatomical criteria for assessing the severity of the disease in these patients.

For functional information about the severity of venous insufficiency, direct pressure measurements are sometimes taken. They are described here because they demonstrate the pathophysiology of chronic venous insufficiency in which the physiological abnormality is *ambulatory venous hypertension*. This usually results from incompetence of the deep venous system, but it sometimes follows obstruction, especially in the ilio-femoral segment.

Figure 32.5 shows the pressure measured in a vein on the dorsum of the foot in a standing patient. During the time marked 'Exercise' the patient performs the repetitive manoeuvre of standing on tiptoe approximately once per second for 10 s.

Two parameters are measured:

1. the fall in pressure with exercise (normally to < 40 mmHg);

2. the refilling time, i.e. the time taken for the pressure to return to the resting level after ceasing exercise (normally > 25 s). The normal response is demonstrated in the lowest line on the figure. In a patient with superficial venous incompetence the fall in pressure is less, indicating inefficiency of the calf muscle pump, and the refilling time is short, as the veins fill by reflux. The response can be restored to normal by placing a tourniquet to occlude the superficial veins. In a patient with deep venous insufficiency the pressure may not fall at all (or may even rise in the presence of venous obstruction).

Information about the refilling time can be obtained non-invasively by the technique of *photoplethysmography*. A light-emitting diode is placed on the skin of the dorsum of the foot. The signal output is proportional to the amount of haemoglobin in the tissue. This falls more or less in proportion to the venous pressure, and rises again at the end of the exercise, allowing measurement of the refilling time. The pressure changes cannot be estimated reliably using this technique.

The incompetence can be relieved by reconstructive surgery which replaces or repairs valves. Obstruction in the iliofemoral segment can be bypassed by a graft from one femoral vein to the other.

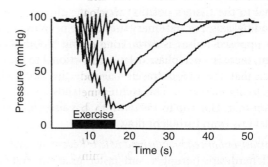

Figure 32.5 Venous pressure measurements (composite figure): lowest line, normal patient; middle line, superficial venous incompetence; upper line, deep venous incompetence.

Cardiovascular haemo-dynamics and assessment

David G. Hill

Introduction

Major surgical procedures, operations on the elderly or operations on patients with known cardiac disease will inevitably result in a proportion who develop peri-operative cardiovascular complications, with a number of cases becoming very unstable. The underlying principles of haemodynamics and management are similar in all patients who have cardiovascular dysfunction, but can be more confusing in the surgical setting. Post-operative patients who develop cardiovascular instability are a high-risk group and are more safely managed in a coronary-care or high-dependency unit.

CARDIOVASCULAR HAEMODYNAMICS

The measurement of cardiac output is important and reflects the status of the entire circulatory system, not just the heart, since it is governed by mechanisms which regulate tissue perfusion. Cardiac output (CO) is the product of stroke volume (SV) and heart rate (HR): (CO = SV × HR). Preload, afterload, heart rate and myocardial contractility combine to determine the cardiac output, and an understanding of the interrelationships between these factors is fundamental to the management of cardiovascular haemodynamics. Normal cardiac output in a resting supine man averages 5.0 L/min. Expressed in relation to body surface area (SA) as cardiac index (CI = CO/SA) the normal values are 2.8–4.2 L/min/m². A CI of < 2.5 L/min/m² is of concern, and a value of below < 2.0 L/min/m² is inadequate for satisfactory tissue perfusion. The thermodilution method using a pulmonary artery catheter (PAC) is the method of choice for measuring cardiac output in the clinical situation. This technique involves injecting a bolus of cold fluid into the right atrium, and the resulting change in temperature is detected by a thermistor in the pulmonary artery. This can also be performed automatically with a special catheter using a heat bolus, which gives regular measurement of cardiac output, providing valuable information about trends as well as sudden events.

The initial length of a myocardial sarcomere determines its force of contraction. On the basis of this premise, the Frank–Starling relationship describes ventricular filling (or preload) as directly proportional to the force of contraction. Ventricular preload is measured as left ventricular end diastolic volume (LVEDV), and is directly proportional to stroke work and ultimately cardiac output. For clinical applications it is not feasible to measure LVEDV regularly, and therefore pulmonary capillary wedge pressure (PCWP) provides a measure of left ventricular end diastolic pressure (LVEDP) and infers LVEDV. In clinical practice, PCWP is extremely useful for the assessment of left ventricular filling, as it equates to left atrial pressure and is obtained by advancing the PAC (Swan Ganz) into a distal branch of the pulmonary artery until the catheter is wedged (when the cardiac pulsations are lost). The normal mean value for PCWP is 10 mmHg (range 5–15 mmHg).

Afterload refers to the resistance against which the left ventricle must eject blood, and is expressed as systemic vascular resistance or the systemic vascular resistance index (SVRI) when related to body surface area. SVRI is a derived calculation from pressure = resistance × flow, i.e.

$$SVRI = \frac{(MAP - CVP) \times 0.80}{CI}$$

where MAP = mean arterial pressure, CVP = central venous pressure and CI = cardiac index.

The normal range for SVRI is 1500–2400 dynes/s/cm^5/m^2. Peripheral arterioles are the main determinants of SVRI, and therefore their degree of constriction or dilatation will determine the amount of afterload present. Clinically if there is general arterial vasoconstriction and the SVRI is raised, vasodilator agents may be given to decrease SVRI and so increase the cardiac index. In critically ill patients this situation often arises and it is best to aim at an SVRI of < 1500 dynes/s/cm^5/m^2 in order to ensure that cardiac work is reduced and the best possible tissue perfusion is achieved. Conversely, if there is a high cardiac index with low blood pressure and SVRI, then vasoconstrictor agents may be used to increase the mean arterial pressure (e.g. in cases of sepsis).

There is a second component of myocardial contractility independent of ventricular filling. The contractile state of the myocardium and the force of contraction increase with increasing availability of intracellular calcium ions. Factors which increase myocardial contractility are said to be positively inotropic, and those which decrease it are referred to as negatively inotropic. The catecholamines and their derivatives exert their inotropic effect by increasing levels of cyclic adenosine monophosphate (cyclic AMP), which causes calcium channels to spend more time in the open state and also increase the active transport of calcium into the myocardium. These agents are commonly used to increase myocardial contractility.

When managing patients with severely compromised cardiovascular haemodynamics, the measurement of cardiac output/cardiac index is vital. When the cardiac index is low, i.e. < 2.5, the degree of cardiac filling (preload) should first be determined by measuring the PCWP, and increased if it is low. Next the SVRI (afterload) should be assessed and vasoconstrictors or vasodilators given as indicated. Finally, if preload and afterload are satisfactory, then it is necessary to consider myocardial contractility. Echocardiography (see below) is also useful in this estimation. If myocardial contractility is reduced, then inotropes may be required.

CLINICAL EXAMPLES

Case 33.1 Two hours after coronary artery surgery a patient is hypotensive with a mean arterial pressure of 52 mmHg. The following measurements are obtained.

CI = 2.1 L/min/m^2.
PCWP = 6 mmHg.
SVRI = 2010 dynes/s/cm^5/m^2.

Comment: The patient is hypovolaemic, and administration of volume will improve the cardiac index. Measure the haemoglobin, and if the patient is anaemic a blood transfusion will be necessary.

Case 33.2 Three days after transurethral resection of the prostate, a patient collapses and, after resuscitation, the following measurements are obtained.

CI = 1.8 L/min/m^2.
PCWP = 16 mmHg.
SVRI = 2800 dynes/s/cm^5/m^2.

Comment: This patient has increased afterload and is vasoconstricted. In the first instance a vasodilator agent may be prescribed (e.g. hydralazine).

Case 33.3 After abdominal aortic aneurysm repair a patient experienced chest pain and became hypotensive (BP = 70/40 mmHg) with shortness of breath. The following measurements were obtained.

CI = 1.6 L/min/m^2.
PCWP = 15 mmHg.
SVRI = 1800 dynes/s/cm^5/m^2.

Comment: It is likely that this patient has decreased myocardial contractility. Investigations should include ECG, echocardiography and myocardial enzymes. The preload and afterload appear to be within normal limits, and if the echocardiogram confirms decreased left ventricular contractility an inotrope is required. In this instance an inotrope with vasodilator properties (e.g. dobutamine) should be used in order to reduce afterload.

CARDIOVASCULAR ASSESSMENT

CLINICAL PRESENTATION

The first action that a medical officer must take when called to see a surgical patient with chest symptoms is to ascertain whether there has been a significant cardiac event. A carefully taken history and meticulous physical examination remain the cornerstones of initial evaluation. Occasionally, however, it may be difficult to balance the need for detail against the need for early and decisive action. Surgical patients who have suffered a myocardial infarction need immediate investigations, specialized consultation, transfer to a coronary-care unit and rapid treatment. *Note that thrombolytic agents may be contraindicated following surgery, but angioplasty remains an option.*

Approximately two-thirds of patients with acute coronary occlusion present with chest pain. Frequently this is classical, but in surgical patients it may be confused with post-operative pain, or altered by analgesics. Other cardiac symptoms include dyspnoea, syncope and collapse, palpitations, nausea and vomiting, diaphoresis and hiccups. *A common mistake is to treat a post-operative patient who is restless and hypotensive with sedation and increased intravenous volume. This is dangerous if the patient has suffered a myocardial infarction.*

The initial physical examination targets conscious state, extent of haemodynamic disturbance and cardiac arrhythmias. A more complete examination will involve a detailed assessment of the cardiovascular system, including pulse, blood pressure, jugular venous pressure, precordial inspection and palpation, cardiac auscultation and signs of congestive heart failure. Hourly measurement of urine output provides a guide to renal perfusion.

INVESTIGATIONS

Electrocardiography

Despite difficulties with interpretation, the 12-lead electrocardiograph (ECG) is the most useful investigation, because it can be performed simply and quickly. In post-surgical patients, myocardial ischaemia and infarction are the most important diagnoses to consider. These are reflected in the ECG by changes in the ST-segments, T-waves and the development of Q-waves, and it is valuable to compare with a pre-operative ECG if this is available.

ST changes The ST-segment may be either depressed or elevated. The depressed ST-segment is typically horizontal or down-sloping. ST depression of $> 1\,mm$ is significant for transient ischaemia but needs to be distinguished from the constant depression seen in left ventricular hypertrophy or the digitalis effect. ST elevation occurs within 1 or 2 min of an acute coronary occlusion, usually in a convex upward pattern. The number of leads with ST elevation and the height of the ST-segment are usually directly proportional to the degree of ischaemia. An exercise ECG may reveal ST changes that were not previously present.

T-wave changes Tall, peaked T-waves may represent the hyperactive phase of acute myocardial infarction. It is usually transient and may be missed. This appearance can also be due to hyperkalaemia. Deep T-wave inversion may develop as part of the pattern of necrosis in acute myocardial infarction, and often resolves over a period of several weeks.

Q-waves Abnormal Q-waves may develop as early as 2 h after the onset of chest pain, and are regarded as an indication of necrosis. It is now clear that both Q-wave and non-Q-wave infarctions are heterogeneous conditions, but patients with non-Q-wave infarctions are more likely to have a patent infarct-related vessel, and represent an unstable state with increased risk of recurrent angina or infarct extension.

Arrhythmias as well as abnormal QRS complexes, including left bundle branch block and right bundle branch block, may be associated with myocardial ischaemia and require investigation.

Biochemical markers of myocardial necrosis

Measurement of creatine kinase isoenzymes (CKMB) is widely used for the diagnosis of myocardial infarction. Skeletal muscle contains less than 3% CKMB, while cardiac muscle contains 15–20% CKMB. Following irreversible ischaemic necrosis, the myocardial cells leak creatine kinase into the interstitial space, which then passes via the lymphatics to the circulation. During passage through the lymphatics, oxidation occurs so that only 15–20% of the creatine kinase returns to the circulation. This accounts for the delay of 3–4 h before the enzyme appears in the blood. The enzyme is cleared by the reticulo-endothelial system. Typical plasma concentration curves for CKMB after myocardial infarction begin to rise at 3–4 h, peak at 20–24 h and decrease over 3–4 days. When coronary reperfusion occurs before myocardial necrosis is complete, there is a shift to the left with early peaking and rapid wash-out of the enzyme. Other enzymes used in the diagnosis of acute myocardial infarction are lactate dehydrogenase (LD) (five isoenzymes), aspartate aminotransferase (AST), myoglobin and troponin.

Radiology

When the cardiovascular system is compromised the chest X-ray may show increased heart size and changes in the lung fields (pulmonary oedema). However, the chest X-ray has limitations for the diagnosis of myocardial infarction or ischaemia unless there is severe dysfunction. The main reason for a chest X-ray in a surgical patient who has chest symptoms is to exclude other important diagnoses (e.g. pneumothorax, pneumonia).

CT scans and magnetic resonance imaging (MRI) are at present of limited value in post-surgical patients with cardiovascular problems. However, they are important modalities for the evaluation of other diagnoses (e.g. aortic dissection), and techniques are being developed to assess myocardial function using MRI.

Echocardiography

The field of cardiac ultrasound has undergone numerous and dramatic changes which have contributed to its growing importance. Two-dimensional image acquisition (colour flow Doppler) is currently widely available, but three-dimensional ultrasound and intravascular imaging are developing rapidly.

Although not routinely required, echocardiography (ECHO) is beneficial in the initial diagnosis after a cardiac event. Percutaneous transthoracic echocardiography is standard, and the sites for transducer location are parasternal, apical, subcostal and suprasternal. Classical planes are described for all areas, and may be either long-axis or cross-sectional short-axis views. It should be noted that many intermediate planes are possible.

Transoesophageal echocardiography (TOE), although more invasive, has important advantages and is particularly useful intra-operatively and in intubated patients. There is usually better imaging of the left-sided cardiac structures (e.g. left atrium, mitral valve and left ventricle) as well as of the thoracic aorta.

The long-axis view of the left heart and the short-axis view of the left ventricle at papillary muscle level are the planes most commonly used when assessing left ventricular function. The long-axis view encompasses most of the structures on the left side of the heart, and there is a good view of the left ventricular wall motion (see Figure 33.1). The short-axis view of the left ventricle at papillary muscle level shows regional wall function, displaying myocardium perfused by the three main coronary arteries (see Figure 33.2). In this view the image is subdivided into four quadrants, namely posterior, anterior, septal and lateral. Initial changes in acute myocardial ischaemia result in abnormal inward motion and thickening of the affected myocardial region. Later changes show systolic wall motion abnormalities (SWMA) measured visually from a fixed central reference point in the left ventricular lumen. SWMA are graded from mild to severe hypokinesia, akinesia and dyskinesia. Normal contraction is defined as > 30% shortening of the radius from

the centre to the endocardial border. Mild hypokinesia is defined as radial shrinking of 10–30%, and severe hypokinesia is defined as < 10% shrinking. Akinesia refers to the absence of wall motion or no inward movement, and dyskinesia is paradoxical or outward motion during ventricular systole.

Other information obtained from echocardiography includes measurements of valve function and the diagnosis of structural abnormalities of the heart, together with pericardial problems (including tamponade).

Echocardiography is also used to measure LVEDV, which is derived from the short-axis view at the level of the papillary muscles and is thought to be more accurate than PCWP for the measurement of preload.

Haemodynamic monitoring

The decision to introduce haemodynamic monitoring, particularly the more invasive methods, requires expert judgement together with a knowledge of the dangers and

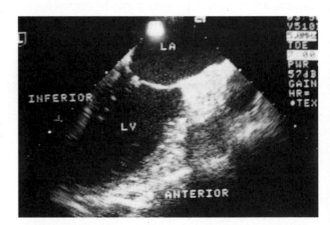

Figure 33.1 Transoesophageal echocardiogram: long-axis, two-chamber view of the left side of the heart showing left ventricle, left atrium and the mitral valve closed.

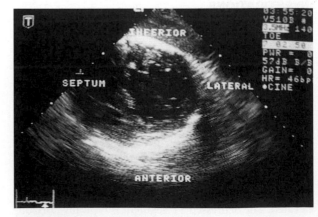

Figure 33.2 Transoesophageal echocardiogram: short-axis view of the left ventricle at papillary muscle level showing four quadrants (interior, anterior, septal and lateral).

limitations. The following are the more commonly used monitoring systems.

Arterial pressure This is an important clinical indicator and can be measured by non-invasive and invasive techniques. The invasive method provides a continuous recording, usually from a catheter in the radial artery. In addition, the arterial line can be used to obtain arterial blood-gas measurements.

Central venous pressure (CVP) This is measured with a central venous catheter (CVC) and estimates blood volume, venous return and right ventricular filling. The normal CVP in healthy individuals is 2–8 mmHg. Higher levels of up to 15 mmHg or more are required in patients with less compliant ventricles. Central venous pressure is a useful parameter when treating hypovolaemia. However, it should be pointed out that it may be misleading as an estimate of left ventricular filling if there is cardiopulmonary dysfunction.

Pulmonary artery catheter (Swan-Ganz catheter) This is a more invasive system and carries a small risk of complications (e.g. pulmonary haemorrhage, infection). However, when the patient is unstable the information obtained from this monitoring system may be critical. The most important measurements are cardiac output, pulmonary capillary wedge pressure and SVRI. The value of these measurements has been discussed previously, and serial observations enable the assessment of important trends in the patient's condition.

Cardiac catheterization including coronary angiography For full cardiological assessment, cardiac catheterization and coronary angiography may be required. At cardiac catheterization, the chambers of the heart and valve function can be visualized by cine angiography. Left ventricular dimensions and contractility can be seen and left ventricular ejection fraction measured. Pressure measurements are made in the relevant chambers and across valves. Coronary angiography outlines coronary anatomy, and identifies any stenoses and the quality of the distal vessels prior to undertaking interventions (e.g. coronary angioplasty or coronary artery surgery).

Nuclear imaging

Additional information can be obtained from nuclear scans, and the following methods are most commonly used.

Gated heart pool scan Radioactively labelled red cells are injected intravenously, and their passage through the left ventricle is scanned. Ejection fraction measured in this way is more accurate than that assessed by echocardiography and angiography.

Thallium and Tc Sestamibi scans The radionuclide enters the coronary circulation and is extracted by normally perfused myocardium, so areas of underperfusion can then be identified. Scans are made both at rest and after exercise, differentiating viable or non-viable muscle tissue. These scans are useful for determining whether a questionable coronary artery lesion seen on angiography is significant.

Positron emission tomography (PET) scan PET imaging is the best non-invasive method for evaluation of cardiac metabolism, but is very expensive and only available in major centres.

FURTHER READING

Kaplan JA. 1999: *Cardiac anesthesia*, 4th edn. Philadelphia, PA: W.B. Saunders.

Oh TE. 1997: *Intensive care manual*, 4th edn. Oxford: Butterworth-Heinemann.

Schlant RC, Alexander RW. 1994: *Hurst's the heart*, 8th edn. McGraw-Hill.

Weyman AE. 1994: *Principles and practice of echocardiography*, 2nd edn. Media, PA: Lea & Febiger.

Pre-operative assessment and consent

D. Wynne L. Davies

Introduction

Pre-operative patients require a consultation with an anaesthetist to assess their suitability for the operation and the type of anaesthetic that is appropriate. It is preferable that the anaesthetist who is going to administer the anaesthetic conducts the assessment, but this is not always possible. Not only is it courteous to do so, but it is also a measure of the quality and standard of care being offered to the patient, and should be expected by all patients. The principle of safety remains paramount, with the need to balance the risk of anaesthesia with the anticipated benefits of the procedure. This chapter aims to cover the assessment of anaesthetic risk, measures that may improve the risk, and the consent that is required from the patient before submitting them to the proposed procedure.

PRE-OPERATIVE ASSESSMENT

The initial anaesthetic consultation is usually performed within hours of the procedure about to be undertaken, unless a specific request has been sought for an anaesthetic opinion on additional measures that may be deemed necessary to prepare the patient for operation. The objectives of this consultation are as follows:

- to assess the medical condition of the patient;
- to anticipate difficulties associated with the proposed surgery and anaesthesia;
- to ensure that the patient is in optimum condition for their surgery;
- to provide information about anaesthesia and peri-operative care, and to allay any fears and anxieties perceived by the patient;
- to prescribe appropriate premedication.

Pre-operative communication, and a 'team approach' between the surgeon who is performing the procedure and the anaesthetist who is administering the anaesthetic, reduce the likelihood of misunderstandings in the timing and nature of the procedure! Successful patient care results from both surgeon and anaesthetist being aware of the range of techniques available to each other, so that they can be harmonized to the patient's best advantage. This communication between the surgeon and the anaesthetist is vital, and some degree of flexibility in approach by both parties, according to the clinical needs of the individual patient, is essential for providing patient satisfaction.

Assessment of medical condition It is invaluable to have a concise summary of the patient's relevant medical history and examination, together with the results of requested investigations available for anaesthetic assessment prior to seeing the patient. Early identification of potential problems is the key to appropriate investigations and to assessing the relative risk for an individual patient. In day surgery, where time may be even more limited, pre-operative questionnaires completed by the patient with the assistance of the nursing staff may aid the selection of patients who require an in-depth assessment. Ideally, these questionnaires should be completed well before the appointment for surgery and anaesthesia, so that any patient with risk factors may be fully assessed before the date of the procedure at an Anaesthetic Assessment Clinic. Early referral for anaesthetic assessment will enable appropriate medical referral and investigations to be performed as an out-patient. An example of such a questionnaire is shown in Table 34.1.1. All patients should have a full clinical history and physical examination. There is little place for routine haematological, biochemical or radiographic screening; appropriate investigations should be based on the clinical history and physical findings. Review of the patient's medical notes is prudent, as this may well avoid duplication of investigations performed in the recent past. The American Society of Anesthesiologists classification of physical status is widely used to classify patients into five risk assessment groups. This classification is commonly used to quantify illness for comparative purposes (Box 34.1.1).

Optimization If an abnormal finding is discovered during the pre-operative assessment, it is important to determine whether this abnormality can be corrected or improved. 'Optimization' of the patient with an acute or chronic disease process is important for reducing the incidence of complications peri-operatively. Ideally, in elective surgery, patients should be presented for surgery in the best medical condition that can be achieved for that patient. The concept of 'fitness' for anaesthesia is a relative one, and depends on whether a particular condition can be improved or 'optimized' in the time available before surgery is planned. There should be time to refer, investigate, treat, follow up and review each and every condition that has been found that could be improved. In urgent or emergency surgery, the time available for 'optimization' may be limited to hours or minutes, but this does not mean that it cannot be achieved. However, there may be limitations on the investigations, which may be performed at short notice.

Minimalization To decrease risk and increase safety, attention must be paid to the risk factors associated with the general medical condition of the patient. Factors such as the condition requiring surgery, age, weight, presence of coexisting disease, previous anaesthetic history and previous medical history are extremely valuable indicators. Of paramount importance is the safety of the patient. The best interest of a 'sick' patient may not be served by cancellation, and calculated risks must be taken with the agreement of the patient or their relatives. Operations are postponed because of a remedial condition, because of inadequate pre-operative investigation or because of the perceived relative risk arising from the poor general condition of the patient. The question to ask yourself is whether there is any way in which the

---

BOX 34.1.1 THE AMERICAN SOCIETY OF ANESTHESIOLOGISTS CLASSIFICATION OF PHYSICAL STATUS

Class I:
The patient has no organic, physiological, biochemical or psychiatric disturbance. The pathological process for which surgery is to be performed is localized, and does not entail a systemic disturbance
Examples: a fit patient with an inguinal hernia; a fibroid uterus in an otherwise healthy woman

Class II:
Mild to moderate systemic disturbance caused either by the condition to be treated surgically or by other pathophysiological processes
Examples: slightly limiting organic heart disease; mild diabetes; essential hypertension or anaemia

Class III:
Severe systemic disturbance or disease from whatever cause, even though it may not be possible to define the degree of disability with finality
Examples: severely limiting organic heart disease; severe diabetes with vascular complications; moderate to severe degrees of pulmonary insufficiency; angina pectoris or healed myocardial infarction

Class IV:
Severe systemic disorders that are already life-threatening, not always correctable by operation
Examples: organic heart disease showing marked signs of cardiac insufficiency; persistent angina; active myocarditis; advanced degrees of pulmonary, hepatic, renal or endocrine insufficiency

Class V:
The moribund patient who has little chance of survival but is submitted to operation in desperation
Examples: ruptured abdominal aneurysm with profound shock; major cerebral trauma with rapidly increasing intracranial pressure; massive pulmonary embolus. Most of these patients require operation as a resuscitative measure with little, if any, anaesthesia

---

patient's present condition can be improved. If the answer is 'yes', then every effort should be made to refer, treat and stabilize that condition prior to surgery. If the answer is 'no', then the next question is whether the risks of anaesthesia are justified by the benefits of the operation. If the answer to this question is 'no', then the operation should be postponed, or preparations made to undertake the procedure with the support of a higher level of expertise and facilities, such as an intensive-care unit. It is never justifiable to undertake surgery or any procedure involving anaesthesia when the risk outweighs the benefit.

Table 34.1.1 Questionnaire for assessment for care in the day unit (general anaesthetic)

Will you:

1. be able to be driven home by private car?
2. have someone to take you home?
3. have a telephone at home?
4. have easy access to a lavatory?
5. have someone at home able to look after you for 24 h?

Have you ever suffered from any of the following:

6. chest pain on exercise or at night?
7. breathlessness?
8. asthma or bronchitis?
9. high blood pressure?
10. heart murmur?
11. fainting easily?
12. convulsions or fits?
13. jaundice (yellowness)?
14. indigestion or heartburn?
15. kidney or urinary trouble?
16. anaemia or other blood problems?
17. excessive bleeding or bruising?
18. arthritis?
19. muscle disease or progressive weakness?
20. diabetes?

Have you ever had:

21. a serious illness?
22. allergy or reaction to medicines, Elastoplast, etc.?

Do you:

23. take any medicines (tablets, patches, injections, inhalers)?
24. smoke?
25. drink more than 1½ pints of beer or 3 shorts a day?
26. have any questions about the procedure?
27. If you are female, are you pregnant or taking the 'contraceptive pill'?
28. Is there anything else you think the surgeon or anaesthetist should know?
29. What operations have you had before, if any? (please list them)
30. Did you have any anaesthetic or surgical complications? (please list them)
31. When was your last local or general anaesthetic?
32. Has any member of your family had problems with anaesthetics?
33. How long will it take you to travel home?
34. Do you have any of the following? (please circle)

    Dentures   Crowned teeth   Contact lenses   Hearing-aid   Pacemaker

---

FURTHER ENQUIRY IF 'NO' FOR QUESTIONS 1–5, OR IF 'YES' FOR QUESTIONS 6–28:

1. If not possible to arrange transport	NOT SUITABLE
2. If not possible to arrange escort	NOT SUITABLE
3. If reasonable access cannot be arranged	NOT SUITABLE
4. Depending on circumstances and procedure	MAY NOT BE SUITABLE
5. If not possible to arrange	NOT SUITABLE

Table 34.1.1 *(Continued)*

6. If pain occurs at rest	NOT SUITABLE
If pain occurs when walking on the flat	NOT SUITABLE
If pain is normally well controlled and occurs only in exceptional circumstances, *request ECG and chest X-ray:*	
If ECG and/or chest X-ray are abnormal	NOT SUITABLE
7. If breathlessness occurs when walking on the flat	NOT SUITABLE
If breathlessness occurs on greater exertion, *request chest X-ray and spirometry:*	
If chest X-ray is abnormal or FEV_1 or FVC is < 70% of predicted value	NOT SUITABLE
8. If patient's normal activity is limited	NOT SUITABLE
If well controlled, *request chest X-ray and spirometry:*	
If chest X-ray is abnormal or FEV_1 or FVC is < 70% of predicted value	NOT SUITABLE
9. If blood pressure is taken regularly and well controlled, *take blood pressure:*	
If > 160/100 mmHg (or > 180/100 mmHg if 60–70 years of age) *repeat;*	
If it remains greater	NOT SUITABLE
10. If there is a clear history of heart murmur	NOT SUITABLE
11. *Record what causes fainting*	
If on exercise or if patient is over 60 years	NOT SUITABLE
12. If epileptic and well controlled on medication	SUITABLE
If there has been an epileptic fit within last year or with an anaesthetic	NOT SUITABLE
13. If jaundice was due to gallstones or infectious hepatitis	SUITABLE
If jaundice was possibly due to hepatitis B, *request hepatitis B screen:*	
If positive	NOT SUITABLE
14. If due to hiatus hernia reliably diagnosed,	
but consider use of H_2 antagonist over pre-operative night	SUITABLE
If there is possible myocardial ischaemia, *request a medical opinion*	NOT SUITABLE
15. If the reason for treatment	SUITABLE
If not the reason for treatment, *request urea and electrolytes*	
If abnormal	NOT SUITABLE
If there is severe difficulty with micturition	NOT SUITABLE
16. If recently anaemic, *request FBC:*	
If Hb is < 10 g/dL	NOT SUITABLE
If haemophiliac	NOT SUITABLE
If known to have sickle-cell trait *(not disease)*	SUITABLE
If of Caribbean, East Mediterranean, Middle or Far Eastern origin and result of sickle-cell test is unknown, *request sickle-cell test:*	
If there is sickle-cell disease	NOT SUITABLE
17. If required hospital treatment	NOT SUITABLE
Has bleeding been excessive following tooth extraction, or bruising occurred without a known cause? If yes, *request clotting screen;*	
If normal	SUITABLE
Is there a family history? If so, or if there is any doubt, *request clotting screen:*	
If normal	SUITABLE
18. If the patient is severely disabled	NOT SUITABLE
If the neck is involved *inform anaesthetist*	SUITABLE
19. If normal activity is compromised (e.g. multiple sclerosis, motor neurone disease)	NOT SUITABLE
If the patient has myasthenia gravis	NOT SUITABLE
If there is a family history of cataracts	NOT SUITABLE
If there is a history of poliomyelitis which required assisted ventilation or was associated with swallowing difficulties	NOT SUITABLE
Otherwise, including ME syndrome	SUITABLE
20. If poorly controlled or insulin-dependent diabetic	NOT SUITABLE

Table 34.1.1 *(Continued)*

21. *Record list of serious medical illnesses*		
22. *Record all allergies*		
23. *Record nature of medication, dose and duration*		
If on steroid or anticoagulation treatment	NOT SUITABLE	
24. *Record number of cigarettes/ounces of tobacco smoked*		
Discourage smoking until after operation		
25. *Record average consumption of alcohol*		
It is recommended that the upper limit for men is 3 units and for women is 2 units per day. Advise patient of this if above limit		
If there is reason to believe patient is abusing alcohol, *order LFTs:* If normal	SUITABLE	
26. Try to answer the question(s). If concerned, *inform surgeon or anaesthetist*		
27. Pregnancy: establish that referring clinician is aware of this. If not, *refer back*		
Pill/HRT: oestrogen-containing pills should be stopped for 6 weeks pre-operatively in patients having operations on legs or of long duration		
Note: advise alternative contraception		
28. If concerned, *inform surgeon or anaesthetist*		
29. If you suspect these may affect suitability for day-case surgery, *seek a medical opinion*		
30. *Record any serious complications*		
31. *Record when last anaesthetic was given*		
32. If a family history of malignant hyperthermia	NOT SUITABLE	
If a family history of scoline or suxamethonium sensitivity, *inform anaesthetist*		
If other significant problems, or if in doubt as to suitability of day-case surgery, *seek a medical opinion*		
33. No more than 1 hour's journey is desirable		
34. *Record*		

IF CONSIDERED UNSUITABLE FOR DAY SURGERY, THE PATIENT SHOULD BE TOLD THE REASON AND BE REFERRED BACK TO THE SURGEON. THE GENERAL PRACTITIONER SHOULD BE INFORMED.

SPECIFIC CONDITIONS AFFECTING RISK

GENERAL HEALTH

The age, weight and blood pressure of the patient should be clearly recorded. They should be asked about any medication that they might be taking, whether physician- or self-prescribed. The question 'Are you taking any drugs?' has specific connotations and usually results in a negative answer (the occasional *user* does, however, spring to light!). It is therefore better to specify what you mean by asking 'Are you taking any medication, i.e. medicines, pills, tablets, potions, lotions, creams or any other drugs?' This usually yields a much greater affirmative response. It is also important to document allergies at this stage, and to elucidate what actually occurred with a particular medication or food. Many apparent allergies are well-described pharmacological actions of specific compounds! Patients should be asked about tobacco and alcohol use, as both of these substances may cause an

adverse peri-operative outcome. The condition of the teeth and oral hygiene will be of particular interest to the anaesthetist, and the presence of capped, crowned, bridged or false teeth should be documented. Poor oral hygiene, which is a potential source of infection, may be detrimental to the outcome of many operations in which artificial prostheses are being inserted. This is of particular importance in some branches of surgery, as poor oral hygiene may be the focus of infection, particularly in endocarditis and prosthetic heart valves.

Specific problems associated with previous anaesthesia together with any family history of anaesthetic problems should be noted. A small number of specific inherited diseases have important anaesthetic implications (e.g. malignant hyperpyrexia, cholinesterase abnormalities (suxamethonium apnoea), porphyrias, the haemoglobinopathies, the myotonic dystrophies and some musculoskeletal disorders, rheumatoid arthritis, ankylosing spondylitis, etc.). Many of these conditions have a major effect on the choice of anaesthesia to be employed.

CARDIOVASCULAR DISEASE

There is a high prevalence of coronary artery disease in patients undergoing anaesthesia and surgery. Almost all anaesthetic agents have an effect on the cardiovascular system. Of particular importance are the symptoms and signs of congestive heart failure. In 1977, Goldman produced a risk index scale for patients with heart disease undergoing anaesthesia and non-cardiac surgery. The strongest predictors of risk were signs associated with heart failure, myocardial infarction during the preceding 6 months, or the presence of atrial or ventricular dysrhythmias (i.e. a rhythm other than sinus rhythm, or premature ventricular ectopic beats at a rate of > 5 beats/min). The more risk factors that are present, the greater the risk of a life-threatening peri-operative cardiac event and the greater the risk of peri-operative death. Coronary artery disease and its consequences are the main cause of death following anaesthesia and surgery. The mortality rate after peri-operative myocardial infarction is high (Table 34.1.2).

Cardiac assessment may be aided by exercise electrocardiography, radionuclide isotope scanning, echocardiography and coronary angiography. Assessment of the ejection fraction, i.e. the stroke volume divided by the end-diastolic volume, expressed as a percentage, provides a good non-invasive assessment of ventricular function. In coronary artery disease an ejection fraction of > 55% is associated with minimal risk of an adverse cardiac event. An ejection fraction of > 35% but < 55% is associated with an increased but small risk of peri-operative cardiac morbidity. However, patients who present with an ejection fraction of less than 35% carry a high risk of a peri-operative cardiac event (e.g. myocardial infarction). Patients with coronary artery disease present clinically with either stable angina (i.e. no change in precipitating factors, frequency or duration of pain during the previous 2 months) or unstable angina (i.e. angina with a changing pattern – more frequent, longer duration, or pain unrelieved by nitrate administration). In the light of a history of unstable angina,

surgery should be postponed and further cardiological investigation requested. Previous successful percutaneous balloon angioplasty (PTCA) and/or coronary artery bypass grafting may well lower the peri-operative mortality rate associated with non-cardiac surgery to around 1.2%. Thoracic, upper abdominal, major aortic or other major vascular surgery increases these risks by approximately two- to threefold.

Patients with valvular heart disease require antibiotic cover and treatment of pre-operative infections prior to anaesthesia and surgery. They may also be taking anticoagulant therapy. Valvular heart disease causes either abnormal pressure or abnormal volume loads on the heart. Pressure loads (e.g. in aortic stenosis) cause concentric hypertrophy of the myocardium with a greatly increased ventricular wall thickness. While there is a considerable increase in the myocardial muscle mass, the overall size of the heart is not increased. This type of hypertrophy imposes an increased demand on the systolic function of the heart. In contrast, volume loads cause an eccentric hypertrophy when the heart becomes grossly dilated (e.g. in mitral and aortic regurgitation). During diastole an increased volume of blood flows through the regurgitant valves. This imposes an increased demand on diastolic function. Safe anaesthesia in patients with valvular heart disease depends on an understanding of the abnormal volume and pressure loads on the heart muscle caused by the abnormal valve. The secondary effects of these changes on the heart and on other organs, particularly the lungs, and the compensatory mechanisms adopted by the heart, require appropriate management during anaesthesia. If risk factors are present which can be treated, anaesthesia and surgery should be delayed unless the indications for surgery are life-threatening. Definitive assessment of valvular heart disease is by echocardiography and cardiac angiography.

The presence of an implanted cardiac pacemaker should be noted. If present, it should be reprogrammed by the cardiac department pre-operatively, usually to a fixed rate, to protect both the patient and the pacemaker.

Table 34.1.2 Incidence of peri-operative myocardial infarction following non-cardiac surgery

Overall incidence	0–0.7%
With known coronary artery disease	0–1.1%
With known three-vessel disease: left anterior descending, circumflex and right coronary stenoses (> 70%)	6%

History of previous myocardial infarction
    > 6 months ago
    > 3 months and < 6 months ago
    < 3 months ago
	
	6%
	10–15%
	20–37%

Hypertension

The World Health Organization definition of hypertension is systolic blood pressure of >160 mmHg and diastolic blood pressure of > 95 mmHg). Hypertension requires assessment pre-operatively. Steps should be taken to look for evidence of end-stage organ damage (e.g. left ventricular hypertrophy, cardiac ischaemia or renal damage). Ideally, patients should be rendered normotensive prior to elective surgery. In patients with a diastolic blood pressure in the range 95–110 mmHg, with no evidence of end-stage organ damage, it is probably safe to proceed to elective surgery. Patients with a diastolic blood pressure of 110–120 mmHg require detailed assessment of end-stage organ damage, and a decision balancing the urgency of surgery against the potential risks considered. Patients with a diastolic blood pressure > 120 mmHg should have surgery postponed, and must have their blood pressure controlled for 4–6 weeks before surgery is reconsidered, unless the indication for surgery is life-threatening. Patients with a normal diastolic blood pressure but systolic hypertension (> 160 mmHg) are usually suffering from arteriosclerosis. Consideration should be given to maintaining this blood pressure peri-operatively, as hypotension may well result in end-stage organ hypoperfusion.

PULMONARY DISEASE

The vast majority of anaesthetic agents are respiratory depressants, i.e. anaesthetic agents affect the reflex mechanisms controlling the body responses to hypoxia and hypercarbia. Breathing is primarily controlled by excretion of carbon dioxide, and the alveolar minute ventilation is directly proportional to carbon dioxide production. There is currently no commercially available accurate non-invasive monitor of arterial carbon dioxide in the non-ventilated, non-anaesthetized patient. Post-operative respiratory depression remains a significant cause of post-anaesthetic morbidity and mortality. The advent of pulse oximetry has made bedside assessment of oxygenation extremely simple. However, it must be remembered that a patient who is breathing an increased inspired concentration of oxygen may well be suffering from severe respiratory depression in the face of normal peripheral oxygen saturation. A non-invasive accurate monitor of arterial carbon dioxide would be a major advance with regard to the safe monitoring of a patient post-operatively.

During anaesthesia, the functional residual capacity (volume of gas in the lung at the end of a normal expiration) is reduced, and the closing volume (volume of the lung at which small airways close spontaneously) is increased. When the closing volume is greater than the functional residual capacity, small-airway collapse occurs during tidal ventilation. This leads to an increased alveolar-arterial PO_2 difference because of atelectasis with resultant hypoxaemia. There is potential for pulmonary collapse in dependent lung areas, and there is an increase in ventilation perfusion mismatch. Volatile anaesthetic agents inhibit reflex pulmonary hypoxic vasoconstriction, whilst intravenous agents generally do not inhibit this reflex. There is therefore a need to increase the inspired concentration of oxygen during general anaesthesia. The need for pre-operative pulmonary function tests is assessed from the pre-operative history of breathlessness, cough, sputum production, presence of cyanosis and exercise limitation. Investigation of patients with pulmonary disease should include a chest X-ray, an ECG, lung function tests and an arterial blood gas analysis, remembering to record the inspired concentration of oxygen at the time when the sample is taken. The FEV_1 should be >1 L and the FEV_1/FVC ratio should be > 0.7. Patients with an FEV_1/FVC ratio of < 0.5 and an FEV_1 of <1 L, have an increased risk of post-operative morbidity. The best pre-operative predictors of the need for post-operative ventilation are the pre-operative arterial oxygen and carbon dioxide levels, together with the presence of dyspnoea at rest. In patients with asthma, elective surgery should not be undertaken unless the asthma is well controlled, with peak flow values of > 250–300 L/min. Consideration should be given to a short course of systemic steroids in patients with intractable airway obstruction. Chest physiotherapy will be needed after all but very minor surgery, and consideration should be given to starting this pre-operatively in patients with severe disease or a productive cough. Good post-operative analgesia, preferably with little respiratory depression, will be required if respiratory complications are to be avoided. Control and treatment of pre-existing respiratory infection will also be needed.

GASTROINTESTINAL DISEASE

It is of paramount importance that a patient who is to be rendered unconscious does not aspirate gastrointestinal content into their lungs. Bowel obstruction, ileus or conditions in which there is gastroparesis (e.g. diabetes), particularly if the stomach contents are acid (e.g. gastrin-secreting tumours), represent particular hazards for the anaesthetist. Consideration should be given to pre-operative nasogastric aspiration and careful correction of fluid and electrolyte imbalance. Drugs such as H_2-blocking agents or proton-pump inhibitors are helpful in reducing the acidity of residual gastric contents.

Many drugs used in anaesthesia are at least partially metabolized in the liver, and pre-existing hepatic disease may have a profound effect on the metabolism of these agents. Serum albumin levels, which are a guide to the severity of liver disease, may be reduced, and a reduced plasma cholinesterase level may affect the degradation of some anaesthetic drugs, thus prolonging their action. Patients with jaundice are at particular risk of developing oliguric renal failure, particularly if the bilirubin concentration is > 200 mmol/L. Patients should be well hydrated and have an established diuresis before undertaking anaesthesia and surgery. Preservation of the urine output with crystalloid or colloid solutions is preferable to the use of specific agents such as mannitol or dextran, which may dehydrate the patient by their osmotic action. Diuretic agents (e.g. frusemide), when given in low doses as an infusion, may be of value provided that the level of hydration is adequate and maintained. The hepatorenal syndrome is usually associated with advanced cirrhosis and ascites. The uraemia is characterized by the absence of proteinuria and a urine sodium excretion rate of < 10 mmol/day. Hypovolaemia must be avoided, as the kidneys are intrinsically normal, and the use of colloid solutions such as plasma protein solution or salt-poor albumin is encouraged. A coexistent coagulopathy, if present, requires correction before anaesthesia, particularly if regional anaesthesia is being considered.

RENAL DISEASE

Patients with renal disease may be anaemic, hypertensive, immunosuppressed and prone to infections. An abnormal fluid and electrolyte content is common, and venous access may be difficult. The presence of shunts and fistulae needs to be noted, and these should be well cared for peri-operatively. This includes the placement of non-invasive blood-pressure cuffs only on limbs with no fistulae or shunts present. Care should be taken when establishing venous access, as peripheral veins may be needed in the future for the formation of further shunts or fistulae. As a general rule of thumb, access should be sited below the wrists and ankles. Measurement of electrolytes, full blood count and coagulation would be prudent in these cases.

NEUROMUSCULAR DISEASE

Patients with neuromuscular disorders may respond to muscle relaxants in an unusual way, e.g. in myasthenia gravis, the myotonic dystrophies, spinal cord injury, etc. Such patients may also have an associated cardiomyopathy. There is a high incidence of difficult airways, and management of these patients needs to be planned. It may include elective ventilation in an intensive-care unit, even for relatively minor surgery.

METABOLIC DISEASE

Familial porphyrias and malignant hyperpyrexia are hereditary, metabolic disorders associated with high anaesthetic morbidity and mortality. Phaeochromocytoma and carcinoid syndromes are associated with severe anaesthetic complications due to their unpredictable effects on the cardiovascular system, and all of these conditions require specific pre-anaesthetic planning.

Diabetes is the commonest metabolic disorder that requires forethought for anaesthesia and surgery. Patients maintained on diet alone generally require no special management prior to surgery. The blood glucose should be monitored and maintained in the normal range (i.e. 4–8 mmol/L) peri-operatively. Most non-insulin-dependent diabetics secrete sufficient insulin to maintain their glucose homeostasis during minor surgery. Oral hypoglycaemic agents should be discontinued prior to fasting and the blood glucose monitored accordingly, bearing in mind that some of the longer-acting agents may produce hypoglycaemia if patients are fasted for a prolonged period. They should be restarted when an oral diet is recommended post-operatively. For insulin-dependent diabetics, an intravenous infusion of glucose with an intravenous infusion of soluble insulin is necessary for all but those undergoing very minor surgery. Close monitoring of the blood glucose level will be required. In practice, for accuracy of blood glucose levels it is beneficial to maintain a steady and constant infusion of glucose (5 or 10%) throughout the 24-h period. This allows a constant infusion rate of soluble insulin to be delivered, limiting frequent changes of the rate of infusion of insulin. The circulating volume and electrolyte balance may then be maintained through another intravenous channel with an infusion of saline, colloid or blood as required. Whatever type of diabetic control is in use pre-operatively, the goals of management are to avoid hypoglycaemia, severe hyperglycaemia, protein catabolism, electrolyte imbalance and ketoacidosis.

Patients who are receiving or who have received adrenocortical steroids in the preceding 3 months will require supplemental hydrocortisone peri-operatively. Morbid obesity, defined as a body mass index of > 30 kg/m², is associated with complications that increase the likelihood of peri-operative morbidity and/or mortality.

SICKLE-CELL DISEASE AND HAEMOGLOBINOPATHIES

Sickle-cell syndromes are inherited haemoglobinopathies in which the dominant haemoglobin is the unstable haemoglobin S (HbSS, HbSC, HBSThal). In sickle-cell trait the dominant haemoglobin is HbA, and significant sickling under adverse conditions is rare. Haemoglobin electrophoresis will determine the relative proportions of haemoglobins present, and should be requested in all susceptible groups in whom there is a positive sickledex test. In the sickle-cell disease states, HbSS, HbSC or HBSThal, hypoxia, hypothermia, dehydration and acidosis should be avoided at all costs, as significant sickling may occur under these conditions. Consideration should be given to pre-operative exchange transfusion in cases of major surgery where significant blood replacement is expected. Tourniquets should generally be avoided.

The thalassaemias are an inherited group of disorders in which there is deficient synthesis of globin chains. There are four genes controlling α-chain production (two on each chromosome 16) and two genes controlling β-chain production (one on each chromosome 11). The type and severity of disease depend on the number and type of these genes which are deleted. In α-thalassaemia trait, two genes are deleted, and there is little discernible effect. In α-thalassaemia intermedia, three genes are deleted, and there is resultant stimulation of erythropoietin and an excess of β-chain production. Insoluble tetramers (HBH) are formed from the excess β-chains. There is a moderately severe anaemia, and red-cell haemolysis. α-Thalassaemia major (four-gene deletion) is incompatible with life. β-Thalassaemia minor heterozygotes have mild iron-resistant hypochromic anaemia, but little disability, whereas homozygotes have β-thalassaemia major, and are unable to produce normal β-chains. Fetal haemoglobin production leads to a total haemoglobin level of 30–50% of normal adult levels. This condition is associated with a severe, chronic, transfusion-dependent anaemia. In clinically significant thalassaemias, bone-marrow hyperplasia is prominent as a result of excess erythropoietin. Difficult intubation, cardiomyopathy and left ventricular failure should be looked for in these cases.

COEXISTENT MEDICATION

Patients often present for surgery while taking medications that may have the potential for anaesthetic interaction. Some examples of interactions with anaesthetic agents are given below.

Monoamine oxidase inhibitors

Monoamine oxidase inhibitors primarily interfere with the metabolism of monoamines e.g. dopamine, tyramine, etc.). However, they may also affect the biotransformation of other drugs. In particular, there is a dangerous interaction between these drugs and pethidine. There appears to be an accumulation of the main metabolite norpethidine, and a possible increase in the CNS levels of 5-hydroxytryptamine. Signs of mental confusion, CNS excitation, hyperpyrexia and either hypertension or circulatory collapse may ensue. This type of reaction has also been observed with the selective type-B monoamine oxidase inhibitor, selegiline. Interactions with other opiate analgesics appear to be much less common. Ideally, monoamine oxidase inhibitors should be discontinued for a minimum of 2 weeks prior to anaesthesia and surgery. Psychiatric consultation should be considered in this situation.

Lithium therapy and anaesthesia

Lithium carbonate is used in the management of manic-depressive disorders. It is absorbed well from the gastrointestinal tract, is water soluble, and relies almost exclusively on renal excretion. Lithium clearance correlates well with creatinine clearance. Its mode of action is unknown. In the body it is handled like sodium and potassium ions, and can therefore have profound effects on electrolyte balance and metabolic processes. The therapeutic range is 0.8–1.2 mmol/L. Toxicity can occur above 1.5–2.0 mmol/L. The therapeutic window is therefore small, and levels should be monitored closely. Side-effects and signs of early toxicity include gastrointestinal symptoms (e.g. nausea, vomiting and diarrhoea), fine tremor, polyuria and polydipsia, and weight gain. These progress to muscle weakness, slurred speech, sleepiness and confusion. Severe toxicity results in convulsions and life-threatening coma. Reduced fluid intake (e.g. from pre-operative starvation, vomiting and obtunded states), combined with the lithium-induced inability to compensate by concentrating urine output, can cause dehydration and precipitate toxicity. Renal function can be disturbed either by pre-operative events or by surgery itself, and this too may cause lithium toxicity by accumulation. Lithium is potentiated by NSAIDs and thiazide diuretics. Conversely, lithium can potentiate the action of neuromuscular agents by inhibiting presynaptic synthesis of acetylcholine. In the elective situation, lithium should be stopped 48–72 h prior to surgery, and pre-operative intravenous therapy should be considered.

Dehydration must be avoided with appropriate fluid management. Lithium should be restarted as soon as feasible (to prevent acute mania), provided that renal function and fluid and electrolyte balance are normal. In emergency situations, signs of toxicity should be sought on a clinical basis. The use of neuromuscular agents should be carefully monitored, but nevertheless it may be necessary to provide a period of respiratory support post-operatively until power is regained. Minor toxicity should be treated with rehydration and mannitol to increase excretion. Loop and thiazide diuretics are contraindicated. Haemodialysis may be required in cases of severe coma-inducing toxicity. Care is needed in the peri-operative management of patients who are taking lithium, and consideration should be given to discontinuation of therapy prior to surgery after psychiatric consultation.

Anticonvulsant drugs

Many anaesthetic agents alter the protein binding of anticonvulsant drugs. This may result in subtherapeutic levels or toxicity of these agents. Patients may also have hepatic microsomal enzyme induction, and larger doses of hypnotics, sedatives or anaesthetic agents may be required. Care should be taken with this group of drugs to ensure a safe environment for the patient.

Anticoagulant therapy

Warfarin should be converted to heparin therapy pre-operatively for at least 3–4 days so that the INR is reduced to < 1.5. Continuation of anticoagulation may be achieved with heparin, and this may be given either intravenously or subcutaneously, depending on local preference.

Oral contraception

Oral contraceptives containing oestrogen should normally be discontinued 4–6 weeks prior to surgery. In practice this is difficult to achieve. Patients who present for surgery on oestrogen-containing contraceptives should therefore routinely receive heparin prophylaxis against venous thrombo-embolism, together with elasticated stockings.

Discussion of the options with regard to anaesthetic technique and anaesthetic risk are ideally best left to the anaesthetist who will provide the anaesthetic. If the surgeon prefers a specific technique, this is best communicated to the anaesthetist directly rather than being recommended to the patient. The anaesthetist must determine the development of the anaesthetic.

PRE-OPERATIVE FASTING

The order 'nil by mouth' from midnight is obsolete. Patients should have their surgery planned, and their fasting time should be related to their planned time of surgery. Of course, aspiration of stomach contents is a cause of anaesthetic morbidity, but excessive starvation does not guarantee an empty stomach! Solid food should be withheld for at least 6 h pre-operatively. However, clear fluids (defined as the ability to read print through the glass) may be administered unrestricted up to 2 h pre-operatively in healthy adults, provided that gastric emptying is normal and the patient has not been premedicated.

PREMEDICATION

The reasons for prescribing premedication are as follows:

- to reduce fear and anxiety;
- to reduce secretion of saliva;
- to prevent vagal reflexes caused by surgical stimulation;
- as part of the anaesthetic technique to provide analgesia and/or sedation;
- to reduce the amount of anaesthetic agents required during induction of anaesthesia;
- to produce amnesia;
- for specific therapeutic effects (e.g. H_2-blockers, beta-blockers, beta-agonists, analgesics, anti-emetics, nitrate patches, etc.).

Premedication will vary greatly depending on the nature of the surgery, together with individual patient and anaesthetic preference. Nowadays patients are most often admitted on the day of their surgery, and consequently are not premedicated.

INTENSIVE CARE AND HIGH-DEPENDENCY UNITS

Intensive care and high-dependency care consist of the care of patients who are deemed to be recoverable, but who require continuous supervision, and who need or are likely to need specialized techniques carried out by experienced skilled personnel. Such techniques and experience are unavailable continuously on a general ward. The decision to admit patients to an intensive care unit (ICU) or a high-dependency unit (HDU) will depend on many factors, and will vary according to local guidelines, but certain broad groups may be defined:

- patients requiring mechanical ventilation or renal dialysis;
- patients requiring continuous monitoring of vital signs;
- patients with severe metabolic or electrolyte disturbances;
- patients with a requirement for heavy or specialized nursing care;
- patients at risk of a lethal complication.

High-dependency units are advocated as being the best place for the medical and nursing care of patients who require more facilities than are usually available on a general ward, but are not 'sick' enough to require intensive care.

CONSENT FOR SURGERY AND ANAESTHESIA

THE RIGHT TO CONSENT

The competent adult patient has a fundamental right to give or withhold consent to examination, investigation or treatment. This right is founded on the moral principle of respect for autonomy. An autonomous person has the right to decide what may or may not be done to him or her. Any treatment, investigation or, indeed, even deliberate touching that is carried out without consent may amount to battery. This could result in an action for damages, or even criminal proceedings, and in a finding of serious professional misconduct by the health-care professional's registration body.

TYPES OF CONSENT

Implied consent

For many of the physical contacts between practitioner and patient, consent is implied. It can be assumed that a patient has consented, for example, to abdominal palpation when they voluntarily undress and lie on a couch, or when they offer an arm for venepuncture.

Express consent

Express (i.e. oral or written) consent should be obtained for any procedure that carries a material risk. The patient's specific agreement (oral or written) must be obtained before the procedure is contemplated.

Oral consent

Oral consent is valid, but it is usual to obtain written consent for major procedures. If, for whatever reason, it is only possible to obtain oral consent, it is appropriate to make an entry in the patient's clinical records confirming what advice was given to the patient and the fact that consent was given.

Written consent

Written consent is not absolutely necessary to defend an action for assault and/or battery, but it may afford documentary evidence that consent has been obtained. An action may be brought several years after the event, and a judge may prefer a patient's evidence to that of a practitioner if a signed and witnessed consent form cannot be produced.

Obtaining consent

When should consent be obtained?

Consent should be obtained before the proposed procedure, and before any sedation is given. For elective surgery, where no change in the basic condition requiring operative treatment is expected, the patient's signed consent could be obtained during an out-patient consultation. This would allow a reasonable interval (a 'cooling-off' period) between the consent being obtained and the actual procedure, thereby enabling the patient to consider the matter further and/or to take advice.

If the patient's condition alters between the out-patient appointment and their admission to hospital, so that there is some material change in the nature, purpose or risks of the procedure, then consent should be obtained again. A further explanation should be given and a new consent form should be signed. Similarly, if a considerable time period has elapsed between the out-patient appointment and admission, consent should be obtained again.

In any event, many practitioners prefer to confirm consent with the patient before sedation for the procedure, even if there have been no significant changes in the patient's condition or in the proposed procedure.

Explanation by a knowledgeable practitioner

In hospitals, consent is usually obtained by a doctor or dentist, although in some circumstances valid consent may be obtained by another health-care professional.

It is important that the person who discusses the procedure with the patient should, whenever possible, be the same person who will carry out the procedure. If this is not possible, then consent should be obtained by someone who is appropriately qualified and familiar with all the details and risks of the proposed procedure and any alternatives. As a result, the task should not routinely be delegated to a junior colleague, especially if a complicated or specialized procedure is contemplated, nor is it appropriate to ask a student to obtain consent.

Duress

Consent must be freely given, and it may not be valid if it is obtained under any form of duress. As well as obvious coercion, failure to allow a patient sufficient time to consider the relevant information before making a decision might mean that they do not really consent at all. It may be advisable to allow a reasonable interval, even if it is only short, between obtaining consent and an elective procedure, to enable the patient to consider the matter further and/or to take advice.

Material risks

Material risks are defined as those to which a reasonable person in the patient's position would be likely to attach significance (see below).

The legal position on whether or not a doctor or other health-care professional is negligent in failing to mention a risk to a surgical patient was determined in the UK in the case of Sidaway. The House of Lords confirmed that the test to be applied is the same as that used in deciding whether a doctor has been negligent in any other aspect of his or her work. This is known as the Bolam test. A practitioner can expect to avoid liability if the court finds that a reasonably competent practitioner in a similar position would not have mentioned the risk, and that such a decision was supported by a responsible body of relevant professional opinion. While a doctor's duty to respond to a patient's direct questions is limited by the Bolam test, doctors should answer questions as truthfully and as fully as possible.

In the Sidaway case, the court retained the right to overrule medical opinion if disclosure was obviously necessary for an informed choice by the patient. In some cases a practitioner may reasonably omit to mention a material risk if, after proper consideration of the patient's condition, he or she believes that a warning would be harmful to the patient's health (therapeutic privilege).

In deciding whether to warn of a particular risk, the practitioner must be mindful of all relevant factors, including the severity and likelihood of the risk compared to the need for the procedure. It may be appropriate to warn of a relatively rare risk for a non-therapeutic procedure, such as sterilization or a screening test, whereas a similar risk for an important therapeutic procedure may not require specific warning because of the possibility of deterring a patient inappropriately from receiving a necessary treatment.

Notwithstanding this legal principle, practitioners should be aware that there is an increasing view among health-care professionals, lawyers and the public that patients should be advised of all possible risks.

Alterations to the consent form

No alterations should be made to the consent form after it has been signed by the patient. If, after the form is signed, there is a change in the planned procedure the patient must be consulted and a new consent form should be signed.

Do not exceed the authority given

Consent is obtained on the basis that the patient understands 'that any procedure in addition to the investigation or treatment described ... will only be carried out if it is necessary and in my best interests and can be justified for medical reasons'.

This covers only what becomes necessary during the operation for the preservation of the patient's life or health. It does not allow a surgeon to contravene the expressed wish of the patient and undertake additional, albeit well-meaning procedures for which the patient has not given consent. The patient is entitled to be told what procedures may reasonably be expected to be carried out. For example, it would be wise to tell a patient who consents to a general anaesthetic if an analgesic suppos-

itory is to be inserted, and failure to do so may result in an allegation of battery.

The consent form

The primary purpose of the consent form is to provide confirmation that the patient gave consent to the procedure in question, and that this was obtained with due care and formality. It cannot be over-emphasized that it is the explanation given to the patient, and the manner in which the patient's questions are answered, that are of paramount importance.

In 1990, the Department of Health in the UK issued new advice on consent (HC(90)22) (the Consent Circular). Model consent forms were revised in 1992 in the document HSG(92)32, and are also available in Bengali, Gujerati, Hindi, Punjabi, Urdu, Cantonese, Vietnamese, Turkish and Greek. The doctor or dentist is required to complete a section of the form that specifies the type of operation, investigation or treatment, and to confirm that this has been explained to the patient, together with such appropriate options as are available, and that the type of anaesthetic (general/local/sedation), if any, has been discussed. This may apparently put the surgeon or one of his or her team in the position of being required to explain the anaesthetic. However, it is generally accepted that a separate discussion should take place between the anaesthetist and the patient, and that the anaesthetist should make a note of this discussion.

The doctor or dentist should also enter full details of the proposed procedure, including the site and, where appropriate, the side, on the form. Abbreviations, especially for 'left' and 'right', should not be used.

The right to refuse treatment

A competent adult has a right to refuse treatment even if others, including doctors, believe that the refusal is neither in his or her best interests nor reasonable.

Unconscious patients

When a patient presents who is acutely unconscious because of injury or illness, a clinician may undertake whatever treatment is necessary to ensure the patient's life or health, without waiting to obtain consent. A note should be made in the clinical records to explain the absence of formal consent. It is good practice to involve relatives or other carers in decision-making. However, in an emergency the desirability of this should not delay the clinician taking such actions as the best interests of the patient demand, but it is important that the clinician restricts him- or herself to providing only the necessary treatment.

Patients on life-support

Difficult issues arise about decisions as to whether to commence or continue life support in severely ill or injured patients who lack the capacity to consent, and have not shown their wishes in an advance directive.

Here the best-interests principle should apply – there is no duty upon doctors to commence or continue futile treatment that would subject the patient to discomfort or indignity. However, such decisions have to be made with great care, and will involve consultation with relatives, other individuals close to the patient, and health-care professionals, as well as appropriate specialist consultations or second opinions.

'Do not resuscitate' decisions

The need to make a 'do not resuscitate' decision may arise in the case of a patient who is competent to make his or her wishes clear, or who had previously done so when competent. Often, however, the clinician is faced with a seriously ill patient who is not known to have expressed any wish about resuscitation, and is currently unable to do so. The overall responsibility for a 'do not resuscitate' decision rests with the consultant in charge of the patient's care. This decision should be made after appropriate consultation and consideration of all aspects of the patient's condition. The perspectives of other members of the medical and nursing team, and of the patient's relatives or close friends, may all be valuable in determining the consultant's decision. Any decision should be reviewed periodically.

Many hospitals may wish to institute a policy for these situations, and the guidelines on cardiopulmonary resuscitation from the BMA and the Royal College of Nursing may be helpful in formulating such a policy.

Post-mortem examination and removal of human tissue

Post-mortems

The law concerning possession of a human corpse is a complex issue. A coroner's order gives the pathologist complete authority to perform a post-mortem examination. In the UK, hospital post-mortems come under Section 2 of the Human Tissue Act 1961. Under the terms of this Section, the authority of 'the person lawfully in possession of the body' should be obtained before a hospital post-mortem is carried out, and before tissue is removed from a body after death. The managers of the hospital are in lawful possession of the body from the moment of death until a near relative or executor comes forward to claim the body. The hospital managers normally delegate this authority to one or more individuals. In an Armed Services hospital, the commanding officer is in lawful possession of the body.

Removal of human tissue or organs

Any doctor who wants to remove human tissue under Section 1 of the Act must obtain authority from those in lawful possession of the body. They in turn must ensure that the necessary procedural steps have been taken (e.g. that a signed consent or kidney donor card exists).

Without such a card, the person lawfully in possession of the body may authorize the removal of tissue only if, after making reasonable enquiries, he or she has no reason to believe that the deceased would have objected, or that the surviving spouse or any relative objects. Specific consent is not necessary – a lack of objection is sufficient. Even if there is a donor card, it would be unwise to act against the relatives' wishes.

If there is any reason to believe that the coroner will require an inquest or post-mortem, the coroner's consent is necessary before authority can be given for the removal of tissue.

It is often convenient to remove human tissue for diagnosis, treatment and research during a routine hospital post-mortem. Although the Act does not require a written agreement from relatives for this, it may be desirable to obtain one.

Surgical implants

A device or prosthesis implanted in a body becomes the property of that person and, on his or her death, part of the person's estate, unless there is specific provision to the contrary. A 'surgical implants' form may serve two purposes – it is a form of consent to the operation, and it vests the rights of ownership of the implant in the hospital's proprietors.

[The text in this section Consent for surgery and anaesthesia up to this point is taken from the MDU's booklet *Consent to treatment* by Dr John Gilberthorpe. © The MDU 1996. All rights reserved.]

THE GENERAL DUTY OF CARE OF SURGEONS

General moral and legal duties

For surgery to be successful there must be a relationship of trust and confidence between surgeon and patient. To achieve this, the surgeon must be sensitive to the vulnerability of the patient and respect their human dignity – their ability and right to plan for their own future. Morally, therefore, surgeons should always act towards patients as they would wish other surgeons to treat them, their families and friends.

The surgeon's clinical duties of care are based on an understanding of the rights of the patient.

Patients are entitled to the following:

- to have their life and health protected to an acceptable professional standard. In the UK, acceptable practice will legally be that which a responsible body of medical opinion would deem appropriate in the clinical circumstances in which such practice occurs;
- to have their autonomy respected – to consent to or refuse surgery on the basis of correct and adequate information about proposed treatments, and

generally to control who has access to personal information about themselves which is revealed during clinical consultation;

- to be treated fairly according only to their needs, and without discrimination or prejudice.

These principles can be expressed in further detail against the background of their interpretation by the professional organizations of both medicine and surgery, together with the courts.

Protecting the life and health of patients

It is the surgeon's obligation at all times to take reasonable care to act in the patient's best interests. In so doing the surgeon should:

- respect both the vulnerability and the dignity of the patient;
- diagnose and treat the patient within acceptable limits of established skill and competence;
- treat for no other purpose than to meet the clinical needs of the patient or to enable the patient to help others in legally acceptable circumstances (e.g. transplantation);
- not subject the patient to painful and distressing procedures of no or little known benefit;
- utilize the knowledge and skills of other clinicians when appropriate;
- maintain accurate records of clinical findings, diagnoses, treatments and results;
- ensure that the patient receives adequate post-operative care, including ensuring that relevant information is effectively communicated both to the patient and to those responsible for their ongoing care;
- respect the right of the patient to obtain a second clinical opinion about diagnosis and treatment;
- maintain and develop his or her professional skills and expertise.

AUTONOMY AND CONSENT – COMPETENT ADULTS

The moral unacceptability of anyone exercising unlimited power over others is at the heart of many of our liberal values. Our capacity for reasoned choice is one of the attributes that differentiates humans from other creatures. Respect for this capacity, especially our right to determine what happens to our own bodies, is an indication of the seriousness with which we respect the humanity and dignity of others.

Therefore, before surgery, the surgeon and members of the surgical team should strive for a well-balanced relationship with the patient through intelligent dialogue and an honest, realistic and sensitive discussion of the facts about the options for treatment.

For consent to treatment to be valid, the patient must be competent to provide it. The surgeon should ensure that the choice of the patient is the result of understanding and deliberation about information provided concerning diagnosis and treatment. The patient should also be able to remember such information, and they should believe that it applies to them.

After these steps have been taken, the surgeon should:

- inform competent adult patients aged 16 years or over of the nature of their condition, together with the type, purpose, prognosis, common side-effects and significant risks of any proposed surgical treatments. Where appropriate, alternative treatment options (including non-surgical treatment) should also be explained, together with the consequences of having no treatment. This information should be provided in the degree of detail required by a reasonable person in the circumstances of the patient to make a relevant and informed judgement. The patient's first language and ability to understand English should be taken into account in the provision of this information;
- attempt to establish that the patient understands the site and size of the incision, and has some insight into the pain and discomfort which sometimes follows surgery, together with the analgesic and other measures available to minimize it;
- determine any special aspects of the life and employment of the patient which require more detailed information for consent to be given acceptably (e.g. risks of loss of specific movement, extent of scarring at the operative site, or social consequences of a stoma);
- outline briefly in the patient's record or on the consent form what appropriate information has been communicated, especially recording the nature of the risks explained. The surgeon is advised to make a note of perceived difficulties in understanding;
- record consent in writing – usually on the consent form – after appropriate information has been communicated;
- recognize that all competent patients aged 18 years or older are legally entitled to refuse life-saving or any other surgical treatment;
- in the absence of a properly drafted and legally binding advance directive stating otherwise, act in an emergency to do what is necessary to save the life

or to prevent permanent and serious disability of adults who are unconscious or otherwise unable to give consent. A valid advance directive is clear about the clinical conditions under which specific treatments are rejected;

- not perform elective surgery (i.e. surgery which is not immediately required to save life or to prevent serious and permanent injury) on adult patients who are unconscious or otherwise unable to give consent. Such surgery should be postponed until explicit consent can be given;

- recognize that, in the UK, no adult – including the next of kin – can consent to surgical treatment on behalf of another adult (aged 18 years or older) who for whatever reason is incapable of providing such consent. Generally speaking, in such circumstances clinicians can lawfully provide treatments which they believe are justified in the patient's best interests. Relevant carers should be consulted with a view to ascertaining what the patient's best interests may be. (In Scotland, there is provision to apply to the Court to be appointed Tutor Dative to a patient. A Tutor Dative can validly give consent on the patient's behalf.)

AUTONOMY AND CONSENT – CHILDREN

The moral duty to respect the life and health of children and to treat them fairly is exactly the same as that for adults. In general, surgeons should obtain explicit consent for any proposed treatment of a child under the age of 16 years from the person with parental responsibility. Such consent should be written unless circumstances make this impossible.

Children can display wide variation in the maturity and understanding required to make decisions for themselves. The competence of children to make decisions should be decided in the same way as for adults. Children under 16 years of age may be competent to consent to treatment, and they should participate in decisions about their surgical treatment.

The dignity and legal rights of young children who are not competent to consent to surgical treatments should also be respected. Such children should still be consulted about their treatment, and should not be ignored in the presence of their parents or others with parental responsibility. Where possible, their views should be recorded in the notes and they should be addressed directly in the process of such a consultation.

The surgeon should:

- inform those with parental responsibility and/or all competent child patients of the nature of their condition, together with the type, purpose, prognosis, common side-effects and significant risks of any proposed surgical treatments. This information should be provided in the degree of detail that would be required by a responsible person, who is in the circumstances of the parents and/or the child, to make a relevant and informed judgement. This does not require communicating with the parents and the child in the same way about such information. A note should indicate that appropriate information has been communicated to the child;

- respect the right of competent children to seek and receive surgical advice and treatment without the knowledge of their parents, provided that the child is encouraged to communicate with their parents and that the treatment is in the child's best interests. Under these circumstances, the confidentiality of the child should be respected;

- recognize that if children of any age are competent to do so, they have the right to consent to treatment;

- recognize that where a competent child (even up to the age of 18 years) refuses treatment, and the refusal is considered not to be in the child's best interests, a parent or the Court may consent on the child's behalf;

- recognise that where the child (even up to the age of 18 years) is at risk of death or permanent and serious disability and treatment is refused by the parents, the ultimate arbiter should be the Court. In such situations the hospital administration or legal adviser should be consulted;

- in an emergency, act to save the life or preserve the health of a child. This should be done in cases where the parents or the child refuse consent and there is not time to obtain a Court Order or where, if the child is not competent, the parents' consent cannot be given in time. In such circumstances the consultant in overall charge of the patient should be involved at as early a stage as possible. There is special provision for patients under the age of 16 years in Section 2(4) of the Age of Legal Capacity (Scotland) Act 1991, which states that 'a person under the age of 16 years shall have legal capacity to consent on his own behalf to any surgical, medical or dental procedure or treatment where in the opinion of a qualified medical practitioner attending him he is capable of understanding the nature and possible consequences of the procedure or treatment'.

AUTONOMY AND CONSENT – PSYCHIATRICALLY ILL OR MENTALLY IMPAIRED PATIENTS

Surgeons should always remember that it does not follow that because a patient is psychiatrically ill or mentally impaired they also lack the autonomy necessary to make informed decisions about specific aspects of their lives, including surgical treatment. Incompetence in some respects does not automatically indicate universal incompetence.

The surgeon should:

- respect the right of competent voluntary psychiatric patients to consent to or refuse surgical treatment. Their rights are the same as those of other competent patients;

- respect the right of patients who are being given compulsory psychiatric treatment under the Mental Health Act to consent to or refuse necessary surgical treatment. The one exception is when, because of their psychiatric condition, they are unable to understand, retain, deliberate upon and believe the information relevant to making an informed choice, and the proposed treatment is necessary to save their life or to prevent serious or permanent injury. Such incompetence should be judged by those responsible for the patient's psychiatric care and, if necessary, by the Court;

- not perform elective surgery on detained patients who are temporarily incompetent to provide valid consent. Treatment should wait until the patient regains sufficient competence to give valid consent;

- perform both elective and necessary surgery on mentally impaired patients who are permanently incompetent to give informed consent, if the treatment is in the patient's best interests;

- recognize that as a matter of law, no adult can give or refuse consent to treatment on behalf of an incompetent adult patient. If relatives are asked to sign consent forms under these circumstances, it should be made clear to them that they are doing so in order to give their advice, i.e. to 'assent', and not actually to provide consent. Asking relatives or carers to provide such 'assent' is an indication of their potential importance in helping to determine the best interests of the patient;

- use minimal necessary force in an emergency, to protect the life and health of a patient whose competence is in doubt until a formal diagnosis of competence can be made by an appropriate clinician (in a non-psychiatric hospital, usually the duty psychiatrist). Further information about the use of

the Mental Health Act and use of restraints can be found in the Code of Practice of the Mental Health Act 1983.

AUTONOMY AND CONSENT – DECISIONS NOT TO BEGIN OR TO WITHDRAW LIFE-SAVING OR LIFE-PRESERVING TREATMENT

According to their general duty of care, surgeons have the responsibility to use their expertise to protect life and health to a professionally acceptable standard. Decisions not to provide or to continue life-saving or life-preserving treatment must therefore be consistent with this duty to act in the best interests of the patient. This may be the case for one of two reasons.

First, competent adult patients have the moral and legal right to refuse life-saving or life-preserving treatment, whether or not their clinician believes it to be in their best interests (e.g. Jehovah's Witnesses), unless there is evidence of coercion. Such patients should be informed as to why their clinician believes that life-saving or life-preserving treatment is in their best interests – if this is the case.

Secondly, life-saving or life-preserving treatment does not have to be given to, or may be withdrawn from, incompetent adults or children in cases where this action is believed by the clinical team – in consultation with relatives – to be in the patient's best interests. In these circumstances, the final decision and responsibility rest with the clinician in charge of the patient's care.

Accordingly, there are three clinical circumstances where non-treatment decisions can be considered to be in the patient's best interests:

1. agreement by the clinical team that any further treatment would be futile, i.e. would not save or preserve life;

2. cases where the patient is irreversibly and imminently close to death and treatment will not improve their condition;

3. cases where the patient already has devastating and permanent neurological injury that is so incompatible with any form of conscious self-directed activity as to represent, in the circumstances of the patient, a demonstrably awful life. There should be a consensus about such incompatibility among the health-care team and, if indicated, with the relatives. Here there is sufficient potential moral and legal debate to necessitate that a decision to withhold or withdraw life-saving or life-preserving treatment should only be taken by the consultant in charge (who may wish to seek legal advice, in addition to obtaining the advice and support of colleagues).

Any non-treatment decision which has been made on the basis of the preceding criteria should be made without prejudice to the clinical duty to provide effective palliative care.

The following points should also be noted.

- Active euthanasia – a clinical choice directed at killing the patient – is illegal in the UK, Ireland, Australia and New Zealand.

- Incompetent adult patients may have made their wishes known in advance while still competent, expressing their decision to refuse specific life-saving or life-preserving treatment(s). Such advance directives should be respected provided that the treatments which are rejected are clearly specified together with the clinical conditions under which they might be offered. Treatments which have not been explicitly refused in relation to clearly stated clinical conditions should always be given if clinically appropriate.

- In the case of children, those with parental responsibility should be informed about any proposal not to provide life-saving or life-preserving treatment. Provided that such treatment is not in the child's best interest and this decision fulfils above criteria, life-saving or life-preserving treatment may be withheld or withdrawn. The views of the parents should be taken into account by the surgeons making this decision. In cases where there is unresolvable conflict, the hospital management should be informed and the appropriate court consulted.

- If a patient is incompetent due to a diagnosis of permanent vegetative state, then artificial nutrition and hydration (e.g. intravenously) should also be regarded as a form of life-preserving medical treatment. Properly formulated advance directives can forbid their use, as well as other life-saving or life-preserving treatments. At present, artificial nutrition and hydration should only be withdrawn after the hospital management has been informed, and with the agreement of the appropriate court. (Surgeons may wish to consult guidelines on the diagnosis and management of permanent vegetative state, published by the Royal College of Physicians and endorsed by the Academy of Medical Royal Colleges and Faculties.)

AUTONOMY AND THE RIGHT OF PATIENTS TO CONFIDENTIALITY

Adults (and sometimes also children in the circumstances already described) usually have the right to determine who has access to personal medical information about themselves. In general, surgeons should respect this right. Apart from the fact that they would wish to be shown such respect themselves, there is an important public interest in medical information remaining confidential to the patient. Confidentiality is central to the clinical relationship of trust. Without it, patients who may pose a threat to the public without clinical care might not seek treatment.

However, there are exceptions where:

- disclosure is to other members of the health-care team participating in the patient's treatment, who also have a strict professional duty to maintain confidentiality;

- disclosure is necessary to obtain information for the purposes of effective clinical care which the patient is unable to provide;

- disclosure can be justified in the public interest, or because of the threat of serious and imminent physical harm to an identified individual;

- disclosure is necessary to comply with a statutory requirement (e.g. informing the relevant authority that a patient has a notifiable disease);

- disclosure is required by a court order;

- disclosure is for the purposes of research, consent cannot reasonably be obtained and there is no intention to make further contact with the patient (e.g. some epidemiological research involving the use of medical records). In such circumstances the potential benefits of the research should be significant, and disclosure to researchers should be strictly authorized and regulated by the Local Research Ethics Committee;

- disclosure is necessary for the purposes of teaching the principles and practice of emergency medicine and surgery, and consent cannot reasonably be obtained (e.g. from patients whose temporary or permanent brain damage makes them incapable of consultation). In such circumstances, students must be advised of their duties concerning confidentiality. Clinical teachers will be professionally responsible for any violation of these duties.

Patients should give their written consent for the retention of any information concerning their condition and treatment that is held on film or video which is to be used for any purpose other than their own treatment. This consent should be based on information about the specific future use for which the material is required.

Surgeons should be aware that disclosure of information about a patient to a specific party (e.g. a court) may be legally justified, but that this does not relieve them of their general obligation to respect the patient's right to confidentiality. Disclosure should never go beyond the requirements of the particular situation. Competent patients should normally be told beforehand of the need/desire for disclosure and agree to it.

APPENDIX

SUGGESTED PROTOCOL FOR ORDERING PRE-OPERATIVE INVESTIGATIONS

Full blood count

A pre-operative full blood count should only be performed if:

- the patient is clinically anaemic;
- the patient has a systemic disease;
- the patient is on any medication (including drug and alcohol abuse);
- surgery dictates this (i.e. group and save or cross-match needed);
- the patient is at either of the extremes of age;
- the patient is on haemodialysis, in which case a post-dialysis full blood count must be available.

Urea and electrolytes

A pre-operative level should only be obtained if:

- the patient is aged 60 years or over;
- the patient has the following systemic disease:
  - renal disease or renal tract disease;
  - severe liver disease;
  - diabetes insipidus/mellitus;
  - inappropriate ADH secretion;
- the patient is on the following drugs:
  - diuretic;
  - digitalis or any other cardiac drug;
  - corticosteroids;
  - any nephrotoxic drug;
- recent large fluid shifts (e.g. persistent vomiting or diarrhoea) have occurred;

- the patient is on dialysis, in which case a post-dialysis urea and electrolytes must be available. The serum potassium level should be < 6 mmol/L on the day of surgery.

Chest X-ray

A pre-operative chest X-ray should only be carried out for anaesthetic reasons if:

- there are acute respiratory symptoms;
- admission to intensive care for further management is planned;
- the type of surgery indicates this (i.e. intrathoracic or major head and neck surgery and suspected or established cardiorespiratory disease, and no recent chest X-ray is available for inspection within the last year);
- major vascular surgery is planned.

ECG

A pre-operative ECG should only be carried out if:

- the patient is aged 60 years or over;
- the patient has a history or physical signs of heart disease;
- the patient has systemic disease associated with cardiac involvement (e.g. hypertension, peripheral vascular disease, diabetes, collagen vascular diseases or rheumatic fever);
- the patient is on potentially cardiotoxic drugs;
- surgery is associated with cardiac complications;
- the patient is at risk of major electrolyte abnormalities;
- an abnormality is found on clinical examination.

Patients who are adequately and appropriately investigated and who have been 'optimized' with regard to control of pre-existing disease are unlikely to have their surgery postponed. Blanket investigations that are not based on sound clinical indications are not cost-effective and should be discouraged.

Anaesthesia: techniques and drugs

D. Wynne L. Davies

Introduction

Anaesthesia is required to allow a surgeon to perform a particular procedure on a particular patient, while at the same time providing a pain-free, comfortable and safe environment for the patient. The function of anaesthesia is therefore to provide surgeons with a safe 'operative field' in which they can operate for the benefit of the patient. This initial goal may be achieved in a number of ways.

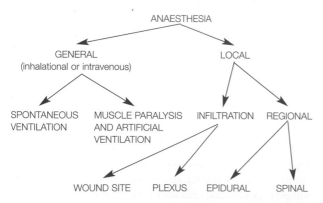

Anaesthesia consists of narcosis, analgesia, relaxation, amnesia and reflex suppression. With 'balanced anaesthesia' it is possible to selectively block each of these components to a greater or lesser degree. An operative field may be provided with major differences in the way it is achieved. Traditionally, the administration of anaesthesia consists of pre-operative assessment of risk, appropriate premedication, induction of anaesthesia, maintenance of anaesthesia, reversal of paralysis, a recovery period and post-operative care.

Many factors influence the choice of anaesthesia, and they depend on anaesthetists', patients' and surgical preferences for a particular procedure. Controversy exists as to the advantages of regional vs. general anaesthesia. The decision to use one technique instead of another is most often based on techniques learned in training, institutional tradition, medico-legal, fears, and perceived time constraints, rather than on factual data supported by the method. There is evidence of direct benefits of regional anaesthesia in the following situations: there are fewer haemodynamic changes in hypertensive patients; there is reduced surgical blood loss; there is a reduced incidence of thrombo-embolism; there is reversal of ischaemic events in patients with ischaemic heart disease; and the technique is safe for patients with malignant hyperpyrexia. The ability to compare outcome of anaesthetic technique is limited by the remarkable safety of both methods. In the healthy, elective surgical patient undergoing non-body-cavity surgery, the risk of dying from a primary anaesthetic cause is probably less than 1:100 000. There is therefore an element of individual preference based on perceived advantages and disadvantages of a particular technique, together with an assessment of the problems of interaction of anaesthetic agents with coexisting medical disease or drug therapy. The primary aim must be to provide an operating environment that is safe for the patient.

Patients often present for surgery while taking a drug which may have the potential for anaesthetic interaction. Some examples of the interaction of drugs with anaesthetic agents have been described in the previous chapter.

Discussion of the options of anaesthetic technique and anaesthetic risk are best left to the anaesthetist who will provide the anaesthetic. If the surgeon prefers a specific technique, this is best communicated to the anaesthetist directly rather than being recommended to the patient. The anaesthetist must determine the development of the anaesthetic.

TECHNIQUES OF ANAESTHESIA

GENERAL ANAESTHESIA

General anaesthesia results in central depression of consciousness and central reflexes. This occurs in a dose-dependent manner. However, central depression does not occur in isolation, as cardiopulmonary and motor function are affected in a similar way. General anaesthesia may be provided with volatile inhalational agents, usually halogenated ethers and hydrocarbons (e.g. halothane, enflurane isoflurane, desflurane, sevoflurane). Unfortunately, the effects of volatile inhalational anaesthetic agents are not confined to the central nervous system. The majority of the volatile anaesthetic agents have detrimental effects on cardiovascular and respiratory function, again in a dose-dependent manner. They are also generally regarded as triggers for 'malignant hyperthermia'. The potency of inhalational agents is measured by the 'minimum alveolar concentration' (MAC_{50}), which is the inhaled concentration of anaesthetic agent required at equilibrium to prevent movement in 50% of the population undergoing a standard surgical incision (i.e. skin incision). The MAC_{95} is the prevention of movement in 95% of the same population, and is about 1.3 times the MAC_{50}. It is a guide to the concentration of inhalational agent required to produce unconsciousness, amnesia and reflex suppression. One of the main advantages of using inhalational anaesthesia is that the inhalational agent may be rapidly removed by reversing the concentration gradient in the inspired ventilatory gas mixture (i.e. it does not rely on metabolism for the termination of action). In comparison, drugs that provide intravenous anaesthesia show wide variation in chemical structure, and rely heavily on redistribution and metabolism for cessation of anaesthetic effect (e.g. propofol etomidate, ketamine, barbiturates). Inhalational and intravenous anaesthetic agents may be used for both induction and maintenance of anaesthesia, and their use may be supplemented with muscle relaxants. Very few of the inhalational or intravenous agents possess significant analgesic properties. With both inhalational and intravenous anaesthetic agents, loss of consciousness and airway reflexes are rapid, and facilities for airway maintenance must be available whenever use of these agents is considered. A mixture of oxygen and nitrous oxide is commonly used to provide the maintenance carrier gas for inhalational agents, although there is an increasing trend towards use of oxygen-enriched air as the detrimental effects of nitrous oxide become more apparent. Modern inhalational anaesthetic agents are generally non-explosive and non-flammable, and are not associated with nephrotoxicity or autoimmune jaundice. Total intra-venous anaesthesia (TIVA) avoids the use of inhalational anaesthesia. Propofol is the commonest agent used for this purpose, as its effects are rapidly reversible on discontinuation of the intravenous infusion. This technique avoids atmospheric pollution and is particularly suitable for patients with a history of malignant hyperpyrexia or familial porphyria. General anaesthesia provided by inhalational or intravenous means does not necessarily provide analgesia. Analgesia is usually provided with an opiate or synthetic opioid, or in combination with a local or regional anaesthetic technique. Opiate or opioid analgesia is still the current 'gold standard' for analgesia both pre- and post-operatively. However, opiate analgesia is far from ideal. The associated sedation, nausea, vomiting and dizziness are minor side-effects in comparison to the potential for life-threatening respiratory depression. It is fear of this last complication that so often limits the dose regime of this group of drugs. This problem is compounded by the fact that we are unable to diagnose respiratory depression accurately without recourse to arterial blood gas analysis.

During general anaesthesia, respiration may be spontaneous or controlled, depending on the degree of relaxation required and the need to protect the airway from aspiration. Artificial ventilation may be facilitated by the use of muscle relaxants. These drugs may be either competitive or non-competitive inhibitors of the neurotransmitter acetylcholine at the neuromuscular junction. The only non-competitive inhibitor in clinical usage is suxamethonium. Suxamethonium acts rapidly, within 30–60 s, depolarizes the neuromuscular junction and produces short-lived, profound muscular relaxation. Its action is terminated by hydrolysis by plasma cholinesterase, normally within 5–10 min. Familial lack of plasma cholinesterase leads to prolonged relaxation (suxamethonium apnoea), and may require prolonged artificial ventilation which may exceed the duration of surgery. All other clinically useful neuromuscular blocking agents are competitive inhibitors at the neuromuscular junction (e.g. curare, pancuronium, atracurium, vecuronium, mivacurium, rocuronium). They do not cause initial depolarization, generally have a slower onset (3–5 minutes), but have a duration of action in the range 30–60 min. There is a wide range of relaxants, all of which have slightly different properties in terms of onset time, length of action and metabolism. They also possess varying degrees of autonomic stimulation or inhibition. Raising the concentration of acetylcholine may reverse residual competitive neuromuscular block. This is usually achieved by administering an anticholinesterase (e.g. neostigmine). However, the level to which anticholinesterase drugs can raise the concentration of acetylcholine is limited, and therefore high levels of competitive neuromuscular blocking agents cannot be adequately reversed by this method. Moreover, raising acetylcholine levels by this method does not confine the effects of acetylcholine to the neuromuscular junction. There is widespread release of acetylcholine throughout the autonomic nervous system as well as at the neuromuscular junction. Fortunately, these adverse effects may be limited by the prior or concurrent administration of an anticholinergic agent (e.g. atropine). *Neuromuscular blocking drugs have no anaesthetic, hypnotic or analgesic properties and therefore it is of the utmost importance to ensure that patients are adequately anaesthetized when this group of drugs is being used.* However, there is no commercial monitor currently available to determine the 'degree' or 'depth' of anaesthesia. Anaesthetists rely very heavily on the extrapolation of calculated levels of anaesthetic agents when muscle relaxants have *not* been used, to determine whether a patient is asleep or not in situations where muscle relaxants are used. 'Awareness' of intra-operative events during surgery in cases where neuromuscular blocking agents have been employed is a *real* problem. In the non-paralysed patient for whom neuromuscular blocking agents have not been used, assessment of anaesthesia becomes very much easier, as reflex movement at the spinal level precedes recovery of central reflexes (consciousness) in terms of depth of anaesthesia. Therefore, reflex movement will be seen before recovery of conscious recall of operative events. A peripheral nerve stimulator may be used to check the degree of neuromuscular block during surgery, and its reversal by neostigmine.

Ketamine is an unusual drug in that it provides intense analgesia and amnesia, together with an altered level of consciousness, but not necessarily hypnosis. Muscular tone is increased and the sympathetic nervous system is enhanced. In large doses it will produce apnoea, and airway reflexes are not guaranteed. However, it is associated with unpleasant auditory and visual hallucinations, and it is not commonly used as a sole agent in this country. It is a very useful induction agent in patients with hypovolaemic shock.

The opiate/opioid group of drugs has agonist or partial agonist activity at opioid receptors. The relative actions at mu, kappa, delta and sigma receptors vary depending on the agent being used. Naloxone is a non-specific antagonist at all receptors. To date, the analgesic effects of opiate drugs have not been successfully separated from the respiratory depressant, sedative, emetic and hallucinatory effects. However, they remain one of the most important groups of drugs for analgesia.

Non-steroidal anti-inflammatory drugs (NSAIDs) inhibit the enzyme cyclo-oxygenase, which converts aracadonic acid to cyclic endoperoxidases, thus preventing formation of prostaglandins and thromboxanes. Prostaglandins are involved in the sensitization of peripheral pain receptors to noxious stimuli. They may also inhibit the lipo-oxygenase pathway by an action on hydroperoxy-fatty acid peroxidase. NSAIDs should be used with caution in patients with platelet dysfunction, renal impairment, proven peptic ulcer disease or coagulopathies.

LOCAL AND REGIONAL ANAESTHESIA

Local anaesthetic agents constitute a group of drugs that reversibly inhibit nerve conduction. Many agents possess local anaesthetic activity if applied to nervous tissue, e.g. pethidine, beta-blockers and local anaesthetics. There are two main groups of drugs that are commonly used as local anaesthetics:

1. the ester group of drugs, (e.g. cocaine, procaine, amethocaine); and

2. the amides (e.g. lignocaine, bupivacaine, prilocaine, and ropivacaine).

The ester group of local anaesthetics produces metabolites that are related to para-aminobenzoic acid, and these have been associated with allergic reactions. The amides, in contrast, are rarely associated with allergic reactions. Esters are rapidly metabolized by plasma esterases and therefore their duration of action is generally short. Currently their use is generally restricted to topical anaesthesia of mucous membranes. However, the amide local anaesthetics are metabolized in the liver by N-dealkylation, and their duration of action is limited by hepatic metabolism. Local anaesthetic drugs reversibly block the transmission of peripheral and neuraxis nerve impulses, by blocking membrane depolarization. The amide group of local anaesthetics may be injected locally into tissue to produce a field block, into a nervous plexus to produce a more widespread plexus block (e.g. brachial plexus) or into the spinal canal to produce a central regional block (e.g. spinal/epidural). All local anaesthetic blocks are limited by the relative toxicity of the local anaesthetic used. Local anaesthetics in solution are weak bases, and their mechanism of action is to inhibit reversibly the sodium channels in the conducting tissues, thereby preventing propagation of an axonal impulse. There is complete block of axonal function, which results in intense, complete anaesthesia of the area supplied by the nerves involved. Local anaesthetic toxicity is related to the pharmacological effects of local anaesthetics on other excitable tissues (e.g. the cardiac and central nervous systems). Local anaesthetic agents exist in solution in equilibrium between their parent base compound and the ionized cation. It is likely that the uncharged base form is responsible for the diffusion of the drug through tissues and cell membranes, but it is the ionized cation that is responsible for 'blocking' the sodium channel. Factors that affect the pH of the solution in which the local anaesthetic is dissolved or present will therefore affect the relative concentrations of the ionized base and ionized cation (e.g. preservatives which may be present to prolong the shelf-life of adrenalin will reduce the pH of the resultant solution). In situations where there is tissue inflammation, there may be poor local anaesthesia, as the proportions of free base and cation are altered due to the acidic nature of the tissues. Inadvertent intravenous administration may result in acute overdosage, with severe central nervous system and cardiac toxicity. The amount of local anaesthetic drug being injected should always be recorded, together with the site of injection. Cardiac arrest as a result of local anaesthetic toxicity may require prolonged resuscitation to ensure that local anaesthetic is metabolized to a level that will allow return of normal cardiac function. The toxicity of local anaesthesia is related to the actual drug. The volume, concentration and speed of injection, together with the site of administration, all play a part in the development of local anaesthetic toxicity. Safe levels of local anaesthetics on a mg/kg basis are therefore provided for guidance only. The onset and duration of conduction blockage are related to the pK_a, lipid solubility and extent of protein-binding of the individual drugs. A low pK_a and a high lipid solubility are associated with a rapid onset time, and a high degree of protein-binding is associated with a long duration of action (e.g. the pK_a of lignocaine is 7.7, of bupivacaine is 8.1, and of ropivacaine is 8.1). The newest agent for clinical use is ropivacaine, which is reported to have a long duration of action, to be less cardiotoxic, and to have a direct vasoconstrictor effect. However, it is slower in onset than lignocaine.

CENTRAL NEURONAL BLOCKADE (CNB)

Spinal block (subarachnoid)

In a subarachnoid or spinal block, local anaesthetic is placed into cerebrospinal fluid at a point below the level of termination of the spinal cord. It will produce a profound motor and sensory anaesthetic block, dependent on the dose of drug injected. The spinal anaesthesia produced is complete, and a sensory level will be produced below which there is complete anaesthesia. Anaesthesia is produced with a small volume of local anaesthetic because the cerebrospinal fluid is confined within the dural sac. If the dose or volume of local anaesthetic is incorrect, it is possible to produce a 'total spinal' if enough local anaesthetic is given. Provision must be made for artificial ventilation of the patient should this occur. Most spinal anaesthesia is performed as a single puncture technique, and therefore the duration of action

is limited (usually 2–3 h) and depends on the type of local anaesthetic used.

Epidural

In epidural anaesthesia, local anaesthetic is placed between the ligamentum flavum and the dural sac (i.e. it is outside the dura and is therefore not confined by an enclosed space). Local anaesthetic diffuses freely up and down the spinal column, as well as traversing the intervertebral foramina and gaining access to the paravertebral spaces. The volume of local anaesthetic needed to produce an equivalent block to a spinal anaesthetic is about fivefold larger. The potential for toxicity is therefore much greater with an epidural than with a spinal anaesthetic. Toxic doses of local anaesthetic are related to peak plasma levels, which are proportional to the total dose of drug given and the route of administration. For guidance, safe doses of local anaesthetic are quoted as follows: lignocaine, up to 3 mg/kg (7 mg with adrenalin); bupivacaine, up to 2 mg/kg (with or without adrenalin); ropivacaine, up to 7.5 mg/kg (with or without adrenalin). An epidural block is segmental, i.e. there will be an upper and a lower sensory level, depending on the volume and amount of drug administered. In between the two sensory levels there will be a 'band' of anaesthesia.

The advantages of a spinal block are that it is easier to perform, quicker in onset, produces more profound anaesthesia and there is little risk of local anaesthetic toxicity. However, breaching the dura runs the risk of introducing infection, bleeding into the cerebrospinal fluid and producing a post-dural puncture headache. An epidural uses a larger dose of local anaesthetic, takes longer to perform, is technically more difficult, has a higher rate of failure and runs the potential risk of local anaesthetic toxicity. However, provided that the dura is not breached during insertion, post-dural puncture headache should not be a problem, the placement of an epidural catheter allows the anaesthesia to be continued via 'top-ups', and this can be used to produce excellent post-operative analgesia. Access to the sacral epidural space may be achieved by an injection through the sacro-coccygeal membrane. Its main use is to supplement general anaesthesia and to provide very effective early post-operative pain relief. It is a widely used technique in paediatric surgery. Common complications of central neural blockade (epidural and spinal) include hypotension, post-dural puncture headache, urinary retention, nausea and vomiting. Opiate drugs may also be administered via the central spinal route. It is possible to produce analgesia at a spinal cord level with a lower dose of opiate drug compared to the parenteral route. The advantage of providing analgesia via the spinal route, rather than using local anaesthesia, is that there is no motor block and very little hypotension associated with this technique. Unfortunately, rostral spread of the opiate is inevitable and the risk of respiratory depression is still present. It would appear that the risk of profound, late (up to 24 h) respiratory depression is particularly high if there has been concurrent administration of opioids or other sedatives by another route. Vigilant monitoring of the patient who has received opiates by any route is of the utmost importance.

Local anaesthetics used in central neural blockade produce anaesthesia of sensory, motor and autonomic nerves. The loss of sympathetic tone results in peripheral vasodilatation and venous pooling. This will reduce venous return initially and result in a fall in cardiac output. The resultant fall in systemic vascular resistance also leads to a lowered systemic blood pressure. Care should be taken in the management of patients with cardiac disease who are dependent on their blood pressure for coronary perfusion (e.g. in those with aortic stenosis). The degree of hypotension is related to the degree of sympathetic blockade. Obviously, anaesthetic block limited to below the level of L2 (sympathetic outflow ends at L2) is unlikely to affect the blood pressure. Epidural catheters may be left in place for a number of days post-operatively to provide excellent post-operative pain relief. However, great care must be taken with pressure areas (e.g. heels, buttocks), as during this time analgesic pressure sores are not uncommon and the lack of mobility may be a major drawback.

Much rarer complications of central neural blockade include spinal haematomas as a result of bleeding, spinal abscess formation as a result of infection, or permanent neurological damage. Each of these complications is extremely rare, but usually disastrous should it occur. Contraindications to central neural blockade are therefore coagulopathies, anticoagulant therapy, sepsis, hypovolaemia, raised intracranial pressure and patient refusal.

Local and regional anaesthetic techniques provide an alternative to general anaesthesia. They are safe techniques but do require anaesthetic expertise. They may be used successfully to provide prolonged post-operative pain relief. Only local anaesthetics, opioids, and non-steroidal anti-inflammatory agents have a clearly defined role in post-operative analgesia.

FURTHER READING

Aitkinhead AR, Jones RM. 1995: *Clinical anaesthesia.* Edinburgh: Churchill Livingstone.

Atkinson RS, Rushman GB, Davies NJH (eds). 1992: *Lee's synopsis of anaesthesia,* 11th edn. Oxford: Butterworth-Heinemann.

Goldstone JC, Pollard BJ (eds). 1996: *Handbook of clinical anaesthesia.* Edinburgh: Churchill Livingstone.

McClure JH, Wildsmith JAW. 1991: *Conduction blockade for postoperative analgesia.* London: Edward Arnold.

Medical Defence Union. 1997: *Consent to treatment.* London: Medical Defence Union.

Nimmo WS, Rowbotham DJ, Smith G. 1994: *Anaesthesia.* Oxford: Blackwell Science.

Royal College of Surgeons of England. 1992: *Report of the Working Party on Guidelines for Daycase Surgery.* London: Royal College of Surgeons of England.

Sasada M, Smith S. 1997: *Drugs in anaesthesia and intensive care,* 2nd edn. Oxford: Oxford Medical Publications.

Senate of Surgery of Great Britain and Ireland. 1997: *The surgeon's duty of care. Guidance for surgeons on ethical and legal issues.* London: The Senate of Surgery of Great Britain and Ireland.

Wildsmith JAW, Armitage EN. 1993: *Principles and practice of regional anaesthesia.* Edinburgh: Churchill Livingstone.

Post-operative care

David J. Leaper

Introduction

Surgical practice continues to expand and specialize, and alongside the increasing complexity of surgical procedures there is an equivalent increase in the demands of post-operative care. We have an ageing population in whom there is an increasing expectation of intervention. Their post-operative care demands more time, high standards and pressures on nursing and medical time, and sophisticated monitoring.

Technologies allow more interventions with safer peri-

operative care. Consequently, we are seeing a growing proportion of older, sicker patients on surgical wards. Despite specialization, general post-operative complications are common to all patients, and their prediction, prevention, prompt identification and early effective treatment follow similar guidelines. In this chapter the post-operative care of pain, the chest, venous thrombo-embolism, and the management of pyrexia and stomas will be addressed.

PAIN AND ITS MANAGEMENT

The post-operative management of pain begins pre-operatively. Patients need preparation and an understanding of the discomforts they may face, and this pre-emptive, preventative approach should be part of obtaining consent for an operation. Inadequate control of pain has serious consequences. Poor respiratory effort caused by pain is attended by sputum retention, atelectasis and subsequent infection or pneumonia. The metabolic response to trauma may be enhanced by inadequate pain relief, with increased cardiac demands and inappropriate fluid, electrolyte and nutritional needs. A multimodal approach to pain relief gives the best results, using a combination of methods with a protocol based on pain scoring and algorithmic rules. The optimal approach is to use a trained team to assess, score and recommend pain relief. Post-operative pain relief methods are listed in Table 34.3.1.

Intramuscular opioids given on demand 4-hourly are associated with poor pain relief even when administered in combination with oral preparations, using pain scores and established protocols. Intravenous opioids are far more effective, but are more likely to cause respiratory depression. Their use is optimized when given as patient-controlled analgesia (PCA), but pumps and the expertise of a team are required. The patient must clearly understand their use, and the background dose and 'lockouts' must be explained.

Epidurals (and to a lesser extent spinal anaesthetics) give outstanding pain relief, but again require expertise in management and skill in placement. They are invasive, may cause hypotension, and if an opioid as well as a local anaesthetic agent is used, they may cause nausea, vomiting and respiratory depression. The high-dependency unit (HDU) is advocated for this type of post-operative analgesia. Such patients have probably undergone major surgery which justifies HDU monitoring.

Enteral analgesics are suitable for day-case surgery

(Table 34.3.1). Many non-opioid (mostly non-steroidal anti-inflammatories) and opioid single and combined preparations exist. Oral and rectal preparations, such as diclofenac (Voltarol), can be used effectively after hernia repair, particularly if the wound edges are infiltrated with local anaesthetic. Field blocks for operative surgery also give good post-operative analgesia.

The effective management of pain requires monitoring, recording and auditing. Pain teams, often led by nurse practitioner specialists, using established protocols and pain-scoring systems, not just in theatre recovery but on the ward as well, give optimal results. Nevertheless, if a patient complains of pain in any circumstance, analgesia must be reviewed and an appropriate analgesic given.

POST-OPERATIVE CHEST CARE

Post-operative chest care accounts for two parts of the airways, breathing, circulation (ABC) algorithm. Pulmonary complications are common, and are easily overlooked as a cause of post-operative confusion related to atelectasis (requiring physiotherapy and humidified oxygen) or impending respiratory failure with pneumonia. Whenever there is doubt, arterial blood gas measurement reveals a rising $PaCO_2$ or falling PaO_2 and indicates the need for active treatment. Respiratory failure relates to air-flow obstruction (e.g. in chronic obstructive pulmonary disease or asthma) or a fall in functional residual capacity and lung volume (e.g. in sputum retention, pneumonia or weakness following sedation) with ventilation/perfusion mismatch (e.g. in adult respiratory distress syndrome (ARDS), pulmonary embolus or left ventricular failure).

The peri-operative care of the chest involves recognition of risk and monitoring. From the history and examination, an idea of respiratory ability can be obtained. Clearly a patient who cannot walk up a flight of stairs or walk a few yards is a risk. Respiratory function tests, peak expiratory flow (PEF), vital capacity and forced expiratory flow in 1 s (FEV_1) can help to predict risk. Chest X-rays should be reserved for patients who have a specific respiratory disease or malignancy – there is no place for routine X-rays, and help can be obtained from a radiologist. To identify patients who retain CO_2, blood gas analysis may be helpful. Patients who are at risk may benefit from having their operation postponed (if possible) to improve their reserve, stopping smoking for 6–8 weeks, or having active physiotherapy and antibiotics, if indicated for purulent sputum.

When patients have post-operative chest complications, remember the ABCs. Clear the airway, use a Guedal airway if necessary, and give oxygen by mask at full rate (15 L/min). Check breathing by the look, listen and feel technique, and supplement this with attention to circulation. ECG, full blood count and electrolytes

Table 34.3.1 Methods for post-operative pain relief

Route of administration	Type of analgesic
Enteral	Non-opioid analgesics (and combined preparations): • paracetamol • NSAIDs (e.g. aspirin, ketorolac, diclofenac)
Oral and per rectum preparations exist	Opioid analgesics (and combined preparations): • dextropropoxyphene (combined coproxamol) • tramadol • codeine preparations
Local anaesthesia (LA)	Lignocaine, bupivacaine: • local wound edge block • field and ring block • EMLA cream (children)*
Parental	Intramuscular opioid (on demand) Intravenous opioid (optimized as PCA) Epidural (LA or opioid) Spinal anaesthetic
Cryoanalgesia	Probably only Accident and Emergency use
Trans-epidermal nerve stimulation	Only chronic pain

*Eutectic mixture of local anaesthetic.

may be helpful in cases of cardiac overload. Consider the underlying cause of problems and treat it, and consider opiate-reversal naloxane if the response to simple airway and oxygen therapy is poor. Further deterioration requires a higher inspired oxygen (FiO_2) using a rebreathing or Hudson mask which gives an FiO_2 of 0.6. Oxygen should be humidified and bronchodilators may be useful. Continued physiotherapy is effective, and continuous positive airways pressure (CPAP) with a valve may be tried before ventilation.

Post-operative respiratory complications are listed in Table 34.3.2. Atelectasis is common with poor basal air entry, and is increased when chronic obstructive airways disease or poorly controlled pain occur. There may be a progressive ventilation/perfusion mismatch if untreated by physiotherapy. It is responsible for a low-grade pyrexia (37.4–38.0°C) in the first 1–2 days post-operatively, but sputum remains clear and antibiotics are not indicated. Aspiration of gastric contents is another early post-operative chest complication which may follow induction of anaesthesia, and is a risk in intestinal obstruction, particularly when a nasogastric tube has been forgotten. An acute chemical pneumonitis follows which requires antibiotics and often ventilation. Pneumonia and lung abscess may follow.

Fat embolus is rare but can follow fractures. A pneumonitis which progresses to ARDS may present with the classical skin haemorrhages and cerebral complications. Pneumothorax can follow trauma, and is associated with fractured ribs, either singly or as a flail chest with haemopneumothorax. It is also a complication of central line insertion and the barotrauma of ventilation in non-compliant lungs. Early recognition with insertion of an underwater chest seal is necessary.

Pulmonary oedema is probably overdiagnosed in surgical patients. It follows fluid overload and left ventricular failure; pre-existing cardiac disease is likely and a myocardial infarct should be considered. Jugular venous pressure (JVP) is not as reliable as CVP measurement for recognition and management. Oxygen therapy, diuretics and ventilation may be required. Pneumonia presents with classic chest signs, purulent sputum and a temperature much higher than atelectasis

Table 34.3.2 Post-operative respiratory complications

Atelectasis
Aspiration
Fat embolus
Pneumothorax
Pulmonary oedema
Pneumonia
Adult respiratory distress syndrome
Venous pulmonary embolism

(≥ 38°C) 4 or 5 days post-operatively. Appropriate antibiotics and physiotherapy are needed – the empirical choice of antibiotic may need to be changed depending on the microbiological results.

ARDS presents after multiple trauma and burns, sepsis and severe acute pancreatitis. It can occur after large blood replacements, and requires early recognition. CPAP and ventilation are needed, but increasing poor compliance and increasing peak expiratory end pressure may lead to risk of barotrauma and pneumothorax. Successfully treated ARDS is still a risk factor for pulmonary fibrosis.

Pulmonary embolus follows venous thrombosis, which may not be evident in the legs. Patients at risk may not be protected by stockings, intermittent compression therapy or anticoagulation. DVT is confirmed by venography or duplex Doppler (radiolabelled fibrinogen is no longer used), and treatment requires anticoagulation. Cardiac catheterization with lytic therapy or embolectomy may be indicated.

DEEP VEIN THROMBOSIS (DVT) AND PULMONARY EMBOLUS

DVT is preventable using thrombo-embolic deterrent (TED) stockings, intermittent compression therapy, heparin (given subcutaneously as unfractionated heparin or the more expensive but probably more effective fractionated heparin) or full anticoagulation. The choice is based on risk (see Table 34.3.3). Risk factors include obesity, smoking, hypercoagulable status (e.g. polycythaemia), cardiac failure and, in particular, a past history of DVT/pulmonary embolus, pelvic or cancer surgery and fractures (mainly involving limbs, especially neck of femur). The risk caused by taking the oral contraceptive pill or hormone replacement therapy (HRT) is small and not clearly quantified, but probably justifies stopping therapy for 4–6 weeks prior to surgery.

The diagnosis of DVT is made on clinical grounds, but Homan's sign is unreliable and possibly dangerous to elicit. It should be looked for daily in in-patients. Classically, DVT presents at 7–8 days post-operatively and may be heralded by a low-grade pyrexia (37.5–38.0°C). There may be tenderness, swelling and warmth over the calf only, or an extensive phlegmasia caerulia dolens which implies an extensive iliofemoral DVT. Confirmation is obtained by venography (injecting contrast into a dorsal foot vein with two tourniquets to prevent superficial vein filling and to fill the deep veins) or duplex Doppler (which is made easier with colour imaging). Duplex Doppler is probably as accurate as venography, with the exception of diagnosis of calf vein thrombus, and is not invasive. Full anticoagulation with

Table 34.3.3 Risk factors for type of DVT prophylaxis

	Example	Type
Low risk	Herniorrhaphy	TED stockings or intermittent compression, consider subcutaneous heparin
Medium risk	Open cholecystectomy	TED stockings with or without intermittent compression and subcutaneous heparin
High risk	Pelvic cancer surgery Previous DVT/PE	TED stockings with or without intermittent compression and high-dose low-molecular-weight heparin

heparin for 7–10 days and then warfarin for 3–6 months is required.

Pulmonary embolus can present in three ways. The first is sudden death (when PE is diagnosed at autopsy) or profound cardiopulmonary collapse. The patient may respond to cardiac resuscitation quite quickly if the embolus breaks up and moves distally into the lung. If they remain severely compromised, cardiac catheterization to confirm the diagnosis should be followed by lytic therapy, or open pulmonary embolectomy may be indicated.

The second way presents a clinical picture of pleuritic pain and haemoptysis with unexplained poor cardiopulmonary performance. Chest X-ray and ECG may support a clinical suspicion, but a V/Q isotope scan is usually diagnostic. Treatment involves anticoagulation with heparin followed by warfarin, and should be instituted if there is any doubt.

The third presentation is multiple pulmonary emboli with increasingly poor pulmonary performance. The source of emboli may be unclear, but a caval filter placed infrarenally may be indicated, and percutaneous placement is preferred.

POST-OPERATIVE PYREXIA

Post-operative pyrexia is common. When observed on the daily ward rounds, a cause should be sought and treatment considered. The blind use of antibiotics should be resisted. The causes can be anticipated by consideration of the type of surgery (e.g. a urinary infection follows the temporary use of a urinary catheter during and after abdominoperineal excision of rectum) and the pattern of pyrexia (e.g. a spiking, church-spire temperature up to 39 or 40°C) may herald an intra-abdominal abscess following an anasto-

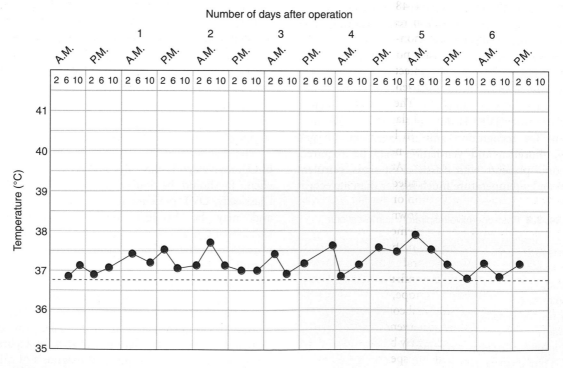

Figure 34.3.1 Grumbling pyrexia.

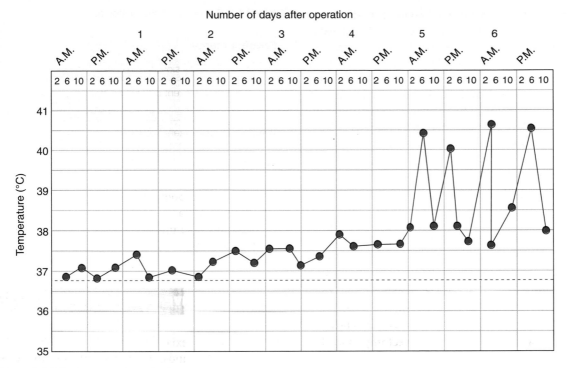

Figure 34.3.2 Church-spire temperature.

motic leak after total gastrectomy, whereas a 'grumbling' pyrexia of 37.5–38°C indicates early atelectasis, or later perhaps a wound infection (see Figures 34.3.1 and 34.3.2).

The time post-operatively when pyrexia is observed may give a clue to the cause. At 24–48 h post-operatively, consider atelectasis, a transfusion reaction or pyrogen-containing IV fluids, or the non-specific metabolic response to trauma. At 2–7 days post-operatively consider a chest infection, urinary infection (particularly if there is a urinary catheter), intravenous or central line infection or wound infection. The median time to develop a wound abscess is 7–10 days (usually seen in primary health care rather than in hospital), although a β-haemolytic streptococcal or necrotizing spreading infection may occur earlier. At 7–10 days post-operatively a DVT should be excluded, and after 10 days there may be an infected collection or anastomotic leak.

The sites to consider are shown in Table 34.3.4. Clinical examination can be supplemented by microbiological analysis of urine, sputum, blood, wound discharge and the tips of central venous catheters. Venography or duplex Doppler confirms DVT and imaging (plain X-ray, ultrasound, isotope, CT or MRI scanning) can localize intra-abdominal collections.

Imaging may also allow intervention to drain an abscess percutaneously. Surgery may be needed if it fails. Antibiotics must be reserved for specific treatment of infection.

STOMAS

The care of stomas begins pre-operatively and should be shared with the stoma nurse. Help should be sought with gaining consent and marking stomas for optimal positioning. The use and indication for feeding stomas can be shared with a nutritionist/dietitian. Feeding can be achieved by percutaneous endoscopic gastrostomy (PEG), or by a jejunostomy placed at operation to avoid the use of nasogastric feeding.

Table 34.3.4 Sites to consider as a cause of post-operative pyrexia

Site	Cause of pyrexia
Wound	Cellulitis, abscess
Legs	DVT
Urinary tract	Is there a catheter?
Chest	Atelectasis, aspiration, pneumonia
IV lines	Peripheral or central
Leak	Anastomotic
Abscess	Intra-abdominal, pelvic or retroperitoneal

The function of the majority of stomas is to divert or bring intestinal contents to the anterior abdominal wall. Stomas may be temporary (usually loop ileostomy or end colostomy – which may be temporary after a Hartmann's procedure). Temporary loop stomas are used to divert intestinal contents and to protect a distal anastomosis. The right transverse loop colostomy is bulky and difficult to manage post-operatively, as well as being prone to complications, and should be avoided, but it is usually easier to reverse than a loop ileostomy. The end ileostomy should be formed into a spout so that the intestinal contents are kept away from the skin. The stomatherapist will look after stomas in the early post-operative days and advise the patient on stoma care. The ileostomy is usually managed with a two-piece device (a flange to go around the spout to help to protect the skin, and a clip-on bag which can be left in position with the flange, sometimes for several days). Good seals not only protect the skin but give good psychological support in the early days post-operatively. End colostomies are made flush with the skin. Because faeces are dehydrated there is less risk to the skin, and semisolid and solid material is easily collected in a bag. Changing flanges or bags too often can damage the skin. Bags are emptied when required whilst in place through a dependent opening closed by a clip, or else they are disposable.

Complications of stomas are listed in Table 34.3.5. Intolerance of feeding and inadequate nutrition need re-evaluation of the feeding regimen and may require supplementary intravenous feeding. Antidiarrhoeal agents may help with diarrhoea. Perforation and leakage are associated with poor fixation of the feeding catheter.

Table 34.3.5 Complications of stomas

Feeding stomas
Leakage, perforation and peritonitis
Intolerance of feeds, diarrhoea, and inadequate nutrition
Problems in removal of feeding line

Diverting stomas
Early necrosis separation, retraction, infection
Later skin damage
Fistula (e.g. Crohn's)
Perforation (after irrigation)
Stenosis
Prolapse
Hernia

Diverting stomas may separate or retract, but this can usually be treated conservatively. A resulting stenosis is unusual, but normally responds to simple dilatation. Gangrene or strangulation which extends for more than 1–2 cm requires refashioning. Transverse loop colostomies are prone to prolapse, which is easily reduced, but closure is the only method of prevention. Parastomal hernias may require surgery when their necks are tight and risk obstruction or strangulation of herniated small bowel or omentum. Management of protuberant stomas becomes difficult when they are large and not cosmetically acceptable, and may need revision. Surgery may be a major procedure for an elderly patient.

Chapter 34.4

The operating room (theatre)

Bryony E. Lovett

Introduction

The term 'operating theatre' is derived from the Latin *opus operis* (work) and *theatrum* (place for assembly, for the performance of plays). The first surgical theatre recorded was that of William Harvey's teacher Heironymus Fabricius of

Aquapedente in Padua *c.* 1600. This was purely for educational purposes, and surgery was performed in the patient's home.

THE THEATRE SUITE

The nucleus concept of theatre suites appropriate to a district general hospital was introduced by the Department of Health and Social Security. Local variations are inevitable, but generally operating theatres are grouped together for ease of management of the specialist theatre staff and equipment. As the range of specialist procedures that can be performed widens to include approaches varying from the laparoscopic to the MRI guided, the requirements of individual operating theatres differ.

Operating theatres are ideally situated away from the mainstream hospital corridor but easily accessed from the surgical wards, intensive-care units, high-dependency units, Accident and Emergency Department, labour ward and X-ray department. The sterile services department should be incorporated into the theatre suite. In many hospitals the day-surgery suite is also closely linked to the main theatre area.

Following Department of Health recommendations, most hospitals have a multidisciplinary users' committee to optimize the efficiency and safety of the operating theatre. This committee should include surgeons,

anaesthetists, operating theatre and anaesthetic nurses, microbiologists, a manager and a finance officer.

OPERATING THEATRE DESIGN

The operating theatre is a highly artificial environment designed to minimize the risk of patients acquiring infections during the course of operations, while at the same time providing a safe environment for both patient and staff.

Operating theatre design is influenced by a number of mandatory external factors, including Planning Acts, building regulations, the Fire Precautions Act, the Health and Safety at Work Act, Control of Substances Hazardous to Health (COSHH) regulations, and the Chronically Sick and Disabled Persons Act. British and International Standards are advised in conjunction with Codes of Practice, building research publications, manufacturer's technical literature and Department of Health guidelines.

The Department of Health norms recommend 50 surgical beds per 100 000 members of the population and one operating theatre per 40–45 beds.

The design of theatre suites is increasingly complex. There are a number of basic requirements for all operating suites.

- Each suite should be set up with a holding area for patients about to enter for surgery, where essential patient details may be checked and the patient handed over to the care of the theatre team.
- Traditionally each theatre has an anaesthetic room attached, although anaesthesia may be induced in the main operating room, or in an anaesthetic area with one consultant supervising a number of junior anaesthetists.
- Patients then move into theatre for the procedure and subsequently out to the recovery area.

OPERATING THEATRE LAYOUT

There are many local variations in the layout of the operating theatre (Figure 34.4.1). However, the general principles are the same.

In the 1930s Paul Nelson and Jean Walter described functional zones within the theatre suite. The *outer, protective, clean, sterile* and *disposal zones* are recommended by the Medical Research Council.

- The *outer zone* includes the rest of the hospital and the reception area.
- Patients and staff enter the suite via the *protective zone*, which includes the changing room, administrative offices and teaching rooms.
- The scrub room, anaesthetic room and sterile store are *clean*.
- The laying up of instruments and the operation take place in the *sterile zone*.
- Instruments and refuse for incineration are passed to the disposal corridor in the *disposal zone* through a hatch system.

THE ANAESTHETIC ROOM

The anaesthetic room has been a part of British hospital design since St Georges's Hospital London opened in 1896 with an adjoining room for anaesthesia attached to each operating theatre. However, anaesthetic rooms are

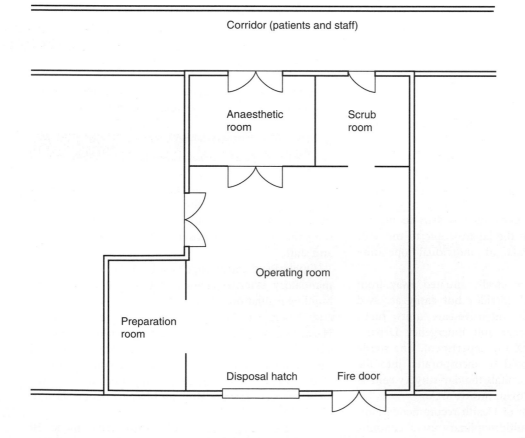

Figure 34.4.1 Typical operating room layout.

not universal world-wide, and few hospitals in the USA have this facility. Arguments in favour of the continued use of separate rooms for the induction of anaesthesia include the following: shielding of the patient from the 'shocks which await in the operating theatre'; patient privacy and comfort; ease of access to familiar equipment and drugs for the anaesthetist; improvement in patient turnover; access for patients' relatives; and use for regional anaesthesia. Arguments against the continued use of the anaesthetic room relate to increased running costs and risk to the patient. A separate room requires duplication of monitoring equipment, disconnection of the patient to enable transfer, and loss of continuous monitoring. If patients are anaesthetized on the operating table they can position themselves, so avoiding the risks of transferring an unconscious patient. Two-thirds of anaesthetists questioned at an Association of Anaesthetists meeting induced anaesthesia in emergencies ASA grade 3–5 in theatre, whereas only one-third would induce elective patients of the same grade in theatre. Financial constraints may result in the demise of the anaesthetic room from future theatre suites, although the increased use of regional methods of anaesthesia may prove their saving grace.

VENTILATION

Each operating theatre has independent control of ventilation which provides:

- control of the direction of air movement within the theatre suite;

- control of sepsis, by diluting the operating theatre air with filtered air to reduce the amount of contaminating bacteria-bearing particles, for the safety of the patient;

- climate control for the safety and comfort of the patient and staff.

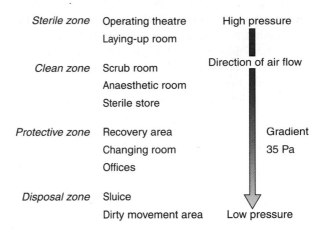

Figure 34.4.2 Operating room air movement.

Air movement

In general, theatres are divided into access zones (Figure 34.4.2), with filtered air passing from the aseptic area (requiring the highest sterility) to the outer zone (requiring the least sterility).

Air filtration

Bacterial standards are available for both plenum and ultraclean theatres, but these have never been validated in clinical trials. Government guidelines outline acceptable air quality as < 35 colony-forming units (CFU)/m^3 when the theatre is empty and < 180 CFU/m^3 during a surgical procedure. The threshold for ultraclean air is 10 CFU/m^3.

Filtered air is supplied to the operating theatre by the theatre plant. Air is drawn in from outside the hospital, the air intake being located away from refuse or kitchen areas, and car exhaust fumes, and protected from prevailing winds and direct sunshine.

A wire mesh prevents the entry of larger debris and birds. The fan draws air through a pre-filter into the negative-pressure side of the plant (Figure 34.4.3). This

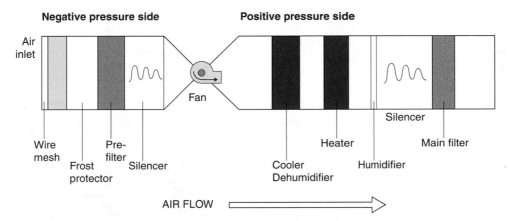

Figure 34.4.3 Air filtration system.

eliminates heavy particles which would shorten the life of the main filter. Air passes the fan and enters the positive-pressure side. Air is then pushed through the dehumidifying, cooling and heating batteries and is subsequently humidified prior to passing through the main filter, which removes particles larger than 5 μm in diameter.

Air change

Charnley recognized the need to provide an aeromicrobiological environment to reduce wound infection. Each person in the operative theatre sheds 10 000 viable bacteria/min, and this increases to 50 000/min with activity. Bacterial counts are reduced by dilution.

Theatre air change is continuous, and there are usually 20–40 changes/h throughout a 24-h period even when the theatre is not in use. Ultraclean theatres may employ up to 400 changes/h during surgery.

Each air change reduces the level of contamination present by a factor of $1/E$ ($E = 2.718$), i.e. by approximately one-third. Two air changes reduce contamination by a factor of $1/E^2$.

Air flow

Traditionally, clean air was mixed with existing room air to reduce bacterial contamination by dilution. Modern ventilation systems use a plenum positive-pressure ventilation system with filtered air supplied at the ceiling or wall and evacuated at floor level.

Plenum turbulent systems rely on downward or lateral displacement of operating room air, with up to 30 changes/h at a velocity of 3–12 m/min. This turbulent air flow stirs up any colony-forming particles, depositing them on surgeons' gloves, instruments and in the wound.

The plenum laminar system provides unidirectional air flow with up to 300 changes/h at a velocity of 0.3 m/s.

However, *horizontal laminar flow* systems rely on there being no obstruction between the air supply and the operative field, as this would cause turbulence. To avoid horizontally flowing air rising due to convection, a minimum velocity of 0.6 m/s is required. This results in rapid drying of exposed tissue and hypothermia.

Vertical laminar flow can be supplied at a lower velocity of 0.3 m/s. The air is warmed as it flows downwards over the operative field. This warm air rises, carrying colony-forming particles either side of the downward air flow, and is drawn into the flow. This process is known as entrainment.

Radial exponential flow of up to 500 changes/h at 2 L/min enclosed within perspex shields provides vertical displacement of 'old air' without entrapment of contaminated air (Figure 34.4.4).

An alternative is the *upward displacement system* in which cool filtered air is supplied at low velocity at floor level and evacuated through ceiling-mounted exhaust devices as it is warmed and rises by convection. A comparison study has shown superiority in the evacuation of gases, smoke and dust particles with the upward displacement system, but the conventional system was more efficient for the elimination of CFU.

The open door

When a person passes through an open door, their movement and the movement of the door allow the transfer of air between the areas separated by the door. This air movement is exacerbated if the door is left open, or if there is a temperature gradient across the door.

If the operating theatre door is kept open, each square metre of opening requires an additional 10 m³ of air flow/min to maintain air flow. Opening the double door to permit entry of a bed requires an additional 35 m³ of air flow/min.

In order to maintain the pressure gradient within each theatre when the door is opened, hinged weighted dampers are built into the operating theatre walls,

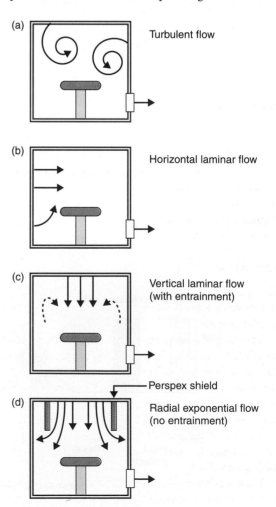

Figure 34.4.4 Ventilation systems.

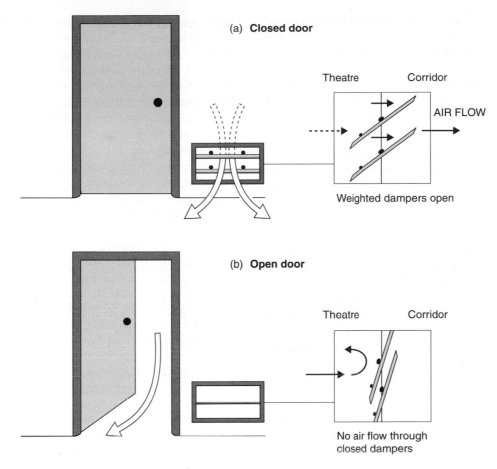

(a) **Closed door**

Theatre   Corridor

AIR FLOW

Weighted dampers open

(b) **Open door**

Theatre   Corridor

No air flow through
closed dampers

Figure 34.4.5 The open door.

between the theatre and the anaesthetic room and corridors. When the operating room door is opened, the pressure gradient between the theatre and the corridor falls, and the weighted flaps close to reduce air flow (Figure 34.4.5). When the door is closed, the pressure gradient rises and the flaps swing open.

Air testing

The government guidelines outlining acceptable air quality have already been mentioned in the section on air filtration.

Sampling of operating theatre air by settle plates or air samplers is required during commissioning of theatres, during outbreaks of infection, or after mechanical breakdown of the ventilation system. Regular sampling of plenum theatres is not generally required. Annual sampling is recommended for ultraclean theatres.

Studies of the movements of patients through the operating theatre have shown two peaks of bacterial levels (Figure 34.4.6).

Many operating theatres utilize movement sensors to detect increased numbers of personnel in theatre and automatically adjust air flow to maintain air quality.

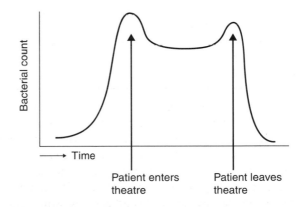

Bacterial count

Time →

Patient enters
theatre

Patient leaves
theatre

Figure 34.4.6 Effect of patient movement on bacterial count.

Climate control

Control mechanisms integral to the ventilation system should maintain steady temperatures at 20–22°C for the comfort of both staff and patients. The temperature may need to be higher to prevent hypothermia in neonates, children and the elderly, although heat loss may be minimized by the use of warming blankets, warm air covers and the infusion of warmed intravenous fluids. (Normal basal heat production requires 1 kcal/kg/h; to warm 1000 mL of intravenous fluid from 20°C to 37°C requires 17 kcal.)

The relative humidity of the theatre is usually in the range 50–60%, and generally the relative humidity of the hospital environment is kept at 45–60%.

ULTRACLEAN OPERATING THEATRES

These theatres are now used for joint replacement surgery where sepsis may not manifest for several years. Joint sepsis rates of *c.* 1% at 2 years carry a high morbidity and can still be reduced.

Ultraclean theatres employ exponential air flow systems in conjunction with body exhaust systems to reduce the CFU count to < 1/m³. Operating personnel wear an encompassing suit and helmet made of material that is impervious to bacteria-carrying liquids. Clean air is drawn into the suit and exhaust gases are removed via a negative pressure system. The suits are designed to capture, contain and remove the continuously generated warm convection currents on which CFU emitted from the body are transported. These suits have been shown to reduce infection rates in ultraclean theatres, but are rarely used as surgeons do not like wearing them.

In a classic study, the post-operative joint sepsis rate for operations performed in conventionally ventilated theatres was compared with the rate for those performed in ultraclean enviroments. The results suggested that a 50% reduction in sepsis could be obtained if the number of bacteria-carrying particles was < 10/m³, and by 75% if it was < 1/m³.

STERILIZATION

All instruments and equipment introduced into the operative field must be sterile. Sterilization is the process of ridding an object or substance of all forms of microorganisms, including bacterial spores and viruses. (Disinfection is intended to remove pathogenic bacteria with the exception of bacterial spores.) Cleanliness is the first step in the process, and mechanical washing and removal of dirt are required prior to sterilization.

Liquids are sterilized by *filtration* through a 2-μm filter.

High-vacuum autoclaves are used to sterilize air-trapping loads, instruments, swabs, drapes and hollow equipment. Modern machines have an automatic cycle which lasts 30 min. Initially air contained in the chamber and within wrapped packs is extracted. The pressure in the chamber is reduced to 20 mmHg, and high-pressure steam is then introduced which, because of the vacuum, rapidly penetrates the packs of equipment. Once the entire load has reached the same temperature (134°C), that level of heat is maintained for 3.5 min. The steam is withdrawn by vacuum and replaced with filtered air.

Hot-air ovens are used for the sterilization of instruments that are sensitive to steam (e.g. ophthalmic instruments). The instrument load is uniformly heated to 160°C, maintained for 1 h and then cooled. A fan ensures even temperature distribution.

Low-temperature steam and formaldehyde is one method used to sterilize heat-sensitive instruments such as endoscopes. A modified vacuum autoclave admits steam at subatmospheric pressure at a temperature of 80°C. This is maintained for 30–120 min. Formaldehyde (38% weight/volume) may be injected to increase the efficiency of sterilization.

Gamma-irradiation is used to sterilize commercially supplied items. Gamma-rays penetrate packs up to 30 cm thick. Automated plants minimize operator exposure whilst each pack receives 2.5 million rads (recommended by the International Atomic Agency of the United Nations Working Party).

Glutaraldehyde may be used for the sterilization of endoscopes and laparoscopes when rapid re-use is required. Each instrument should be immersed for 20–30 min and then rinsed three times in sterile water. Glutaraldehyde (2% w/v) at a pH of 7.5–8.5 is active against Gram-positive and Gram-negative bacteria. Acid-fast bacteria are moderately susceptible, and fungi and bacterial spores vary in sensitivity. In common with other alkylating agents, glutaraldehyde is potentially carcinogenic, and precautions are needed to prevent unnecessary inhalation. The vapour is irritant to the respiratory tract, and contact dermatitis has been reported.

Indicators of sterilization are available for the various sterilization techniques. Chemical indicators (Browne's tubes and Bowie-Dick tape) undergo colour changes if sterilization conditions have been maintained for the appropriate length of time. They may be inserted into packs and removed to test penetration, or applied externally for easy viewing. Commercially packaged single items may bear imprinted patterns which change colour after sterilization.

Biological indicators are standardized preparations of bacterial spores which are exposed to the sterilization process. After sterilization the spores are grown in nutrient broth to exclude surviving growth potential.

THEATRE LIGHTING

Theatre illumination must:

- be bright without producing glare;

- provide even light without shadowing (scialytic 'shadow-free' lamps are used);

- render natural colour.

Three lighting zones are identified:

- the central operative field;
- the table surround;
- the peripheral area.

Light reflectance from the ceiling should be 100%, with 60% from the walls and 30% from the floor. Matt surgical drapes reflect less than 30% of light.

Fluorescent lighting employed around the theatre suite is power efficient, producing 50 lumens (units of light flux) per watt of power, and little heat. Emitted light has a bluish tinge and reduces the fidelity of colours at the blue end of the spectrum.

Tungsten lights used for the operating field produce 18–24 lumens per watt of power, and more heat per watt. They emit colour at the red end of the spectrum and have high fidelity for colours at the blue end. Thus cyanosis is more obvious under tungsten light than under fluorescent light.

OTHER CONSIDERATIONS

Flooring

Theatre flooring must be capable of withstanding heavy wear, frequent washing and scrubbing with machines, and must be slip resistant when wet. Flooring is usually speckled to ensure minimal reflectance of light (*c.* 30%).

Walls

Theatre walls must be easy to clean, and may be covered with ceramic tiles, plastic skin with sealed joints, or simply gloss paint to reflect 60% of light. The wall edges should be protected from impact damage by metal or plastic edging. Window ledges and narrow horizontal surfaces should be avoided, and where possible should be sloped.

Storage

Minimal amounts of surgical equipment should be stored in the operating theatre or in corridors, and adequate space must be available in the theatre suite. Obsolete equipment should be regularly removed. Shelving in the operating theatre should be kept to a minimum and regularly cleaned with hypochlorite and phenol to kill both viruses and bacteria.

OPERATING PERSONNEL

The main source of bacterial infections in operating rooms is bacteria shed from the operating room person-nel. Infection rates are reduced if the numbers of personnel are kept to a minimum, and infected individuals should be excluded from the theatre suite.

SCRUBBING UP

Contamination of the wound through accidental punctures in surgical gloves is a potential source of surgical wound infection. Thorough washing of the hands and forearms with an antiseptic agent (4% chlorhexidine gluconate or 5% povidone iodine) before donning sterile gown and gloves will reduce the number of micro-organisms present on the skin for the duration of the operative procedure. Experimental evidence has established a required scrubbing time of 5 min, with 3 min for consecutive scrubs. The use of a brush should be confined to the fingernails.

A recent Australian study has concluded that a brief 2.5-min initial scrub with 4% chlorhexidine gluconate, followed by a 30-s application of 70% isopropanol with 0.5% chlorhexidine or 70% ethanol with 0.5% chlorhexidine and a subsequent 30-s application of the alcohol-based antiseptic is an effective alternative to the 5-min, 3-min regime.

CLOTHING

Dress

Operating room dress is significant in preventing bacterial shedding from theatre personnel. Clean, closely woven polycotton tunics tucked into trousers with elasticated cuffs minimize bacterial shedding. Impermeable barrier operating gowns are used for scrubbed personnel.

Masks

The use of masks is not essential for conventional surgery, but they should be worn if the surgeon or nurse has an upper respiratory tract infection, if the patient is susceptible to infection, or for the insertion of a prosthesis. Theatre masks with visors attached are available for high-risk patients and procedures where an aerosol of blood or bone fragments is likely.

Hat

The omission of a theatre hat has been shown to increase the risk of infection in a laminar-flow theatre by a factor of four.

Footwear

Theatre footwear is a matter of personal choice. Rubber boots are deemed safest for high-risk cases, while clogs are usually considered more comfortable. All theatre footwear must have closed toes. Antistatic footwear is no longer a legal requirement.

Eye protection

Goggles are recommended for all personnel who are at risk of inoculation by spraying blood or tissue, and when dealing with high-risk patients.

Gloves

Surgical gloves have advanced considerably since their introduction by William Halstead in 1890. In general, surgical gloves are made of latex, and they are now powder free to prevent post-operative adhesions secondary to starch. Various types of hypoallergenic gloves are also available.

- Double-glove techniques for high-risk procedures are commonplace and do reduce the incidence of needlestick injuries, but are perceived by surgeons to impair comfort, sensitivity and dexterity.

- New puncture-resistant materials are being developed for protection against disease and needlestick injuries, in addition to finger-guards and glove-liners. However, currently available systems offer limited protection over the hand, and in clinical trials have been shown to reduce dexterity of suture and instrument handling.

PERSONNEL MANAGEMENT STRUCTURE

Staff from a variety of disciplines are required for the efficient functioning of an operating theatre suite. Figure 34.4.7 outlines the basic management structure. The National Association of Theatre Nurses recommends a minimum of two qualified staff for each operating room.

NUMBER OF PERSONNEL

In order to minimize the risk of infection and maximize safety, the minimum number of personnel should be present in the operating theatre.

HAZARDS TO STAFF

The safety of the patient in the operating room is discussed elsewhere in this book. It is important that the safety of operating room personnel is maintained at all times.

HIGH-RISK PATIENTS

Operating room staff are at risk from a number of serious and potentially fatal viral diseases, including viral hepatitis, cytomegalovirus (CMV) and human immunodeficiency virus (HIV).

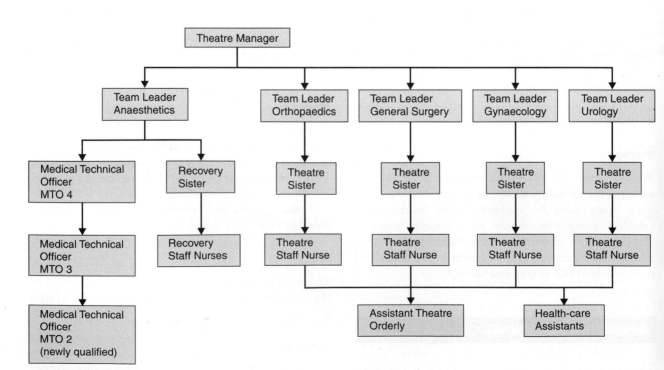

Figure 34.4.7 Operating room management structure.

Viral hepatitis

Viral hepatitis is the commonest liver disease worldwide. Hepatitis may result in death in the acute phase from fulminant liver failure, or lead to chronic active hepatitis, cirrhosis, a carrier state or, in the case of hepatitis B, to the development of primary liver cancer. The Department of Health requires that all operating-room staff are immunized against hepatitis B. However, there is no vaccine available for hepatitis C. There is evidence that post-exposure intervention with interferon is helpful in acute hepatitis C.

Cytomegalovirus

Between 60 and 70% of the population are seropositive for CMV by the age of 60 years. In the normal adult, the symptoms of fever, sore throat and hepatosplenomegaly are similar to those of glandular fever. In the immuno-compromised patient, serious infection may result in pneumonia or hepatitis. Placental transmission to the fetus may result in intrauterine death or spontaneous abortion.

Human immunodeficiency virus

For each patient with AIDS, there are an estimated 24–100 carriers of HIV. Seroconversion following a hollow needlestick injury occurs within 12 weeks in 1 in 280 cases and inevitably leads to AIDS within 8–10 years, with death usually within 1 year. There are no figures available for the risk of infection from 'aerosol' effects of orthopaedic surgery.

Equipment and procedures for the management of high-risk cases in the event of exposure should be established in all operating theatres. Universal precautions recommended by the Occupational Health and Safety Administration (OHSA) include the following:

- double gloves;
- impermeable gowns;
- waterproof footwear;
- safe procedures for passing sharps;
- safe disposal in 'sharps bins';
- no resheathing of needles;
- reporting of needlestick injuries to Occupational Health.

These universal precautions should be practised by all personnel who handle the patient or are likely to come into contact with body fluids. Potential innoculum includes blood, bloodstained fluids, CSF, synovial, peritoneal, pericardial, amniotic and pleural fluids, urine, semen and vaginal secretions. Operating room practice should reflect the possibility that all patients are potentially 'high risk'.

SHARPS

Sharps injuries are the primary route through which health-care workers acquire blood-borne diseases. Recent research suggests that a percutaneous injury occurs in 6.9% of surgical procedures. During high-risk procedures the use of sharps may be kept to a minimum by employing cutting and coagulation diathermy for the skin incision and any intra-abdominal dissection. Where possible the hands-free technique of passing sharps should be practised, whereby the scrub nurse places the sharp instrument in a kidney dish, and the dish is then passed to the surgeon who picks up the instrument him- or herself.

The majority of glove punctures are to the non-dominant glove, most commonly during closure of the abdomen. While the use of blunt-tipped needles does not eliminate the risk of puncture, their use in association with a 'no-touch techinque', whereby the wound edge is manipulated with instruments, is recommended in abdominal closure both for the abdominal wall and for the skin.

Laundry workers are at high risk of needlestick injuries from incorrect sharps disposal. It is imperative that all personnel are aware of the sharps disposal procedure (usually polypropylene containers with tamper-proof lids which are incinerated).

Needlestick injuries 'sharps accident policy'

- Immediate action should be taken to promote bleeding, and the injury should be washed under running water. If the eye is involved, wash with copious amounts of water.

- All needlestick injuries should be reported to the nearest supervisor and to Occupational Health.

- An accident form should be completed.

- Donor details are required.

The aim of the needlestick procedure is to identify individuals who are at risk and to initiate treatment with antiviral therapy as required.

HAZARDOUS SUBSTANCES

Anaesthetic agents

Volatile anaesthetic agents used in the operating theatre have been perceived as a serious hazard to operating staff, reportedly increasing the risk of abortion, decreasing fertility and affecting performance and concentration. Studies to date have not confirmed these suspicions.

UK legislation enacted in the Control of Substances

Hazardous to Health (COSHH) Act in 1990 now requires regular assessment of the level of pollution in the theatre environment. Methods of reducing anaesthetic gas levels are now commonplace, including active and passive scavenging systems, circle-absorber systems, low-flow and closed-circuit techniques, and the use of total intravenous anaesthesia or regional anaesthetic techniques when appropriate.

Cleaning materials

Any substances that are considered hazardous must be appropriately stored in a locked facility in line with guidelines for the storage of hazardous materials.

FIRE AND EXPLOSION

The decline in the use of volatile inflammable anaesthetic gases has reduced the risk of fire and explosion in theatres. It is no longer a requirement that all staff wear antistatic shoes, although most operating rooms are still equipped with antistatic flooring.

The main risk is from the use of diathermy and lasers in the operating room, particularly in association with alcoholic skin preparations.

STRESS

The operating room may be a highly stressful place. It is essential that staff are allowed breaks in duty, and suitable facilities are required for breaks where drinks and food should be readily available. Ideally, rest areas should have access to natural light. A relaxed stress-free atmosphere is conducive to both the well-being of staff and the care of their patients. False windows in the operating theatre are considered unnecessary by some, as they do not provide adequate light and may increase the risk of infection due to condensation, but natural light is preferred by staff. Daylight bulbs may alleviate this problem.

Music in the operating room is a matter of personal taste. Noise levels in operating theatres often exceed acceptable limits, making communication difficult and contributing to stress levels. Surprisingly, the addition of appropriately selected music may decrease overall noise levels. There have been few objective measurements of the effects of music on operating personnel. However, one study showed significantly greater speed and accuracy when surgeon-selected music was played.

LATEX ALLERGY

Cotton liners and spray-on barrier creams are available for the approximately 20% of health-care workers who suffer from latex allergy of type IV (eczema and dermatitis). More recently, severe type I anaphylactic (immunoglobulin E-mediated, urticaria, asthma) hypersensitivity reactions have been reported. Staff who suffer from this allergy may not be able to continue working in the operating room.

FURTHER READING

Department of Health and Social Security. 1983: *Ventilation of operating departments: a design guide.* London: Department of Health and Social Security.

Khan PCA, Thompson JF. 1997: Latex allergy: an emerging health hazard for operating theatre staff. *British Journal of Surgery* **84,** 289–90.

Meyer-Witting M, Wilkinson DJ. 1992: A safe haven or a dangerous place – should we keep the anaesthetic room? *Anaesthesia* **47,** 1021–2.

Whyte W, Lidwell OM, Lowbury EJL, Blowers R. 1983: Suggested bacteriological standards for air in ultraclean operating rooms. *Journal of Hospital Infection* **4,** 133–9.

Wounds and wound healing

Donald G. MacLellan

Introduction

Wound healing is an absolute prerequisite for survival. Without the ability to heal wounds, the body will succumb to haemorrhage or infection. Thus it is not surprising that interest in wound healing practices has extended from the time of the Smith Papyrus in 1700 BC to the present day.

Wound management has seen dramatic developments over the past decade, and the future promises even more. Since the discovery of the first growth factor (epidermal growth factor) in 1962, the science of wound repair and regeneration has advanced enormously. In 1962, the moist wound concept of healing also evolved. These two major developments have led to a rethinking of the management of wound repair and to the spawning of an exponential growth of new wound dressings.

However, it is a sobering fact that, despite these clinical and scientific advances, the management of both acute and chronic wounds remains a major health problem and consumes a significant amount of the health budget. Wound care practices can and must be optimized, but improved wound management does not rely solely on the use of modern wound dressings. It is vital that the clinician understands wound repair processes and adheres to the basic principles of wound management.

INCISIONS

The skin incision is the route to deeper structures and cavities, and should therefore be well planned to achieve optimal access. The following considerations in the choice of incisions are important:

1. *orientation of skin tension lines (Langer's lines)* – these lines are determined by the orientation of the dermal collagen fibres. If the incision is parallel to these lines, the resultant scar is less evident;

2. *strength and healing potential of the tissues* – the site where the incision is created should take into account the healing properties of the underlying tissue;

3. *anatomy of the underlying structures* – when placing an incision, the position of nerves and other major structures must be known and the incision placed to minimize their potential for damage;

4. *cosmesis* – there is only one major sign that the patient sees to remind them of their surgery, and that is the post-operative scar. A poor cosmetic result will detract from surgical brilliance, which unfortunately remains hidden!

TYPES OF HEALING

It is customary to divide the types of wound healing into primary, secondary and delayed primary (tertiary) healing. *Primary intention* healing occurs when tissue is able to be approximated with sutures, tapes or tissue glue. Repair involves minimal new tissue formation, and the wound is sealed within days. *Secondary intention* healing is the healing of an open wound through formation of granulation tissue, wound contraction and epithelialization. Considerable new tissue formation is required and, depending on the size of the wound, takes from weeks to months to epithelialize. *Delayed primary healing (tertiary intention)* is chosen when there is a high probability of bacterial contamination of the wound, and thus an increased potential for wound infection if the wound is closed primarily. The wound is allowed to heal by secondary intention for a few days, and is then closed to complete healing by primary intention. Closure of a wound by skin graft is another example of tertiary intention healing.

WOUND REPAIR

The response of tissue to injury has five major components:

1. inflammatory response;
2. fibroblast proliferation;
3. blood vessel proliferation (angiogenesis);
4. connective tissue synthesis;
5. epithelialization.

The healing process translates the mechanical injury into cellular and biochemical signals which attract the appropriate cells to the site, stimulate replication of fibroblasts and endothelial cells, increase collagen synthesis, organize wound contraction and stimulate epithelial cell replication and migration. The sequence of wound repair includes signals which initiate the host response to injury and terminate the process once repair is complete. The repair process is usually described as a continuum commencing with the *inflammatory* phase, and moving through the *proliferative* phase to the *maturation* phase. The cellular relationships within these phases are depicted in Figure 34.5.1.

The inflammatory phase commences at the moment of injury. Surgical or traumatic injury disrupts tissue architecture and causes haemorrhage. Blood is exposed to collagen, which activates Hageman factor and causes degranulation of platelets and the release of platelet-derived growth factor (PDGF). Subsequently, four major biochemical amplification systems are activated:

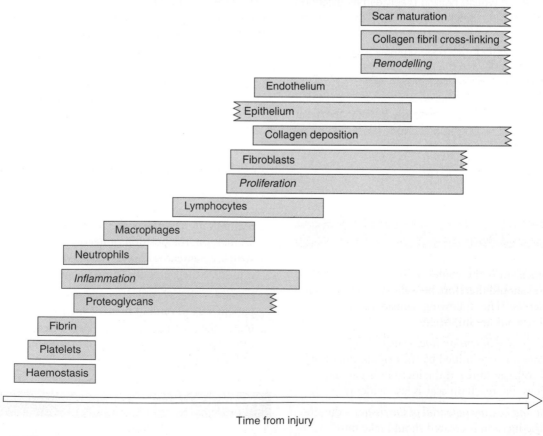

Figure 34.5.1 Sequence of events in wound healing. (Reproduced with permission from Greenfield LJ, Mulholland MW, Oldham KT, Zelenock GB. 1993: *Surgery. Scientific principles and practice.* Philadelphia, PA: Lippincott, p. 86.)

1. complement cascade;
2. clotting mechanism;
3. kinin cascade;
4. plasmin generation.

Each is a series of enzymes that amplifies the original injury signal and produces mitogens and chemoattractants.

Within a few hours, there is a major influx of poly-morphonuclear neutrophils (PMNs) and lymphocytes recruited by complement chemotactic factors. Mono-cytes soon follow, also recruited by fibrin degradation products, and become tissue macrophages. Macrophages remain the predominant leucocytes in the wound until repair is complete.

The wounding process disrupts and thromboses cap-illaries. Kinins cause vasodilatation in the surrounding intact vessels, producing the typical inflammatory ery-thema. The actively metabolizing leucocytes create a wound milieu which is acidotic, hypoxic, hypoglycaemic and hyperlactic. This environment appears to be the source of signals for fibroplasia, collagen synthesis and migration of fibroblasts and endothelial cells.

The duration and nature of the healing response are determined by the amount of dead space that must be replaced by connective tissue. If the wound is precisely approximated, a very small amount of dead space results, and new capillary circulation can cross the wound in 3–4 days. By days 4 to 5, the proliferative phase develops with an orderly progression of tissue growing in from the edge of the wound, consisting of dividing fibroblasts, sprout-ing capillary networks and newly synthesized collagen, fibronectin and proteoglycans, all orchestrated by macrophages. This process continues until the dead space is obliterated.

The fibroblast, probably stimulated by the high lac-tate environment and fibroblast growth factor (FGF), produces collagen. Lysis of old collagen occurs simultan-eously. An imbalance of either process may contribute to dehiscence. While the laying down of collagen occurs within a relatively short period of time, its realignment and remodelling take months. Thus the breaking strength of a wound will increase gradually over a period of 6–9 months, during which time no net collagen pro-duction is evident.

Contraction via the myofibroblasts is independent of collagen content and heralds the maturation phase. Epithelialization commences very early after injury, and stems from the wound edge and the remnant hair folli-cles. The wound must be moist during healing or else the cellular advance will cease. Epithelialization is 30–40% more rapid in a moist environment than in a dry envi-ronment or scab.

During the past few decades, the importance of growth factors in tissue repair has increasingly been rec-ognized. These growth factors are peptides produced by a variety of cells in the wound, and are designed to act on specific cell receptors to stimulate migration, collagen synthesis, proliferation and metalloprotease activity. Most growth factors act in an autocrine manner (on cell membrane of cell of origin) or paracrine manner (on adjacent cell membrane).

PDGF is one of the growth factors that initiates heal-ing, and is released from platelets. A cascade of events follows PDGF release, including inflammatory cell influx and proliferation, migration of fibroblasts and a chemo-tactic stimulus for macrophages. The macrophage is responsible for wound repair. It produces TGF-β which induces fibroblast migration, proliferation and collagen production as well as inhibition of collagenase activity. Epidermal growth factgor (EGF) is a reasonably non-specific stimulant of epithelial cell proliferation, and it suppresses collagen synthesis. FGF stimulates epithelial-ization, collagen synthesis and angiogenesis. Much research is currently in progress to discover more about the specific roles of these growth factors (Table 34.5.1) as well as their interactions.

PRINCIPLES OF WOUND HEALING

Before commencing the treatment of any wound, it is essential to determine the underlying aetiology and to establish what other patient factors might mitigate against wound healing, as well as deciding what wound dressing is most appropriate. These are the well-defined principles of wound healing, which should be followed whenever a patient presents with any kind of wound (Box 34.5.1).

BOX 34.5.1 PRINCIPLES OF WOUND HEALING

1. *Define* the aetiology.
2. *Control* the factors that affect healing.
3. *Select* an appropriate moist wound dressing and bandage.
4. *Plan* for maintenance of the healed wound.

DEFINING THE AETIOLOGY

It is remarkable how infrequently attempts are made to define the aetiology of wounds, particularly chronic wounds. Consequently, optimal wound healing rates are not achieved. The major causes of wounds are well rec-ognized (Table 34.5.2), and thus should be accurately diagnosed by most clinicians.

A systematic and rational approach to defining wound aetiology is achieved by taking a careful history,

Table 34.5.1 Peptide factors that affect wound healing

Factor	Abbreviation	Source	Functions regulated
Platelet-derived growth factor	PDGF	Platelets and macrophages	Fibroblast proliferation, chemotaxis and collagenase production
Transforming growth factor β	TGF-β	Platelets, polymorphonuclear neutrophil leucocytes, T-lymphocytes and macrophages	Fibroblast proliferation, chemotaxis, collagen metabolism and action of other growth factors
Transforming growth factor α	TGF-α	Activated macrophages and many tissues	Similar to EGF functions
Interleukin-1	IL-1	Macrophages	Fibroblast proliferation
Tumour necrosis factor	TNF	Macrophages, mast cells and T-lymphocytes	Fibroblast proliferation
Fibroblast growth factor	FGF	Brain, pituitary, macrophages and many other tissues and cells	Fibroblast proliferation, stimulation of collagen deposition and angiogenesis
Epidermal growth factor	EGF	Saliva, urine, milk and plasma	Stimulation of epithelial cell proliferation and granulation tissue formation
Insulin-like growth factor	IGF	Liver, plasma and fibroblasts	Stimulation of synthesis of sulphated proteoglycans, collagen and cell proliferation
Human growth factor	HGF	Pituitary and therefore plasma	Anabolism

Table 34.5.2 Major causes of wounds

Acute	Trauma
	Burns
	Crushing injuries
	Lacerations
Chronic	Leg ulcers
	Arterial
	Venous
	Vasculitic
	Neoplastic
	Neuropathic
	Pressure ulcers
	Traumatic wounds
	Surgical wounds
	Neoplastic ulcers

undertaking a complete physical examination and directing investigations as appropriate. Many wound protocols exist to ensure that the proper diagnosis is concluded in an expeditious manner (Table 34.5.3).

FACTORS AFFECTING WOUND HEALING

Both intrinsic and extrinsic factors will affect wound healing rates (Table 34.5.4). Optimizing their control ensures that the overall health status of the patient is improved, which will in turn be beneficial to wound healing.

Intrinsic factors

The general health status of the individual has important implications for wound healing. Many medical conditions adversely affect wound healing rates, and some of them cause specific wound-healing problems in their own right. For example, wounds in diabetics have a poor inflammatory response, higher infection rate and a higher rate of arterial degeneration. The vascular changes in association with neuropathy make the feet of the diabetic patient particularly susceptible to injury. Optimizing diabetic control improves wound healing.

The nutritional status of the patient can often be overlooked during their clinical assessment. An adequate intake of calories is needed to meet the energy demands of the normal reparative process. Certain vitamins and

Table 34.5.3 Wound management protocol

1. History
Initiating factors
Past medical history
Family history
Drug history
Ulcer treatment history

2. Physical examination
Document wound site, size, colour and character
Peripheral pulses
Neurological status
Stigmata of venous, arterial, connective tissue disorders
Nutritional status

3. Initial investigations
FBE
Nutrition
    Weight
    Serum albumin
    Diet chart
Serum glucose
Vasculitic screen
    ESR
    ANCA
Vascular
    Doppler
    ABI
    Duplex
Radiology/bone scan
Wound biopsy

Table 34.5.4 Factors that affect wound healing

Intrinsic factors	Extrinsic factors
Health status	Mechanical stress
Diabetes	Debris
Circulation	Temperature
Anaemia	Desiccation
Immune status	Infection
Age	Chemical stress
Nutritional status	Medication

trace elements (vitamins C, A, K and B, zinc and copper) are also essential for wound healing. These are mostly available in a well-balanced diet containing plenty of fresh fruit and vegetables. Wound pain can also cause vasoconstriction and a decrease in tissue oxygen levels. If the wound is causing the patient discomfort, this problem must be addressed or it will delay wound healing.

Extrinsic factors

Mechanical stress
Unrelieved pressure on a pressure ulcer will contribute to ongoing destruction. Any patient who is immobile in bed or in a chair is particularly susceptible to the development of pressure ulceration.

Debris
Wounds that contain necrotic tissue will not heal. Debris and necrotic tissue must be removed, and surgical, enzymatic and autolytic debridement are essential components of wound healing.

Temperature
As cells and enzymes function optimally at body temperature, a temperature fall of 2°C is sufficient to affect biological processes. A simple dressing replacement can decrease the wound temperature for 4 h before it returns to normal. The wound should therefore be insulated and not left exposed for any significant length of time.

Desiccation
Cells, enzymes and growth factors cannot function in a dry environment. Wounds should not be 'dried out' by exposure to the air or the sun, exposure to certain chemicals or dry bandages, as this kills the surface cells and increases the reparative requirements. Granulation tissue is fragile and easily damaged, particularly on removal of dry dressings, thus disrupting the wound healing process and returning it to an earlier (inflammatory) phase of healing. The moist wound concept of healing enhances the healing process.

Clinical infection
Clinical infection must be controlled by appropriate systemic antibiotic therapy. The clinical features of infection include increasing pain and pus at the wound site, lymphangitis, lymphadenopathy and systemic features (e.g. fever, rigors, etc.). There is considerable overuse of wound swabs for microbiological assessment of chronic wounds. Wound swabs should be confined to ulcers that show clinical evidence of infection, where slough or tissue can be gathered by the wound swab. As wound swabs generally remove the surface bacteria, the information obtained is usually only the identification of the non-pathogenic colonizing organisms on the wound surface. If there is infection, the pathogenic bacteria are in the tissue and can be accessed by biopsy. Too often the use of wound swabs leads to the inappropriate prescribing of antibiotics.

Chemical stressors
All antiseptics are cytotoxic! They have been shown to damage cellular elements and the wound microcirculation. Although antiseptics may have a role in the topical management of heavily contaminated acute traumatic

ulcers, they are often inappropriately used for long periods of time on chronic ulcers. The need to sterilize a leg ulcer to achieve healing is unproven, and there is thus little evidence to support the use of antiseptics on a continuing basis for chronic wounds.

Drugs

Many medications have side-effects which interfere with or delay wound healing. For example, steroids and anti-inflammatory drugs are immunosuppressive and reduce the effect of the inflammatory phase of wound healing. Although many of these drugs are essential for the patient's continuing health, it is important to realize that they can have a deleterious effect on wound healing. Many older patients are on multiple drugs, many of which can affect wound healing. Thus it is important for the clinician to assess the need for some of these medications.

SELECTING AN APPROPRIATE WOUND DRESSING

Before selecting a dressing, the wound must firstly be accurately assessed.

It is important to emphasize that a wound passes through several stages of healing before the process is complete. Therefore no single dressing will be suitable for the management of a chronic or slow-healing wound from the time of injury until the time of complete healing. A system of wound assessment which is simple but effective is the colour, depth and exudate (CDE) system.

Colour is a well-recognized method of determining the phase of wound healing:

- black – dehydrated dead tissue (inflammatory stage of healing);
- yellow – sloughy tissue (inflammatory stage of healing);
- red – granulation tissue (proliferative stage of healing);
- pink – epithelialization (maturation stage of healing).

The *depth* of the wound denotes the level of tissue damage. A partial-thickness (superficial) wound involves damage to the epithelium and some dermis, whereas a full-thickness (cavity) wound involves epidermal, dermal and even subdermal damage.

The *exudate volume* determines to a large extent the type of dressing chosen. Proper selection will avoid maceration of the surrounding skin or the possibility of the dressing sticking to a relatively dry wound. Before choosing a specific dressing, several other features should be noted.

1. Documentation of wound size is essential in healing by secondary intention. Tracing or photography (if available) provide objective data on wound progress, and aid determination of the success or failure of the treatment.

2. Pain can be charted using the 1–10 analogue pain scale scoring system.

3. Signs of clinical infection should be determined. Infected wounds require a daily dressing change and systemic antibiotics.

4. Malodorous wounds can be treated with metronidazole gel applied to the wound daily for 1 week. This will remove the Gram-negative anaerobic bacteria which grow on the slough. Frequent dressing changes are recommended. This treatment can be supplemented with charcoal-impregnated dressings which are designed to absorb odours. Debridement of the slough will also assist in controlling the problem in most cases.

CLASSIFICATION OF DRESSINGS

Modern wound dressings can be divided into five 'families' or categories, namely films, foams, alginates, hydrogels and hydrocolloids.

FILMS

These dressings consist of a thin polyurethane membrane coated with a layer of acrylic adhesive. They are gas and water vapour permeable, and impermeable to micro-organisms. They provide a moist wound environment and encourage autolysis. However, they do not have the ability to absorb exudate, so their use is limited to clean superficial wounds with little exudate, as secondary dressings, or in the prevention of skin breakdown in pressure areas.

FOAMS

Polyurethane foams meet many of the criteria for standard dressings in that they allow the passage of exudate through the surface layer to the main body of the product, thereby maintaining a moist environment. These products are highly absorbent of exudate, and can be used in moderate/heavy exuding wounds, including leg ulcers, donor sites and minor burns. Foams are also useful as secondary dressings to alginates and amorphous hydrogels. While there are no contraindications, they would not be considered appropriate for dry wounds or wounds with eschar.

ALGINATES

Alginates are the calcium salts of alginic acid, obtained from seaweed. When applied to a wound, the sodium salts present in the wound exudate exchange with the calcium in the alginate to form sodium alginate, which is a hydrophilic gel. This gel has the ability to absorb exudate into itself while maintaining a moist environment at the surface of the wound. These products also have haemostatic qualities and are therefore useful in acute trauma, donor sites and for lightly packing cavities (e.g. nasal packing in epistaxis). These dressings are contraindicated for dry and low-exudate wounds because they are reliant on an exudate to form a gel.

HYDROGELS

Hydrogels are composed mainly of water with varying amounts of propylene glycol as a preservative and humectant. This broad class of polymers will rehydrate dry tissue and absorb a certain amount of fluid. Therefore they are efficient in rehydrating sloughy wounds and necrotic debris to encourage autolytic debridement.

Hydrogels are available in two forms, namely *amorphous* (i.e. free flowing) hydrogels, which will fill a cavity wound, and *sheet* hydrogels, which consist of a cross-linked polymer and water held on a wafer backing. These products are particularly useful in the management of superficial burns, post-radiotherapy skin trauma, and to aid the removal of necrotic tissue or slough.

HYDROCOLLOIDS

Hydrocolloids are familiar to most clinicians as they were originally introduced as stomahesive to protect good skin around ileostomies and colostomies. They are composed of a combination of polymers held in a fine suspension. When placed in contact with a wound, the polymers combine with the exudate to form a soft moist gel which encourages autolysis and aids the removal of slough in the wound.

Hydrocolloids are available in two forms. The wafer forms are occlusive, making them impermeable to gases and water vapour. They form an excellent barrier to micro-organisms, and are waterproof. The thick hydrocolloids are used in moderately exuding wounds (e.g. chronic leg ulcers, donor sites and pressure ulcers). They are not suitable for dirty or infected wounds, and are contraindicated for deep wounds down to the level of muscle and bone.

The thin hydrocolloids have a polyurethane backing and are not occlusive. They are suitable for lightly exuding wounds and can be used to prevent skin breakdown in pressure areas. They are also very useful as post-operative dressings.

COMBINATION DRESSINGS

New products have been released which combine two of these 'families' of dressings (e.g. alginates have been added to some hydrocolloids to increase absorbency). These dressings are also useful in routine wound management.

With over 60 dressings available on the market, clinicians have a considerable responsibility to be familiar with the products that they are using. The special features of many dressings will assist wound healing greatly if used appropriately. However, considerable damage can be caused by use of the incorrect product. Trial and error should be avoided, as it is a time-consuming and wasteful practice.

Chapter 34.6

Principles of anastomoses

Michael C. Pietroni

Introduction

Decisions made by surgeons determine outcomes. Constructing an anastomosis involves making decisions about the healthiness of tissues, their vascularity, the absence of tension and the choice of suture material and sewing technique to be used. How surgeons make decisions and what factors influence the way in which they make them are just as important as the final decision itself. Successful outcomes will depend on the following:

- having the right attitudes;
- seeing what you are doing;
- thinking about what you wish to achieve;
- thinking about the problems you wish to avoid;
- practising perfect surgical technique.

Remember that complications do not 'happen', but are the direct result of sometimes foreseeable circumstances.

HAVING THE RIGHT ATTITUDE

Education is about attitudes. Skills develop with training and experience.

An anastomosis is a join between two tubes that is created by a surgeon. The most important factor determining success is the surgeon's attitude to the decision-making process. Anastomoses must remain secure after the wound has been closed, and must present no long-term physiological or pathological problems.

Why, then, do some anastomoses leak, stenose or present problems when they are apparently well constructed? Where does judgement over these matters let the surgeon down? Careful, precise, unhurried accurate surgery with unimpaired access and view is vital. You should ask yourself whether you are the right surgeon to do the job, whether this is the right time and whether this the right hospital environment.

Good surgeons, regardless of their level of experience or seniority, recognize their own limitations. Do not be afraid to ask for help and advice from surgeons senior to yourself. Always ask yourself whether an operation should be postponed (in order to ensure more experienced help), or whether transfer to a more appropriate hospital environment is advisable.

Better surgeons achieve better results. Operations performed in the middle of the night can often be postponed. Certain specialist procedures (e.g. vascular and colonic surgery) are better performed in specialist centres if time allows. An experienced surgeon is needed before considerations about blood supply, freedom from tension and secure surgery can be entertained (Figure 34.6.1).

How does experience become expertise? Wisdom in decision-making requires thought as well as experience and knowledge. A store of experience by itself does not necessarily confer wisdom. For this to occur, there must be a phase of reflection that analyses the bearing of each new experience on previous knowledge and experience.

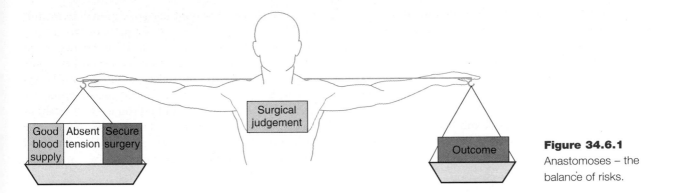

Figure 34.6.1
Anastomoses – the balance of risks.

Reflect on your experience, audit your results, and be conscientious about your own responsibility for continuing to learn. Keep an unhappy experience in proportion. You can only learn lessons if the analysis is performed with careful review of all the facts. Difficult decisions are made not only in the light of knowledge and science, but also in the light of what will work given all of the prevailing circumstances. Decisions between alternative strategies require skill in risk analysis. If you know the facts, then this will help you to minimize risks.

It is difficult to argue with success, and no surgeon has ever been sued when a successful outcome followed an unwise decision. However, beware of being tempted by success when wisdom and experience suggest that an alternative decision might have been correct. A successful anastomosis under such circumstances may lull you into a false sense of security, exposing your next patient to another unwise decision and perhaps a different outcome. Do not be seduced by the glamour of possible spectacular success by choosing the risky option. Second laparotomies, fistulous Crohn's disease, disseminated malignancy, obstruction, perforation and peritonitis are hazardous fields for difficult anastomoses.

SEEING WHAT YOU ARE DOING

Always ensure that your incision is large enough for you to see. Use your assistants and your retractors with careful thought and in such a way as to establish and maintain an adequate exposure. Often a better view is obtained by the liberal use of stay sutures. You need to be free to perform the anastomosis unhindered by the need to keep re-establishing the exposure. Ensure that you display the problem in its entirety, as only then can you formulate a plan. Once you have decided what to do, only then should you proceed with carrying out the plan. Remember:

- display the problem;
- decide what to do;
- carry out the plan.

Insist on having a good view of things. Vascular anastomoses require a bloodless field, and gut anastomoses require the ends to be free of intestinal contents. Use clamps appropriately. All anastomoses must be constructed without any other organs impinging on the view. These factors have an important bearing on the application of the principles for safe anastomotic surgery.

THINKING ABOUT WHAT YOU WISH TO ACHIEVE

When it is finished, an anastomosis must appear to the naked eye to be secure. There must be obviously demonstrable luminal continuity and no apparent scope for leaks. In the gut you should not be able to see mucosa protruding. Generally, therefore, there is a tendency to produce inversion of the edges. In the vascular tree you should not be able to see wide gaps between adjacent stitches. There must not be any internal irregularity facing the flowing blood; therefore there is a tendency to produce eversion of the edges.

AVOIDING SHEAR FORCES

Security is achieved by sewing together tubes of equal diameter in such a way as to produce an equal distribution of the two circumferences. Unequal distribution results in the development of shear forces. If there are episodic changes in luminal pressure, then the shear forces induced at particular points will be unequal, and this may produce leaks. The danger of this is of course exaggerated when sewing tubes of unequal diameters. When faced with this problem, ensure that you have distributed the inequality evenly throughout the circumference of the anastomosis. In these circumstances you may decide to use stay sutures at the four quadrants of the circle of your anastomosis in order to ensure that you have distributed this inequality evenly. The shear forces will then also be equally distributed.

In vascular surgery, shear forces can also develop where there is a compliance mismatch (because of differences in elasticity) between tissues that have been sewn together. This can happen in cases where polytetrafluoroethylene (PTFE) meets arterial wall. Precautions must be taken to distribute tensions evenly around the circumference of the anastomosis. Because these issues are so important, and because you need to distribute the sutures very carefully at the heel of an end-to-side PTFE anastomosis, the parachute technique is recommended (Figure 34.6.2).

This compliance mismatch arising from differences in elasticity may nevertheless lead to long-term fibro-endothelial hyperplasia and narrowing of the anastomosis. Many vascular surgeons recommend an interposition cuff of vein wall between the artery and the PTFE graft when the anastomosis is below the knee.

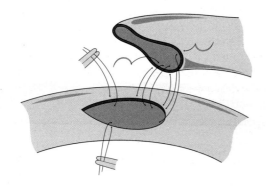

Figure 34.6.2 The parachute technique.

ESTABLISHING HEALTHY TISSUE MARGINS

You must sew together what appear to be healthy tissues, i.e. tissues that look normal to the naked eye, and appear to be free from disease and have a good blood supply. Do not allow any of these considerations to be compromised. Sometimes you may be concerned about cutting back to more normal tissue because you fear that the tubes may not then meet. You should separate in your mind the two tasks that you face, namely the gaining of healthy tissues and the establishment of an anastomosis free of tension. The first goal is to achieve healthy tissue ends. Only then can you address the problem of establishing a tension-free join. Unfortunately, it may be necessary that for the sake of 5 cm or so free of tension you have to mobilize or even resect 30–60 cm of bowel. Your ultimate objective is a satisfactory operation, not a short one. Be meticulous in achieving both healthy bowel ends and freedom from tension. The ends of the tubes should be free of fibrosis (common bile duct), calcium (blood vessels), cancer and inflammatory disease (gut). Do not use tissues that have been crushed by an

intestinal clamp. The limit of cancer growth in the tube itself is easy to recognize in some parts of the gut (e.g. colon, rectum) and more difficult in others (e.g. stomach, oesophagus). The naked eye is not always a good judge of this, and you may have to call on your knowledge of the pathology of the disease and its propensity for submucosal spread in guiding you towards establishing entirely healthy cancer-free tissues. This may be especially important in cases where a bypass anastomosis is contemplated without resection of the underlying tumour.

AVOIDING TENSION

Relieving tension is an exercise in itself. It is not usually a problem in the small bowel but, if it is, the solution lies in dividing the vessels that feed the mesenteric arcades. This may sometimes be a problem in preparing a Roux loop for an oesophago-jejunal or biliary anastomosis, or in preparing the distal ileum for a colonic or ileo-rectal anastomosis. Take care to fan out the mesentery and arrange for a light to shine through so that the arcades are clearly displayed. When you have decided how to relieve the tension, place soft clamps on the vessels which you propose to divide before doing so. Spend a little time ensuring that the vascularity will not be compromised before you actually divide the vessels. When you do divide the vessels, this must be done between ligatures with the vessel in continuity. Do not use haemostats on the vessels with the intention of dividing between them. You cannot risk the haemostats slipping and producing a mesenteric haematoma.

Achieving a tension-free anastomosis is more of a problem in the colon, especially on the left side. Ensure that you have mobilized the splenic flexure. Sometimes, despite this manoeuvre, the agent that appears to prevent the release of tension is the leash of vessels from the inferior mesenteric artery. Division of vessels here appears to commit you to cutting back the bowel to a level that is satisfactorily perfused by the left branch of the middle colic artery. It also appears to lengthen the operation by 15 min or so. Do not be afraid to do this. Freedom from tension is more important than the length of colon that remains.

Because two loops of bowel just meet, this does not automatically mean that there is no tension. You are observing the situation with the bowel in a flaccid state in the open abdomen. Once vigorous peristalsis occurs, muscle action can have a tendency to pull the loops apart. Allow for this by sewing together floppy rather than tight loops.

Mobilization of the bowel often produces freedom from tension and an increase in length. Unfortunately, you cannot gain length by mobilizing the oesophagus, the common bile duct or the ureter. Mobilization merely interrupts the blood supply to these tubes. To obtain freedom from tension, you need to mobilize the organ you wish to bring up to these tubes (the Roux jejunal loop or urinary bladder, respectively). You cannot gain length in a divided blood vessel by mobilizing the ends. When dealing with trauma, it is important not to sew disrupted arterial ends under tension. In such circumstances you need to accept that an interposition graft will be required.

AVOIDING DISTAL OBSTRUCTION

There must always be freedom from distal obstruction (potential or actual). Naturally you will not attempt an anastomosis proximal to an unresected lesion that has the potential to obstruct. However, do not forget that strong muscle action distal to your anastomosis may result in the same effect. Similarly, a sphincter distal to your anastomosis can also produce intraluminal pressures which your anastomosis may be unable to withstand.

THINKING ABOUT THE PROBLEMS YOU WISH TO AVOID

The main complications are leakage, stenosis and pathological complications. Ask yourself what is the complication you fear most and what is the commonest complication of the procedure you propose to adopt. Then ask yourself whether you have minimized the likelihood of these complications occurring.

AVOIDING LEAKS

Anastomoses leak because of a failure to appreciate the existence of a problem that should have been foreseen. In the absence of distal obstruction and tension, and in the presence of a good blood supply and healthy tissues, then an anastomosis cannot help but heal, provided that perfect surgical technique has been practised. A leaking anastomosis indicates that at some point judgement was faulty. Sometimes sutures are pulled too tightly. A continuous suture technique that looked perfect in the collapsed bowel may produce a purse-string effect when the bowel is distended.

In the vascular tree, leakage can sometimes be contained by the surrounding tissues. However, persistence of the connection with the arterial lumen will in time lead to a false aneurysm. If this leakage occurs at the upper end of an aortic graft, then this may lead to serious problems with an aorto-duodenal fistula. Therefore

it is important to take precautions. Do not tie your knots in the middle of the front wall of the aorta, where they can rub against the posterior wall of the duodenum. If possible, insert a portion of the old aortic wall or a portion of omentum between the aortic suture line and the duodenum.

AVOIDING STENOSIS

If you attempt to avoid leaks by taking large bites of the bowel wall, the amount of tissue that is inturned is large. You may consider that you have reduced the likelihood of leakage. However, the blood supply is correspondingly obstructed, leading to an anastomosis which, when it heals, will produce an unyielding fibrous ring. It is important to bear in mind the healing process. Healing by primary intention, not by fibrosis, is the aim. This is especially relevant in the biliary system.

If you are encountering difficulties because you are dealing with narrow tubes (e.g. in children), consider using interrupted suture techniques rather than continuous ones. These have the further advantage of allowing not only for distension but also for growth.

AVOIDING PATHOLOGICAL COMPLICATIONS

It is important to avoid cancer cells seeding themselves in the gut on granulations around unabsorbed suture material. You do not want stones to form on the surface of an irregularly constructed join in the urinary or biliary system, or in one where suture material persists on the luminal surface. Therefore you must take appropriate precautions.

In the vascular tree, your aim is to have an endothelial surface that is as smooth as possible. You do not want platelets to accumulate and produce either thrombosis or distal embolization, and you want the minimum amount of suture material to show on the endothelial surface. Again appropriate precautions must be taken.

Immunosuppressed patients and those whose tissues have been irradiated pose special challenges before the likelihood of healing can be assumed. It is important to take all necessary precautions.

PRACTISING PERFECT SURGERY

The principles of perfect surgery are as follows:
1. mobilize;
2. resect to healthy tissues;
3. ensure a good blood supply;
4. ensure that there is freedom from tension;
5. then sew together securely.

SUTURE TECHNIQUE

Having achieved tubes free of tension with what appears to be healthy tissue on either side, you now need to sew them together securely. You need to ask two questions.

1. Where does the strength in the tube lie?
2. Can I rotate this tube so as to see an outside surface over 360°?

Ask yourself whether your knowledge of the anatomy of this tube tells you where the strength in this tube lies. Bowel that is covered by serosa has a strong seromuscular coat and a strong collagenous layer in the submucosa. The mucosal lining itself does not contribute much to the strength. Although the serosa is absent on most of the rectum, the muscle wall is very strong and the collagenous layer of the submucosa also contributes. However, in the oesophagus the muscle layer is often of poor quality, and of course there is no serosa. Oesophageal anastomoses demand good strong bites through the only layers that count for strength (i.e. the mucosa and submucosa). That is why it is recommended that oesophageal anastomoses involve suturing the whole thickness of the wall. However, in the rest of the bowel, you can safely exclude the mucosal lining (but not the submucosa).

Arteries always require full-thickness bites. This is because separation of the adventitia and the endothelial layer is undesirable. Where it occurs, an endothelial flap can easily develop, and if this is downstream it may lead to the accumulation of platelets and embolism or eventual occlusion of the vessel.

When the needle traverses the arterial wall it should enter from within outwards (Figure 34.6.3).

As a general rule, continuous sutures of prolene are used in vascular surgery, ranging from 3/0 to 6/0 depending on the thickness of the vessel wall.

The following general rules apply to vascular anastomoses:

1. keep the lumen free of blood;
2. choose a vessel site free of calcium;
3. match the graft and vessel carefully;
4. pass the needle from inside out;
5. avoid shear forces;
6. use prolene or similar material.

When dealing with bowel, ask yourself whether you can rotate these tubes around their long axes so that you can always see the external aspect throughout 360°. You will always be able to do this with small bowel, and often with the colon. If you can rotate the tubes, the eye will always see the outside surface. Use a double-armed suture and place an extramucosal suture for the whole circumference of the anastomosis. Start at the point on the bowel where the mesentery is attached, ending up with the knot on the outside. You will need to slip one of the needles under the knot. This way you will do the most dangerous part first. Finish at the antimesenteric point working clockwise and anticlockwise from the mesenteric point (Figure 34.6.4).

If you cannot rotate the bowel fully, as in the duodenum and the rectum, then a different strategy is required. The eye will see the posterior wall from its mucosal aspect and the anterior wall from its external aspect. Under these circumstances it is better to use a posterior mattress suture in the posterior wall (Figure 34.6.5) and an extramucosal suture for the anterior wall. This permits more careful apposition of the walls. However, it is important to be careful at the corners (at the junctions of the two methods of suturing), as it is here that leaks may occur if adequate precautions are not taken.

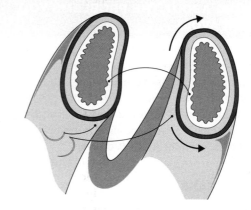

Figure 34.6.4 The extramucosal suture technique on rotatable bowel.

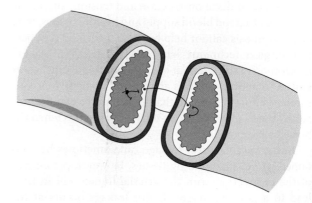

Figure 34.6.5 The posterior wall mattress suture on non-rotatable bowel.

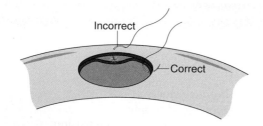

Figure 34.6.3 Vascular suturing.

It is also easier if all of the posterior wall sutures are placed with the two ends of the bowel widely apart. Use interrupted sutures, securing these sequentially in carefully placed haemostats so that they do not cross each other. When all of the sutures have been inserted, approximate the bowel ends and then knot the sutures carefully.

Sometimes in a very low anterior resection, or in an anastomosis to the hepatic bile ducts, completing the posterior wall in this manner makes it very difficult to place the anterior wall sutures accurately. Under these circumstances, the anterior wall sutures are placed first (in the rectum or in the hepatic duct) from outside in, and the needles retained. Once the posterior wall is finished, the needles can then be placed through the anterior wall of the bowel from inside out, and knotted on its outer surface (Figure 34.6.6).

SUTURE MATERIAL

Almost any suture material can be used to ensure *initial* security of almost any anastomosis. However, the aim is to *maintain* security. Sutures are used to hold together tubes that have a natural propensity to heal. However, tissues vary widely in their propensity to heal. For this reason you should have a very clear idea of how long healing takes. In general, healing in the urinary tract occurs very rapidly, and even a rapidly absorbed suture material such as catgut is sufficient in these areas. However, in areas where healing may take longer (e.g. in the oesophagus) it is wise to use suture material that remains strong and unabsorbed for a longer period of time. It was for this reason that in former years surgeons used two layer suturing methods, or absorbable material on the inside and non-absorbable material on the outside of the gastrointestinal tract. Modern suture materials are so reliable and predictable in their behaviour that, provided the right choice of material is made, there is now rarely any need for a two-layered approach to any anastomosis.

Just as tissues vary in their propensity to heal, so do patients. Hypoxia, low-output heart failure, poor nutrition, steroids, immunosuppression and previously irradiated tissues all contribute adversely to healing rates. In these circumstances it is important to take extra precautions with your choice of suture material and suture technique.

Once healing has taken place, persistence of the suture serves no purpose and may in fact be harmful (see above). Ask yourself what the effect of the suture material you propose to use will be on the tissue and its flowing contents.

Joins between artificial material (Dacron and PTFE) and arterial wall never heal securely and predictably in the absence of persistent suture material. We know this because when silk was the strongest suture material available, it unfortunately disintegrated after 5 years or more, and patients began to develop late false aneurysms at arterial joins that had previously appeared to be sound. Prolene®, which is inert, runs smoothly through tissues and remains strong and unabsorbed for an indefinite period. It is the ideal suture material for vascular anastomoses.

Surgeons generally have preferences for particular suture materials, which are dictated by the handling characteristics of the latter. Braided materials are easier to knot than monofilament materials. However, they do not run as smoothly through tissues and they may cut through unless they are carefully handled. The choice today appears to be between Vicryl® and Dexon® on the one hand and PDS® and Maxon® on the other. Newer suture materials, such as Biosyn® and Monocryl®, are intermediate in their *in-vivo* strength and absorptive characteristics. An experienced surgeon will select the suture material that is appropriate to the objectives of achieving initial security, ensuring continuing security and producing no long-term consequences. The choice will be dictated not only by the tissues but also by co-existing disease which may adversely affect healing rates.

PROTECTING THE ANASTOMOSIS

A well-constructed anastomosis generally requires no protection. However, in the presence of factors which may adversely affect healing, or in cases where an anastomosis has been created near a previous fistula (e.g. recto-vaginal or colo-vesical), it may be wise to mobilize omentum and wrap this around the join. On occasion you may wish to protect an anastomosis from raised intraluminal pressures by creating a proximal temporary colostomy or ileostomy.

Surgeons vary in their attitudes to the use of drains.

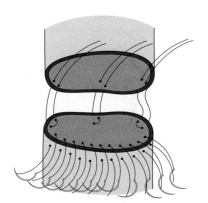

Figure 34.6.6 The anterior wall sutures are placed first in the rectum in a difficult low anterior resection.

There does not appear to be incontrovertible evidence that draining an anastomosis makes any useful contribution. Moreover, there is some evidence that certain rigid plastic drains may actually predispose to leakage. Therefore drainage is not recommended.

Some surgeons believe that the integrity of the anastomotic suture line should be tested at the end of the procedure. In the colon and rectum this is achieved by insufflation from below through the rectum. This practice has not gained general acceptance.

STAPLING DEVICES

Stapling devices are used by many surgeons as a substitute for hand-sewn techniques. Staplers undoubtedly save time in pouch surgery, and many surgeons believe that they may make certain difficult anastomoses (e.g. low anterior resection) easier to construct. The same general principles apply to the use of staplers as to hand-sewn anastomoses. However, it is important to be careful when using linear staplers not to telescope a length of bowel wall. When using circular staplers, ensure not only that the purse-string suture encompasses the whole circumference in an even manner, but also that when the knot is tied the bowel wall is distributed evenly between successive throws. Always check the doughnuts at the end for completeness. A stapled anastomosis cannot distend to the same extent as a hand-sewn join, so it is important to bear this in mind when dealing with narrow tubes.

Patient safety in the operating room

Kingsley Faulkner

Introduction

All surgical operations have their own specific hazards, as well as the general hazards that are inherent to all patients as they enter the operating room. It is incumbent upon surgeons, anaesthetists, nurses, technicians and other assistants to be constantly aware of these risks and to minimize their potential to cause harm to patients.

This chapter will address the specific hazards of positioning, electrical earthing and diathermy equipment, temperature control, tourniquet usage and wound care. Other factors which are relevant to the patient's safety include the construction and mechanical reliability of all equipment used.

POSITIONING

The objective of positioning of the patient is to provide the best surgical access for a particular procedure whilst also allowing the anaesthetist to have ready and safe control throughout the course of the operation.

Surgical access may be compromised by a patient's excessive body bulk, musculoskeletal problems or fragile physiology. Positions which limit good exposure of the operative field usually prolong and complicate the surgical procedure. Positions that exceed the limits of a patient's tolerance whilst under anaesthesia may cause physical injury or dangerous physiological disturbance.

The positioning must be such that no harm is done to the patient and the highest level of comfort and safety is achieved. Careful pre-operative assessment by both anaesthetist and surgeon will do much to achieve that objective. Positioning of a patient requires well-drilled teamwork and routines.

Transfer to and from the operating table must proceed with the utmost care. Special care will, of course, be needed if the patient has certain specific injuries, such as a cervical spine fracture or fractured limb. Care must be taken not to abduct the upper limbs beyond 90° for any period because of the potential to injure the brachial plexus, an injury which could be permanent.

The safe positioning of the patient should achieve the following goals.

- There should be no redness or change in skin integrity over bony prominences, pressure areas and the electrosurgical earthing pad site.

- There should be no subsequent complaints by the patient of strained muscles or ligaments, altered range of movement, compression or other injury to nerves post-operatively.

- The circulation in the extremities should not be impaired by the operation.

- Haemodynamic changes related to positioning should be carefully monitored and corrected and lead to no long-term problems. If any such problems are observed, they should be documented in the post-operative record.

The pre-operative assessment should entail a clear understanding of the surgical procedure to be embarked upon, and a careful enquiry into any positioning problems encountered during previous operations. Extreme obesity or congestive cardiac failure are factors which could predictably cause problems if the supine position is chosen or a head-down tilt is necessary during the procedure.

If on raising the arms above the head pre-operatively the thoracic outlet syndrome is provoked, then that position will need to be avoided during any operation. Freedom of neck movement and other musculoskeletal restrictions also require pre-operative assessment. Patients who are ill or who have electrolyte disturbance and vasomotor instability are certainly at increased risk during movement and positioning on the operating table.

Protective padding is of vital importance, especially over the bony prominences if neuropathies and decubitus ulcerations are to be prevented.

Special care should be directed towards the ulnar nerve at the medial aspect of the elbow and the peroneal nerve at the lateral aspect of the upper fibula on each occasion. Injury to the ulnar nerve is five times more likely in male patients undergoing the same types of surgical procedures, possibly because the condylar groove is shallower. Any sharp or rigid projection on the operating table or adjacent equipment should have sufficient padding to prevent injury both at the commencement and during the course of the operation.

Increased cardiovascular demands can occur, not only with the induction of anaesthesia and during the operation itself, but also during the course of changing the patient's position (e.g. tilting the operating table). While awake, a healthy individual rapidly regulates systemic blood pressure and tissue perfusion by pressoreceptor reflexes. In the presence of disease, injury or anaesthesia, postural changes that would not normally elicit stress are able to cause significant decreases in both arterial pressure and tissue perfusion. Respiratory excursion can be affected by positioning or in circumstances where there is any factor restraining diaphragmatic or chest movement.

Even if correct positioning has been established at the commencement of the procedure, other factors may cause problems. The patient's stability on the operating table needs to be ensured if subsequent tilting does occur. Self-retaining retractor systems should be installed with care to avoid pressure at unintended points. The Mayo table should be positioned high enough to avoid pressure, and the surgical staff should be alert to the danger of leaning on the patient's torso, head or limbs.

Shearing forces can readily cause dermal injury, especially in the elderly and malnourished. Vascular impairment will add to the risk of decubitus injury during prolonged operations, and may be minimized by the use of waterbeds or similar cushioning devices.

If the arms are to be positioned by the side during the operation, they need to be secured in position by armrests or some form of sheeting, taking particular care to avoid nerve compression injury.

A variety of useful accessories, such as pillows and other forms of padding, are available to assist in the positioning of the patient in a secure and comfortable manner. Care should be taken to avoid direct contact of the patient with any metallic surface on the operating table which could cause electrical burns.

There should be no obstruction to venous drainage from the lower limbs or, for example, of the inferior vena cava during Caesarean section (for which operation the patient should be tilted to her left).

Operating room tables can be adjusted in height and length and should be ergometrically efficient. They can be tilted from side to side and also head up and head down. They are generally divided into three sections to facilitate flexion and extension, and both head and foot sections are usually removable. Various other rests are available.

X-ray and fluoroscopy-compatible tables are available, and the table orientation may need to be altered when X-rays are to be used during a particular procedure (e.g. operative cholangiography).

STANDARD POSITIONS

The three basic positions are supine, prone and lateral, although each can be modified for a specific purpose.

Supine position

In the supine position, the patient should lie in a straight line on a well-padded mattress with the head well supported. The arms may be placed alongside the body with the palms down and the fingers slightly extended, and held in position by sheets passed around them and then beneath the torso. Alternatively, the arms may be placed out on arm-boards which are fixed at the same height as the mattress. The degree of abduction should be less than 90° and the palms placed upwards.

The hips and lower limbs should be parallel, with the heels slightly separated and carefully padded. Some adjustments may be necessary with variations in body habitus.

Respiratory function can be compromised in the supine position by lessening diaphragmatic excursion, particularly in the obese patient. If the head needs to be turned or the neck extended (e.g. for thyroid surgery), it should be supported comfortably in that position. The eyes should be protected at all times.

Variations of the supine position include the head-down (Trendelenburg) position which is used, for example, in pelvic surgery. This position allows better exposure, but can cause vascular engorgement of the head and neck. The patient needs to be secured to avoid slipping, and care must be taken to prevent compression or stretching injuries against restraints. The brachial plexus is certainly at risk.

The lithotomy position is another variation, in which the legs are raised on two level supports in unison and abducted to expose the perineal region. A small soft lumbo-sacral support is usually added. Modern leg-holders are a major advance over earlier mechanisms. The position of the legs must be carefully secured in a comfortable position with some antithrombotic prophylaxis, such as thrombo-embolic disease stockings (TEDS).

Special care must be taken not to over-stretch joints, including those of the spine, or to cause any neuropathy by compression or stretching. The obturator, femoral, sciatic and common peroneal nerves, as well as the lumbosacral plexus, are all potentially at risk. The risk is increased by prolonged duration in this position and by a thin body habitus.

The leg supports should be as low as possible and tilted slightly outwards, if appropriate, during the lithotomy position. The arms cannot be placed by the side when using this position because the hands will be endangered. They should be spread out on arm-boards or folded loosely across the abdomen. Lowering the legs at the end of the procedure should be performed simultaneously and slowly.

If a sit-up (modified Fowler's) position is used, extra support under the buttocks and the small of the back is required. Sciatic nerve damage from pressure and air embolism are potential hazards of this position. The head will require extra support, and hyper-extension of the shoulder region must be avoided. Thrombo-embolic stockings or intermittent compression should be used to facilitate venous return.

Prone position

The prone position poses extra risks of access and function of general anaesthesia. Careful pre-operative assessment is necessary. Gradual pooling of blood in the lower extremities may lead to hypotension, but this problem can be minimized by the use of compressive stockings. Temperature control may also be a problem.

Pillow support beneath the chest and hips is necessary to allow free abdominal diaphragmatic movement and to protect female breasts and male genitalia. Specially designed support frames may be used instead. The arms are brought down and forward to rest on arm-boards with the elbows comfortably flexed and the hands pronated. Padding is placed under the ankles.

The jackknife (Kraske) position is a modification of the prone position and is used for some anorectal procedures. The patient is flexed at the hips with the bottom up, and much of the weight is borne by the knees. A small pad beneath each shoulder will protect the brachial plexus, and some padding will be needed beneath the shins and ankles as well as the knees.

Lateral position

If the lateral position is used, the patient is placed on the unaffected side and supported on that side by padding of various types, including air-mattresses. Modern visco-elastic materials are also very useful. Care must be taken to establish comfortable alignment and to avoid over-stretching of the body or limbs in any direction.

Care must be taken to secure the unconscious patient, and sufficient staff should be available to perform the tasks smoothly and safely. One pillow is placed under the patient's head and another is placed beneath their legs, with the bottom leg flexed at the hip and knee and the top leg straight or slightly flexed. It is very important to pad the lateral side of the bottom knee, to avoid pressure on the peroneal nerve.

The lateral position is usually well tolerated, but cardiovascular changes can occur, as can compressive injuries to nerves and skin overlying bony prominences.

For surgery on the kidney, for example, the contra-lateral loin should be over the break in the table. The bridge (kidney rest) can be used and the bed flexed so that the space between the twelfth rib and the iliac crest is opened up.

The lateral chest position allows good access to the thoracic cavity. The arm on that side is supported by a special arm-rest and raised above the head. The lower shoulder is brought slightly forward to prevent pressure on the brachial plexus, and the arm is flexed at the elbow.

The torso needs to be stabilized by padding and strapping, which are placed so that respiratory movement is not impaired and surgical access is not compromised.

There are many other variations of positions and devices available for specific procedures. For example, the orthopaedic fracture table allows the patient to be well positioned for hip fracture surgery and for closed femoral nailing. The patient is positioned supine with the pelvis stabilized against a vertical perineal post, and well padded to avoid pressure on the genitalia and injury to the pudendal nerves. Traction is achieved by restraining the injured leg in a well-padded boot-like device to protect the foot and ankle. The lower limb may be manipulated safely with this mechanism, and it allows good access for taking X-rays.

PNEUMATIC TOURNIQUETS

Pneumatic tourniquets are often used on the extremities to facilitate operating in a relatively bloodless field. The limb is initially exsanguinated by elevating it and then usually by applying either some form of rubber bandaging (e.g. an Esmarc bandage) or using a compressive sleeve before inflating a previously applied tourniquet with compressed gas or air.

Most modern tourniquets are controlled by a microprocessor for regulation of pressure and time applied, and have auditory and visual feedback.

There are certain relative and other absolute contraindications to their use, including the compartment syndrome, peripheral vascular disease, hypertension and McArdle's syndrome.

The time of application is important. As a rough guide, the tourniquet should not be applied to the upper limb for more than 1 h and to the lower limb for more than 1.5 h.

The cuff should be over a minimum width of 7.5 cm and a maximum of 15 cm and should be positioned to avoid pinching skinfolds. The equipment should be checked regularly to ensure accurate function. The pressure of the tourniquet during its active use should be 50 mmHg above the recorded systolic blood pressure for the upper limb and 100 mmHg above that level for the lower limb.

ELECTROSURGERY

Modern electrosurgical units provide considerable scope for cutting tissues and for the coagulation of blood vessels and raw surfaces. Bipolar units offer precise coagulation ability with more precise protection of adjacent structures as required, for example, in neurosurgery. All such units can be dangerous both for the user and for the patient. The equipment must be correctly installed, used and maintained with regular checks of safety aspects.

The patient's skin must be assessed before and after usage, particularly at positional pressure points and at the point of application of the dispersive pad (earthing electrode).

After positioning of the patient, the earthing pad should be applied to a clean, dry, hairless region. It should be as close to the operation site as is reasonable, and overlie a large muscle bulk, if possible, avoiding bony prominences, pressure points, skin over metal prostheses and scar tissue. Most earthing pads require a gel to facilitate conduction. Placement should be even across the entire surface of the pad.

The active electrodiathermy (usually a pencil) should be placed in a well-insulated quiver when not in use, and power settings should be kept as low as possible for each particular procedure. The settings should be confirmed orally by the circulating nurse before activation.

The current is dispered through the body by the active electrode via the earthing electrode and back to the power source. If there is a fault in the system, the current can travel via alternative pathways and cause burns at points of contact. If the electrocoagulation is ineffective at normal settings, then there is probably a fault in the electrical circuit. Some modern electrosurgical units have a patient-monitoring system which increases efficiency and safety.

If an ECG monitor is being used, the electrodes should be placed as far away as possible from the operation site. Care must also be taken in patients with indwelling cardiac pacemakers or similar electrical devices. Modern pacemakers have protective mechanisms, but the use of diathermy equipment will be contraindicated in some instances.

WOUND CARE

This subject has been discussed in Chapter 34.5. The only additional point to emphasize is the need to protect pre-existing wounds on patients as they are being transferred to and from the operating room, and while they are being positioned on the operating table.

The revolution in minimally invasive surgery has highlighted the degree to which the surgical wound contributes towards the morbidity of each operation, and these wounds must be treated with great care and gentleness in order to reduce the impact of surgical trauma.

TEMPERATURE CONTROL

It is becoming increasingly apparent that temperature control during operations is of major importance. Hypothermia can readily occur peri-operatively because of the inhibition of thermoregulation by anaesthetic agents, and exposure of the patient to a cool environment when there is an absence of voluntary corrective measures because of the unconscious state. Hypothermia may lead to many complications, including coagulopathy, morbid cardiac events and a decreased resistance to surgical wound infections.

There is evidence that the threshold for response to warmth (sweating and active vasodilatation) normally exceeds the threshold for the first defence against cold (vasoconstriction) by only 0.2°C in core temperature. This precision of thermoregulatory control is similar in men and women but declines in the elderly.

Anaesthetics inhibit thermoregulation, primarily centrally, in a dose-dependent manner, and inhibit vasoconstriction and shivering about three times as much as they inhibit sweating. General anaesthetics raise warmth response thresholds in linear proportion to increased dosages. They widen the inter-threshold range to a value of approximately 20 times the normal range, and consequently the anaesthetized patient is poikilothermic with their body temperature determined by the environment over a temperature range of about 4°C in core temperature.

During general anaesthesia, there is a redistribution of body heat from the core to the periphery, resulting in a decline in core temperature during the first hour of 1–1.5°C, whilst the loss of heat to the environment during this period is relatively small. After the first hour, with vasodilatation in the skin, heat is lost to the environment, 90% of this loss occurring through the surface of the skin, with radiation and convection (usually) contributing far more of the loss than conduction or evaporation.

After 3 to 5 h of anaesthesia, the core temperature often stops decreasing, especially if the patient is well insulated or warmed. If the patient is sufficiently hypothermic, the halt in core temperature decline is due to thermoregulatory vasoconstriction, but the mean body temperature and the total heat content continue to decrease, and may reach dangerously low levels, with the core temperature decline being insufficient to trigger shivering.

Regional anaesthetics impair both peripheral and (indirectly) central thermoregulation, and hypothermia is therefore common in patients who have spinal or epidural anaesthetics. The core temperature can drop significantly even though the patient does not usually feel cold. Most of the body heat loss is caused by the peripheral inhibition of thermoregulatory vasoconstriction.

There are some operations where there is a definite advantage in reducing the core temperature. Cardiac surgery performed at around 28°C does offer some protection to the myocardium and central nervous system. Reduced temperatures may have advantages during operations where cerebral ischaemia is a definite risk, such as carotid endarterectomy and neurosurgery. Core temperatures near 34°C also appear to aid recovery from adult respiratory distress syndrome.

However, there are significant disadvantages to even mild hypothermia. There is a reduction in resistance to surgical wound infection as a result of decreasing cutaneous blood flow (thereby reducing oxygenation of tissues), directly impaired immune function (especially oxidative killing by neutrophils) and decreased collagen synthesis.

Mild hypothermia may decrease coagulation function and increase blood loss. Core hypothermia of 1.5°C causes a threefold increase in the incidence of ventricular arrhythmias and morbid cardiac events.

There are a number of measures which nurses, anaesthetists and surgeons can take to reduce heat loss during operations. The ambient temperature of the operating room should be maintained in the range 22–25°C, above which it may be too uncomfortable whilst working beneath the hot operating lights. Infusion of cold fluids can significantly decrease the body temperature, and such fluids (especially in major and prolonged cases), should be warmed to about 37°C. Inhaled gases should be humidified, although less than 10% of metabolic heat loss is through respiration. Insulated mattresses (sometimes warmed), surgical drapes, blankets or modern insulating sheets are useful, and forced air-warming systems for prolonged operations, especially when these are performed on the elderly or other high-risk groups, can be invaluable. The objective is to maintain the core temperature at about 36°C.

The surgeon can also assist by performing the operation expeditiously, avoiding prolonged exposure of bowel, using warm lavage fluids, and limiting fluid soaking of the drapes.

If the core temperature can be maintained, then a smoother, more comfortable and safe post-operative period will ensue, and the period of hospitalization should not be prolonged.

FURTHER READING

Martin JT, Warner MA. 1997: *Positioning in anaesthesia and surgery*, 3rd edn. Philadelphia, PA: W.B. Saunders.

Meeker MH, Rothrock JC (eds). 1995: *Alexander's care of the patient in surgery*, 10th edn. St Louis, MO: Mosby.

Sessler DI. 1997: Mild perioperative hypothermia. *New England Journal of Medicine* **336**, 1730–7.

Sutures, staples and knots

William E.G. Thomas

Introduction

Following any operative procedure, careful approximation of the tissues will allow healing to occur as long as there is no tension and a good blood supply is present. The method for the approximation of the tissue edges varies depending on the site and tissue concerned, but for cen- turies the mainstay of such approximation has been the suture. Other methods have now become available, such as 'Steristrips', tissue glue, clips and staples, but the suture with its many forms and characteristics remains the predominant method for wound closure.

SUTURES

There is no such product as the ideal suture. Surgeons have sought to define certain characteristics that are highly desirable, including the following:

- easy to handle;
- secure knotting;
- predictable tensile strength and performance;
- sterile;
- should not shrink in the tissues;
- pulls through tissues easily;
- non-electrolytic;
- non-capillary;
- non-allergenic;
- non-carcinogenic;
- does not promote tissue reaction or infection;
- inexpensive.

There is no suture material that will fulfil all of these cri- teria, and furthermore certain procedures place specific requirements on suture material (e.g. vascular anasto- moses require a smooth, non-absorbable suture mater- ial, while gastric anastomoses require an absorbable material). For absorbable sutures, the length of time needed for wound support varies in different tissues (e.g. subcutaneous tissues or muscular aponeuroses). Therefore, in closing any wound the surgeon needs to define clearly the requirements for closure, bearing in mind the tissues involved, and then to select the suture material and method of suturing that will most effec- tively achieve the desired objective.

SUTURE MATERIALS

For any suture material the following characteristics need to be considered:

- physical nature;
- strength;
- tensile behaviour;
- absorbability;
- biological behaviour.

Physical nature

Suture material can be monofilament or multifilament. A monofilament suture such as polypropylene (Prolene®) is smooth and slides well in the tissues, but requires very careful knotting techniques. Furthermore, it can be easily damaged by gripping it with the needle holder or forceps. Such damage can predispose towards fracture of the suture. Multifilament sutures, or braided materials, are more rough on the tissues and have a surface area several thousand times that of monofilament sutures, resulting in capillary action and the potential for the interstices of the braided material to become colonized with bacteria. However, such sutures are easy to handle and have good knotting qualities.

Strength

The strength of a suture depends on its thickness, the material of which it is made, and its behaviour in the tissues. Manufacturers classify suture thickness according to diameter in tenths of a millimetre. However, the figure assigned to each suture is also dependent on the nature of the material (Table 34.8.1). It is also important to recognize that loss of tensile strength and mass absorption are two separate events, in that a suture may support the wound for only a few days but it may remain as a foreign body for a much longer period. The *ideal* suture, which would disappear

Table 34.8.1 Suture sizes

Metric number (diameter of suture in tenths of a mm)	Catgut	Non-absorbable
0.2	–	10/0
0.3	–	9/0
0.4	–	8/0
0.5	8/0	7/0
0.7	7/0	6/0
1	6/0	5/0
1.5	5/0	4/0
2	4/0	3/0
3	3/0	2/0
3.5	2/0	0
4	0	1
5	1	2
6	2	3 + 4
7	3	5
8	4	6

completely as soon as its work was done, does not yet exist. Even for non-absorbable sutures, strength is not always constant. Although these materials do not absorb, those of biological origin (e.g. silk) lose strength without initially showing any change in the mass of the suture, and even fragment over time. However, other non-absorbable materials, especially those of synthetic origin, never lose tensile strength and do not change in mass in the tissues. These materials are particularly useful in cases where permanence is required (e.g. vascular anastomosis).

Tensile behaviour

Some suture materials have more plastic characteristics, while other may be more elastic. Deformability and flexibility are important for ease of handling, while many of the synthetic materials demonstrate 'memory', i.e. they keep curling up in the pattern in which they were packaged. A sharp but gentle pull on the material helps to diminish this memory. More memory results in less knot security. Thus knotting also plays a role in a suture's tensile strength, and it is important to note that most sutures lose 50% of their strength at the knot.

Absorbability

Suture materials tend to be either absorbable or non-absorbable. Absorbable sutures provide temporary wound support over a period of time, but this period depends on the nature of the material (Table 34.8.2). Man-made, non-absorbable sutures tend to maintain their strength indefinitely, but natural protein materials such as silk, although officially classified as non-absorbable, lose most of their tensile strength in about 1 year, fragment and usually cannot be found after 2–3 years.

Biological behaviour

The biological behaviour of a suture in tissues depends on the origin of the raw materials. Man-made or synthetic materials are more predictable, elicit minimal tissue reaction and tend to be inert, which is an important non-carcinogenic property. Biological or natural sutures tend to produce a much greater tissue reaction, and can cause local irritation and even rejection. The handling of the suture materials by the body also varies, with absorption taking place by proteolysis (enzymic activity) for substances such as catgut, and by hydrolysis for materials such as glycolide and lactide. Such activity is rendered even more unpredictable in the presence of infection, urine or faeces.

NEEDLES

In the past, needles had eyes in them and suture material had to be loaded into these, which was not only time-consuming, but also meant that the needle holes in tissues were

Table 34.8.2 Suture characteristic

Suture	Trade name	Type	Raw material	Tensile strength
Plain catgut	–	Absorbable monofilament	Purified animal intestines (sheep or beef)	At least 21 days
Chromic catgut	–	Absorbable monofilament	Purified animal intestines (sheep or beef)	At least 28 days
Glycolide and lactide	Coated Vicryl (Polyglactin 910)	Absorbable braided, coated	Copolymer of lactide and glycolide coated with polyglactin 370 and calcium stearate	28 days
Glycolide and lactide	Vicryl *rapide* (Polyglactin 910)	Absorbable braided, coated	Copolymer of lactide and glycolide coated with polyglactin 370 and calcium stearate	10–14 days
Glycolide	Dexon	Absorbable braided, coated	Polymer of glycolic acid	30 days
Polydioxanone	PDS II (Polydioxanone)	Absorbable monofilament	Man-made polymer	56 days
Poliglecaprone	Monocryl	Absorbable monofilament	Copolymer of glycolide and caprolactone	21 days
Silk	Mersilk	Non-absorbable braided	Natural protein fibre of raw silk spun by silk-worm	Loses most or all in about 1 year
Polyester	Mersilene Ethibond	Non-absorbable braided	Man-made	Indefinite
Braided polyamide	Nurolon Surgilon	Non-absorbable braided	Polyamide polymer	Loses 15–20% per year
Monofilament polyamide	Ethilon	Non-absorbable monofilament	Polyamide polymer	Loses 15–20% per year
Polypropylene	Prolene	Non-absorbable monofilament	Polymer of propylene	Indefinite

considerably larger than the suture material being used. Currently needles are eyeless or 'atraumatic', with the suture material being embedded within the shank of the needle. The needle has three main parts (Figure 34.8.1):

1. shank;
2. body;
3. point.

The needle should be grasped by the needle-holder approximately one-third of the way back from the rear of the needle, avoiding both the shank and the point.

The body of the needle is either round, triangular or flattened. Round-bodied needles gradually taper to a point, while triangular needles have cutting edges along all three sides. The actual point of the needle can be

Table 34.8.2 *(Continued)*

Mass absorption rate	Contraindications	Frequent uses
By 90 days	Should not be used in tissues that heal slowly and require support	Ligation; subcutaneous and other fast-healing tissues; ophthalmology
By 90 days	Being absorbable, should not be used where prolonged approximation of tissues under stress is required	Ligation; ophthalmology
56–70 days	Being absorbable, should not be used where prolonged approximation of tissues under stress is required	Ligation or suturing of tissues where absorbable suture is desirable, except where approximation under stress is required; ophthalmology
42 days	Should not be used in tissues that heal slowly and require support beyond 7 days	For closure of skin and mucosa (e.g. minor surgery, paediatric surgery, perineal repair, oral mucosa, scalp wounds, wounds under plaster
60–90 days	Being absorbable, should not be used where prolonged approximation of tissues under stress is required	Ligation or suturing of tissues where absorbable suture is desirable, except where approximation under stress is required
180 days	Being absorbable, should not be used where prolonged approximation of tissues under stress is required	Abdominal and thoracic closure; subcutaneous tissue; colon and rectal surgery
90–120 days	Should not be used in neural tissue, cardiovascular tissue, microsurgery, ophthalmology (except strabismus) or where extended support is required	Subcuticular skin ligation; gastrointestinal, muscle
Usually cannot be found after about 2 years	Should not be used for placement of vascular prostheses or artificial heart valves	Most body tissues for ligation and suturing; general surgery; ophthalmology
Non-absorbable; remains encapsulated in body tissues	None	Cardiovascular; general surgery; retention
Degrades at a rate of about 15–20% per year	None	Most body tissues for ligating and suturing; general closure; neurosurgery
Degrades at a rate of about 15–20% per year	None	Skin closure; retention; plastic surgery, ophthalmology
Non-absorbable; remains encapsulated in body tissues	None	General surgery; plastic surgery; cardiovascular; skin closure, ophthalmology

round with a tapered end, *conventional cutting* with the cutting edge facing the inside of the needle's curvature, or *reversed cutting* with the cutting edge on the outside. Round-bodied needles are designed to separate tissue fibres rather than to cut through them, and are commonly used in intestinal and cardiovascular surgery. Cutting needles are used when tough or dense tissue needs to be sutured (e.g. skin and fascia). Blunt-ended needles are now being advocated in certain situations such as closure of the abdominal wall, in order to reduce the risk of needlestick injuries in this era of virally transmitted disorders.

The choice of needle shape tends to be dictated by the accessibility of the tissues to be sutured, and the more confined the operative space, the more curved is the ideal

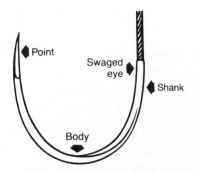

Figure 34.8.1 Parts of an atraumatic suture needle.

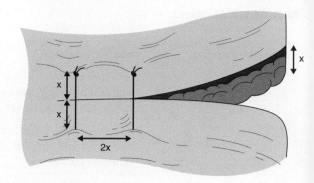

Figure 34.8.2 The principles of interrupted sutures.

needle. Straight needles may be used on skin, while half-circle needles are commonly utilized in the gastrointestinal tract. 'J'-shaped needles, quarter-circle needles and compound-curvature needles are used in special situations such as the vagina, eye and oral cavity, respectively. The size of the needle tends to correspond to the gauge of the suture material, although it is possible to obtain similar sutures with differing needle sizes.

SUTURE TECHNIQUES

There are four frequently used suture techniques:

1. interrupted sutures;
2. continuous sutures;
3. mattress sutures;
4. subcuticular sutures.

Interrupted sutures

Interrupted sutures require the needle to be inserted at right angles to the tissue and pass through both aspects of the suture line and exit at right angles, taking care not to drag the needle through the tissues, but to follow the curve of the needle. As a guide, the distance from the entry point to the edge of the wound should be approximately equal to the thickness of the tissue being sutured, and successive sutures should be placed at twice this distance apart (i.e. approximately double the thickness of the tissues) (Figure 34.8.2). All sutures should be placed at right angles to the wound, the same distance apart, and each suture should reach into the depth of the wound.

Continuous sutures

Continuous sutures should be inserted in an identical manner to interrupted sutures but, after tying the first suture, the rest of the sutures are inserted in a continuous manner until the far end of the wound is reached. The suture material should then be knotted either using an Aberdeen knot or tying the free end to the loop of the last suture inserted. In order to maintain a constant tension along the wound, it is vital to have an assistant who

can 'follow' the suture, keeping it at the correct tension at all times. If this does not occur, then there is a danger either of 'purse-stringing' the suture, or of leaving the suture line too lax. There is a greater risk of producing too much tension by using too little suture length than of leaving the suture line too lax. Post-operative oedema will often take up any slack.

Mattress sutures

Mattress sutures may be either vertical or horizontal (Figure 34.8.3). They may be useful in awkward sites or for ensuring eversion or inversion of a wound edge. They appose the wound edges accurately, but should not be tied too tightly. The initial suture is placed as for an interrupted suture, but then the needle should be reversed in the needle-holder and the needle taken back either vertical to the previous traverse or horizontal to it and then ligated.

Subcuticular sutures

When the wound edges can be approximated easily with no tension, then a subcuticular suture results in a very

(a)

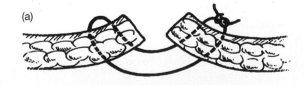

(b)

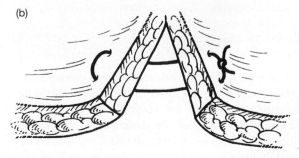

Figure 34.8.3 Mattress sutures: (a) vertical and (b) horizontal.

neat scar. The suture material may be absorbable or non-absorbable and, depending on the material used, the initial fixation at one end of the wound is by means of either beads for non-absorbable sutures or a buried knot for absorbable sutures. Small bites of the subcuticular tissues are taken on alternate sides of the wound (Figure 34.8.4), and are then pulled gently together and fixed at the far end either by a further crushed bead, or by a 'Z' sequence of passes of the needle.

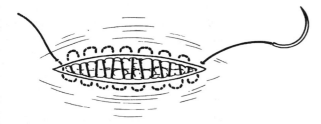

Figure 34.8.4 Subcuticular suture.

OTHER TECHNIQUES

Steristrips

An alternative to skin sutures consists of self-adhesive tapes or 'Steristrips'. These cannot be used if there is any tension on a wound or if there is significant moisture. However, they are very suitable for superficial lacerations of the face and fingers. It is vital that good adhesion is achieved on application of the strips, and this may be enhanced by painting the skin with Tincture benzoin compound prior to applying the strips. When using such strips on the fingers or toes, it is important to ensure that the digit is not encircled entirely, to avoid producing a tourniquet effect.

Tissue adhesive

Tissues adhesives or 'glue' are now available and tend to be based on a solution of *n*-butyl-2-cyanoacrylate monomer. When applied to a wound, this material rapidly polymerizes, forming a firm and adhesive bond. The wound should be clean, dry and able to be approximated without tension. The wound edges should be approximated accurately *before* applying the adhesive, as the polymerization is very rapid and mistakes can occur.

STAPLES

Staples tend to be made of stainless steel and thus confer the advantages of high tensile strength combined with low tissue reaction. They can either be applied individually as for skin closure, or form part of a stapling device that can be used to fashion an anastomosis during either open or laparoscopic surgery.

CLIPS

Skin clips produce a very neat scar with good wound eversion and a minimal cross-hatching effect. They can be placed faster than suture insertion, and have a lower predisposition to infection, as they do not penetrate entirely through the wound and do not produce a complete track from one wound edge to the other. However, they can be uncomfortable for the patient, and they require a special instrument to remove them. Furthermore, they tend to be a more expensive method for wound closure than simple suture techniques.

STAPLING DEVICES

Stapling devices are widely used, particularly in the gastrointestinal tract. They usually apply two rows of staples, offset in relation to each other to produce a sound anastomosis. Many of them also divide the bowel or tissue that has been stapled, while other devices merely insert the staples and the bowel has to be divided separately. For all stapling devices it is crucial that the surgeon understands the principles of each device and has a detailed knowledge of the mechanism and function of the instrument.

End-to-end anastomoses (EEA)

Circular stapling devices allow tubes to be joined together, and such instruments are commonly used in the oesophagus and lower rectum. The detached stapling head/anvil is introduced into one end of the bowel, usually being secured within it by means of a purse-string suture. The body of the device is then inserted into the other end of the bowel, either via the rectum for a low rectal anastomosis, or via an enterotomy for an oesophago-jejunostomy, and the shaft is either extended through a small opening in the bowel wall or secured by a further purse-string suture. The head/anvil is re-attached to the shaft and the two ends are approximated. Once the device is fully closed, as indicated by the green indicator in the window, the device is fired, and after unwinding three half turns the stapler is gently withdrawn. It is important to assess the integrity of the anastomosis by examining the 'doughnuts' of tissue excised for completeness. It is essential that no extraneous tissue is allowed to become interposed between the two bowel walls on closing the stapler.

Transverse anastomoses (TA)

These instruments, which are available in different sizes, simply provide two rows of staples for a single transverse anastomosis. They are useful for closing bowel ends, and the larger sizes have been used to create gastric tubes and gastric partitioning, etc. One important technical point is that the bowel should be divided before the instrument is reopened after firing, as the instrument is designed with a ridge along which to pass a scalpel to ensure that the correct length of cuff of bowel remains adjacent to the staple line. Down in the pelvis it may be helpful to use such a device with a movable head (roticulator).

Intraluminal anastomoses (IA)

These instruments have two limbs which can be detached. Each limb is introduced into a loop of bowel, the limbs are reassembled and the device is closed. On firing, two rows of staples are inserted on either side of the divided bowel, the division occurring by means of a built in blade that is activated at the same time as the insertion of the staples. Such an instrument may be used to fashion a gastro-jejunostomy or jejuno-jejunostomy, and is also used in ileal pouch formation.

Other devices

Other devices are available that will staple/ligate and divide blood vessels. Skin closure may also be undertaken using hand-held stapling devices rather than individually picking up staples/clips and inserting them as described above. Many of the intestinal stapling devices are now adapted to be inserted down cannulas during laparoscopic surgery, and although they look very different, the principles of function are identical to the open-surgery variety.

KNOTS

Knot tying is one of the most fundamental techniques in surgery, and yet is often poorly performed. The principles behind a knot are poorly understood by many surgeons, and sadly a poorly constructed knot may therefore jeopardize an otherwise successful surgical procedure. The general principles behind knot tying are as follows.

- The knot must be tied firmly but without strangulating the tissues.

- The knot must be unable to slip or unravel.

- The knot must be as small as possible to minimize the amount of foreign material.

- The knot must be tightened without exerting any tension or pressure on the tissues being ligated (i.e. the knot should be bedded down carefully, only exerting pressure against counter-pressure from the index finger or thumb).

- During tying, the suture material must not be 'sawed', as this weakens the thread.

- The suture material must be laid properly during tying, otherwise tension during tightening may cause breakage or fracture of the thread.

- When tying an instrument knot, the thread should

only be grasped at the free end, as gripping the thread with artery forceps or needle-holders can damage the material and again result in breakage or fracture.

- The standard surgical knot is the reef knot, with a third throw for security.

THE REEF KNOT

A standard reef knot may be tied using two hands, in a similar manner to tying shoe-laces, but most surgeons find it more flexible and versatile to use the one-handed technique.

The one-handed reef knot technique

1. Hold the end of the short end of the suture between the thumb and middle finger of the left hand with the loop over the extended index finger (Figure 34.8.5a). Hold the remainder of the suture material with the right hand.

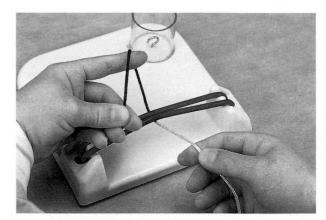

Figure 34.8.5(a)

2. Bring the remainder of the suture material in the right hand over the left index finger by moving the right hand away from the operator (Figure 34.8.5b).

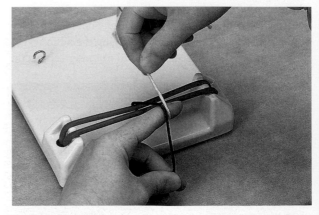

Figure 34.8.5(b)

3. Use the distal phalanx of the left index finger to pass under the thread held in the left hand in preparation for pulling it through the loop (Figure 34.8.5c).

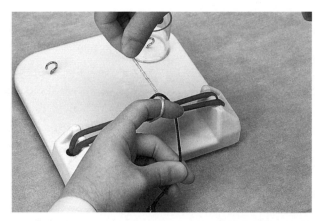

Figure 34.8.5(c)

4. Pull the thread through and complete the throw by drawing the left hand towards the operator and the right hand away from the operator (Figure 34.8.5d).

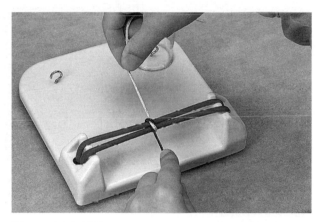

Figure 34.8.5(d)

5. Continue to hold the short end of suture in the left hand between the thumb and index finger, looping the thread around the other three fingers (Figure 34.8.5e).

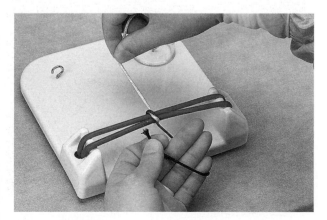

Figure 34.8.5(e)

6. Bring the strand held in the right hand across towards the operator to cross the left-handed thread as shown (Figure 34.8.5f).

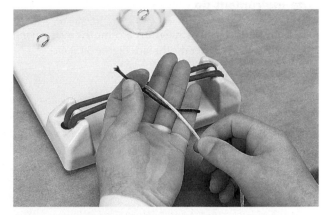

Figure 34.8.5(f)

7. Use the distal phalanx of the left middle finger to bring the left-handed strand under the right-handed strand (Figure 34.8.5g).

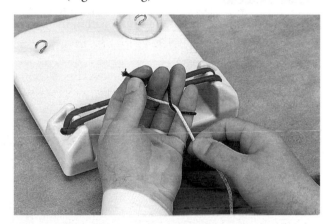

Figure 34.8.5(g)

8. Bring the strand through and then tighten it by drawing the right hand towards the operator and the left hand away from the operator.

9. On completion of the reef knot, the classical pattern of the knot can be clearly seen (Figure 34.8.5h).

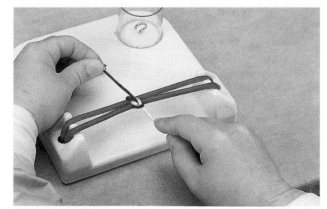

Figure 34.8.5(h)

10. For security, another index finger throw is usually applied.

The instrument tie

1. Loop the long end of the suture around the instrument, which is placed over the thread (Figure 34.8.6a).

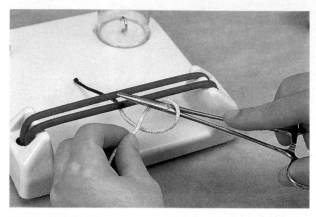

Figure 34.8.6(a)

2. Grasp the short end of the suture within the jaws of the instrument (Figure 34.8.6b).

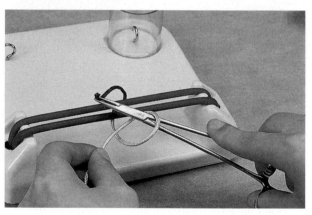

Figure 34.8.6(b)

3. Complete the first hitch (Figure 34.8.6c).

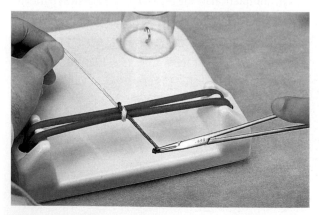

Figure 34.8.6(c)

4. Now form a loop around the instrument, this time with the instrument placed under the thread (Figure 34.8.6d).

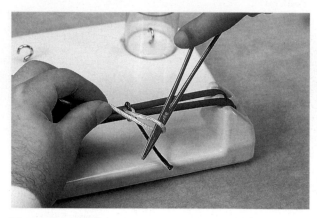

Figure 34.8.6(d)

5. Grasp the short end again within the jaws of the instrument (Figure 34.8.6e).

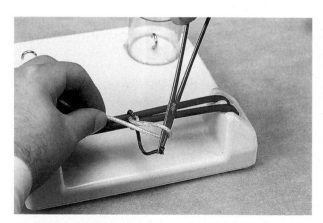

Figure 34.8.6(e)

6. Pull through to complete the classical reef knot (Figure 34.8.6f).

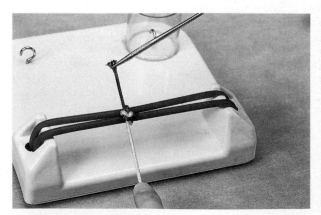

Figure 34.8.6(f)

The 'Aberdeen' knot

1. This knot is useful when, having finished a continuous suture, you are left with a loop and a free end (Figure 34.8.7a).

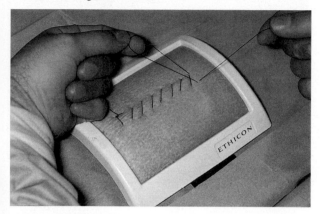

Figure 34.8.7(a)

2. Holding the loop open with your left hand (Figure 34.8.7b), grasp the free end between the thumb and

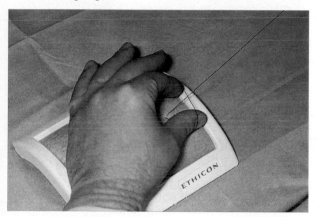

Figure 34.8.7(b)

index finger and pull it through the loop (Figure 34.8.7c). Tighten by pulling on the thread, thus

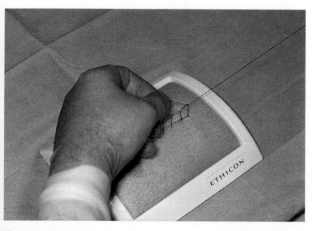

Figure 34.8.7(c)

eliminating the old loop. Keep hold of the free end, thus creating a further loop (Figure 34.8.7d).

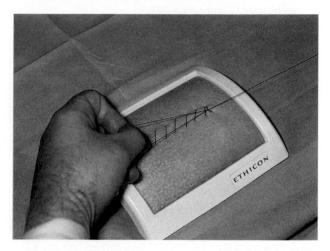

Figure 34.8.7(d)

3. Repeat this exercise six times.
4. Finally, pull the free end through entirely (Figure 34.8.7e)

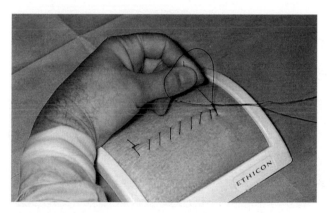

Figure 34.8.7(e)

and tighten down (34.8.7f).

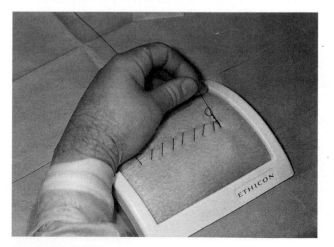

Figure 34.8.7(f)

The surgeon's knot

1. A single throw is placed using a one- or two-handed technique (Figure 34.8.8a).

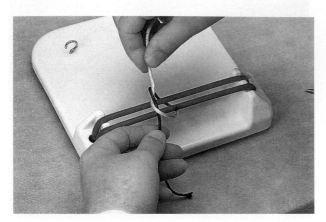

Figure 34.8.8(a)

2. A further throw is placed in the same manner (Figure 34.8.8b).

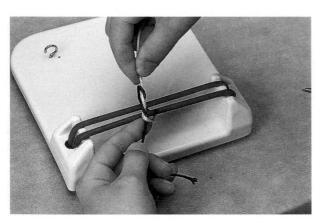

Figure 34.8.8(b)

3. The double throw is tightened in a conventional manner (Figure 34.8.8c).

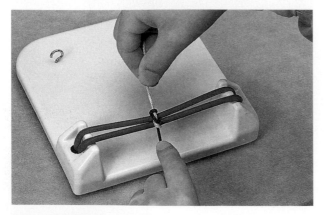

Figure 34.8.8(c)

4. A further throw is now fashioned in the same manner as for a reef knot (Figure 34.8.8d), but is not tightened.

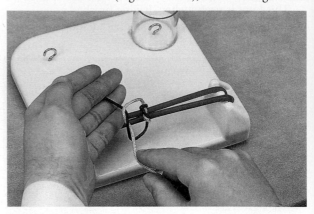

Figure 34.8.8(d)

5. A similar throw is again fashioned, producing a double throw as before (Figure 34.8.8e).

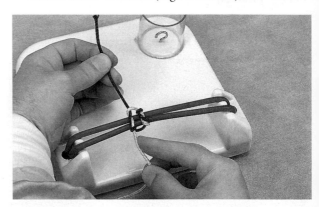

Figure 34.8.8(e)

6. The double throw is now tightened. The result may not look very pretty, but is very secure as long as the final throw is tightened as horizontally as possible.

Tying at depth

1. The thread should be placed around the object to be ligated with the right index finger or using an instrument such as a haemostat (Figure 34.8.9a).

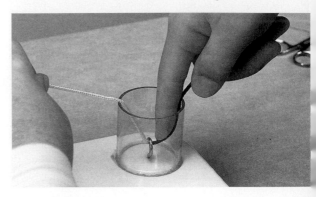

Figure 34.8.9(a)

2. Fashion a classical throw for a reef knot on the surface (Figure 34.8.9b).

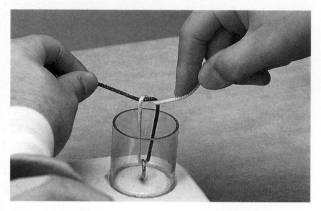

Figure 34.8.9(b)

3. Advance the knot down into the cavity using the right index finger (Figure 34.8.9c).

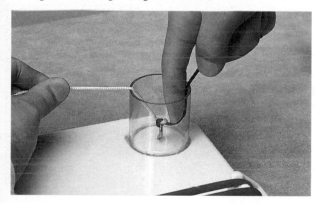

Figure 34.8.9(c)

4. Snug the knot down using tension on the long strand against the index finger of the right hand, ensuring that no tension exists on the structure being ligated.

5. Fashion a further throw on the surface in the manner of a reef knot (Figure 34.8.9d).

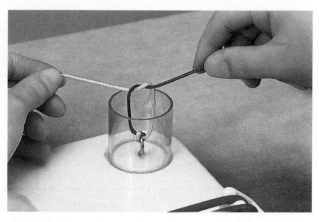

Figure 34.8.9(d)

6. Advance into the cavity and snug down with the right index finger as before (Figure 34.8.9e).

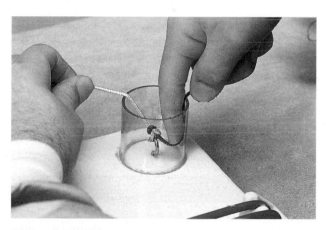

Figure 34.8.9(e)

FURTHER READING

Brown JS. 1997: *Minor surgery*. London: Chapman & Hall Medical.

Kirk RM. 1994: *Basic surgical techniques*. Edinburgh: Churchill Livingstone.

ACKNOWLEDGEMENTS

The illustrations are reproduced from the participants handbook of the Basic Surgical Skills Course with kind permission of the Royal College of Surgeons of England and Ethicon Limited.

Diathermy

Raja L.A. Jayaweera

Introduction

Diathermy is the use of electricity to cut, coagulate, incise, divide or otherwise deal with tissues during operative surgery. 'Diathermy', a term coined by Nagelschmidt around 1910, literally means 'heat goes through'. However, in the context of its use in surgery this is terminologically incorrect, for it is the *current* that goes through the body. The heat produced is confined to the site of application of the electrosurgical instrument. Nevertheless, the use of the term is hallowed by tradition, and it may legitimately be so employed as long as the physical phenomenon of the process is correctly understood.

CAUTERY

Another related term that must be clearly understood is 'cautery' as, for instance, in the phrase 'cautery to cervix'. Here, too, as in diathermy, the electric current (in this case a DC current) is made to produce heat to 'treat' tissues. However, in contrast to diathermy, the current does not enter the body and therefore the latter does not form part of the electrical pathway. It is the heat alone that impinges on the body tissue, the electrical current being confined to the conducting cable (Figure 35.1.1a).

PHYSICS OF DIATHERMY

If ordinary AC mains current, at a frequency of 50–60 Hz, is passed through the human body, certain effects can occur, ranging from the minor and almost imperceptible to the extremely dangerous or indeed fatal. The nature of the effects depends on the strength of the current (see Table 35.1.1).

An increase in the frequency of the mains alternating current will lead to a progressive decrease in the electrical effects *per se* of the current on the human body, and at higher frequencies (400 kHz – 3 MHz) the effects are those of heating alone (see Table 35.1.2). However, if the frequency is increased further to 4 MHz or higher, phenomena such as 'capacitive coupling' and 'inductance' may occur, which can reintroduce the harmful effects of electricity by inducing potentially dangerous currents in

Table 35.1.1 Effects of mains current (50–60 Hz) on the human body

1 mA	Threshold of perception
5 mA	Pain
15 mA	'Let-go' current, severe pain
50 mA	Respiratory muscle spasm (death from asphyxia)
80–100 mA	Ventricular fibrillation (death from myocardial failure)
> 1A	Sustained myocardial contraction (death from cardiac asystole)

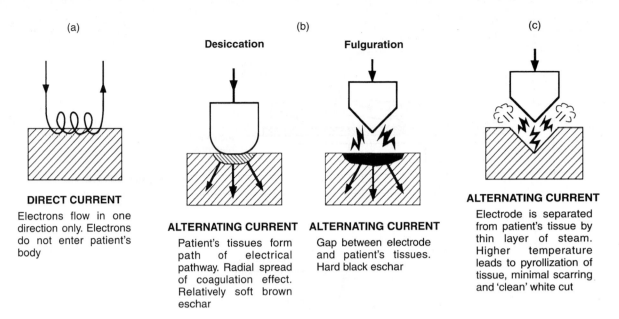

(a)

DIRECT CURRENT

Electrons flow in one direction only. Electrons do not enter patient's body

(b)

Desiccation

ALTERNATING CURRENT

Patient's tissues form path of electrical pathway. Radial spread of coagulation effect. Relatively soft brown eschar

Fulguration

ALTERNATING CURRENT

Gap between electrode and patient's tissues. Hard black eschar

(c)

ALTERNATING CURRENT

Electrode is separated from patient's tissue by thin layer of steam. Higher temperature leads to pyrollization of tissue, minimal scarring and 'clean' white cut

Figure 35.1.1 Modalities of thermal ablation of tissues. (a) Cautery. (b) Coagulation. (c) Cutting.

all nearby conductive objects, even though they may not be in physical contiguity with the high-frequency current cable. Therefore, by confining the frequency of the current to the 'intermediate' range of 0.4–3 MHz, the benefits of 'burning' can be obtained without the harmful effects of 'electrocution'.

When an electric current is passed through a poor conductor, energy is lost (in the form of heat) as the current attempts to overcome the resistance of its pathway. This leads to heat production and a rise in temperature. The amount of heat produced is equal to the resistance multiplied by the square of the current (watt-seconds = ohms × amperes^2). The amount of heat generated at the site of application of the diathermy point depends on 'current density', i.e. the current flow per unit area, which in turn depends on the resistivity of the tissues (see Table 35.1.3).

DIATHERMY MACHINE: 'GROUNDED' AND 'ISOLATED' UNITS

The diathermy current used for the purposes of electrosurgery is produced by a machine which is essentially a high-frequency electricity generator. The latter may be 'grounded', i.e. the return current passes to 'ground' via the return electrical pathway and the generator machine (Figure 35.1.2). However, if an alternative return electrical pathway is available, then depending on the impedance of this, the current may find its way back to 'ground' without passing through the generator (Figure 35.1.3). If, in addition, the normal return pathway to the generator is interrupted, then the only possible pathway to 'ground' is via that part of the patient's body which is

'earthed', and this may cause a burn at the site of contact (Figure 35.1.4). The danger is that if during the use of electrosurgery any part of the patient is inadvertently 'connected to earth' through a conductive pathway (e.g. the metal operating-table or a drip stand), then this will act as a return pathway for the current to the current-originating station. If this contact between the patient and the conductive pathway is of high resistance, then heat will be produced (in accordance with the equation: watts-seconds = resistance (ohms) × current

Table 35.1.2 Effects of increasing frequency of mains alternating current on the human body

50–60 Hz	Harmful
1 kHz	Minimal
100 kHz	Negligible
400 kHz–3 MHz	Heating effects only
> 4 MHz	Capacitive coupling and induction currents

Table 35.1.3 Resistivities of body tissues (expressed in ohms/cm) at 50–60 Hz

Bone	500–6000
Fat	2500–3000
Lung	1275
Cardiac muscle	750
Blood	150
Skin (variable resistivity)*	c. 300

*Dry skin has high resistivity; wet skin has low resistivity.

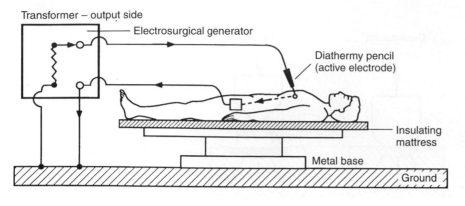

Figure 35.1.2 Grounded monopolar electrosurgery.

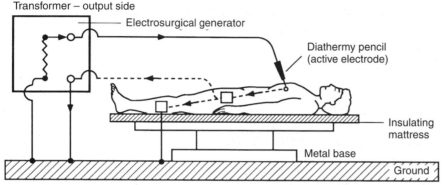

Figure 35.1.3 Grounded monopolar electrosurgery: extraneous return pathway.

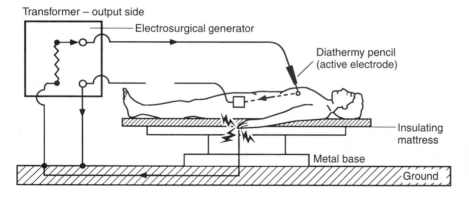

Figure 35.1.4 Grounded monopolar electrosurgery: interrupted normal return pathway. Patient's body is 'earthed' via operating table.

(amperes^2)), and the patient will receive a diathermy burn.

For these reasons, among others, grounded diathermy units have now been replaced by 'isolated' generators. In this system the 'primary' generator, which is earthed, induces a current in a 'secondary' generator, which is not earthed (Figure 35.1.5). Therefore, if any part of the patient's body is touching a grounded object, such as the operating-table or a drip stand, an electric current from this type of generator cannot complete the electric circuit necessary to cause a current to flow, and therefore the patient is not at risk of a diathermy burn at the site where their body is touching the grounded object.

MONOPOLAR AND BIPOLAR ELECTROSURGERY

In the monopolar electrode mode there is only one pole (hence the term 'monopolar') at the intended site of electrosurgical effect. Since electricity can only flow when there is a completed circuit, there must be a return pathway for the current back to the generator. This is provided by the patient's body, the diathermy plate and the return electrode cable (see Figure 35.1.6).

In the bipolar mode both the active electrode and the return electrode are at the site of intended electrosurgical activity, and the electrical pathway is completed by the

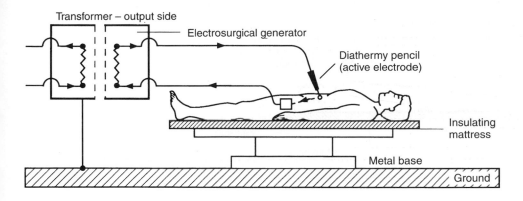

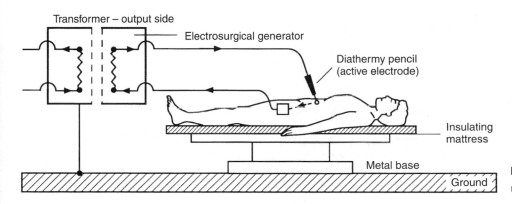

Figure 35.1.5 Isolated monopolar electrosurgery.

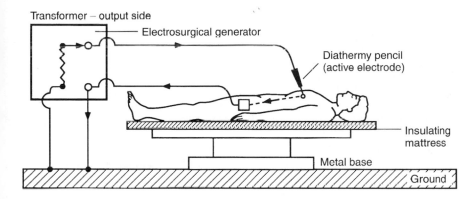

Figure 35.1.6 Monopolar electrosurgery.

tissue grasped between the two tines of the surgical forceps. Thus the patient's body is not required to form part of the electrical pathway, and therefore there is no need for a diathermy plate (Figure 35.1.7). However, in this mode it is essential that sufficient tissue is gripped between the tines of the forceps to make the current application effective. Simply holding the two tines of the forceps together while enabling the current pathway to be completed will not necessarily effect proper coagulational haemostasis.

COAGULATING AND CUTTING DIATHERMY

These two modes of electrosurgery purport to do precisely what the terms suggest, namely to 'coagulate'

bleeding vessels and to 'cut' tissues. Their respective modes of action are produced by adjusting the phasic activity of the electric current as follows. An AC current consists of a large number of electrons passing along a conductor at high speed, changing direction at a frequency which, in the case of conventional mains electricity, is 50–60 Hz. The high-frequency current in electrosurgery is at a frequency ranging from about 0.4 to 3 MHz. When the machine is in cutting mode this alternation is maintained continuously as a continuous wave form, i.e. the 'duty cycle' of the current is 100%. However, when the machine is in coagulation mode the current is active for only a fraction (about 6%) of the time, as a pulsed wave form; for the rest of the time it is quiescent. The 'duty cycle' is thus about 6%. When the

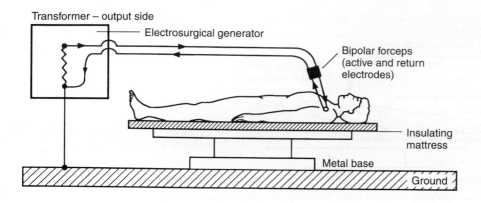

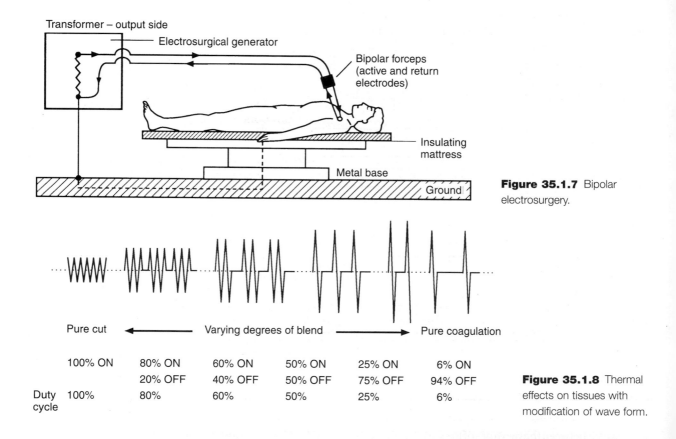

Figure 35.1.7 Bipolar electrosurgery.

Figure 35.1.8 Thermal effects on tissues with modification of wave form.

electrosurgical unit is in blend mode, the duty cycle is modified, and the degree of modification can be varied from one extreme to the other so as to alter the relative intensities of cutting and coagulation (Figure 35.1.8).

As a result of their different duty cycles, the coagulating and cutting modalities have different properties. Since a coagulating mode is produced by a lower duty cycle, it requires a higher peak voltage and also produces less heat (*c*. 150 W). As a result, such a mode produces maximal haemostasis with minimal vaporization of tissues. The effect is therefore of a firm coagulum leading to a dark brown to black eschar. In the case of the pure cutting mode, because the duty cycle is 100%, there is

less need for the same high-peak voltage to produce the desired effect. Nevertheless, the 100% duty cycle produces a higher degree of heat (*c*. 400 W). The result is a much higher tissue temperature, in fact so high that not only the water in the tissues but even the semi-liquid proteins are vaporized, a phenomenon known as *pyrollization*. Since most of the heat in this process is expended in providing the latent heat of vaporization of the proteinaceous materials of cells, relatively little heat is left to 'char' the adjacent tissues. Thus the effect of the cutting mode of diathermy is to produce a clean 'white' cut with minimal adjacent charring (Figures 35.1.1b and c).

RISKS OF DIATHERMY

Historically, the main risks of diathermy were explosions resulting from the use of inhalational anaesthetic agents (e.g. diethyl ether and cyclopropane) and electrocution caused by grounded and faulty diathermy machines. Both types of occurrence are now extremely rare. The use of potentially explosive anaesthetic agents in the UK has virtually ceased, and the modern diathermy machine is not only electrically isolated but also conforms to additional extremely stringent safety standards.

However, there are three other important sources of risk – first, fires associated with the use of surgical spirit, collodion, mastiche, etc., secondly, the potential for a diathermy burn of the skin at a site or sites other than that of intended application of diathermy and, thirdly, 'channelling'. The decrease in the use of inflammable cleansing agents has reduced the likelihood of the first, but the second and third risk factors are ever present.

If when a diathermy pad is applied to the skin the degree of contact is relatively low, the diathermy current can nevertheless pass through at the skin–pad interface and, in so far as the system is concerned, coagulation can be satisfactorily effected at the surgical site. However, if the contact is less adequate, the electrical impedance at the interface increases and more heat is likely to be generated at the skin site, with the possible risk of a diathermy burn. This will not be recognized until the pad is removed at the end of the surgical procedure. To eliminate this risk, the return electrode monitoring plate has been introduced.

In this system the diathermy plate consists of two plates separated by a conducting tab whose resistivity is monitored by a separate interrogation current of 3 mA at a frequency of about 140 kHz. If the impedance at the plate–skin interface is higher than a critical value, then the interrogating current circuit 'senses' this and not only sounds an audible alarm but also deactivates the generator and thereby prevents a diathermy pad burn (Figure 35.1.9).

THERMO-ELECTRICAL BURNS

These may be:

1. intended (active electrode at site of intended action); or

2. unintended:

   - active electrode (unintended action at 'extraneous' site);

   - return electrode site (inadequate or poor physical contact, tenting, gel drying, moisture invasion, scar tissue, displacement during patient repositioning, bony prominences, excess hair, excessive adiposity).

Channelling is another risk during the use of monopolar diathermy. Sometimes the patient-tissue component of the return electrical pathway is attenuated either by its inherent nature or as part of the intended surgical manipulation. This commonly occurs during operations such as orchidopexy, especially in children, where the spermatic cord has to be mobilized and its containing structures delineated as part of the operative procedure, and it may then become attenuated (Figure 35.1.10). Since the (monopolar) diathermy current must necessarily use the cord as its return current pathway, it is very likely that the resistivity in it will rise, leading to heat coagulation and subsequent devitalization of the cord

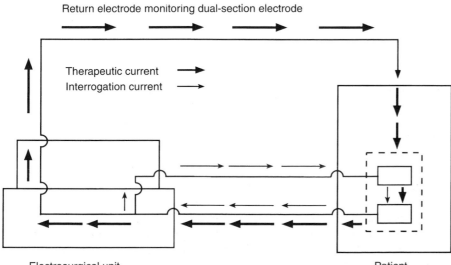

Return electrode monitoring dual-section electrode

Therapeutic current →
Interrogation current →

Electrosurgical unit

Patient

Figure 35.1.9 Electrosurgery.

and, in particular, the blood supply to the testis. It can also occur during minimally invasive intra-abdominal endoscopic procedures, where diathermy coagulation and divisions of bands and adhesions are performed. In such circumstances, high tissue resistivity can lead to excessive heat production and devitalization of tissues acting as the return pathway for the diathermy current. This can be prevented by the use of the bipolar mode or, where feasible, by decreasing tissue resistivity through the use of saline-soaked packs to accentuate the return electrical pathway when using monopolar diathermy (Figure 35.1.11).

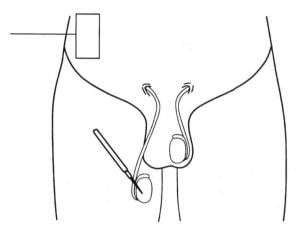

Figure 35.1.10 Electrosurgery. Channelling effect.

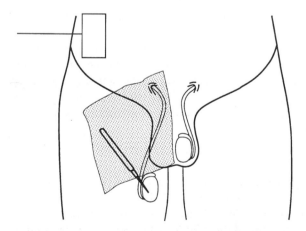

Figure 35.1.11 Electrosurgery. Channelling effect: prevention.

NEW ALTERNATIVES TO CONVENTIONAL DIATHERMY

Apart from the use of lasers to achieve some of the cautery and coagulatory effects of diathermy, argon flow and ultrasonic beams are now in vogue. In the former, a stream of argon gas is used. Argon is an inert and non-combustible rare gas, and is easily ionized by an electric current. Once ionized, the gas forms an effective current pathway and creates a glowing stream of ionized gas. The electric current in the electrode travels via the stream of argon gas to the site of action and thereby cuts and coagulates tissues. The advantages of this method are that there is less tissue damage, and lower volumes of smoke are generated.

The 'harmonic scalpel' utilizes ultrasonic energy and converts it into a frequency of 55.5 kHz which vibrates a mechanical blade. At this high frequency, tissue protein is denatured, producing a firm coagulum and thus bringing about sealing of tissues. The advantage of this technique is that there is no flow of electric current through the patient, and therefore all the risks of patient contact with electricity are eliminated.

FURTHER READING

Battig CG. 1968: Electrosurgical burn injuries and their prevention. *Journal of the American Medical Association* **204**, 91–5.

Becker CM, Malhotra IV, Hedley-White J. 1973: The distribution of radio-frequency current and burns. *Anesthesiology* **38**, 106–22.

Corson SL, Patrick H, Hamilton T, Bolognese RJ. 1973: Electrical considerations of laparoscopic sterilization. *Journal of Reproductive Medicine* **2(4)**.

Mitchell JA. 1978: *A handbook of surgical diathermy*. Bristol: Wright & Sons.

Lasers

Douglas E. Whitelaw and Stephen G. Bown

Introduction

Lasers produce an extremely intense, narrow beam of single-wavelength light. Most medical applications of lasers rely on the heat produced when laser light is absorbed to vaporize, coagulate or cut tissue. Laser light can usually be delivered via optical fibres, allowing treatment of organs during endoscopy or laparoscopy. The main non-thermal application of clinical lasers is photody-namic therapy (PDT), in which a pre-administered photo-sensitizing drug is activated by low-power light to produce tissue necrosis. Lasers are convenient light sources for PDT because, by selecting a laser wavelength which is strongly absorbed by the photosensitizing drug, an optimal tissue effect can be achieved.

LASER PHYSICS

A laser produces a unique form of light which is *mono-chromatic*, *coherent* and *collimated*. This means that the light is of a single wavelength and is configured in a narrow, highly directional beam.

When energy is supplied to a light-emitting medium, a small proportion of the atoms absorb energy by moving an electron from an inner orbit (ground state) to an outer orbit (excited state). At a variable time thereafter, the atoms revert to the ground state and the extra energy is released as light. This is known as *spontaneous emission*.

By contrast, when a lasing medium is supplied with energy, the *majority* of the atoms or molecules attain the excited state. This is known as a population inversion. Emitted light from an excited atom now has a high probability of bombarding another excited atom. If it does so, it stimulates a further emission, resulting in a pair of electromagnetic waves that are identical in wavelength, phase and direction. This process is known as *stimulated emission*. The lasing medium (which can be solid, liquid or gaseous) is usually constructed into a cylinder with a total reflector at one end and a partial reflector at the other. All light emitted along the axis of the cylinder is reflected back and forth along its length, stimulating increasing numbers of atoms to emit in this axis. This longitudinal reflection within the cylinder is known as light amplification, and any light emitted in other directions escapes. The light transmitted through the partially reflective end of the cylinder is the laser beam. The entire process is therefore known as **l**ight **a**mplification by **s**timulated **e**mission of **r**adiation (LASER).

LASER–TISSUE INTERACTION

Only when light is absorbed by tissue is heat produced. This may cause the tissue to vaporize, desiccate or coagulate. Coagulation occurs with relatively slow heating, and is due to denaturing of the cellular and structural proteins. More rapid heating drives off water, causing desiccation, while vaporization occurs when intense heating causes intracellular water to boil. The cell then explodes, throwing off steam and organic debris which ignites in the laser beam.

Tissue absorption of light is wavelength dependent. The carbon dioxide laser (wavelength 10 600 nm) is very strongly absorbed and penetrates tissue and water by only a fraction of a millimetre. The blue argon laser (wavelength 514 nm) penetrates water readily but is absorbed by pigments such as haemoglobin, so it only reaches a depth of 0.5–2 mm in tissue. The neodymium:YAG laser (wavelength 1064 nm) penetrates tissue to a depth of 6–8 mm. Strongly absorbed wavelengths are useful for vaporizing and cutting tissue, because a high power density can be created within a tiny tissue volume. With less strongly absorbed wavelengths, less energy is absorbed per unit volume, allowing tissue coagulation. Conduction of the heat away from an absorbing tissue takes a finite time. Very precise cutting can be achieved using a pulsed laser, such as an excimer, because a high-powered beam (but one with low total energy) can be delivered to the target tissue in a microsecond pulse, preventing conduction of heat to adjacent tissue.

The advantages of lasers in clinical practice include:

- delivery down optical fibres;
- precise control of power and energy delivered to tissue;
- the availability of a range of lasers and tissue interactions;
- endoscopic or percutaneous access to any tissue;
- rapid tissue healing.

LASERS USED IN MEDICINE AND SURGERY

CARBON DIOXIDE LASER

The carbon dioxide laser produces a beam with a wavelength of 10 600 nm. This infra-red beam is invisible, so a red or green aiming beam is usually added coaxially. Tissue vaporization and cutting are possible because the beam penetrates tissue by less than 1 mm. Carbon dioxide lasers are used in surgery as cutting tools, and in otolaryngology and gynaecology to ablate benign or premalignant tissue. Power settings up to 100 W are commonly used. The carbon dioxide laser is the only medical laser which cannot be transmitted down an optical fibre, because it is highly absorbed by the fibre itself. The beam is therefore steered towards the patient by a series of mirrors inside an articulated arm. Attachments such as micro-manipulators or sterile hand-held 'scalpels' can be connected to the arm as required.

ARGON LASER

Argon lasers consist of a tube of argon gas which ionizes when subjected to a high electrical current. These lasers produce wavelengths of visible green/blue light at 488 or 514 nm. These wavelengths are strongly absorbed by haemoglobin and melanin, and one of the main uses of these lasers is to ablate abnormal blood vessels and pigmented lesions in the skin. The other important application is the treatment of diabetic retinopathy, where the periphery of the retina is targeted to reduce oxygen demand, thereby minimizing neovascularization near the macula. Modern argon lasers use an attenuated beam for aiming, with up to 15 W power available with the full beam.

NEODYMIUM:YTTRIUM ALUMINIUM GARNET LASER

The neodymium:yttrium aluminium garnet (Nd:YAG) laser is widely used in clinical practice, and produces an infra-red beam with a wavelength of 1064 nm which passes through water without absorption (Figure 35.2.1). Power settings of up to 100 W are available which can coagulate tissue to a depth of 6–8 mm. This type of laser is commonly used endoscopically for non-contact coagulation, in which the laser fibre is cooled by gas flowing down a coaxial sheath. However, contact cutting and vaporization are also possible using tips made of ruby, sapphire or ceramic. An electronic modification of the Nd:YAG laser, known as a Q-switch, produces a pulsed wave output which is used for lithotripsy and ophthalmic surgery. The holmium:YAG (Ho:YAG) laser produces a different infra-red wavelength and is naturally pulsed giving tissue effects which overlap with those of the Nd:YAG and carbon dioxide lasers.

POTASSIUM TITANYL PHOSPHATE LASER (KTP OR 'FREQUENCY-DOUBLED YAG LASER')

This is a Nd:YAG laser combined with a potassium titanyl phosphate (KTP) crystal which doubles the frequency (and halves the wavelength) of the emerging beam. Residual 1064-nm light is filtered out, leaving a green laser which behaves like an argon laser. Modern devices are available which can be switched between 1064 and 532 nm according to the required tissue effect.

DIODE LASER

Diode lasers use semiconductors such as gallium-aluminium-arsenide as the lasing medium. In a similar

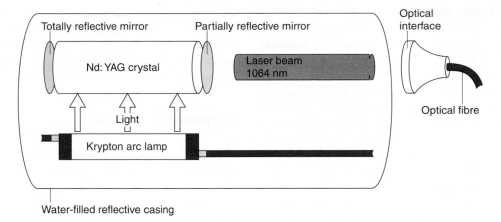

Figure 35.2.1 Neodymium:yttrium aluminium garnet (Nd:YAG) laser consisting of neodymium in a crystal (or garnet) of yttrium and aluminium. A krypton arc lamp provides the input energy and 'pumps' the laser. The crystal and lamp are enclosed in a reflective cavity which is continuously cooled by water.

manner to the light-emitting diodes (LED) found in domestic electronics, the light amplification is produced by highly polishing the sides of the diode. Devices are currently available containing arrays of multiple diodes which can produce up to 60 W of infra-red light (e.g. 805 nm). These lasers are highly portable and require no special power supply or water cooling. Difficulties in coupling diodes to an output fibre have prevented the development of high-power diode lasers at other wavelengths. However, low-power diode lasers (up to 2 W) specifically designed for photodynamic therapy are now available, with wavelengths of 653 and 630 nm in the visible red spectrum.

DYE LASER

The lasing medium of a dye laser is a mixture of organic dyes such as rhodamines, which produce a band of laser wavelengths. The versatility of this laser is due to the ability to 'tune' the emerging beam by removing unwanted wavelengths using a diffraction prism and filters. Dye lasers are ideal for photodynamic therapy, because the wavelength can be matched to the photosensitizing drug, and also for dermatology, where the laser can be tuned for maximum absorption by unwanted pigment in skin lesions. The energy input for a dye laser is provided by a strong light source such as a copper vapour laser.

EXCIMER LASER

'Excimer' is short for 'excited dimer', which refers to the lasing medium, which is stable in its excited dimeric state and unstable in its component parts (ground state). The xenon-chloride laser is the most widely used type, and produces ultraviolet light (308 nm). It is used for coronary angioplasty and corneal resurfacing. Excimer lasers produce tissue ablation with virtually no adjacent thermal damage, because their light is naturally pulsed and very strongly absorbed.

CLINICAL APPLICATIONS OF LASERS

GENERAL SURGERY

Nd:YAG, Ho:YAG and argon lasers can be used for laparoscopic surgery in contact or non-contact mode. However, it is now apparent that there is little to choose between laser and electrocautery in terms of complications, bleeding and operative time. As laser purchase and running costs are high, their use has been largely abandoned. Some specific open operations, such as non-anatomical liver resections and partial nephrectomies, may benefit from the haemostasis afforded by the laser, but these techniques are limited to centres with a special interest in lasers. On the body surface, carbon dioxide lasers and contact Nd:YAG lasers have been used to produce precise surgical incisions. However, apart from slightly superior haemostasis, they are indistinguishable from traditionally created incisions. Much recent research has focused on the technique of interstitial laser photocoagulation (ILP), in which laser light is delivered to lesions within solid organs via optical fibres placed percutaneously under image guidance. Relatively low power (typically about 3 W per fibre) from a Nd:YAG or diode laser is then used to destroy the tissue by coagulation rather than by vaporization, leaving the resulting debris to be organized by the normal healing mechanisms. This technique has been most widely used for solitary hepatic metastases, but clinical trials of ILP for treating uterine fibroids and breast tumours are also in progress.

GASTROENTEROLOGY

Palliation of malignant dysphagia is effective and safe using the Nd:YAG laser delivered during flexible endoscopy. When combined with dilatation, swallowing can be improved in most patients. Haemostasis is ensured because the surface of the tumour is vaporized while deeper tissue is coagulated. Laser endoscopy is often performed as a day-case procedure, but is relatively labour-intensive initially, and must be repeated every 4–6 weeks to maintain swallowing. However, combining Nd:YAG laser with adjuvant intra-lumenal brachytherapy may reduce the need for subsequent endoscopies. For rectal and colonic tumours, Nd:YAG laser treatment effectively reduces blood loss and the need for palliative colostomies, while minimizing symptoms. At one time lasers were used to treat bleeding duodenal ulcers. This technique has been replaced by injection sclerotherapy, but the Nd:YAG laser remains useful for coagulating vascular lesions such as water-melon stomach and angiodysplasia. The metaplastic epithelium of Barrett's oesophagus may be photo-ablated using the KTP laser, but the effect on long-term malignant potential is unknown.

UROLOGY

For 10–15 years attempts have been made to treat benign prostatic hypertrophy (BPH) with lasers. Side-firing transurethral fibres delivering Nd:YAG laser energy were introduced in the 1990s, with one type (TULIP) incorporating transurethral ultrasound guidance. The advantages of laser prostatectomy over electrosurgical resection (TURP) include a lower incidence of haemorrhage and post-TURP syndrome, but these must be weighed against prolonged catheterization times and more severe irritative symptoms. Recent randomized trials have shown laser prostatectomy to be inferior to TURP both in reducing the symptoms of BPH and in objectively improving urinary flow. The Nd:YAG laser has been used to coagulate superficial bladder tumours during cystoscopy. Ureteric and bladder calculi may be fragmented using pulsed Ho:YAG lasers or dye lasers. High-energy laser pulses produce shock waves which shatter the stone, allowing the pieces to be retrieved transurethrally.

OTOLARYNGOLOGY

The carbon dioxide laser is the workhorse of ENT surgery. In conjunction with an operating microscope it is used as a cutting tool for laryngeal resections such as arytenoidectomy. Juvenile laryngeal papillomatosis and other vocal cord lesions can be controlled by regular

laser treatment. Special precautions must be taken when intubated patients undergo laryngeal laser surgery. Flexible metal or foil-covered endotracheal tubes must be used to prevent plastic 'flaming' in the oxygen-rich atmosphere.

ORTHOPAEDIC SURGERY

Many orthopaedic centres now perform percutaneous laser disc decompression (LDD) using KTP, Nd:YAG or Ho:YAG lasers. The laser fibre is inserted via a needle into the prolapsed disc, which is then coagulated. Significant cost savings are claimed, as the majority of these operations are performed as day-case procedures. Most series have reported success rates of up to 70%. Holmium:YAG lasers are used for arthroscopy and allow haemostatic cutting of cartilage and capsular tissue.

PLASTIC SURGERY

Lasers have been used to treat most cutaneous vascular malformations and pigmented lesions at some time. The argon laser was used originally, because its beam (514 nm) passes through the epidermis with little absorption, but is well absorbed by haemoglobin in ectatic dermal vessels. Currently, pulsed dye and copper vapour lasers are used for these lesions, and produce a more selective ablative effect. 'Excellent' results are obtained in 30–40% of patients with port-wine stains, with darker lesions generally responding better than lighter ones.

Tattoos may be removed using pulsed dye or Q-switched ruby lasers. The laser wavelength is selected according to the colour of the tattoo, so that there is maximal absorption in the tattoo ink.

CARDIAC AND VASCULAR SURGERY

The use of lasers in peripheral vascular occlusion was widely promoted in the 1980s, but the results were rarely better than those obtained with balloon angioplasty alone, and the technique was largely abandoned. However, recent attention has focused on laser percutaneous translumenal coronary angioplasty (PTCA), with the xenon:chloride excimer and the Ho:YAG lasers attracting most interest. Early results suggest that laser PTCA is useful for complex stenoses which are not readily amenable to traditional PTCA. For short uncomplicated stenoses, complications occur slightly more frequently with laser PTCA, and as yet there is no firm evidence that patency rates are prolonged.

Trans-myocardial laser revascularization (TMLR) is an experimental treatment in which ischaemic myocardial muscle is revascularized by creating minute channels in the myocardial muscle with a laser, to allow direct contact between the muscle cells and oxygenated blood from the left ventricle.

NEUROSURGERY

Lasers are used as cutting tools in neurosurgery. The carbon dioxide laser is used in open operations, and the Ho:YAG and Nd:YAG lasers are used for stereotactic and trans-sphenoid surgery.

GYNAECOLOGY

The carbon dioxide laser is widely used for cone resection of the cervix and vaporization of premalignant lesions of the cervix and vagina. Carbon dioxide and KTP lasers have been used for laparoscopic ablation of endometriosis.

PHOTODYNAMIC THERAPY (PDT)

In PDT, a photosensitizing drug is taken up by cells in the body. Tissue necrosis occurs when the photosensitizer and oxygen react on exposure to low-power light. Using a laser as the light source allows a wavelength to be selected which is maximally absorbed by the photosensitizing drug, thereby producing optimal conditions for tissue necrosis. Initial hopes that selective uptake of photosensitizers by tumour cells would lead to a selective tumour kill have not been realized and, in practice, the light must be accurately targeted on the tumour. However, because photodynamic therapy is a non-thermal process, it has the potential to destroy cells with less damage to surrounding tissue than alternative thermal or surgical methods. In addition, there is no cumulative toxicity, so treatment can be repeated as necessary.

Several photosensitizing drugs are now in clinical use, including porfimer sodium, 5-amino-laevulinic acid (ALA) and meta-tetra hydroxyphenylchlorin (mTHPC). Porfimer sodium and mTHPC are synthetically modified porphyrin rings, while 5-amino-laevulinic acid is a naturally occurring prodrug which is converted into the active photosensitizer protoporphyrin IX (PPIX) by most cells. ALA has the advantage of skin photosensitivity lasting only 48 h, while mTHPC and porfimer sodium cause skin photosensitivity that lasts for 2–3 weeks and 2–3 months, respectively. PPIX and porfimer sodium are optimally activated by light with a wavelength of 630–635 nm, while mTHPC has an absorption peak at 652 nm. Until recently, these wavelengths could only be produced by unwieldy pumped dye lasers. However, portable diode lasers have now been developed for these wavelengths, greatly increasing the geographical accessibility of PDT.

Applications

PDT with ALA produces very superficial effects when used in the gastrointestinal or urinary tract, so most recent research has focused on its use for premalignant lesions such as *in-situ* oral and bladder carcinoma and Barrett's oesophagus. Encouraging short-term results have been obtained, and efforts are now being directed towards producing uniform effects over entire dysplastic surfaces. PDT with topically applied ALA for basal-cell carcinoma and acne is at an advanced stage of investigation.

Porfimer sodium PDT has been used in the gastrointestinal and respiratory tract for a number of years, and tumours of the oesophagus, colon and bronchi have been treated. A variable degree of success has been reported, but with prolonged skin photosensitivity and sunburn as frequent side-effects. PDT using porfimer sodium has been compared to Nd:YAG laser treatment for obstructing oesophageal carcinoma in a randomized controlled trial, with little evidence of superiority.

mTHPC is a powerful photosensitizing drug, and trials using it to treat oesophageal, oral and bronchial cancer are in progress. In addition, trials using interstitially placed laser fibres and mTHPC for the treatment of pancreatic and prostate cancer are yielding encouraging early results. PDT with mTHPC can produce necrosis up to 1.5 cm deep using red light. KTP laser light is more strongly absorbed by mTHPC than red light, but penetrates tissue less well. This has led some investigators to use green KTP light to obtain more superficial lesions with less risk of perforation.

SUMMARY OF APPLICATIONS

Laser treatment is unrivalled for:

- treatment of vascular and pigmented skin lesions and tattoos;
- treatment of diabetic retinopathy and haemorrhage;
- corneal resurfacing;
- photodynamic therapy.

Laser treatment is approximately equivalent to other modalities for:

- recanalization of malignant dysphagia;
- treatment of benign prostatic hypertrophy;
- tissue cutting during endoscopic ENT operations;
- lumbar disc decompression;
- treatment of premalignant cervical lesions.

FURTHER READING

Absten GT, Joffe SN. 1993; *Lasers in medicine and surgery – an introductory guide.* London: Chapman & Hall Medical.

Bown SG. 1998: New techniques in laser therapy. *British Medical Journal* **316**, 754–7.

Bown SG, Millson CE. 1997: Photodynamic therapy in gastroenterology. *Gut* **41**, 5–7.

Haddad NG, Fleischer DE. 1994: Endoscopic laser therapy for esophageal cancer. *Gastrointestinal Clinics of North America* **4**, 863–74.

Hecht J. 1992: *The laser guidebook.* New York: McGraw-Hill.

te Slaa E, de la Rossette JJMCH. 1996: Lasers in the treatment of benign prostatic obstruction – past, present and future. *European Urology* **30**, 1–10.

Intra-operative ultrasound

Christian H. Wakefield and O. James Garden

Introduction

The use of ultrasonography is now well established as an important non-invasive diagnostic tool in a variety of surgical conditions. Conventional extracorporeal ultrasonography is limited by the impedance of anatomical structures such as the abdominal wall, costal margins and overlying bowel gas. To overcome the interference of these tissue structures, low-frequency ultrasound is required which allows greater penetrative depth, but at the expense of loss of the resolution and fine detail seen with high-frequency ultrasound. Operative ultrasound (OUS) overcomes this compromise by allowing the organ of interest to be examined by placing it in direct contact with a high-frequency ultrasound probe, thereby producing images of far superior resolution.

Operative ultrasound was first reported in the literature in the 1960s in relation to its use in the location of renal calculi, bile duct calculi and attempts to localize cerebral mass lesions during neurosurgical procedures. However, enthusiasm for the technique was tempered by difficulties in interpreting A-mode scanning images, which were represented by blips on a monitor screen. The development of ultrasound technology brought B-mode, 'real-time' scanners whose images' relative ease of interpretation rekindled interest in OUS. A decade after its inception, the use of real-time intra-operative ultrasound scanning was described not only in urological and biliary surgery and neurosurgery, but had also expanded into the fields of hepatic, pancreatic, endocrine, vascular and cardiac surgery. Over the last 15 years, high-resolution real-time ultrasound has become the gold standard for OUS. Newer modalities, such as colour Doppler imaging, have further enhanced its functionality, particularly in the fields of cardiac and vascular surgery. In the minimally invasive era, laparoscopic ultrasound has evolved from OUS and has resulted in an increased acceptance of the use of operative ultrasound in surgical practice.

TECHNICAL ASPECTS OF ULTRASONOGRAPHY

Central to the physics of ultrasonography are the electro-mechanical properties of piezoelectric crystals. The application of an electric current across such a crystal results in a conformational change, which in turn generates a high-frequency sound wave. Similarly, deformation of the crystal by incident sound waves produces an electrical current whose magnitude is proportional to the amplitude of the waveform. In diagnostic ultrasound, the frequency of the waveform is in the range 3.5–10 MHz, and the velocity of the wave depends on the medium in which it propagates, being lowest in air and highest in bone (the velocity through soft tissues is identical to that through water). The two main types of diagnostic ultrasound used in current clinical practice are imaging reflective ultrasound and Doppler ultrasound.

The Doppler effect is a change in the apparent frequency of a sound when either the source or the detector moves in relation to the other. Doppler ultrasound utilizes two fixed piezoelectric units, one acting as a source and the other as a receiver. Because these units are fixed in relation to each other, any frequency shift of a sound wave reflected from a target object is proportional to the velocity of that object. This frequency shift will increase as the object approaches the receiver and decrease as the distance between the object and the receiver increases. The Doppler effect allows the measurement of both blood flow rate and its direction relative to the ultrasound probe.

Imaging reflective ultrasound utilizes a piezoelectric unit which acts as both a transmitter and a detector for alternating time periods. The transmission and reception of a sound wave contain qualitative information about the reflected signal or echo, its amplitude (or intensity), the time between transmission and reflection, whether the echo source is in motion, and the rate of change of this duration. The amount of sound that is reflected at the interface between two media will depend on the difference in their acoustic impedances. If there is a substantial difference between the acoustic impedances of the two media, as would occur, for example, with a gallstone within the gall bladder, more sound will be reflected back, resulting in a 'bright' echoic signal. Conversely, two media of similar acoustic impedance will reflect little ultrasound at their boundary, as would occur, for example, when a tumour of similar echogenicity to the liver is being examined. This would result in poor distinction of the boundaries of the tumour within the liver parenchyma.

B-mode imaging provides a two-dimensional image, consisting of an aggregation of dots whose brightness corresponds to the amplitude of the reflected sound wave. Current B-mode imaging is in real time, in which a linear array of transducers or a mechanical or electrical sector scan produces an image in near instant time.

probes allows the visualization of lesions as small as 1-mm gallstones, 4-mm tumours and 2-mm cysts.

The ultrasound probe should be compact enough to allow manipulation within confined operative fields. Linear-array probes are either cylindrical, flat, I- or T-shaped. Flat probes are ideal for examining large organs such as the liver, whereas front-viewing sector probes lend themselves to scanning of small structures deep in the operative field. I-shaped transducers and front-viewing probes are the ideal configuration for laparoscopic ultrasound probes, which have to be passed through laparoscopic ports of 10 mm diameter. Colour Doppler imaging, although less frequently used by general surgeons, allows the mapping of blood flow in real time on conventional B-mode images. Blood flow rates as low as 4 mm/s can be detected and displayed in colour (normally blue or red depending on the direction of flow in relation to the probe), the colour becoming brighter with higher flow rates. The use of colour Doppler is particularly useful for rapidly distinguishing between blood vessels and other tubular structures.

Ultrasound probes used in surgery may be sterilized by either standard cold gas sterilization or immersion in 2% glutaraldehyde. Modern ultrasound machines are now sufficiently compact and mobile to allow them to be positioned close to the operating table without hindering theatre staff. The ultrasound unit is connected to the probe by a sterile cable, or by a cable in a sterile plastic sleeve. During the operative procedure the surgeon runs the probe in direct contact over the organ. Lubricant gel is not required, but acoustic coupling and therefore image quality can be improved by instilling sterile saline into the operative field. As with all forms of ultrasound examination, the diagnostic value of the examination is user dependent, and the information obtained should complement rather than replace pre-operative investigations and clinical assessment.

ULTRASOUND EQUIPMENT

Both linear-array and sector-ultrasound probes may be used in OUS. Sector probes have the advantage of being able to scan through a narrow window. This is usually not a concern for the operative ultrasonographer who has relatively easy access to the organ to be examined. This enables a linear-array probe to be used, allowing structures near the transducer to be visualized and the simpler orientation of the image in relation to the anatomy of the examined organ. Transducer frequencies for OUS are in the range 5–10 MHz, with 7.5 MHz being most commonly used. This gives a tissue penetration of approximately 6–8 cm, which should be sufficient for most operative examinations. The use of high-frequency

ULTRASONOGRAPHY IN BILIARY SURGERY

The major early use of OUS was for the detection of extrahepatic lithiasis, as an alternative to operative cholangiography. Early prospective studies comparing the two modalities at open surgery have shown that OUS has a greater overall accuracy in detecting common bile-duct stones compared to conventional cholangiography (Figure 35.3.1). The widespread enthusiasm for laparoscopic surgery has meant that less open gall bladder surgery is being performed, with a concomitant move away from operative cholangiography. A number of studies have confirmed that laparoscopic ultrasound is as accurate as cholangiography in detecting common bile

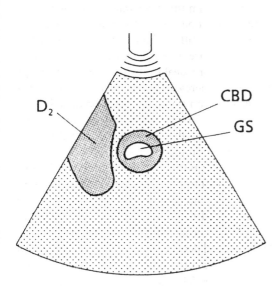

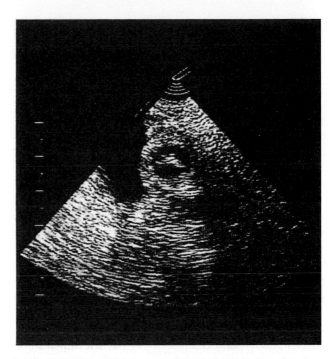

Figure 35.3.1 Laparoscopic ultrasound image of an impacted gallstone (GS) in the distal common bile duct (CBD). D_2 = lumen of second part of the duodenum.

duct stones, albeit with a lower sensitivity than that reported in studies of ultrasonography at open cholecystectomy (Table 35.3.1). Operative ultrasonography may be quicker to perform than cholangiography, and has the advantage of being able to image the intrahepatic biliary tree. Intrahepatic stones and associated segmental dilatation of the biliary tree can be clearly visualized. The principal disadvantages of OUS are the lack of information about the function of the sphincter of Oddi and demonstration of anatomical anomalies, for which cholangiography is distinctly superior.

Patients with cholangiocarcinoma often present with advanced disease, and OUS enables the careful evaluation of the tumour and its resectability without subject-

ing the patient to the potential morbidity and mortality of a trial dissection. Ultrasonographic information may be crucial in the approach to difficult malignant strictures in the biliary tree. Lesions at the hilus and in the gall bladder may be locally invasive to the liver parenchyma, portal vein and hepatic arteries, and thus be unresectable. The presence of lymph-node involvement and hepatic metastases may also be determined using OUS. When the nature of a biliary stricture is in doubt, ultrasound-guided biopsies may allow accurate tissue determination. In the event of a patient requiring a biliary bypass, the identification of dilated ducts by ultrasonography provides a ready target for hepatico-enteric bypass.

Table 35.3.1 Comparative studies of operative cholangiography and operative ultrasound examination of the common bile duct during cholecystectomy

Author (year)	Number of cases	Accuracy of OUS (%)	Accuracy of operative cholangiography (%)
Jakimowicz et al. (1993)	145	97.5	94.4
Machi et al. (1993)	401	98.5	94.2
John et al.* (1994)	60	93	94

* Laparoscopic US vs. laparoscopic operative cholangiography.

ULTRASONOGRAPHY IN LIVER SURGERY

Advances in radiological techniques have resulted in improvements in the pre-operative evaluation of liver lesions. Despite this, however, lesions may not be defined with sufficient accuracy to allow the surgeon to perform a safe, curative resection of a tumour involving the liver. Operative ultrasound has become well established in liver surgery because it allows the precise location of a lesion in relation to portal pedicles and hepatic veins, defining the lesion's segmental boundaries and thus overcoming the lack of surface landmarks on the liver, a potential pitfall in hepatic resectional surgery (Figure 35.3.2).

Having accurately located the position of a hepatic lesion, abnormalities whose pre-operative CT or ultrasound features may not be typically characteristic may be biopsied under ultrasound guidance. Needle placement also allows aspiration of cavity lesions, injection of contrast materials and cannulation of bile ducts, and more recently ultrasonography has been used to direct probes for cryosurgery. When there is doubt as to whether a small nodular lesion in a cirrhotic liver represents a hepatocellular carcinoma or a regenerating nodule, biopsy may be valuable in the management of such a condition. OUS may further distinguish between haemangiomata and metastatic deposits, averting inappropriate resections in cases where occult non-palpable tumour deposits are present.

OUS is more accurate than more conventional methods of screening for colorectal liver metastases (clinical studies report that an additional 10% of patients with otherwise unrecognized metastatic lesions are detectable by OUS). It has been shown that OUS provided additional information in one-third of patients undergoing hepatic resections, and that this information led to a modification in the intended surgical procedure in 50% of cases. The principal route of dissemination of hepatocellular carcinoma is by the portal venous system, and OUS delineates tumour thrombi accurately, thereby ensuring that the excision margins contain the susceptible portal territory. This translates into a long-term benefit by reducing the incidence of tumour involvement at resection margins when OUS is utilized. An extension of the capabilities of OUS has allowed the surgeon to perform anatomical resection of segments and sub-segments, which was not previously thought to be feasible (Figure 35.3.3).

OUS may aid the management of benign liver conditions such as hydatid disease, liver cysts and abscesses. Although currently the majority of liver abscesses are treated by percutaneous drainage, in those patients who require surgery, OUS allows the relationship of the abscess cavity to major vessels and biliary radicals to be determined. In addition, small adjacent loculi may be detected, whose adequate drainage is required for effective control of infection.

Laparoscopic ultrasonography has been used to stage hepatic tumours, and in some studies has been shown to provide additional information in up to 40% of patients assessed by conventional radiological means. None the less, it has perhaps had less impact in the pre-operative assessment of liver lesions than in the pancreaticobiliary field.

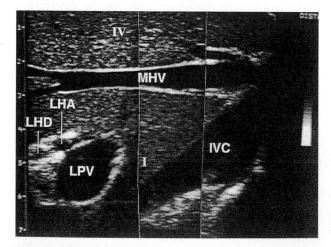

Figure 35.3.2 Laparoscopic ultrasound image of the left hemi-liver in the parasagittal plane. The successive cuts show the convergence of the middle hepatic vein (MHV) with the inferior vena cava (IVC). The hilar structures – left portal vein (LPV), left hepatic artery (LHA) and left hepatic duct (LHD) – are shown, surrounded by the hyperechoic Glissonian sheath. I, segment I; IV, segment IV.

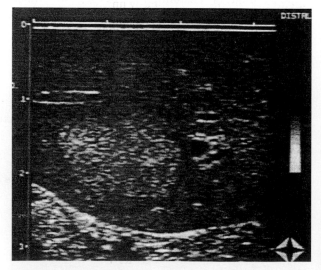

Figure 35.3.3 Laparoscopic ultrasound image of a hyperechoic metastasis within the liver. The lesion is surrounded by an anechoic 'halo'.

ULTRASONOGRAPHY IN PANCREATIC SURGERY

Operative ultrasonography has been shown to be beneficial both in aiding the management of inflammatory disease of the pancreas and (particularly with the advent of laparoscopic ultrasound) in the evaluation of neoplastic pancreatic disease. The pancreas is a difficult organ to examine radiologically because of its retroperitoneal position. For this reason, staging and the assessment of resectability of pancreatic cancers pre-operatively can be difficult, resulting in an unacceptably high rate of laparotomy without pancreatic resection. It may be impossible pre-operatively (and even at laparotomy) to distinguish between chronic pancreatitis and carcinoma of the head of the pancreas, and these conditions may even coexist. At open surgery, OUS allows the safe collection of tissue samples from suspicious areas with minimum risk to adjacent structures and maximum potential diagnostic yield. Unnecessary dissection may be avoided by the detection of vascular encasement, occlusion or invasion of the portal vein with ultrasonography. In experienced hands, OUS is more specific in detecting portal vein invasion than pre-operative US, CT and angiography. In patients for whom trial dissection is considered to be an option, the dissection is greatly facilitated by OUS with the clear identification of anatomical landmarks.

In the management of complications of acute pancreatitis, OUS allows clarification of the extent of pseudocyst formation and indicates into which organ the cyst is best drained. Such drainage procedures (either pseudocyst or abscess) may be guided by OUS in order to avoid adjacent vascular structures. Operative ultrasound may also detect previously undiagnosed gallstone disease. The role of OUS in chronic pancreatitis is less clear. However, it may facilitate pancreatic drainage procedures by identifying the position and extent of pancreatic duct dilatation.

The introduction of laparoscopy and laparoscopic ultrasound has become a major recent development in the staging of pancreatic cancer, and has greatly reduced the number of open-and-close laparotomies. Laparoscopy has the same advantages as laparotomy in being able to visualize peritoneal and visceral surfaces for metastatic deposits. When combined with contact ultrasonography, this minimally invasive technique allows local resectability to be more accurately assessed than by any non-invasive imaging technique. The use of a high-resolution transducer allows the precise size of the tumour to be determined together with its relationship to the major vessels. The presence of lymphadenopathy may also be assessed (Figure 35.3.4).

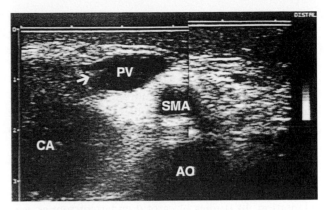

Figure 35.3.4 Laparoscopic ultrasound image taken during the staging of a pancreatic malignancy. A hypoechoic carcinoma (CA) extends to invade the lateral wall of the portal vein (PV), and the irregularity in the vein wall is indicated (arrow). The superior mesenteric artery (SMA) and aorta (AO) are clear of tumour.

ULTRASONOGRAPHY IN ENDOCRINE SURGERY

Operative ultrasound has been used in thyroid and adrenal surgery. However, its main use has been described in the assessment of parathyroid and pancreatic islet cell tumours. Over 50% of insulinomas and gastrinomas are not adequately delineated pre-operatively, but high-resolution ultrasonography is able to detect lesions of 3–4 mm in diameter, and is therefore more effective than detecting lesions at laparotomy by simple palpation. Detection rates of 100% for insulinomas have been reported utilizing OUS, and of 95% for pancreatic gastrinomas, with the detection rate falling to 58% for extrapancreatic gastrinomas. Peroperative imaging studies are not normally required during parathyroid surgery, the exception being for reoperations in parathyroid disease. Parathyroid adenomas appear as hypo-echoic areas compared to the surrounding tissue, and their localization by OUS minimizes dissection, detecting adenomas accurately in 80% of cases. The sensitivity of OUS is greater than pre-operative CT, ultrasound and technetium-thallium, particularly with intrathyroidal lesions.

ULTRASONOGRAPHY IN VASCULAR SURGERY

The main role of OUS in vascular surgery is the evaluation of vessels after reconstruction. Early ultrasonography in vascular surgery utilized Doppler velocity analysis. However, since the advent of B-mode imaging probes, reconstructed vessels can be examined for intimal flaps, thrombi and strictures. Early correction of these defects during the same procedure reduces postoperative complications and morbidity. In both experimental models and clinical studies, OUS is as accurate as angiography in detecting such defects, and is considerably quicker to perform.

The patency and quality of vascular reconstructions can be assessed in a number of surgical procedures, in peripheral revascularization, and during organ transplantation. In studies of carotid endarterectomies, vascular defects were detected by OUS in 30% of procedures, and of these defects one-third were deemed to be significant enough to require surgical correction. Operative colour Doppler provides additional information on blood flow, enhancing the efficacy of OUS so that on-table angiography may be used selectively for the distal vascular tree or when OUS evaluations are inconclusive.

ADDITIONAL APPLICATIONS OF OPERATIVE ULTRASONOGRAPHY

The experience of contact ultrasonography developed for the detection of gallstones has been modified and utilized by urologists for locating renal calculi during nephrolithotomy. Although the majority of renal calculus disease is managed by minimally invasive techniques, OUS allows the identification of avascular routes to renal calculi, enabling the surgeon to make incisions without renal artery clamping. Neurosurgeons continue to use ultrasonography for localization of intracerebral abscesses, tumours and arteriovenous malformations. Surgical gastroenterologists are exploring the potential of laparoscopic ultrasound for staging oesophageal and gastric malignancy, although the laparoscopy is perhaps more useful for detecting overt peritoneal and hepatic spread than the transducer's ability to assess local extension of tumour. In the evaluation of patients with lung cancer, mediastinal ultrasonography is proving to be a useful adjunct for assessing mediastinal lymphadenopathy, and it allows safer biopsy of affected lymph nodes in close proximity to the great vessels. Gynaecologists are able to assess the adequacy of endometrial curettage, and in this setting ultrasonography may improve the diagnostic yield of the procedure. More recently, anaesthetists have utilized transoesophageal echocardiography as a non-invasive means of performing continuous cardiac output monitoring during surgical procedures.

CONCLUSION

Although the concept of intra-operative ultrasonography has been recognized for over 30 years, its acceptance into surgical practice beyond that of the specialist pancreatic and hepatobiliary surgeon has been hesitant. This is partly as a consequence of the limited user-friendliness of the hardware. However, it is mainly due to the reluctance of surgeons to transgress into the field of the radiologists using unfamiliar technology. If the experience of surgeons in subspecialties is any guide, these difficulties can be overcome, allowing the general surgeon to adopt operative ultrasonography as an established part of his or her diagnostic armamentarium.

FURTHER READING

Barnes R, Garrett WV. 1978: Intraoperative assessment of arterial reconstruction by Doppler ultrasound. *Surgery, Gynecology and Obstetrics* **146**, 896–900.

Bismuth H, Castaing D, Garden OJ. 1987: The use of operative ultrasound in surgery of primary liver tumors. *World Journal of Surgery* **11**, 610–14.

Boldrini G, de Gaetano AM, Giovannini I, Castagneto M, Colagrande C, Castiglioni G. 1987: The systematic use of operative ultrasound for detection of liver metastases during colorectal surgery. *World Journal of Surgery* **11**, 622–7.

Charnley RM, Hardcastle JD. 1990: Intraoperative abdominal ultrasound. *Gut* **31**, 368–9.

Garden OJ. 1995: *Intraoperative and laparoscopic ultrasonography*. Oxford: Blackwell Science.

John TG, Greig JD, Crosbie JL, Miles WFA, Garden OJ. 1994: Superior staging of liver tumors with laparoscopy and laparoscopic ultrasound. *Annals of Surgery* **220**, 711–19.

John TG, Greig JD, Carter DC, Garden OJ. 1995: Carcinoma of the pancreatic head and periampullary region: tumor staging with laparoscopy and laparoscopic ultrasonography. *Annals of Surgery* **221**, 156–64.

Knight PR, Newell JA. 1963: Operative use of ultrasonics in cholelithiasis. *Lancet* **i**, 1023–5.

Machi J, Sigel B. 1989: Overview of benefits of operative ultrasonography during a ten year period. *Journal of Ultrasound in Medicine* **8**, 647–52.

Sigel B, Coelho JCU, Nyhus LM, Donahue PE, Velasco JM, Spigos DG. 1982: Comparison of cholangiography and ultrasonography in the operative screening of the common bile duct. *World Journal of Surgery* **6**, 440–44.

Operating magnification: loupes and the operating microscope

David A.R. Bessant and D. John Brazier

Introduction

In 1921 Nylen used an operating microscope in the treatment of patients with chronic otitis. By the early 1950s, Carl Zeiss had introduced the first series-produced, stereoscopic microscope, and otological microsurgery became an established practice. Since then, the use of magnifying systems (operating microscopes and loupes) in surgery has become widely accepted by surgeons in many disciplines, including hand surgery, neurosurgery, obstetrics, ophthalmology, otolaryngology, plastic surgery and urology.

BASIC PRINCIPLES

A surgical magnifying system is designed to produce an enlarged image of the operating field. As an absolute minimum, the enlarged image must be upright and unreversed to prevent the surgeon having to perform unnecessary reorientation, and stereoscopic (three-dimensional) adjustment for satisfactory depth perception. To enable adequate access for microinstruments to be utilized, the minimum working distance between the front surface of the magnifier and the operating field needs to be 150 mm.

MAGNIFICATION

SIMPLE MAGNIFIER

For practical purposes, the magnifying power (M) of a single lens can be defined as the ratio between two angles of sight, namely the angle which the object subtends with the optical system, compared to the angle as seen with the naked eye, at a constant distance (D). This gives rise to the magnification formula $M = D/F$, where F is the focal length of the lens. Since the near point of the unaided human eye is 250 mm, the distance D used in this formula is 250 mm. The working distance (WD) of a single lens is equal to its focal length.

Therefore, according to this formula, a simple magnifying glass with a focal length of 50 mm will provide $5\times$ magnification. However, it will be of no use as a surgical magnifier, as it will have a WD of only 50 mm.

SURGICAL MAGNIFIERS

To produce magnifying systems with a useful working distance, a telescope based on either the Galilean lens system or the Kepler prism system must be adopted. A Galilean telescope consists of a convex objective lens which determines focal length, and a concave eyepiece lens, the two lenses being separated by the difference of their focal lengths.

The Kepler roof prism system is familiar in the form of field-glasses (binoculars). This system consists of a combination of two prisms situated between the objective and eyepiece lenses of a telescope, which serve to erect and reverse the inverted and reversed image created by an astronomical telescope. The optics of both systems can be adapted for either distance or close viewing. The Galilean system is the more compact and lightweight of the two, but offers a smaller-diameter field of view.

FIELD OF VIEW AND DEPTH OF FOCUS

In any operating system, magnification of the image is not without penalty. As the level of magnification increases so the diameter of the field of view decreases. This is demonstrated by the diminishing field of view provided by loupes of increasing magnification power (Table 35.4.1). In addition, when magnification increases at a given working distance, the depth of the field in the viewing direction in which object structures remain clearly visible (the depth of focus) is also reduced. Outside this range objects appear blurred and are of low contrast. Finally, as magnification increases, so all movements of the surgeon's instruments, the operating field and the magnifying system will be equally magnified. Thus with 8× loupes a 1-mm/s movement of the operating field will be apparent as a movement of 8 mm/s, and with a microscope set at 30× magnification this movement will become 30 mm/s.

LOUPES VS. OPERATING MICROSCOPES

Operating loupes are available with magnifying powers ranging from 2× to 8×, whilst operating microscopes can provide magnifications ranging from 2× to 40×. Loupes are compact, lightweight and relatively inexpensive. They are therefore a good option when lower levels of operating magnification are sufficient, when cost is an important factor, and in circumstances where the surgeon is called upon to operate in several different locations. Loupes follow every movement of the surgeon's head, necessitating the maintenance of a steady head-neck position during surgery. This frequently limits their use to procedures with a duration of less than 1 h.

As well as increased magnification, the microscope also has the advantages of a wider field of view, the ability to change magnification quickly during a surgical procedure, and better depth of focus. Microscopes offer the surgeon's assistants excellent views, identical in some cases to that of the principal surgeon, and provide the opportunity for high-quality documentation in the form of 35-mm slide and video photography. However, since the microscope does not move with the surgeon's head, the patient, surgeon and microscope must be correctly positioned at the outset of the surgical procedure.

LOUPES

These small low-power Galilean or Kepler telescopes are designed to be mounted on spectacle frames or attached to a headband (see Figure 35.4.1). Correction of ametropia in an individual surgeon can be achieved by the use of prescription spectacles. Since these telescopes would normally produce a distant image, they are adapted for near vision by the incorporation of an additional lens of suitable focal length adjacent to the objective.

The use of these telescopes is influenced by working distance, magnification, field of view and source of illumination. The working distance of loupes, which ranges from 145 mm to 420 mm, depends on the desired magnification, and should be determined by the nature of the procedure. A working distance of 350 mm is frequently the most comfortable. Although magnifying powers range from 2× to 8×, the optimum magnification is often of the order of 3×. The field of view decreases markedly with increasing magnification. With a 2× loupe it may be 95 mm, whilst with an 8× magnifier the field of view is restricted to 22 mm (Table 35.4.1).

Illumination during operations in which loupes are used may be provided by an overhead illuminator (operating-room lights) so long as the wound is wide and shallow. However, if the wound is particularly deep or cavernous, additional illumination will be required, usually in the form of head-mounted fibre-optic systems. Once they are perfectly aligned, these will provide full,

Table 35.4.1 Loupes – magnification, working distance and field of view

Type	Galilean telescope			Kepler prism		
Magnification	2×	2.5×	3×	3.5×	4×	6×
Working distance (mm)	420	420	420	420	340	340
Field of view (mm)	95	85	52	65	50	38

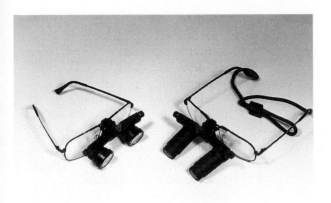

Figure 35.4.1 Spectacle-mounted Galilean and Kepler prism loupes. Loupes may also be mounted on a headband.

concentric, cool, even and shadow-free illumination. The fibre-optic headlight can be mounted on the same headband as the loupes and connected to a distant light source by a flexible fibre-optic cable. This avoids tissue desiccation, which may be a problem with light sources that are placed too close to the wound, and prevents the light source from interfering with the surgeon's access to the wound.

OPERATING MICROSCOPES

As the sophistication of microsurgical techniques and instruments has increased, so higher magnifications of the operating field and instruments, of the order of 10× to 40×, have become necessary. The microsurgeon frequently needs to change magnification power, using lower powers for preliminary dissection and higher powers for manipulation of delicate structures such as nerves and blood vessels. As a result, all operating microscopes are fitted with a magnification changer.

The operating microscope essentially consists of a pair of prism binoculars viewing the operating field through a single additional objective lens (see Figure 35.4.2). The magnification changer is interposed between the prism binocular and the objective lens. As with loupes, the functioning of the microscope is dependent on magnification, working distance, field of view and illumination. Complex high-quality lens systems are in fact used in place of individual thin lenses to minimize the effect of optical aberrations (distortion, chromatic aberration, spherical aberration and field curvature) and produce the clearest possible image.

MAGNIFICATION

The total magnification provided by an operating microscope is a product of all its components, i.e. the power of the eyepiece lens, the focal length of the binoculars, the power of the magnification changer and the focal length of the objective lens.

Eyepieces

Eyepieces are available in powers of 6.3×, 10×, 12.5×, 16× and 20×. Of these, the 12.5× eyepiece is most popular. Eyepieces are provided with adjustable settings, commonly ranging from −5 to +5 dioptres, which should be set according to the refractive error of the surgeon to ensure parfocality (maintenance of focus during changes in magnification) throughout the operation. The correct interpupillary distance (IPD) for the surgeon should also be set before surgery commences by altering the distance between the two binocular tubes. The refractive correction and the IPD may need to be reset if a different surgeon takes over during the procedure.

Binocular tubes

Binoculars are available in different focal lengths. Longer focal lengths provide greater magnification but a narrower field of view. The tubes can also be straight, inclined or smoothly inclinable. Straight tubes allow the operator to view the operative field directly through the microscope, and are favoured by otolaryngologists and endodontists. The patient must be correctly positioned in order for the surgeon to use direct vision. Inclined tubes are offset at 45° to the head of the microscope, whilst inclinable tubes can be angulated to any position between 0° (straight) and 60°. Inclinable tubes are used by ophthalmologists, who position the eye to be operated on facing upwards, and must therefore approach from the side whilst the microscope axis remains vertical.

Magnification changers

Magnification changers consist of either a wheel of selectable Galilean telescopes (three- and five-step manual changers) or a zoom Galilean telescope (power-zoom changer). A three-step changer has a pair of lenses mounted on a rotating turret and a vacant position on the turret which produces magnification solely from the other components of the microscope (eyepieces, binoculars and objective lens) (see Figure 35.4.2a). Two fixed powers of magnification can then be obtained from a single pair of magnifying lenses, according to which lens of the pair lies adjacent to the objective lens. In one position the lens pair will enlarge the image (e.g. 2.5×) whilst with the lenses in reverse there will be a reduction in image size (the magnification factor will be 1.0/2.5 = 0.4×). A five-step changer has two pairs of lenses mounted on the turret and can provide magnification factors of 0.4×, 0.63×, 1.0×, 1.6× and 2.5×. Manual

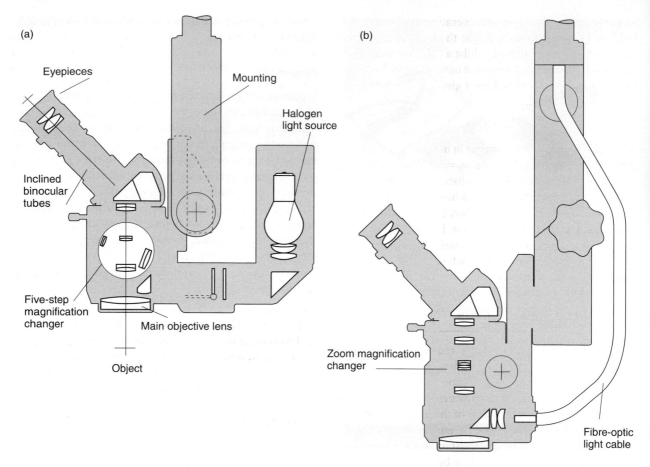

Figure 35.4.2 (a) Design principle of an operating microscope with a five-stage manual magnification changer and halogen-bulb illumination system. (b) Operating microscope with a zoom magnification system and integral fibre-optic illumination. (Modified with permission from Lang WH, Muchel F. 1981: *Zeiss microscopes for microsurgery*. Berlin: Springer-Verlag.

changers have the disadvantage of a limited number of fixed magnification powers, and require the surgeon to stop operating momentarily in order to change the magnification.

Many microscopes are now fitted with an automatic, foot-controlled power-zoom changer incorporating a series of lenses that move back and forth on a focusing ring (Figure 35.4.2b). This system allows smooth control of a continuous and wide range of magnification powers. A power zoom with a ratio of 1:5 could provide magnification in the range 0.5× to 2.5×. The foot pedal which controls magnification can also include controls for focusing and X–Y movement of the microscope head.

Objective lenses and working distance

Without an objective lens the microscope would act as a pair of field binoculars and focus at infinity. The focal length of the objective lens determines the working distance (WD) between the microscope and the surgical field, and working distances of between 150 and 400 mm can be achieved simply by changing this lens. The optimal WD for a microsurgical procedure (usually around

200 mm) is determined both by the magnification and field of view required and by the need for an adequate distance between the microscope and the operative field for the introduction of surgical instruments.

Total magnification

The total magnification of a complete operating microscope can be represented by the following equation:

$$m_T = f_T/f_O \times m_C \times m_E$$

where m_T = total magnification, f_T = focal length of the binocular tube, f_O = focal length of the objective, m_C = magnification factor of the magnification changer and m_E = magnification factor of the eyepieces. This information can also be derived from tables and nomograms supplied by the manufacturer.

FIELD-OF-VIEW DIAMETER AND DEPTH OF FOCUS

Increasing the magnification power of a microscope decreases the field-of-view diameter in exactly the same way as it does with loupes. An operating microscope utilized at 5× magnification might therefore have a field-of-view diameter of 40 mm, whilst at 25× magnification this would be reduced to just 8 mm. The field-of-view diameter can be calculated for a given microscope from the following formula:

$$d_F = x/m_T$$

where d_F = field-of-view diameter in millimetres, x is an instrument constant (e.g. 200) and m_T = total magnification.

As noted above, the depth of focus is also diminished by increasing magnification, and in some circumstances it may be necessary for the surgeon to reduce the level of magnification during an operation in order to bring all the relevant objects in the operating field into clear focus. This may be important when documenting the procedure photographically.

ASSISTANTS' MICROSCOPES

Many microsurgical procedures require two or more surgeons to co-operate. This can be achieved by attaching a separate assistant's microscope to the main microscope. The axis of these microscopes forms an angle of between 8° and 27° with the axis of the main microscope, giving the assistant a slightly different view to that of the principal surgeon. However, assistants' microscopes do have the advantage that they can be turned through a wide range around the axis of the main microscope.

In order to perform microsurgery in deep narrow cavities it may be necessary for the assistant to have an identical, coaxial field of view. This is achieved by the installation of a stereo beam splitter between the binocular tubes and the magnification changer, where the imaging rays are parallel. The stereo beam splitter contains a large complex prism arranged above the beam paths, which relays equal quantities of light to each of two pairs of eyepieces. The surgeon and assistant then have exactly the same stereoscopic view of the surgical field. This instrument is popular in hand surgery and neurosurgery.

When assistants' microscopes are in use it is important that all surgeons set their refractive corrections and IPD readings, and then ensure correct focusing of their microscope at the highest magnification setting before surgery commences, to ensure that the entire operating team remains parfocal throughout the procedure.

ACCESSORIES FOR CO-OBSERVATION AND DOCUMENTATION

The use of a much simpler beam splitter, consisting of a pair of prism cubes, permits monocular co-observation and photographic equipment to be attached to the operating microscope. In this device, 50% of the light from each of the stereo beam paths is reflected 90° laterally, whilst the remaining 50% is available for direct observation of the operating field. The beam splitter has two portholes located on its body, situated at 180° to each other, through which this reflected light can be directed to cameras or co-observer tubes (see Plate 35.4.1 in the colour plate section). Because extremely bright illumination is available, the loss of 50% of the available light is hardly noticeable to the operator, but it may become important when utilizing an attached 35-mm camera. Although the relative light sensitivity of photographic film has improved, electronic flash units mounted over the objective lens may be necessary to supplement the microscope's lighting system in some instances.

In contrast, commercial video cameras are extremely sensitive and, due to reductions in their size and weight, can now be easily mounted directly on the operating microscope. This allows colour television pictures to be fed to monitors both within and outside the operating theatre, and permits simultaneous recording of the procedure on videotape for teaching, patient education and medico-legal purposes. Standard VHS videotape records only 230 lines of resolution, whilst S-VHS tape records more than 400 lines, and is preferable for high-quality documentation.

ILLUMINATION

Overhead theatre-lighting systems are of inadequate intensity when using an operating microscope, and are further compromised by shadows produced by the microscope itself. As the magnification is increased, the effective viewing aperture of the microscope is decreased, and more light is required. Fan-cooled xenon or quartz halogen bulbs provide the integral light source in most modern microscopes, with light intensity controlled by a rheostat. Halogen lamps are preferable because they emit a higher percentage of blue light than do incandescent (tungsten) lamps, increasing the contrast between objects of different colours and producing a more pronounced gradation of colours.

Classically, the bulb of an operating microscope is situated adjacent to the observation system and its light is relayed through a condenser, via a deflecting prism and a colour filter to the heat filter, and thence via a second deflecting prism through the microscope objective to the operation site (Figure 35.4.2a). The illumination path of this system remains adjacent to the observation paths and is not therefore strictly coaxial. This is in fact desirable, since the off-centre arrangement of the illuminating beam is of great importance in suppressing direct reflections.

Fibre-optic illumination systems offer greater light intensity, and the advantage that the lamp housing can be installed at a distance from the microscope, which permits rapid changes of failed bulbs and prevents heat transfer to the microscope body (Figure 35.4.2b). Fibre-optic systems can be attached to the lower portion of the microscope to give either quasi-coaxial or oblique illumination.

SURGEONS IN TRAINING

Learning to operate satisfactorily using a microscope takes considerable time, and until the necessary depth perception and co-ordination have been achieved, the trainee should practice with micro-instruments and sutures under simulated operation conditions.

Additional information about the technical principles of operating microscopes, their illumination systems and accessories can be obtained from texts published in association with the major microscope manufacturers. Details of the applications of operating microscopes within different surgical specialities are available in the appropriate specialist literature (see Further Reading section below).

FURTHER READING

Barraquer JI. 1980: The history of the microscope in ocular surgery. *Journal of Microsurgery* **1**, 288–99.

Buncke HJ. 1986: Microsurgery – retrospective. *Clinics in Plastic Surgery* **13**, 315–18.

Edwards WG. 1980: The versatility of the basic microscope system in otolaryngology. *Journal of Microsurgery* **1**, 387–93.

Henderson SR. 1984: The reversibility of female sterilization with the use of microsurgery: a report on 102 patients with more than one year of follow-up. *American Journal of Obstetrics and Gynecology* **149**, 57–65.

Krampe C. 1984: Zeiss operating microscopes for neurosurgery. *Neurosurgical Review* **7**, 89–97.

Lang WH, Muchel F. 1981: *Zeiss microscopes for microsurgery.* Berlin: Springer-Verlag.

McLoughlin MG. 1980: The role of microsurgery in male infertility. *Clinical Obstetrics and Gynaecology* **23**, 1293–9.

Meyer V. 1987: The place of the microscope in hand surgery. *Journal of Hand Surgery* **12**, 155–7.

Nylen CO. 1954: The microscope in aural surgery: its first use and later development. *Acta Oto-laryngologica* **116**, 226.

Rubinstein R. 1997: The anatomy of the surgical operating microscope and operating positions. *Dental Clinics of North America* **41**, 391–413.

Principles of the use of 'foreign materials' in surgery

Stephen G.E. Barker

Introduction

The use of 'foreign materials' throughout surgical practice is increasing rapidly, with both new applications being found for materials that have already been developed, and entirely new materials being produced for either specific or generic use in a variety of medical situations. Autogenous materials (derived from the patient), such as the long saphenous vein, are usually deemed to be the 'gold standard' against which the results of use of a synthetic material are compared. However, in many cases a suitable autogenous material does not exist, although it is not always a straightforward matter to place a 'foreign material' instead and expect it to function perfectly without complications and stand the test of time.

Foreign materials may be natural products (e.g. a pig's heart valve used to replace a diseased human aortic valve), semi-synthetic (e.g. the Dardik® human umbilical vein graft, where a natural product has been chemically altered and subsequently covered in a synthetic mesh) or synthetic (e.g. a polytetrafluoroethylene (PTFE) patch used to widen a stenosed blood vessel). Categorization could also be made under a number of other headings, such as whether the foreign material is biodegradable (e.g. a collagen sponge acting as a temporary haemostat, or carbon fibres used to replace damaged ligaments around the knee) or whether the material is made from metal, plastic or fabric (e.g. a stainless-steel hip prosthesis, a silicone finger-joint replacement or a Dacron® graft used to perform a femoro-popliteal bypass). Regardless of which classification is employed, the principles of use applicable to all classes of foreign materials should be understood (see Box).

Any foreign material that is placed within (and often on)

COMMON PRINCIPLES FOR USE OF FOREIGN MATERIALS

- Access to implant
- 'Length of stay'
- Fixation
- Consideration of the complications of use
- Cost and benefit

---

the body will have previously been subjected to an extensive series of evaluations prior to gaining appropriate regulatory body approval for its clinical use. In the UK, such materials are likely to carry the 'CE' mark awarded by the European Commission and have approval from either the Medicines Control Agency (MCA) or the Medical Devices Agency (MDA). In the USA, Food and Drug Administration (FDA) approval is the benchmark standard, and in Australia the Therapeutic Goods Administration (TGA) (a division of the Department of Health and Family Services) will have given permission for product usage. Materials that are not involved in widespread commercial development may not have national regulatory body approval, but will still have been granted either local Ethics Committee approval, supplemented by a Doctors' and Dentists' Exemption (DDX), or a Clinical Trials Exemption (CTX) certificate, for trial use or use on a 'named patient' basis.

Commercial research and development groups undertaking bioengineering or biomaterials work need to meet appropriate standards for manufacture and production. These aspects are covered in the award of either Good

Laboratory Practice (GLP) or Good Manufacturing Practice (GMP) certificates. Once a newly developed foreign material has been formulated and tested as necessary (in laboratory tests, *in vitro* or *in vivo*), it will be required to be trialled for clinical use. Usually, a phase I trial will be initiated, the aim of which is to study and assess the effects of the material on the patient and, indeed, the effects of the patient on the material. A full series of histological and toxicological assays is necessary, usually conducted by a third-party organization which may, for example, investigate inflammatory responses produced in the area immediately adjacent to where the material is placed, or determine the serum levels of any chemical agent that is impregnated into the material. Once satisfactory data have been obtained, approval will be sought for a phase II clinical trial. The purpose at this stage is to test in the actual clinical setting, that the new material does indeed achieve what it sets out to do. For example, the aim may be to test whether a solid Vicryl® sheet used to rebuild the floor of the orbit can function to support the eye physically, or whether a gelatin-coated vascular graft does in fact obviate the need to pre-clot the graft, so as to prevent massive blood loss through the weave of the graft material itself. During a phase II trial, modifications to the original design of the material can be made based on the clinical findings to date. Finally, a phase III trial continues on from the phase II study, using what should be the final pre-marketed product on a far larger number of patients. This routine developmental schedule can take many years to complete, and incur considerable expense. Failure of the new foreign material can occur at any stage.

All surgical specialities now implant foreign material routinely into patients (see Table 36.1). The list given in the table is by no means exhaustive, and new indications for old materials are often found to bolster the increasing number of new materials designed for a specific purpose.

THE USE OF POLYPROPYLENE MESH IN HERNIA REPAIR

Currently, one standard repair of an inguinal hernia is with mesh using the Lichtenstein technique. The mesh is constructed of 'woven' monofilamentous polypropylene. It is inert and does not biodegrade, and is designed, therefore, to last the lifetime of the patient. Inherently it is very strong and does not 'give' or deform to any great extent, even with time. It is provided either as a large (> 50 × 50 cm) or small (perhaps 6 × 15 cm) sheet, or pre-cut to the shape that is considered to be best suited to the inguinal canal. It is provided in a sterile package that has been gamma-irradiated. Although the original meshes were quite stiff, meshes with a softer feel are increasingly widely available.

The monofilamentous design helps to minimize the potential for bacterial colonization (which is found to be more of a problem with multifilamentous materials). Once placed, the 'repair' gains greater strength with the ingrowth of fibrous tissue into the weave of the mesh, thereby 'incorporating' the mesh far more substantially.

Access is usually via a direct incision in the groin to expose the inguinal canal. The mesh is laid along the back wall of the inguinal canal, with the cord structures placed anteriorly. Other approaches to hernia repair using mesh are commonplace, including its use in sheet form from a pre-peritoneal approach (using a slightly higher anterior abdominal wall incision), or laparoscopically, passing the folded mesh down a port, and approaching the hernial defect from either a pre-peritoneal approach (using 'balloons' to create a working

Table 36.1 Foreign materials used in different surgical specialities

Surgical speciality	Foreign material and usage
General surgery	Polypropylene mesh for inguinal hernia repair
	Latex T-tubes for bile-duct drainage
	Silicone breast implants
Vascular surgery	Dacron for arterial bypass grafts
	PTFE for vascular patches
	Stainless steel or Nitinol® wire for endoluminal stents
Cardiac surgery	Stainless steel for heart valves
	Porcine heart valves
	Nylon fabric patches for septal defects
Urology	Latex indwelling urinary catheters
	Silastic ureteric catheters and stents
	Silicone testicular implants
Orthopaedic surgery	Cobalt-chrome joint prostheses
	Nylon joint replacements
	Carbon-fibre ligament replacements
ENT/ophthalmic and maxillofacial surgery	Plastic auditory ossicles Plastic intra-ocular lenses
Obstetrics and gynaecology	Stainless-steel clips for sterilization
	Plastic and copper coils for contraception

space) or a trans-peritoneal approach, which many consider to be optimal for simultaneous, bilateral hernia repair or recurrent hernia repair.

After placement by whatever means of access, the mesh may be held in position by either simply onlay (using gravity and 'anatomy'), suturing or stapling. An important principle for hernias is a tension-free repair (i.e. local tissues are not brought together and held as such forcibly, which is thought to cause prolonged postoperative discomfort and predispose the patient to recurrence). Most surgeons accessing with a direct approach tend to fix the mesh in position using nonabsorbable sutures in either a continuous or an interrupted fashion, joining the bottom edge of the mesh to the innermost part of the inguinal ligament and the upper edge to the conjoint tendon. Staples are used by some surgeons, particularly those who gain access by laparoscopic means.

A new variation on hernia repair with mesh involves the use of a mesh plug, resembling a flower with layers of petals (Figure 36.1), which is simply placed in an advantageous anatomical pocket sited adjacent to the cord structures as they come through the weakened deep inguinal ring. The shape of the plug and gravity keep the hernial sac and its contents within the abdominal cavity, later reinforced by ingrowing fibrous tissue. A second onlay piece of mesh (Figure 36.1) rests in the usual place. Theoretically, no suturing at all is required, providing the ultimate tension-free repair.

To date, with the Lichtenstein repair the failure rate of the operation (expressed as percentage recurrence after a 5-year period) is < 5%, compared to a recurrence rate of < 2% for the traditional Shouldice repair (the 'gold standard' operation). The considerations for the 'successful' use of the mesh as a foreign material concern the time saved per operation, the reduction in post-operative discomfort experienced by the patient, and their earlier return to 'normal' activity.

Implantation of mesh material is not without potential complications. Recurrences can and do occur, usually because the mesh has been cut too small and placed insufficiently medially, beyond the pubic tubercle, where most recurrences are usually found. Cord and testicular oedema can occur if the hole cut for the cord structures to pass through is too tight. Migration of an onlay patch can occur, but does not appear to be a major problem. Sutures placed right through the periosteum of the pubic tubercle to hold the mesh can cause prolonged pain, as can sutures that inadvertently 'bind down' the ilio-inguinal nerve. However, the complication feared most with regard to any implanted foreign material is infection.

Many surgeons give a prophylactic dose of IV antibiotic at the commencement of mesh hernia repair (although there is no proven requirement for this). The mesh itself is originally sterile, and most surgeons would try to minimize its handling prior to implantation and aim to avoid it resting for lengthy periods on the outer skin surface. The basic principle of 'coverage' of foreign material is achieved by completely enveloping the mesh behind the reconstituted external oblique aponeurosis. Few surgeons give post-operative antibiotics, but some either pre-soak the mesh in antibiotic or antiseptic solution (although of unproven benefit) or use iodine-based sprays directed into the wound at the end of the operation. Infection is usually from a skin commensal such as *Staphylococcus aureus*. The presence of a haematoma encourages infection, and hence haemostasis at the time of surgery is particularly important. In this context, it is often worth ligating vessels (usually veins) formally, rather than making injudicious use of diathermy. Infection usually manifests with pain, swelling, heat and redness of the overlying skin. Often a serious wound discharge heralds a more unpleasant purulent discharge. Antibiotic therapy is unlikely to 'sterilize' infection around placed foreign material, and the usual requirement is for surgical removal. Early post-operative infection is met with easy removal of 'unincorporated' graft material, whereas late infection (which may occur as a result of blood-borne bacterial spread) results in the far more difficult removal of a fully incorporated mesh, often presenting as a discharging sinus.

Mesh material does cost considerably more than the simple sutures used alone in the more traditional forms of hernia repair. In the UK, a pre-cut polypropylene mesh costs approximately £60, whereas two sutures as used beforehand would cost approximately £4. As companies spend more on research and development and ever more on advertising and marketing, newer foreign materials are likely to become increasingly expensive, impinging further on often cash-limited health services.

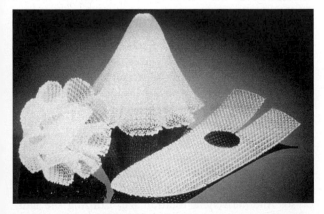

Figure 36.1 A polypropylene mesh 'plug' and pre-cut onlay patch for inguinal hernia repair. (Photograph courtesy of Impra, a subsidiary of C.R. Bard Inc.)

THE (CEMENTED OR UNCEMENTED) HIP PROSTHESIS

Currently, there are more than 60 varieties of hip prosthesis available for either single- or double-component repair of damaged hip joints. Many are engineering variants designed to cater for different stress loads caused by, for example, fractures that are either more proximal or more distal to the femoral head. They are usually manufactured from stainless steel, titanium or one of a number of alloys (e.g. cobalt-chrome). Acetabular cups, although originally made of metal, are nowadays composed of ultra-high-molecular-weight polyethylene, although metal cups are again in vogue, the so-called 'metal-on-metal' prosthesis, due to improved wear characteristics.

Hip replacement is undertaken on either an emergency or an elective basis (the former usually following a fracture, and the latter commonly associated with osteoarthritis). Access to replace the joint is by means of a muscle-splitting lateral or posterior approach. There then follows disarticulation of the hip and excision of the native femoral head. The prostheses are designed to last the patient's lifetime, but in reality tend to function for about 15–20 years. The components used must be fixed securely into position. Taking the femoral part only, it can be sited using either a cementing or non-cementing technique. With the former, following appropriate reaming of the femur, the cement is prepared and placed into the femoral shaft. The reagents used to form the cement produce a marked exothermic reaction. The cement is pressurized into the femoral canal using a cement gun. When no cement fixative is used, it is the shape and length of the prosthesis stem that wedges it firmly in place and holds it there. In either case, incorrect alignment may result in early loosening or, if very severe, dislocation.

Occasionally, prosthesis designs have prompted unexpectedly early problems with excessive wear, sometimes associated with metal fatigue. Topically, the 3M device (Capital) in use since the late 1980s has been shown in many cases to be unsatisfactory, with more than one-third of patients requiring early revision surgery to date. However, there can be no doubt whatsoever that hip prostheses overall have been extremely successful, bringing relief (usually from extreme pain) to many hundreds of thousands of patients, and at present being implanted at a rate of over 45 000 per annum in the UK alone.

There are two main complications of use, of which once again infection is the most feared. At operation, prophylactic antibiotics are given at induction, and at 8 and 16 h post-operatively. Handling of the prosthesis is kept to a minimum. Orthopaedic surgeons often work in 'ultraclean' environments, using 'Charnley tents' or personal, all-enveloping sterile suits. During placement, antibiotic-impregnated cement containing gentamicin is almost always used. Prosthesis infection usually manifests with pain and immobility (together with any systemic manifestations). Sterilization of foreign material is again unlikely, and hence revision surgery is required.

The second major complication is loosening, which can occur secondary to infection, but commonly develops simply with time. Again this causes pain, which is made worse on walking, and revision surgery is necessary. Other complications may include femoral shaft fracture (either at the time of prosthesis placement or later), and recurrent dislocation of the hip if there is prosthesis misalignment.

Hip prostheses are expensive. However, the cost benefit to health services can be immense when patients who have repeatedly attended out-patients and undergone innumerable investigations are finally discharged from hospital following hip replacement. Morever, younger patients can at last return to work. In the UK, the cost of a hip prosthesis can range from £300 to over £2000. There is now a tendency to try to limit the number of new variants of prosthesis that come on to the market, which may help to reduce overall costs. Any significant advance in technology will, of course, be passed on from the developer to health-care providers.

SILICONE BREAST IMPLANTS

Breast implants have two major categories of use, namely reconstruction following mastectomy and cosmesis (Figure 36.2). A broad size range is available, usually measured by volume (cm³). The prosthesis aims to mimic the texture (when implanted) of normal breast tissue. The majority of breast implants are made from 'medical-grade' silicone, although new varieties may be filled with saline or agents such as soya oil.

Breast reconstruction may be undertaken at the time of mastectomy, or as a second-stage procedure at a time when the wound has fully healed, and any adjuvant treatment courses have finished. In this situation, the prosthesis is not simply placed behind the mastectomy scar, lying anterior to the pectoralis major, but is placed in a 'pocket' created behind the pectoralis major, and held in place by the action of the muscles on the underlying chest wall. Usually there needs to be some degree of stretching of the skin and muscle first, using a tissue expander that is gradually filled with saline over a month or so. Alternatively, a rotation flap utilizing the latissimus dorsi muscle can be used to 'bulk' the breast area, with a prosthesis placed posteriorly. However, cosmetic augmentation procedures usually involve placing the

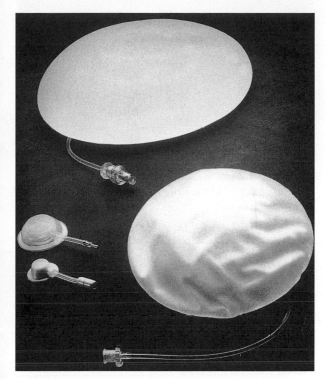

Figure 36.2 A silicone breast prosthesis (saline filled) and a tissue expander used before its' implantation. (Photograph courtesy of Ms Christobel Saunders MS FRCS.)

prosthesis behind the mammary disc in front of the pectoralis major.

Breast prostheses are designed to last the patient's lifetime. Over the past few years, however, it has become apparent that the prosthesis may degrade after several years, often leaking its contents, which can promote local fibrosis, distorting the shape of the breast and significantly altering its texture. This phenomenon is termed capsular contraction. Lumps may form which can be confused with the development of recurrent (or new) carcinoma.

There is no doubt that, when placed satisfactorily, breast prostheses can restore body shape and image and help, therefore, to enhance the self-esteem of the patient. The cost in the UK of a standard implant prosthesis is approximately £400 to £800.

The principles of use of this particular foreign material once again relate directly to complications. Incorrect sizing has obvious implications for asymmetry between the reconstructed side and the remaining breast, as has malpositioning (often with the prosthesis lying very high). More fundamentally, if it is misplaced or fixed incorrectly, the breast prosthesis can migrate from its 'pocketed' space and come to lie very laterally, often in the axilla. Infection is a major problem and warrants surgical removal. Significant infection will tend to promote scar tissue formation, which in itself causes a textural change in the surrounding native tissues. Full psychological counselling is needed before embarking on breast reconstruction, so that the patient is aware of the potential problems and has realistic expectations of the end cosmetic result. There is increasing litigation associated with breast implants, and it is incumbent upon surgeons who are implanting such devices to be fully up to date in their knowledge of the newer biomaterials that are available.

With the above three examples I have attempted to outline the basic principles of use of foreign materials placed within the body. Although it is reassuring to know that each material has undergone rigorous pre-clinical and clinical trials testing, it is often the case that problems only come to light after many years of 'routine' usage. Thus careful audit of usage is essential, with long-term records kept of those patients who have been implanted, and with what materials. Short-term, future development will see current products being used in different circumstances. For example, vascular endoluminal stents will be used in the carotid arteries. These same types of stents (albeit of larger size) are used to hold open biliary or colonic strictures. Collagen sponges, currently used for haemostasis, will be developed into sheets for use in the peritoneal and pleural cavities to prevent adhesion formation. Biopolymers linked with various drugs will be used for local delivery of these agents in high concentrations. In each case, the same basic principles of use will apply, namely access to implant, 'length of stay', fixation, complications of use and, finally, cost in relation to benefit.

FURTHER READING

Davis JM, Shires GT. 1991: *Principles and management of surgical infections.* Philadelphia, PA: J.B. Lippincott.

Kogel HC (ed.). 1991: *The prosthetic substitution of blood vessels.* Munich: Quintessenz-Verl.

Morris PJ, Malt RA (eds). 1994: *Oxford textbook of surgery.* Oxford: Oxford University Press.

Poston GJ. 1996: *Principles of operative surgery.* Edinburgh: Churchill Livingstone.

Sabiston DC, Lyerly HK (eds). 1994: *Sabiston – essentials of surgery.* Philadelphia, PA: W.B. Saunders.

Chapter 37.1

Applied clinical pharmacology for surgeons

Julia M. Potter and John E. Payne

Introduction

In the practice of modern surgery, it is necessary for there to be a significant understanding of the scientific basis of all of the tools which are available to aid the surgeon in every aspect of his or her work. Pharmacological tools as aids to the practice of surgery are as old as the use of drugs to induce stupor and to dull pain (in modern parlance, anaesthesia and analgesia), or as modern as the triple therapy to treat *Helicobacter pylori* or the antiviral therapy of HIV. Some drugs are day-to-day companions (e.g. in the treatment of the aged patient with cardiac failure, or the antibiotics used prophylactically in bowel surgery). Others are more exotic, and appear at first glance to be the purview of research laboratories and academic institutions. However, the latter have a habit of becoming available for use in the general community. Although it may seem unlikely that a surgeon would be called upon to prescribe such a drug, he or she is very likely to care for patients who are receiving such medication.

Given this broad general picture, what should a modern surgeon know about pharmacologically based therapy? The era of molecular medicine has dawned, and with it an increasing knowledge of the mechanism of action of many drugs at a cellular if not subcellular level. With this knowledge has come a better understanding of general principles. Whilst in the early days of therapeutics much of the use of drugs was pragmatic, and the rote learning of side-effects was a necessity, now that the different classes of drugs are better understood one should be able to predict substantial likely outcomes of related drugs – both efficacious, desirable outcomes and undesirable toxicities.

As with every discipline in medicine, pharmacology has its own particular language. To be able to converse and discuss with one's colleagues, the knowledge and use of this language are prerequisites of informed practice. This is true whether the discussion is within the field of surgery, or with a physician whom one consults for one's patient, or with a pharmaceutical company representative who wishes to persuade you of the virtues of a new product or a reformulation of an old product. Just as an anatomical term (e.g. porta hepatis) or the name of a surgical instrument (e.g. artery forceps) conjures up a very specific image, so should the basic language of therapeutics. The material within this chapter has been selected to provide a 'skeleton' on which subsequent practice and experience can build. Much of the material should be familiar, for the intention is to concentrate on widely used drugs or drug groups. Some less familiar drugs are included as an indication of the potential direction in which drug development may be moving. Some drugs are being reclassified in the light of recent pharmacological and physiological knowledge, and the long-term outcome should be improved therapy for the patient, with better drugs and better outcomes.

The material is presented in two major sections. The first part is a summary of the mechanisms of action of drugs and drug groups as they can be classified currently. This section also serves to cover many of the major therapeutic areas with which a surgeon should be familiar. The second part explores the principles of pharmacokinetics. The aim of this section is to provide an overview of the factors which influence drug utilization, such as routes of administration and drug clearance. The result should be a practical understanding of the dosing intervals and how and why significant pathological processes may influence a patient's response to medication.

PRINCIPLES OF DRUG ACTION

Pharmacology and its application to therapeutics are firmly based on the principle that the majority of drugs act by influencing target molecules or binding sites. Most identified binding sites are proteins, and can be classified as enzymes, carrier molecules, ion channels or receptors, with DNA and RNA a historically recent development. The nature and characteristics of the binding form part of the signature of any drug.

In this section, examples are given of the individual classes of proposed mechanisms of action of drugs. In each case, where possible, the mechanism of action is considered together with the clinical outcome and major side-effects which are also related to this mechanism. Binding to or occupancy of an effector site will produce a change which may either be the initiation of an event (in which case the drug is said to be an *agonist*), or it may involve decreasing or stopping an event (i.e. the drug is an *antagonist*). The mode of interaction between the acting drug or compound (known as the *ligand*) and the effector site can be classified as competitive or non-competitive. A competitive ligand binds to the site in a reversible manner, and may be displaced from the site by a mass of alternative ligand (e.g. acetylcholine is a competitive, naturally occurring agonist of muscarinic receptors; atropine is a competitive antagonist at that site, and its inhibition may be overcome by increasing the local concentration of acetylcholine). Occupation of a binding site by a non-competitive ligand results in a physical change in or around the receptor (e.g. succinylcholine binding to nicotinic receptors with depolarizing neuromuscular blockade).

ENZYMES AS TARGETS OF DRUG ACTION

As shown in the examples below, the principles of this type of drug effect can be summarized by the following questions.

1. Is the inhibition competitive or non-competitive?
2. Is there a pharmacologically active metabolite?

Competitive enzyme inhibition

Warfarin is an orally active anticoagulant whose mechanism of action is competitive inhibition of vitamin K reductase. Vitamin K-dependent coagulation factors (II, VII, IX and X) must be carboxylated to achieve maximal potential efficacy. In the continual provision of these factors, vitamin K is cycled from a reduced to an oxidized form, reduced vitamin K being the state necessary for its cofactor function. Vitamin K reductase activity ensures that sufficient cofactor is available for continued synthesis. Anticoagulation due to a vitamin K antagonist will take several days to become effective. Even though the enzyme inhibition is rapid, in the patient with normal synthetic liver function and normal vitamin K status, there are already circulating and intrahepatic coagulation factors which have been carboxylated. Effective anticoagulation will only occur when there has been a significant decrease in the concentration of all four carboxylated factors. The effect of warfarin can be reversed by giving a large parenteral dose of vitamin K. However, short-term reversal for minor surgery can be achieved by replacing the coagulation factors with fresh frozen plasma (FFP), similar to the supplementation which may be necessary in patients with severe liver dysfunction.

Simvastatin is one member of a family of drugs which competitively inhibit the enzyme 3-hydroxy-3-methyl-glutaryl-coenzyme A reductase (HMG-CoA reductase). These are widely used in the treatment of hypercholesterolaemia. Inhibition of HMG-CoA reductase, which is the rate-limiting enzyme in cholesterol synthesis, results in decreased cholesterol production. There is a compensatory upregulation (increased synthesis) of LDL-receptors, which in turn results in a secondary increase in the clearance of low-density lipoprotein (LDL). The fall in plasma cholesterol is dose dependent, and is of the order of 30–40% in high-dose therapy. The serious side-effects of HMG-CoA reductase inhibitors are myositis and rhabdomyolysis, the cause of which is not understood. It must be remembered that patients who are homozygous for familial hypercholesterolaemia do not respond to simvastatin, as they lack the ability to synthesize normal LDL-receptors.

Hypertension is a major contributor to the morbidity and mortality of ischaemic heart disease and cerebrovascular disease. The angiotensin-converting enzyme (ACE) inhibitors are among the most widely used antihypertensive drugs. The octapeptide angiotensin II is a potent vasoconstrictor in the vascular beds such as the kidney, heart and brain. It also contributes to hypertension and has a role in the genesis of cardiac failure in its role in the renin–angiotensin system, with aldosterone secretion and sodium and water resorption. Synthesis of the active angiotensin II depends on the activity of ACE, a carboxypeptidase which cleaves off a pair of amino acids from the precursor angiotensin I. The ACE inhibitors (e.g. captopril) bind to the active site of the carboxypeptidase and produce a fall in blood pressure, particularly in patients with high circulating renin concentrations. However, in patients with bilateral renal artery stenosis or in those with one kidney (e.g. following transplantation), glomerular filtration may be dependent on vasoconstriction of the efferent arteriole maintained by angiotensin II. In these patients, the use of captopril may precipitate renal failure. ACE is also one of the enzymes which metabolizes bradykinin, and use of ACE inhibitors is often accompanied by a dry cough (and occasionally worsening asthma), due to accumulation of bradykinin. The newer members of this group (e.g. enalapril, lisinopril) produce more prolonged effective inhibition, and therefore the dosing intervals are longer.

One of the earliest examples of competitive inhibition was the use of neostigmine to reverse competitive neuromuscular blockade by drugs such as *d*-tubocurarine in anaesthesia. Neostigmine is a competitive antagonist of cholinesterase, with a plasma half-life of 1–2 h. Acetylcholine released from nerve terminals is usually hydrolysed very rapidly by *in-situ* cholinesterase. Acetylcholine is the natural ligand of both the nicotinic receptors of the neuromuscular junction (see section below on receptors as targets of drug action) and cholinesterase. Therefore inhibition of cholinesterase allows accumulation of acetylcholine, which can now compete with *d*-tubocurarine, causing its displacement and restoration of normal muscle contraction. Acetylcholine will also accumulate within the synapses of parasympathetic nerve terminals and neuronal ganglia, resulting in side-effects such as bradycardia (via the vagus nerve) and sweating. These muscarinic symptoms can be prevented by pretreatment with atropine.

Methotrexate is one of the established cytotoxic drugs which are also being used as immunosuppressive drugs in the treatment of autoimmune disease such as rheumatoid arthritis, as well as in transplantation. Its mechanism of action is via competitive inhibition of dihydrofolate reductase. Dietary folate requires intracellular conversion into tetrahydrofolate, in which form it is an essential cofactor in *de-novo* synthesis of purines and pyrimidines. If availability of the bases for DNA and RNA synthesis is severely restricted, then the drug is cytotoxic. If the availability of nucleotide bases is restricted to a lesser degree, the influence is more subtle, with RNA and protein synthesis being limited, and immunomodulation is the clinical outcome. This same dose–reponse relationship is seen with the toxicity profile of methotrexate, with severe potential toxicity including bone-marrow suppression and gastrointestinal mucosal loss. Following high-dose intravenous methotrexate, it is standard practice to measure the concentration of methotrexate at defined times post-infusion. If the concentration exceeds the known defined threshold for toxicity, then the potential toxicity can be limited by administration of large intravenous doses of folinic acid. The latter is a synthetic tetrahydrofolate which bypasses the immediate need for dihydrofolate reductase (so-called 'rescue'). Folate (via tetrahydrofolate as a cofactor) also has a pivotal role in the metabolism and interconversion of some amino acids, such as homocysteine. Homocysteine is an independent risk factor for arteriosclerotic disease, and one of the most

important causes of morbidity and mortality among transplant recipients is cardiovascular disease.

The mechanism of action of heparin is an extension of the concept of enzyme inhibition. The coagulation cascade is effectively a series of reactions whereby at each step a previously inactive protein is transformed into an active enzyme (a serine protease). The final end-product of the coagulation pathway is fibrin derived from fibrinogen. Under normal physiological conditions, antithrombin III inactivates factor Xa and thrombin by binding to the active serine site on the enzyme. These two enzymes are the key points in the reaction cascade. In the presence of heparin the rate of this interaction is vastly increased. Heparin is a member of the glycosoaminoglycan family, and any particular pharmaceutical preparation contains a wide range of molecular weights. Low-molecular-weight heparins are cleaved products of heparin, having more closely defined molecular weights. Compared to heparin, they have a greater effect on the antithrombin III interaction with factor Xa than the other potential sites, and a more predictable biological effect on a dose basis. Both heparin and the low-molecular-weight products require parenteral administration.

Non-competitive enzyme inhibition

Non-competitive inhibition occurs when there is covalent binding between the enzyme and the inhibitor or a part thereof. Restoration of enzyme activity requires synthesis of new protein. The most practical example of this type of inhibition is the important action of aspirin (acetylsalicylic acid) in the prevention and control of vascular occlusive disease and in the treatment of acute myocardial infarction. Aspirin acetylates one of the serine residues in the active site of cyclo-oxygenase (COX-1). COX-1 activity in the cell can only be restored by synthesis of new enzyme, a possibility that is denied to platelets, for they lack a nucleus, and hence any cohort of platelets that is circulating and exposed to aspirin will be unable to synthesize thromboxane A2 (which promotes platelet aggregation). Endothelial cells, on the other hand, are able to synthesize more COX-1, and prostacyclin (PGI_2) production will be restored. The net effect is a change in the balance in the vascular bed, with decreased platelet aggregation and relative promotion of vasodilatation.

Production of an active metabolite

Drugs which depend on continued enzyme activity with production of a pharmacologically active metabolite can be subdivided into two groups. In the first, the analogue of a natural substrate is metabolized to an active compound whose properties differ from those of the natural metabolite. In the second group, an increased amount of substrate is made available and there is enhanced production of an active (natural) metabolite.

An example of the first group can be found in cancer chemotherapy, with analogues of both the pyrimidine and purine bases. The analogues are metabolized *in vivo* to their active forms, namely the phosphorylated nucleotides. These compounds control cell growth in several ways. Inhibition of enzymes in the nucleoside pathway (substrate inhibition, with decreased base nucleoside availability) and substitution of analogues into DNA and RNA cause misreading of genetic information. For instance, in the pyrimidine pathway, 5-fluorouracil is converted to fluorodeoxyuridine monophosphate, which inhibits thymidylate synthesis. Inhibition of thymidylate synthetase effectively inhibits DNA synthesis, but both RNA and protein production continue. This disparate effect of active cell growth in the presence of decreased cell division is one of the conditions which leads to apoptosis, and inability to repair DNA (because of decreased amounts of natural base) will further contribute to this. In the purine pathway, the analogues 6-mercaptopurine and thioguanine are both phosphorylated *in vivo*, at which stage they may either decrease *de-novo* purine synthesis (by negative feedback) or be incorporated into DNA or RNA. Therefore the antiproliferative actions of the cytotoxic drugs can be regarded as a combination of changes in the cell cycle as well as promotion of apoptosis. These effects are seen in both neoplastic and normal rapidly dividing tissue. The latter are side-effects and include changes in bone marrow (particularly decreased leucocyte production), loss of hair, damage to gastrointestinal mucosa (with mouth ulceration and diarrhoea), decreased fertility and teratogenicity.

The best known clinical example of enhancement of existing enzymatic activity concerns the use of L-dopa in the treatment of Parkinson's disease. In this disease there is progressive loss of the dopaminergic cells of the basal ganglia, resulting in loss of fine motor control and increasing muscle tone mediated via the unopposed cholinergic pathways. By increasing the amount of dopa available for the enzyme dopa decarboxylase, maximal intraneuronal stores and release of dopamine are achieved, with a better balance restored between the two pathways. Dopamine itself does not cross the blood–brain barrier, nor is it well absorbed from the gastrointestinal system. If the precursor L-dopa is given orally, still only 1% of it may reach the CNS. However, this percentage is increased by simultaneous administration of a competitive inhibitor of dopa decarboxylase (e.g. carbidopa), decreasing the peripheral utilization of L-dopa. This strategy also decreases the peripheral symptoms of excess dopa.

Nitric oxide is the product of the reaction between molecular oxygen and L-arginine. Its synthesis is enzy-matically controlled by nitric oxide synthase, of which several isoforms have been described. Nitric oxide appears to act as a paracrine agent, diffusing into cells adjacent to its site of synthesis and activating guanylate cyclase. Among the physiological consequences of the raised cGMP which is produced are vasodilatation and decreased platelet aggregation, as well as effects on neuronal development. Inhaled nitric oxide is being used to treat adult respiratory distress syndrome. The controlled hypotension produced by sodium nitroprusside during cardiopulmonary bypass is due to spontaneously released nitric oxide. A similar pathway is involved in the anti-anginal function of glyceryl trinitrate.

There are, of course, examples of enzyme inhibition in which the one drug has more than one mechanism of action. Allopurinol is one such complex inhibitor that displays both competitive and non-competitive inhibition. It is widely used in the prophylaxis of gout, which may occur secondary to high purine turnover and hyperuricaemia. Allopurinol is an analogue of hypoxanthine and inhibits xanthine oxidase, the final enzyme in the metabolic pathway, which catalyses the conversion of soluble hypoxanthine and xanthine to insoluble uric acid. Allopurinol itself is metabolized by xanthine oxidase to alloxanthine, which is an effective non-competitive inhibitor of xanthine oxidase. The inhibition will be maintained for the life of the enzyme, and any newly synthesized enzyme will be inhibited so long as allopurinol (half-life 2–3 h) and alloxanthine (half-life 18–30 h) are present. Xanthine oxidase is also a significant metabolic pathway for clearance of the cytotoxic purine analogues (e.g. 6-mercaptopurine,) and the toxicity of these drugs is increased by the concurrent use of allopurinol. Similarly, it is one of the pathways of clearance for the methylxanthines (caffeine and theophylline), whose toxicity will be enhanced in the presence of allopurinol.

CARRIER MOLECULES AS TARGETS FOR DRUG ACTION

Many polar molecules, such as ions and small organic molecules, are unable to diffuse easily across the predominantly lipid content of cell membranes. They utilize carrier molecules to gain access to or be excreted from cells. Examples of such systems include glucose and amino acid transport into cells, the excretion of organic acids and bases in the kidney, the maintenance of ion disequilibrium across cells (a high K^+ concentration intracellularly and a high Na^+ concentration in the extracellular fluid), the uptake of neurotransmitters into neuronal and non-neuronal tissues, and the proton pump of the gastric mucosa.

Digoxin has an important place in the history of therapeutics. William Withering's description of the beneficial effects of foxglove on certain sufferers of the 'dropsy' (oedema) was published in 1785. Digoxin and the cardiac glycosides bind to the Na^+/K^+-ATPase on the external cell surface of the myocardial cell. In an electrically active cell, such as the myocardium, Na^+/K^+-ATPase restores the disequilibrium after the cell has repolarized; there is active extrusion of three Na^+ ions into the extracellular fluid in exchange for two K^+ ions. If the ionic balance is not restored, the resting membrane potential of these cells will start to drift towards the threshold for depolarization. This will produce significant changes in cardiac function due to altered conduction, and dysrhythmias may arise. The binding of digoxin on the outside of the membrane is competitive with that of K^+, and therefore digoxin's effect and potential toxicity are increased if there is hypokalaemia. One of the most common causes of hypokalaemia is the use of potassium-losing diuretics, such as thiazides, and therefore there is a significant potential interaction between these diuretics and digoxin. Some of the extra-cardiac side-effects of digoxin are due to inhibition of Na^+/K^+-ATPase in other tissues (e.g. in the eye, causing peripheral colour changes, and in the brain, causing psychosis).

The proton pump in the gastric mucosa is also an ATPase, namely H^+/K^+-ATPase. The net effect of the complex ion-exchange system within gastric parietal cells is the secretion of H^+ (via the proton pump) and Cl^- (via a symport, i.e. a parallel, linked system) into the gastric lumen, while HCO_3^- is exchanged for Cl^- across the basal membrane. Omeprazole, a proton-pump inhibitor, binds irreversibly via sulphydryl groups to the proton pump. Because the binding is irreversible, a single daily dose will affect acid secretion for 2–3 days, whilst the plasma half-life is only 1 h.

The organic acid and base pathways in the proximal renal tubules both depend on specific carrier mechanisms. Both pathways transport compounds against an electrochemical gradient and have very high rates of clearance across the kidney. For example, the organic acid pathway is a target in the treatment of gout. High-dose probenicid competes with both the active resorption and secretion of uric acid, resulting in a net increase in uric acid excretion. Probenicid is also used to decrease the renal excretion of penicillins to improve antibiotic efficacy (e.g. in subacute bacterial endocarditis). Competition down these pathways can cause significant drug toxicity (e.g. use of one of the non-steroidal analgesic drugs such as aspirin or indomethacin will decrease the renal excretion of methotrexate and increase its potential toxicity).

Diuretics are among the most widely used drugs. The primary targets of both the loop and thiazide diuretics are carrier molecules within the nephron. Frusemide acts in the luminal membrane of the ascending (thick) limb of the loop of Henlé, where it inhibits the co-transporter which moves ions from the lumen of the nephron into the tubular cells (in the proportions of $Na^+/K^+/2Cl^-$ used). The thiazide diuretics (e.g. chlorothiazide), acting in the diluting (or early) segment of the distal convoluted tubule, decrease active Na^+ absorption by binding to the chloride site of the Na^+/Cl^- transporter on the luminal membrane. Both groups of drugs produce an intraluminal urine which has a relatively increased Na^+ content as it passes via the distal tubule and collecting duct. On a mass-action basis, some of this Na^+ is exchanged for K^+ or H^+, resulting in a hypokalaemic alkalosis in the patient (i.e. these drugs are potassium-losing by definition).

ION CHANNELS AS TARGETS FOR DRUG ACTION

An ion channel is an ionophore which passes through the full thickness of the cell membrane and allows the passage of specified ions through the channel, or potential channel, contained therein. They are another solution to the problem of transport of ionized molecules, and tend to be used for more rapid mass transit than the systems described in the above section on carrier molecules as targets for drug action. Channels which allow the passage of cations are lined by negative charges, and conversely chloride channels are positively charged. Further specificity is given to the channels by their physical dimensions, so that when they are activated or opened, their diameter is slightly larger than that of the hydrated specified ion. The pharmacological effects on ion channels can be divided into those in which the channel is physically blocked by occupation by a drug molecule (e.g. local anaesthetics), and the more complicated mechanism in which the drug binds to a component of the channel and modulates the gating of the channel (e.g. calcium-channel blockers).

Local anaesthetics (e.g. lignocaine) block the fast Na^+ channels in electrically active membranes and prevent both the initiation and propagation of action potentials. All electrically excitable cells will be affected by local anaesthetics. Both sensory and motor axons will be affected, so temperature sensation as well as pain will diminish, as will motor function. The blockade is terminated by diffusion of the local anaesthetic away from the site of administration. The major predictable side-effects of these drugs are due to their actions on other electrically excitable tissues. For example, in the CNS they can produce agitation, convulsions and loss of consciousness, and in the cardiovascular system they produce myocardial depression (a direct effect), vasodilatation (due to effects on smooth muscle as well as autonomic nerves) and a net resultant hypotension.

Benzodiazepines (e.g. diazepam, nitrazepam and

midazolam) increase the affinity of $GABA_A$ receptors for gamma-amino butyric acid (GABA), an important inhibitory neurotransmitter. The $GABA_A$ receptor is a post-synaptic ligand-gated chloride ion channel which consists of several different subunits surrounding a central channel. The subunits display some structural polymorphism, and different combinations of the subunits help to explain the varying properties of the benzodiazepines at therapeutic doses (e.g. why diazepam is more anxiolytic than clonazepam, which is anticonvulsant at lower concentrations). Flumazenil is a benzodiazepine antagonist which is able to reverse the effects of a benzodiazepine, i.e. it will competitively displace diazepam off its binding site, and the enhancement of GABA will be reversed. In the case of a benzodiazepine overdose, the CNS depression should decrease.

The CNS effects of the barbiturates and of ethanol are also produced by enhancing the action of GABA. However, these compounds bind to different sites on the $GABA_A$ receptor/Cl^- channel, and their effects are much less specific than those of the benzodiazepines. Their CNS depressant effects are not reversed by flumazenil.

Calcium-channel blockers are also known as calcium-channel antagonists or calcium antagonists. They prevent the opening of voltage-gated calcium channels, thereby inhibiting Ca^{2+} entry, mainly in heart and smooth muscle. Verapamil is relatively more active in the heart, i.e. it is cardioselective (and is therefore useful as an anti-arrhythmic drug), nifedipine is relatively active in smooth muscle (so useful for reducing vascular tone and hence reducing cardiac afterload and hypertension), and diltiazem is intermediate (and is often used in angina pectoris). The main side-effects in the cardiovascular system can be attributed directly to decreased Ca^{2+} availability in the cell (e.g. resulting in decreased cardiac contractility and hence in cardiac failure).

RECEPTORS AS TARGETS OF DRUG ACTION

In this discussion the term receptor is reserved strictly for structural units which interact with compounds classified as neurotransmitters and hormones including the cytokines and growth factors. Some of the ion-channel examples above could also be classified as receptor effects. There are four main types, based on their molecular structure and mechanisms of action.

Receptors coupled directly to an ion channel

Receptors for fast neurotransmitters are coupled directly to an ion channel (e.g. nicotinic acetylcholine receptor, $GABA_A$ receptor, 5-HT$_3$ receptor, glutamate receptor). Oligomeric proteins (with several subunits) are arranged around a central aqueous channel (see previous section). Minor variations in binding account for differences in

tissue response and the response to blocking drugs. In addition to these differences in affinity, CNS receptors may be 'protected' in terms of exposure, because the drug may not cross the blood–brain barrier.

At synapses where nicotinic receptors are found (i.e. neuromuscular junctions and autonomic ganglia), acetylcholine is hydrolysed rapidly by acetylcholinesterase (within 1 ms), so that only a single post-synaptic action potential is usually generated in response to the agonist effects of acetylcholine. However, if the acetylcholine or a nicotinic analogue continues to stimulate the excitatory post-synaptic receptors, a depolarizing block will occur. Suxemethonium (succinyldicholine) is a highly charged molecule which does not cross the blood–brain barrier, and whose effects are therefore confined to the peripheral nervous system. It causes a depolarizing, non-competitive neuromuscular block. The initial stimulation (producing skeletal muscle fasciculation) persists, and there is sustained depolarization and leakage of K^+ ions out of the cell. Although the membrane repolarizes, the receptor is desensitized and is unable to respond to further agonist stimulation (flaccid paralysis). Recovery is time dependent and also requires removal of the agonist. The activity of suxemethonium is prolonged because it is hydrolysed by plasma cholinesterase (not the synaptic enzyme), and the usual effective duration of action is 3–5 min. If there is decreased plasma cholinesterase activity (sometimes called pseudocholinesterase), due to an atypical variant (autosomal recessive inheritance), diminished synthesis in chronic disease, or chronic organophosphate exposure, prolonged neuromuscular paralysis will occur (so-called 'Scoline apnoea'). Administration of neostigmine will deepen the block. Organophosphate poisoning produces a depolarizing blockade similar to that created by suxemethonium by causing accumulation of released acetylcholine.

Non-depolarizing neuromuscular blockers (e.g. *d*-tubocurarine, vecuronium, pancuronium, mivracurium) are competitive antagonists at the nicotinic receptors. As well as causing flaccid paralysis, they block nicotinic receptors in autonomic ganglia and cause hypotension. Gallamine also blocks cardiac muscarinic receptors (i.e. it is not a pure nicotinic antagonist) and may produce tachycardia (see below). The newer competitive blocker mivracurium is metabolized by plasma cholinesterase and can cause prolonged blockade in patients with pseudocholinesterase deficiency.

5-HT$_3$ receptors are also directly linked to ion channels. Selective 5-HT$_3$ receptor antagonists (e.g. ondansetron, tropisetron) are efficacious anti-emetic drugs, and in particular are used to reduce nausea and vomiting associated with cancer chemotherapy and radiotherapy. The target 5-HT$_3$ receptors for the anti-emetic effects are located both in the gut and in the chemoreceptor trigger zone in the hypothalamus, but lying outside the blood–brain barrier. Some of the anti-emetic properties of metoclopramide are also due to 5-HT$_3$ antagonist properties.

Receptors coupled to G-protein

Many hormones and slow neurotransmitters depend on so-called 'second messengers' in their effector systems, the receptor being linked to the effector system by a G-protein (e.g. muscarinic acetylcholine receptors, adrenergic receptors, dopamine, 5-HT, peptides, purines). The response time of a G-protein-dependent event tends to be of the order of seconds, rather than milliseconds as for fast neurotransmitters. The basic structure of all of these receptor proteins is a single polypeptide chain which is folded into seven transmembranous alpha-helices. Four possible effector systems have been described, namely guanylate cyclase, adenylate cyclase, phospholipase C and phospholipase A2, with their respective second messengers (e.g. cyclic GMP, cyclic AMP, inositol triphosphate, diacylglycerol or arachadonic acid).

Selectivity and specificity are endowed by changes in the extracellular part of the peptide (i.e. the receptor itself) and the effector system to which it is coupled. Muscarinic cholinergic receptors serve as a practical example of this. They have three functional subclasses, with small changes in the ligand binding site coupled to different second messengers. Although the receptor differences are subtle, it has been possible to produce relatively specific muscarinic antagonists. Pirenzepene is M1-selective (affecting gastric parietal cells and postsynaptic neural tissue), but its use in the treatment of peptic ulcer disease has now been superseded by more efficacious drugs such as the H$_2$-antagonists or proton-pump inhibitors. Benztropine, used prophylactically to prevent the Parkinsonism which accompanies the older antipsychotic phenothiazines (e.g. fluphenazine), has less peripheral (M2 and M3) effects in relation to central ones (M1) than does atropine. This means that a patient on benztropine will not display, for example, the tachycardia that an equivalent dose of atropine would cause.

In traditional terminology, antihistamines referred to H$_1$-antagonists (e.g. diphenhydramine, promethazine) used to treat allergic reactions such as rhinitis. As a group they often have other receptor activity; diphenhydramine is also antimuscarinic. They had considerable sedative effects, readily crossing the blood–brain barrier, and these properties made them useful as anti-emetics. Newer H$_1$-antagonists such as terfenadine are selective for H$_1$-receptors and do not have the associated sedation. H$_2$-receptor antagonists such as cimetidine or ranitidine are widely used in the symptomatic treatment of peptic ulcer disease. They competitively inhibit histamine- and gastrin-stimulated acid secretion. Their role in the long-term treatment of ulceration has been revised in the light of the probable contribution of *Helicobacter pylori* to ulceration.

All adrenoreceptors are coupled to G-proteins. The major adrenoreceptor subgroups (α and β) show different functional responses and anatomical distributions. In practical terms, few agonist drugs have been successfully developed to exploit structural differences for β-receptors. Often routes of administration are used to give relative specificity. For instance, when inhaled to treat asthma, isoprenaline will produce less stimulation of cardiac receptors (β_1), allowing significant agonist effects on bronchial receptors (β_2), than if equivalent doses were given intravenously. Although noradrenalin has more α-receptor activity than β-agonist effects, it must be remembered that noradrenalin is the natural transmitter of the β-receptor. If it is used to limit the use of local anaesthetic for instance, or to control bleeding, a significant amount may be absorbed into the circulation. The net effect could be an increase in blood pressure due to a combination of peripheral vasoconstriction (α_1) and tachycardia (β_1), as well as CNS-induced anxiety. The dose dependency of catecholamines is well demonstrated by the use of dopamine. When used as a low-dose infusion (1–5 μg/kg body weight/min) to improve renal perfusion, it causes renal vasculature dilatation (dopamine receptors). At higher rates of infusion, α_1 receptors in other vascular beds are recruited (vasoconstriction), and finally there is a β_1-agonist effect on the heart, with increased force of contraction. Although the development of specific catechol agonists has not been very successful, the development of specific adrenoreceptor antagonists has been more so. For instance, prazosin is a selective α_1 antagonist used in the treatment of hypertension. A more recent role for α-blockade and prazosin is in the control of some of the urinary symptoms of benign prostatic hyperplasia. It has fewer side-effects than the non-specific α-blocker hydralazine. Similarly, atenolol is a specific β_1 antagonist used in hypertension which has fewer side-effects than propranolol, a non-selective β antagonist which is more likely to cause bronchoconstriction in an asthmatic subject. Traditional teaching has been that β-blockers may precipitate or worsen congestive cardiac failure. However, carvedilol (a non-selective β-blocker with vasodilatory and possible free-radical-scavenging properties) has produced significantly improved patient survival in congestive cardiac failure.

The opioids are a chemically disparate group of compounds which include the naturally occurring peptides of the CNS (e.g. endorphins), the alkaloids of the poppy *Papaver somniferum* and their derivatives (e.g. morphine, heroin), and the synthetic compounds with structures unrelated to morphine (e.g. pethidine, methadone; see Chapter 1.10). The opioid receptors differ from other

G-protein receptors in that the main agonist effects seem to link the G-protein directly to ion channels, without an apparent need for second messengers. Opioid agonists cause K^+ channels to open (with hyperpolarization of the membrane) and decrease neurotransmitter release (due to decreased calcium entry into the cell). This difference is potentially important in explaining the mechanism of tolerance and addiction to opioids.

G-protein receptors coupled through tyrosine kinase

Proteins which have a role in cell growth and differentiation, and which act by regulating gene transcription, have a common homology in their receptors which are linked intracellularly to tyrosine kinase (e.g. insulin and cytokines stimulating mitosis, such as interleukin-2 (IL-2), tumour necrosis factor).

Inhibitors which act on the extracellular binding domain of the large cytokine receptors have been developed. The best-known such inhibitor is OKT3 (Muromonab-CD3), the monoclonal antibody raised against the CD3 antigen on the T-lymphocyte. Binding of OKT3 to CD3 prevents T-lymphocyte receptor activation. The earlier-generation polyclonal antibodies, antithymocyte globulin (ATG) and antilymphocyte globulin (ALG), have similar effects. In contrast, the immunosuppressant cyclosporin A inhibits clonal expansion of T-lymphocytes by decreasing production of IL-2 and other cytokines and inhibiting the expression of IL-2 receptors on the surface of maturing T-lymphocytes. The immunosuppressant tacrolimus also inhibits gene transcription, but its inhibition is at a different point to that of cyclosporin.

Synthetic analogues of many of the haemopoietic growth factors are now in clinical use. These include recombinant erythropoietin, which is used in patients with chronic renal failure. Granulocyte-colony-stimulating factor (G-CSF) acts on neutrophil stem cells, and is used increasingly to limit or treat leucopenia which occurs secondary to high-dose cytotoxic chemotherapy. It also has a role in preparation for harvesting peripheral (blood) stem cells for later autotransplantation. Granulocyte-macrophage-CSF (GM-CSF) acts on several stem-cell lines, including neutrophils, monocytes and megakaryocytes. Both G-CSF and GM-CSF cause bone pain in 10–20% of recipients (related to intense marrow expansion). At high doses, GM-CSF may produce a symptom complex similar to influenza (hypotension, tachycardia, breathlessness), probably due to excess cytokine release from newly synthesized cells, and venous and pulmonary embolism (excess platelet synthesis). As all of these analogues are glycoproteins; they require parenteral administration.

Nuclear receptors

Nuclear receptors regulate DNA transcription in response to steroid hormones, thyroid hormones, retinoic acid and vitamin D. The receptor is a large nuclear protein, the C-terminal end of which contains the binding domain. In the case of steroids, the genomic response may be either increased or decreased transcription of mRNA, depending on the particular genome. Production of mRNA occurs within minutes of steroid binding, but the biological result, which is due to altered protein production, may take hours or days to become apparent. For instance, cortisol or prednisolone given for bronchospasm in severe asthma attack will not show a significant clinical benefit for at least 4 h. All nuclear receptor agonists and antagonists are lipid soluble and diffuse into the nucleus. The biological half-life of these compounds will depend on the half-life of the synthesized protein as well as their affinity for the receptors. Because the receptors are present in all cells, there is a high incidence of side-effects, and these are particularly seen clinically with steroid use.

If the steroid is an antagonist (e.g. spironolactone and its metabolite, canrenone), the antagonist–receptor complex does not bind to DNA, so mRNA and protein synthesis stops. In the case of aldosterone antagonists such as spironolactone, the onset of clinical effect (diuresis) will depend on the half-life of the proteins previously caused to be synthesized by circulating aldosterone. One would not expect a significant diuresis before 36–40 h post-dose, and furthermore the largest response would be in (primary or secondary) hyperaldosteronism.

Tamoxifen is known as an 'anti-oestrogen'. It is more correctly a weak partial agonist, which in breast tissue competes with natural oestrogen for binding to oestrogen receptors. It binds with high affinity but inhibits transcription at the oestrogen-responsive genes in breast tissue. It is used as adjunctive therapy in oestrogen positive carcinoma of the breast. However, its partial agonist properties are apparent in post-menopausal women, in whom there are significant decreases in LDL-cholesterol and increases in HDL. The result is a plasma lipoprotein profile more like that of premenopausal women, and possibly conferring some of the cardiovascular protection of the premenopausal group.

Cyproterone is a partial agonist at androgen receptors as well as being a progestogen. It competes with dihydrotestosterone (the active metabolite of testosterone) in androgen-sensitive tissues such as the prostate. In treatment of carcinoma of the prostate, cyproterone can be used in association with one of the gonadotrophin-releasing-factor analogues, such as gosorelin or leuprorelin.

PHARMACOLOGY AND PHARMACOKINETICS

We shall now consider the major principles governing drug use, such as the bioavailability and pharmacokinetics of drugs. Although the different mechanisms of action which have been described above are important, a novel drug with a unique and specific mechanism of action may be of no practical value if its bioavailability is so low that it is not absorbed from the gastrointestinal system. If its rate of clearance is so high that it requires constant infusion to be effective, or if it is so unstable that a pharmaceutical formulation appears to be unattainable, the drug may not come into use. There are numerous examples of these 'what-ifs', and in each case, if the drug really does offer a unique advance, there may be a solution which we accept for therapeutic benefit. For instance, in the first example given, of poor bioavailability, aminoglycoside antibiotics (e.g. gentamicin) are a case in point, and the solution is parenteral administration. In the second example, of very high clearance, the drug could be fentanyl, the solution being constant infusion or administration of small repetitive doses. The third example is the province of the medicinal chemist, with solutions such as the storage of drugs protected from light (e.g. halothane), or solubilizing drugs immediately prior to administration (e.g. hydrocortisone). In other cases, preparation of a soluble salt from a relatively insoluble drug may be required to facilitate administration (e.g. aminophylline is the soluble parenteral formulation of theophylline), or development of a pro-drug may be necessary to achieve clinical efficacy (e.g. mycophenylate mofetil is the pro-drug for mycophenylate). These examples are not exclusive, but are selected to demonstrate a range of possibilities, all of which the practitioner takes for granted, but of which it is important to be aware.

DRUG ABSORPTION AND EXCRETION

Absorption of a drug into plasma from the site of administration will be determined by the physico-chemical properties of the drug itself, as well as by a number of factors which include the formulation of the drug, the pH of the environment, the nature of the barriers which exist between the drug and plasma, and the blood flow through the tissue. The barriers between the aqueous compartments of the body all have their own particular properties, but there are some general principles. In general, molecules cross cell membranes in one of four ways. They may diffuse through lipid (e.g. steroid hormones such as cortisol), they may diffuse through aqueous pores or channels (e.g. Na^+ through very fast sodium channels), they may combine with a specific carrier (e.g.

Na^+/K^+-ATPase), or they may undergo pinocytosis after binding to a specific receptor (e.g. insulin).

Movement across vascular endothelium may be through the intercellular gaps, or it may require passage of the drug across the endothelial cells themselves. In the CNS, under normal circumstances the capillary endothelium can be regarded as a continuum, allowing little diffusion of non-lipid-soluble molecules across the blood–brain barrier. Similar tight endothelial junctions exist in the placenta. Special transport processes are very important in these tissues for the supply of normal nutrients and maintenance of fluid and electrolyte balance. In many tissues the intercellular gaps are usually wide enough to permit diffusion across the capillary walls of molecules of molecular weight less than approximately 30 kDa. In inflammation, the intercellular gaps increase, and there is exudate formation. This increase in the presence of inflammation changes the characteristics of the capillary endothelium, so that antibiotics which are usually excluded by the blood–brain barrier will cross into cerebrospinal fluid and brain tissue in meningitis and encephalitis.

Diffusion through lipid requires the compound to be lipid soluble, non-polar and non-ionized. Net movement will be down a concentration gradient. A good clinical example of this is seen with the benzodiazepines, which are very lipid soluble. When diazepam or clonazepam is administered as an intravenous bolus in the treatment of status epilepticus, the drug crosses the blood–brain barrier very rapidly from the high plasma concentration to zero or low intracerebral concentration. Rapid delivery of the drug to the brain is further helped by the high proportion of cardiac output, which is distributed to the CNS. This favours the early delivery of drugs to the brain, almost in a preferential manner. As soon as the concentration in the plasma starts to fall, the drug will diffuse out of the CNS down the now opposite concentration gradient, and be redistributed into other high lipid-containing sites (e.g. other membranes in the periphery and adipose tissue). If the cerebral concentration falls below that required, fitting may recur.

Many drugs are either weak acids or weak bases, and will exist in the body in both ionized and non-ionized forms in equilibrium. For any given drug in aqueous solution, the degree of ionization will depend on the pH of the environment, which is governed by its pK_a. Only the non-ionized form can potentially move into or across the cell membrane. Local anaesthetics (e.g. lignocaine) have a pK_a of 8–9 and tend to be ionized at physiological pH. However, in their function as local anaesthetics or anti-arrhythmics, the binding site which they occupy in the fast Na^+ channel is at the intracellular end of the ion channel. They can only access this site by crossing the axon sheaths and neuronal membranes while they are non-ionized and lipid soluble. On reaching the cytoplasm, the pH favours re-ionization and the drug becomes pharmacologically active, binding to the fast sodium channel. In addition, the lignocaine is effectively 'trapped' within the cytoplasm.

There are many other examples of ionization and pH entrapping drugs in different body compartments. Acidic drugs (e.g. aspirin and salicylate, with a pK_a of 3.5) will tend to remain in urine of pH 8 compared to plasma of pH 7.4. This has been exploited in the treatment of aspirin or salicylate overdose, with alkalinization of the urine used to increase the urinary excretion of the parent drug. Omeprazole is a weak base (with a pK_a of 3.97) which tends to accumulate in an acid environment such as that associated with the mucosal crypts and gastric parietal cells, where it binds to the proton pumps.

Carrier-mediated transport is widespread throughout the body. Examples of drug absorption from the gastrointestinal system include levo-dopa being absorbed via the phenylalanine transport system, and 5-fluorouracil utilizing the pyrimidine uptake system. Carrier-mediated transport has a prominent role in drug excretion in the liver and kidney, and in drug transport across the blood–brain barrier. A characteristic of all carrier-mediated transport systems is that they are subject to saturation and competitive inhibition. For instance, the active transport systems in the kidney are carriers for drugs (e.g. the organic acid pathway for excretion of penicillins). They are also targets for therapeutic strategies (e.g. frusemide inhibiting the co-transporter for Na^+ and Cl^- in the ascending limb of the loop of Henlé).

PLASMA PROTEIN BINDING

At therapeutic concentrations the majority of drugs are bound to some extent to proteins in plasma. However, the degree of binding varies widely between different drugs (Table 37.1.1). The protein to which a particular drug will bind is determined by its chemical characteristics. For example, acidic drugs bind primarily to albumin (e.g. salicylate), basic drugs bind to α_1-acid glycoprotein (e.g. lignocaine), and highly lipid-soluble drugs dissolve

in lipoproteins (e.g. cyclosporin A). In addition, there may be binding to immunoglobulin (e.g. antibody production stimulated by porcine insulin). A further specialized case is that of a hormone (or its analogue) binding to the naturally occurring binding protein (e.g. cortisol to corticosteroid-binding globulin, thyroxine to thyroxine-binding globulin and pre-albumin). In almost all circumstances it is considered that the bound drug is biologically inactive, and only the free, unbound drug will have access to receptors or be available for uptake into cells. Secondly, the same free, unbound moiety is subject to clearance (e.g. filtration in the kidney or hepatic uptake and metabolism). As the binding to protein is reversible in most cases, the bound portion will be a pool of stored drug with equilibrium at steady state between the bound and free moieties. The concentration of plasma protein will also influence the mass of drug that is bound.

For a small number of drugs a significant proportion of the drug concentration may bind to or be taken up into cellular components of blood. Clinically important examples of this are the immunosuppressant drugs cyclosporin A and tacrolimus, antimalarial drugs such as chloroquine, and toxins such as lead. In all of these cases, measurement of the drug or toxin in the plasma compartment alone will seriously underestimate the patient's total exposure, and the whole blood concentration should be measured. Just as for drugs that are bound to plasma proteins, the moiety which is contained within the erythrocytes is in equilibrium with the free, unbound drug in plasma, and will become available as the free concentration tends to fall. In addition, it will be released if the cell should undergo lysis or die.

A large number of drug interactions and effects have been ascribed to plasma protein binding. However, at steady state, protein binding is only considered to be clinically important when the percentage of drug bound is very high (usually considered to be > 90%; Table 37.1.1) and/or when the capacity of binding is limited (i.e. saturable). The examples which are important to remember are those in which potentially serious clinical consequences arise, such as binding of phenytoin

Table 37.1.1 Plasma protein binding at therapeutic concentrations

Percentage of drug bound			
>95	90–95	50–90	<50
Amitriptyline	Cephalothin/cefoxitin	Aspirin/salicylate	Aminoglycosides
Cyclosporin A	Chlorpromazine	Carbamazepine	Cefotaxime
Diazepam	Glibenclamide	Lignocaine	Digoxin
Thyroxine	Indomethacin	Penicillin	Paracetamol
Warfarin	Phenytoin	Sulphonamide	Phenobarbitone
	Valproate		

(anticonvulsant), tolbutamide (hypoglycaemic), salicylate (analgesic), warfarin (anticoagulant) and unconjugated bilirubin (particularly in the neonate). There is another factor to be considered, too. If there is a decrease in protein binding, is there a mechanism which could effectively result in the increase in unbound drug being reduced to the pre-existing concentration? This would limit both the duration of any decreased binding and its potential toxicity. Phenytoin is very lipid soluble, so for the excess free drug to be accommodated it might bind to alternative sites (e.g. tissue proteins), or be taken into potential stores (e.g. adipose tissue). If the additional free phenytoin is to be metabolized, there must be excess capacity in the metabolic pathway. If the pathway is saturated, then the free moiety will remain elevated, and clinical toxicity will become apparent.

When considering individual patients in whom the total plasma phenytoin concentration is the same, but there are differing albumin concentrations, the lower the albumin level, the higher the free fraction is likely to be. Toxicity may therefore occur when total plasma drug concentrations are within the normal therapeutic concentration range, but if the albumin concentration is low, there are higher free concentrations. A similar effect has been shown for uptake of cyclosporin A into red blood cells, so toxicity can occur within the therapeutic blood reference range if there is significant anaemia.

If more than one drug binds at a particular binding site (or domain) of a molecule, then a drug interaction may occur. If the drug which is displaced from the protein is usually highly protein bound, then the net result will be similar to that discussed above, i.e. if there is limited clearance and limited redistribution, there will be a sustained increased free fraction. One of the best recognized clinical examples is the interaction between sulphonamides and warfarin, where the sulphonamide in cotrimoxazole displaces warfarin, with a resulting increase in anticoagulation. Another example is the interaction between unconjugated bilirubin and salicylate in neonates. In these examples the important end result is determined by whether there is a limited clearance (sulphonamide–warfarin interaction with a resulting increase in anticoagulation and a raised prothrombin time), or whether movement of the displaced ligand elsewhere may pose a threat (e.g. unconjugated bilirubin moves into the CNS and kernicterus may result).

Drug metabolism

The most active site for drug metabolism is the liver. However, many of the reactions described also occur in other tissues, such as gut wall and kidney, and may be important in influencing bioavailability, for example. The underlying principle of hepatic metabolism is the modification of the parent drug to produce a compound which is more polar and more water soluble than the parent. The reactions are classified as phase I and II reactions. Phase I reactions include oxidation, hydroxylation, dealkylation and deamination. The enzymes include the microsomal mixed-function oxidases, which include the haem proteins of the cytochrome P450 (CyP) families. Drugs may undergo single or multiple transformations (e.g. benzodiazepines) and the metabolites may be pharmacologically active. Other oxidative systems include xanthine oxidase (in the metabolism of purines), monoamine oxidase (in the intracellular metabolism of catecholamines and serotonin) and alcohol dehydrogenase. Reductive reactions are much less common than oxidative ones (e.g. conversion of prednisone to its active form prednisolone). Phase II or conjugation reactions result in compounds which are much less lipid soluble and more water soluble than either the parent or phase I products. Some drugs are conjugated without any prior modification. The most common conjugates formed are the glucuronides, but others include sulphate, methyl, acetyl, glycyl and glutamyl derivatives. Following metabolism in the liver, many compounds are actively transported out of the hepatocyte. Competition for the transport mechanism may cause side-effects (e.g. cholestasis secondary to rifampicin). Phase II (conjugation) reactions occur in the lungs and kidneys as well as in the liver. An additional metabolic pathway is enzymatic hydrolysis, which occurs in many tissues. It may be intracellular or extracellular, the latter utilizing enzymes synthesized by the liver (e.g. succinylcholine is hydrolysed by plasma pseudocholinesterase). Clinically important drug interactions arise from competition between different drugs for metabolism. This type of interaction is said to be pharmacokinetic (e.g. cimetidine or erythromycin inhibiting CyP 3A4 and decreasing theophylline or cyclosporin A metabolism).

Pharmacogenetics

There is increasing awareness that there are genetically determined differences in the activity of the enzymes involved in drug metabolism. These are important contributors to the differences in clearance which have been observed between some individuals. Table 37.1.2 lists examples of some important clinical consequences of these variations. The general principle is that rapid metabolic clearance may be associated with decreased efficacy, because the dose of drug required may be greater than that usually prescribed. The same increased metabolic clearance may give rise to side-effects if the metabolic derivative is pharmacologically active. Slow rates of metabolism tend to lead to toxicity associated with parent drug accumulation. The other group of side-effects related to genetics is often referred to as 'idiosyncratic'. In this latter group, pharmacokinetics

Table 37.1.2 Pharmacogenetics: clinical examples of identified genetic influences in drug response

Pathway/enzyme	Drug	Clinical outcome
Acetylation	Procainamide	Slow acetylation associated with autoimmune disease e.g. Lupus erythematosus
	Isoniazid	Slow acetylation and peripheral neuropathy
		Fast acetylation and hepatotoxicity
	Sulphonamides	Fast acetylation and crystalluria
Pseudocholinesterase	Succinylcholine Mivracurium	Autosomal recessive inheritence, slow metabolism and prolonged apnoea
Cytochrome P450 super family		
2C9/19	Phenytoin	Slow metabolism and saturable pathway with likely toxicity
2D6	Codeine	Slow metabolism and poor analgesic response, as morphine not produced
Thiopurine methyl transferase	6–mercaptopurine Azathioprine	Slow metabolism and increased cytotoxicity, with bone marrow aplasia etc
Aldehyde dehydrogenase	Acetaldehyde (ethanol)	Autosomal dominant inheritance; flushing, tachycardia, anxiety due to acetaldehyde accumulation; cf response to disulfiram in alcohol avoidance programmes
Glucose-6–phosphate dehydrogenase	Sulphonamides Primaquine	Sex-linked recessive inheritance; exposure results in intravascular haemolysis
Porphobilinogen deaminase*	Barbiturates Phenytoin Oestrogens	Autosomal dominant inheritance; exposure may precipitate attack of acute intermittent porphyria
?Ryanodine receptor of sarcoplasmic reticulum	Halothane Succinylcholine	?Dominant inheritance; exposure may precipitate malignant hyperthermia

*as an example of one of the enzyme defects in the porphyrias.

per se are not altered, but there is a drug-induced response which is deleterious and may appear spontaneous and unexpected.

Induction

Some drugs (e.g. phenobarbitone), when administered repeatedly, increase the activity of the microsomal oxidases and conjugating enzymes. The net result may be increased metabolism of the agent itself (auto-induction) as well as of other compounds. Each agent has a characteristic profile of induction. For instance, phenobarbitone has a wide spectrum of effects, while benzopyrene, which is carcinogenic, is more selective in the pathways that it affects. The most frequent clinical reflection of induction is the increased activity of biliary enzymes such as gamma-glutamyl transpeptidase seen in the liver function testing profile of patients in whom these anticonvulsants (e.g. phenytoin) are being – or have been – used. Ethanol produces the same effect. The dose requirements of the anticonvulsants and of some other drugs will be increased in these cases.

Stereoisomers

Although many drugs exist as optical isomers (e.g. adrenalin, warfarin), they are currently most often administered as racemic mixtures. The isomers differ not only in their pharmacodynamic effects and efficacy (i.e. binding to the receptor), but also have different affinities for metabolic enzymes. In some cases there can be metabolic transformation of one isomer to another in vivo, but in general this is not yet well understood. In the future there is every likelihood that drugs which exist as stereoisomers will be available in pharmaceutical preparations as the pure stereoisomer.

Activation

Drug metabolism should not be considered only in its role as one of the mechanisms of drug clearance. A significant number of drugs require modification in order to become pharmacologically active (e.g. metabolism of codeine to morphine, azathioprine to 6-mercapto-purine, prednisone to prednisolone), the parent compound being known as a pro-drug. Many metabolic products have significant pharmacological activity themselves (e.g. morphine and morphine-6-glu-curonide, diazepam and oxazepam). In some cases the metabolite's activity is responsible for major toxicity (e.g. metabolism of pethidine to norpethidine, the latter causing fits if there is accumulation, and paracetamol giving rise to paracetamol epoxide, a highly reactive molecule with potential hepatotoxicity; Table 37.1.3).

Drug-induced liver disease

To complete this section, brief consideration should be given to the influence which drugs may have on liver function other than the induction discussed above. Drugs may cause changes which mimic all types of liver pathology. Table 37.1.3 lists a few examples of drugs which produce significant abnormalities of liver function. These liver abnormalities may be temporary, with full recovery following cessation of exposure to the drug, or there may be sustained damage and, for example, cirrhosis.

RENAL EXCRETION

Compounds of molecular weight $< 20\,kDa$ pass into the glomerular filtrate at a rate which is governed by renal blood flow, perfusion pressure and the number of functional glomeruli. The protein-bound moiety of drugs will not be filtered in a normal glomerulus. As well as being filtered in the glomerulus, drugs are actively secreted and resorbed in the tubules – acidic compounds via the organic acid pathway and basic compounds down that designed for their configuration. Both systems are subject to saturation and competition. This can be used

therapeutically to good effect. For example, probenecid inhibits the excretion of penicillin, resulting in increased plasma levels of penicillin and improved efficacy in the treatment of bacterial endocarditis. However, it may cause major side-effects (low-dose aspirin or thiazide diuretics inhibit uric acid, with resultant hyperuricaemia and precipitation of gout). Any diffusion and resorption from the glomerular filtrate will depend on the lipid solubility of the drug and its polarity, as well as the pH of the glomerular filtrate (e.g. aspirin, as discussed earlier).

Drugs that are excreted almost exclusively by the kidneys (Table 37.1.4) will be significantly affected if there is renal impairment (e.g. in the elderly or in renal disease). Drugs themselves can also cause renal pathology (Table 37.1.5), the mechanisms of which are very varied.

BIOAVAILABILITY

This is the percentage of drug dose which is available to the systemic circulation following its administration. By definition, an intravenous dose is 100% bioavailable. Following oral administration, bioavailability is the amount of the dose which is absorbed from the gastrointestinal system and not metabolized in either the intestinal mucosa or the liver, i.e. which does not undergo first-pass or presystemic metabolism. Although there is a tendency to consider bioavailability in terms of orally administered drugs, the same principles should be applied for drugs which are applied topically to the skin or eyes, or inhaled. In all cases, any drug which is absorbed and produces systemic effects is bioavailable. These effects may be undesirable and responsible for much of the side-effect profile (e.g. inhaled steroids in the treatment of asthma).

Table 37.1.3 Examples of drug-induced liver disease

Effect	Drug
Elevated enzyme activity	Phenytoin, rifampicin, alcohol
Hepatocellular damage, necrosis	Halothane, isoniazid, paracetamol (large dose)
Cholestasis	Chlorpromazine, erythromycin, anabolic steroids, oestrogens
Neoplasia	Anabolic steroids, oestrogens, aflatoxin

Table 37.1.4 Examples of drugs with significant renal excretion

Cardio-active	Diuretics	Antibiotics	Miscellaneous
Atenolol	Amiloride	Penicillins	Lithium
Digoxin	Chlorothiazide	Aminoglycosides	Chlorpropamide
Disopyramide	Frusemide	Sulphonamides	Methotrexate
Procainamide	Mannitol	Vancomycin	Morphine-6–glucuronide

Table 37.1.5 Examples of drug-induced renal disease

Effect	Drug
Acute tubular necrosis	Aminoglycoside antibiotics, vancomycin, amphotericin B, non-steroidal anti-inflammatory drugs (high dose), cisplatin, lithium
Papillary necrosis	Phenacetin (chronic), ?paracetamol and other NSAIDs
Acute interstitial nephritis, arteritis, vasculitis	Penicillins, sulphonamides, allopurinol, non-steroidal anti-inflammatory drugs
Glomerular damage	D-penicillamine, gold salts
Crystalluria	Sulphonamides, methotrexate
Uric acid nephropathy	Cytotoxic drugs (tumour lysis syndrome)
Myoglobinuria	Opioids (overdose), clofibrate, simvastatin

ROUTES OF ADMINISTRATION

Oral administration

With the majority of drugs, little absorption occurs in the gastrointestinal tract until the drug passes into the small intestine. Numerous factors within the lumen of the gut influence the bioavailability of drugs, and these will now be discussed.

Absorption will be slowed by decreased gastrointestinal motility; gastric emptying is decreased post-operatively (due to endogenous endorphins and/or administered opioids). Severe nausea has a similar effect (e.g. in patients with severe migraine). Absorption is accelerated by drugs such as metoclopramide and cisapride, which increase the rate of gastric emptying. These relatively simple interactions have practical consequences. In a patient with migraine, analgesics such as paracetamol or salicylates may be made more efficacious if metoclopramide is given first, and thus the administration of parenteral analgesics is avoided. The profound gastric stasis that precedes or accompanies migraine makes 'simple' analgesics ineffective because they are not absorbed.

Gastric pH has three separate effects which must be considered. First, some drugs are acid labile. Such drugs are either not given via the oral route (e.g. benzylpenicillin) or are administered in sufficient doses for some drug to retain activity (e.g. omeprazole), or are given between meals, at a time when the pH is less acidic (e.g. phenoxymethylpenicillin). Alternatively, the drug may be formulated in a gelatine capsule and so be protected until it passes into the small intestine. The second effect of pH is the potential for ion trapping. The aminoglycoside antibiotics (e.g. gentamicin) and vancomycin are highly polar and are very poorly absorbed from the gut. This property is exploited therapeutically, with neomycin being used for bowel preparation or oral vancomycin in the treatment of *Clostridium difficile* in patients with pseudomembranous colitis. In both cases

the drugs have no systemic effects. For systemic use, the drug must be given parenterally. The third consequence of pH is related to changes induced by therapy, by administration of either antacids or drugs used to decrease acid secretion. The most common antacids are the hydroxide salts of aluminium and magnesium. Apart from the direct effects which Al^{3+} and Mg^{2+} may have on smooth muscle (producing constipation and diarrhoea, respectively), they can form insoluble complexes that decrease the bioavailability of drugs such as iron and tetracycline. Bacterial overgrowth of the gut can occur in patients who become profoundly achlorhydric.

Bile salts are critical to the formation of micelles and, in turn, the absorption of fat-soluble compounds is dependent on normal micelle formation. Decreased bile acid availability in the gut secondary to either cholestatic jaundice or drainage of bile to the exterior via a T-tube will markedly decrease the absorption of fat-soluble vitamins (vitamins A, D, E and K).

The activity of pancreatic amylase and lipase secreted into the duodenum is important in the digestion of carbohydrates and lipids. In patients with cystic fibrosis or other forms of chronic pancreatic insufficiency, oral supplementation of these enzymes is necessary. If the level of supplementation is not sufficient, steatorrhoea will occur and give rise to problems similar to those associated with bile acid deficiency.

With regard to drug binding within the lumen, the formation of complexes between drugs and other contents of the gut will influence bioavailability (e.g. digoxin binding to cholestyramine, tetracycline binding to calcium, ferrous iron binding to dietary phosphates and phytates). With such drugs, in order to maximize or have relatively reproducible absorption, administration should take place at least 2 h before or after other drugs or food, unless there are contraindications. For example, in patients with a peptic ulcer, iron preparations can exacerbate symptoms when taken alone, so administration with food is a practical alternative in this situation.

An additional factor which is now gaining recognition is the presence of P-glycoprotein. This protein was first identified as being responsible for acquired drug resistance to cytotoxic drugs that were being used in the treatment of malignancy. Within the gut, P-glycoprotein is important in the active secretion of drugs out of mucosal cells back into the intestinal lumen. Blockade of this system with drugs such as diltiazem will increase the oral bioavailability of drugs such as cyclosporin or phenytoin. This mechanism is additional to the decrease in bioavailability due to the same compound (diltiazam) inhibiting the metabolism of certain drugs within the gastrointestinal mucosa itself.

In summary, the influence of food in the gut on drug absorption is complex. Although drug delivery into the small intestine may be delayed (and thereby drug absorption may also be delayed), and admixing of the drug with food may decrease its exposure to the gut wall (decreasing the rate of and possibly total absorption), the presence of fat and bile acids will enhance micelle formation and improve absorption of lipid-soluble compounds, and postprandial splanchnic blood flow may increase absorption. However, the presence of food may result in the binding of specific compounds and acid hydrolysis may reduce the absorption of certain biologically active drugs.

The lining of the small intestine has a very large surface of thin mucosa covering the microvilli and the crypts. In diseases involving villous atrophy, such as coeliac disease or tropical sprue, the surface area is markedly reduced. Chronic effects on nutrient absorption are well recognized (e.g. folate deficiency causing macrocytic anaemia). Malabsorption affects drugs such as digoxin and thyroxine, and bowel resection may give rise to specific malabsorption states depending on the anatomical site of resection (e.g. vitamin B_{12} deficiency secondary to either gastrectomy or resection of the terminal ileum).

If splanchnic blood flow is decreased, whether due to hypovolaemia or cardiac failure, absorption of nutrients and drugs alike will be decreased. In patients with clinical signs consistent with diminished splanchnic perfusion, intravenous administration of drugs should be considered. For example, a patient may be apparently unresponsive to oral diuretics, but in fact may not be absorbing them, and an intravenous dose may markedly improve cardiovascular function and indirectly improve subsequent absorption as well. Similarly, the absorption and efficacy of analgesics may be influenced.

Laxatives and purgatives

Purgatives are drugs which increase the rate of passage of food through the gut. In the context of drug administration, if the rate of transit of gut contents is increased too much, drug absorption may be decreased. This is utilized in the treatment of overdose, when an oral fructose solution is given to increase the rate of removal of the drug from the gut (e.g. following paracetamol overdose). The purgatives can be classified into four groups which differ in practical terms.

1. *Bulk laxatives* (e.g. methylcellulose and bran) are polysaccharide polymers that are resistant to digestion. They act osmotically, retaining water within the lumen, and the increased bulk promotes peristalsis. These laxatives will not be functional if the myenteric plexus is interrupted or blocked, and therefore they are not useful if the constipation is due to opioid use.

2. *Osmotic laxatives* are poorly absorbed solutes which maintain large volumes of water within the lumen. The main examples are fructose (described above), magnesium salts and lactulose. Lactulose (a disaccharide of fructose and galactose) is hydrolysed by colonic bacteria and metabolized within the lumen to acetic and lactic acids. As well as being osmotically active, the resultant decrease in gut pH inhibits ammonium production within the gut. It has thus become an integral component of the management of hepatic encephalopathy.

3. *Faecal softeners* (e.g. docusate sodium) are similar to detergents.

4. *Stimulant purgatives* (e.g. senna, bisacodyl) act by initiating local gut reflexes which are transmitted through intramural plexuses to the gut smooth muscle. They may induce cramping pain, and long-term use produces altered gut function and atonic colon. Senna-containing anthracene derivatives are administered orally, and bisacodyl is more often given as a suppository.

Drug formulation

In general, drug formulation is an important determinant of absorption across any surface. Pharmaceutical chemistry can manipulate particle size to allow rapid dissolution of a tablet for fast absorption, giving high peak concentrations if required. The particles may be made larger, or coated or encapsulated, in order to give a slowed or 'sustained' absorption, with fewer fluctuations in plasma concentration (e.g. lithium, diltiazem). The 'ultimate' preparations contain microspheres of differing volumes. These are designed to release drug at different rates and throughout the length of the small intestine, so that the smoothest possible concentration–time curve will be obtained, and in some cases single daily dosing is the outcome even for a drug with a relatively short plasma half-life. Coatings (made of wax or sugar) or gel capsules may also protect an acid-labile compound and delay release of the drug until the pH of the lumen is more favourable. In addition, such coatings may limit local mucosal damage by slower release (e.g. salicylate and gastric mucosa). Apart from these changes in the physical conditions of the formulation, drugs may be prepared as derivatives in order to improve their bioavailability, i.e. they are prepared as pro-drugs. For instance, the immunosuppressive agent mycophenylate mofetil (MPA) is a salt of mycophenolic acid. MPA is the active moiety, but it has such a high presystemic elimination that it was could not be given orally.

Bioavailability is an important criterion when a drug formulation is described and the preparation is licensed for therapeutic use. All new drugs and formulations that are released require stringent testing to define their bioavailability. When a drug patent lapses prior to release on to the market, any generic or alternative product preparation is required to have demonstrated bioequivalence. This means that under Australian licensing arrangements, for example, the bioavailability of the generic product must be within 25% of that of the brand-name drug.

Sublingual administration or buccal administration

This can be a useful route of administration if the drug is unstable at gastric pH, or if a rapid response is required for a drug with a high presystemic elimination. Nitroglycerin is the classic example. Other drugs which have been formulated to be administered in this way include an opioid (butyrophenone) and certain preparations of antibiotics for children. It must be noted that, because of the high surface area of the mucosa and absorption directly into venous blood, the drug is not subject to first pass in the liver. Therefore there is a higher bioavailability than for oral administration. Toxicity may result if dose differences are not taken into account (e.g. if used in an emergency, the sublingual dose of the calcium-channel blocker verapamil is very similar to that given intravenously, 2.5–5 mg, whereas the smallest oral dose is 40 mg). In general, drug formulations that have been prepared for one route of administration should not be used for another route.

Rectal administration

The rectal mucosa has a large surface area. The drugs most often administered via this route have been glucocorticosteroid enemas (used for high-dose local treatment of ulcerative colitis) and the overnight indomethacin suppository (for rheumatoid arthritis). Drugs administered via the rectal route are subject to presystemic clearance, the majority of the venous blood ultimately passing via the portal vein to the liver.

Conjunctival administration

Systemic absorption of drugs following topical application of eye drops or ointments is an important cause of side-effects. The drug is absorbed locally through the mucous membrane of the conjunctiva, and excess drug will flow down the nasolacrimal duct and be absorbed from there or from the mucosa of the posterior nasopharynx (as for buccal absorption). The drugs are not subject to first-pass metabolism, and systemic effects may be large. An example of an important side-effect resulting from this route is asthma precipitated by beta-blocker eyedrops used for the treatment of glaucoma (timolol). In a patient who is sensitive to beta-blockers, the amount of timolol absorbed from the overflow down the nasolacrimal duct is sufficient to precipitate bronchoconstriction and cause asthma.

Nasal administration

The mucous membrane of the nose is also highly vascular. It has been used as the route of administration for drugs such as desmopressin (an analogue of antidiuretic hormone) and gonadotrophin-releasing hormone (GRH). The absorbed drug is not subject to a first-pass effect. However, the percentage absorption can be very variable, and will be affected by factors such as excessive mucous secretion in upper respiratory tract infections or allergic rhinitis. It is the preferred route for administration by users of cocaine and snuff, with chronic administration of the former leading to mucosal damage and necrosis of the cartilage of the nasal septum.

Administration by inhalation to the lungs

This route is used in two specific circumstances. The time-honoured example is for the administration of gaseous (e.g. nitrous oxide) and volatile (e.g. isofluorane) anaesthetics. The second is the now very common application of drugs used in the treatment of respiratory disease (e.g. bronchodilators in the treatment of asthma). This topical administration is accompanied by a reduction in systemic side-effects compared to that which would be observed if the drug was given systemically, i.e. the drug has been rendered relatively specific in its action (e.g. isoprenaline). By modification of the drug's structure, the systemic response can be limited even further (e.g. using ipratropium, which is a quaternary derivative, instead of atropine, and thereby markedly decreasing absorption). However, side-effects do occur. It should be remembered that 'puffers' deliver only a portion of their metered dose to the airway, the remainder being sprayed on to the oropharynx or swallowed with subsequent absorption. Fluticasone propionate is an inhaled steroid for which a reduced side-effect profile is claimed, due to a very high rate of presystemic elimination compared to beclamethasone, for example.

Topical application to the skin

Traditionally, topical application of drugs to the skin has been primarily for local effects, and side-effects due to systemic absorption have been regarded as troublesome (e.g. topical use of glucocorticoids for dermatitis with hypothalamic–pituitary–adrenal axis suppression). However, the application of drugs in transdermal preparations is becoming more common. These may be either creams (e.g. nitroglycerine – 'rub over your heart') or incorporated into patches which are applied to an area of thin skin (e.g. nicotine for control of withdrawal symptoms, hyoscine (for prevention of motion sickness) stuck behind the ear or worn in a bracelet, oestrogen (for hormone replacement) hidden on the abdomen). Creams are absorbed more quickly and completely if the area is warm and covered with an occlusive dressing, or if the dermis has been abraded. Patches have a major advantage in that their removal immediately stops absorption.

Parenteral administration

This route is used in circumstances where it is imperative that there is no uncertainty about the absorption of a drug from its site of administration, particularly in the case of an unconscious patient, or when a drug is poorly or erratically absorbed. The choice of whether the injection should be intravenous, intramuscular or subcutaneous is sometimes dictated by matters of humanity as well as pharmacology. For example, is the volume large and the dosing frequent? Does the patient have sufficient muscle or subcutaneous tissue mass? Is a constant plasma concentration required, i.e. would an infusion be more appropriate? Is the rate of absorption from muscle or fat unpredictable (e.g. diazepam)? Is there any coagulopathy, or is the patient on anticoagulants?

Intrathecal injection (i.e. into the subarachnoid space)

This route is utilized when the blood–brain barrier represents too great a barrier to access of drugs (e.g. methotrexate in cerebral leukaemia), or when administration may give some relative specificity or more effective response (e.g. opioids in palliative care, or epidural analgesia). As a general rule, antibiotics do not need to be given intrathecally, as in the presence of meningeal inflammation most antibiotics are able to penetrate the blood–brain barrier in sufficient amounts.

CONCEPTS OF POTENCY AND EFFICACY

If the drugs that are being compared all produce the same maximal response (i.e. irrespective of the mass of drug used), then the drugs are all equally efficacious. If the response is the maximum that can be produced in that tissue or organ, then the drugs are full agonists. If the mass of drug which is required to give the maximum response differs between compounds, then one drug is said to be more potent than another (for examples see

Chapter 1.10). If a drug is apparently acting through the same receptor, but the greatest response elicited is always less than maximal, then the drug is said to be a partial agonist. If partial agonists and full agonists are mixed, then there will be potential competition between the two, and the partial agonist may act as a competitive inhibitor or antagonist. If an antagonist is competitive, then increasing the concentration of the agonist will overcome the inhibition.

PHARMACOKINETICS

This refers to the concentration–time relationships between the administration of a drug and its absorption, distribution and elimination from the body. Basic principles can be defined which allow quantitative conclusions to be drawn about the likely time-courses of a drug's action. In turn, these can be used to define some practical characteristics for drug utilization in individual patients (e.g. dosing regimes).

The term 'compartment' in pharmacokinetics does not necessarily refer to tangible anatomical entities, but is a mathematical concept. In general the body may be regarded as a central (vascular) compartment, which consists of the circulating blood volume and tissues of organs which receive a high percentage of the cardiac output (e.g. heart, liver, kidneys). A second compartment generally consists of the tissues of the remainder of the body (e.g. muscle, adipose tissue) (Figure 37.1.1). There are some tissues (e.g. the brain) which, because of specific characteristics (e.g. the blood–brain barrier), must be regarded as being outside and separate from the general schema.

Practically, the concepts of compartments are most useful in explaining clearance of drugs. Clearance is the volume of blood that is cleared of drug per unit time, e.g. mL/min or L/h. It refers to the irreversible elimination of a drug from the body, and may concern processes as

(a)

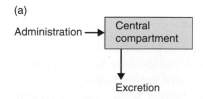

(b)

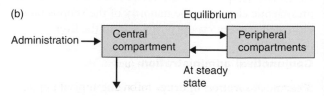

Figure 37.1.1 (a) A single-compartment model. (b) A two-compartment model.

varied as the metabolism of a drug to other active constituents (e.g. procainamide to N-acetylprocainamide) or to inactive products (e.g. oxazepam to oxazepam-glucuronide), or it may refer to the diffusion of a gas into the alveolar air (e.g. nitrous oxide following an anaesthetic). Clearance may be expressed in terms of an individual organ (e.g. liver, kidney, skin, lungs) or of the whole body (i.e. the sum of individual contributions).

Following bolus intravenous administration of a drug, the decreasing blood and plasma concentration plotted against time is described by a curvilinear plot (see Figure 37.1.2). The same data can be expressed with drug concentration on a logarithmic scale and the time axis on an arithmetic scale. The initial short-lived decline will remain curvilinear, and the terminal decline will be described by a single straight line.

If the original curve (Figure 37.1.2a) can be resolved mathematically into one terminal component (straight line), then the drug distribution and elimination are said to follow a one-compartment model (Figure 37.1.2b). In practice (as discussed below), most studies of drugs are confined to the central (blood) compartment. The rate of elimination of the drug from this central compartment is described by the half-life ($t_{1/2}$) of the drug in this compartment and shown as the slope of this straight line (known variously as the terminal or elimination phase). If multiple and frequent samples are collected in the first 15–20 min after IV administration, the initial part of the curve is the distribution phase, and describes the time taken for a drug to 'mix' in this compartment. It is also described in terms of its $t_{1/2}$. The $t_{1/2}$ of a distribution phase will be short (usually $< 20\,\text{min}$) for a drug which has only one compartment, for it represents the admixing of the drug in the circulating blood pool.

The half-life of the drug is the time taken for the drug concentration in plasma or blood to decrease by 50%. It is dependent on drug clearance (which is in turn influenced by factors such as protein binding). The clearance of the drug can be calculated mathematically as $0.693/t_{1/2}$. Extending the straight line to the abscissa gives the theoretical concentration (C_0) in the compartment at time zero (t_0) and is used to define the apparent volume of distribution (V_{d0}) (see below).

If the terminal phase can be resolved mathematically into two or more components (e.g. by using curve-peeling techniques), then the drug is behaving as though it were in a two- or even three-compartment model (Figure 37.1.3). The clearance from each compartment

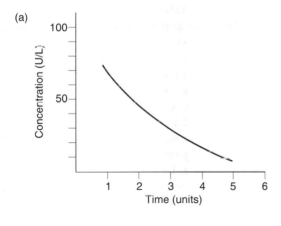

(a)

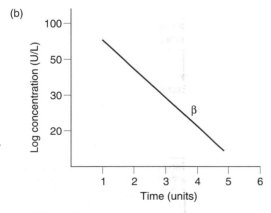

(b)

Figure 37.1.2 Plasma concentration of a drug with single-compartment kinetics following intravenous administration. (a) Exponential clearance. (b) Logarithmic transformation.

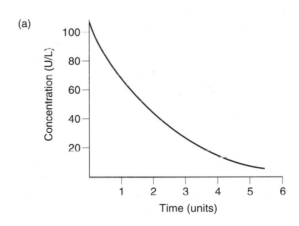

(a)

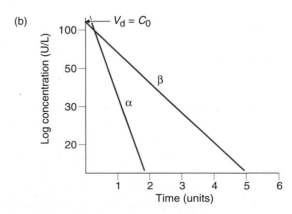

(b)

Figure 37.1.3 Plasma concentration of a drug with bi-exponential clearance following intravenous administration. (a) Bi-exponential clearance. (b) Logarithmic transformation.

can be calculated using its derived $t_{1/2}$. Implicit in the understanding and working of the two-compartment model is that there is movement of drug between compartment 1 (the central compartment) and the components of compartment 2 (Figure 37.1.1) and compartment 3, etc. When a drug first enters the central compartment following absorption or injection, its relatively high concentration will favour its movement to the peripheral compartments. This movement will be seen as the distribution phase, the $t_{1/2}$ of which will reflect the rate of movement of drug. With time, however, movement into and out of the peripheral compartments will become equal (i.e. equilibrium is established). If drug is removed from the central compartment (by excretion or metabolic conversion), then the concentration falls, and drug will tend to move from the periphery (i.e. the net movement will always be in the direction of the lowest unbound (free) concentration). Drugs are cleared from the central compartment, and although metabolism may occur in peripheral tissues, such metabolism constitutes only a small proportion of the total clearance, i.e. the liver, kidney and lungs are all defined as part of the central compartment.

The rate and ease of movement of drug between compartments will be determined by the properties of the individual drug, such as protein binding, tissue uptake, etc. Once equilibrium or steady state is established between the central (1) and peripheral (2) compartments, at a time removed from the distribution phase, the concentration of unbound drug in the central compartment will be the same as, or closely approximate to, the concentration in the peripheral tissue compartment (Figure 37.1.1). This concept is important when these principles are used to define the timing of samples for therapeutic drug monitoring (TDM). Identifying the time post-dose when this equilibrium may have been achieved is also critical, particularly in the case of orally administered drugs. In the latter case, the early distribution phase is occurring simultaneously with absorption of the drug (Figure 37.1.4).

In the majority of cases, the empirical solution is to take blood samples from the central compartment immediately prior to taking the next dose (i.e. a so-called 'trough concentration'). In terms of TDM, if these data are to be clinically relevant, then an association must have been demonstrated between the drug concentration and a clinical event (e.g. phenytoin and control of epilepsy or the appearance of toxicity, digoxin and control of atrial fibrillation, cyclosporin and prevention of acute transplant rejection).

If a third compartment can be defined mathematically, there is a significant (in terms of size) tissue or binding site which has even slower equilibrium constants. In practice, few drugs are considered to have third compartments in terms of guiding dosing requirements,

for example, and the concept of the third compartment is often regarded as being more important in the area of toxicology. However, very strong binding to structural/skeletal elements is well recognized (e.g. tetracycline or lead to teeth and bone). The absence of a demonstrated third compartment does not negate binding, but simply means that leaching from this compartment is so slow as to be very difficult to measure. The examples cited above both have very high apparent volumes of distribution, i.e. the volume of distribution reflects the binding of a drug in its defined various compartments.

The volume of distribution (V_d) may be used to describe the case for either the whole body or a compartment within the body. It is another mathematical concept that is used to summarize a drug's characteristics. Drugs with a low apparent V_d are often found to be largely confined within the circulating blood volume or extracellular space, whereas drugs with a high V_d tend to be highly bound (i.e. have a high affinity) to structural elements with a low turnover. The V_d is expressed in litres (or L/kg), i.e. as though the drug throughout the body or compartment was equally distributed and soluble in water. It is a calculation of the theoretical volume

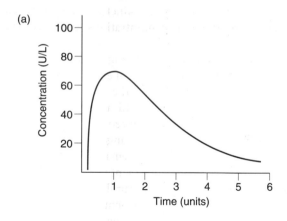

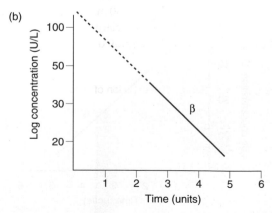

Figure 37.1.4 Plasma concentration of a drug following oral administration. (a) Absorption and clearance. (b) Logarithmic transformation.

of water (or volume/kg) which would be necessary to give the calculated concentration (C_0) at t_0 (Figure 37.1.3). If the drug is distributed predominantly within the vascular space, then the V_d will be low (< 0.15–0.2 L/kg), i.e. approximate to the circulating blood volume (e.g. gentamicin). If it is distributed throughout the total body water, the V_d will approximate to the volume of that space (0.5–0.7 L/kg) (e.g. theophylline). If it is highly bound (e.g. to bone or protein or in lipid stores), then the value will exceed this (> 1.0 L/kg) (e.g. chlorpromazine) (Table 37.1.6).

Saturation kinetics

The clearances of the drugs which have been illustrated in Figures 37.1.2, 37.1.3 and 37.1.4 follow exponential or bi-exponential time-courses, i.e. the excretion or metabolism is proportional to the drug concentration. This is referred to as first-order kinetics and describes the clearance of the majority of drugs. However, with a small number of drugs, plasma clearance is independent of drug concentration and the rate of clearance is apparently fixed. This is referred to as zero-order or saturation kinetics. Drugs which obey saturation kinetics include ethanol, phenytoin, salicylate and methadone. As the plasma concentration falls, the kinetics of clearance may change, and at lower concentrations clearance may become first order.

The practical importance of drugs which obey saturation kinetics is that the duration of effect of the drug will be dependent on the dose of the drug. For example, compare an individual with clinical phenytoin toxicity and a plasma phenytoin concentration of 30 mg/L (120 mmol/L) (therapeutic range 10–20 mg/L or 40–80 mmol/L). He or she may remain toxic for 4–5 days after the drug is stopped. A patient with carbamazepine toxicity (which may produce similar cerebellar symptoms) should show improvement within 1–2 days (plasma carbamazepine 18 mg/L or 65 mmol/L) (therapeutic range 4–12 mg/L or 15–50 mmol/L). Both drugs are elevated to the same degree relative to their respective therapeutic ranges, but the quoted half-life for carbamazepine is 6–14 h, and that for phenytoin is 6–24 h depending on plasma concentration.

Dosing

Although the half-life has been discussed in connection with timing of sample collections in TDM, the half-life of a drug may also be important in determining the dosing interval of a drug, and in calculating the time to steady state of a drug. For a drug with first-order kinetics, if the dosing intervals are constant, steady-state plasma concentrations will be approached in a time which approximates to five half-lives of the drug (Figure 37.1.5).

In the example shown, the same drug has been given, but twice the dose was used in A as in B. The same dosing interval (equal to the expected half-life) has been used in both cases, and the drug has been given intravenously. Clearly the use of an initial 'loading dose' will alter this relationship, and this approach can be used to good effect therapeutically. However, if the drug has a narrow therapeutic range, caution is necessary with regard to the rate of administration of this loading dose, in order to avoid or limit toxicity (e.g. theophylline, phenytoin). It is important to note that changes in formulation will also influence these parameters, particularly the use of the increasingly popular 'slow-release' preparations (e.g. diltiazem). Slow-release formulations also pose a particular problem if they are the vehicle used in an overdose. If they are not removed from the gastrointestinal tract, and depending on the dissolution properties of the preparation, the ingested tablets will be a potentially prolonged source of the drug. Secondly, if the formulation is designed to have an initial slow dissolution followed by a more rapid phase, then this second stage may cause a sudden rapid absorption of drug. This is potentially more dangerous if such a delayed effect is not anticipated (e.g. theophylline slow-release absorption is well documented, and overdose cases are well described). Not all drugs require administration according to a regular dosing pattern. For example, so-called 'hit-and-run' drugs are administered differently (e.g.

Table 37.1.6 Volume of distribution of some representative drugs

V_d < 0.2 L/kg	V_d 0.5–0.8 L/kg	V_d > 1 L/kg
Aspirin/salicylate	Aciclovir	Amiodarone
Amoxycillin/gentamicin	Azathioprine	Amitriptyline/chlorpromazine
Atracurium	Ethanol	Chloroquine
Chlorothiazide/frusemide	Lithium	Cyclosporin
Probenecid	Phenytoin	Diazepam
	Theophylline	Digoxin
		Morphine

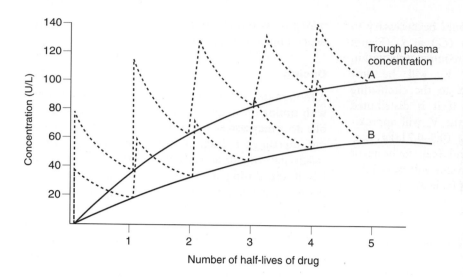

Figure 37.1.5 Effect of drug half-life on achievement of steady-state plasma concentrations. Twice the dose was used in A as in B.

cytotoxic drugs used cyclically), and drugs with a very long biological half-life compared to the plasma/blood half-life are often used differently (e.g. parenteral vitamin B_{12} to replenish liver stores given monthly or 3-monthly). It must also be remembered that one of the other consequences of zero-order kinetics is that the relationship between steady-state plasma concentration and dose is not predictable. Particularly if the rate of dosing approaches or exceeds the rate of clearance, then a steady-state concentration will not be achieved, and theoretically the concentration could increase indefinitely. Usually, of course, signs and symptoms of toxicity intervene.

PHARMACOKINETIC DRUG INTERACTIONS

Pharmacokinetic drug interactions occur as a result of changes in the kinetics of drugs induced by the presence of a second drug. The common mechanisms for interacting drugs are either competition for metabolism or transport via the same pathway (with one drug tending to inhibit clearance of the second drug), or by induction of the pathway (with increased clearance of one drug occurring in the presence of the second drug). Examples of clinically important interactions are shown in Tables 37.1.7 and 37.1.8. In principle, the clinically important drug interactions are those in which there is a narrow therapeutic range for the affected drug, and the concentration–response curve of the drug is steep, so that a small change in plasma concentration may produce a significant change in response. The common theme throughout relates to the nature of the side-effect or the disease being controlled. Little latitude is allowed in the prevention of thrombosis, for example, whilst the risk of haemorrhage in the post-operative patient is the balance to be considered. Similarly, the occurrence of increased fitting may be the prodrome of status epilepticus, or a

significant arrhythmia may precede cardiac failure or cardiac arrest.

Changes in bioavailability and drug absorption have already been discussed, as have effects on protein binding. Drugs which are cleared by active secretion in the renal tubules also give rise to pharmacokinetic drug interactions.

Paracetamol toxicity is an important example which demonstrates the importance of individual patient attributes and drug interaction, as well as the inherent toxicity of the drug. It is greatly enhanced in patients in whom there is either reduced hepatocellular tissue mass and/or induction of cytochrome P450. At normal therapeutic doses, paracetamol is metabolized primarily by glucuronidation and sulphation. A relatively small fraction is metabolized to a highly reactive compound by the cytochrome pathway, and this is usually rapidly conjugated with glutathione. If a very large dose is taken (usually in excess of 10 g), the proportion that is metabolized via cytochrome P450 increases, and the concentration of glutathione may not be sufficient for its detoxification role. If it is not conjugated, the reactive epoxide binds to tissue, with consequent damage. A similar phenomenon occurs in an induced liver, in which the proportion of paracetamol moving down CyP 1A2 is increased (Table 37.1.7), or if there is a reduced liver mass the glutathione will be depleted rapidly. In these examples, toxicity and liver failure may occur with therapeutic doses of paracetamol.

APPLIED CLINICAL PHARMACOLOGY OF ANTIBIOTICS

This section will provide a brief overview of pharmacokinetic principles and clinical pharmacology as applied to antibacterial, antiviral, antifungal and antiprotozoan

Table 37.1.7 Pharmacokinetic drug interactions due to changes in metabolism

Pathway/enzyme	Common drug	Inhibiting drug	Inducing drug
CyP 1A2	Theophylline Paracetamol Amitriptyline Ethanol	Cimetidine Erythromycin Mexilitene Moclobamide	Rifampicin Ethanol (chronic) Omeprazole
CyP 2C9/19	Amitriptyline Moclobamide Diclofenac Warfarin	Cimetidine Omeprazole Itraconazole Fluoxetine	Rifampicin Barbiturates Phenytoin
CyP 2D6	Haloperidol Propranolol Codeine Amitriptyline	Cimetidine Fluoxetine Haloperidol	
CyP 3A4	Lignocaine Carbamazepine Cortisol Cyclosporin A	Itraconazole Erythromycin Cimetidine Diltiazem	Rifampicin Barbiturates Phenytoin Carbamazepine
Monoamine oxidase	Pethidine	Moclobamide	
Xanthine oxidase	6–mercaptopurine Azathioprine	Allopurinol	
Pseudocholinesterase	Succinylcholine	Ecothiopate (organophosphates)	

Table 37.1.8 Pharmacokinetic drug interactions caused by changes in renal clearance

Drug inhibiting renal excretion	Drug with extended half-life
Probenecid Salazopyrine Aspirin and NSAIDs Thiazide diuretics	Penicillin Azidothymidine Methotrexate
Diuretics	Lithium
	Digoxin
Verapamil Amiodarone	

compounds. In general the greatest protection that the mammalian system has against unwanted side-effects of these drugs is that their mechanism of action is targeted against specific pathways or structures which are not shared by mammalian systems, or which are sufficiently different as not to have overlapping effects. As will be seen, whilst this is the ideal, and achievable to some extent, with the development of many compounds significant potential problems are encountered.

ANTIBACTERIAL DRUGS

Interference with folate synthesis and metabolism

Sulphanilamide, the parent sulphonamide, is a structural analogue of *p*-aminobenzoic acid, which is an essential precursor of folate in bacteria. Bacteria are unable to transport folate across their cell wall. Trimethoprim is a dihydrofolate reductase inhibitor. The bacterial enzyme is much more sensitive to trimethoprim than the human form. However, its use may precipitate folate deficiency when used in high doses, particularly in patients such as those with human immunodeficiency virus (HIV) and acquired immunodeficiency syndrome (AIDS), who often have pre-existing malabsorption and are at risk of folate deficiency. This group of patients is most likely to be receiving high-dose cotrimoxazole, a combination of suphamethoxazole and trimethoprim, as treatment for *Pneumocystis carinii* pneumonia.

The clearance of sulphonamides (e.g. suphamethoxazole, sulphapyridine) is by acetylation within the liver (Table 37.1.2) with renal excretion of the conjugated metabolite. Their major side-effect is hypersensitivity, which ranges from a mild rash to Stevens-Johnson syndrome. This potential risk has severely restricted their clinical utility in recent times, as alternatives have become available. Trimethoprim is a weak base which is renally excreted.

β-lactam antibiotics (e.g. penicillins, cephalalosporins, carbapenems)

These drugs interfere with the synthesis of the bacterial cell wall peptidoglycan. They do not enter mammalian cells, and only cross the blood–brain barrier when it is inflamed. Penicillins have varying oral bioavailability (e.g. benzylpenicillin is acid labile and best used parenterally). Most of them are actively secreted in the kidney, although there is significant biliary secretion of cloxacillin and flucloxacillin, both of which can cause cholestatic jaundice. The most common side-effect of the group is hypersensitivity due to hapten formation between the penicillin and a host protein. The resulting antigen is the basis of immune reactions, including anaphylaxis. As a group they also show significant nephrotoxicity. Reference has been made to increasing the efficacy of penicillins by co-administration of probenicid. Other approaches used to enhance their efficacy include the use of clavulinic acid, which is a non-competitive inhibitor of bacterial β-lactamase. Another example is the use of cilastatin, which is administered with imipenem. Cilastatin inhibits the proximal renal tubular enzyme dihydropeptidase, which metabolizes imipenem.

Drugs affecting bacterial protein synthesis (e.g. tetracyclines, chloramphenicol, aminoglycosides, macrolides)

The tetracyclines, which are usually given orally, have variable bioavailability. Complexing to food and divalent cations in the gastrointestinal system has already been discussed. Their high affinity for calcium results in their deposition in bones and teeth, with staining of the latter and potential alteration in dentition if they are used during tooth formation. For this reason they are contraindicated in pregnancy, in children and in nursing mothers. Tetracyclines are excreted via the kidney and biliary system. They accumulate in renal failure, and may worsen the latter. Their effect on renal function is well illustrated by demeclocycline, which is used to treat the hyponatraemia of chronic secretion of antidiuretic hormone, such as may occur in some malignancies. This is the so-called syndrome of inappropriate ADH secretion (SIADH).

Chloramphenicol acts at the same site on the bacterial ribosome as do the macrolide antibiotics and clindamicin. It is orally active and widely distributed in all compartments of the body. It is metabolized in the liver, and in the neonatal liver immaturity of conjugation may give rise to the 'grey baby syndrome'. Its most important side-effect is the potentially fatal bone-marrow toxicity and aplastic anaemia, an idiosyncratic reaction, not yet adequately explained. Two scenarios are recognized as being related to aplastic anaemia – one is its occurrence after very low-dose exposure (hypersensitivity), and the second is related to a cumulative dose over approximately 2 weeks.

The aminoglycoside antibiotics (e.g. gentamicin, tobramycin, amikacin) are highly polar molecules which are not absorbed from the gut. Following parenteral administration they are generally confined to the extracellular space in humans, and although they do not cross the blood–brain barrier, they may cross the placenta. Clearance is by glomerular filtration, and with normal renal function the half-life is approximately 2 h. As a group they are nephrotoxic and ototoxic, and there is synergy with drugs such as cyclosporin A and loop diuretics, respectively.

The macrolide antibiotics (e.g. erythromycin, clarithromycin, roxithromycin) are orally bioavailable, but they do not cross the blood–brain barrier. They are metabolized via the cytochrome P450 system and excreted in the bile. The drug interactions arising from inhibition of the cytochrome P450 system are clinically important. In addition, erythromycin may result in cholestatic jaundice.

Drugs affecting topoisomerase II

These include quinolones (e.g. nalidixic acid) and fluoroquinolones (e.g. ciprofloxacin). In their antibacterial action these drugs prevent the formation of the bacterial DNA double helix from the existing DNA. Their oral bioavailability is reduced by binding to divalent cations (e.g. calcium and magnesium antacids). As a group they are excreted by both kidney and liver. They can cause renal impairment and photosensitivity.

Glycopeptide antibiotics (e.g. vancomycin, teicoplanin)

This group is similar to the aminoglycosides in both pharmacokinetics and side-effect profile.

Treatment of *Mycobacterium tuberculosis* and *M. leprae*

Isoniazid has good oral bioavailability and is widely distributed throughout the body. It crosses cell membranes and is therefore effective against intracellular bacteria as well. Metabolism is via acetylation in the liver, and it may inhibit clearance of many anticonvulsants. It can precipitate neuropathy due to complexing with pyridoxine (vitamin B$_6$), particularly in slow acetylators in whom there will be higher concentrations of isoniazid. Rifampicin is also given orally. It has an enterohepatic circulation, which extends its plasma half-life. It stains secretions (including tears, saliva and urine) an orange colour. Its most important side-effect is its induction of many liver enzymes and the consequent drug interactions (Table 37.1.2). It may also cause jaundice (both cholestatic and hepatocellular).

With regard to ethambutal, although side-effects in general are uncommon, it is important to be aware of optic neuritis, which is reversible if recognized early. Its occurrence is related to plasma concentration, and is more likely in patients with renal failure.

Dapsone is chemically related to the sulphonamides, and its side-effects are similar. This includes methaemoglobinaemia and intravascular haemolysis.

With the resurgence of mycobacterial infections in immunocompromised individuals, alternative treatment strategies have been sought. One of these is the use of thalidomide, most specifically for Hansen's disease (leprosy). One must never forget the lesson of thalidomide as a teratogen and the occurrence of phocomelia.

ANTIVIRAL DRUGS

Inhibitors of DNA polymerase

This is the first of the group of drugs all of which ultimately decrease viral nucleic acid synthesis.

Most inhibitors of DNA polymerase are analogues of the nucleotides or nucleosides (Table 37.1.9). Their bioavailability tends to be poor, and thus in most cases parenteral administration is required. However, aciclovir, despite having a bioavailability of $< 20\%$, is widely used orally. The majority of this group of drugs are excreted via the kidney, both filtered in the glomerulus and actively secreted in the tubule. Renal impairment results in accumulation. The group may also precipitate renal dysfunction. The potential for alteration of DNA in the host cell is reflected by the observed mutagenicity and carcinogenicity of some of the drugs.

Inhibitors of reverse transcriptase

This group of drugs has formed the basis for the treatment of HIV.

These analogues affect the activity of the gamma-DNA polymerase in the mitochondria of the host's cells. The resultant alteration in the mitochondrial DNA may underlie many of the documented side-effects, the most important of which are listed in Table 37.1.10.

Protease inhibitors (e.g. saquinavir mesylate, ritinavir, indinavir sulphate)

HIV-1 protease has a role in the final maturation of the virion. This maturation occurs following the virion's release into plasma from the infected cells. The protease inhibitors competitively inhibit the active site of the pro-

Table 37.1.9 Pharmacological properties of some of the DNA polymerase inhibitors

Drug	Structural analogue	Route of administration	Clearance	Major side-effects
Aciclovir	Guanosine	Oral, IV, topical	Renal	Encephalopathy, renal dysfunction
Ganciclovir	Guanosine	IV	Renal	Bone marrow depression, carcinogenic
Vidarabine	Adenine arabinoside	IV, topical	Renal after deamination	Neurotoxic (high dose), Bone marrow depression, mutagenic, carcinogenic
Idoxuridine	Thymidine	Topical (eye)		Mutagenic
Foscarnet	Pyrophosphate	IV	Renal	Nephrotoxic (serious)

Table 37.1.10 Pharmacological properties of some of the reverse transcriptase inhibitors

Drug	Structure	Route of administration	Clearance	Major side-effects
Zidovudine (AZT)	Thymidine analogue	Oral (60–80% bioavailable)	80% Liver – glucuronidation 20% Renal (Probenicid)	Bone marrow depression Myopathy Flu-like syndrome
Didanosine (ddI)	Purine deoxynucleoside analogue	Oral (taken with antacid)	Renal (active secretion)	Peripheral neuropathy Pancreatitis (5–10%)
Zalcitabine (ddC)	Thymidine nucleoside analogue	Oral	Renal	Neuropathy

tease, which is effectively at the centre of a dimeric enzyme. Some of the important properties of the protease inhibitors are summarized in Table 37.1.11. There is a significant potential for drug interactions in this group of drugs, and there are major differences in dosing requirements due to differing bioavailability.

Inhibition of viral entry

This category incorporates two subgroups, namely drugs which inhibit attachment to the cell wall and drugs which may prevent penetration of the cell wall. Amantadine is one of the earliest antiviral drugs. It is of interest both in that historical context and because of its mechanism of action in acting prophylactically against influenza A. Gamma-globulins with their role in passive immunity also fit into this category (e.g. hyperimmune pooled gamma-globulin against hepatitis B or varicella).

Immunomodulators: interferon

The interferons are cytokines produced as part of the normal immune response. The recombinant proteins used therapeutically must be given either intravenously or intramuscularly. The major side-effects are a flu-like syndrome including fever, malaise, headache and myalgia. These symptoms are reminiscent of the responses which accompany the use of many of the cytokines.

ANTIFUNGAL DRUGS

Orally active drugs

As a group there are significant drug interactions which both result from and influence the use of these drugs. Griseofulvin is an inducer of the cytochrome P450 system, via which it is metabolized. Clinically, the most

apparent consequences of this interaction are decreased efficacy of oral contraceptives and warfarin, and precipitation of acute porphyria. The azoles (e.g. ketaconazole, fluconazole, itraconazole, minazole) are also metabolized in the liver in the cytochrome system, but they can produce significant inhibition of the CyP 2C9/19 and 3A4 pathways. A further interaction is the inhibition by ketaconazole of adrenosteroidogenesis. This side-effect may be used therapeutically in the suppression of cushingoid symptoms in inoperable malignancy secondary to ectopic ACTH or adrenal neoplasia. In addition to these interactions, ketaconazole is potentially hepatotoxic, and Stevens-Johnson syndrome is a recognized complication of drugs belonging to this group.

The remaining member of this orally administered group of antifungal agents is flucytosine, which is used in the treatment of yeast infections such as candidiasis. It is renally excreted, with dose reduction recommended in the presence of renal impairment. Toxicity is due to accumulation of its toxic metabolite, 5-fluorouracil (an analogue of uracil), which may result in depression of bone-marrow stem-cell activity, slowed replacement of gut wall mucosa, and alopecia, all of which are common symptoms of cytotoxic drugs.

Amphotericin and nystatin

Both of these drugs are polyene antibiotics which bind primarily to ergosterol in fungal cell walls. When bound to the cell wall, the antibiotic acts as an ionophore, allowing intracellular electrolytes to escape. These drugs are poorly absorbed, and amphotericin is administered parenterally as a slow intravenous infusion. The major side-effect is renal toxicity, with 80% of all recipients

Table 37.1.11 Pharmacological properties of the protease inhibitors

Protease inhibitor	Oral bioavailability	Clearance	Side-effects
Saquinavir	Very low (4%) Improved by taking with fatty food	Liver – CyP 3A Half-life decreased by rifampicin, increased by ketoconazole and ritinovir	Nausea, diarrhoea
Ritinovir	Taken with meals	Liver – CyP 3A Inhibits CyP 3A* Induces CyP 2C9/19*	Nausea, diarrhoea Altered taste ?myopathy concentration related
Indinavir	Taken between meals	Liver – CyP 3A Induced by rifampicin Inhibited by ketoconazole and ritinovir 20% renal clearance	Nephrolithiasis (precipitation in collecting ducts)

* see Table 37.1.7.

showing some degree of renal impairment, some of which will be permanent. In addition, hepatic dysfunction and anaemia or thrombocytopenia are not uncommon. The development of a liposomal amphotericin preparation is said to reduce toxicity, but it is much more expensive. Use of nystatin is essentially confined to topical use (skin, vagina and gut contents).

ANTIPROTOZOAN DRUGS

Antimalarial drugs

All effective antimalarial drugs used to treat the acute attack must pass into either the erythrocyte (e.g. quinine, mefloquine, chloroquine, doxycycline) or liver cells (e.g. primaquine). Drugs used prophylactically generally act to block the link between the hepatic and erythrocytic stages, thus preventing an attack (e.g. mefloquine, chloroquine, doxycycline, dapsone). Several general principles must be noted. First, drugs related to quinine may have significant cardiac effects (e.g. decreased atrioventricular conduction, so-called 'quinidine-like' effects). Secondly, the biological half-life of the drug may be very long (e.g. for chloroquine it is 50 h). Thirdly,

during chronic administration retinopathy may occur due to accumulation, as a result of either short-term high-dose treatment or chronicity of treatment.

Amoebiasis

Metronidazole, which is also used to treat anaerobic bacterial infections, depends on liver clearance and cytochrome P450. Its most dramatic reported drug interaction is with alcohol, producing a reaction similar to that between disulfiram and alcohol.

FURTHER READING

Grahame-Smith DG, Aronson JK. 1992: *Oxford textbook of clinical pharmacology*, 2nd edn. Oxford: Oxford University Press.

Laurence DR, Bennett PN. 1992: *Clinical pharmacology*, 7th edn. Edinburgh: Churchill Livingstone.

Melmon KL, Morrelli HF, Hoffman BB, Nierenberg DW (eds). 1992: *Clinical pharmacology. Basic principles in therapeutics*, 3rd edn. New York: McGraw-Hill.

Antimicrobial agents

John M.B. Smith and John E. Payne

Introduction

Antimicrobial therapy demands an initial clinical evaluation, including the significance of any underlying compromise, the nature and extent of the infective process, and knowledge of the likely causative microbe(s). With many surgery-related infections, the causal microbes are part of the indigenous or normal flora (see Table 37.2.1). Where possible, the clinical assessment should be supported by laboratory investigations aimed at establishing the microbial aetiology and the sensitivity of the microbe(s) involved to possible therapeutic choices (see Chapter 29.4). In most cases, the causal microbe(s) will likely be susceptible to a variety of antimicrobial agents. The choice of one or more of these depends on a variety of drug and patient factors, including the preferred route and frequency of administration, known adverse effects, the drug's pharmacological and kinetic features (including its likely penetration and activity at the site where the microbe is growing), the age and clinical state of the patient, and cost.

The exact role of antibiotics in curing infections is largely unknown, although it seems that in most situations the mere deceleration of microbial growth and multiplication will allow the host defences to eradicate the causal microbes. Antibiotics alone seldom rid tissues and fluids of the offending pathogen. With many surgical infections, the cornerstone of therapy is therefore appropriate surgical intervention (e.g. debridement or abscess drainage) and empirical antimicrobial therapy.

SELECTED ANTIBACTERIAL GROUPS

Antibacterial therapy is based on the use of drugs that are active against some part of the prokaryotic bacterial cell that is absent or different to that found in eukaryotic mammalian cells – so-called selective toxicity. The most obvious bacterial target site is the cell wall, with other more significant targets being the protein-building ribosomes and the DNA (see Figure 37.2.1)

The bacteria that are associated with surgically relevant infections consist of representatives of the normal flora (see Table 37.2.1) and a few environmental microbes, such as *Pseudomonas aeruginosa*, which may occur as transients on the skin or in the intestinal tract.

Treatment of infections by these relevant bacteria can be accomplished using a limited range of antibiotics, although escalating problems of resistance to some of these agents are of growing concern. The therapeutic options for important pathogens are listed in Table 37.2.2, while important properties and characteristics of the surgically more significant antibacterial agents are summarized below.

β-LACTAMS

The β-lactams are compounds that are active on the cell wall, and include the penicillins (penams), cephalo-

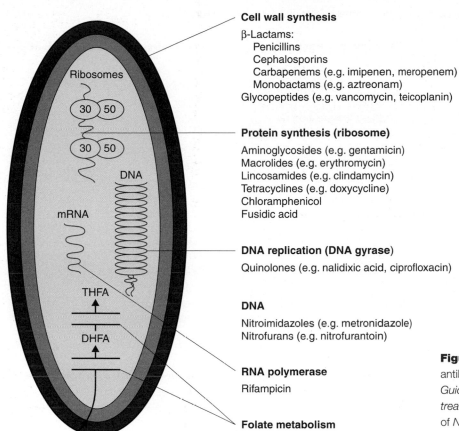

Cell wall synthesis

β-Lactams:
    Penicillins
    Cephalosporins
    Carbapenems (e.g. imipenen, meropenem)
    Monobactams (e.g. aztreonam)
Glycopeptides (e.g. vancomycin, teicoplanin)

Protein synthesis (ribosome)

Aminoglycosides (e.g. gentamicin)
Macrolides (e.g. erythromycin)
Lincosamides (e.g. clindamycin)
Tetracyclines (e.g. doxycycline)
Chloramphenicol
Fusidic acid

DNA replication (DNA gyrase)

Quinolones (e.g. nalidixic acid, ciprofloxacin)

DNA

Nitroimidazoles (e.g. metronidazole)
Nitrofurans (e.g. nitrofurantoin)

RNA polymerase

Rifampicin

Folate metabolism

Trimethoprim
Sulphonamides

Figure 37.2.1 Site of action of antibacterial agents. (Adapted from *Guide to pathogens and antibiotic treatment 1998*, with kind permission of *New Ethicals*, Adis International and Dr Selwyn Lang, Medlab Auckland, New Zealand.)

sporins (cephems), carbapenems (e.g. meropenem), monobactams (e.g. aztreonam) and β-lactamase–inhibitor combinations (e.g. coamoxyclav). In all cases, the target sites are enzymes associated with the cross-linking of the newly formed linear peptidoglycan strand to the existing cell wall. These enzymes have been termed penicillin-binding proteins (PBPs).

Most β-lactam antibiotics are poorly absorbed from the gastrointestinal tract, and their absorption is delayed by the presence of food; only a few are available as oral formulations. In general, they are widely distributed in the body and cross the placenta. However, only a few reach significant concentrations in bile, cerebrospinal fluid or milk. Most have short plasma half-lives, and this should be considered when proposing their use as prophylactic agents for prolonged surgical procedures. A large proportion show significant protein binding (e.g. 96% with flucloxacillin). Excretion is mainly by renal tubular secretion, and blood levels may be increased in renal failure or by administration of probenecid.

Penicillins

Since the advent of penicillin G in the early 1940s, the penicillins have gone through a remarkable series of changes. Early penicillins were natural products with a relatively narrow antibacterial spectrum aimed primarily at streptococci and clostridia (and initially staphylococci). Subsequent manipulation of the biologically active 6-aminopenicillanic acid nucleus has resulted in a range of semisynthetic penicillins, including the broad-spectrum ampicillin/amoxicillin range and more recently the extended spectrum or antipseudomonal penicillins (e.g. ticarcillin and piperacillin). Most strains of *Staphylococcus aureus* now elaborate penicillinases capable of inactivating all of these penicillins. However, since the early 1960s a range of penicillinase-stable or antistaphylococcal penicillins have emerged on the market, of which flucloxacillin, dicloxacillin and nafcillin are the most commonly used examples.

The main disadvantage of penicillin use is the risk of allergy – the most frequent complication of therapy is penicillin hypersensitivity (in up to 2% of patients). Mild reactions may consist of only a morbilliform or scarlatiniform rash on the trunk and extremities, which may disappear spontaneously during treatment. Such skin reactions are common after amoxycillin treatment, and may be associated with viral diseases such as infectious mononucleosis. Urticarial or oedematous skin rashes, with or without fever and sometimes accompanied by joint swelling, laryngeal oedema, conjunctivitis or other symptoms, should be taken more seriously.

Table 37.2.1 Important bacterial pathogens, their normal habitat and antibiotic considerations

Microbe	Predominant habitat	Antibiotic(s) for serious infections
Obligate anaerobes		
Bacteroides species	Intestines, female genital tract	Metronidazole, meropenem*
Bilophila wadsworthia	Intestines	As for *Bacteroides*
Clostridium species	Intestines (transient on skin of lower body)	Metronidazole, penicillin
Fusobacterium species	Intestines/oral cavity	As for *Bacteroides*
Peptostreptococcus species (anaerobic cocci)	Intestines, external genitalia, oral cavity, skin	Meropenem*, penicillin, metronidazole
Porphyromonas species	Oral cavity, intestines	As for *Bacteroides*
Prevotella species	Oral cavity, female genital tract	As for *Bacteroides*
Gram-positive cocci		
Enterococci (e.g. *Enterococcus faecalis*)	Intestines	Amoxycillin with or without gentamicin
Staphylococcus aureus	Nasopharynx (transient on skin)	Flucloxacillin or similar penicillinase-stable penicillin, fusidic acid
Staphylococcus epidermidis	Skin	Teicoplanin†
Streptococcus anginosus (milleri)	Oral cavity, intestines	Penicillin, cefuroxime
Streptococcus pyogenes	Oral cavity	Penicillin, cefuroxime
Gram-negative bacilli		
Escherichia coli and related coliforms	Intestines	Gentamicin, cefotaxime, ciprofloxacin
Pseudomonas aeruginosa	Environment (transient on moist skin and intestines)	Tobramycin plus piperacillin

* Or related imipenem.
† Or related vancomycin.

Anaphylactic shock is fortunately rare but is extremely serious, and lethal in around 10% of cases. Other more relevant adverse effects include diarrhoea (including pseudomembranous colitis), haematological abnormalities and (rarely) seizures. Of increasing concern is the association of flucloxacillin with severe and debilitating cholestatic hepatitis after extended use in elderly patients.

Cephalosporins

Since the production of the first-generation cephalosporins (e.g. cephalexin) in the early 1960s, a steady stream of second-, third- and fourth-generation compounds has become available. Second-generation compounds (e.g. cefamandole, cefuroxime) retain the excellent antistaphylococcal and antistreptococcal activity of the first-generation drugs, and have improved activity against some Gram-negative bacilli and, in the case of cefoxitin and cefotetan, against some anaerobes. The latter two compounds are not true second-generation cephalosporins, but 7-methoxycephalosporins or cephamycins. The third-generation group (e.g. cefotaxime, ceftriaxone, ceftazidime) has excellent activity against Gram-negatives, including most Gram-negative

enteric bacilli. A few (e.g. ceftazidime) have therapeutic antipseudomonal activity, while the excellent activity of most third-generation drugs against streptococci and to a lesser extent *Staphylococcus aureus* is often overlooked. The fourth-generation cephalosporins (e.g. cefepime, cefpirome) have enhanced (compared to third-generation compounds) antibacterial activity against Gram-negative bacilli, including *Pseudomonas aeruginosa*, and against Gram-positive bacteria such as staphylococci and streptococci. However, a continuing problem with cephalosporins has been their universal lack of activity against enterococci, as well as (apart from the cephamycins) their subtherapeutic activity against obligate anaerobes.

The most common systemic adverse reaction seen with cephalosporins is hypersensitivity, although this is an uncommon event compared to the frequency with which it is seen with penicillins. Cross-reaction with penicillin allergy is rare, and its incidence has been estimated at 3–7%. In general, cephalosporins can be used with reasonable safety in patients who exhibit *mild* penicillin allergy. Other uncommon adverse events include haematological reactions (e.g. hypoprothrombinaemia following prolonged use of extended spectrum com-

Table 37.2.2 Characteristics of commonly used antibiotics in surgery

Group	Name	Half-life (h)	Usual dosing interval (h)	Useful therapeutic spectrum
β-lactams	Penicillin G	<1	4–6	Streptococci, clostridia
	Flucloxacillin	<1	6	*S. aureus* (except MRSA)
	Amoxycillin	1	8	Enterococci, streptococci
	Coamoxyclav	1	6–8	Enterococci, *S. aureus*, anaerobes
	Piperacillin	1	4	Gram-negative enterics, pseudomonads
	Piperacillin/tazobactam	1	8	Most aerobes/anaerobes
	Cephalexin	<1	6	Streptococci, staphylococci
	Cephazolin	2.0	6–8	
	Cefuroxime	1.3	8	Staphylococci, streptococci,
	Cefamandole	<1	4–6	some Gram-negative bacilli
	Cefoxitin	<1	6	Anaerobes, *S. aureus*,
	Cefotetan	3.5	12	some Gram-negative bacilli
	Cefotaxime	1.2	6–12	Gram-negative bacilli, streptococci,
	Ceftriaxone	8	24	*S. aureus*
	Ceftazidime	1.8	8–12	Gram-negative bacilli, pseudomonads
	Cefpirome	2.0	12	Gram-negative bacilli, pseudomonads, streptococci, *S. aureus*
	Meropenem	1	8	Most aerobes/anaerobes
	Imipenem	1	6–12	
Aminoglycosides	Gentamicin	1.5	8–24*	Gram-negative vacilli, *S. aureus*
	Tobramycin	1.5	8–24*	Gram-negative bacilli, pseudomonads
Nitroimidazoles	Metronidazole	7	8	*B. fragilis* and other obligate anaerobes
Others	Vancomycin	6	6	Most Gram-positives, including MRSA
	Teicoplanin	>50	8–24	
	Fusidic acid	4–6	6–8	*S. aureus*
	Rifampicin	3	24	*S. aureus*
	Ciprofloxacin	4	12	Gram-negative bacilli, pseudomonads, *S.aureus*

*24-h dosing interval feasible in most surgical settings.

pounds), antibiotic-associated diarrhoea (which is most common following the use of cephalosporins with biliary excretion or poor oral absorption, e.g. cefuroxime), sludge in the gall bladder and common bile duct (with ceftriaxone), nephrotoxicity (which has limited the use of some earlier cephalosporins) and disulfiram-like alcohol reactions (with cefotetan).

Carbapenems

Two carbapenems are currently in use, namely imipenem and meropenem. Both have a similar and extremely wide spectrum of activity, being lytic for most aerobic and anaerobic bacteria. They provide useful monotherapy for serious nosocomial infections.

As imipenem is hydrolysed by renal dehydropeptidase to form inactive and toxic compounds in urine, it is administered in equal amounts with cilastatin, which inhibits the action of the peptidase. Apart from the adverse reactions common to most β-lactams, the most serious problem associated with imipenem use is seizures – a side-effect most often seen in those with underlying central nervous system pathology, or with impaired renal function. Meropenem, which is less epileptogenic, is unaffected by renal dehydropeptidase, and is slightly more active against Gram-negative bacteria and less active against Gram-positive bacteria than imipenem.

β-Lactamase inhibitor combinations

A number of β-lactams with weak antibacterial properties exist which are potent inhibitors of many plasmid-encoded and some chromosomal β-lactamases. These so-called β-lactamase inhibitors include clavulanic acid and several penicillanic acid sulphone derivatives (e.g. sulbactam and tazobactam). β-Lactamase inhibitors have been combined with an active β-lactam, usually a penicillin, as a companion agent. The antibacterial activity of the resulting β-lactam combination is largely determined by the companion antimicrobial, which may have its β-lactamase susceptibility reversed by the concurrent presence of the inhibitor. As the two components are not chemically joined together, the *in vivo* activity of the combination relies on both compounds possessing similar pharmacokinetic properties. The potential for one component to diffuse without the other should be borne in mind when proposing the use of these compounds for life-threatening infections.

The most commonly used β-lactam/β-lactam inhibitor combination is amoxycillin/clavulanate or coamoxyclav (Augmentin®). In the surgical arena, it has been used predominantly as an antistaphylococcal agent for minor skin and soft-tissue infections. It is also effective against many anaerobes. Other examples include ticarcillin/clavulanate (Timentin®) and the very broad-spectrum piperacillin/tazobactam.

AMINOGLYCOSIDES

It is unfortunate that aminoglycosides (e.g. gentamicin, tobramycin, amikacin), which are cheap, safe and effective, share the potential for nephrotoxicity, ototoxicity and (rarely) neuromuscular blockade. This fact, coupled with their low therapeutic index, has tended to restrict their use in some countries, although the introduction of once-daily dosing regimens has gone some way towards addressing these problems. Aminoglycosides also display synergy with cell-wall-active antibiotics. However, as aminoglycosides and β-lactams are physically and chemically incompatible, they should not be mixed for any length of time before infusion. For optimum results, they should be infused 20–30 min apart.

Aminoglycosides are virtually not absorbed at all from the gastrointestinal tract, and there may be some patient variation in absorption from intramuscular injection sites; the preferred route is intravenous. The drugs have long half-lives, and they display concentration-dependent killing and a marked post-antibiotic effect. They show little protein binding, and are widely distributed in the extracellular fluid; passage across the placenta is poor. As with most antibiotics, diffusion across the blood–brain barrier is poor. Although they are found in pus, they are rapidly inactivated in such an environment and are not active against anaerobes. Excretion is renal, and rapid accumulation may occur even with minor renal impairment. This effect may be of some advantage in chronic renal failure, when administration may be required only after each haemodialysis.

The side-effects reported with aminoglycosides include allergic reactions, rashes, gastrointestinal upsets, drug interactions, vestibular and acoustic nerve damage, nephrotoxicity, and neuromuscular blockade following the use of muscle relaxants during anaesthesia. A significant proportion of injected aminoglycoside becomes sequestered in the lysosomes of the tubular epithelial cells, and prolonged accumulation can lead to acute tubular necrosis, although this is reversible as the basement membrane remains intact. Pre-existing renal disease may exacerbate the problem. Nephrotoxicity is increased when aminoglycosides and certain other drugs (e.g. vancomycin, cyclosporin) are used in combination. This may be exacerbated by shock or by the simultaneous administration of powerful diuretics.

Failure of aminoglycoside therapy against susceptible bacteria is primarily attributable to a failure to achieve sufficiently high blood and/or tissue antibiotic levels, and this is particularly problematic in trauma and septic patients. Increasing evidence supports the use of a single daily dose of aminoglycosides in many patients. Clinically this appears to be as effective as divided doses, and clearly it is less nephrotoxic. It is certainly worth consideration in many surgical situations, and has major benefits for the surgeon and the patient, and for hospital antibiotic costs. With gentamicin or tobramycin, each 24-h dose of 5–7 mg/kg is in reality a loading dose, and peak serum levels of 15–25 mg/L are far in excess of the 5 mg/L therapeutic minimum. To avoid renal toxicity and ototoxicity, trough levels should be maintained below 0.5 mg/L (see Chapter 29.4). When trough levels are found to exceed this safe level, increasing the time between doses is mandatory. Recent studies have shown that the increased susceptibility of some patients to aminoglycoside ototoxicity is associated with a specific mutation in mitochondrial DNA.

ANTI-OBLIGATE ANAEROBE AGENTS

A variety of antimicrobials exhibit therapeutic activity against obligate anaerobes. By far the most effective is metronidazole, followed by imipenem and meropenem (β-lactams), clindamycin, chloramphenicol, β-lactam combinations (e.g. coamoxyclav and piperacillin/tazobactam), the cephamycins cefoxitin and cefotetan, and penicillin.

Metronidazole is effective against most obligate anaerobes, including *Bacteroides fragilis* and *Clostridium perfringens*. Of the significant anaerobes, it seems least effective against peptostreptococci and more aerotolerant species. It is well absorbed by both oral and rectal routes, but the rate is decreased when it is administered with food. Adequate blood levels of metronidazole are maintained following rectal administration; initial loading doses should be given intravenously. The drug is universally distributed (including the cerebrospinal fluid) and is less than 20% bound to plasma proteins. It has a long half-life, which may be prolonged further when hepatic function is impaired. It is removed by haemodialysis but not by peritoneal dialysis.

The most frequent side-effects are gastrointestinal. Metronidazole may produce neurotoxicity, blood dyscrasias, hypersensitivity and genito-urinary effects. The drug has been reported to be carcinogenic in mice and rats, a finding which initially restricted its use in the USA. It should therefore be avoided in pregnancy. It may interact with coumarins, alcohol (disulfiram-like effect), phenobarbital and certain other drugs.

GLYCOPEPTIDES

Vancomycin and teicoplanin are relatively expensive cell-wall-active glycopeptide antibiotics, and their site of action is at an earlier stage of cell-wall synthesis than that affected by the β-lactams. They are the drugs of choice for many methicillin-resistant strains of *Staphylococcus aureus* (MRSA), and for other Gram-positive bacteria that are resistant to β-lactams (e.g. penicillin-resistant pneumococci). They have no activity against Gram-negative bacteria, being unable to pass through the outer membrane of the Gram-negative cell wall.

With vancomycin, ototoxicity and nephrotoxicity are most likely to occur in patients with renal failure, although no clear and concise relationships between serum concentrations and toxicity are evident from the literature reviews. When used in combination with an aminoglycoside, nephrotoxicity has been reported to be common. In patients receiving prolonged (> 48 h) vancomycin therapy, serum monitoring should be carried out. Pre-dose or trough levels should be maintained in the range 5–10 mg/L. Levels of 12–15 mg/L indicate that accumulation is occurring, although some clinicians regard trough levels approaching 15 mg/L as acceptable in serious staphylococcal infections.

Vancomycin is given by slow intravenous infusion – rapid administration causes histamine release and 'red-neck' syndrome, hypotension and even cardiac arrest. This drug must not be given intramuscularly. Teicoplanin is said to be somewhat safer in all of these respects, perhaps in part because it is given in lower doses. Teicoplanin is available for intramuscular as well as intravenous administration, and can be given over 3–5 min. The half-life of vancomycin is 6 h, but that of teicoplanin is almost 10 times longer, allowing once-daily use (and out-patient use). Given orally, vancomycin is a useful alternative to metronidazole for the treatment of severe pseudomembranous colitis.

FLUOROQUINOLONES

Ciprofloxacin is the most potent of the generally available fluoroquinolones, with excellent bioavailability after oral administration and good activity against most Gram-negative bacilli, including pseudomonads. It is also effective against *Staphylococcus aureus*, including some methicillin-resistant strains. Because monotherapy with ciprofloxacin has a tendency to select resistant strains of staphylococci, it should be combined with a second antistaphylococcal agent wherever possible. Some newer fluoroquinolones (e.g. trovafloxacin) retain the Gram-negative activity of ciprofloxacin, but have enhanced therapeutic activity against most Gram-positive cocci, including *Staphylococcus aureus*, vancomycin-resistant enterococci and penicillin-resistant pneumococci, and obligate anaerobes such as *Bacteroides fragilis*.

PROBLEMS OF ANTIBACTERIAL RESISTANCE

Resistance to commonly used first-line antibacterial agents (see Table 37.2.2) is an emerging global problem.

Metronidazole, chloramphenicol and probably imipenem/meropenem still have excellent efficacy against the important obligate anaerobes, although increasing levels of resistance to drugs such as clindamycin, cefoxitin/cefotetan and β-lactamase inhibitor combinations are being encountered.

Methicillin (flucloxacillin)-resistant strains of *Staphylococcus aureus* (MRSA) are now common in many hospitals and, where appropriate investigations have been carried out, in the community. In hospitals where MRSA are present or anticipated, empirical therapy for serious staphylococcal sepsis should utilize a penicillinase-stable penicillin (e.g. flucloxacillin) together with an appropriate agent to cover possible methicillin-resistant strains. The choice of the second antimicrobial agent depends on local sensitivity patterns and also to some extent on the seriousness of the infection. Alternatives include vancomycin, gentamicin, fusidic acid, rifampicin, cotrimoxazole and ciprofloxacin. More specific monotherapy or combined therapy can be initiated when sensitivity results become available.

For enterococci that do not show high-level resistance to gentamicin or penicillins, ampicillin (or amoxycillin) plus gentamicin is the therapy of choice. In cases where sensitivity patterns suggest that these agents may be ineffective, vancomycin or teicoplanin are logical alternatives. The therapeutic options for vancomycin-resistant enterococci (VRE) may be limited. In cases where strains do not reveal high-level ampicillin resistance (i.e. minimum inhibitory concentrations (MICs) $\leqslant$ 32 mg/L), a combination of high-dose ampicillin and imipenem has been suggested, while streptogramin combinations (e.g. quinupristin/dalfopristin, Q/D) have been used experimentally for the treatment of severe infection due to multiresistant strains of *Enterococcus faecium* (strains of *Enterococcus faecalis* are resistant to streptogramins). Some of the newer fluoroquinolones (e.g. trovafloxacin) appear to have excellent *in-vitro* activity against multiresistant VRE, and have been suggested as possible therapeutic alternatives.

About 2% of Gram-negative enteric bacilli (e.g. *Klebsiella pneumoniae*, *Escherichia coli*) express extended-spectrum β-lactamases (ESBLs), implying resistance to extended-spectrum penicillins and third-generation cephalosporins. The genes responsible are plasmid encoded and often coexist with genetic elements that confer gentamicin resistance. The therapeutic options for ESBL-producing Gram-negative bacteria include meropenem (and imipenem) and ciprofloxacin.

Of increasing concern in nosocomial infections (e.g. sternum/mediastinum infections following thoracic surgery) are *Enterobacter cloacae* and *Enterobacter aerogenes*. These microbes are often resistant to 'older antimicrobials', with treatment options consisting of combinations of third-generation cephalosporins and aminoglycosides, cotrimoxazole with or without a cephalosporin or aminoglycoside, fluoroquinolones and meropenem.

OTHER SELECTED ANTIMICROBIAL AGENTS

ANTIVIRAL AGENTS

Virus replication is so intimately associated with the host cell that it has been difficult to develop agents which act selectively against viruses without being unduly toxic to mammalian cells. Potential antiviral targets are associated with the entry, reproduction, assembly and release of new virus from the infected cell. Of the antiviral agents currently in use, most are nucleoside analogues. These are phosphorylated within the host cell and, after incorporation into the elongating nucleic acid chain, they result in chain termination, i.e. they inhibit nucleic acid synthesis. In recent years, no doubt fuelled by the global HIV epidemic, novel antiviral agents which inhibit the activity of viral proteases (enzymes which cleave precursor polyproteins to generate essential viral structural proteins and enzymes) have been developed. These are the so-called protease inhibitors.

Anti-herpes-virus agents

A number of nucleoside analogues (e.g. aciclovir (aciclo-guanosine), valaciclovir, penciclovir (famciclovir), ganciclovir) are available for the treatment and/or prophylaxis of infection by various herpes viruses e.g. herpes simplex virus, cytomegalovirus (CMV). Serious CMV infections can also be treated with foscarnet, which is not a nucleoside analogue and has a number of toxic side-effects (e.g. nephrotoxicity, renal failure, hypocalcaemia, penile ulceration).

Anti-HIV agents

Nucleoside analogues, which have only modest antiviral activity, have also been used in the treatment and prophylaxis of infections by human immunodeficiency virus (HIV) (e.g. zidovudine (azidothymidine or AZT), didanosine (ddI), zalcitabine (ddC), stavudine (d4T), lamivudine (3Tc)). These are reverse-transcriptase (RT) inhibitors. All of them have varying toxicity profiles (e.g. dose-related but reversible bone-marrow toxicity with AZT). Prolonged use of any one agent is associated with the emergence of less-susceptible strains of HIV, although cross-resistance between the compounds is uncommon. The differing properties of these drugs have led to the use of combined or alternating treatment regimens formulated to reduce the emergence of resistant strains or intolerable side-effects.

There are also a number of non-nucleoside reverse-transcriptase inhibitors (NNRTIs) which have limited availability but have been used as part of combination therapy in clinical trials. These include efavirenz, delavirdine, loviride and nevirapine, which are all taken by mouth. NNRTIs appear to lower the viral load dramatically.

During the drive to develop more potent drugs that target other stages in the HIV-virus life cycle, a new class of compounds that inhibit HIV-1 protease activity has been discovered. These protease inhibitors appear to suppress HIV replication to a far greater extent than was previously considered possible. Unlike the nucleoside inhibitors, they seem to be capable of reducing the production of infectious virus particles from chronically infected cells. As these may constitute a major reservoir of virus within the body, this is an important advance. Four such agents, namely saquinavir mesylate, ritonavir, nelfinavir and indinavir sulphate, are currently available and undergoing clinical investigation, while others seem to be imminent. Combinations of various protease inhibitors with nucleoside and NNRTIs have been studied extensively in the laboratory. In all cases, the combinations have been at least additive and usually synergistic in their action.

There is no doubt that all protease inhibitors are extremely potent inhibitors of viral replication, and in combination with two nucleoside analogues they produce profound and sustained inhibition of viral replication. The major disadvantage of the present protease inhibitors, which are all peptide mimetics, is their individual and cross-class toxicities (e.g. renal stones with indinavir, diarrhoea with ritonavir, and cytochrome P450-associated drug interactions). The present protease inhibitors also have a complex effect on intermediary metabolism, with a small incidence of diabetes and an almost invariable rise in the mean cholesterol and triglyceride levels, which may be serious in a small number of patients. In addition, some individuals have developed an increase in visceral fat, with an accompanying loss of fat from the face and limbs (lipodystrophy); this is often associated with more serious metabolic disturbances. Other problems with combination therapeutic regimens are the sheer number of pills that have to be taken daily, and the complexity of the dosing regimen. In this respect, the use of NNRTIs has some advantages.

While North American and some European authorities favour a triple combination of two nucleoside analogues (e.g. AZT, 3Tc) together with a protease inhibitor (e.g. indinavir) for the treatment of HIV infection, many Europeans favour a combination of one or two nucleoside analogues (e.g. AZT, ddI) plus an NNRTI (e.g. nevirapine) as initial therapy when the viral load is low (less than 50 000 copies), saving protease inhibitors for those patients with more aggressive and pronounced disease. Unfortunately, the development of a rash and rapid emergence of resistance (single mutation) make NNRTIs less robust than protease inhibitors. However, whatever the combined therapy, the aim is to reduce the viral load to undetectable levels, with a parallel rise in CD_4 numbers.

ANTIFUNGAL AGENTS

Both fungal and mammalian cells are typically eukaryotic. Therefore the formulation of antifungal agents that are free from human toxicity has been a problem. However, while fungi do possess a cell wall composed of a polysaccharide matrix in which glucans appear to be structurally important, most of the current systemic antifungal agents act by interfering with the synthesis and function of the cytoplasmic membrane and, in particular, the membrane sterol, ergosterol. Ergosterol is the primary sterol in the fungal cell, as opposed to cholesterol in the mammalian cell membrane. Alterations in membrane porosity and permeability, as well as impair-

ment of cytochrome P450-dependent enzyme activities, appear to be important. Unfortunately, cytochrome P450 is reasonably well conserved throughout the biological world, and is important in some human metabolic pathways (e.g. adrenal androgen biosynthesis), which has resulted in a number of significant drug interactions and adverse events with some antifungal agents. Other potential sites of antifungal activity are the nucleic acids and protein synthesis.

Of the currently available systemic antifungal agents, two are of importance to surgeons – amphotericin B and fluconazole. The major disadvantage of the conventional formulation of amphotericin B is the high incidence of adverse reactions. The most commonly observed such reactions are chills, fever, vomiting, generalized pain, thrombophlebitis and pain at the infusion site, abnormal renal function (e.g. azotaemia, renal tubular damage, hypokalaemia) and anaemia. Most patients who are receiving the drug experience at least one side-effect. When total doses exceed 4 g (around 6–7 weeks of therapy), renal tubular damage is predictable. Although it has not been possible to prevent renal side-effects, infusion of 500–1000 mL of normal saline before the administration of amphotericin B appears to ameliorate renal toxicity. In this respect, the expensive lipid formulations (e.g. liposomal complexes, lipid-stabilized amphotericin B aggregates or ABLC, amphotericin B colloidal dispersion or ABCD) appear to be less nephrotoxic. Concurrent use of other antimicrobials and drugs with known renal toxicity (e.g. aminoglycosides, the diuretic chlorothiazide, cyclosporin) should be avoided. Amphotericin B is cidal to many fungi, and is currently regarded as the treatment of choice for most serious systemic mycoses, including invasive candidosis, aspergillosis and zygomycosis. Wherever feasible, surgical resection of involved tissues (e.g. lung lesions with aspergillosis) is an important surgical adjunct.

For many of the invasive or mucocutaneous yeast infections encountered by surgeons, the fungistatic agent fluconazole is an excellent and more patient-tolerable alternative to amphotericin. Fluconazole has excellent water solubility, permitting both intravenous and oral administration. Clinically it has excellent penetration into CSF (> 50% serum concentration) and other sites such as peritoneum, a feature not shown by other systemic antifungals apart from flucytosine. It also has a relatively prolonged half-life (> 24 h) and is largely excreted unchanged via the kidneys, which also makes it potentially useful in urinary tract infections. Fluconazole is an excellent oral alternative for the treatment of infections by many common *Candida* species in surgical patients, and in the prophylaxis of yeast infections in bone-marrow transplant patients. Interactions with cytochrome P450-metabolized drugs (e.g. cyclosporin) may occur.

ANTIHELMINTHIC AGENTS

There is really no effective chemotherapy for hydatid disease, although claims have been made for success with prolonged courses (e.g. 3 months) of benzimidazoles, including mebendazole and albendazole, with non-calcified liver cysts. Reported cure rates have been in the range 50–70%.

ANTIBACTERIAL PROPHYLAXIS IN SURGERY

It is now generally accepted that surgical-site infection rates are influenced by the degree of wound contamination during surgery, the duration of surgery exceeding 2 h, and the pathophysiological status of the patient as measured by the American Society for Anesthesiologists (ASA) or Acute Physiology and Chronic Health Evaluation II (APACHE II) scores. In addition, where hair removal is necessary, the use of a depilatory or clipping device immediately prior to skin incision is clearly better than early clipping or any form of razor shaving. Some surgical wound infections occur several weeks after patients have been discharged from hospital.

For most elective procedures, it now seems that prophylaxis is used without obvious reference to the known risk factors. This is reasonable when microbial contamination is a readily predictable factor. Thus prophylactic antibiotics are undoubtedly beneficial in all contaminated procedures (e.g. colon resection). Antibiotic prophylaxis is also indicated in 'high-risk' patients underoing gastric surgery. In this case, many of the documented risk factors (e.g. malignancy, concurrent acid reduction therapy) result in what should be a relatively microbe-free environment becoming heavily contaminated and/or colonized with a microbial flora.

Appendectomy is an emergency procedure involving an infected organ, so antibiotic use is not strictly prophylactic. While the level of infection is low in non-perforated cases, the situation changes markedly if perforation has occurred. In the absence of perforation, the use of prophylactic regimens and/or principles appears satisfactory, bearing in mind the likely dominance of obligate anaerobes. In cases where perforation has occurred and/or the appendix is markedly gangrenous, more prolonged therapeutic antibiotic regimens are justified.

In the case of biliary surgery, there is a close correlation between 'infected' bile (bactibilia) and post-operative septic complications, especially wound infections. Although bile cultures are more often positive in 'high-risk' patients (e.g. those with acute cholecystitis, jaundice, choledochal stones, diabetes mellitus, a non-functional gall bladder, or aged over 70 years) it is apparent that bile colonization cannot be accurately predicted pre-operatively using such associations. It is therefore unreasonable to restrict prophylaxis to high-risk patients only, and most patients undergoing biliary surgery now routinely receive prophylaxis. In cases of acute cholecystitis, antibiotics are used as adjuncts to cholecystectomy to reduce the incidence of post-operative septic complications thought to be related to bactibilia.

It is universally accepted that prophylactic antibiotics are beneficial in patients undergoing clean operations with a foreign-body implant (e.g. many vascular, cardiac and orthopaedic operations), or in cases where subsequent sepsis has horrendous repercussions (e.g. cardiac surgery, transplant surgery). Prophylaxis could also be supported by the extended duration of operation in many of these situations. General agreement suggests that this list should be extended to include patients undergoing a number of clean procedures without foreign implants (e.g. breast surgery, hernia repair, central nervous system operations, transurethral prostatectomy). This is because all infections produce physical and psychological disability and stress, and some of them may result in recurrence of the original problem requiring that the operation be repeated.

It is also prudent to use prophylactic antibiotic cover in patients who are undergoing various invasive investigational procedures known to be accompanied by a high prevalence of transient bacteraemia – especially in individuals who, because of pre-existing problems (e.g. foreign-body implant), are at serious risk from bacteraemic episodes. The more common investigational procedures include endoscopy, percutaneous abscess drainage, abdominal exploration for penetrating abdominal trauma with no observed gastrointestinal leakage, and placement of a chest tube to correct a pneumothorax associated with chest trauma.

Most institutions now have in place a series of proven and acceptable regimens (see Table 37.2.3), which have a number of features in common. These can be summarized as follows.

1. High concentrations of antibiotic should be present in target tissues at the time of incision, and should be maintained until completion of wound closure.

2. The optimal timing for prophylaxis by parenteral administration is at the time of induction of anaesthesia, i.e. about 20 min prior to incision.

3. The timing of any oral regimen is critical. Before commencement of the operation, the antibiotic(s) used must reach maximum levels at the operation site as well as at the skin incisional site (oral regimens employing only non-absorbed antibiotics do not fulfil this requirement).

Table 37.2.3 Examples of antibiotics used in surgical prophylaxis

Type of surgery	Important post-surgery infecting bacteria†	Antibiotics*	Relative cost
Appendicectomy	Anaerobes, coliforms	Cefotetan, or ceftriaxone, or ciprofloxacin, *each plus* metronidazole	++ ++++ ++++
Biliary	Coliforms, enterococci, anaerobes (with obstruction)	Coamoxyclav, or cephazolin, or ceftriaxone	+ + ++++
Cardiovascular	Staphylococci	Cefamandole, or teicoplanin‡	++ ++++
Colorectal	Anaerobes, coliforms	Cefotetan, or coamoxyclav, or cefuroxime plus metronidazole	++ + +++
Gastric (for malignancy)	Coliforms, anaerobes	Coamoxyclav, or cephazolin plus metronidazole	+ ++
Gynaecological	Coliforms, anaerobes, streptococci	Cefotetan, or coamoxyclav	++ +
Orthopaedic: Artificial hip	Staphylococci, coliforms	Cephazolin§ or cefamandole, or teicoplanin‡	+ ++ ++++
Amputation Ischaemic lower limb	Clostridia, staphylococci, streptococci	Coamoxyclav, or flucloxacillin with or without metronidazole	+ ++
Transplant	Coliforms, pseudomonads, staphylococci	Ciprofloxacin, or ceftazidime	++++ ++++
Urological	Coliforms	Coamoxyclav, or gentamicin	+ +

*In most cases a variety of equally effective alternatives are available.
†In addition to *Staphylococcus aureus* in skin incisional wounds.
‡Where MRSAs are prevalent, teicoplanin or vancomycin may be required for adequate cover.
§Cephazolin has better bone penetration and a longer half-life than similar cephalosporins (e.g. cephalothin).

4. For elective procedures lasting 2 h or less, a single dose of prophylactic antibiotic is sufficient. Prophylactic courses continued after wound closure should be restricted because of unproven benefit and the risk of selection of resistant bacteria.

5. For procedures lasting more than 2 h, or where there is pronounced blood loss, one or two further doses given at intervals of two times the plasma half-life (i.e. around 2-hourly for most antibiotics) may be

required. In such cases, a good time for the final dose is just prior to wound closure. The use of antibiotics with longer half-lives is a consideration for operations expected to exceed 2 h, as this may negate repeat dosing.

6. Complete cover of all possible microbes likely to be encountered is unnecessary. The antibiotic(s) chosen must be active against the microbes most likely to result in surgical-site infection following the

operation, and should always possess *S. aureus* cover. In complex situations such as colon resection for cancer, cover of skin (e.g. staphylococci) and bowel (e.g. obligate anaerobes, coliforms) flora with parenteral and oral antibiotics may be optimal.

7. In cases involving an emergency, the likelihood of active infection, an obstruction, unusual blood loss, trauma, a high-risk patient or other very special circumstances, the antibiotic regimen may be prolonged and composed of maximal doses of the drugs that are most likely to reach extravascular spaces. In reality this is therapy, not prophylaxis.

SUMMARY

The development of antimicrobial drugs has been one of the most important achievements of medicine in the twentieth century. Antimicrobials have enabled the provision of a scope of surgical therapy that is only limited by technology and that is attended by morbidity and mortality no longer mostly related to sepsis or septic complications. There has been a remarkable evolution in surgical infection for the betterment of patient outcome, which has only recently been tempered by the emerging problems of antimicrobial resistance. For optimal treatment to be initiated and for informed evaluation of the current and future numbers of anti-infective drugs, a surgeon should fully understand the microbiological and pharmacological principles in the clinical perspective.

FURTHER READING

Clunie GJA, Tjandra JJ, Francis DMA (eds). 1997: *Textbook of Surgery*. Asia: Blackwell Science.

Greenwood D (ed.). 1995: *Antimicrobial chemotherapy*, 3rd edn. Oxford: Oxford University Press.

Smith JMB, Payne JE, Berne TV. 1999: *The surgeon's guide to antimicrobial chemotherapy*. London: Edward Arnold.

Chapter 38

Common surgical procedures

Matthew A. Clark and John P.V. Collins

Introduction

This chapter outlines the commonly performed surgical procedures, some of which may be life-saving. A knowledge of the safe and effective use of such techniques is crucial to the training of a surgeon. Ideally one would read about a procedure, seek out an opportunity to observe a mentor performing the technique, and then attempt it oneself under supervision. If in doubt about competence in a particular procedure, *ask for help*.

For any procedure, a number of different methods may be in use. Only one is generally presented here, but other methods may be equally useful (or even more so) depending on the operator's experience, training and available equipment. Be prepared to evaluate critically alternative methods in order to determine which is most appropriate for a particular situation.

LEARNING FROM EXPERTS

When it is available, tuition from experts is invaluable. Training in specific techniques may be available. For example, the Advanced Trauma Life Support® (ATLS®) course is strongly recommended for all surgical trainees, and provides hands-on practice in many of the skills discussed here. Anaesthetists and intensivists place central venous lines regularly, and they should be observed and teach the correct ways to do this. Videotapes of some procedures are available from Colleges or Departments of Surgery, Emergency Medicine or Intensive Care. Many excellent models and mannequins are now available to aid the learning of specific techniques, such as urinary catheterization.

UNDERSTANDING RELEVANT ANATOMY AND POTENTIAL COMPLICATIONS

Much of surgery deals with anatomy. A thorough knowledge of the anatomy underlying these (and other) procedures leads to improved confidence in the techniques, and minimizes the risk of potential complications.

As with any procedure performed in medicine, the possibility of complications exists, especially in the emergency situation where environmental and patient-related factors are frequently suboptimal. As a general rule, anyone who attempts emergency procedures should also be competent to deal with the common complications that attend them – such as the development of a pneumothorax with central venous line insertion, which may require chest drain insertion.

GENERAL PRINCIPLES OF ALL PROCEDURES

The patient should first be informed about the reasons for a particular intervention. The effect of this information in reassuring an anxious patient should not be underestimated. However, in emergency situations and with an unconscious patient this may not be possible, but if a relative or caregiver is available they should be kept informed of the situation.

The principles of aseptic technique have been discussed in previous chapters, and should be adhered to except in the most extreme emergency. Sterile gowns and gloves are recommended for all but the simplest procedures, and double-gloving is encouraged (the advantages of this include better protection for the doctor against blood-borne pathogens, familiarity with the 'feel' of double-gloving, the experience of which is transferable to the operating theatre, and the ability to remove the outer gloves when a procedure is completed and still have a barrier underneath to continue with dressings or cleaning a trolley, etc.). Eye protection is also strongly encouraged.

Hospitals often differ from each other with regard to available equipment, staff skills and expertise, and guidelines or protocols for many procedures. Familiarization with these before the need arises is well worthwhile.

CRICOTHYROIDOTOMY

> **Case 38.1** A 19-year-old man is involved in a head-on car crash, and is ejected from the vehicle. Severe facial injuries are present in this unconscious patient, and an attempt by an experienced anaesthetist to place an endotracheal tube is unsuccessful. You are asked to place an emergency surgical airway.

Emergency access to the airway may be obtained by a number of methods, depending on the urgency of the situation. An experienced anaesthetist or intensivist is often able to control the airway with endotracheal intubation, but rarely this is not possible. Options such as bag-mask ventilation, laryngeal mask airway or fibre-optic intubation may be considered, but in the true emergency a surgical airway should be provided.

The two emergency surgical options to consider are *needle cricothyroidotomy* or *surgical cricothyroidotomy*. Tracheostomy, either open or percutaneous, should not be considered in the emergency situation unless considerable expertise is available.

NEEDLE CRICOTHYROIDOTOMY AND INTERMITTENT JET INSUFFLATION

This is only a temporary measure, which can oxygenate the patient for up to 30 min. Hypercarbia may occur rapidly due to hypoventilation. Further assistance should be swiftly obtained during this time.

The necessary equipment consists of high-flow oxygen tubing, a 14-G angiocath connected to a 10 mL syringe, a Y-connector and skin preparation.

With the patient supine, identify the cricothyroid membrane (between the thyroid and cricoid cartilages in the midline). Stabilize the trachea between the thumb and forefinger of the left hand. Insert the angiocath and attached syringe through the cricothyroid membrane, directed 45° caudally, while maintaining a negative pressure on the syringe plunger. Aspiration of air confirms entry to the tracheal lumen. Advance the angiocath forwards 2–3 mm, and then remove the needle. Attach the oxygen tubing and Y-connector to the angiocath hub. The patient is ventilated by occlusion of the Y-connector lumen for 1 s, followed by release for 4 s. Verify that lung inflation is occurring and that breath sounds are heard. Then tape the angiocath securely to the neck.

SURGICAL CRICOTHYROIDOTOMY

The necessary equipment consists of a scalpel with a number 11 blade, an appropriate-sized cuffed endotracheal or tracheostomy tube (usually size 5 or 6) and skin prep.

With the patient supine, identify the cricothyroid membrane (between the thyroid and cricoid cartilages in the midline). Stabilize the trachea between the thumb and forefinger of the left hand. Infiltrate 5 mL of 1% lignocaine with adrenalin over the area if the patient is conscious. Make a transverse skin incision over the cricothyroid membrane, and carry this through the membrane itself. An air leak often results. Use the handle of the scalpel or an artery forceps to open the incision by placing it into the wound and rotating through 90°. Insert the endotracheal or tracheostomy tube into the trachea, directing it caudally. Inflate the cuff of the tube and ventilate the patient. Verify that lung inflation is occurring and that breath sounds are heard. Then tape the tube securely to the neck.

CHEST DRAIN INSERTION

> **Case 38.2** A 72-year-old male pedestrian is hit by a vehicle at low speed, and complains of severe shortness of breath *en route* to hospital by ambulance. Initial examination confirms a patent airway but severe dyspnoea. The patient's right chest wall is moving poorly and has a resonant percussion note. Mild subcutaneous emphysema is present. The trachea is deviated to the left. A clinical diagnosis of tension pneumothorax is made, and needle thoracentesis is performed.

Chest drains are inserted to drain air or blood from the pleural cavity, or occasionally on suspicion of such findings when the risk of ventilatory compromise is high (e.g. for positive pressure ventilation, air ambulance transfer, etc.). *A chest drain should not be inserted for tension pneumothorax as it takes too long. On clinical suspicion of this entity, needle decompression should be performed immediately.*

NEEDLE THORACOCENTESIS

The necessary equipment consists of a 16-G angiocath and skin preparation.

Identify the second intercostal space on the side of the suspected tension pneumothorax. The mid-clavicular line is the usual insertion site. If time permits, the skin over this area is infiltrated with 5 mL of 1% lignocaine with adrenalin, and the skin is then prepared. Insert the angiocath through the skin and immediately above the rib (to avoid the main neurovascular bundle) to puncture the parietal pleura. If tension pneumothorax is present, an immediate escape of air under pressure will occur. Remove the needle from the angiocath and secure the open catheter with tape. A chest drain is usually inserted as definitive management of the pneumothorax, and the decompression angiocath may be removed after this has been done.

> **Case 38.3** The pedestrian's dyspnoea improves dramatically. A supine chest radiograph performed subsequently shows a 40% simple pneumothorax, with fractures to the 8th, 9th and 10th ribs laterally. A decision is made to insert a chest drain.

CHEST DRAIN INSERTION

The necessary equipment consists of a size 32 Fr chest drain (with trocar removed), heavy monofilament suture on a curved cutting needle (e.g. 1 nylon), 20 mL of 1% lignocaine with adrenalin, sterile drapes and a chest drain bottle system (many hospitals have pre-prepared chest drain packs).

Ask an assistant to abduct the arm away from the chest wall (imagine the patient giving a salute). The nipple level is around the fifth intercostal space, and here (or above), just anterior to the mid-axillary line, is a good position for chest drain insertion. (This should place the insertion site anterior to the latissimus dorsi and posterior to the pectoralis major.) In an obese patient, landmarks may be difficult to identify. Go as high into the axilla as is practicable. Draw a 4 cm line along the top of the rib with a skin-marking pen. Infiltrate 10 mL of anaesthetic around this area, down to the periosteum. Prepare the skin and drape the site. Make a 4 cm skin incision at the marked site with a scalpel, and bluntly dissect down to the intercostal muscles by repeatedly opening an artery forceps in the subcutaneous tissues. Under direct vision, infiltrate the remaining 10 mL of anaesthetic into the intercostal muscles at the insertion site, including the parietal pleura. Puncture the intercostal muscles and parietal pleura with the tip of a large artery forceps, and open slightly. Usually an escape of air (or blood) results. Immediately insert a finger into the thoracic cavity to verify entry and clear any adhesion or clots from the site. Place the chest drain (*without* trocar) into the thoracic cavity, directed posteriorly, and superiorly for air or inferiorly for blood. (Exact placement is difficult and probably irrelevant – capillary action and the closed drainage system will usually clear the pleural space.) Ensure that all drainage holes are within the pleural space. Correct placement is verified by fogging of the tube or audible air movement, or by drainage of blood. Suture the drain into position.

A vertical mattress suture of heavy non-absorbable material may be used to close the wound in the middle, with subsequent attachment of the drain to the ends of this. Each end of the suture is wrapped around the base of the drain twice and tied; this procedure is then repeated. A 'roman sandal' arrangement is not encouraged, as this has a tendency to work loose. Two further sutures are placed laterally. A purse-string is not left *in situ*. If the chest drain is removed within a few days, an occlusive dressing is placed over the wound for 2 days, by which time the wound is completely sealed. If the requirement for chest drainage is prolonged, a simple suture closure of the site is performed under local anaesthetic on removal.

PERIPHERAL VENOUS CUTDOWN

> **Case 38.4** A 54-year-old woman who has been started on NSAIDs for back pain is admitted with haematemesis and impalpable blood pressure. Initial attempts at percutaneous venous access have been unsuccessful. You are asked to perform a peripheral venous cutdown.

In haemorrhagic shock, more lives have been saved by prompt provision of vascular access by venous cutdown than by central lines. Furthermore, complications are less common. Act swiftly.

The necessary equipment consists of a scalpel, skin prep, 5 mL of 1% lignocaine plain, an angiocath and a braided absorbable tie (2/0 polyglactic acid).

Identify the site of the vein. The usual site is the long saphenous vein, 2 cm anterior to and above the medial malleolus. If this is unsuitable, the medial basilic vein in the antecubital fossa is found in the elbow crease 2.5 cm lateral to the medial epicondyle. Prepare the skin and infiltrate local anaesthetic over the site. Make a 2.5 cm full-thickness skin incision transversely over the selected site. Identify the vein by blunt dissection using an artery forceps, and free this up over a 2 cm length. It is important to avoid injury to the saphenous nerve, which is closely related to the long saphenous vein. Tie off the vein distally. Place a tie loosely around the vein proximally, and make a transverse venotomy in the vein. Introduce the angiocath through this, and tie the proximal suture around the angiocath and vein. Consider drawing blood for haematology, biochemistry and cross-matching if this has not been done. Attach intravenous tubing to the angiocath and secure it. Close the incision with interrupted sutures, and apply a dressing to cover it.

CENTRAL VENOUS LINE (CVL) INSERTION

> **Case 38.5** A 61-year-old woman with non-insulin-dependent diabetes is being treated with intravenous antibiotics for osteomyelitis for an extended time period. A decision is made to insert a subclavian CVL to facilitate this.

Access to the central venous compartment may be needed for a number of reasons. Some drugs are potentially dangerous when ·given peripherally (e.g. inotropes, potassium, calcium). Hyperosmotic agents such as intravenous nutrition may irritate peripheral vessels. Patients on long-term antibiotics may eventually have poor peripheral access. Central venous pressures may require monitoring in some situations.

Shock is not generally an indication for a CVL. In hypovolaemia, the central veins may be poorly filled and difficult to find. Furthermore, although lumens may be large, the length of the catheter means that resistance to fluid flow is high, precluding fast volume resuscitation.

Sites chosen for central venous lines may include the internal jugular vein, the subclavian vein or the femoral vein. Internal jugular lines are very conveniently inserted intra-operatively by anaesthetists. Subclavian lines have the advantage of ease of dressing and minimal interference with neck movement. Femoral venous lines have traditionally been used as a last resort, as dressings are more difficult and there may be a higher risk of line infection and deep venous thrombosis. If used in the short term, these risks are minimal. However, the consequences of introducing infection via any CVL should not be underestimated. Insertion should always be undertaken as a sterile procedure.

The necessary equipment consists of a central venous line, skin prep, heparinized saline, skin suture (e.g. 3/0 nylon on a curved cutting needle) and sterile dressings (many hospitals have pre-prepared CVL packs).

SUBCLAVIAN VENEPUNCTURE (INFRACLAVICULAR APPROACH)

Place the patient about 15° head down to distend the upper body veins. Optimize the position with the head turned slightly away and a rolled-up towel behind the spine and between the shoulders. Prepare the skin (after a shave if necessary) and drape the area. Mark an area 1 cm below the clavicle just lateral to the midpoint. Infiltrate with 5 mL of 1% lignocaine with adrenalin. Consider using a 22-G 'seeking' needle to verify the position of the vessel. Using the needle supplied with the CVL kit, attached to a 10 mL syringe containing 2 mL of heparinized saline, puncture the skin over the marked point. The needle is aimed medially and slightly cranially and posteriorly towards a finger placed in the suprasternal notch. Advance the needle while aspirating until blood appears in the barrel, and then advance 2 mm further. Remove the syringe and insert the guide-wire; occlude the hub of the needle in between to minimize the risk of air embolus (some CVL kits have a Raulerson syringe which allows passage of the guide-wire through the hub of the syringe). The guide-wire should advance without resistance. If any resistance is encountered, reapply the syringe and verify that there is free flow of blood. Remove the needle when the guide-wire is placed. Enlarge the skin entry point adjacent to the guide-wire with a scalpel. Pass the supplied dilator over the guide-wire, and then remove the dilator. Pass the catheter itself over the guide-wire and remove the latter once the CVL is positioned. Verify that there is free flow of blood from the lumen (or lumens) of the catheter, and then 'lock' with heparin. Suture the catheter into position with 3/0 nylon and apply a sterile dressing. Tape the intravenous tubing in place to minimize the risk of traction on the entry site. Obtain an erect chest radiograph to confirm the placement of the line and exclude complications before use (optimally, the tip of the catheter should lie just above the junction of the superior vena cava and right atrium).

INTERNAL JUGULAR VENEPUNCTURE

Note: Many different approaches to the internal jugular vein have been described.

Place the patient about 15° head down to distend the upper body veins. Optimize the position with the head turned slightly away. Prepare the skin (after a shave if necessary) and drape the area. Mark an area in the centre of the triangle formed by the sternal and clavicular heads of the sternocleidomastoid and the clavicle. Infiltrate with 5 mL of 1% lignocaine with adrenalin. Consider using a 22-G 'seeking' needle to verify the position of the vessel. Using the needle supplied with the CVL kit, attached to a 10 mL syringe containing 2 mL of heparinized saline, puncture the skin over the marked point. The needle is aimed caudally, parallel with the sagittal plane, and 30° posteriorly. Advance the needle while aspirating until blood appears in the barrel, and then advance 2 mm further. If the vein is not encountered, withdraw to the skin level and redirect the needle slightly *laterally*. Once the vein is entered, proceed as for subclavian venepuncture.

FEMORAL VENEPUNCTURE

With the patient lying on their back, prepare the skin (after a shave if necessary) and drape the area. Identify the femoral artery; the femoral vein is immediately medial to this structure (remember *nerve, artery, vein, lymphatics*). Infiltrate with 5 mL of 1% lignocaine with adrenalin. Consider using a 22-G 'seeking' needle to verify the position of the vessel. Using the needle supplied with the CVL kit, attached to a 10 mL syringe containing 2 mL of heparinized saline, puncture the skin directly over the femoral vein while aiming at 45° upwards and in the frontal plane. Advance the needle while aspirating until blood appears in the barrel, and then advance 2 mm further. Once the vein is entered, proceed as for subclavian venepuncture.

URINARY CATHETERIZATION

Case 38.6 A 67-year-old man is recuperating from an elective inguinal hernia repair performed earlier that day. It is noted that he has not passed urine, and is now uncomfortable with a palpable bladder. A diagnosis of acute urinary retention is made, and a urinary catheter is inserted.

Catheterization of the urinary bladder is used to drain the bladder of urine or to measure urinary output accurately. Indications for this procedure include acute urinary retention, or operations in the pelvis where access is needed (including anterior resection or diagnostic laparoscopy).

Contraindications to urinary catheterization include suspected urethral injury (major trauma with pelvic fracture, blood at the urethral meatus, or a high-riding prostate on digital rectal examination) or known urethral strictures. One should be cautious in cases with a history of prostatism or recent prostatic surgery. In either of these situations percutaneous suprapubic catheterization should be considered.

The necessary equipment consists of size 16 Fr and 20 Fr Foley balloon catheters (size 14 Fr for women), sterile anaesthetic lubricant, non-irritant skin prep, 10 mL of saline, a urine collection bag and sterile guards (most hospitals have pre-prepared catheterization packs).

MALE CATHETERIZATION

Prepare the skin of the penis, glans and meatus with preparation solution. Place sterile drapes under and around the penis. If the foreskin will not stay retracted, use the left thumb and index finger over a gauze swab for this, and re-prepare the glans and meatus. The left hand should now be considered unsterile. Inject the sterile anaesthetic lubricant slowly into the urethra, and then occlude the urethra with the left thumb and index finger immediately behind the glans. It is important to allow 1 min for anaesthesia to be obtained. With the catheter on the sterile drapes, insert the catheter into the urethra with a spiral motion (invagination of the meatus is uncomfortable for the patient, and can be avoided with adequate lubricant around the meatal opening). Continue until the catheter is completely inserted. If urine starts to flow from the catheter, inflate the balloon with 10 mL of saline and connect to the collection bag. The foreskin should be reduced at the end of the procedure.

If resistance to passage of the catheter is encountered,

maintain a gentle steady pressure on the catheter for 30 s. Sometimes a hold-up at the urogenital diaphragm may be overcome in this manner. If unsuccessful, perform the same manoeuvre with a 20 Fr catheter (which has less lateral flexibility and will sometimes – paradoxically – pass when the 16 Fr catheter fails to do so). *Undue pressue may cause false passage and should be avoided.* If it is still not possible to pass the catheter urethrally, seek help from someone more experienced or consider suprapubic catheterization. Do not be tempted to use a catheter introducer – this is a two-part instrument, the second part being a doctor with urology experience!

If urine fails to flow from the catheter, the most common cause is occlusion by the lubricant. Try to aspirate urine with a syringe. If no urine is obtained, the bladder may be empty. Rarely, a blood clot may occlude urine flow. If no resistance to the passage of the catheter has been encountered, it is generally safe to inflate the balloon.

FEMALE CATHETERIZATION

Female patients should be positioned supine with their heels together and knees wide apart. The urethral meatus should be clearly identified and prepared with antiseptic solution while the labia are held apart by the thumb and index finger of the left hand. Insertion of the catheter is otherwise as described above for male catheterization.

ARTERIAL PUNCTURE FOR BLOOD GAS DETERMINATION

Case 38.7 A 42-year-old man with severe gallstone pancreatitis has undergone an ERCP and basket extraction of impacted common duct stone. His clinical state is deteriorating, with falling blood pressure and oxygen saturation by pulse oximetry. An arterial blood gas determination is requested.

Analysis of arterial blood gases can provide information on oxygenation, ventilation and systemic acid–base balance. This information is crucial for the assessment of seriously ill patients.

The traditional site of arterial puncture is the radial artery. *Allen's test* is often performed to ensure that any intimal damage to the radial artery does not result in a threatened hand. (After occlusion of both radial and ulnar arteries at the wrist, ask the patient to clench their fist vigorously to drain venous blood. This results in blanching of the hand, and release of the ulnar artery should result in an immediate flush of blood, indicating an intact palmar arterial arch). Following this logic, the non-dominant radial artery should be sampled. In shock states the radial pulse may be impalpable. In this case, consider using the brachial artery at the elbow, or the femoral artery at the groin.

The necessary equipment consists of a 22-G needle, arterial blood gas syringe and skin prep.

Palpate the artery with two fingers separated by a gap, and prepare the skin in between. Introduce the needle with attached syringe at a 45° angle to the artery, and advance it slowly. Entry to the lumen is verified by spontaneous pulsatile flow into the barrel. Collect 3 mL of arterial blood (or the amount specified by the laboratory). On withdrawing the needle, apply firm pressure to the site for *at least* 5 min.

FINE-NEEDLE ASPIRATION (FNA) CYTOLOGY

Case 38.8 A 27-year-old woman without risk factors for breast carcinoma presents with a 2 cm mobile firm lump in the upper outer left breast. Clinically and on ultrasound examination this has the appearance of a fibroadenoma. To complete 'triple assessment' of this breast lump, an FNA is thought to be appropriate.

Biopsy by aspiration cytology of accessible lumps is easily performed, and is frequently the first (and sometimes only) investigative procedure. Common lesions investigated in this manner include breast lumps, dominant thyroid masses and other head and neck lesions. If a cytopathologist is present at a clinic, immediate answers may sometimes be available. If the material is insufficient for diagnosis then the FNA may be repeated without delay.

The necessary equipment consists of 21- and 25-G needles, a 10 mL syringe (and syringe-holder if desired), skin prep and a glass slide (pre-labelled with identifying details).

In most instances the use of a 25-G needle without an attached syringe will be appropriate, and it is recommended for the first attempt. If the specimen obtained is inadequate, then a second pass with an attached syringe should be used. With experience it may be possible on clinical examination to identify certain characteristics of a lump – such as hardness – where the use of a syringe may improve the diagnostic yield. Both techniques are described here.

Local anaesthetic is not required. The lesions should be fixed between the fingers and thumb of one hand

and the overlying skin prepared. Allow time for the skin to dry if an alcohol-based preparation has been used, to avoid stinging. After the needle has been inserted into the lesion it is withdrawn and inserted repeatedly within the lesion over a distance of a few millimetres, similar to a 'sewing-machine' motion. Use two or three different trajectories if the lesion is of an appropriate size. Capillary action will fill part of the needle with cells. Withdraw the needle and attach the syringe, which has been pre-filled with air. Express the aspirated material without force on to the glass slide and using a second slide, spread as for a blood smear. Allow the specimen to air-dry or fix it as directed by the pathologist. If a syringe is attached to the needle in order to obtain the specimen, the needle should be inserted into the lesion as before. Apply gentle suction as each pass is made. After releasing the suction, the needle is withdrawn and is then detached from the syringe. The syringe is then filled with air and a slide made as described above. An appropriately prepared and pack-aged air-dried slide will transport well to the laboratory even if this is at some distance from the clinic.

Note: If a cyst is encountered, some units recommend that the fluid is centrifuge examined. If a bloody aspirate occurs, proceed normally. In many cases, diagnostic specimens are obtained despite the blood-staining.

FURTHER READING

American College of Surgeons Committee on Trauma. 1997: *Advanced Trauma Life Support® student manual*, 6th edn. Chicago: American College of Surgeons Committee on Trauma.

McMinn RMH. 1994: *Last's anatomy, regional and applied*, 9th edn. Singapore: Churchill Livingstone.

Morris PJ, Malt RA (eds). 1994: *Oxford textbook of surgery*. New York: Oxford University Press.

Chapter 39

Ethics in surgery

Grant Gillett

Introduction

The context of any medical relationship has several key features of which we need to remind ourselves before we tackle the common problem areas that arise. These include care, trust, professionalism and partnership (Figure 39.1). If these features are made part of every clinical encounter, then very few ethical problems will arise, but they represent a departure from the traditional ways in which many of us learned to practise.

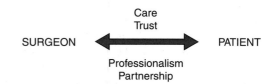

Figure 39.1 Key features of the relationship between the surgeon and the patient.

CARE, TRUST, PROFESSIONALISM AND PARTNERSHIP

The first feature, namely *care*, requires a genuine concern for how things are with the patient and an appreciation of the cause of their present or future suffering. These two aspects provide a basis on which the surgeon can undertake appropriate investigations to reveal further the cause of that suffering. The second feature, namely *trust*, arises from the patient's sense that the doctor does care and is being open about the problem she has presented with. Notice that this is a trust which is born of openness and a recognition that the surgeon has taken the trouble to ascertain what is important to the patient, not a blind trust arising merely from the fact that the surgeon is who he is. If the surgeon openly provides information and communicates the fact that he is taking the problem seriously, then *professionalism* results from an efficient and competent way of proceeding. Professionalism gives space for the kinds of skills and

procedures that a good professional would exercise, and prevents the surgeon from descending into mere sympathy or sentimental intentions to do the best he can. An important but sometimes overstated aspect of professionalism is a measure of distance between the patient and the surgeon. This does not mean that the surgeon deliberately draws back from care or openness, but rather that he recognizes that there is an appropriate level of involvement which allows surgical skills to be exercised but does not entangle him in such a way as to distort judgement in crucial clinical situations. *Partnership* is a concept that allows the surgeon and the patient to adopt the attitude that they have a mutual problem to solve and must work together on it. This requires maximum information sharing so that the intelligence of the patient is fully engaged, as well as clinical acumen on the part of the surgeon.

If the doctor–patient relationship has these features, then significant disputes between patients and doctors after the event become quite uncommon and the profession can concentrate on the genuine ethical issues that need to be addressed, rather than being driven into 'defensive medicine' mode.

MAJOR ISSUES AND BASIC VALUES

The major ethical issues that arise in surgery can be summarized as follows:

1. informed consent;
2. confidentiality;
3. telling bad news;
4. decisions at the end of life;
5. clinical research;
6. innovative treatment;
7. dealing with malpractice.

In each of these issues, certain basic values need to operate. These include a standard of reasonable medical practice and the desire to act in the best interests of the patient. A standard which reflects reasonable medical practice is based on the conduct and required skills of competent members of the specialty group relevant to a clinical situation. Our patients are entitled to expect this from us, and it includes two main components, namely *competence* and the *recognition of limitations*. Competence is fundamental, and entails the ability to do those things that one has been trained to do. When the surgical challenge outstrips one's personal competence, then the surgeon must involve a suitable colleague who can do what is required.

The desire to act in the best interests of the patient rather than to serve any other agenda arises from the care and partnership discussed above, and is the second value on which our ethical standards rest. Notice, however, that the best interests concerned must truly be those of the patient, and therefore we need to develop a fairly clear idea of what would count as significant benefit for our patients. A definition is in order here: 'A significant benefit is an outcome that now or in the future the patient would regard as worthwhile' (Campbell *et al.*, 1997, p. 10).

This is a patient-centred standard of benefit rather than being tied to survival, correction of a medical or pathological problem, or anything else of that kind.

INFORMED CONSENT

The idea of informed consent is based on the fact that every individual of sound mind has the right to make decisions about their own body and what will be done to them. The question then arises as to what standard of information is required to allow an individual to make an informed decision. This has changed over the last few years as a result of some key court decisions. However,

the difference between *spontaneous* and *responsive* disclosure is sometimes not reflected in ethical discussion of these decisions. Spontaneous disclosure concerns the information that is given spontaneously in either spoken, written or video form. It should tell the patient what their problem is, what its natural history is likely to be, what the aim of the intervention is, and convey the risks of the intervention. The risks that must be conveyed are determined by a combination of frequency and severity, and the crucial test is *material risk*. A material risk is one that would be taken into account by a reasonable person. In effect this means that a serious but low-probability risk (e.g. quadriplegia or incontinence) would count, as would a more probable but less serious risk (e.g. wound infection or bone-graft pain). The fact that it refers to a reasonable patient rather than this particular patient means that it is what is often called an *objective patient standard*, as distinct from a *subjective patient standard*. Under either standard it is clear that the patient's questions must be answered honestly and with the accuracy of information to be expected of a qualified specialist in the area, so the standard for responsive information giving is fairly clear (here the Sidaway decision is pivotal). The subjective patient standard ties the giving of information to the level of disclosure dictated by a particular patient's concerns and worries, and is to be found in the famous Whittaker decision. In this decision, an eye surgeon did not disclose the risk of blindness in the contralateral eye (estimated as 1 in 14 000) when his patient clearly had a major concern about her vision in that eye and gave every indication of that concern. Despite the fact that any caring professional would have realized that she had this concern, the surgeon involved in this case did not tell her of the risk of sympathetic ophthalmoplegia and she became blind. The court ruled that the surgeon should have realized that the risk of contralateral blindness was of material concern to this patient despite its very low probability, and should therefore have been mentioned.

The aim of informed consent is to enable the patient to make a reasoned decision in the light of an adequate understanding of the facts of her predicament. If the surgeon puts himself in the patient's shoes, the important factors affecting that decision are easily appreciated. She needs to know what is wrong, what is proposed to be done, what is the natural history of the disorder if it is not done, what are the likely benefits to accrue from the proposed intervention, what are the chances of success and what are the material risks. Information that is given to the patient should cover all of these aspects with a clear indication of the options open to the patient. It is then the patient's choice as to what will happen, although the New Zealand Code of Patient Rights makes it clear that the doctor has an obligation to make a recommendation. Note that this is a *recommendation* and not a prescription, and the patient should always be aware that the decision is hers and hers alone to make.

This leads directly to the other factor that ought to be mentioned in any discussion of informed consent, which is that the patient should not feel coerced to make any particular decision. Coercion can take many forms apart from direct pressure by the surgeon to go along with his recommendation. Some patients feel coerced by the fact that they have waited for a long time to get their assessment, and they worry that if they show hesitation or need time to think about things they will be moved to the bottom of the waiting-list. Other patients feel that they have to make a decision then and there in the surgeon's consulting room or clinic because that is expected of them. Yet others feel uncertain but are afraid that the surgeon will be offended if they want to discuss the decision with someone else or seek a second opinion. The surgeon should put the patient at ease about any of these hesitations and make them feel comfortable about taking as long as they need to make an informed and careful decision, while of course giving a clear indication of the risks that are associated with a delay in treatment. It is often helpful to send the patient a copy of the letter that is sent to the referring doctor so that they can see exactly what is being proposed and obtain as clear an idea as possible of the decision that has to be made.

Therapeutic privilege is a concept that is used when treatment is required without consent. It refers to the fact that, in a situation where the patient's wishes cannot be ascertained, the doctor ought to do those things that clearly would be done were the best interests of the patient to be the sole consideration. However, the onus is on the surgeon, in the event of questions being raised, to prove that he had no alternative but to proceed with the treatment in question and that, given the facts available to him, what he did seemed to be in the best interests of the patient. Legitimate questions would then be asked about the soundness of the surgeon's clinical judgement in reaching his clinical conclusions and the attempts made to ascertain the true wishes of the patient.

Provided that the intervention is defensible on these grounds, the concept of therapeutic privilege applies. Clinical research and innovative treatment are also bound by these same principles of informed consent. Here it is mandatory for the surgeon to disclose the fact that certain interventions are part of a research trial or are innovative in some way and therefore depart from standard clinical practice. Generally, a fairly comprehensive written information sheet about the nature of the research or innovation will be required so that the patient is aware of the situation in which they are getting involved.

Any surgeon who abides by these guidelines in determining the nature and quality of information required to obtain adequately informed consent should not have any serious worries about the adequacy of their practice in this area.

The key concepts can be summarized as follows:

- objective patient standard;
- spontaneous and responsive disclosure;
- material concern;
- surgical recommendation;
- patient's choice;
- non-coercion.

CONFIDENTIALITY AND THE USE OF INFORMATION

Confidentiality is often treated as an absolute principle in medical ethics, although this has never been the case in practice. Even the Hippocratic Oath states that: 'Whatever, in connection with professional practice or not in connection with it, I see or hear, in the life of men, which ought not to be spoken of abroad, I will not divulge, as reckoning that all such should be kept secret.'

This divulgence of information is here linked to a clinical judgement about the propriety of sharing that information (as is the case with most codes of practice world-wide). There are a number of well-established exceptions to the rule of confidentiality for communicable diseases such as tuberculosis and syphilis, and other exceptions in clinical situations where people other than the doctor or the patient are involved in the patient's care. One such exception is where communication with another health-care professional is required for good clinical care, and another is where the police can obtain details of a patient's treatment (e.g. after an accident). In each of these cases an ethical analysis quickly establishes that more than one person has a right to the information, given their position *vis-à-vis* the patient and the illness. On occasion the patient has a right to veto the use of the information and, in cases of doubt, clarification should be sought from an appropriate person such as a hospital administrator or medical lawyer. In most cases a fairly common-sensical approach based on what the doctor would want to happen if the information was about him provides the answer to any question that might be asked.

There is a great deal of confusion about the entitlement of patients to information that is contained in their own medical records, and about the use of information recorded in those notes. This confusion is not helped by discussing the issue in terms of who owns the notes. It is much better approached by considering the content of what is recorded in the notes, the purposes for which the information is being recorded, the proper interests of various parties in that information, and the clinical needs for clarity of communication and access to information. The right of patients to have free access to their own notes is the norm in most commonwealth countries, and is likely to become so in the very near future in Australia.

Contents of the notes

The notes contain information about the patient and the conduct of the surgeon, and professional opinions about the patient's problems. If we consider the features of a good doctor–patient relationship, then an attitude of care allows the surgeon to derive from the clinical interview the information that is needed to make a good diagnosis and management plan. This information is only properly obtained in an atmosphere of trust and partnership in which the patient feels that she has a duty to give the surgeon the best possible understanding of the problem so that he is not hampered in any way in making a sound clinical assessment of the situation. We shall comment on situations in which this is not the working assumption at the end of this section.

At this point we should probably deconstruct the artificial distinction between information revealed to the doctor by the patient and information gained about the patient by examination and testing. Both types of information are obtained by the doctor through the exercise of clinical skills (history-taking, physical examination and interpretation of test results) but are made available by the patient through her compliance in the clinical procedures concerned. They are therefore ethically on a par with each other, and on that basis a legal distinction is unlikely to be maintained in any robust or enduring manner. Legal challenge is usually dependent on a sense of natural justice or the ethics of the situation concerned, so that dubious or ethically unsound distinctions, while they may have a brief moment of importance, are usually abandoned under the weight of case law (which determines how statute law is applied).

Once information has been given and received, the standards of reasonable care become important in the way in which the surgeon responds to the information by ordering investigations, discussing the problem with the patient, and so on. It is after this response has been made that the surgeon records the interview for his own future reference and corresponds with the referring doctor or writes a report. Here professionalism is of supreme importance. It may be that the patient is almost certainly malingering, but the evidence to hand only allows the judgement that a pathological cause for the patient's suffering cannot be identified. This is the restrained conclusion that should enter the notes together with some kind of differential diagnosis and check-list of the tests or points of history and examination that have led to the conclusion. Relevant factors such as financial strain, the likelihood of a generous settlement if the suffering is attributed to some or other event, and so on, may enter

into the opinion but should always be stated fairly dispassionately and in the spirit of a reasoned assessment, rather than in the guise of a dismissive or high-handed judgement about the patient. The meaning of such restrained and weighed professional opinions is not lost on the informed reader, but it does avoid some of the indignation and conflict that arise if the patient gets hold of the report. It is important to ask how well grounded one's conclusions are and to be fastidiously professional in the way in which they are stated. If these simple rules are followed, then the issue of who gets to see the reports in question is not highly charged, as there is nothing contentious or offensive contained in them. Most patients who are 'trying it on' on the health system recognize a 'fair cop' and can appreciate the professionalism with which the opinion is given when that is the case.

Who owns the notes?

It should now be clear why this is a silly question. The crucial questions should be couched in terms of rights of access, control over the use of the information, accountability for what is in the medical records, and responsibility for the maintenance of the records in a fit condition to serve the purposes for which they have been prepared.

The patient has an ethical right to access to the notes because it is information about her that affects her future care and that is based, in part, on material that she has freely given during an interview. The doctor also has a right to have access to what is in the notes because he has written them and needs them to manage the patient in an adequate manner. The doctor also has rights to use the information in the notes because they are a record of his professional conduct and therefore they are about him as well as about the patient. However, the patient should also have some control over what is done with the notes, given that they may contain intimate and sensitive information about her. She should therefore be able to rest assured that the notes will be used for the purpose for which the patient has given the information (i.e. her own clinical care), but only for other purposes (such as clinical case reports or lectures) with the patient's permission.

Accountability and responsibility for the notes shift the focus to the doctor's ethical duties. He must make notes that reflect his clinical judgement and competence, and he is therefore accountable for what they contain. He also has the clerical backing to ensure that the notes are maintained in an adequate and up-to-date condition so that they can serve their primary purpose, and so the doctor is responsible for them in that sense.

For these reasons it would be inappropriate to claim that the notes were owned either by the patient or by the doctor. Clearly both doctor and patient have certain rights and responsibilities in order for the records to function as part of the clinical management of the patient's problem. We can summarize this by saying that the patient and the doctor both have rights to access and use of the information contained in the notes, but that the doctor also has duties to ensure that the notes are adequate to fulfil their purpose as a record of his dealings with the patient and any significant findings which form part of good patient care. In New Zealand these issues are clearly spelt out in the Privacy Act, and any questions can be resolved by enquiries directed to the office of the Privacy Commissioner. In Australia the situation is slightly less clear, with a difference in status accorded to records held by a public health care institution as distinct from those held by a private practitioner. The patient does have access to publicly held records, but not to privately held records. In fact this distinction is difficult to defend ethically, and the best advice one can give is to make sure that all information conforms to the ethical desiderata given above.

Conflicts over the use of information

On occasion there is a conflict between respect for a patient's request for confidentiality and the doctor's duty of care. For instance, this situation could arise if the patient does not want some fact recorded in the notes, but the doctor believes that that omission might prejudice future care. This might happen, for example, if the doctor was to obtain a history of a sexually transmitted disease. Given that the use of information here is supposed to be in accordance with the doctor's duty of care, then the decision to contravene the patient's wishes would need to be in accordance with the judgement of a reasonable practitioner and the existence of reasonable grounds for that action. The test would be that it would be unreasonable for a doctor possessing the information in question not to enter it in the notes in view of its potential later importance to the management of the patient's present or future condition.

There are situations in which the non-communication of a certain piece of information about the patient would be in conflict with a duty to others, including other doctors. The most obvious situations where this circumstance arises are in relation to the care of AIDS patients and in relation to child abuse or other violent crime. In such cases the doctor has to recognize his wider duties as well as his responsibilities to the particular patient before him. For instance, if a patient with AIDS will not tell a partner or a future medical caregiver, then that person is indicating that they are prepared to jeopardize the life of another in order to preserve their own privacy. One can argue that this is wrong not only on consequential grounds but also in terms of the moral values operating in the relationships concerned. On con-

sequential grounds, it is evident that the potential harm (the loss of an innocent life) far outweighs the potential benefit (the preservation of privacy.) However, were one to eschew consequential reasoning and pay attention to the moral values operating in the relationships involved, then the non-disclosure emerges as equally vicious. The patient is asking the doctor to collude in the introduction of a lie (that the patient has not got AIDS or HIV infection) into a relationship which should be based on trust and partnership (an intimate partnership or another doctor–patient relationship). This is an unethical demand in that it runs counter to a basic moral feature of the relationship in question.

In the case of child abuse or violent crime it is the consequential calculation that is most obvious in deciding what the doctor should do, but here also there is the question of collusion with an immoral relationship in which the patient's relationship to their family or to society in general is founded on exploiting an ill-grounded assumption that they are a decent and trustworthy participant in the relationships concerned. Given that the relationships in question are grounded on consensual non-violent interactions, the doctor can, with some justification, claim that the same double standard applies here as it does in the AIDS case. In either case the patient could be said to have undermined the values according to which they expect the doctor to act, and therefore cannot call on those values to constrain their action. In the New Zealand Privacy Code there are explicit exceptions for situations in which confidentiality would impact upon the well-being of others.

There are other situations where the non-disclosure of certain information about a patient conflicts with a duty to society in general. These include communicable diseases and driving while in an unfit condition. In either case the patient may be happy to be left to go about her life without having to take any care with regard to the potential harm to other members of society, but the doctor should not be asked to collude in that judgement or course of action. Again the New Zealand Privacy Code makes explicit provision for this exception to the respect for confidentiality.

Computerization and access to information

Computerization does not really affect the use of clinical information or its accessability by a wide range of people, and therefore does not really affect the ethical issues that arise in this area. In fact, medical records are quite insecure in terms of privacy and confidentiality, with all of the information recorded therein available to anyone who manages to get their hands on them. The use of clinical information is based on therapeutic need, and this always has to be weighed against reasonable privacy for the individual. It is particularly a problem in small towns where everybody knows somebody who knows someone else. In general, the body of information in medical records is widely available to members of the health-care team, and this must be so to allow adequately informed care. If anything, the computerization of medical records should allow much more controlled access to patient information than in the case for written notes bound together in a file. On a computer one can specify grades of access to certain details on a 'need-to-know' basis. Codes can be assigned and automatic records can be kept of who accesses the patient's file and what information they have downloaded from it. Bars can be put in place so that inappropriate usage is difficult if not impossible, and irregularities can be monitored. This should make individuals in general feel more rather than less secure about the confidentiality with which their medical information is treated. I suspect that much of the current anxiety in this area arises because people have traditionally not known how insecure the privacy of their sensitive health-care information really was.

There are aberrant relationships where malingering or conflicts of interest disrupt the eliciting and sharing of the information required for good clinical care. In such cases the trust and openness of the doctor–patient relationship are missing and the surgeon must rely on his skill and wisdom to overcome the resulting problems. Malingerers often give themselves away, and the patient with a conversion reaction or who somatizes all of her complaints can usually be diagnosed as such. In these cases the doctor must still abide by the principles of care and professionalism and be particularly judicious about the recording and use of information. Apart from those qualifications, the basic principles still apply. In fact it is in cases of conflict or misleading presentations that openness and the sharing of clinical problems can come to the doctor's aid in avoiding problems. For instance, if the patient is malingering it is often helpful to put the problem you face squarely to the patient by saying something like the following:

> I would like you to understand my problem. Your story sounds a bit like you might have X or Y or Z, but when I examine you and look at your tests, that is clearly not the problem. That means that I cannot find a physical basis for your suffering and an operation will not help you. Can you help me any further?

Or even:

> What do you suggest we do at this point? How shall we manage this problem of yours?

This kind of approach puts the relationship on the footing of a partnership solving a problem, rather than the surgeon sitting in judgement on the patient. It also enables the surgeon to be quite open about the contents of any report to a third party such as an insurance company, a compensation scheme or a court.

The key concepts can thus be summarized as follows:

- openness;
- truth-telling and sharing of clinical dilemmas;
- responsibility in the composition of opinions and the use of information;
- shared control of clinical information;
- shared rights of access to that information;
- an open partnership in clinical care.

TELLING BAD NEWS

This is something many of us do not do well. My formative experience in this area occurred in a surgical ward when I was attending teaching round. We were invited to examine the axillary glands of a woman who had disseminated breast cancer. I can still remember the sickening feeling as we went to leave the room and she asked the surgeon what was wrong with her. Unfortunately he did not respond to her request for information but turned his back on her. She persisted, and we left the room as she desperately pleaded with him to tell her what was wrong with her and what was going to happen to her.

Patients are not very demanding in the area of bad news. They require only that we communicate compassionately to them and tell them the truth. If they do not want details, they will not ask for them. They may be upset by what we tell them, but that is only natural given the gravity of their situation, and they have usually guessed what we are going to say before we ever say it. In fact it is usually our honesty that is in question when we share the news about their pathology, and not the news at all. There are certain things that most people want to know, such as how long they have to live and what they can expect in terms of suffering and symptoms. These facts can usually be conveyed sympathetically, and with reassurance that appropriate management of symptoms is part of our ongoing care.

We must, of course, try to be as frank as possible about the uncertainties surrounding prognosis, and my own practice is to mention the exceptions which allow a small glimmer of hope in an otherwise fairly bleak outlook. It is best to temper one's mention of these with fairly realistic probabilities, but such an approach at least allows the patient to pick up the aspects of the prognosis that they need in order to hold things together in the time they have left. Life is grim enough with a fatal prognosis, and we should not perceive our role to be that of unrelenting harbingers of doom. The world abounds with cancer patients who have proved their doctors' confident prognoses wrong, and it is best not to add to the problem by making overly definite predictions about the uncertain business of death and dying.

The general rule in this area is to be as realistic as possible about a patient's prospects, but to allow a window of hope based on the real and ever present clinical uncertainty that must be part of any prognosis. Thus the key concepts here are:

- honesty;
- hope;
- the need to cope.

DECISIONS AT THE END OF LIFE

Decisions at the end of life arise in cases where the imperative to save life is in question and we must accept the responsibility for wise management of a potentially terminal state. For some of us the decisions arise with depressing frequency (e.g. in the management of severe head injuries), while for others they are infrequent. In cases where life and death are critically poised there are certain concepts which should be clarified if sound decisions are to be made. In using these concepts we must be aware of the need to deal with the *uncertainty* which is a pervasive feature of acute care situations. We need to be very open about the difficulties of prognosis, update people on when they can expect to hear more news, and treat the management plan as a plan in evolution, rather than a rigid programme from the outset with all the weight of medical authority behind it.

The first ethical concept that must be factored in is that of *a life worth living*. Here we are attempting to understand what kind of life the patient would want to live. We must be careful that we accept a non-elitist standard in this area, as several publications by disabled rights groups have reminded us. It is important that it is a patient-centred standard as to what kind of life is worth living, and that it is our responsibility to use what sources we can to find out what the patient would want. Relatives and friends are an important source of this information, but we should not make the mistake of regarding them as the decision-makers in such cases. It remains the responsibility of the clinical team to make a decision in the best interests of the patient about life and death issues, rather than shifting that responsibility onto the relatives. The relatives can, of course, object that the clinical team or the surgeon in charge made no attempt to find out or act on a reasonable judgement of what the patient would regard as worthwhile, but they cannot object on the basis that the clinical team did not follow their orders, as they have no legal role, except as informants, in the decision being made.

The situation is not so clear-cut with regard to children, although even here the clinical team is responsible for making a decision in the best interests of the child. In the case of children, the adult caregivers of the child are usually considered to be the individuals best placed to determine what is in the child's best interests, but one can think of cases where that is clearly not so. Situations can arise where child abuse has occurred or where a parent for reasons of religious faith will not sanction treatment that most parents would consider to be in the best interests of the child. In such situations a clinical team may have to act directly counter to the parents' wishes. If they do so, they must later be prepared to defend their actions as being reasonable in the light of an objective assessment of the child's interests, and not just in line with their own opinion. The same proviso applies to a decision made about an adult patient, and again the surgeon must be able to show that he made a decision which a reasonable person or a court would regard as being in the patient's best interest, as far as that could be ascertained at the time when the decision was made.

The second concept is related to the first, and is that of *substantial benefit*, which is usually contrasted with *futility*. Narrow or physiological futility depends on the assessment that the intervention is unlikely to do what it sets out to do in narrowly medical terms. This might apply to cardiopulmonary resuscitation of a patient with heart failure or disseminated cancer, where one is unlikely to return the patient to a stable cardiorespiratory state, but it is not the most important sense of futility, which is the obverse of substantial benefit. Substantial benefit is best defined as: 'an outcome which now or in the future the patient would regard as worthwhile'.

A further important concept in this area is the *RUB* (the *risk of unacceptable badness*). This acronym is taken from Hamlet, who could not abide death if the sleep of death meant unending guilty and tortured dreams about his choices in life. In a clinical situation the RUB is predicated on two factors, namely the values of the patient and the medical probabilities. It is easy enough to grasp in principle but sometimes difficult to assess in practice. One can find out what the values and attitudes of the patient are in terms of various possible outcomes of an intervention or a clinical event and then assess the risks that the patient will or will not fall into the group with a given outcome. For instance, if the patient has given clear indications that a life as a bedridden and brain-damaged individual dependent on others for daily care and basic needs would not be acceptable to her, then the risk of that state coming about is, for this patient, a risk of unacceptable badness. What then remains is to define that risk. For instance, if the patient, should they survive a particular procedure, would have a 90% chance of being in an unacceptably bad state, then the RUB is 9 to 1. With this chance of ending up in a state which the patient would regard as unacceptable, it would be reasonable not to take that risk. Often when we face a life-and-death decision we spell out the chances of survival but we do not spell out the RUB. If we did, then the comment that any chance is better than none at all would not be so persuasive, as a 9 to 1 risk of unacceptable badness should one survive is not to be taken lightly.

The RUB makes clear the need for informed participation by the patient if possible, or otherwise the relatives, in deciding how to proceed in a critical emergency. The relatives, as mentioned above, cannot make a binding decision but should be consulted, where appropriate, in order to decide what the best interests of the patient might be (in the light of the patient's conceptions of substantial benefit and the RUB).

Here the related concepts of *substituted judgement* and *best interests* are often mentioned. A substituted judgement is a judgement about what the patient would opt for if, *per impossibile*, she were able to be consulted. A judgement on the basis of best interests is just that – an assessment of what a reasonable person would regard as being in the patient's best interests. Here, as in informed consent, there is an objective and a subjective standard, where the former involves a judgement about what any reasonable person in the position in which the patient finds herself would want to happen. The latter (a subjective best interests standard) is very similar to a substituted judgement in that it is an attempt to gauge what this particular patient, in the light of her values and attitudes, would regard as being in her best interests.

It is at this point that the idea of a *trial of treatment* becomes important, in that it tends to undercut debates about the relative ethical merits of withholding treatment as opposed to withdrawing it. Both withholding and withdrawing involve a recognition that treatment is no longer justified in the light of the best information available, but there is a difference in the amount of information involved. In the case of withholding treatment, one has not had the opportunity to gauge response to initial measures, the clinical course of the problem, and so on, whereas the withdrawal of treatment follows the initial interventions which allow those factors to be assessed and therefore sounder decisions to be made. Both of these practices involve a decision to allow the patient to die, but the difference in information is crucial, and implies that it is ethically much more sound to withdraw than to withhold life-saving treatment.

All such decisions should also be relativized to a conception of *reasonable practice* or the measures that would be taken by an appropriately qualified and well-motivated specialist in the clinical discipline concerned.

There is a separate step involved when we contemplate active euthanasia for a patient, because that involves a decision that this patient should die now, when that would not happen without our actively bringing about the death. Most doctors feel hesitant about such a decision on ethical grounds, quite apart from the fact that it contravenes existing law in Australia, New Zealand and elsewhere.

The key concepts with regard to decisions at the end of life can be summarized as follows:

- dealing with uncertainty;
- a life worth living;
- substantial benefit;
- the RUB;
- informed participation;
- trial of treatment;
- reasonable practice.

DEALING WITH MALPRACTICE

Deficient practice by a colleague is extremely unpleasant to deal with. Nevertheless, we must preserve standards of care so that patients do not suffer from bad management, and the profession as a whole does not fall into disrepute. This requires of each of us that we give opinions in such cases which reflect an orthodox and yet sympathetic view of the care that was actually given. Some mistakes are inexcusable, either through reasons of competence or because the patient's rights and interests were completely ignored. An expert witness in such cases is not required to pass judgement on a colleague but to state as clearly as possible what the limits of reasonable practice are, and whether the case in hand falls within his or her understanding of those limits. The surgeon called as expert witness has an unenviable task, and must approach the problem mindful of his Hippocratic duty to treat his colleague as a brother or sister but also mindful of the need to give a fairly objective view of what constitutes good practice. We are not all perfect – in fact, one might safely say that none of us are, and those who think that they are perfect are probably suffering from some kind of mild delusion. It is very important that we approach discipline as we do all of the other problems in ethics, with a clear eye to safeguard the best interests of patients, and wisdom about clinical life and its challenges. Any opinions that are expressed must be well reasoned and carefully grounded in the facts. Ethical issues, particularly concerning the adequacy of consent, must be judged on the basis of sound principles so as not to be biased in favour of either party, and our attitude should be that the practitioner concerned probably did his or her best under the circumstances unless the facts clearly indicate otherwise (this equates to the innocent-until-proven-guilty rule in the criminal courtroom).

We might finally venture a comment on systems of medical malpractice regulation and surveillance. Here again one must bear in mind the real consequences for the various parties concerned. In most litigation-based systems the doctor is sued by the patient and it must be proved that he acted deficiently in relation to professional standards in order for the patient to be compensated. The penalty for the doctor is minimal apart from the angst of going through the hearing and subsequent events. The settlement is extracted from malpractice insurance, and only indirectly affects the doctor (by an increase of shared premiums). For this reason a somewhat less capricious system in which patient compensation is detached from doctor fault, and the deficiencies of doctors are dealt with by professional disciplinary hearings, has somewhat better ethical credentials. The latter impose real penalties, including restriction of practice, and only do so on the basis of true fault uncontaminated by sympathy for the patient, who otherwise receives nothing. This is clearly an issue on which professional bodies such as Colleges need to do some ethical work in relation to their own and government policy.

The key concepts can be summarized as follows:

- careful and sympathetic judgement;
- assessment of clinical competence shown;
- awareness of ethical duties.

A SIMPLE APPROACH TO AN ETHICAL DECISION

I will finish this chapter by outlining a methodical approach to actual ethical problems in a clinical setting.

Once these questions have been answered and the points made above attended to, it is usually possible to achieve a solution that can be lived with by all of the individuals concerned.

A doctor facing a possible ethical dilemma should ask the following questions.

1. What is the factual situation?
2. What are the interests of the people concerned?
3. Are there significant cultural issues at stake?
4. Are all of the people concerned aware of the relevant facts?
5. What is the conflict?
6. Are the interests of the most vulnerable participants being respected?
7. Are there relevant legal constraints?
8. Can a negotiated solution be reached?

FURTHER READING

Campbell AV, Charlesworth M, Gillett G, Jones DG. 1997: *Medical ethics.* Melbourne: Oxford University Press.

Charlesworth M. 1993: *Bioethics in a liberal society.* Cambridge: Cambridge University Press.

Faulder C. 1985: *Whose body is?* London: Virago.

Gillon R (ed.). 1994: *Principles of health care ethics.* Chichester: John Wiley & Sons.

Jonsen A, Siegler M, Winslade W. 1992: *Clinical ethics.* New York: McGraw-Hill.

Index